INTERNATIONAL ENCYCLOPEDIA OF
PHARMACOLOGY AND THERAPEUTICS

Executive Editor: A. C. Sartorelli, *New Haven*

Section 141

ANTICANCER DRUGS: REACTIVE METABOLISM AND DRUG INTERACTIONS

Some Recent Volumes

DENBOROUGH
The Role of Calcium in Drug Action

WEBBE
The Toxicology of Molluscicides

GRUNBERGER and GOFF
Mechanisms of Cellular Transformation by Carcinogenic Agents

TIPPER
Antibiotic Inhibitors of Bacterial Cell Wall Biosynthesis

CORY
Inhibitors of Ribonucleoside Diphosphate Reductase Activity

HAYASHI
Ornithine Decarboxylase: Biology, Enzymology, and Molecular Genetics

BALFOUR
Psychotropic Drugs of Abuse

SCHÖNBAUM and LOMAX
Thermoregulation: Physiology and Biochemistry

SCHÖNBAUM and LOMAX
Thermoregulation: Pathology, Pharmacology, and Therapy

ORME
Anti-Rheumatic Drugs

HARVEY
Snake Toxins

BELL
Novel Peripheral Neurotransmitters

FILE
Psychopharmacology of Anxiolytics and Antidepressants

TAYLOR
Intracellular Messengers

GRAM
Metabolic Activation and Toxicity of Chemical Agents to Lung Tissue and Cells

INTERNATIONAL ENCYCLOPEDIA OF PHARMACOLOGY AND THERAPEUTICS

Section 141

ANTICANCER DRUGS: REACTIVE METABOLISM AND DRUG INTERACTIONS

SPECIALIST SUBJECT EDITOR

Garth Powis
Arizona Cancer Center
University of Arizona
Tucson, AZ, U.S.A.

PERGAMON PRESS
Oxford • New York • Seoul • Tokyo

U.K.	Pergamon Press Ltd, Headington Hill Hall, Oxford OX3 0BW, England
U.S.A.	Pergamon Press, Inc, 660 White Plains Road, Tarrytown, New York 10591-5153, U.S.A.
KOREA	Pergamon Press Korea, KPO Box 315, Seoul 110-603, Korea
JAPAN	Pergamon Press Japan, Tsunashima Building Annex, 3-20-12 Yushima, Bunkyo-ku, Tokyo 113, Japan

First edition 1994

Library of Congress Cataloging in Publication Data

Anticancer drugs: reactive metabolism and drug interactions,
Garth Powis—1st ed.
p.cm.—(International encyclopedia of pharmacology and therapeutics; section 141)
Includes bibliographical references and index.

British Library Cataloguing in Publication Data

A catalogue record for this book is available from the British Library.

ISBN 0 08 0423353

The paper used in this publication meets the minimum requirements of American National Standard for Information Sciences—Permanence of Paper for Printed Library Materials, ANSI Z39.48–1984

Printed in Great Britain by BPCC Wheatons Ltd, Exeter

PREFACE

There are over 50 clinically approved anticancer drugs, as well as numerous steroidal agents, and in addition there are many new anticancer drugs in various stages of preclinical and clinical development. Cancer drug treatment has had a mixed success. Nearly 12% of cancers are now curable, including acute lymphocytic leukemia, Hodgkin's disease and testicular cancer. Unfortunately, the majority of human cancers, including most of the slow growing solid cancers, such as lung, colon, breast and prostate cancer, remain refractory to chemotherapy. There is a critical need for new approaches to treating cancer and it is certain that we will see an increasing number of new drugs with exotic chemical structures used for chemotherapy in the future. To understand the mechanisms of action of any drug it is important to know how the drug is transformed in the body, either into active metabolites or inactive products to be excreted. With this information the success or failure of a drug in arresting cancer cell growth can be assessed, and perhaps more effective drugs designed.

Another reason for understanding the metabolism of anticancer drugs is to explain their toxicity. Cancer drugs are, arguably, the most toxic class of chemical agents given with therapeutic intent to human subjects. Almost all forms of anticancer chemotherapy are associated with some form of toxicity, sometimes even life threatening toxicity. It is possible that different metabolites may be responsible for the therapeutic and toxic effects of anticancer drugs. Moreover, there are marked inter-individual differences between patients in their response to the toxic effects of anticancer drugs. Understanding the causes of this variability in toxicity can go a long way toward individualizing treatment regimens and increasing the acceptability of anticancer drug therapy to patients.

The anticancer drugs embody a diverse array of chemical structures. The purpose of this two volume publication is to provide a comprehensive review of the metabolism of anticancer drugs. The authors, each expert in their fields, have attempted to emphasize the relation of metabolism to the therapeutic and toxic effects of anticancer drugs, drawing whenever possible on human studies. By the time this work becomes outdated it is hoped that there will be new classes of cancer drugs with dramatically improved efficacy for previously intractable human cancers. Medical science has taken the first important steps toward controlling cancer. The use and study of current chemotherapeutic drugs has taught us much about how toxic chemicals can be employed to treat human cancer; comprehending the underlying metabolism of these drugs should facilitate even better modalities of treatment for the future.

Garth Powis
Tucson, Arizona

CONTENTS

LIST OF CONTRIBUTORS

Jarle Aarbakke
Department of Pharmacology
Institute of Medical Biology
University of Tromsø
Tromsø
Norway

M. D'Incalci
Instituto de Richerche Farmacologiche "Mario Negri"
Milan
Italy

John M. Erikson
Department of Medicine
The University of Texas Southwestern Medical School
Dallas TX, U.S.A.

Peter B. Farmer
MRC Toxicology Unit
IRC for Mechanisms of Human Toxicity
Leicester, U.K.

S. Garattini
Instituto de Richerche Farmacologiche "Mario Negri"
Milan
Italy

Andreas Gescher
Cancer Research Campaign Experimental Chemotherapy Group
Pharmaceutical Sciences Institute
Aston University
Birmingham, U.K.

P. Ghezzi
Instituto de Richerche Farmacologiche "Mario Negri"
Milan
Italy

John S. Lazo
Department of Pharmacology
University of Pittsburgh School of Medicine
Pittsburgh PA, U.S.A.

Francis Y. F. Lee
Pharmaceutical Group
Bristol-Myers Squibb Company
Wallingford CT, U.S.A.

Charles L. Litterst
Developmental Therapeutics Branch
Division of AIDS
National Institute of Allergy and Infectious Diseases
Bethesda MD, U.S.A.

Garth Powis
Arizona Cancer Center
University of Arizona
Tucson AZ, U.S.A.

Russell A. Prough
Department of Biochemistry
University of Louisville School of Medicine
Louisville KY, U.S.A.

Donald J. Reed
Department of Biochemistry and Biophysics
Oregon State University
Corvallis OR, U.S.A.

Said M. Sebti
Department of Pharmacology
University of Pittsburgh School of Medicine
Pittsburgh PA, U.S.A.

N. E. Sladek
Department of Pharmacology
University of Minnesota
Minneapolis MN, U.S.A.

Lars Slørdal
Clinical Pharmacology Laboratory
The Norwegian Radium Hospital
Oslo
Norway

Michael D. Threadgill
School of Pharmacy and Pharmacology
University of Bath
Bath, U.K.

Donald J. Tweedie
Drug Metabolism Department
Pfizer, Inc.
Groton CT, U.S.A.

Paul Workman
Department of Medical Oncology
University of Glasgow
Glasgow, U.K.

Garth Powis, editor.
(1994) *Anticancer Drugs: Reactive Metabolism and Drug Interactions*,
Pergamon Press Ltd, pp. 1–77
Printed in the United Kingdom

CHAPTER 1

METABOLISM AND REACTIONS OF ALKYLATING AGENTS

PETER B. FARMER

MRC Toxicology Unit, Hodgkin Building, University of Leicester, P.O. Box 138, Lancaster Road, Leicester LE1 9HN, U.K.

1. INTRODUCTION

Although alkylating agents were the first compounds to be used in cancer chemotherapy, dating from the introduction of nitrogen mustard in 1946, they still hold a central position today in cancer treatment. An alkylating agent may be defined as a compound whose chemical reactivity involves the transfer of an alkyl group to a second molecule. Typically an alkylating agent's molecule will contain an alkyl group with an electron-deficient centre, bound to a leaving group; reaction with an electron rich centre in a second compound results in the displacement of the leaving group and the formation of a covalent bond with the alkyl group ('alkylation'). The biological activity of alkylating agents is thought to be due to alkylation reactions with intracellular molecules and in particular with nucleic acids. Amongst the consequences of such alkylations are cytotoxicity, mutagenicity, teratogenicity and carcinogenicity.

The application of alkylating agents in cancer chemotherapy naturally involves their use at doses which are cytotoxic, although clearly there must be some selective aspect of this toxicity in order to produce a useful anti-tumour agent. Cell killing by alkylating agents requires the cell to be in cycle and consequently these compounds are toxic not only to rapidly dividing tumour cells but also to many normal proliferating tissues. Additionally, they are less effective against the quiescent or slowly dividing tumour cells which occur in many tumours. Since the introduction of alkylating agents to cancer treatment there has therefore been a continued effort to develop novel agents that possess some extra selectivity towards tumour cells.

Listed below are summaries of the mechanism of action, metabolism, pharmacokinetics and therapeutic effectiveness of the leading alkylating agents that have been used for cancer treatment over the past 40 years. Three additional and highly important classes of compounds that also possess alkylating activity, the oxazaphosphorines, the nitrosoureas and the triazenes are covered in separate chapters.

2. NITROGEN MUSTARD (MECHLORETHAMINE)

Nitrogen mustard (Fig. 1, I) (*N*,*N*-bis(2-chloroethyl)methylamine) has the simplest chemical structure of the clinically used mustard compounds and was the first of these to be introduced into cancer treatment (Gilman and Philips, 1946). It is a powerful alkylating agent, now used generally in combination with other drugs. The compound was also produced in the past as a chemical warfare agent.

Reaction of nitrogen mustard with nucleophiles is rapid. Studies of the reaction kinetics in

Abbreviations—AUC, area under curve; AZQ, 3,6-diaziridinyl-2,5-bis(carboethoxyamino)-1,4-benzoquinone; BCH, 2-amino-bicyclo[2,2,1]heptane carboxylic acid; BZQ, 3,6-diaziridinyl-2,5-bis(hydroxyethylamino)-1,4-benzoquinone; CCNU, *N*-(2-chloroethyl)-*N*′-cyclohexyl-*N*-nitrosourea; CLL, chronic lymphocytic leukaemia; CSF, cerebrospinal fluid; DOH, 4-[bis(2-hydroxyethyl)amino]-L-phenylalanine; ECD, electron capture detection; GC, gas chromatography; MAP, microtubule associated protein; MOH, 4-(2-hydroxyethyl)-4-(2-chloroethyl)amino-L-phenylalanine; MS, mass spectrometry; TEM, 2,4,6-tris(1-aziridinyl)-1,3,5-triazine; TEPA, tris(1-aziridinyl)phosphine oxide; thio-TEPA, tris(1-aziridinyl)phosphine sulphide.

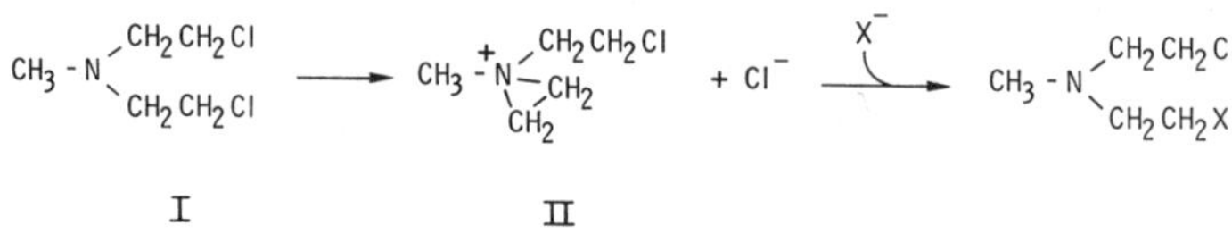

FIG. 1. The alkylation mechanism of nitrogen mustard.

aqueous media indicate that the reaction proceeds via a unimolecular first-order process leading to a relatively stable aziridinium ion (Fig. 1, II), which is subsequently ring-opened by S_N2 reactions with nucleophiles (Fig. 1). In unbuffered water the half-life for chloride production at 25°C has been reported to be 7 min (Hanby et al., 1947); a similar value was observed by Cohen et al. (1948) for the ring-closing reaction at pH 8.8. The half-life for loss of alkylating ability in pH 7.4 0.1 M phosphate buffer (37°C) is ca. 60 min (Williamson et al., 1966). (The test for alkylating ability used in this experiment (nitrobenzylpyridine assay—see below) will detect both uncyclized and cyclized nitrogen mustard and to a lesser extent any monofunctional alkylating agents derived therefrom.) The presence of serum accelerated the alkylating activity loss to a half-life of 9 min.

Reaction of nitrogen mustard with other nucleophilic centres and in particular with those in nucleic acids has been well studied (Wheeler and Skipper, 1957; see review by Price, 1975). Alkylation occurs extensively at the N-7 positions of guanine residues in nucleic acids (Brookes and Lawley, 1961a). Such N-7 alkyl adducts are unstable products and decompose by both chemical and enzymic processes. For example the half-life of the nitrogen mustard-deoxyguanosine adduct is 0.65 hr in aqueous conditions at pH 7.4, 27°C (Kallama and Hemminki, 1986). 7-Alkylated guanines are excised from nucleic acids, leaving 'apurinic sites'. The resulting damaged section of a DNA strand may then be repaired, following ligation at the apurinic site and synthesis of a repair patch. (Monofunctional alkylations of DNA are thought to be of particular significance with regard to induction of mutations and cancer by alkylating agents, as the presence of the alkylation may promote mispairing of bases between two DNA strands.)

Following an alkylation of DNA by one of the chloroethyl groups of nitrogen mustard it is also possible for the second alkylating centre of the mustard to interact with another nucleophile, resulting in a cross-link being formed between two sites in DNA or between DNA and protein. Cross-linking of DNA strands represents a much greater threat to cell survival than monofunctional alkylations and is believed to be responsible for the cytotoxic effects of bifunctional alkylating agents (Goldacre et al., 1949; Brookes and Lawley, 1961b; Hansson et al., 1987). These alkylations may occur at any stage of the cell cycle, but will not be recognized as hazardous until the cell enters DNA synthesis (S) or premitotic (G_2) phases, where progression through the cell cycle is blocked. Unbalanced synthesis of protein and of RNA may result and the cell may become enlarged. In synchronized Chinese hamster ovary cells, populations enriched in G_1 were most sensitive to nitrogen mustard (Murray and Meyn, 1986).

Cross-linking of DNA has frequently been demonstrated in in vitro experiments (Rutman et al., 1969; see review by Kohn, 1979). For example, during the reaction of L5178Y lymphoblast chromatin with nitrogen mustard, up to 25% of the reaction products were guanines cross-linked as bis(2-guanin-7-yl-ethyl)methylamine (Yerushalmi and Yagil, 1980). Protein cross-linking to DNA was similarly observed. The chemical identity of the guanine–guanine cross-link produced by nitrogen mustard has recently been confirmed by fast atom bombardment mass spectrometry (MS) (P. B. Farmer and P. D. Lawley, unpublished data). The relative reactivity of guanines in a DNA sequence varies towards nitrogen mustard. Runs of guanines are particularly susceptible to mustard attack. Using a modification of the Maxam and Gilbert DNA sequencing technique the parameters involved in the selectivity in DNA attack have been partially characterized (Mattes et al., 1986; Kohn et al., 1987, 1988). A significant one appears to be the molecular electrostatic potential induced at the guanine N-7 position by the nearest neighbour base pairs. To evaluate the biological consequences of interstrand cross-links a human shuttle vector, which contains a synthetic duplex cross-linked oligonucleotide, has recently been constructed (Ojwang et al., 1989; Grueneberg et al., 1991).

As a result of the dependence upon cellular proliferation for the cytotoxic effects of nitrogen mustard, many rapidly dividing tissues (e.g. bone marrow, intestinal mucosa, hair forming cells) are damaged during treatment in vivo. Quiescent cells, such as those in the liver, are therefore relatively resistant to alkylating agent treatment. Furthermore, in slowly proliferating cells DNA repair systems will have more chance to be effective in removing the lesion before it is recognized as being toxic.

2.1. Analysis

Nitrogen mustard may be determined colorimetrically by its reaction with 4-(4′-nitrobenzyl)pyridine (Friedman and Boger, 1961). This reaction is sensitive to all alkylating agents and therefore will not distinguish between parent drug and any mono- or bifunctional alkylating metabolites or partial hydrolysis products. However, it is readily applicable to biological samples and has a sensitivity of 0.5 μg/mL for nitrogen mustard.

The high reactivity of nitrogen mustard has limited the application of chromatographic techniques for its determination, although paper chromatography and TLC have both been attempted (Sakurai and Ito, 1960). A sensitive spectrophotometric method for quantitating nitrogen mustard after TLC has been reported by Norpoth et al. (1973). The plate is sprayed with 4-pyridine carboxaldehyde 2-benzothiazolyl hydrazone and heated over acetophenone. Spots (red) are developed with triethylamine and assayed at 530 nm. The sensitivity of the method for nitrogen mustard is ca. 1 nmol. The high sensitivity of fluorimetry has also been used (Mellett and Woods, 1960a) to detect nitrogen mustard at concentrations down to 0.02 μg/mL. Because of its high electrophilic chemical reactivity nitrogen mustard may be effectively trapped in biological systems by the addition of nucleophiles. Such a reaction was used by White et al. (1989), using diethyldithiocarbamate as the trapping agent, as the basis of a sensitive capillary gas chromatographic method for the analyis of nitrogen mustard. The compound is quantitated by the use of an internal standard, the analogous diethyldithiocarbamate adduct of nornitrogen mustard.

2.2. Transport and Resistance

The in vitro accumulation of nitrogen mustard into cells has been shown to be via a temperature sensitive, active transport process. In murine leukaemia L1210 cells uptake of nitrogen mustard was rapid, even at 0°C, reaching a cell-medium distribution ratio of 1 within 3 min (Kessel et al., 1969). In Ehrlich ascites tumour cells Wolpert and Ruddon (1969) demonstrated that uptake was temperature dependent and inhibited by metabolic inhibitors which affect membrane function (e.g. ouabain). Concentration of the drug occurred in the cells; in resistant cells, however, the accumulation of nitrogen mustard was only half that of sensitive cells, suggesting that decreased membrane permeability might be a contributing cause for development of resistance. A similar conclusion had previously been reached by Rutman et al. (1968), who observed a decreased permeability of nitrogen mustard into Lettre–Ehrlich ascites tumour cells that had been made resistant to the drug after treatment in vivo to high doses (3–80 mg/kg). Decreases in DNA alkylation and cross-linking have also been observed in resistant Ehrlich ascites tumour cells treated with nitrogen mustard in vivo (Chun et al., 1969).

A kinetic analysis of nitrogen mustard uptake by sensitive and resistant L5178Y lymphoblasts (Goldenberg et al., 1970) confirmed that a transport carrier was involved in nitrogen mustard uptake, which was found to proceed uphill against a concentration gradient up to 35-fold. Competitive inhibition of uptake was observed with analogues of nitrogen mustard (dimethyl 2-chloroethylamine and hydrolyzed nitrogen mustard). Resistance to nitrogen mustard could partly, but not entirely, be accounted for by alteration of the transport carrier and resultant decreased permeability. The close structural similarity of nitrogen mustard and choline prompted Goldenberg et al. (1971b) to investigate the interaction of nitrogen mustard with choline transport. The time course of choline uptake into L5178Y lymphoblasts closely parallelled that of nitrogen mustard and the transport was competitively inhibited by the drug and its hydrolyzed derivative. It was concluded therefore that the same carrier is involved in the transport of nitrogen mustard and choline into L5178Y cells. Choline also had a significant protective effect against the cytotoxicity of nitrogen mustard to L5178Y cells in vitro, although no protective effects could be observed in vivo in animals at near lethal levels of choline (Goldenberg and Sinha, 1973a). Choline also increased the survival of mouse haemopoietic and transplantable myeloma stem cells in vitro when these were exposed to nitrogen mustard (Ogawa et al., 1973).

The proliferation rate of the cells is also important, with transport of choline and nitrogen mustard being more active in rapidly dividing cells (Goldenberg et al., 1971a). Uptake of choline and the hydrolyzed form of nitrogen mustard was also shown to be via the same active transport process into normal and leukaemic human lymphoid cells, although as choline did not appear to be a classical competitive inhibitor of the mustard uptake, it was suggested that there was an additional low affinity, choline independent transport system for high doses of hydrolyzed mustard (Lyons and Goldenberg, 1972). In Walker 256 carcinosarcoma cells (Goldenberg and Sinha, 1973b) and in the Yoshida sarcoma cell line (Inaba, 1973) the choline active transport system also appeared to be involved in nitrogen mustard transport. Resistance in the Yoshida cells was again associated with decreased activity of the choline transport carrier (Inaba, 1973). An exception to this mechanism of resistance was observed in rat ascites hepatoma cells, where there was little difference in uptake and binding of nitrogen mustard between sensitive and resistant cell lines (Inaba and Sakurai, 1977). However, in the latter cells DNA repair activity was enhanced.

In recent years the transport system for nitrogen mustard into murine tumour cell lines has been examined in some detail. Incubation with the mustard inhibits potassium influx (Baxter et al., 1982; Grunicke et al., 1982, 1985; Doppler et al., 1985). In L1210 leukaemia cells the inhibition is brought about by a reduction in a diuretic-sensitive component of Rb^+ influx, identified as being mediated by a $Na^+/K^+/Cl^-$ cotransporter (Wilcock and Hickman, 1988; Wilcock et al., 1988). The question of whether or not the inhibition of the cotransporter is alone a lethal lesion remains open.

A variety of other mechanisms have been proposed to explain resistance of cells to nitrogen mustards. Tisdale and Phillips (1978) observed decreased cAMP-binding protein, phosphodiesterase and cAMP-dependent protein kinase in an alkylating agent resistant Walker 256 rat mammary carcinoma cell line. There was no difference in the formation or rate of removal of mustard-induced DNA cross-links between resistant and sensitive Walker 256 cells (Dean et al., 1986b). However the resistant cells showed a loss of guanine-O^6-alkyl transferase activity (Dean et al., 1986a), elevated glutathione-*S*-transferase activity (Butler et al., 1987), lower sensitivity for inhibition of histone acetylation by nitrogen mustard (Helliger et al., 1988) and hypophosphorylation of nuclear matrix lamin (Moy and Tew, 1986). Elevated glutathione-*S*-transferase (and γ-glutamyl transpeptidase) was also observed in a mustard-resistant rat brain tumour cell line (Evans et al., 1987). A Chinese hamster ovary cell line has been made resistant to mustards (Robson et al., 1986) and has been shown to have reduced levels of drug-induced DNA cross-links, but elevated glutathione-*S*-transferase (Robson et al., 1987). In resistant human Burkitt lymphoma cells there were decreased DNA cross-links, increased glutathione content and an increased topoisomerase II activity (Tan et al., 1987, 1988) the latter being postulated as the cause of enhanced mono adduct repair (and consequential decrease of DNA cross-links).

Because of the normal practice of administering nitrogen mustard to patients in combination with other drugs, there has been considerable interest in any effects that these might have on nitrogen mustard transport. In L5178Y leukaemia cells the uptake of hydrolyzed nitrogen mustard and of choline was stimulated by atropine, morphine and cocaine (Goldenberg, 1974). Morphine and cocaine also stimulated transport of hydrolyzed nitrogen mustard in lymphocytes from normal and leukaemic patients; in acute leukaemia cells it was shown that the low dose choline dependent transport system was stimulated preferentially in comparison with that in normal lymphocytes, suggesting possibilities for increasing the therapeutic activity of the nitrogen mustard (Goldenberg, 1976). It has also been suggested (Presant and Carr, 1980) that the resistance of cells to nitrogen mustard could be reversed by administration of amphotericin B, which had been found to stimulate nitrogen mustard uptake in fresh ovarian carcinoma cells and in cultured human colon and epidermoid carcinoma cells. Incorporation of nitrogen mustard into liposomes dramatically increased its transport into cells, as measured by the effects of the drug on macromolecule synthesis by Ehrlich cell mitochondria (Rutman et al., 1977).

Other compounds which increase the activity of nitrogen mustard are ethacrynic acid (which binds glutathione-*S*-transferase) (Nagourney et al., 1990), disulfiram (and its metabolite diethyldithiocarbamic acid) (Valeriote and Grates, 1989) and quercetin (which inhibits protein kinase C) (Hofmann et al., 1988). Protection may be achieved with 5-*N*,*N*-dimethylamiloride, which inhibits the choline transport system used by nitrogen mustard (Doppler et al., 1988). Post-incubation of treated cells with albumin also decreases mustard cytotoxicity, presumably because of removal of intracellular unreacted intermediates (Ritter et al., 1989).

2.3. Distribution and Metabolism

The distribution of nitrogen mustard was first studied by Skipper et al. (1951) in normal and leukaemic mice using [^{14}C]-methyl labelled drug (Foreman et al., 1950). The radioactivity was distributed throughout all tissues, with the intestine having the highest activity in normal mice. Thirty to fifty percent of the activity was found in tissues by 6 hr and in leukaemic mice there was preferential labelling of the lymph nodes, adrenals, thymus and brain. Fifteen to eighteen percent of the radioactive carbon was exhaled as carbon dioxide and 5–7% was excreted in the urine as unidentified products. Nadkarni et al. (1956) reported that [^{14}C]-methyl nitrogen mustard was rapidly lost from the blood of rats and mice; 45–80% of the plasma content was associated with plasma proteins.

Because of interest in the use of nitrogen mustard as an antisickling agent, haemoglobin-binding of the drug has also been investigated. In vitro alkylation of human haemoglobin by nitrogen mustard resulted in two types of adducts, one which was alkali labile and one which was stable (Roth et al., 1981). The alkali-labile adducts are believed to be esterified acidic amino acids within the protein chain and the stable adducts have been shown (partially by X-ray crystallography) mainly to comprise alkylated histidine imidazole rings. Some alkylation of cysteine thiol groups is also thought to occur.

Because of its reactive chemical nature nitrogen mustard will undoubtedly bind to all the nucleophilic sites within a cell and as indicated above the binding (and cross-linking) of DNA is of especial significance to the cytostatic properties of the drug. The nature of the conjugated derivative formed by the interaction of nitrogen mustard with glutathione (which may play a role in drug resistance) has recently been investigated by NMR (Gamcsik et al., 1990). The intermediacy of an aziridinium intermediate in the alkylation reaction was confirmed. Nucleolarphosphoproteins have also been shown to be susceptible to attack by nitrogen mustard. Thus nucleophosmin was shown by Chan (1989) to be cross-linked in treated mouse leukaemia P388 cells.

As an example of the generalized binding of nitrogen mustard it was shown by Inaba and Sakurai (1971) that Yoshiba sarcoma cells exposed to tritiated nitrogen mustard contained similar specific activities (within a factor of 2, measured as disintegrations per minute/mg protein) in the nucleus, mitochrondrion, microsomes and supernatant. The relative specific activities (disintegrations per minute/mg) for protein, DNA and RNA were 1.3:1.0:1.9.

Little information is available concerning metabolic transformations of nitrogen mustard. The evidence for transmethylation metabolic pathways is slight, as only 0.1–0.4% of radiocarbon from [^{14}C]-methyl nitrogen mustard, injected i.v. into rats, could be detected in choline and virtually none in methionine and creatine (Trams and Klopp, 1955). *N*-Demethylation has, however, been observed in in vitro rat liver systems, with the production of formaldehyde (Trams and Nadkarni, 1956).

2.4. Toxicity

Patients treated with nitrogen mustard show typical alkylating agent toxicity. Haemotopoietic suppression is particularly notable with maximal leukopenia and thrombocytopenia at 1–3 weeks after drug administration (Nissen-Meyer and Host, 1960). Other toxicities include nausea and vomiting, testicular germ cell depletion and local skin reactions close to the site of drug injection. Skin toxicity may be alleviated by local treatment with sodium thiosulphate which will react with the mustard and render it ineffective (Dorr et al., 1988). Nitrogen mustard is also mutagenic and clastogenic in a variety of systems (I.A.R.C., 1975b, 1982a; Perticone and Lambert, 1986; Goldstein, 1987; Tokuda and Bodell, 1987; Ehling and Neuhäuser-Klaus, 1989). In yeast all possible types of base pair substitutions as well as deletions and double mutations were observed (Kunz and Mis, 1989). Nitrogen mustard causes aneuploidy in human lymphoblastoid cells (Crespi et al., 1987) and is carcinogenic to mice and rats (Heston, 1949, 1950; Conklin et al., 1965; Schmähl and Osswald, 1970; Zackheim and Smuckler, 1980). It was stated by I.A.R.C. (1982a) that there was inadequate evidence for carcinogenicity in man although many reports have been made of the development of acute nonlymphocytic leukaemia and other tumours in patients treated with nitrogen mustard (Schmähl et al., 1982). The definite association of these secondary malignancies with nitrogen mustard is difficult because of the widespread use of other drugs and radiation in combination with this compound. Schmähl et al. (1982) claim that about 50% of the tumours induced by nitrogen mustard are leukaemias, followed in abundance by carcinoma of the urinary bladder (ca. 15%). Teratogenicity of nitrogen mustard has also been observed in the rat (Murphy et al., 1958) and caution is clearly required when considering the administration of the drug to pregnant women.

3. CHLORAMBUCIL

Chlorambucil (4-[p-bis(2-chloroethyl)aminophenyl] butyric acid, Leukeran) (III) is an aniline mustard derivative bearing a butyric acid side-chain. It was synthesized by Everett et al. (1953) and has become established as a drug of major importance in the treatment of chronic lymphocytic leukaemia, ovarian cancer, Hodgkin's disease, breast carcinomas and other lymphomas and solid tumours. Chlorambucil is a reactive alkylating agent and hydrolyzes in aqueous solution to yield the bis(2-hydroxyethyl) analogue. This hydrolysis is promoted by basic conditions and complete reaction occurs in 120 min at 37°C in 0.025 N sodium hydroxide. At pH 7.5 the rate constant is 4 times lower (Linford, 1961). At 4°C the alkylating action of chlorambucil is very weak, there being no detectable hydrolysis in 10 hr (Linford, 1963). Later, more detailed studies by Owen and Stewart (1979) and Ehrsson et al. (1980b) showed that chlorambucil hydrolysis is a unimolecular process, with a rate of reaction independent of hydroxide ion concentration in the range pH 5–10 (k 0.54 hr^{-1}). Below pH 5, when the amino group becomes protonated, the reaction rate decreases, which suggests that the rate-determining step is the formation of a cyclic ethyleneimmonium ion.

The presence of plasma slows the rate of hydrolysis considerably. The in vitro degradation rate constant determined by Alberts et al. (1979b) for chlorambucil in plasma at 37°C was 0.12 hr^{-1} compared with the rate constant in water of 0.43 hr^{-1}. The half-life for chlorambucil in a 45 mg/mL albumin solution at 37°C was found by Ehrsson et al. (1981) to be 15.8 hr (in comparison to the half-life in pH 7.35 phosphate buffer of 0.45 hr). In plasma the half-life was similar to that in the albumin solution (17.8 hr). Chlorambucil is extensively bound ($98.98 \pm 0.05\%$) to albumin in plasma. In Chinese hamster V79 cell medium the hydrolytic half-life of chlorambucil is 2.5 hr (Hartley-Asp et al., 1986).

For experimental use of the drug Bosanquet and Clarke (1986) recommended that solutions should be stored at −70°C to minimize decomposition. Addition of 10% serum to a chlorambucil solution increased the drug's stability 4-fold. Contact with polyvinylchloride should also be avoided as this adsorbs chlorambucil.

Reaction with other nucleophiles occurs when biological systems are exposed to chlorambucil. For example the drug alkylates red cell membranes and causes them to lyse (Linford et al., 1963). A drug concentration of 1 mg/mL resulted in 90% haemolysis in 2 hr at 37°C, whereas no lysis occurred with the bis(2-hydroxyethyl) analogue. However, lysis did not appear to be solely dependent on the alkylation process as it also occurred with chlorambucil at 4°C when the drug was not active as an alkylating agent (Linford et al., 1969). Nuclear proteins were also attacked by chlorambucil, resulting in their removal from chromatin (Riches and Harrap, 1973). Binding of the drug to these nuclear proteins is both covalent and non-covalent, with more drug protein interaction in sensitive tumours compared to resistant tumours (Riches and Harrap, 1975). The mechanism of the antitumour action of chlorambucil is believed to be associated with its ability to alkylate DNA and in particular to form DNA–DNA cross-links. The presence of these has been demonstrated in yeast cells by Ruhland et al. (1978). Overall tumour nucleic acid binding is prolonged and has been shown in rats to be maximal 24 hr after i.p. injection of chlorambucil (Tew and Taylor, 1978).

As with nitrogen mustard (see above) the relative extent of reaction of chlorambucil with guanine residues in DNA depends on the molecular electrostatic potential induced by the neighbour base pairs (Kohn et al., 1988). Unlike nitrogen mustard, chlorambucil has been shown to produce adenine adducts in DNA, some of which are postulated to be intrastrand cross-linked (Pieper and Erickson, 1990). It was suggested that these may be associated, in vitro, with termination of transcription of DNA.

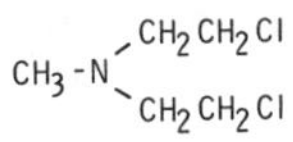

I

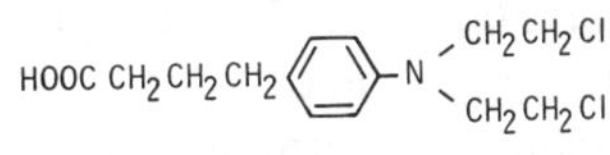

III

3.1. Analysis

The analysis of chlorambucil was initially carried out by the Epstein colorimetric procedure using 4-(4′-nitrobenzyl) pyridine; for example Boyland et al. (1961) used this technique to study the concentration of chlorambucil in regionalized limb perfusion in dogs. An alternative colorimetric procedure was developed by Kozlov and Bernshtein (1968) using nicotinic acid and benzidine. Spectrophotometric determination of chlorambucil was used by Linford (1962) to measure the drug in serum or plasma at concentrations down to 2μg/mL. A fluorescence assay with a lower limit of sensitivity of 100 ng/mL has also recently been described (Bernier et al., 1984a).

Liquid chromatographic techniques have now become established as the optimal method for chlorambucil analysis. Leff and Bardsley (1979) determined chlorambucil as its *n*-propylester derivative in human plasma samples down to concentrations of 10 ng/mL using a reversed phase octadecylsilica column and a mobile phase of water, methanol and ammonium acetate. Methanol, water and acetic acid may also be used as the mobile phase allowing satisfactory analyses to be made down to 15 ng/mL (Newell et al., 1979). Although in both of these analyses the drug is extracted into an organic solvent prior to HPLC, it is also possible to analyze plasma following its direct injection into the HPLC column so long as an appropriate guard column is included in the system (Zakaria and Brown, 1982). A similar sensitivity of detection for HPLC analysis of chlorambucil in plasma (10 ng/mL) was reported by Adair et al. (1985). In this analysis the plasma proteins were precipitated by addition of perchloric acid prior to C_{18} Sep Pak chromatography and isocratic reversed phase HPLC. No internal standard was used. Further reported analyses are those of Workman et al. (1987) using isocratic paired-ion reversed phase HPLC and a fluorinated internal standard (detection limit 60 ng chlorambucil/mL plasma) and Oppitz et al. (1989) using a reversed phase system, with limit of detection 30 ng chlorambucil/mL plasma. Many of these analyses are equally effective for determination of the chlorambucil metabolite phenylacetic mustard (see below).

Chlorambucil may also be subjected to gas chromatography (GC) after chemical derivatization of the carboxylic acid function. Mass spectral selected ion monitoring in combination with GC allows highly sensitive determination of chlorambucil in biological fluids. Thus Jakhammer et al. (1977) developed an analytical procedure, using d_8-labelled chlorambucil as internal standard, for determining plasma chlorambucil (derivatized as its methyl ester) down to a concentration of 8 ng/mL. The trimethylsilyl derivative was used by Chang et al. (1980) in an analogous procedure for determining chlorambucil in plasma or urine. The d_8-labelled internal standard was also used in the GC-MS procedure of Ehrsson et al. (1980a); in this approach the chlorambucil was extracted from the plasma and converted to a thiazane derivative by reaction of the mustard group with sodium sulphide. The carboxylic acid was then esterified, using extractive alkylation with allyl bromide. The detection limit was 1 ng/mL plasma and the relative standard deviation for the analysis at 10 ng/mL was 5%. Chlorambucil and its metabolite phenylacetic mustard may also be determined by capillary GC alone, using a flame ionization detector. The two compounds were determined quantitatively as trimethylsilyl derivatives, with a limit of detection 30 ng/mL plasma, by Lohmar et al. (1989), using phenylpropionic acid mustard as internal standard.

3.2. Uptake, Transport and Resistance

The uptake of chlorambucil by tumour cells appears to be by a simple diffusion process. Sensitive and resistant Yoshida ascites sarcoma cells incorporated a constant fraction of the drug to which they were exposed within 5 min (Harrap and Hill, 1970). The hydrolysis of the mustard in the resistant cells was similar to that in saline controls, but occurred 2.5 times slower in sensitive cells. Additionally the aromatic ring of chlorambucil was more extensively degraded in resistant cells. The combination of these effects was a lower intracellular concentration of active drug in the resistant cells. These studies were later extended to lymphocytes from the blood of chronic lymphocytic leukaemia patients (Hill and Harrap, 1972). The drug was again taken up in 5 min and hydrolyzed at a rate similar to controls, indicating that the mustard group was unmodified by the lymphocytes. However, increases in the aromatic degradation of the drug were seen in two patients who responded favourably.

The synthesis of [^{3}H]-labelled chlorambucil by Hill et al. (1971) allowed the use of much lower concentrations of drug in uptake studies in vitro. At concentrations equivalent to those resulting from treatment in vivo the rate of uptake of [^{3}H]-chlorambucil into sensitive strains of Yoshida ascites sarcoma was twice that of resistant cells. Similar differences were seen in the extent of protein binding. At concentrations greater than 0.33 mM both cell types incorporated equivalent amounts of drug. Hill (1972) showed with labelled drug that uptake into Yoshida cells was not decreased at low temperature (4°C) or by oxidative phosphorylation inhibitors and that the intracellular concentration of the drug was not accumulated against a concentration gradient. At 4°C the differences in uptake between resistant and sensitive cells disappeared, indicating that these were caused not by the transport mechanism but by a metabolic/hydrolytic process. At doses of chlorambucil that are equivalently toxic to sensitive and resistant cells (30-fold greater for the latter) only four times more chlorambucil-derived radioactivity was bound to the nucleic acids and proteins of resistant cells, which reflects the reduced transport of the drug into these cells (Hill, 1975).

In L5178Y lymphoblasts chlorambucil was also taken up rapidly by a simple diffusion process (37 and 4°C). Efflux of the drug was rapid and not by active transport (Begleiter and Goldenberg, 1983). Transport may, however, be affected by pH differences between the outside and inside of the cells. As chlorambucil is a weak acid, its accumulation is enhanced in cells where the extracellular pH is lowered (< 7) relative to the intracellular pH (Mikkelsen et al., 1985), which may be of relevance in the treatment of some solid tumours where the interstitial pH is low.

As is the case with nitrogen mustard (see above) many investigations have been made on mechanisms of resistance. In chronic lymphocytic leukaemia (CLL) cells resistance to chlorambucil does not appear to be related to uptake (Silber et al., 1989; Bank et al., 1989), although drug DNA binding was increased in cells from resistant patients. An inverse correlation was found to exist between cellular glutathione transferase activities and the number of DNA cross-links produced by chlorambucil in a number of CLL cell lines (Johnston et al., 1990), suggesting that glutathione conjugation may be an important determinant of chlorambucil resistance. The conjugate has recently been prepared and mass spectral techniques established for its analysis (Dulik et al., 1990). Resistant Walker 256 cells and Chinese hamster ovary cells contain higher glutathione transferase levels than sensitive cells (Buller et al., 1987; Robson et al., 1987). Inhibition of glutathione transferase in the resistant Chinese hamster ovary cells with indomethacin potentiates the cytotoxicity of chlorambucil (Hall et al., 1989). Ethacrynic acid and piriprost have been used with similar effect in the resistant Walker 256 cells (Tew et al., 1988). Human glutathione transferases have now been expressed in *Saccharomyces cerevisiae* which confers resistance of the yeast to chlorambucil (Black et al., 1990).

Detailed attempts have been made to increase the selectivity of transport of chlorambucil to tumour cells by binding the drug either physically (Ghose et al., 1972) or covalently (Ross, 1975a,b) to an antibody. As insufficient toxicity was obtained by this approach, more active toxins (such as ricin or diphtheria toxin) are now being used in the conjugates (Thorpe and Ross, 1982). Chlorambucil has also been linked to an anti-CEA antibody (Bernier et al., 1984b) and this conjugate may be useful for carrying the drug to colonic cancer cells. More recently Smyth et al. (1986b) have studied chlorambucil, covalently and non-covalently bound to monoclonal antibodies. Potentiation of chlorambucil's cytotoxicity to tumour cells was observed with IgM and IgG2a subclasses of antibodies. Non-covalently bound chlorambucil entered cells independently of the antibody and it was suggested that the antibody was having its effect by altering the properties of the tumour cell or by promoting cell surface alkylation by chlorambucil. Using a covalently bound chlorambucil-monoclonal antibody conjugate specific targetting of the drug to a murine thymoma was achieved (Smyth et al., 1986a).

3.3. Metabolism

One of the first studies on the absorption, distribution and elimination of chlorambucil was that carried out by Hill and Riches (1971) who administered a ring-labelled tritiated drug to rats bearing Yoshida ascites sarcoma. The highest concentration of label was seen in the liver and kidney and was maintained for longest in the kidney. Differences in cellular uptake and nucleic acid binding of the drug were seen in sensitive and resistant tumours, in accord with the authors' postulate that resistant cells have a greater ability to hydrolyze or metabolize the drug (Harrap and Hill, 1970). Chlorambucil labelled with [^{14}C] at one of three positions (mustard side-chain, carboxyl group and the carbon vicinal to the carboxyl group) was administered to rats by Godeneche et al. (1975). The label from the latter two of these analogues, but not that from the mustard side-chain was significantly lost as carbon dioxide, indicating that oxidative metabolism had occurred in the butyric acid side-chain.

The most detailed study of chlorambucil metabolism in rats has been that of Mitoma et al. (1977), using both ring-labelled and mustard side-chain [^{14}C]-labelled drug. Again liver and kidney were found to show the highest concentrations of radiolabel. Metabolites were extracted from urine and characterized by GC-MS after methylation or trimethylsilylation. The metabolic processes (summarized in Fig. 2) involve oxidative degradation of the butyric acid side-chain to give phenylacetic and benzoic acid derivatives, coupled with hydrolytic degradation of the mustard side-chain.

An expected metabolite from β-oxidation of the butyric acid side-chain would be phenylacetic mustard (Fig. 2, IV) (formed via 3,4-dehydrochlorambucil) which was more toxic than chlorambucil and has a lower therapeutic index against Walker 256 carcinoma in rats (McLean et al., 1976, 1980). Phenylacetic mustard has been detected in rat blood (McLean et al., 1976, 1980) and in human plasma (Newell et al., 1979; McLean et al., 1979; Alberts et al., 1979). The major urinary metabolite in the rat was 2-(4-*N*-(2-chloroethyl)aminophenyl) acetic acid (McLean et al., 1980) which is inactive as an antitumour agent. Rats injected with 3,4-dehydrochlorambucil also produced phenylacetic mustard in the blood (McLean et al., 1980) confirming the proposed β-oxidation pathway.

Attempts to improve the therapeutic efficiency of chlorambucil by inhibiting the β-oxidation pathway were made by Farmer et al. (1979). The drug was synthesized with 2 deuterium atoms at the α- or β-positions of the butyric acid side-chain. The deuterium/hydrogen isotope effect caused lower plasma levels of phenylacetic mustard in rats administered chlorambucil-β-d_2, but no difference in therapeutic activity was observed. The effect of β,β-disubstitution with fluorine on chlorambucil's metabolism and activity was studied by Lee et al. (1986). β-Difluorochlorambucil was less potent than chlorambucil but showed a slightly greater therapeutic index to a murine fibrosarcoma. Despite the fluorine substitution it was still β-oxidized, although at a reduced rate. Two new unidentified metabolites were also produced. The amount of non-protein bound drug in plasma was 0.45% for β-difluorochlorambucil, compared to 0.9% for chlorambucil and it was postulated that potency of chlorambucil analogues may be dependent upon this parameter.

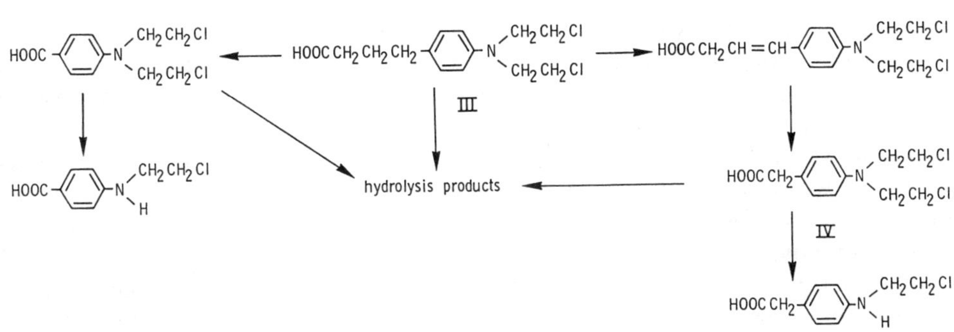

Fig. 2. Metabolism of chlorambucil.

3.4. PHARMACOKINETICS

In the rat, the pharmacokinetics of chlorambucil have been studied following its s.c. administration (Newell et al., 1981). After a dose of 40 mg/kg (2 rats) peak plasma levels (12 μg/mL) occurred within 2 hr. The parent drug was eliminated with a half-life of 2.4 hr which was similar to that of the metabolite phenylacetic mustard ($t_{1/2}\beta$ 2.9 hr). Peak plasma concentration of this metabolite was 7.3 μg/mL.

For human use, chlorambucil is frequently administered orally and is rapidly absorbed from the gastrointestinal tract, before its metabolism to phenylacetic mustard. Four patients with haematological malignancies who were administered chlorambucil in the dose range 38–50 mg (0.6–1.21 mg/kg) showed maximum chlorambucil plasma levels (determined by the GC-MS method of Chang et al., 1980) of 1.1 ± 0.6 μg/mL (Alberts et al., 1979b). The mean terminal phase half-life of chlorambucil was 91.7 ± 19.3 min, but the urinary excretion of chlorambucil in the first 24 hr was only 0.54%. Peak plasma levels of phenylacetic mustard were achieved within 2–4 hr (0.81 ± 0.32 μg/mL). The mean terminal phase half-life of this metabolite was 1.6 times greater than that of chlorambucil with an area under curve (AUC) level 1.9 times larger than chlorambucil. Urine from the first 24 hr contained only 0.25% of the dose as this metabolite, the remaining material being composed mostly of hydrolysis products of the parent drug or metabolites.

Almost complete absorption of oral chlorambucil was observed also by McLean et al. (1979) who studied the fate of the [^{14}C]-labelled compound in advanced cancer patients using TLC and GC-MS techniques. Newell et al. (1983a) determined, by HPLC, the systemic availability of chlorambucil to be > 70% after oral administration of 10 mg doses to 5 patients, with a mean elimination phase half-life of 109 ± 16 min. A much shorter half-life (mean 24 min) was observed by Leff and Bardsley (1979) in a group of 5 ovarian carcinoma patients receiving 5–10 mg oral chlorambucil, although the range of values observed was very large (2–55 min). Doses of 10 mg chlorambucil given to 5 lymphoma and immunocytoma patients by Ehrsson et al. (1983b) were shown by GC-MS techniques to have elimination half-lives in the range 0.55–13 hr. Maximum plasma concentrations were variable (0.26 ± 0.20 μg/mL) as were the AUC values (0.38 ± 0.25 μg.h/mL).

Many drugs administered orally show different absorption if given with food. Such effects could be important for chlorambucil in view of its ready decomposition in aqueous solutions. Under fasting conditions the maximum plasma concentration of chlorambucil (40 mg) was reached in 0.64 ± 0.36 hr ($n = 5$) whereas in the same patients under non-fasting conditions the absorption was slower (1.90 ± 1.19 hr) (Ehrsson et al., 1984). The peak concentration decreased from 1.46 ± 0.74 μg/mL to 0.56 ± 0.21 μg/mL when the drug was given with food. However, the AUC for chlorambucil and for phenylacetic mustard was unchanged by fasting. However Adair et al. (1986), in a larger study, showed that food caused a significant reduction in the bioavailability (AUC) of chlorambucil, together with reduced peak plasma levels and elimination rate constants. Gastrointestinal absorption of chlorambucil in the rat is believed to be by a non energy-dependent system (Adair and McElnay, 1986).

Comparative studies by Alberts et al. (1980a) on the pharmacokinetics of oral melphalan and chlorambucil suggested that the latter should be a more predictable alkylating agent in patients, based on its greater in vitro stability, its low urinary excretion and its more rapid and predictable availability after oral dosing.

Kinetics for intravenous chlorambucil follow a two compartment open model. In three patients treated with [^{14}C]-labelled chlorambucil the plasma radioactivity levels were found by McLean et al. (1979) to have $t_{1/2}\alpha$ 0.32, 0.85 and 0.25 hr and $t_{1/2}\beta$ 20.6, 9.0 and 7.1 hr. However these measurements include *all* drug derived material rather than just chlorambucil itself. A more satisfactory study was that of Newell et al. (1983a), using an HPLC determination of chlorambucil in the plasma of patients ($n = 7$) receiving 10–200 mg i.v. drug. The mean half lives were $t_{1/2}\alpha$ 7.0 ± 1.3 min and $t_{1/2}\beta$ 80 ± 24 min which is similar to the oral terminal phase half life.

In anaesthetized rats, intravenously administered chlorambucil had plasma $t_{1/2}$ of 0.43 hr and the drug was 99.6% plasma protein bound. The brain:plasma AUC ratio was 0.021 (Greig et al., 1988). Attempts have been made to synthesize chlorambucil analogues with greater brain penetration. Seven lipophilic esters were studied by Greig et al. (1990b) but none of the compounds examined delivered and maintained high brain concentrations of chlorambucil. However the t-butyl ester of chlorambucil which is not highly susceptible to hydrolysis in plasma did enter and remain in the brain (rat), (brain:plasma AUC ratio 0.68). The plasma AUC of alkylating agents from the *t*-butyl ester was 5-fold lower and the brain AUC 7-fold higher than those from an equimolar dose of chlorambucil (Greig et al., 1990a). Thus this analogue may have value in the treatment of human brain tumours. An HPLC assay has now been developed for analysis of chlorambucil *t*-butyl ester and its metabolites chlorambucil and phenylacetic mustard (Greig et al., 1990c).

The toxicity and anti-tumour activity of chlorambucil are both enhanced by pretreatment with chemosensitizers such as misonidazole. Lee and Workman (1986) have demonstrated that misonidazole exerts this effect by reducing plasma clearance of chlorambucil and its metabolites and thus increasing the AUC.

3.5. Toxicity and Carcinogenicity

The alkylating properties of chlorambucil give rise to toxicity to rapidly dividing cells such as those in bone-marrow. Drug administration also induces nausea and vomiting, pulmonary fibrosis (Cole et al., 1978) and spermatogenesis (Richter et al., 1970). Jaundice has been observed in ca. 10% of patients treated with chlorambucil (Robert et al., 1968).

The genotoxic effects caused by the alkylation of DNA by chlorambucil are illustrated by its ability to induce chromosome breakages in cultures of human peripheral lymphocytes (Reeves and Margoles, 1974), mutations in *Salmonella,* sister chromatid exchanges in CHO cells (Athanasiou and Arzimanoglou, 1986) and chromosome damage in the lymphocytes of long-term treated patients (Palmer et al., 1985; Reeves et al., 1985). Germ-line mutations induced by chlorambucil in mice have been analyzed (Rinchik et al., 1990).

Teratogenicity has also been reported following i.p. administration of chlorambucil to rats (Chaube et al., 1967; Murphy et al., 1958) and foetal abnormalities were observed in women who were pregnant while receiving chlorambucil treatment (Shotton et al., 1963; Steege and Caldwell, 1980). The embryotoxicity of chlorambucil has been demonstrated in whole mouse embryo cultures (Van Maele-Fabry and Picard, 1987). In mice the teratogenicity is potentiated by caffeine (Fuji and Nakatsuka, 1983).

In rats and mice there is considerable evidence that chlorambucil is carcinogenic. Skin application to mice in the presence of croton oil results in 58% (11/19) development of papillomas (Salaman and Roe, 1956). Intraperitoneal administration caused a significant excess of lung tumours, lymphosarcomas and ovarian tumours (Shimkin et al., 1966; Weisburger et al., 1975). In rats an increase in the incidence of lymphomas was seen in the male but not in the female following i.p. chlorambucil. Oral administration of chlorambucil to BALB/c mice resulted in lung and lymphoreticular system tumours in both sexes and mammary carcinomas in females (Cavaliere et al., 1990).

There is also sufficient evidence to classify chlorambucil as a human carcinogen (I.A.R.C., 1981). Several reports have been published associating the development of leukaemic and other tumours in patients receiving chlorambucil. For example Reimer et al. (1977) observed two acute myelogenous leukaemias and one erythroleukaemia in chlorambucil-treated ovarian cancer patients. Catovsky and Galton (1971) observed myelomonocytic leukaemia in a chlorambucil-treatment CLL patient and Steigbigel et al. (1974) reported on an acute myeloproliferative disorder following long-term chlorambucil treatment. In a randomized trial with 431 polycythemia vera patients chlorambucil treatment was associated with a 13-fold increase in the incidence of acute non-lymphocytic leukaemia (Berk et al., 1981). The occurrence of second tumours following anti-cancer drug treatment has been reviewed by Schmähl et al. (1982), with the conclusion that more than 50% of these tumours were acute leukaemia.

4. PREDNIMUSTINE

Prednimustine (V) (pregna-1,4-diene-3,20-dione,11β,17α,21-trihydroxy-21[4-*p*-(bis-(2-chloroethyl)amino)phenyl butyrate]) is the prednisolone ester of chlorambucil. This was synthesized

(Könyves et al., 1975) in the hope that the steroid would act as a carrier for the cytotoxic function of chlorambucil, allowing it to cross the neoplastic cell membrane more effectively. The clinical efficacy of combinations of prednisolone and chlorambucil against human mammary carcinoma had previously been demonstrated (Freckman et al., 1964). The activity and toxicity of prednimustine has been reviewed by Hartley-Asp (1986).

In the rat Walker 256 carcinoma the therapeutic index (LD_{50}/ED_{50}) of prednimustine was increased in comparison to that of an equimolar mixture of prednisolone and chlorambucil (Könyves et al., 1975). However, later studies by Harrap et al. (1977) on the Yoshida ascites sarcoma in rat showed that, although prednimustine was more effective than chlorambucil in killing the tumour cells, the antitumour effect of chlorambucil could be enhanced to a level similar to that of prednimustine, if prednisolone was also administered 4 hr after chlorambucil treatment. (At 4 hr chlorambucil subcellular binding had previously been shown by Hill and Riches (1971) to be close to maximal.) The mode of action of prednimustine on macromolecule biosynthesis inhibition appeared to be similar to that of chlorambucil and typical of alkylating agents. Some selectivity in the action of prednimustine was seen against a steroid-sensitive lymphoma cell line, which was sensitive to prednimustine (and prednisolone) but resistant to chlorambucil. In testing against the alkylating agent sensitive L1210 leukaemia in mice, prednimustine showed a 23-fold ratio of cell-killing effectiveness for the tumour cells in comparison with resting stem cells, a value considerably greater than that for other alkylating agents tested (Evenaar et al., 1973). The clinical use of prednimustine has included treatment of chronic lymphocytic leukaemia and lymphoma (Pedersen-Bjergaard et al., 1980a; Brandt et al., 1975; Moller et al., 1975; Gandara et al., 1987), ovarian carcinoma (Johnsson et al., 1979; Leonard et al., 1989) and breast cancer (Mouridsen et al., 1980; Rankin et al., 1987).

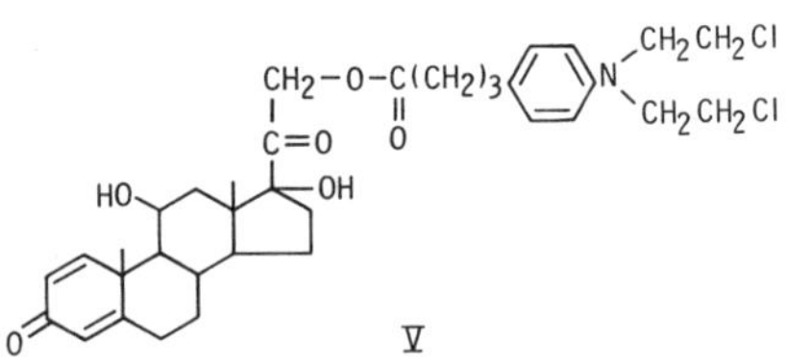

V

The analysis of prednimustine in biological fluids has normally been carried out by HPLC (Newell et al., 1979; Oppitz et al., 1989) or GC-MS techniques (Jakhammer et al., 1977). In HPLC techniques, both chlorambucil, prednimustine and the potential metabolite phenylacetic mustard may be simultaneously determined. However, for the GC-MS method preliminary separation of chlorambucil and prednimustine (by extraction) is required as both compounds are subsequently converted to the same derivative (chlorambucil methyl ester) for determination. The use of octa-deuterated prednimustine as internal standard allows a detection limit of 8 ng/mL in plasma and a relative standard deviation of 5% for prednimustine determinations at the 30–60 ng/mL level.

The ester linkage of prednimustine in vitro is subject to hydrolysis by non-specific esterases (Wilkinson et al., 1978). During incubation with Chinese hamster cells (to which prednimustine is 3–4 times more potent than chlorambucil) the drug is hydrolyzed to chlorambucil and prednisolone, with a reduction to half concentration in 15 hr (Hartley-Asp et al., 1986). The hydrolysis was catalyzed by a serum esterase. With plasma in vitro hydrolysis of prednimustine was demonstrated and an additional metabolite was identified as the cholesterol ester of chlorambucil (Gunnarsson et al., 1984). This was formed by a transesterification process, catalyzed by lecithin:cholesterol acyltransferase.

Hydrolysis of prednimustine appears to be extensive in vivo. In the rat after s.c. administration of prednimustine no parent drug could be detected in the plasma, although chlorambucil and phenylacetic mustard were present at low concentrations ($< 5\ \mu M$) (Newell et al., 1981). Newell et al. (1983a) also showed that none of prednimustine, chlorambucil or phenylacetic mustard could be detected in the plasma of patients administered oral prednimustine (20 mg), suggesting that the drug is poorly absorbed from the gastrointestinal tract. Oral administration of prednimustine (20–100 mg, [^{3}H]-labelled) to mammary carcinoma patients also resulted in variable absorption with faecal excretion of unchanged drug ranging from 0.3–55.2% of the dose administered in 72 hr

(Könyves et al., 1975). Following 40 mg/m^2 oral [^{14}C]-prednimustine Gaver et al. (1983) observed 40–60% excretion of radioactivity in urine in 72 hr. No intact prednimustine was detected in plasma.

Although prednimustine is not sufficiently water soluble for normal intravenous use, Kirdani et al. (1978) administered the drug i.v. as a suspension in ethanol/saline. Comparison with orally administered prednimustine suggested that a cause of variable absorption was sequestration of the drug in certain tissues. Ehrsson et al. (1983b) carried out a comparative study of the absorption of chlorambucil (10 mg) and prednimustine (100 mg) administered orally on two sequential days. No detectable (less than 5 ng/mL) prednimustine could be detected in the patients' plasma. However, chlorambucil was detected with variable peak levels (25–240 ng/mL); the calculated bioavailability was five times lower than that of orally administered chlorambucil. Similar variability was seen in the AUC levels of chlorambucil following prednimustine administration. In a later study Oppitz et al. (1989) compared the bioavailability of chlorambucil and its metabolite phenylacetic acid mustard after administration of oral prednimustine (200 mg) or chlorambucil (30–50 mg)/prednisolone (50 mg) combinations. For prednimustine no unchanged drug was found in plasma. The peak levels of chlorambucil and phenylacetic mustard were reached later than after administration of chlorambucil/prednisolone and the AUCs were lower. In the study of Bastholt et al. (1991) which compared prednimustine (200 mg) with chlorambucil (20 mg) plus prednisolone (20 mg) the relative availability of chlorambucil from prednisolone was 16%. Alkylating metabolites derived from prednimustine (chlorambucil and phenylacetic mustard) had a more prolonged elimination phase than those derived from chlorambucil itself.

In view of the fact that prednimustine has so far remained undetected in patients' plasma and that oral prednimustine appears to be acting as a rather poor prodrug for chlorambucil (and presumably prednisolone) there appears little reason to use the drug in place of a mixture of chlorambucil and prednisolone (Newell et al., 1983b). The long-term carcinogenic effects of prednimustine appear however to be lower than those of chlorambucil (Berger et al., 1986).

5. MELPHALAN

Melphalan (VI) (L-phenylalanine mustard, L-PAM, Alkeran) is a derivative of L-phenylalanine with a bis(2-chloroethyl)amino (mustard) substituent at the *para* position of the aromatic ring. Melphalan was synthesized in 1953 by Bergel and Stock (1953, 1954) in the hope (which was unfulfilled) of gaining some specific transport of the nitrogen mustard into the melanin biosynthetic pathway, so that the drug would be effective for the treatment of melanoma. The D-isomer of phenylalanine mustard (medphalan) was similarly prepared by Bergel and Stock (1953, 1954) but was shown (Schmidt et al., 1965) to be of lower activity than melphalan. Sarcolysin (merphalan) the racemic (D,L-) phenylalanine mustard, synthesized by Bergel and Stock (1953, 1954) and by Larionov et al. (1955), again showed no therapeutic advantage over melphalan. Melphalan has therefore been the isomer of choice for therapeutic use and has proved to be one of the more useful alkylating agents in clinical practice.

Despite the rationale for the melphalan synthesis no evidence exists that the drug is of especial selectivity for melanoma cells. More successful applications of melphalan have been in treatment of primary breast cancer (as an adjuvant to surgery) (Fisher et al., 1979) and in the therapy of multiple myeloma (Costa et al., 1973). Other clinical uses include treatment of cancer of the ovaries (Frick et al., 1968), the testes and the gastrointestinal tract.

5.1. Alkylating Properties

Chemically melphalan behaves as a typical alkylating agent and reacts readily with nucleophiles. In unbuffered water it hydrolyzes sequentially to the monohydroxy derivative (VII) (MOH, 4-(2-hydroxyethyl)-4-(2-chloroethyl)amino-L-phenylalanine) and the dihydroxy derivative (VIII) (DOH, 4-[bis(2-hydroxyethyl)amino]-L-phenylalanine) (Chang et al., 1978b), which have been identified by MS (Furner et al., 1976).

At 37°C the first order rate constant for the loss of melphalan in water is 0.83 hr^{-1} (i.e.

$t_{1/2} = 0.83$ hr), but in the presence of albumin the rate of loss is slowed (e.g. $k = 0.46$ hr^{-1} in 80 mg/mL albumin) (Chang et al., 1978b). In whole blood or plasma the decrease in melphalan concentration due to hydrolysis is 5% during 24 hr incubation at 37°C (Gera et al., 1989). Chang et al. (1978b) and Evans et al. (1982) have determined the rate constant for the disappearance of melphalan in human plasma of 0.3–0.45 hr^{-1} and Ehrsson and Lönroth (1982) have shown a 3-fold increase in stability when melphalan is bound to albumin compared to being unbound in solution. In cell culture medium at 37°C melphalan hydrolyzes to MOH with $t_{1/2}$ 66 min and then to DOH with $t_{1/2}$ 58 min (Bosanquet and Bird, 1988). Melphalan solutions stored at low temperature or in hydrochloric acid solution are more stable; for example Furner and Brown (1980) have shown that solutions in phosphate buffer, serum, or 11 mM hydrochloric acid showed no change in composition over 4 hr at 0°C. Melphalan in a formulation product (kit from Burroughs Welcome, London, U.K.) has a half-life of 3.3 hr at 41°C (equivalent to a first order rate constant of 0.21 hr^{-1}) (Flora et al., 1979), indicating that preheating of formulations should be kept to a minimum. As the decomposition of melphalan follows unimolecular first order kinetics with the production of a carbonium ion and a chloride ion, the decomposition may be reversed by the presence of chloride ions in the hydrolysis medium. Melphalan in 0.156 M sodium chloride (isotonic saline) has been shown to have a disappearance rate constant of 0.28 hr^{-1} (Chang et al., 1979), compared with solutions in pH 7.4 phosphate buffer with a k value of 1.02 hr^{-1}. Bosanquet (1985) has reported that melphalan solutions in normal saline lose only 5% of their activity in 20 hr at 5°C. Retardation of hydrolysis rates of melphalan have also been observed in animal and human bile (Chang et al., 1978c).

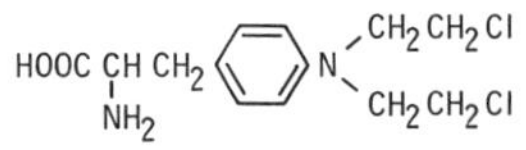

VI

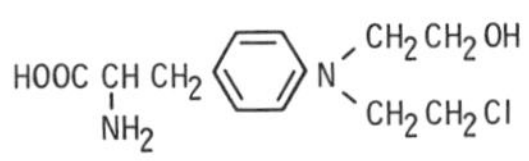

VII

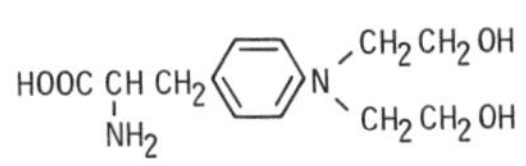

VIII

Melphalan also binds covalently to nucleophilic centres in macromolecules; equilibrium dialysis, coupled with fluorescence measurements, was used by Chirigos and Mead (1964) to show that 60% of melphalan at a concentration of 40 μg/mL was bound to serum proteins. Later studies with [^{14}C]-melphalan (Chang et al., 1978a) suggested that 30% of the drug in a 30 μg/mL solution in human plasma was protein-bound.

Binding in vitro to DNA in L1210 cells, human lymphoblastoid cells, Burkitt lymphoma cells and melanoma cells has also been demonstrated. As is generally the case for bifunctional alkylating agents, cross-linking occurs between two nucleophiles in the DNA strands or between DNA and protein. The alkaline elution technique was used by Ross et al. (1978) to measure cross-links in L1210 cells treated for 30 min with 15 μM melphalan. Cross-link formation increased for 12 hr and was still significant after 24 hr. Later studies by Brox et al. (1980) with human lymphoblastoid cells showed that the cross-links formed after a 1 hr drug incubation at 3.3 μM were between DNA and protein. Repair occurred by 24–48 hr. The significance of cross-links with respect to the cytotoxic activity of melphalan was confirmed by Ducore et al. (1982) who used the alkaline elution technique to quantitate DNA–DNA and DNA–protein cross-links in three Burkitt's lymphoma cell lines treated with 12 μM melphalan. Although the total extent of cross-linking has some relationship with the antiproliferative efficacy of melphalan against the three cell lines, the extent of DNA interstrand cross-linking showed a better correlation, suggesting that interstrand cross-linking is of greater importance than DNA–protein cross-linking with regard to the cytotoxic effects. DNA cross-links have also been measured in lymphocytes from chronic lymphocytic leukaemia patients after treatment with melphalan, using an ethidium bromide fluorescence assay (Panasci et al., 1990). A non-linear dose–response relationship was observed. Association of DNA cross-linking with cytotoxicity has been observed in human melanoma cells (Hansson et al., 1987) and the F_1 variant of B_{16} melanoma cells (Torres-Garcia et al., 1988). The cytotoxicity of melphalan to human lymphoma cells is enhanced by pretreatment with the ornithine decarboxylase inhibitor α-difluoromethylornithine. This results in a longer maintenance of DNA interstrand cross-linking (Ducore and McNamara, 1986). Parsons et al. (1981) have estimated that one interstrand cross-link per 2×10^9 Da is associated with melphalan damage to human melanoma cells at the dose which on average would kill the cells.

Melphalan reacts preferentially with guanine residues in DNA, with specificity according to their molecular electrostatic potential (Shepherd and Sage, 1986; Kohn et al., 1987, 1988). Increased ionic strength and cationic DNA affinity binders inhibit the alkylation (Hartley et al., 1990). Adenine adducts, some of which are intrastrand cross-linked, have also been detected (cf. chlorambucil) (Pieper and Erickson, 1990). DNA damage caused by melphalan may be detected using monoclonal antibodies (Tilby et al., 1987). With the use of synthetic standards it was concluded that the alkylation of guanine bases is the major contribution to the immunoreactivity of melphalan-alkylated DNA and that cross-linkage is required for the highest immunoreactivity (Tilby et al., 1990). A further approach to measuring DNA damage caused by melphalan is to use flow cytometry to detect cells reacting with a monoclonal antibody that was generated against nitrogen mustard treated DNA. Resistance to melphalan results in decreased immunoreactivity (Frankfurt et al., 1990).

5.2. Analysis

Non-specific colorimetric determinations of alkylating drugs may be achieved using the Epstein reagent (4-(4′-nitrobenzyl)-pyridine) (Epstein et al., 1955), which yields a violet coloured product following its alkylation by the drug. This was the first technique used for melphalan determination (Klatt et al., 1960) which allowed detection down to 15 μg/mL blood; in 1966 the Epstein reaction was cited as an appropriate identity test for melphalan (Anon, 1966), even though other alkylating agents (and even the half hydrolysis product (VII) of melphalan) would have given similar colorimetric results. Fluorescence detection as used by Chirigos and Mead (1964) similarly is not totally selective for melphalan.

More sensitive and selective techniques for the drug were rapidly developed in the 1970s (Table 1). GC was first employed by Goras et al. (1970) using the trimethylsilyl derivative of melphalan, although no detection limit was reported. Later GC determinations were combined with MS and Pallante et al. (1980) have developed a GC-chemical ionization MS method using the *N*-trifluoroacetyl methyl ester derivative of melphalan and an octa-deuterated analogue as internal standard. This technique allows the analysis of plasma concentrations as low as 2 ng/mL. Quantitation has also been achieved by direct probe MS determinations using dideuterated melphalan as internal standard (Tattersall et al., 1978).

The analytical method most generally used for determinations of melphalan in biological samples is HPLC and a representative selection of applications is shown in Table 1. The chromatographic conditions should be such that the hydrolysis products (VII) and (VIII) are resolved from the parent drug. This has been achieved in the reported assays by using a reverse phase C_{18} column. The required sensitivity of the assay is dictated by the fact that peak plasma concentrations of melphalan following an oral dose of 10 mg melphalan are in the 50–100 ng/mL range (Pallante et al., 1980; Bosanquet and Gilby, 1982a). This sensitivity has been obtained using either UV or fluorescence detection. As an example Bosanquet and Gilby (1982a) have analyzed melphalan with a limit of detection of 5 ng/mL plasma using a C_{18} reverse phase column eluted isocratically with a mixture of methanol, sodium dodecyl sulphate and sulphuric acid. The method has been used to monitor the pharmacokinetics of oral and i.v. melphalan during treatment of multiple myeloma (Bosanquet and Gilby, 1982a,b). Similar sensitivity has been reported by Egan et al. (1981) using fluorescence detection following chromatography on a C_{18} column with isocratic methanol–water

TABLE 1. *Analytical techniques for melphalan determinations*

	Method	Detection limit	Reference
Colorimetry	Reaction with 4-(4′-nitrobenzyl)-pyridine	15 μg/mL blood	Klatt et al., 1960
Fluorimetry	Excitation 268 mμ, detection 365 mμ	—	Chirigos and Mead, 1964
GC	Trimethylsilyl derivative	—	Goras et al., 1970
GC-MS	*N*-Trifluoroacetyl, methyl ester derivative, CI.	2 ng/mL plasma	Pallante et al., 1980
MS	Direct insertion probe	—	Tattersall et al., 1978
HPTLC	Silica; chloroform/methanol/acetic acid	20 ng/mL plasma	Taha et al., 1981
HPLC (UV detection)	C_{18} column; 2-methoxyethanol/acetic acid	10 ng/mL serum	Furner et al., 1976
	C_{18} column; methanol/water/acetic acid	50 ng/mL plasma	Chang et al., 1978a
			Brox et al., 1979
	C_{18} column; methanol/NaH_2PO_4	1 μg/mL buffer	Flora et al., 1979
	C_{18} column; acetonitrile/acetic acid	100 ng/mL blood	Ahmed and Hsu, 1981
	C_{18} column; acetonitrile/acetic acid	10 ng/mL plasma	Davis et al., 1982
	C_{18} column; methanol/sodium dodecyl sulphate/sulphuric acid	5 ng/mL plasma	Bosanquet and Gilby, 1982a
HPLC (Fluorescence detection)	C_{18} column; methanol/water	<5 ng/mL plasma	Egan et al., 1981
	C_{18} column; *o*-phthalaldehyde derivative; methanol/pH 7 phosphate buffer	10 ng/mL plasma 25 ng/g tissue	Sweeney et al., 1985
	C_{18} column; *N*-acetylcysteine derivative; ethanol, citrate buffer, octanesulphonic acid	5 ng/mL plasma	Ehrsson et al., 1986

mixtures. MOH (VII) and DOH (VIII) can be quantitated down to 30 ng/mL (Osterheld et al., 1988). Later work by Sweeney et al. (1985), utilizing the fluorescence detection of the derivative of melphalan with *o*-phthalaldehyde, allowed detection of the drug down to concentration limits of 10 ng/mL in plasma (100 μL) and 25 ng/g in tissue (50 mg). Derivatization of melphalan with *N*-acetylcysteine was used by Ehrsson et al. (1986) to produce a fluorescent compound which was quantitated by HPLC down to drug concentrations of 5 ng/mL plasma.

5.3. TRANSPORT

As early as 1957 it had been observed that melphalan inhibited incorporation of amino acids into proteins. Crathorn and Hunter (1957) demonstrated that [^{14}C]-phenylalanine incorporation into *Staphylococcus aureus* was markedly inhibited and that this inhibition was lost if hydrolyzed drug was used. Later work by Vistica et al. (1976) showed that the cytotoxicity of melphalan to murine L1210 leukemia cells in culture was reduced in growth medium containing amino acids. An analysis of this inhibition, with single amino acids, revealed that it is largely due to leucine and glutamine. Furthermore deletion of these amino acids from the culture medium increased the cytotoxicity of melphalan to L1210 cells (Vistica et al., 1978d). Uptake of melphalan into these cells was reduced 6-fold when the drug was supplemented by 0.1 mM leucine or 0.1 mM glutamine and inhibition analysis has shown that melphalan was transported into L1210 cells by a high affinity leucine-type (L)-amino acid system (Vistica et al., 1978c). Similarly the uptake of melphalan into L1210 cells taken from a mouse tumour was reduced by leucine (Vistica et al., 1979a). Studies in vivo have shown that injection of leucine with therapeutically effective doses of melphalan dramatically reduced the cure rate for L1210 tumours (Vistica et al., 1978a, 1979a) and that this inhibition of anti-tumour effect could be reversed by simultaneous injection of α-amino-γ-guanidino butyric acid (a compound which has also been shown to promote melphalan cytotoxicity in leucine-protected cells in vitro (Vistica et al., 1978d). Further studies in vitro, using 2-amino-bi-cyclo[2,2,1]heptane carboxylic acid (BCH), a model L-system synthetic amino acid, have suggested that melphalan is transported by two separate leucine carrier systems, one sodium dependent and

BCH insensitive and the other sodium independent and BCH sensitive (Vistica, 1979). The uptake process is temperature and energy dependent and proceeds uphill against a concentration gradient giving a distribution ratio of ca. 10 in L1210 cells (Vistica and Rabinowitz, 1979). Leucine is only partially effective (ca. 6-fold less) at protecting L1210 cells from medphalan cytotoxicity suggesting a separate transport system for this isomer (Vistica et al., 1979b).

A wide variety of drugs have been tested for their effects on melphalan incorporation into L1210 cells. *N,N'*-bis(2-chloroethyl)-*N*-nitrosourea (BCNU) was the only drug that stimulated incorporation; adriamycin, *N*-(2-chloroethyl)-*N'*-cyclohexyl-*N*-nitrosourea (CCNU), methyl-CCNU, mustine and vincristine all inhibited the accumulation of the drug (Martin et al., 1982). In human breast cancer cells the anti-oestrogen tamoxifen was effective at reducing intracellular melphalan concentrations, both by reducing influx and by stimulating efflux (Goldenberg and Froese, 1985).

Melphalan transport into L5178Y lymphoblasts has also been studied in detail (Goldenberg et al., 1977). Again this is temperature sensitive, proceeds uphill (concentration gradient ca. 8-fold) and appears to be equally distributed between two energy-dependent systems, the leucine-L-system and a BCH-insensitive system similar to that used by alanine, serine and cysteine (ASC-system) (Begleiter et al., 1979). Efflux from L5178Y cells occurs by a different mechanism and is stimulated by a variety of amino acids (Begleiter et al., 1982).

Other cell types where melphalan transport has been studied are the MCF-7 breast cells, peripheral blood lymphocytes LPC-1 plasmacytoma cells, BALB/c 3T3 fibroblasts and human medulloblastoma cells. For MCF-7 cells the uptake proceeds uphill against a concentration gradient of ca. 13-fold and for lymphocytes 3-fold and again there are sodium sensitive and BCH sensitive components (Begleiter and Goldenberg, 1979; Begleiter et al., 1980). Higher intracellular concentrations of melphalan were found in breast cells compared to lymphocytes and the V_{max} for the carrier system was some 50-fold greater for the former. There is no significant difference in K_m or V_{max} of melphalan transport in lymphocytes from untreated, treated sensitive and treated resistant patients (Panasci et al., 1988). Interestingly however BCH was without effect on incorporation of melphalan into mononuclear cells from normal human bone marrow (Millar et al., 1989). For LPC-1 plasmacytoma cells (a suggested model for human multiple myeloma) a similar pair of transport mechanisms (sodium-sensitive/BCH-insensitive and sodium-insensitive/BCH-sensitive) exists, with transport proceeding uphill against a concentration gradient of ca. 10-fold (Goldenberg et al., 1979). Similar transport systems exist in BALB/c 3T3 mouse fibroblasts (Blosmanis et al., 1987). Human medulloblastoma cells also show transport systems for melphalan that may be inhibited by both BCH and sodium ion depletion (Friedman et al., 1988). The large amino acid carrier system appears to be involved in transport of melphalan across the rat blood–brain barrier (Greig et al., 1987).

Thus melphalan transport into cells appears generally to involve a double carrier system. The existence of these energy-dependent systems may be of considerable significance both for the selectivity and for the resistance of cells to the effects of melphalan. As indicated above the cytotoxicity and chemotherapeutic effectiveness of melphalan may be reduced in model systems by the coinjection of leucine or glutamine (Vistica et al., 1978a,b, 1979a) and it might therefore be expected that there is potential for increasing the anti-tumour activity of melphalan by the removal of these amino acids. Studies in vitro with L1210 cells showed that *Actinobacter* glutaminase:asparaginase (which depletes glutamine) promoted the uptake and cytotoxicity of melphalan (Vistica et al., 1978b) and this combination of agents has subsequently been tested (i.p.) in vivo on murine tumours and on three patients with i.p. metastatic cancers, with promising results (Holcenberg et al., 1983).

Removal of the amino group of melphalan by acetylation produces a much less toxic drug, presumably because it is not taken up by the amino acid transport system. However activity may be restored in experimental systems by coupling *N*-acetylmelphalan to monoclonal antibodies appropriate for the target cells (Smyth et al., 1987). Phase I trials of this conjugate against colorectal carcinoma have been carried out (Tjandra et al., 1989). Human immunoglobulin conjugates are also being developed (Shiraishi et al., 1989).

5.4. METABOLISM

Attempts to metabolize the drug in vitro with rat liver microsomes led only to the hydrolyzed derivatives MOH and DOH (Evans et al., 1982). Similar products were formed after incubation of the drug in plasma (Evans et al., 1982; Flora et al., 1979). Some evidence for metabolism of melphalan in vitro to a mutagenically active product was obtained by Benedict et al. (1977), who showed a 3-fold increase in mutations in *Salmonella typhimurium* tester strains when a rat liver S-9 fraction was added to the incubation.

Incubation of melphalan with immobilized microsomal glutathione transferases yielded a mixture of products which was separated by HPLC and the major components identified by MS (Dulik et al., 1986). In addition to melphalan, MOH and DOH, the mono- and di-glutathionyl conjugates were characterized. In these conjugates the glutathione had displaced the chlorines on the mustard side chain of melphalan. A similar mixture of products was obtained using cytosolic glutathione transferases. Dulik and Fenselau (1987) later identified a further glutathione conjugate formed by immobilized microsomal glutathione-*S*-transferase as 4-(glutathionyl)-phenylalanine, in which glutathione had displaced the whole mustard moiety. The specificity of the isozymes of murine hepatic glutathione-*S*-transferase for the formation of melphalan conjugates was studied by Bolton et al. (1991). Enzymes of the α class catalyze the formation of the mono-glutathionyl conjugate on the chloroethyl side chain.

Metabolism does not seem to be an important determinant for the disposition of melphalan in vivo. In patients receiving the drug orally or intravenously (Alberts et al., 1979a,c) no identifiable degradation products were seen in plasma or urine. Similarly Tattersall et al. (1978) have shown, by TLC, no significant amount of melphalan metabolites in blood or urine following i.v. administration of the drug. A low level of DOH has been observed in patients' blood long after oral doses of melphalan (Ahmed and Hsu, 1981). The identity of this compound was confirmed by chemical ionization MS and it is likely that DOH is at least partly responsible for the terminal phase in the disappearance of label from plasma of patients receiving oral [^{14}C]-melphalan (see below and Tattersall et al., 1978). Some evidence for metabolism of melphalan in vivo in animals has come from the work of Furner et al. (1977b) and Furner and Brown (1980) who showed by HPLC the presence of several radioactive peaks in urine, serum and bile of the rat, dog, mouse, monkey and shark. The identity of these components is so far unknown. Similarly Ahmed et al. (1982a) have demonstrated the presence of four unknown metabolites in the blood of rats administered oral melphalan.

Some variation appears to exist with regard to the nature of the biliary excretion products; in the dog (orally dosed) 80% of the biliary product was parent compound (Furner et al., 1977a), whereas in rat (i.v. dosed) most of the biliary products were metabolites (Byington et al., 1980). (It is known that melphalan is relatively stable towards hydrolysis in bile in vitro, see above and Chang et al., 1978c.)

5.5. DISTRIBUTION AND PHARMACOKINETICS

The distribution of melphalan has been studied in animals using either [^{14}C]- or [^{3}H]-labelled drug. Initial experiments by Cohn (1957) showed that [^{14}C]-melphalan, administered to rats bearing the Walker carcinoma, distributed evenly between liver, blood and tumour, although the kidney showed the highest specific activity of [^{14}C] protein incorporation. Later studies by Milner et al. (1965) using [^{3}H]-melphalan in the same animal system confirmed the incorporation of radioactivity into liver, kidney, tumour and a variety of other organs, although interestingly virtually no evidence was obtained for covalent binding of radioactivity to DNA in the tumour cells. More detailed investigations by Furner et al. (1977a) and by Furner and Brown (1980) have more completely characterized the distribution of [^{14}C]-melphalan in mice, monkeys and dogs. For example, in monkeys 4 hr after an i.v. dose of 0.75 mg/kg, 51.7% of the total activity was found in the bile, 4.8% in the kidneys, with all other organs studied containing $< 1.0\%$ (Furner and Brown, 1980). HPLC, however, showed that only 7.5% of the activity in bile was melphalan. Similarly in the dog (Furner et al., 1977a,b) rapid biliary excretion occurred, although in this species as indicated above a much larger proportion of the activity was due to melphalan. Renal failure induced in dogs increased the drug's terminal phase half-life and caused correspondingly greater toxic effects to the bone marrow (Alberts et al., 1981).

The pharmacokinetics of uptake and rate of elimination of [^{14}C-ring] melphalan from body tissues of the rat has been determined over a 72 hr period following oral doses of 20 mg/kg (Ahmed et al., 1982b). As expected for this route of administration, the stomach and gastrointestinal tract showed the highest levels of radioactivity, with most tissues showing their highest activity 2–4 hr after administration of the drug ($t_{1/2} < 1$ hr). Elimination was most rapid from gastrointestinal tissues and from the bone marrow. Covalent binding was observed in all tissues and in most it accounted for more than half of the activity remaining after 48 hr. Melphalan also binds covalently in vivo to red blood cells and in particular to the membrane proteins (Ahmed et al., 1982a). Elimination of [^{14}C] from blood was biphasic with $t_{1/2}\alpha$ 7 hr and $t_{1/2}\beta$ 75 hr, with the hydrolyzed drug (DOH) being the main species present after 15 hr.

The pharmacokinetics of melphalan in patients undergoing therapy has been extensively studied (see review by Farmer and Newell (1983)). Following i.v. administration of the [^{14}C]-drug at doses of 0.6 mg/kg it was rapidly cleared from the plasma with mean $t_{1/2}\alpha$ 13 min and $t_{1/2}\beta$ 86 min (Alberts et al., 1977, 1979c). Forty-five percent of the drug-derived radioactivity (including $13 \pm 5.4\%$ as unchanged drug) was excreted in the first 24 hr urine. Tattersall et al. (1978) reported a similar plasma half life of 67 min, with a prolonged terminal phase of $t_{1/2}$ 160 hr. Repeated i.v. doses of 20 mg/m^2 showed mean $t_{1/2}$ of 22 min (Brox et al., 1979). The renal clearance and protein binding of i.v. melphalan (5 mg/m^2) was studied in detail by Reece et al. (1988). The percentage unchanged dose excreted ranged from 2.5 to 92.8% ($n = 9$) and the renal clearance from 4.1 to 188 mL/min/m^2. Following high i.v. doses of 140 mg/m^2 it was not possible to detect concentrations of melphalan in cerebrospinal fluid (CSF) (Ardiet et al., 1986), although in rats the brain:plasma concentration ratio was 0.13 (Greig et al., 1988). The pharmacokinetic parameters for high dose (140–220 mg/m^2) i.v. melphalan administered to children were not significantly different from adult values ($t_{1/2}\beta$ 1.3 hr, Taha et al. (1983); $t_{1/2}\alpha$ 6.6 min, $t_{1/2}\beta$ 3 hr, Ninane et al. (1985); $t_{1/2}\alpha$ 8.8 min, $t_{1/2}\beta$ 43 min, Gouyette et al. (1986)). Very high peak concentrations of the drug (6–115 mg/mL) may be achieved by limb perfusion of melphalan (0.75 or 1.2 mg/kg), which yielded a complete response rate of 81% in a series of melanoma patients (Minor et al., 1985). However Briele et al. (1985) showed that uptake of perfused drug into tissue is saturable, being complete within 30 min. Plasma half-lives for malignant melanoma patients in this study were $t_{1/2}\alpha$ 5–10 min and $t_{1/2}\beta$ 35–50 min and in the study of Benckhuijsen et al. (1986) $t_{1/2}\alpha$ 4.7 ± 0.3 and $t_{1/2}\beta$ 53.0 ± 1.6 min.

Oral administration of melphalan results in very variable and incomplete absorption of the drug. On some occasions no melphalan has been found in plasma or urine following p.o. doses (0.6 mg/kg, Alberts et al., 1979a, 1980a; 9 mg/m^2 Brox et al., 1979). Plasma half-lives following the peak of plasma levels at 3–6 hr were similar to the values for i.v. doses (e.g. $t_{1/2}\beta$ 90 min (Alberts et al., 1979a)) with 28% of the drug-derived radioactivity being excreted in urine during the first 24 hr. On average the melphalan concentration × time in plasma for oral doses was less than 0.6 of that for i.v. doses (Alberts et al., 1980a). For lower p.o. doses (0.15–0.25 mg/kg) peak plasma levels of the drug were seen between 0.7 and 2.3 hr after ingestion (Pallante et al., 1980). Oral doses of 0.12–0.17 mg/kg melphalan given to multiple myeloma patients (also receiving prednisolone) showed variable AUC and variable lag-time for the drug in plasma, with a plasma $t_{1/2}$ of 0.9 ± 0.5 hr (Taha et al., 1982). Pretreatment with cimetidine reduces the bioavailability of oral melphalan by approximately 30% (Sviland et al., 1987). Renal dysfunction results in an increase in AUC of oral melphalan (Osterborg et al., 1989) and there is evidence for saturable absorptive pathways for p.o. melphalan (Choi et al., 1989).

Comparative studies of p.o. and i.v. administration of melphalan by Bosanquet and Gilby (1982b, 1984) have confirmed the variable availability of melphalan. Fasting of multiple myeloma patients increased the absorption of p.o. melphalan to a mean of 93% of the i.v. level compared to 49% for fed patients, suggesting that oral melphalan would best be administered first thing in the morning. A further study by Woodhouse et al. (1983) showed that bioavailability of melphalan administered orally to fasted multiple myeloma patients (10 mg/patient) was 61.5–102% (mean $78.3 \pm 6.3\%$) with peak plasma levels at ca. 1 hr and $t_{1/2}\beta$ 67 min. With oral doses of 5–20 mg (Ehrsson et al., 1989) the bioavailability of melphalan was found to be 29–124% and decreased during the treatment course. Reece et al. (1986) showed a higher AUC for fasting patients and 85%

bioavailability (compared to 58% for fed patients). Experiments with rat tissues have demonstrated that melphalan uptake from the intestine is via an energy-dependent system (Adair and McElnay, 1986) and may be inhibited by the amino acid L-leucine (Adair and McElnay, 1987). In some patients L-leucine reduces plasma melphalan concentrations after p.o. dosing (Reece et al., 1987).

Intraperitoneally administered melphalan was shown by Alberts et al. (1980b) to result in high local concentrations of the drug with only 39% absorption into the systemic circulation and may thus be a suitable treatment for patients with tumours confined to the peritoneal cavity. Peak peritoneal concentrations of nearly one hundred times those obtained in plasma have recently been reported in ovarian and gastrointestinal tumour patients by Howell et al. (1984).

5.6. Toxicity

The toxicity of melphalan is characteristic of alkylating agents and includes damage to the haematopoietic cells and gut epithelial cells, induction of nausea and vomiting and pulmonary fibrosis (see review by Colvin, 1982). Ovarian failure has also been reported (Kellie and Kingston, 1987). Myelosuppression is normally the dose limiting toxicity and may be ameliorated by the use of bone-marrow rescue techniques. For example malignant melanoma patients have been treated by McElwain et al. (1979) at the high dose of 140 mg/m^2 after removal of bone marrow, which is subsequently reinfused 8 hr after melphalan administration, when plasma levels of the drug have declined to a safe level.

Intraperitoneally injected melphalan is carcinogenic in rats (peritoneal sarcomas) (Weisburger et al., 1975) and in mice (lung tumours and lymphosarcomas) (Shimkin et al., 1966; Weisburger et al., 1975). Melphalan is also mutagenic in the Ames *Salmonella* test (Benedict et al., 1977; Matheson et al., 1978). In a shuttle vector system utilizing the plasmid pZ189 the mutations induced by melphalan were mostly base substitutions with A–T to T–A transversions being by far the most frequent (Wang et al., 1990). Melphalan induces sister chromatid exchanges in vitro (Banerjee and Benedict, 1979) and in mouse bone marrow and lymphocytes (Conner et al., 1989). In human subjects in vivo, cytogenetic damage is also seen (Sharpe, 1971; Lambert et al., 1981, 1986; Mamuris et al., 1989) and considerable evidence has been obtained for the drug's carcinogenicity. An increased risk of leukaemia exists in melphalan treated patients (Karchmer et al., 1974; Kyle et al., 1975; Reimer et al., 1977; Law and Blom, 1977; Einhorn, 1978; Greene et al., 1986; Cuzick et al., 1987) and many case reports of second malignancies following treatment have now been reported (I.A.R.C., 1979; Schmähl et al., 1982). Solid tumours have also been observed in ovarian cancer patients subsequent to treatment with melphalan (Einhorn et al., 1988). Melphalan is therefore now classified by I.A.R.C. as one of the compounds for which there is 'sufficient evidence of carcinogenicity to humans'.

5.7. Priming Doses

Priming doses of alkylating agents may protect against the expected toxicity of later doses of these compounds or of other alkylating agents. Thus for example a proportion of mice treated with a toxic dose of busulphan (35–45 mg/kg) may survive if they are treated with cyclophosphamide (200 mg/kg) 1–2 days previously (Millar et al., 1975). Cyclophosphamide (50 mg/kg) given to mice 4 days before a 400 mg/kg dose of cyclophosphamide caused a reduction in the damage to the urothelium caused by the latter dose (Millar and McElwain, 1978). The mechanism of the reduction of busulphan toxicity is thought to be a stimulation of haematopoietic stem cell regeneration. For cyclophosphamide toxicity reduction, the mechanism is unknown. No effects on metabolism have been observed and the combination is still effective against animal tumours.

In the case of melphalan, rats could be protected from a normally lethal dose by treatment 2 days earlier with a priming dose (1 mg/kg) (Jeney et al., 1968). Merophan (1 mg/kg) had a similar effect in protecting against melphalan (or merophan) toxicity. Interestingly however the selectivity of the protection was demonstrated by the facts that a priming dose of melphalan did not protect against merophan toxicity and merophan was inactive at protection of toxicity from another alkylating agent, nitrogen mustard. Mice were similarly protected from high doses of melphalan by pretreatment with cyclophosphamide, cytosine arabinoside or low dose melphalan (Millar et al.,

1978), or methyl-CCNU (Zimber et al., 1988). (Later experiments by Kulkarni et al. (1985) revealed some inconsistencies in the protecting effect of cyclophosphamide in mice.)

The protective effect of priming doses of alkylating agents also extends to γ-irradiation toxicity. Thus protection to lethal doses (1000 rads) of γ-irradiation in mice was achieved by pretreatment with cyclophosphamide (200 mg/kg). Again the timing was critical, with a maximum effect being observed 3 days before irradiation. No protection could be seen by pretreatment with lower doses of irradiation. Again the protective effect caused by cyclophosphamide was thought to be because of enhanced haemopoietic recovery and the antitumour effectiveness of the combination of agents was not decreased.

There is clearly considerable potential for the application of the priming dose regime in patient treatment. For example Hedley et al. (1978) showed in seven malignant melanoma patients that priming doses of cyclophosphamide (500 mg i.v.) protected against the bone marrow toxicity caused by melphalan treatment (140 mg/m^2) 7 days later. In other patients cyclophosphamide priming reduced gastrointestinal toxicity after high dose melphalan (Cornbleet et al., 1983; Selby et al., 1987).

5.8. Drug Interactions

Hypoxic cell radiosensitizers have been shown to enhance the activity of melphalan against a variety of animal tumours (see review by McNally, 1982). Thus Clement et al. (1980) showed that an i.p. dose of misonidazole increased the activity of melphalan against a M5076 ovarian carcinoma in mice. The effectiveness of the drug was increased 2.2-fold against the tumour, while bone marrow toxicity was increased only 1.2-fold. A similar enhancement of melphalan activity against murine tumours (RIF-1 sarcoma) was also seen after prolonged exposure to low doses of misonidazole (of more relevance with respect to the normal clinical use of misonidazole) (Brown and Hirst, 1982).

Experiments in vitro by Twentyman and Workman (1983b) also showed an enhancement of melphalan's activity at clinically achievable concentrations of misonidazole, but no effects were seen in vivo with KHT or RIF-1 sarcomas in mice. Randhawa et al. (1985) showed that there was a threshold for the tumour concentration of misonidazole for murine fibrosarcoma cells and that prolonged exposure to low doses of misonidazole was ineffective for chemosensitization of melphalan. Other radiosensitizers such as benznidazole also increased the antitumour effect (murine RIF-1 sarcoma) of melphalan, but in this case there was a large increase in toxicity, indicating that the clinical benefit of the combination is doubtful (Twentyman and Workman, 1983a). Phase I trials of combinations of misonidazole and melphalan were initiated in 1981 (Coleman et al., 1983). Thirty-five patients were treated with misonidazole 2 hr before melphalan. No effects were seen on the pharmacokinetics of the alkylating agent and both drugs could be given up to their maximum individually tolerated doses without excess haematological toxicity. In a Phase II trial (Coleman et al., 1988) on patients with non-small cell lung cancer, misonidazole increased the response rate from melphalan.

The mechanism for chemosensitization has been investigated in detail. Taylor et al. (1983) showed that a major cause for chemosensitization of Chinese hamster ovary cells to melphalan was an enhanced efficiency of DNA cross-linking. No effect was seen on the rate of removal of these cross-links. Murray and Meyn (1983) similarly showed an increased formation of DNA cross-links in vivo in tumour and normal cells from mice treated with misonidazole followed by melphalan. Glutathione depletion was shown not to be responsible for this effect. The possibility that altered pharmacokinetic parameters could be the reason for the increased extent of cross-linking was investigated by Hinchliffe et al. (1983) and Horsman et al. (1984), who showed that large single doses of misonidazole caused great changes in the disposition of melphalan e.g. greater and more prolonged peak concentrations and delayed plasma clearance. However this effect was not seen with chronic low dosing of misonidazole, such as that used clinically with the drug. Changes in pharmacokinetics and anti-tumour activity of melphalan caused by pretreatment with misonidazole were not due to the reduction of body temperature caused by the latter compound (Hinchliffe et al., 1983; Randhawa et al., 1985). It has been suggested by Mulcahy et al. (1990) that the chemosensitizing agent is a reduced metabolite of misonidazole. Using a model agent, 1-methyl-2-

nitroimidazole, it was demonstrated that the 2-electron reduction product 1-methyl-2-nitrosoimidazole, was a potent chemosensitizer in vitro under either aerobic or anaerobic conditions.

The efficacy of melphalan treatment of tumours may also be enhanced by addition of a perfluorochemical, such as Fluosol-DA, which has good oxygen-carrying properties. The effect is enhanced by the use of atmospheres containing high partial pressures of oxygen (Teicher et al., 1985, 1987a,b).

5.9. RESISTANCE

A variety of mechanisms have been proposed for the development of cellular resistance to melphalan. These include alterations in drug transport, changes in DNA-binding and cross-linking and increases in glutathione levels. Resistance of L1210 cells to melphalan has been partially associated with slower uptake and a lower intracellular accumulation caused by mutation of the lower affinity L-transport system (Redwood and Colvin, 1980). Melphalan-resistant Chinese hamster ovary cells have also been shown to have a lower intracellular concentration of the drug (Elliott and Ling, 1981).

Another well recognized cause for resistance to alkylating agents is the presence of higher than normal amounts of sulphydryl compounds. One of the first melphalan-resistant tumour lines (rat Yoshida sarcoma, Ball et al., 1966) showed a 63% increase in protein-free thiol groups. Later studies by Suzukake et al. (1982) showed that reduction of glutathione levels, by nutritional deprivation of cysteine, sensitized melphalan-resistant L1210 cells. Such resistance was directly related to the intracellular concentration of glutathione and to production of the hydrolyzed dihydroxy derivative (DOH) (Suzukake et al., 1983). Confirmation that reduction of glutathione levels increased the sensitivity of resistant L1210 cells to melphalan was obtained by treating them with buthionine sulphoximine, an inhibitor of γ-glutamylcysteine synthetase and hence of glutathione biosynthesis (Somfai-Relle et al., 1984). In human ovarian cells resistant (4-fold) to melphalan, the glutathione level was twice that of normal cells and although there was no difference in melphalan uptake the levels of DOH derived from it were also increased 2-fold in the resistant cells. Again buthionine sulphoximine removed the resistance to melphalan (Green et al., 1984). Only relatively small changes in glutathione-linked enzyme levels were seen in such resistant ovarian cells, although glutathione transferase was increased by 14% (Hamilton et al., 1985). Chemosensitization of many tumour cells to melphalan may be achieved by coadministration of L-buthionine sulphoximine, e.g. L1210 leukaemia cells (Kramer et al., 1987), human ovarian cancer cells (Andrews et al., 1986; Ozols et al., 1987), human melanoma cells (Hansson et al., 1988) and human medulloblastoma xenografts (Skapek et al., 1988). In mice, buthionine sulphoximine does not enhance organ toxicity of melphalan (Skapek et al., 1991), suggesting that therapeutic use of this combination should be further explored. Human melanoma cells containing high levels of glutathione transferase may be sensitized to melphalan by treatment with the enzyme inhibitor ethacrynic acid, which also results in an increased extent of DNA interstrand cross-links (Hansson et al., 1991).

Elevated glutathione levels have also been observed in cells from resistant human gastric carcinoma (Barranco et al., 1990). Non-protein thiol levels are apparently associated with resistance of human myeloma cells to melphalan (Bellamy et al., 1991). However this was not the case for resistant human CLL (Panasci et al., 1988) or plasma cell lines although a novel glutathione-*S*-transferase was induced in the latter cells (Gupta et al., 1989).

An alternative mechanism for L1210 resistance was investigated by Zwelling et al. (1981), who demonstrated that sensitivity to melphalan in pairs of sensitive and resistant lines was correlated with DNA interstrand cross-linking both in vitro and in vivo. In human melanoma cells resistant to melphalan, the degree of interstrand cross-linking was 50% of that in the parent culture. No difference in melphalan transport was found and it therefore appears that the DNA of resistant cells is more inaccessible to the bifunctional alkylating agent (Parsons et al., 1981).

Cellular glutathione levels modulate the initial degree of DNA cross-linking caused by melphalan (Dorr, 1987). CLL cells resistant to melphalan show a decreased percentage of DNA cross-links compared to sensitive cells (Panasci et al., 1988) and this has been demonstrated to be due to an enhanced removal of cross-links in resistant cells (Torres-Garcia et al., 1989) associated with increased expression of the repair gene ERCC1 and of 3-methyladenine-DNA glycosylase (Geleziunas et al., 1991). Enhanced DNA cross-link removal has also been observed in resistant human breast cancer cells (Batist et al., 1989).

6. ESTRAMUSTINE PHOSPHATE

Estramustine phosphate (Estracyt®, estra-1,3,5(10)-triene-3,17βdiol-3-[bis(2-chloroethyl)-carbamate]17-phosphate) (IX) is a phosphorylated derivative of a complex of nor-nitrogen mustard with oestradiol and has been widely used in the treatment of prostatic cancer (Jönsson et al., 1977; Andersson et al., 1977; Mittelman et al., 1977; Leistenschneider and Nagel, 1980; Madajewicz et al., 1980; Boccardo et al., 1988). Limited use against metastatic melanoma has also been reported (Jönsson et al., 1988). Although the compound contains an alkylating function its mechanism of action has not so far been fully elucidated. Estramustine phosphate was synthesized in the hope that its alkylating group would be transported selectively towards tumours bearing oestrogen receptors, such as those in the prostate.

Estramustine phosphate has a variety of effects on the hormonal system, including an antiprostatic effect, manifested by reduction in 5α-reductase enzyme levels and a decrease in prostate weight and secretion in the rat (Kirdani et al., 1974). Suppression of DNA synthesis in cultured rat ventral prostate results from treatment with oestramustine or oestramustine phosphate, although no enhancements over the effects of oestradiol are seen (Buchanan and Riches, 1987). The oestrogenic properties of oestramustine phosphate are weak with a uterotropic effect one hundred times weaker than that of oestradiol-17β (Fredholm et al., 1974) and the drug does show activity in patients not susceptible to normal oestrogen therapy. However the antiproliferative effect of oestramustine phosphate on a variety of human tumour cell cultures was reported to be related to their cytosolic oestrogen receptors (Pavelic et al., 1991).

The drug is readily dephosphorylated following its administration to rats (Forshell and Nilsson, 1974; Forshell et al., 1976), to dogs (Dixon et al., 1980) or to humans (Dixon et al., 1980; Gunnarsson et al., 1981; Andersson et al., 1981). In the rat, dosing with [^{3}H]-oestramustine phosphate results in accumulation of radioactivity by the prostate, mainly accounted for by dephosphorylated metabolites (Forshell and Nilsson, 1974). This accumulation of radioactivity was also observed with [^{3}H]-oestramustine (Appelgren et al., 1978) and is caused by the presence of an oestramustine-binding protein in the prostate (Forsgren et al., 1979b). This protein accounts for ca. 20% of the ventral prostatic cytosolic proteins and it binds oestramustine with k_D 2×10^{-8} M. Following purification the protein had a molecular weight of 46,000 and was shown to be glycosylated. Antibodies were raised against the purified protein and a radioimmunoassay procedure has been developed for its determination (Forsgren et al., 1979a). An analogous protein with molecular weight ca. 54,000 was found to be present in 22 out of 27 hyperplastic prostatic cytosolic fractions from humans (Björk et al., 1982).

Subcellular fractionation of rat ventral prostate after administration of i.v. [^{3}H]-oestramustine showed that there were two main sites of radioactivity localization, one associated with the endoplasmic reticulum fraction and one associated with the cytosol fraction (Peterson et al., 1983). Transfer of the activity from the former to the latter was observed with time suggesting the secretion of a drug–protein complex to the soluble fraction.

Estramustine binding proteins have also been found in the submaxillary gland of the rat (Pousette et al., 1987), human breast cancer biopsy samples (Ferno et al., 1987a), lung cancer cell lines (Bergh et al., 1988) and malignant glioma cell lines (von Schoultz et al., 1988, 1989). A binding site for oestramustine has also been found in about 20% of metastatic melanoma samples (Ferno et al., 1987b) prompting an evaluation of the activity of oestramustine phosphate towards these tumours.

The mechanism of uptake of oestramustine in human prostatic tumour cells has been studied using a fluorescent dansylated oestramustine (Stearns et al., 1985) or [^{3}H]-oestramustine (Kruse et al., 1988; Kruse and Hartley-Asp, 1989a). Binding to the nuclear protein matrix was observed (Hartley-Asp and Kruse, 1986). RNA synthesis was inhibited by oestramustine, but DNA synthesis was not (Kruse and Hartley-Asp, 1989b).

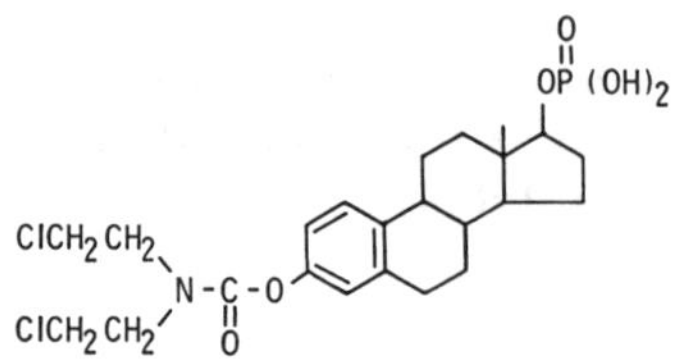

IX

6.1. METABOLISM

As indicated above, oestramustine phosphate is rapidly dephosphorylated in vivo. This hydrolysis is catalyzed by a variety of tissue extracts, including prostatic and intestinal (Kadohama et al., 1978; Gunnarsson et al., 1983) and by human glioma cell lines (von Schoultz et al., 1989). In plasma however oestramustine phosphate is stable although the drug is subject to hydrolysis by serum phosphatases (Tritsch et al., 1974; Dixon et al., 1980). Following the release of oestramustine, further metabolism involving the oxidation of the 17-position to the estrone derivative, estromustine, occurs. Thus in rat or human plasma (Dixon et al., 1980; Kadohama et al., 1979; Gunnarsson et al., 1981) or in rat ventral prostate (Peterson et al., 1983) estromustine is the major metabolite of oestramustine. In the dog both oestramustine and oestromustine were abundant in the plasma (Dixon et al., 1980). A second metabolic route is the hydrolysis of the carbamate from the steroid (Gunnarsson et al., 1983), which results in elevated plasma levels of both oestradiol and oestrone (Kadohama et al., 1979; Dixon et al., 1980; Gunnarsson et al., 1981; Andersson et al., 1981).

Only limited data are available on the excreted metabolites of oestramustine phosphate. Kirdani et al. (1975, 1977) and Forshell et al. (1976) administered a mixture of [^{3}H]-oestramustine phosphate (labelled in the oestradiol) with [^{14}C]-oestradiol to humans, baboons, dogs and rats. In humans and baboons 10–15% of the [^{3}H] oestramustine phosphate was converted to [^{3}H]-oestradiol which was conjugated and excreted. Ready hydrolysis was also seen in the dog, with both [^{3}H] and [^{14}C] being excreted together. In the rat however the [^{3}H] was excreted in the urine much slower than the [^{14}C] label. Doubly labelled oestramustine phosphate ([^{3}H] in the oestradiol and [^{14}C] in the carbamate) gave much slower excretion of [^{14}C] (2–25%) than [^{3}H] (9–34%) in the urine of human subjects, again indicating that the carbamate function was hydrolyzed and metabolized independently of the steroid nucleus. Hartley-Asp and Gunnarsson (1982a) showed that there was little ester cleavage of oestramustine during experiments in vitro with a human prostatic carcinoma cell line. Furthermore, oestramustine was active against a hormone resistant cell line to a greater extent than the possible hydrolysis product nor-nitrogen mustard, indicating that it is oestramustine itself that is responsible for the cytotoxicity.

6.2. MICROTUBULE INHIBITION

The biological effects of oestramustine phosphate are in part characteristic of mitotic inhibitors. In human prostatic cells in culture it is cytotoxic (Hartley-Asp and Gunnarsson, 1982b) induces mitotic arrest at metaphase (Hartley-Asp, 1984), coupled with a depletion in intracellular glutathione (Tew et al., 1986). Specific effects of oestramustine phosphate, which were not shown by nor-nitrogen mustard or oestradiol 17β-phosphate, have been observed with brain microtubules (Kanje et al., 1985) and this is thought to be due to the binding of the drug to microtubule proteins (Wallin et al., 1985, 1986). This leads to disturbance of the cytoskeleton which has been demonstrated in a variety of systems (Stearns and Tew, 1985; Tew and Stearns, 1987; Wang et al., 1987; Mareel et al., 1988) (see review on mechanism of action of oestramustine by Tew and Stearns, 1989). Two of the best characterized microtubule associated proteins (MAPs) are MAP-1 (molecular weight 330,000) and MAP-2 (300,000) and the binding of oestramustine to these (and consequent disruption of microtubule assembly) has been demonstrated in human prostatic cells and rat brain extracts, respectively (Stearns et al., 1988; Stearns and Tew, 1988). Friden et al. (1987) showed that tau and the tubulin-binding part of MAP-2 had binding sites for oestramustine phosphate in common. Specific binding of oestramustine to MAP-1A and inhibition of type IV collagenase secretion has recently been detected (Stearns et al., 1991). Collagenase secretion had previously been shown to be blocked by oestramustine during tumour cell invasion (Wang and Stearns, 1988). Although the anti-microtubule effect appears to be a leading mechanism for oestramustine toxicity it has also been suggested that active oxygen damage to DNA may be involved (Henriksson et al., 1990).

7. BUSULPHAN

Busulphan, (myleran, L,4-dimethylsulphonyloxybutane) (X) was first reported by Timmis (1950) and its use in the treatment of chronic myeloid leukemia was rapidly established (Haddow and Timmis, 1953; Galton, 1953). Because of its selectivity of action towards bone marrow, busulphan has remained the drug of choice for this disease (Korbitz and Reiquam, 1969; Dunn, 1974). The use of busulphan for solid tumours has been more limited, although Phase I/II trials of high dose therapy, coupled with autologous bone marrow support, have been carried out (Peters et al., 1987).

Busulphan is a bifunctional alkylating agent which reacts with nucleophiles by an S_N2 mechanism, i.e. the rate determining step involves both the drug and the nucleophile. Thus the nature and concentration of the nucleophile are important to the rate of covalent bound formation between busulphan and cellular constituents. (This is in contrast to some nitrogen mustards where the rate determining step is the unimolecular formation of an ethylene immonium ion.) In biological systems, sulphur nucleophiles are generally the most powerful reactors in S_N2 processes and it has been shown (see below) that the major urinary metabolite of busulphan is a sulphur adduct. Hydrolysis of busulphan also occurs in biological fluids (e.g. $t_{1/2}$ 8.7 hr in blood, Ehrsson and Hassan, 1983). In contrast to the behaviour of chlorambucil and melphalan, busulphan is more stable in buffer solution (pH 7 phosphate, $t_{1/2}$ 16 hr).

DNA alkylation similarly occurs and the production of cross-links was first suggested by Brookes and Lawley (1961b). However, DNA cross-linking by busulphan was not observed by caesium chloride gradient centrifugation and renaturation studies following alkaline treatment (Verly and Brakier, 1969; Mitchell and Walker, 1972). Mitchell and Walker (1972) additionally failed to find any chromatographic evidence, on paper, for the production of cross-links in DNA by busulphan. Similarly Alexander and Lett (1960) showed by centrifugation studies that busulphan was very ineffective at cross-linking DNA in sperm head suspensions. More recently, however, Tong and Ludlum (1980) have synthesized the guanine–guanine cross-linked product, 1,4-di(7-guanyl) butane, by reaction of busulphan with guanosine and confirmed its structure by mass and ultraviolet spectrometry. Reaction of DNA with busulphan was shown to give a product, in low yield, with identical HPLC properties to the synthetic cross-linked guanine. Bedford and Fox (1982), using the more sensitive technique of alkaline elution, also identified DNA cross-links in Yoshida lymphosarcoma cells following busulphan treatment, at a level of 0.04 ± 0.01 per 10^9 Da (Bedford and Fox, 1983). In L1210 cells, against which busulphan is relatively ineffective, no interstrand cross-linking of DNA could be found, although DNA–protein cross-links were produced (Pacheco et al., 1989).

Analogues of busulphan of greater or smaller carbon chain length have also been synthesized and subjected to anti-tumour (Haddow and Timmis, 1953; Bedford and Fox, 1983), immunosuppressive (Berenbaum et al., 1967) and neutrophil-depressing (Elson, 1951, 1958) activity testing and it has been of some interest to study the rationale for selection of busulphan for clinical use. Historically, the first antitumour tests (Walker 256 carcinoma in the rat, Haddow and Timmis, 1953) showed maximal activity for chain lengths C_4–C_6. Maximal activity on circulating neutrophils in the rat was seen with C_4, which also showed the greatest effect on haemopoietic colony forming units in the rat (Dunn and Elson, 1970). The rate of hydrolysis of busulphan in aqueous acetone (which might be taken as an indication of its chemical reactivity) had k 1.79×10^{-5} sec^{-1}, but this did not differ significantly from the rates of hydrolysis of the C_5–C_8 chain length diesters (Hudson et al., 1959), suggesting that the electrophilic activity of busulphan was not the most important parameter governing its activity. The distribution of the drug may be important however as the lipid–water partition coefficient (measured by the ratio of ether:water solubilities) was highest for busulphan (5.7) compared to other members of the series (Hudson et al., 1959).

Detailed studies on this homologous series of drugs have also been carried out on the Yoshida lymphosarcoma in vitro and in the rat by Bedford and Fox (1983). There was no peak of anti-tumour activity for the C_4 compound (busulphan) and the C_8 compound exhibited twice the therapeutic ratio of busulphan. However, for the C_8 compound, a correlation was seen between cytotoxicity in vitro and DNA–DNA cross-link formation, although the C_6 compound was the most active. Clearly distribution in vivo and other pharmacokinetic parameters must be of considerable significance to the anti-tumour activity of these dimethanesulphonic acid esters.

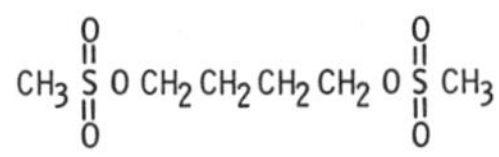

X

7.1. ANALYSIS

Radiochemical techniques were first used to quantitate busulphan and its metabolites in biological fluids ([^{14}C], [^{35}S], Nadkarni et al., 1959; [^{3}H], Vodopick et al., 1969). A more selective technique for monitoring plasma levels of the drug by GC-MS has recently been developed by Ehrsson and Hassan (1983). In this method plasma is first spiked with an internal standard (1,5-pentanediol dimethane sulphonate) and the drug and standard then both extracted with methylene chloride. The dimethane sulphonates are converted to the diiodocompounds, 1,4-diiodobutane and 1,5-diiodopentane, by treatment with sodium iodide in acetone and the products subjected to packed column GC-MS selected ion recording. Analyses can be carried out down to low ng/mL concentrations of busulphan in plasma, the standard deviation for the determination at 10 ng/mL being $\pm$ 4.3%. Vassal et al. (1988) later used an analogous analytical method except that the internal standard was the stable isotope labelled analogue d_4-busulphan. Quantitation was by capillary GC-MS multiple ion recording.

In a development of the method of Ehrsson and Hassan (1983) the derivatization and extraction of busulphan from plasma was carried out in a single step and the drug quantitated by capillary GC and electron capture detection (ECD) (Hassan and Ehrsson, 1983). The precision of this method at the 10 ng/mL level is $\pm$ 3.9%. GC with ECD was later used in the method of Chen et al. (1988), in which busulphan was derivatized with 2,3,5,6-tetrafluorothiophenol. The internal standard was the homologue 1,8-bis(methanesulphonyloxy)octane and limit of quantitation 10 ng/mL plasma.

Following derivatization with sodium diethyldithiocarbamate busulphan may be determined by HPLC using UV detection (Henner et al., 1987). The method is claimed to be suitable for the monitoring of kinetics during high dose therapy, but could not be validated by later workers (Kazemifard and Morgan, 1990).

The method was subsequently improved by MacKichan and Bechtel (1990), allowing satisfactory analysis of busulphan down to plasma concentrations of 50 ng/mL.

An alternative derivatizing agent that has been used for HPLC quantitation of busulphan is thiocresol (Grochow et al., 1989) which allowed a detection limit of 0.4 μmol/L plasma (100 ng/mL).

Recently post-column photolysis has been used to detect busulphan in a rapid isocratic HPLC analysis (Blanz et al., 1990). In this procedure the drug is converted to its diiodo derivative. Upon photolysis this yields iodide ions which may be detected by UV.

7.2. TRANSPORT

Unlike the situation for nitrogen mustard, the transport of busulphan into L121O cells did not appear to be carrier mediated (Kessel et al., 1969). The uptake of busulphan was temperature insensitive and equilibrium between cellular drug levels and the medium was reached within 1 min. Uptake of busulphan into Yoshida ascites sarcoma cells was also rapid and both sensitive and resistant cells took up the same amount of drug (Harrap and Hill, 1970). Retention of busulphan was also the same in both sensitive and resistant cells.

7.3. Metabolism and Pharmacokinetics

Peng (1957) and Trams et al. (1959) investigated the absorption and excretion of [^{35}S]-labelled busulphan in the rat. Some concentration of [^{35}S] was seen in bone marrow, intestine and spleen. Following i.v. injection of [^{35}S]-busulphan (2 mg/kg), 86% of the label was excreted in urine in 24 hr and 62–68% of this was methanesulphonic acid, identified as its phenylhydrazonium derivative (Trams et al., 1959). Another 25–30% of urinary radioactivity was unchanged busulphan.

For the [^{14}C]-labelled drug, injected i.v., (4 mg/kg) liver, kidney and lungs were heavily labelled (Trams et al., 1959). The [^{14}C] was excreted as expired carbon dioxide (12–14%) and in the urine (22–36%) and faeces (0.8–3.5%) in 24 hr. A large number of metabolites was present in urine, including 1,4-butane diol as a minor component. Unchanged busulphan was also detected. Later studies by Roberts and Warwick (1961) with i.p. injected 2,3-[^{14}C]-busulphan (20 mg/kg) in rat showed 28–35% urinary and 4–8% exhaled CO_2 excretion in 24 hr. A major urinary metabolite, which accounted for at least 60% of the urinary radioactivity, was identified as 3-hydroxytetrahydrothiophene-1,1-dioxide (XI). The same metabolite was produced following injection of tetrahydrothiophene-1,1-dioxide, tetrahydrothiophene and *S*-*β*-L-alanyltetrahydrothiophenium mesylate, suggesting that its route of formation is via bis-alkylation of a protein or amino acid based sulphydryl group, followed by liberation of the tetrahydrothiophene and oxidation to its dioxide.

A more detailed study by Hassan and Ehrsson (1987b) used GC-MS and NMR for metabolite identification. [1,4-^{14}C]-Busulphan (15 mg/kg) was administered i.p. to rats and 70% of radioactivity was excreted in the next 72 hr. At least eight components were separated by HPLC, including busulphan, which accounted for 6%, XI (39%), tetrahydrothiophene-1-oxide (20%) and sulpholane (tetrahydrothiophene1,1-dioxide) (13%). Low binding of busulphan to plasma proteins was observed (9.2 $\pm$ 4.4%); $t_{1/2}$ for elimination of [^{14}C] was ca. 8 hr and for elimination of busulphan 3.1 hr (Hassan et al., 1988). The radioactivity ratio brain:plasma was 0.95 $\pm$ 0.12 (busulphan ratio 0.74 $\pm$ 0.05) and most of the above mentioned [^{14}C] metabolites of busulphan were found in brain.

The glutathione sulphonium ion adduct (*γ*-glutamyl-*β*-(*S*-tetrahydrothiophenium) alanylglycine) has been identified by time of flight mass spectrometry (^{252}Cf-plasma desorption) as a biliary metabolite of busulphan in a perfused rat liver (Hassan and Ehrsson, 1986, 1987a), but was not found in rat urine (Hassan and Ehrsson, 1987b). However 26% of the dose of busulphan (i.v., 1 mg/kg) was excreted in the bile as a conjugate which released tetrahydrothiophene on hydrolysis (Marchand et al., 1988). HPLC co-chromatography was used to demonstrate that this was the glutathione sulphonium conjugate.

In man, Vodopick et al. (1969) found rapid absorption of oral [^{3}H]-busulphan (6–10 mg/patient), with maximal plasma activity within the first hour. The clearance showed a $t_{1/2}$ for the first phase of 1.3–3.3 hr although this was affected (increased $t_{1/2}$) by the existence of a second phase where plasma levels rose again. Similar values were obtained for i.v. doses. Urinary excretion totalled ca. 30% of the administered radioactivity by both routes of administration. Later exponential decreases of plasma activity were also observed ($t_{1/2}$ 1 day, 5 days) although the significance of these is unknown (in view of the likely widespread distribution of tritium within the body). Nadkarni et al. (1959) using [^{14}C] and [^{35}S]-busulphan showed that over 90% of the radioactivity was removed from the blood in less than 5 min. (Insignificant reversible protein binding occurs (Ehrsson and Hassan, 1984).) Following this loss a steady level of radioactivity (1–3%) remained in the blood for 2 days. Eighty-eight to 93% of the blood radioactivity was associated with plasma and there was an indication that it was associated with the protein fraction. Total urinary excretion of [^{14}C] from [^{14}C]-busulphan was 25–30%, whereas 45–60% of [^{35}S] was excreted. The major metabolite of [^{35}S]-busulphan (>95% of the excreted activity) was identified as methane sulphonic acid. [^{14}C]-Busulphan yielded twelve radioactive urinary components (all unidentified). No unchanged compound was found.

Detailed pharmacokinetic studies on the unchanged drug in chronic myelocytic leukaemia patients have been carried out by Ehrsson et al. (1983a), using the GC-MS analytical method on the diiodo-derivative of the drug (see above and Ehrsson and Hassan, 1983). Following oral doses of 2, 4 and 6 mg, busulphan was eliminated with $t_{1/2}$ of ca. 2.5 hr (k 0.27 hr^{-1}). The area under the curve was linearly related to the dose of the drug and zero-order absorption kinetics were followed. In this case a trace of busulphan (1.2 $\pm$ 1.3% the dose, range 0.04–3.0%) was found in the urine. At an oral dose of 1 mg/kg Grochow et al. (1989) found a first order absorption of the drug and $t_{1/2}$ 58–433 min. Peak concentrations of busulphan were variable in the range 1.2–10.4 μmol/L (295–2558 ng/mL).

In children at the same dose (1 mg/kg) the mean C_{max} was 3.3 ± 0.93 μmol/L (804 ± 229 ng/mL) with an elimination $t_{1/2}$ of 2.33 ± 0.51 hr (Vassal et al., 1989). Repetitive doses did not significantly alter the pharmacokinetic parameters. The passage of busulphan into the CSF was observed, with a CSF:plasma ratio of 0.95 ± 0.25. The maximum tolerated dose of busulphan in a series of adult patients with solid tumours was 16 mg/kg and plasma drug levels were achievable in the range 2–10 μmol/L (492–2460 ng/mL) (Peters et al., 1987).

Following oral doses of 1 mg/kg every 6 hr steady state plasma concentrations of 1080 ng/mL were achieved (Hassan et al., 1989). Over 4 day treatment $t_{1/2}$ increased from 2.3 to 3.4 hr. Plasma protein binding was 7.4% and the CSF:plasma ratio 1.3. Urine contained 1.7% of the dose as unchanged drug, plus sulpholane, XI and tetrahydrothiophene-1-oxide. Hassan et al. (1991) found that during conditioning therapy with busulphan (1 mg/kg × 4 for 4 days) there was an age-related variation in pharmacokinetics, with children showing a shorter elimination half-life (2.05 hr) compared to adults (2.59 hr). A circadian rhythm for busulphan concentrations, with a 3-fold variation between daytime and night-time levels, was also observed.

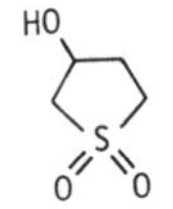

XI

7.4. TOXICITY

Patients treated with busulphan show bone-marrow depression and decreased leucocyte counts. In some cases pulmonary fibrosis or 'busulphan lung' (Sostman et al., 1977) or cataract formation (Ravindranathan et al., 1972) are also observed. High dose busulphan is associated with neurotoxicity which may be alleviated with clonazepan (Vassal et al., 1990). In experimental systems phenytoin and phenobarbital offered protection from the neurotoxic effects of busulphan but also reduced the myelosuppressive effects (Fitzsimmons et al., 1990).

Busulphan can sterilize mice (Bucci and Meistrich, 1987) and induce specific locus and dominant lethal mutations (Ehling and Neuhäuser-Klaus, 1991). Busulphan is mutagenic in short term tests and causes chromosomal aberrations and sister chromatid exchanges in vitro and in vivo in man (for review see I.A.R.C., 1982b). The cytogenetic effects of busulphan have been compared in normal bone marrow and Philadelphia chromosome positive cells from chronic myeloid leukaemia patients (Beccher and Prescher, 1988). Although chromosome aberrations were similar the Philadelphia positive cells showed lower sister chromatid exchanges, indicating less sensitivity to DNA damage by busulphan. Sufficient evidence has also been obtained for the carcinogenic effect of busulphan in man. For example, 243 patients were treated with busulphan after bronchial carcinoma resection; after 5 years 69 were still alive, but 4 died of acute non-lymphocytic leukaemia (Stott et al., 1977). There were no comparable deaths amongst patients treated with placebo or with cyclophosphamide.

8. TREOSULPHAN

Treosulphan (dihydroxybusulphan, L-threitol-1,4-dimethanesulphonate) (XII) is a bifunctional alkylating agent, first synthesized by Feit (1961), in the hope that its alkylating mechanism might be different from that of busulphan because of the hydroxyl groups adjacent to the dimethanesulphonyloxy groups. An improved synthesis, (from L-(+)-tartaric acid) suitable for large scale preparation of the compound, was also reported by Feit (1964). Because of its structural similarity to busulphan, early emphasis was placed on its activity against chronic myeloid leukaemia (Loeb, 1964). However, more recently the drug has been used in the treatment of ovarian cancer (Fennelly, 1977).

The drug is subject to hydrolysis and also may undergo intramolecular displacement of its sulphonyloxy groups by the adjacent hydroxyl groups. Such a reaction was first demonstrated for treosulphan by Davis and Ross (1963) who suggested that the mono- and diepoxides (XIII) and (XIV) should be formed, but that the monoepoxide (XIII) would not accumulate in view of its rapid conversion to (XIV). The diepoxide (XIV) (L-diepoxybutane) is itself an active bifunctional alkylating agent and could therefore be the active chemotherapeutic principle following administration of treosulphan. The rate of epoxide formation is pH-dependent, with little conversion below pH 7. Matagne (1967) showed that at pH 7 the loss of treosulphan at 25°C was 4.2% over 3 hr, whereas at pH 8.5 the conversion was 80.9%. Clearly therefore the drug for clinical use should be in neutral or acidic solution.

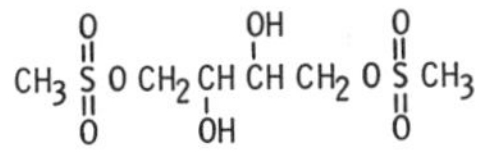

XII

8.1. Analysis

The only analytical method described for monitoring treosulphan is GC (Welsh et al., 1982). The compound was analyzed after its extraction from the biological fluid on a packed column (15% Carbowax 20 M + 2% potassium hydroxide on chromosorb W), using cyclohexanol as internal standard. Because of the basic nature of the stationary phase it was assumed that the drug would be instantly converted on the column to diepoxybutane.

8.2. Distribution and Pharmacokinetics

Treosulphan may be administered orally or intravenously to patients; the drug is well absorbed from an oral dose with a bioavailability approaching 100% (Welsh et al., 1982). Plasma decay of treosulphan concentration followed first order kinetics with $t_{1/2}$ 1.8 hr (oral) or 1.5 hr (i.v.). The drug was also detected in tear, saliva and urine samples.

8.3. Toxicity

Characteristic alkylating agent toxicities are observed with treosulphan, with leucocyte and platelet depressions occurring within 4 weeks of therapy (oral, 10–25 mg/kg) (Loeb, 1964). The development of an Addisonian Syndrome has also been associated with treosulphan therapy in a single patient (Prior and White, 1978) and skin pigmentation has often been observed (Fennelly, 1979).

Treosulphan is mutagenic in *Salmonella typhimurium*, with a pH dependence suggesting that diepoxybutane is the responsible agent (Zeiger and Pagano, 1989). In mice it has been shown to be capable of inducing micronuclei in bone marrow or peripheral blood cells (Shelby et al., 1989; Gulati et al., 1990). A detailed study of 553 patients with ovarian cancer treated with treosulphan has revealed that the drug is leukaemogenic (Pedersen-Bjergaard et al., 1979, 1980b). Between 21 and 58 months after the chemotherapy 7 cases of acute non-lymphocytic leukaemia were observed (normal expected number 0.04). There is no evidence for acute non-lymphocytic leukaemia in untreated ovarian cancer patients (Reimer et al., 1977).

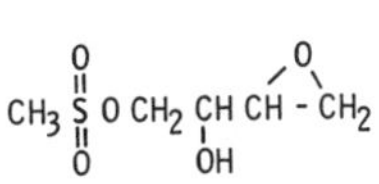

XIII

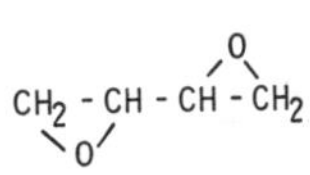

XIV

9. AZO-MUSTARDS

The azo-mustards (XV) are a class of alkylating agents which have low chemical activity but which can be activated in vivo by reduction of the azo-linkage to yield *p*-phenylene diamine derivatives (Fig. 3). Initially the concept of using azo-mustards as latent anti-cancer alkylating agents (Ross and Warwick, 1955) was to obtain selective reduction and hence a localized cytotoxic effect in the tumour. 4-(*N*,*N*-Bis(2-chloroethyl)-amino-2-methylazobenzene-2′-carboxylic acid (CB 1414, Ross Azo-mustard) (XVI) was particularly effective against tumours in animals (Ross and Warwick, 1956a; Duvall, 1961) and was submitted to clinical trial in 1960 (Israels and Ritzmann, 1960). As this compound is stable towards hydrolysis in vitro (less than 1% hydrolysis in 30 min at 66°C in 50% aqueous acetone) it was assumed that it is activated by reduction in vivo. The likelihood of such a reductive process was supported by in vitro experiments using chemical reducing agents (Ross and Warwick, 1956b) or enzyme systems (Connors et al., 1972). The reduced product was confirmed to be the cytotoxic 4-bis(2-chloroethyl)amino-2-methylaniline after trapping of the latter as a thiazane derivative which was identified by mass spectrometry (Connors et al., 1972).

When it was found that the levels of the activating enzyme were not solely associated with the tumour but were also high in the liver, a further series of azo-mustards was synthesized, in the hope of producing an agent of selective toxicity towards hepatocellular carcinoma (Bukhari et al., 1973). For this purpose the active alkylating agent produced by reaction of the azo-mustard would need to be of exceptionally high reactivity, so that any material that escaped the liver would be rapidly hydrolyzed to harmless products. The following structure–activity relationships were established by Bukhari et al. (1973). No reduction of the azo-mustard occurred if there was no substituent *ortho* to the azo-linkage and a 2′-carboxyl group appeared essential. An increase in reduction was seen with methylation at the 2-position, but the nature of the alkylating function was without effect on the reduction. However, the reactivity of the phenylenediamine mustard produced by the reduction could be increased by replacing the bis(2-chloroethyl)amino group with a bis(2-bromo-*n*-propyl)amino group, the half life for hydrolysis of the latter being 12 times smaller than that of the former. Thus, the compound chosen for further study as a hepatoma-specific alkylating agent was *N*,*N*-bis(2-bromo-*n*-propyl)-amino-2-methylazobenzene-2′carboxylic acid (CB 10-252) (XVII) (Bukhari et al., 1973). In rats CB 10-252 cured the Walker tumour in the liver (Connors et al., 1973b) and its reduction has been demonstrated in rat, mouse, baboon and human liver and by rat and human hepatocellular carcinoma cell supernatants (Autrup et al., 1974). Other tissues where azo-reductase activity has been observed include bone marrow and spleen (Curt et al., 1977). Clinical testing by Murray-Lyon et al. (1978) showed no significant activity for CB 10-252 on primary hepatocellular carcinoma, with myelosuppression rather surprisingly being observed. The possibility of other non-liver localized enzymes being responsible for the reduction of azo-mustards was raised by Kitamura and Tatsumi (1983) who showed that aldehyde oxidase had azo-reductase activity.

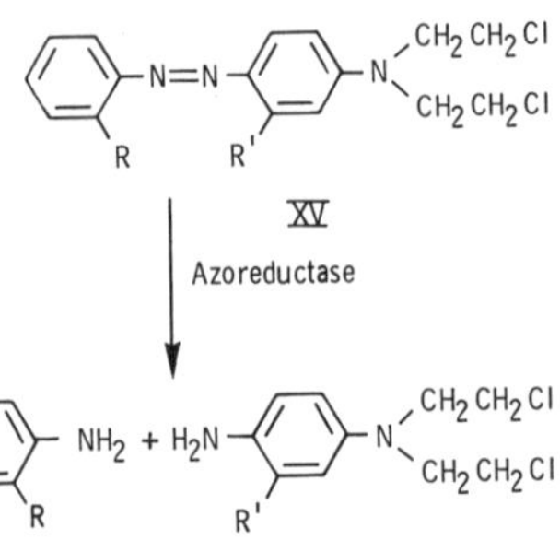

FIG. 3. Metabolism of azo-mustards.

10. ANILINE MUSTARD

Aniline mustard (*N,N*-di-(2-chloroethyl)aniline) (XVIII) was initially synthesized by Robinson and Watt in 1934, but was later prepared as part of a series of potential anti-cancer agents by Ross (1949). Aniline mustard is uniquely effective in curing mice bearing advanced ADJ/PC5 plasma cell tumours (Whisson and Connors, 1965a,b). These tumours have high levels of the enzyme β-glucuronidase (Connors and Whisson, 1966) which led to the hypothesis that the selective action of aniline mustard is related to the metabolic scheme shown in Fig. 4. The postulate is that the drug is metabolized in the liver to 4-hydroxyaniline mustard which is rapidly converted to the β-glucuronide. This conjugate is then hydrolyzed back to 4-hydroxyaniline mustard in areas of high β-glucuronidase activity. As 4-hydroxyaniline mustard is 10 times more toxic in mice than aniline mustard and as the glucuronide is of comparable or lower toxicity than aniline mustard (Bukhari et al., 1972; Workman et al., 1976b), the metabolic route shown in Fig. 4 would represent a tumour specific activating process for the drug.

The involvement of glucuronidase is further supported by the observations that other tumours with high β-glucuronidase levels (e.g. mouse ADJ/PC6A, (Connors and Whisson, 1966), mouse HT67 (Double and Workman, 1977) and rat mammary tumours induced by 7,12-dimethylbenz[a]anthracene (Benckhuysen et al., 1981)) are sensitive to aniline mustard and that tumours with low enzyme levels (e.g. sarcoma 180 and NK lymphoma) are resistant to the drug. Furthermore the β-glucuronide conjugate of 4-hydroxyaniline mustard was synthesized (Bukhari et al., 1972) and shown to be highly active against the ADJ/PC6A plasma cell tumour in mice.

The postulated mechanism of action for aniline mustard was validated by metabolic studies in rat liver homogenates; the glucuronide was isolated and identified by MS (Connors et al., 1973a). In rats the glucuronide was a major metabolite in the bile and in the serum; in the latter, smaller amounts of *N*-(2-chloroethyl)-4-hydroxyaniline were also identified. The glucuronide has been shown to undergo entero-hepatic circulation in the rat although it was suggested, on the basis of experiments in rabbit where aniline mustard metabolites are not abundant in bile, that human entero-hepatic circulation would be negligible (Chipman et al., 1980).

It has also been considered possible that the 4-*O*-phosphate or 4-*O*-sulphate of aniline mustard might be latent anti-tumour agents which could liberate the cytotoxic 4-hydroxy-aniline mustard in regions of high phosphatase or sulphatase activity. These conjugates were also synthesized by Bukhari et al. (1972). The sulphate is of low activity against the ADJ/PC6A tumour and is refractory to hydrolysis by aryl sulphatases (Ball and Double, 1974). The 4-*O*-phosphate is a substrate for phosphatases (Ball and Double, 1974; Workman et al., 1976a) and shows significant activity against the ADJ/PC6A tumour in mice (Bukhari et al., 1972). Additionally the phosphate was cytotoxic towards HeLa cells, which was ascribed to the cells' content of alkaline phosphatase (Workman et al., 1976a). The hydrolytic conversion of the 4-*O*-phosphate of aniline mustard to 4-hydroxyaniline mustard is however catalyzed by acid and alkaline phosphatases found in the bone marrow, small intestine mucosa and serum of mice and such a widespread distribution of these enzymes does not strongly support the hypothesis of a tumour-selective production of 4-hydroxyaniline mustard from the phosphate (Workman and Double, 1978). However as human prostatic tissues may contain high levels of acid phosphatase, it was of interest to investigate the susceptibility of 4-hydroxyaniline mustard phosphate to this enzyme. Unfortunately, the enzyme is inhibited by the compound, presumably because of its alkylation, which suggests that the prostate may not be a selective target for aniline mustard phosphate (Workman, 1978).

In clinical trials, Young et al. (1976) found a partial correlation between tumour tissue β-glucuronidase activity and patient response. However out of 78 patients only 6 (5 prostate cancer and 1 renal cancer) patients responded significantly. Two patients who relapsed were found to have lost their enzyme activity and became insensitive to aniline mustard.

11. SPIROHYDANTOIN MUSTARD

Spirohydantoin mustard (3-[2-[bis(2′-chloroethyl)amino]-ethyl]-5,5-pentamethylene-hydantoin, spiromustine) (XIX) is a covalent complex of nor-nitrogen mustard with a substituted hydantoin. The compound was synthesized by Peng et al. (1975) in an attempt to achieve selectivity for

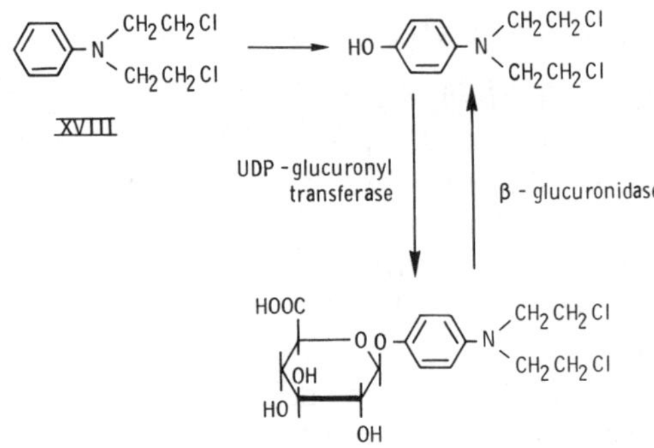

FIG. 4. Metabolism of aniline mustard.

treatment of tumours of the CNS; it was known that other hydantoins, such as the anticonvulsive drug phenytoin (5,5-diphenylhydantoin) crossed the blood–brain barrier and distributed preferentially to brain tumours (Rosenblum and Stein, 1963). Some other mustards linked to hydantoins had been previously prepared by Mauger and Ross (1962), although the rationale of these investigators, (which was subsequently disproved) was that the hydantoin might be selectively hydrolyzed in the tumour to an amino acid, which could act as a carrier for the cytotoxic function.

Spirohydantoin mustard has only limited solubility in water. Its rapid decomposition in aqueous solutions has prevented determination of the octanol:water partition coefficient (p) although Levin (1980) has calculated that log p should be 2.47. Hydrolytic studies for this drug have been carried out in solutions in 10% dimethylacetamide in buffers; the rate of reaction was monitored by chloride determination and by GC after freeze-drying and derivatizing the samples with a trimethylsilylating reagent (Flora et al., 1982). Both the mono- and bis-hydroxylated hydrolysis products were detected by GC-MS. The first order hydrolysis half-time at pH 6 was 14 min, but the rate of decomposition could be considerably decreased by dissolving the drug in a 10% fat emulsion, when a zero order decomposition was observed with 10% decomposition occurring in 49 min. (Such fat emulsions have been acceptable for administration to humans of other lipid soluble substances.) Further mathematical treatment of the data of Flora et al. (1982) by Chan et al. (1985) gave first order kinetic rate constants of 0.0414 min^{-1} for the hydrolysis of spirohydantoin mustard to the mono-hydroxy derivative and 0.00625 min^{-1} for the hydrolysis of this to the bis-hydroxyspirohydantoin mustard. Analogues of spirohydantoin mustard containing more methylene groups between the nitrogen mustard and the hydantoin ring were of greater hydrolytic instability and somewhat lower activity against murine P-388 leukaemia (Haces et al., 1986). Spirohydantoin mustard was shown by Hilton et al. (1977) to be a DNA cross-linking agent in intracerebral rat glioma 9L and in rat bone marrow.

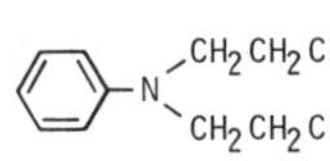

XVIII

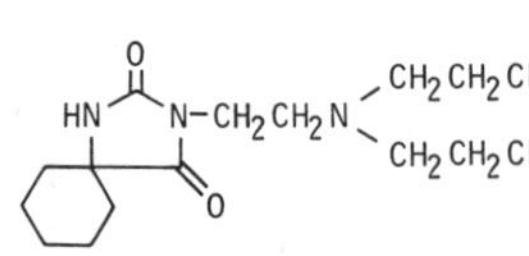

XIX

Rose et al. (1982) formulated the drug in 10% fat emulsion, in preparation for preclinical toxicology and found that the GC method of Flora et al. (1982) was unreliable, necessitating the development of an assay method utilizing HPLC. Analysis of ethyl acetate extracts of spirohydantoin formulations in 10% fat emulsion again demonstrated its stability in this medium.

The passage of spirohydantoin mustard across the blood–brain barrier was confirmed in rats by Kobayashi et al. (1979) and in dogs by Plowman et al. (1977) who demonstrated the presence of the drug in the CSF using GC-MS. Later studies by Plowman and Adamson (1979) using [^{14}C]-ethyl and [^{14}C]-hydantoin-labelled drug showed that concentrations in the brains of rats and dogs, following i.v. injection, were comparable. After oral dosing to rats, the plasma level of radioactivity from the [^{14}C]-ethyl drug was 2.6 times greater than the brain concentration. The distribution of both labelled forms of the drug into the brain over 4 hr was similar, suggesting that no major metabolism of spirohydantoin mustard occurred before binding in the brain. In the bile, however, two major metabolites of spirohydantoin mustard were found, which were believed to be conjugates with cysteine or acetylated cysteine. Only a trace of unmetabolized drug was found in the bile. Metabolism in vitro by mouse liver supernatant yields a single non-polar product (Suling et al., 1983), which is mutagenic in the Ames test with *S. typhimurium* (Ames et al., 1973) after i.p. injection of spirohydantoin mustard. As spirohydantoin mustard is not mutagenic this metabolic process may represent an activating mechanism and further studies of the nature and existence of this metabolite in vivo are clearly required.

Treatment of 9L brain tumour cells with spirohydantoin mustard showed that exponentially growing and plateau phase cells were equally responsive (Deen et al., 1979). Degradation of the drug within 30 min was seen in the cell culture medium. In vivo the survival of rats bearing the intracerebral 9L tumour was surprisingly not increased and this was ascribed to the presence of cells that were not cycling and could repair the drug-induced damage before DNA synthesis started (Sano et al., 1983). This clearly has implications regarding dosing protocols for the drug. The growth delay of 9L rat brain tumour multicellular spheroids was greater after a split dose of spirohydantoin mustard (2 or 4 hr apart) compared to a split dose control (Jostes et al., 1985). Effectiveness against the murine ependymoblastoma model had previously been demonstrated by Peng et al. (1975). The anti-tumour activity of spirohydantoin mustard against other animal tumour systems has been reviewed by Shoemaker et al. (1983).

Preclinical toxicological studies have been reported (Meeks, 1983; Meeks and Frick, 1983; Liao et al., 1983); dose-related and reversible effects were seen on the haematopoietic tissues. In a Phase I study neurotoxicity was the dose-limiting toxicity (Brown et al., 1986; Pazdur et al., 1987) and a split-dose schedule was suggested for further trials. Neurotoxicity was again a problem (though partially reversible with physostigmine), in a pediatric Phase I evaluation (Heideman et al., 1988). Interestingly though the penetration of the drug to the CSF was low (concentration ratio to plasma 4.7%). Some evidence of activity of spirohydantoin mustard against recurrent malignant gliomas has been observed (Prados et al., 1987).

12. AZIRIDINYL COMPOUNDS

As indicated above the alkylating mechanism of many nitrogen mustards involves the intermediacy of positively charged aziridinium ions (see e.g. (II)). These ions are subject to nucleophilic attack which results in their ring opening and the alkylation of the nucleophile. For this reason there has been considerable interest in the synthesis and anti-tumour testing of other aziridinyl compounds which might alkylate cellular molecules in a similar fashion (see e.g. Hendry et al., 1951 for early animal studies). Several di- or tri-functional compounds have reached clinical practice, although their impact on cancer chemotherapy is currently not very significant.

12.1. 2,4,6-Tris(1-Aziridinyl)-1,3,5-Triazine

2,4,6-Tris(1-aziridinyl)-1,3,5-triazine (TEM, triethylenemelamine) (XX) was one of the first aziridinyl drugs studied in cancer treatment (Gellhorn et al., 1952; Rundles and Barton, 1952; Wright et al., 1952; Axelrod et al., 1953). TEM was originally used in the treatment of chronic leukaemia, lymphomas, Hodgkin's disease and retinoblastoma, but its use is now restricted in view of the powerful bone-marrow depressing and other toxic effects caused by the drug.

The drug is a powerful alkylating agent, especially under acidic conditions when the aziridine ring becomes protonated. For example in pH 7.5 aqueous solution at 25°C little degradation of TEM occurs in 24 hr; at pH 3 immediate degradation occurs and at pH 5 approximately half of the drug is lost in 4 hr (Beroza and Borkovev, 1964). TEM also interacts with deoxyguanosine and with DNA to yield a product with spectral characteristics of an *N*-7 alkylguanine (Doskocil, 1965; Lawley and Brookes, 1967). Tomasz (1970) confirmed that *N*-7-alkylation of guanine occurred by studies of the labilization of a tritium label at the C-8 position of the purine.

12.1.1. *Analysis*

No quantitative gas or liquid chromatographic methods have been reported for TEM. Colorimetric determination of the compound is, however, possible using the 4-(4′-nitrobenzyl) pyridine test (Epstein et al., 1955) which is general for all alkylating agents. Titrimetric methods, based on the reaction of the aziridine with thiosulphate (Allen and Seaman, 1955; Beroza and Borkovec, 1964) have also been established for this drug.

12.1.2. *Distribution and Metabolism*

The tissue distribution and excretion of TEM in normal and tumour-bearing mice was studied by Nadkarni et al. (1954), using the [^{14}C] triazine-labelled drug. Seventy-one to 87% of the radioactivity was excreted in urine in 24 hr, with up to 5% in the faeces. Less than 2% of the activity was excreted as exhaled carbon dioxide and the major urinary metabolite was identified by cocrystallization as cyanuric acid, indicating that the triazine ring remained essentially intact during metabolism of the drug. No significant differences were seen between normal and tumour-bearing animals in the uptake of radioactivity to body organs. Later studies by Goldenthal et al. (1958) using aziridine [^{14}C]-labelled drug again showed little excretion of the label as exhaled carbon dioxide or in the faeces, with 68–73% of the radioactivity being excreted in the urine in 24 hr. The loss of drug from blood was rapid with greater than 80% of the radioactivity being lost within 1 min. Attempts were made to separate the urinary metabolites, which numbered at least 16, but only creatinine (8–13% of urinary radioactivity) and urea (less than 1% of urinary radioactivity) could be identified.

Similar observations were made on the metabolism of [^{14}C]-aziridinyl-labelled drug administered to cancer patients (Nadkarni et al., 1956, 1959, 1961). Blood levels of radioactivity decreased to less than 10% within 5 min (i.v. dose), with ca. 90% of the radioactivity being associated with plasma. Urinary excretion amounted to 25–30% of the dose in 24 hr and of the 14 separated metabolites, 2 (totalling 8% of the total radioactivity) were identified as urea and creatinine.

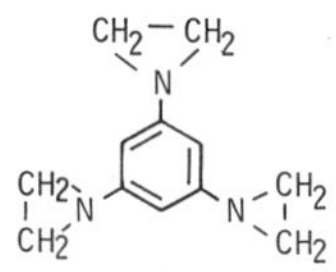

XX

12.1.3. *Toxicity*

As indicated above TEM produces pronounced alkylating agent-related toxicities to bone marrow and to other proliferating tissues. Additionally it is mutagenic and causes chromosomal aberrations in cultured human leucocytes (Hampel et al., 1966). Sister chromatid exchanges have been shown to be induced by TEM in mouse and Chinese hamster cells in vivo (Nath et al., 1988; Neft et al., 1989). TEM also shows genotoxic activity in mouse spermatogonial cells (Nagao and Fujikawa, 1990). Its carcinogenicity to mice (Roe and Salaman, 1955; Hendry et al., 1951; Shimkin, 1954; Conklin et al., 1965) and rats (Walpole, 1958) has also been demonstrated.

12.2. TRIS(1-AZIRIDINYL)PHOSPHINE OXIDE AND TRIS(1-AZIRIDINYL)PHOSPHINE SULPHIDE

Although both tris(1-aziridinyl)phosphine oxide (TEPA, triethylenephosphoramide) (XXI) and tris(1-aziridinyl)phosphine sulphide (thio-TEPA, triethylenethiophosphoramide) (XXII) showed anti-tumour effectiveness in animals, thio-TEPA had less unfavourable toxicological characteristics in man and its use in the clinic has therefore been preferred to that of TEPA. Thio-TEPA has been used to treat lymphomas, breast and ovarian adenocarcinomas, leukemias, malignant melanoma, carcinoma of the bladder and many other tumours (Wright et al., 1958; Hart et al., 1981; National Bladder Cancer Cooperation Group, 1977; Lazarus et al., 1987; Lokich et al., 1989); the limited use of TEPA has been in the treatment of Hodgkin's disease, lymphosarcoma, chronic lymphatic leukaemia, neuroblastoma and malignant melanoma (Farber et al., 1953; Sykes et al., 1953). There has recently been a resurgence of interest in thio-TEPA because of its use at high doses, made possible by autologous bone marrow transplantation.

Thio-TEPA is a directly acting alkylating agent and forms adducts with DNA. Liquid chromatography thermospray MS analysis of the supernatant after incubation of thio-TEPA with calf thymus DNA revealed the presence of 7-(2-aminoethyl)guanine and 7-(2-aminoethyl)adenine (Musser et al., 1989). Cohen et al. (1991) have recently demonstrated, using the alkaline elution technique that thio-TEPA produces interstrand cross-links in DNA, but that the lesions produced by TEPA are alkali-labile, consistent with mono-functional adducts. Reaction of thio-TEPA also occurs slowly with water, but the rate of hydrolysis is promoted by salt, increased drug concentration, or decreased pH (Pyatigorskaya et al., 1987).

12.2.1. *Analysis*

Both TEPA and thio-TEPA have been assayed by colorimetric techniques using the reaction with 4-(4′-nitrobenzyl)pyridine (Epstein et al., 1955). Titrimetric methods involving reaction with thiosulphate (Allen and Seaman, 1955; Raine, 1962) have also been employed. The fluorescence characteristics of TEPA and thio-TEPA were used by Mellett and Woods (1960b) in the development of an assay sensitive down to concentrations of 0.05 μg/mL drug in plasma or urine. Differential extraction procedures allowed the estimation of each compound separately from mixtures of TEPA and thio-TEPA. More recently methods of greater selectivity and sensitivity have been developed using GC. Grochow et al. (1982) and later Hagen et al. (1985) reported a method utilizing a nitrogen-phosphorus GC detector sensitive down to thio-TEPA concentrations of 0.5 ng/mL in cerebrospinal fluid or plasma. This method was unable to quantitate TEPA, the proposed major metabolite of thio-TEPA (see below), because of its cochromatography with the internal standard (diphenylamine) and because of its poorer extraction from the biological fluid than thio-TEPA. Variations to the method were therefore made by Egorin et al. (1985), using diphenhydramine as internal standard, allowing simultaneous detection of both drugs at limits of detection of 0.01 μg/mL thio-TEPA and 0.1 μg/mL TEPA in plasma and by McDermott et al. (1985), who achieved a slightly higher sensitivity utilizing a capillary GC column, nitrogen detection and hexaethylphosphoramide as internal standard.

Thio-TEPA and TEPA may also be quantitated by HPLC, with limits of determination 10 ng/mL and 20 ng/mL respectively (Sano et al., 1988). In this method the compounds are reacted with sodium sulphide and the products then condensed with *o*-phthalaldehyde and taurine to yield a fluorescent product. Underivatized thio-TEPA may be determined down to 25 ng/mL plasma by using a low wavelength (200 nm) UV detection (Tinsley et al., 1989).

12.2.2. *Transport*

Thio-TEPA is accumulated into L1210 cells by a two stage process (Egorin et al., 1989). The first stage is rapid and compatible with simple diffusion. The second phase is slower and it was originally postulated that this may reflect alkylation of cellular nucleophiles, or accumulation of a polar metabolite. The second phase is not observed with red blood cells, which lack nucleic acids. It was subsequently demonstrated that during the second phase of accumulation into L1210 cells there was extensive (80–85%) accumulation of phosphatidylethanolamine, indicating that thio-TEPA may undergo a decomposition pathway leading to aziridine and thence ethanolamine (Egorin and Snyder, 1990). The second slow phase of accumulation of radioactivity from [^{14}C]-thio-TEPA was reduced by the addition of unlabelled ethanolamine to the system (Egorin et al., 1990), consistent with this hypothesis.

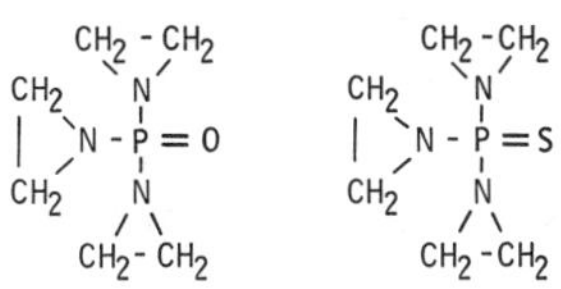

XXI XXII

12.2.3. *Metabolism and Pharmacokinetics*

Incubation of thio-TEPA with microsomes results in the formation of TEPA (Ng and Waxman, 1990; Cohen et al., 1991). This is associated with a suicidal inactivation of the P450 by reactive metabolites produced in this process (Ng and Waxman, 1990, 1991). Metabolism of thio-TEPA in rat liver S-9 homogenate enhances its cytotoxicity, which could not be accounted for by production of TEPA (Teicher et al., 1989).

Species variation has been observed in the in vivo metabolism of TEPA. In the rat over 80% of the injected (i.p.) dose of [^{32}P]-TEPA was excreted in the urine within 24 hr and the major constituent (50–70%) was unchanged drug (Craig and Jackson, 1955). Similar results were obtained in the dog with 24–34% of the administered dose (i.v.) excreted as intact drug in urine (Mellett and Woods, 1960b). In the mouse however, no unchanged TEPA was detected in urine following i.p. administration of [^{32}P]-labelled drug (Nadkarni et al., 1957). Similarly in man, although ca. 25% of the administered radioactivity was excreted in the urine, there was no detectable TEPA present (Nadkarni et al., 1959). The major urinary metabolite in mice, rats and man was inorganic phosphate, although minor proportions of an organic phosphate, thought to be an intermediate in the hydrolysis of TEPA to phosphate were found in the mouse and man (Nadkarni et al., 1957, 1959). No localization of activity was associated with any particular tissue of normal or tumour-bearing animals.

Thio-TEPA has been found to be extensively metabolized to TEPA in all species studies. In rat after administration of [^{32}P]-thio-TEPA (2 mg/kg, i.v.), urinary radioactivity was almost entirely associated with TEPA and the plasma 30 min after injection of drug contained approximately equal amounts of TEPA and thio-TEPA (Craig et al., 1959). In contrast, [^{14}C]-TEPA was excreted by the rat following 9 mg/kg i.v. injections of [^{14}C]-thio-TEPA to the extent of 20–30% leaving 70–80% of the drug unchanged (Boone et al., 1962). Ninety-five percent of the administered radioactivity was excreted within 8 hr, with some minor retention of activity in haemoglobin and the liver.

In the mouse further degradation to phosphate occurred, as observed following TEPA administration (see above). Thirty minutes after injection of [^{32}P]-thio-TEPA, mouse plasma contained TEPA and phosphate, but only traces of unchanged drug. The urine contained mostly phosphate (Craig et al., 1959). In mice bearing a series of colon tumours the tumour to plasma concentration ratio of thio-TEPA after a 20 mg/kg i.p. dose ranged from 0.87 to 1.17 (Bibby et al., 1987). The concentration range in spleen was lower (ratio 0.73–0.80).

Dog and rabbit excreted TEPA as the major metabolite of thio-TEPA (Craig et al., 1959; Mellett and Woods, 1960b; Mellett et al., 1962), although other unidentified metabolites were present. Maximal plasma levels of TEPA were seen 90–120 min after i.v. injection of thio-TEPA to dogs, with concentrations at this time up to 10 times greater than those of thio-TEPA.

Human metabolism of thio-TEPA was also extensive, with less than 1% of an oral dose ([^{14}C]-labelled) excreted intact in the urine (Mellett et al., 1962). In a patient administered 20 mg thio-TEPA i.m., a first order decrease in plasma concentration, determined by GC, was observed, with an elimination half-life of 1.2 hr (Hagen et al., 1985). Again less than 1% of the thio-TEPA was recovered in urine. More detailed studies using the GC procedure of Egorin et al. (1985), with a breast cancer patient receiving 12 mg/m^2 i.v. thio-TEPA showed $t_{1/2}\alpha$ 3.4 min and $t_{1/2}\beta$ 74 min. Substantial quantities of TEPA found in the plasma remained at a stable concentration (0.7 μg/mL) from 30 to 240 min after injection. Urinary thio-TEPA levels were extremely low, although TEPA could be detected at 1–3 μg/mL (0.3 mg/kg).

In a series of breast cancer patients receiving 12 mg/m^2 (0.3 mg/kg) i.v. thio-TEPA (in combination chemotherapy) an average $t_{1/2}\alpha$ of 7.7 $\pm$ 1.2 min and $t_{1/2}\beta$ 125 $\pm$ 21 min was observed (Cohen et al., 1986). TEPA persistence in plasma was more prolonged than thio-TEPA. Urine contained 1.5% of dose as thio-TEPA, 4.2% as TEPA and 23.5% as unidentified alkylating material. Roughly similar results were obtained by Hagen et al. (1990) following single therapy of ovarian cancer patients with i.v. thio-TEPA (less than 2% excretion of thio-TEPA and TEPA and 13% alkylating activity). The pharmacokinetics of high dose thio-TEPA (1.8–7.0 mg/kg, i.v.) also appear to be similar (Ackland et al., 1988). Serum protein binding of thio-TEPA is small (ca. 10%) (Hagen and Nilson, 1987). During repeated treatments the elimination half-life of thio-TEPA has been reported as ca. 90 min and large interindividual variation was noted in AUC (Hagen et al.,

1987). Doses of 20 and 30 mg produced no observable effects on pharmacokinetics (Hagen et al., 1988). The pharmacokinetics of i.v. thio-TEPA in children has been studied by Heideman et al. (1989). Following doses of 25–75 mg/m^2 $t_{1/2}\alpha$ was 8.4–19.2 min and $t_{1/2}\beta$ 80–120 min; clearance decreased with increasing doses. TEPA $t_{1/2}$ ranged from 4.3 to 5.6 hr. Both thio-TEPA and TEPA penetrated well into the cerebrospinal fluid.

A recent reevaluation of the pharmacokinetics of thio-TEPA was carried out with an i.v. dose range of 30–75 mg/m^2. The results were similar to those described above (thio-TEPA $t_{1/2}$ 52–212 min, TEPA $t_{1/2}$ 3.0–21.1 hr, decrease in thio-TEPA clearance with increasing dose) (O'Dwyer et al., 1991). Other routes of administration of thio-TEPA where pharmacokinetics have been studied are i.p. (Lewis et al., 1990) and intravesical (Masters et al., 1990). Following administration of thio-TEPA by ventricular reservoir, maximal plasma concentrations were seen after 1–3 hr, at levels of 0.5% of the cerebrospinal fluid concentrations of drug. The cerebrospinal fluid elimination half-life was 8 $\pm$ 5 hr suggesting that therapeutically useful concentrations of thio-TEPA could be maintained for meningeal diseases (Grochow et al., 1982).

12.2.4. *Toxicity*

Thio-TEPA causes severe toxicity to the bone marrow. Additionally it has been shown to be teratogenic in mice and rats (Tanimura, 1968; Murphy et al., 1958). The drug also causes chromosomal aberrations in cultured human lymphocytes (Hampel et al., 1966) and is carcinogenic in mice (i.p. injection) where it produces lung tumours in a dose-related fashion (Stoner et al., 1973). Carcinogenicity in rats has also been demonstrated (Schmähl and Osswald, 1970). Although several examples of acute leukaemia have been seen in patients treated with thio-TEPA (I.A.R.C., 1975a) there is no unequivocal evidence for its human carcinogenicity.

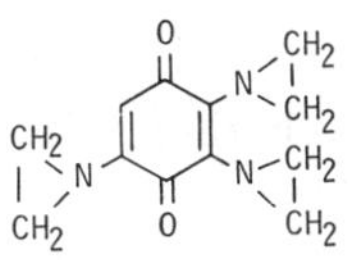

XXIII

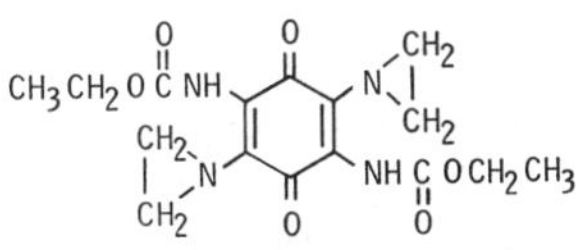

XXIV

13. AZIRIDINYL BENZOQUINONES

A variety of di- and tri-functional aziridinyl benzoquinones have been introduced to clinical practice, the most widely used being 2,3,5-tris(1-aziridinyl)-1,4-benzoquinone (triaziquone, trenimon) (XXIII) and 3,6-diaziridinyl-2,5-bis(carboethoxyamino)-1,4-benzoquinone (diaziquone, AZQ) (XXIV).

13.1. Triaziquone (Trenimon)

The synthesis of triaziquone was first reported by Gauss (1958) and the drug was initially used in the treatment of a wide selection of tumours, including leukaemias, polycythemias, carcinoma of the colon, breast and bronchus and in ovarian cancer. The drug shows typical alkylating agent toxicities, particularly towards the haematopoietic system. In view of its potency (i.e. low dose-requirement relative to that of other currently available alkylating agents) triaziquone was extensively applied in the 1960s, but its use has subsequently considerably diminished.

The aziridine rings of triaziquone are subject to hydrolysis with an increase in rate under acidic conditions, when the aziridine ring becomes protonated. Under neutral conditions (0.001 M phosphate, pH 7.5, 37°C) triaziquone is stable for 24 hr (Linford, 1973). However, Froese et al. (1969) showed, using thiosulphate as a model nucleophile, that the rate of reaction at pH 5.5 is 50 times greater than that at pH 7. The first aziridine ring to react has a half-life of 6 min, the second 16 min and the third 27 min when triaziquone (0.43 mM) is reacted with a 10-fold excess of thiosulphate at pH 5.5. At pH 8.0 no reaction occurs and at pH 7.4 only two aziridine residues are attacked with half reaction times of 150 and 280 min. Thus tumours of lower than physiological pH, owing for example to their high glycolytic rate, may be particularly susceptible to the drug.

Triaziquone also reacts by a reduction mechanism with sulphydryl compounds (e.g. cysteine, glutathione) which results in loss of the quinonoid structure and production of a more hydrophilic aromatic structure, which is itself a reactive agent (Linford, 1973). In vitro formation of a triaziquone-glutathione adduct has been demonstrated by Lusthof et al. (1990a). Binding of the drug to haemoglobin and to albumin, presumably by an analogous mechanism with protein cysteine groups, has also been observed (Linford, 1973). For haemoglobin the binding is 1 mol drug:1 mol protein indicating that only one cysteine residue is available for reaction, but with albumin extensive binding of the drug occurs.

DNA alkylation in vitro by triaziquone resulted both in the loss of purine bases (probably as a result of the formation of N-7 and N-3 purine adducts) and in the development of strand breaks (Klamerth and Kapun, 1971). At later times of reaction with triaziquone (14 mM) cross-linking of the DNA chains was observed.

The alkylation of 4-(4′-nitrobenzyl) pyridine has been the basis of quantitative estimations of triaziquone in biological fluids and tissues (Obrecht et al., 1967; Terranova, 1969).

13.1.1. *Transport*

The incorporation of triaziquone (0.87–870 nM) into Ehrlich ascites and Yoshida ascites sarcoma cells proceeded against a concentration gradient (Schmidt and Liss, 1978). This phenomenon is not thought to be due to an active transport system but rather to the intracellular reaction of the drug into a non-excretable adduct. Erythrocytes can similarly incorporate the drug effectively and again intracellular reactions are known to occur (Froese et al., 1969). With L5178Y mouse lymphoma cells approximately half of the triaziquone from a 0.17 mM solution was absorbed within 30 min at 37°C (Linford, 1973). The cysteine adduct of triaziquone was unable to enter these cells and was consequently considerably less toxic to them.

13.1.2. *Conclusion*

Although the clinical use of triaziquone has been effectively discontinued the drug has remained of considerable interest to experimentalists interested in the mechanism of DNA damage caused by alkylating agents (see review of Obe and Beck, 1979). The drug is a powerful mutagen in plants, in cell systems in vitro and in vivo and causes chromosomal damage. Its carcinogenicity has also been demonstrated in rats (Schmähl and Osswald, 1970).

13.2. AZQ (DIAZIQUONE)

In a survey of the anti-tumour effects of quinones by Driscoll et al. (1974) at the National Cancer Institute, the aziridinyl benzoquinones were notable as a compound class that showed high activity against rodent tumours, both intraperitoneal and intracerebral. One of the problems associated with administration of aziridinylquinones, however, is their aqueous insolubility. In view of this Khan and Driscoll (1976) and Chou et al. (1976) synthesized a series of aziridinyl benzoquinones with the intention of producing an agent which retained good activity against CNS tumours, but which also showed improved aqueous solubility properties. AZQ (XXIV) was shown to possess high activity against intracerebral L1210, P388 and ependymoblastoma in animals (Khan and Driscoll, 1976; Driscoll et al., 1979).

Although the solubility of AZQ is still low (0.5 mg/mL) it was considered sufficient for the compound's administration to humans and it was therefore introduced to the clinic, mainly for treatment of CNS tumours (Griffen et al., 1982; Curt et al., 1982; Aroney et al., 1982). The drug partitions well across the blood–brain barrier in monkeys (Gormley et al., 1981) and in man (Schilsky et al., 1982). The CSF:plasma concentrations of the drug in 3 patients ranged from 0.21 to 1.4. Many more tumour types have more recently been subjected to AZQ clinical trials, e.g. head and neck cancer, multiple myeloma, pancreatic cancer, acute myeloid and non lymphocytic leukaemia, ovarian cancer and soft tissue and bone sarcoma.

The mechanism of action of AZQ presumably involves alkylation as the aziridine rings in compounds of this type are known to cross-link DNA bases (Akhtar et al., 1975). Using the alkaline elution technique King et al. (1984a) showed that AZQ produced single strand breaks, DNA–DNA cross-links and DNA–protein cross-links in Chinese hamster ovary cells. The cross-linking effect of AZQ was also demonstrated in vitro with calf thymus DNA and was shown to be dependent upon the presence of a reducing agent, e.g. $NaBH_4$ (King et al., 1984b). Gutierrez et al. (1987) postulated that the antitumour activity of $NaBH_4$-reduced AZQ is largely associated with oxidation of 2-electron-reduced AZQ ($AZQH_2$). Reductive activation of AZQ and other 2,5-bis(1-aziridinyl)-1,4-benzoquinones, may also be achieved electrochemically (Lusthof et al., 1989). Reduction facilitates protonation of the aziridine ring and its subsequent ring opening and alkylation reactions. Alkylation and cross-link formation is thus increased at acidic pH values. Two electron reduction of quinones may be achieved with DT-diaphorase and this enzyme has been shown by Siegel et al. (1990b) to be effective in bioactivating AZQ to genotoxic and cytotoxic metabolites.

In addition to the alkylating activity shown by reduced AZQ there is also the potential for oxygen radical production from the quinone function. One electron reduction of quinones as in AZQ may occur with NADPH-cytochrome C reductase (Gutierrez et al., 1982) or xanthine oxidase (Lusthof et al., 1990b) leading to semiquinone radicals and redox cycling. The production of a semiquinone free radical was also observed when AZQ was incubated with rat liver preparations (Gutierrez et al., 1982) and structure–activity relationships were established for a series of AZQ analogues for their ability to redox cycle with rat liver microsomes (Prins et al., 1989). AZQ semiquinone and hydroxyl radicals are also produced upon irradiation of AZQ with 500 nm visible light (Mossoba and Gutierrez, 1985) and it has been shown to photosensitize L1210 cells (Kessel and Thompson, 1986). The mechanism of reduction of AZQ to such radicals has been well studied using electrochemical and spectroscopic methods (Mossoba et al., 1985; Butler et al., 1987). The correlation between free radical formation and biological activity of bisaziridinylquinones is not clear; thus for cell killing of P388 cells (Nguyen et al., 1988), L1210, K562 cells (Lea et al., 1988) or inactivation of phage DNA (de Mol et al., 1988) toxicity was not solely reflected by free radical production.

Other biochemical effects that have been observed with AZQ include the inhibition of DNA synthesis in cultured cells (Akhtar et al., 1975), the destruction of mitochondria in human glioma cell lines (Oberc-Greenwood et al., 1983) and oxidation of glutathione in isolated hepatocytes (Silva and O'Brien, 1989).

The metabolism and distribution of [^{14}C]-AZQ has been investigated in mice by Spiegel et al. (1982). Within 30 min of an i.v. injection less than half of the radioactivity in the plasma was AZQ. Only 0.2% of AZQ remained in the plasma after 3 hr. [^{14}C] was extensively retained by tissues and again the material present was not AZQ and was unidentified. In the monkey Gormley et al. (1981) similarly found unidentified compounds other than AZQ.

The drug may be monitored by HPLC, using UV absorption at 340 nm for detection and 2,5-diamino-3,6-dichloro-1,4-benzoquinone as internal standard (Schilsky et al., 1982). In treated patients (1–20 mg/m^2 AZQ), plasma decay curves fitted a 2-compartment model, with $t_{1/2}\alpha$ 2.8 $\pm$ 1.3 min and $t_{1/2}\beta$ 33.3 $\pm$ 4.5 min. In the pharmacological study of Lu et al. (1983) patients were administered 1–12 mg/m^2 AZQ daily for 5 days. The plasma disappearance of the drug showed a later phase, with a half-life of 45.5 $\pm$ 3.1 hr. An analogous HPLC method of Kelley and Chong (1981) was used by Tan et al. (1982) to study the pharmacokinetics of AZQ (20–25 mg/m^2) in children; the 2-compartment half lives obtained being 2.6 min and 20.3 min. The amount of intact AZQ excreted in urine was low, reported to be 0–0.2% of the dose administered in 2 hr (Schilsky et al., 1982) or 8.6 $\pm$ 1.4% of the dose in 96 hr (Lu et al., 1983). Following continuous i.v. infusions (10–20 mg) plasma concentrations as high as 1 μg/mL may be achieved with elimination $t_{1/2}$ 37.2 $\pm$ 13.9 min (Bjornsson et al., 1985). The toxicity caused by AZQ is mainly myelosuppression; nausea and vomiting are also occasionally observed. The genotoxic potential of AZQ is illustrated by its ability to induce sister chromatid exchanges in treated patients (Kligerman et al., 1987).

Because of the rather limited water solubility of AZQ, Chou et al. (1976) synthesized BZQ (3,6-diaziridinyl-2,5-bis(hydroxyethylamino)-1,4-benzoquinone, which has similar antitumour activity but is considerably more soluble (2 mg/mL).

Like AZQ, BZQ may undergo one electron reduction, although its reduction potential is -376 mV as opposed to -70 mV for AZQ (Butler et al., 1987). No correlation has been observed between free radical production and cytotoxicity to leukaemic cell lines (Lea et al., 1988). It was concluded by Butler et al. (1989) that the mechanism of action of BZQ is likely to be bifunctional alkylation and that its oxidation or reduction are of lesser importance.

BZQ may be determined by HPLC with a sensitivity of 3 ng/mL, using a reverse phase column and UV detection (Betteridge et al., 1988). Protein binding of BZQ is negligible. After i.v. dosing of 18–60 mg BZQ, the drug was eliminated with $t_{1/2}\alpha$ 6.2 ± 1.5 min and $t_{1/2}\beta$ 24 ± 4 min (Betteridge et al., 1990).

14. HEXITOL DERIVATIVES

Of the many cytostatic hexitol derivatives that have been synthesized, two examples, dibromodulcitol and dianhydrogalactitol, have received extensive clinical testing.

Dibromodulcitol (1,6-dibromo-1,6-dideoxygalactitol, mitolactol) (XXV) has been used against a variety of malignancies, including leukemias, breast cancer and squamous cell carcinomas (Eckhardt et al., 1963; Sellei et al., 1969; Andrews et al., 1971, 1974; Mischler et al., 1979; Chiuten et al., 1981). The bromine atoms in the dibromodulcitol molecule may be displaced in vivo by typical alkylating agent type reactions with nucleophiles (including water), but it is also possible for intramolecular displacement of these atoms by the sugar hydroxyl groups to occur. The initial studies (Institoris et al., 1973) suggested the formation of dianhydrogalactitol (XXVI) with a yield of 47% in pH 7 solution at 35°C. In aqueous solution at 100°C the main product from dibromodulcitol is the 5-membered anhydro-derivative 3,6-anhydro-1-bromo-1-deoxygalactitol (Vidra et al., 1982), whereas at physiological pH or in other mildly alkaline solutions the production of the mono-epoxide 1,2-anhydro-6-bromo-6-deoxygalactitol (XXVII) (Horvath et al., 1979) and the diepoxides 1,2-5,6-dianhydrogalactitol (XXVI) (Elson et al., 1968) and 1,2-3,6-dianhydrogalactitol (XXVIII) (Vidra et al., 1982) have been detected. The tumour inhibitory effect of (XXVII) and (XXVI) is apparent at 20- to 30-fold lower doses than that from dibromodulcitol; however the therapeutic indices (LD_{10}/ID_{50}) are not significantly different (Horvath et al., 1982b).

The hypothesis that dibromodulcitol is acting in vivo via its conversion to these two active epoxides (XXVII) and (XXVI) has been supported by their identification in the plasma of patients treated with the drug (Horvath et al., 1979). Other degradation products isolated were dulcitol and 1,2-anhydrodulcitol. In the urine Belej et al. (1972) found mono-bromodulcitol,1,2-anhydrodulcitol and dulcitol; the epoxides 1,2-anhydro-6-bromo-6-deoxygalactitol and 1,2-5,6-dianhydrogalactitol were later identified in urine by Horvath et al. (1979).

Recent data has indicated that the anti-tumour effect of dibromodulcitol may also be in part due to alkylation by the parent drug. Pretreatment of rats or mice with phenobarbital lowers the toxicity of dibromodulcitol and also decreases its anti-tumour effectiveness (Gati and Somfai-Relle, 1982), suggesting that metabolism by P450 may play a part in the deactivation of the drug. Rat liver 9000-g supernatant actually protects against the decomposition of dibromodulcitol by delaying it for a period of 30 min at 37°C. After this time there is a rapid formation of inactive degradation products such as 3,6-anhydro-1-bromo-1-deoxygalactitol. Neither of the active epoxide metabolites (XXVI) and (XXVII) were found in this system (Csetenyi et al., 1985).

Oral administration of [^{14}C]-dibromodulcitol to patients results in almost complete absorption of the drug, with a plasma $t_{1/2}$ for loss of radioactivity of ca. 8 hr (Belej et al., 1972). Horvath et al. (1982a), using oral dosing of dibromodulcitol labelled with [^{3}H] at C-1 showed an absorption rate constant of 1.7 ± 0.7 hr ($t_{1/2}$ 25 min), with no radioactivity being found in the faeces. The plasma $t_{1/2}$ for the first phase of elimination of [^{3}H] was 4.6 hr but the elimination of active alkylating drug had $t_{1/2}$ 2.2 hr. Total urinary excretion of radioactivity amounted to 47–84% of the dose with 17 ± 3% being effective drug.

In mice treated with 20 or 100 mg/kg i.p. dibromodulcitol no (< 4%) reversible protein binding was observed and the drug was eliminated with a first order elimination constant of 0.92×10^{-2} min (Henner et al., 1985). In this study unlabelled drug was used and plasma concentrations were quantitated (in conjunction with other active bifunctional metabolites) by HPLC, after their reaction with sodium diethyldithiocarbamate. The same procedure was used by Kelley et al. (1986) to monitor dibromodulcitol in a Phase I study. The observed elimination $t_{1/2}$ was 158 ± 106 min and no dose dependent alterations in pharmacokinetic parameters were observed.

Distribution studies in animals have shown a high incorporation of dibromodulcitol into the central nervous system (Institoris et al., 1973). In man dibromodulcitol also crosses the blood–brain barrier and the metabolic degradation and removal of drug from the cerebrospinal fluid is slower than that in the plasma (Horvath et al., 1982a) with a $t_{1/2}$ that may be as long as 24 hr (Csetenyi et al., 1983). About 30% of the drug-derived material in the cerebrospinal fluid is present as active alkylating agents 6 hr after administration of the drug to patients (Horvath et al., 1982a; Belej et al., 1972).

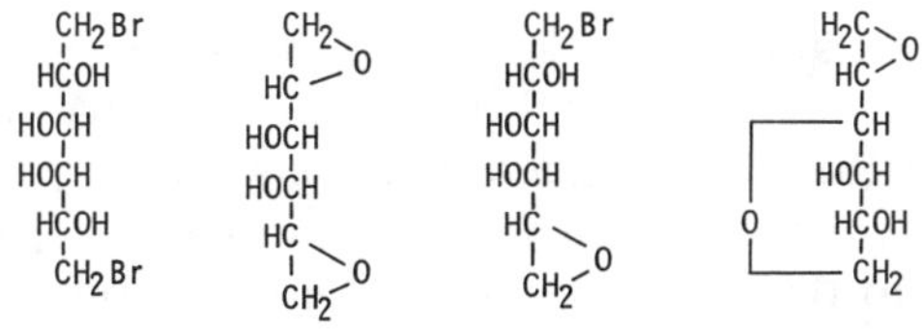

XXV XXVI XXVII XXVIII

Neutron activation analysis was used by Sziklai et al. (1990) to monitor bromine content in brain samples of patients receiving 400–500 mg/m^2 p.o. dibromodulcitol. The incorporation of bromine into tumour and white matter was different than after a control of sodium bromide, suggesting that covalent bonding had occurred with dibromodulcitol.

In both mice and dogs dibromodulcitol has high activity against brain tumours (Geran et al., 1974; Merker et al., 1975) and the clinical use of the compound has therefore included central nervous system tumours. It has been suggested that dibromodulcitol might be preferable to 1,2-5,6-dianhydrogalactitol (see below) for treatment of such tumours in view of its greater hydrophobicity and of its slow release of active metabolites which might allow a more prolonged level of high alkylating activity in the brain (Csetenyi et al., 1983).

1,2-5,6-Dianhydrogalactitol (XXVI) is a hexitol diepoxide, which has undergone Phase I, II and III trials and was considered of potential use for treatment of central nervous system tumours. In mice it was the most active drug against the intracerebral ependymoblastoma (Geran et al., 1974) and it has been shown in combination therapy to be active against other intracerebral tumours (Levin and Wheeler, 1982). It is a bifunctional alkylating agent whose reaction with DNA in vitro yields two main products: 7-(1-deoxygalactit-1-yl)guanine and the cross-linked 1,6-di(guanin-7-yl)1,6-dideoxygalactitol, which were identified by UV and MS by Institoris and Tamas (1980). A third product which was extensively formed when dianhydrogalactitol was reacted with guanosine but not abundant in the DNA reaction was 7-(1-deoxyanhydrogalactit-1-yl)guanine. The formation of this material may partly be caused by the conditions used for the hydrolysis of the nucleoside during its isolation.

Alkylation in vivo of DNA of Yoshida sarcoma cells by [^{3}H]-dianhydrogalactitol in rats yielded the same three alkyl-guanines after hydrolysis of the nucleic acid (Institoris, 1981). Interestingly the alkylated products seem rather stable as the extent of labelling of the DNA did not decrease over the first 24 hr (which is normally a characteristic phenomenon for DNA containing N-7-guanyl derivatives).

Cross-linking of DNA by dianhydrogalactitol has also been detected by measurements of hyperchromicity of renatured DNA (chicken blood) after alkaline denaturation (Ötvös and Elekes, 1975) and in Yoshida sarcoma cells by alkaline sucrose gradient sedimentation centrifugation and DNA-renaturation studies (Institoris and Fox, 1978). No evidence was obtained for protein–DNA cross links in the Yoshida cells.

In mice and rats Institoris et al. (1973) showed that the accumulation of radioactivity within tissues after dosing with [^{3}H]-dianhydrogalactitol was considerably greater than with dibromodulcitol (see above). Transport of radioactivity into the brain was also observed although in this case the difference between dianhydrogalactitol and dibromodulcitol was not marked. The entry of the drug into the brain of rats was confirmed by Levin et al. (1976) using [^{14}C]-dianhydrogalactitol; transport into an intracerebral gliosarcoma was even more rapid. A large nucleic acid bound pool of [^{14}C] was observed, with RNA-binding about 6 times greater than DNA-binding.

In man tritiated dianhydrogalactitol was used for some early pharmacokinetic studies by Eckhardt et al. (1977), which showed a $t_{1/2}\beta$ of 2.05 hr for loss of plasma radioactivity. More detailed studies of the pharmacokinetics of dianhydrogalactitol became possible with the development of chromatographic methods for the drug's estimation. Kimura et al. (1976) converted dianhydrogalactitol, after its extraction from the biological fluid, into its *n*-butane boronate ester, which could be estimated by GC with a sensitivity of 100 ng/mL. Munger et al. (1977) developed an HPLC assay following derivatization of dianhydrogalactitol with diethyl dithiocarbamate, which converts it into a highly UV-absorbing product which can readily be extracted from the biological fluid. The detection limit of this assay is 50 ng/mL in plasma. Using this method Munger et al. (1978) found $t_{1/2}\beta$ of dianhydrogalactitol in rat plasma to be 43.7 min. Eagan et al. (1982) using a slight modification of the method studied patients receiving two infusions of dianhydrogalactitol at 50–80 mg/m^2. The drug was rapidly removed from the plasma with $t_{1/2}\alpha$ 3.9 min and $t_{1/2}\beta$ 31.3 min. It was suggested that the method of administration of dianhydrogalactitol should give greater and more prolonged plasma concentrations (which were only 1.9–5.6 μg/mL in these patients). In the only patient studied, 4.4% of the drug was excreted intact. The pharmacokinetics of dianhydrogalactitol in the CSF were studied by Eckhardt et al. (1977) who reported a half-life of 20 hr.

Using ^{3}H-labelled dianhydrogalactitol Horvath et al. (1986) later completed a detailed study of the distribution and degradation of the drug after i.v. and oral doses to patients. The drug readily entered the cerebrospinal fluid from which it was removed at a slower rate than from plasma. Metabolites in plasma and urine were largely unidentified although galactitol and minor quantities of chloroepoxygalactitol and dichlorogalactitol were shown to be present. The mean residence time of dianhydrogalactitol in the body was 1.9 ± 1.1 hr, some 6 times shorter than that for dibromodulcitol. It was proposed that the faster clearance of the former drug was due to its metabolic processes.

15. MITOMYCIN C

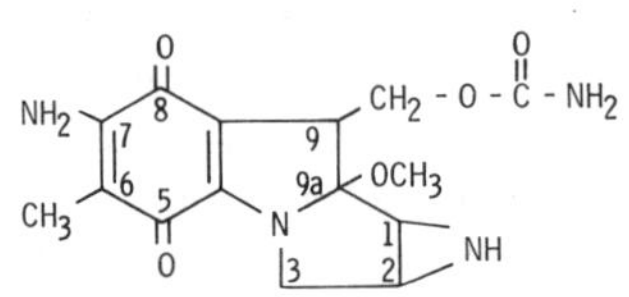

XXIX

Mitomycin C (XXIX) is one of a group of antibiotics isolated from the fungus *Streptomyces caespitosus* (Hata et al., 1956; Wakaki et al., 1958). The structure of mitomycin was elucidated by Webb et al. (1962) and contains two reactive side chains (an aziridine and a carbamate) coupled to a three-ring quinonoid structure. It has a broad spectrum of anti-tumour activity, being used against for example carcinomas of the gastrointestinal tract, breast, bladder, pancreas, lung, liver and head and neck. The role of mitomycin C in the treatment of solid tumours has been reviewed by Sartorelli (1986).

Cross-linking of DNA by mitomycin C was first observed by Iyer and Szybalski (1963) in *Bacillus subtilis* and *Escherichia coli* cells. However no effect was seen on purified DNA in vitro unless a cell lysate was added. The activating process was shown to involve reduction of the quinone function as DNA cross-linking was also observed when chemical reducing agents (e.g. sodium hydrosulphite or sodium borohydride) were added to mixtures of mitomycin C and DNA (Iyer and Szybalski, 1964). These authors postulated that the quinone reduction promoted loss of the methoxy group at position 9 and activated both the aziridine and the carbamate functions towards nucleophilic attack. Release of methanol during the reduction of mitomycin C was shown to be essentially quantitative. It was also suggested that the carbon 7 position might be activated in this process, although the displacement of an amino group in a DNA cross-linking reaction seems chemically unlikely. An analogous conclusion was reached simultaneously by Schwartz (Schwartz, 1962; Schwartz et al., 1963) who showed that mitomycin C was rapidly metabolized under anaerobic conditions with rat liver homogenates, but was unexpectedly stable under

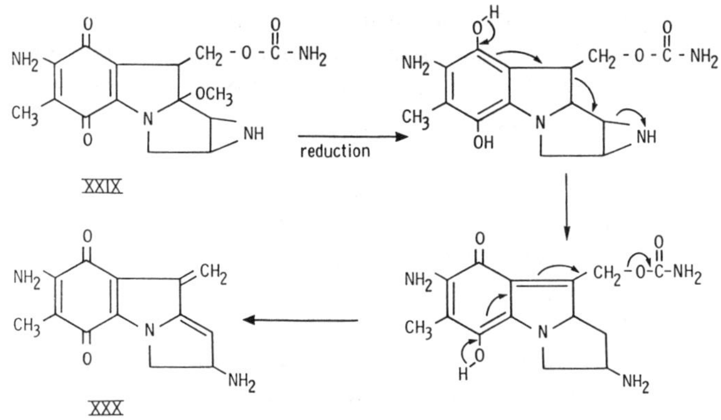

FIG. 5. Proposed activating mechanism of mitomycin C.

aerobic conditions with homogenates and with nucleophilic chemicals (4-(4′-nitrobenzyl)-pyridine, thiosulphate).

Reduction of mitomycin C to the hydroquinone was the basis of the mechanism of action suggested by Moore (1977) (Fig. 5) in which the species (XXX) was proposed as the active bifunctional metabolite. The formation of this quinone methide intermediate would involve firstly the aziridine ring opening (promoted by the hydroquinone structure) followed by loss of the carbamate function.

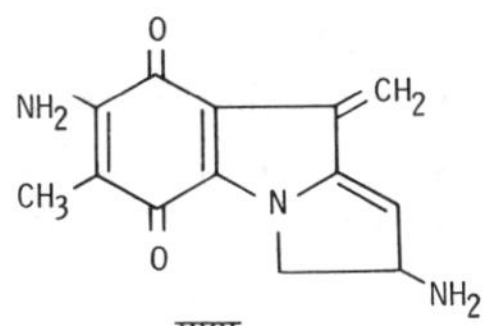

XXX

A modification of this mechanism of activation was suggested by Tomasz et al. (1974) on the basis of in vitro experiments which suggested that a partially reduced mitomycin C (semiquinone radical) was highly active at binding to DNA. Such an intermediate species had previously been detected for mitomycin C analogues by electron spin resonance (ESR) by Patrick et al. (1964) and was later demonstrated for microsomally reduced mitomycin C by Kalyanaraman et al. (1980). Tomasz et al. (1974) also confirmed that the aziridine group was an essential component in the cross-linking process as analogues which did not contain this group, although biologically active, could alkylate DNA only monofunctionally.

Further evidence for the involvement of radicals was the observation that both superoxide (Handa and Sato, 1975; Kalyanaraman et al., 1980) and hydroxyl radicals (Hamana et al., 1985) were generated when mitomycin C was reduced by NADPH-rat liver microsomes or NADPH-cytochrome P450 reductase. The consequent production of H_2O_2 has been observed with both chemically and microsomally reduced mitomycin C and took place even with mitomycin that was bound to DNA (Tomasz, 1976). Hydroxyl and superoxide radicals may be detected by HPLC if they are trapped with 5,5-dimethyl-1-pyrroline *N*-oxide (Pritsos et al., 1985). This technique was used to demonstrate the production of these radicals by mitomycin C activated by NADPH cytochrome C reductase (Pritsos et al., 1985), tumour cell sonicates, xanthine oxidase and mitochondria (Pritsos and Sartorelli, 1986). Spin trapping has been used to demonstrate hydroxyl and superoxide formation in rat cardiac microsomes and isolated perfused rat hearts treated with mitomycin C (Politi et al., 1989).

Investigations using liver subcellular fractions later showed that the reductive activation of mitomycin C occurs both with microsomes and with nuclei (Kennedy and Sartorelli, 1979). In reconstituted enzyme systems the presence of NADPH, NADPH-cytochrome P-450 reductase, phospholipid and cytochrome P-450 were required to metabolize mitomycin C to a reactive intermediate under hypoxic conditions (Kennedy et al., 1982). In the sarcoma 180 or EMT6 mouse mammary tumour cell lines the bioactivation of mitomycin C similarly required hypoxic conditions and pyridine nucleotide reducing equivalents (Kennedy et al., 1980). This dependence on hypoxia has been confirmed in a variety of other cell lines, including Chinese hamster ovary, Chinese hamster V-79 and human HeLa (Rauth et al., 1983).

Purified NADPH-cytochrome P-450 reductase is effective in the reduction of mitomycin C, although less effective than complete microsomal systems (Vromans et al., 1990). Resistance to mitomycin in a Chinese hamster ovary cell line has been associated with a reduced activity of NADPH-cytochrome P-450 reductase (Hoban et al., 1990) and bacteria in which the rat liver reductase is expressed show increased sensitivity to mitomycin C under aerobic (but not hypoxic) conditions (Bligh et al., 1990).

Data consistent with the postulate that the reductive activation of mitomycin C by the nuclei of EMT6 tumour cells is by a one electron reduction pathway came from the studies of Kennedy et al. (1985b), who showed that the process was inhibited by radical trappers (glutathione, *N*-acetylcysteine), but not by ethyl xanthate, which would have interacted with the 2-electron reduction product of mitomycin. Liver cell nuclei, however, could activate mitomycin by either pathway. The possible involvement of the 2-electron quinone-reducing enzyme, DT-diaphorase, which is present in EMT6 cells was initially excluded on the basis of experiments with enzyme inhibitors (Keyes et al., 1984) and it appeared that NADPH cytochrome C reductase is one enzyme responsible for mitomycin C activation (Sartorelli, 1986).

The role of DT-diaphorase in activation of mitomycin has been extensively studied, with varying conclusions on its significance. Dicoumarol, an inhibitor of DT-diaphorase, increases the cytotoxicity of mitomycin to hypoxic cells, but decreases it to aerobic cells (Keyes et al., 1984, 1985; Rockwell et al., 1988). In vivo the antineoplastic effect of mitomycin to EMT6 tumours is enhanced by dicoumarol (Rockwell et al., 1989). Mitomycin C was shown to be a weak inhibitor of human kidney DT-diaphorase, though not a substrate (Schlager and Powis, 1988). However Siegel et al. (1990a) have demonstrated that it *is* possible to metabolize mitomycin C using purified DT-diaphorase from rat liver and human colon cells, if the pH is lowered to 5.8. The metabolism is NADH dependent, inhibited by dicoumarol and yields 2,7-diaminomitosene. It therefore seems likely that DT-diaphorase plays a significant role in mitomycin C bioactivation. A relationship has been suggested recently between DT-diaphorase levels and mitomycin resistance in human cell lines (Marshall et al., 1991).

Chemical studies of the nature of the reduced metabolites are hindered by their instability (Patrick et al., 1964; Hornemann et al., 1976). Tomasz and Lipmann (1981) however suceeded in isolating and identifying 5 major metabolites isolated after microsomal reductive metabolism and aerial oxidation of the product. These compounds (previously characterized as products of acid treatment of mitomycin (Tomasz and Lipman, 1979)) were 2,7-diaminomitosene derivatives indicating that the aziridine ring had been activated and ring opened. Potassium ethyl xanthate was used by Hornemann et al. (1979) to trap diaminomitosenes produced by the chemical reduction of mitomycin. Interestingly the second postulated active centre (the C_{10} carbamate) was inert in this system.

HPLC was used by Pan et al. (1984) to examine the formation of such diaminomitosene derivatives following the reduction of mitomycin C by NADPH-cytochrome P-450 reductase or xanthine oxidase. The proportion of derivatives was pH dependent with 2,7-diaminomitosene being essentially the only metabolite formed when the pH was dropped to 6.5. Electron paramagnetic resonance studies showed that both these enzyme systems produced a radical anion from mitomycin C. The authors postulated that this initially formed metabolite was responsible for the formation of monofunctional alkylation adducts, but that further radical activation was necessary to produce the active bifunctional species. Further investigations of the intermediates in one electron reduction of mitomycin have been carried out using pulse radiolytic techniques (Hoey et al., 1988).

An alternative activating mechanism was noted by Lown et al. (1976), who observed that *unreduced* mitomycin C could cross-link DNA in vitro if the pH was lowered to 4. As indicated above, Tomasz and Lipman (1979) showed that acid treatment resulted in products in which the aziridine ring had been cleaved, with the yield of derivatives being dependent on a group of pK_a 4.0 (i.e. most likely aziridine). Kinetic studies by Underberg and Lingeman (1983) suggested that the first stage in the degradation of mitomycin C in acidic solution was protonation and loss of the 9-methoxyl group to yield a 9-carbenium ion. Subsequent protonation of the aziridine destabilizes this ion resulting in the formation of a double bond and hydrolysis of the aziridine ring.

It is possible therefore that mitomycin C could be activated in vivo in the vicinity of aerobic cells if the pH was low. The toxicity of mitomycin C towards EMT6 cells under aerobic conditions was increased as the pH was reduced from 7.5 to 5.7. Furthermore as the extracellular pH was lowered, alkaline elution profiles revealed that more interstrand DNA cross-links were being formed (Kennedy et al., 1985a).

15.1. DNA Interaction

Following the original observation of Iyer and Szybalski (1963, 1964) that reduced mitomycin C can cross-link DNA, Weissbach and Lisio (1965) synthesized [^{3}H]-labelled drug by exchange labelling with tritium and quantitated the extent of DNA binding. After reduction by sodium hydrosulphite the extent of in vitro reaction of mitomycin C with nucleic acids was up to 1 adduct per 500 nucleotide residues with the alkylations suggested to be mostly monofunctional. DNA modified by mitomycin was less well utilized as a primer by DNA polymerase than control DNA and is also less susceptible to exonuclease action (Pricer and Weissbach, 1965).

Alkylation of nucleic acids by mitomycin is highly guanine-specific (Lipman et al., 1978). Initially this specificity was suggested by difference spectrophotometry (Kodama, 1967) or by in vitro reactions with polynucleotides (Lipsett and Weissbach, 1965; Tomasz et al., 1974). Thus poly(dG) bound mitomycin well whereas little binding was observed with poly(dA), poly(dT) or poly(dC). The preference for guanine adduct formation was confirmed by Tomasz et al. (1983) who suggested initially using data from NMR, Fourier transform infra red and circular dichroism spectra, that the major adduct formed between reduced mitomycin C and d(GpC) was an O^6-(2′-deoxyguanosyl) derivative, linked to the 1-position of the mitomycin structure. This structure was later revised by Tomasz et al. (1986b) to be the N^2-(2′-deoxyguanosyl) derivative. Following reaction of reductively activated mitomycin C with calf thymus DNA, 90% of the adducts were accounted for by the same alkylated N^2-guanine (Tomasz et al., 1986a). These results are in contrast with those of Hashimoto et al. (1983) and Hashimoto and Shudo (1985) who separated by HPLC three major products of the reaction of mitomycin with DNA, after catalytic reduction with H_2 and showed them by NMR, UV and chemical degradation to be 2,7-diaminomitosene adducts to the N^2 of guanine, O^6 of guanine and N^6 of adenine. The same adducts were found in DNA alkylated in vivo (rat) by mitomycin C. The major adduct following interaction of DNA with mitomycin C after its reductive activation by NADPH cytochrome P-450 reductase or xanthine oxidase was proposed by Pan et al. (1986) to be O^6-(2′-deoxyguanosyl)-2,7-diaminomitosene.

Under acidic conditions the interaction products of mitomycin C with d(GpC) or DNA differ from those formed after its reductive activation, being predominantly N-7 guanine adducts (Tomasz et al., 1987b).

DNA adducts of mitomycin C in vivo have not been well characterized. The potential of ^{32}P-postlabelling for detecting mitomycin-induced DNA damage in rats was demonstrated by Reddy and Randerath (1987) and adducts were subsequently detected in treated cancer patients (Kato et al., 1988). The cytotoxicity of mitomycin C to human embryonic cells deficient in the DNA repair enzyme O^6-alkylguanine transferase were greater than that to cells containing the enzyme, suggesting that O^6 alkylation of guanine may be of significance to the cytotoxic process (Dusre et al., 1989).

The cross-links in DNA formed by mitomycin are much more stable than those produced by nor-nitrogen mustard, either to heat or to alkaline conditions (Tomasz et al., 1974), which suggests that they do not involve N-7 guanine alkylation. A similar conclusion was reached by Tomasz (1970) by the use of an alkylation assay using 8-[^{3}H]-guanine. The number of cross-links increased with increasing content of G + C in the DNA (Iyer and Szybalski, 1964; Lown et al., 1976). Single strand cleavage of DNA as well as cross-linking and monoalkylation has also been observed (Lown et al., 1976), this being postulated to be associated with production of a hydroxyl radical from mitomycin C (Hamana et al., 1985).

A cross-linked adduct has been isolated following the reaction of reductively activated mitomycin C with *Micrococcus luteus* DNA (Tomasz et al., 1987a). Two exocyclic 2-amino groups of guanines were cross-linked, the linkage points being the 1 and 10 positions of mitomycin. The same bifunctional adduct was later isolated from digests of oligodeoxyribonucleotides reacted with reductively activated mitomycin and its properties examined in detail (Borowy-Borowski et al., 1990a). (The alkylating ability of the C-10 position, though not readily detectable for monofunctional alkylations with mitomycin C, can be demonstrated with 2,7-diaminomitosene, which upon reduction yields C-10 adducts with 2′-deoxyguanosine (Iyengar et al., 1990).) The mechanism of DNA cross-link formation by mitomycin C is thus believed to involve two activation processes, first at C-1 and then at C-10 (Tomasz et al., 1988). The factors involved in the sequence specificity of mitomycin cross-linking have been extensively investigated (Teng et al., 1989; Cera and Crothers, 1989; Borowy-Borowski et al., 1990b). The favoured sequence for cross-linking appears to be CpG.

Other effects of mitomycin C associated with DNA include inhibition of DNA synthesis (Shiba et al., 1959; Claassen et al., 1986), changes in reversible denaturation of DNA (Matsumoto and Lark, 1963; Iyer and Szybalski, 1964), altered circular dichroism spectra (Mercado and Tomasz, 1977) and increased helix-coil melting temperature (Cohen and Crothers, 1970). Flow dichroism measurements indicate that mitomycin C is not an intercalator but rather binds to one of the DNA grooves (Kaplan and Tomasz, 1982).

15.2. Analysis

Mitomycin C determination in biological fluids is generally carried out by HPLC using UV or ECD. Kono et al. (1979) first reported on the analysis of mitomycin at concentrations down to 40 ng/mL, using a reverse phase separation of an acidic extract of serum, urine or ascites. As indicated above, mitomycin C is unstable in acidic solution and consequently methods involving milder extraction procedures are preferred. For example a neutral extraction procedure was adopted by den Hartigh et al. (1981), Porapak Q extraction by van Hazel and Kovach (1982), Amberlite XAD-2 chromatography by Tjaden et al. (1982) and a reverse phase Sep Pak column by Eksberg et al. (1983). Sensitivities of detection have now been increased and include 0.5–1 ng/mL plasma using reverse phase HPLC and UV detection (den Hartigh et al., 1981, 1983; Tjaden et al., 1987; Dalton et al., 1989) and 50 ng/mL urine using UV or ECD (Tjaden et al., 1982).

The time-consuming extraction steps may be removed from HPLC procedures for mitomycin analysis by the use of on-line extraction using an injector loop packed with Porapak Q (Choi et al., 1985) or Spherisorb octadecylsilica (Czejka et al., 1989). Phase-system switching has been used as a means to introduce mitomycin C into supercritical fluid chromatography columns, which have been used to analyze the drug down to a concentration of 5 ng/mL plasma (Niessen et al., 1988).

Other analytical methods that have been applied to mitomycin C generally have considerably less specificity (e.g. UV detection and bacterial growth inhibition (Schwartz and Philips, 1961)). The results obtained by the *E. coli* cup–plate bioassay, however, correlated well with HPLC determinations of mitomycin concentration in plasma and urine from dogs (Barbhaiya et al., 1984). Serum concentrations of mitomycin C have also been determined by enzyme-linked immunoassay with a limit of detection of 4 ng/mL (Fujiwara et al., 1982).

A mutant Chinese hamster ovary cell line, which is extremely sensitive to mitomycin C has been used to detect the drug in patient plasma at concentrations as low as 1 ng/mL (Marshall et al., 1985).

15.3. Pharmacokinetics and Distribution

The first pharmacokinetic studies on mitomycin were carried out on intravenously injected rats and dogs (Schwartz and Philips, 1961). Although the analytical methods of the time were not sensitive enough to make a detailed analysis it was shown that the drug was lost rapidly from the plasma and that up to one third of the dose was excreted in the urine. Fujita (1971) reported on the rapid loss of human blood concentrations of mitomycin C and later calculations by Reich (1979) suggested elimination half-lives of 30–49 min.

Following development of HPLC methods of determination, detailed investigations of human mitomycin C pharmacokinetics have been carried out (see Verweij et al., 1987a). For example, after an i.v. injection of 10–20 mg/m^2 mitomycin (as a single agent) a 2-compartment model was observed with $t_{1/2}\alpha$ 5.2 min and $t_{1/2}\beta$ 50 min (den Hartigh et al., 1983). Similar values were seen after intra-arterial (i.a.) injection and also by van Hazel and Kovach (1982) on 2 patients receiving rapid i.v. doses of 15 mg/m^2 of mitomycin C ($t_{1/2}\alpha$ 10.3, 13.2 min, $t_{1/2}\beta$ 44.3, 62.0 min) and by Sarna et al. (1982) on high dose mitomycin patients. The use of the drug in combination chemotherapy at 5–10 mg/m^2 reduced these values to 4.6 and 42 min, respectively (den Hartigh et al., 1983). No evidence was found for dose-dependent pharmacokinetics although large inter-individual variations were observed between patients. Urinary excretion of mitomycin C was detectable up to 8 hr after drug injection and varied from 2 to 15% of the dose administered. (Similar observations were made by Tjaden et al. (1982) on a patient receiving 20 mg i.v. who excreted ca. 5% of the dose in 8 hr and by Eksborg et al. (1983) on a patient receiving 0.15 mg/kg who excreted ca. 12% of the dose.) Mitomycin was also detected by den Hartigh et al. (1983) in the bile (possibly with entero-hepatic recycling) and in the ascites. Hu and Howell (1983), in a comparison of i.a. and i.v. infusions, noted steady state plasma levels of the drug within 2 hr consistent with the previously reported elimination rate constants; only limited advantages were seen for the i.a. route.

15.4. Toxicity and Resistance

Mitomycin C shows potent effects on the bone marrow in both animals (Philips et al., 1960) and in man (Reynolds, 1982). The myelosuppressive effects of mitomycin in mice are not altered by administration of the alkylating agent 'trap' diethyldithiocarbamate (Schmalbach and Borch, 1989). Immediate nausea and vomiting and kidney (Verwey et al., 1987) and pulmonary damage (Verweij et al., 1987b) can also be significant. A factor involved in the production of haemolytic uraemic syndrome by mitomycin C may be the inhibition of prostacyclin synthesis by the drug (Duperray et al., 1988). The gastrointestinal damage caused by mitomycin C may be associated with increased permeability to Na^+ and reduced transport of D-glucose and L-alanine across brush-border membrane vesicles (Mizuno et al., 1987). Bowel toxicity is associated with high dose mitomycin C (Sarna et al., 1982).

In human lymphocytes mitomycin induces sister chromatid exchanges in a dose-related manner (Bianchi et al., 1986) and chromosomal aberrations (Ceccherini et al., 1988). A positive dose–response relationship has also been observed for the production of micronuclei in mouse erythrocytes (Sato et al., 1989). Mitomycin C is carcinogenic in rodents, but has not yet been positively associated with human malignancies.

The mechanisms involved in resistance to mitomycin toxicity appear to be varied. Natively resistant human carcinoma cells show a deficiency in activation of mitomycin C and a decrease in phosphorylation of specific nuclear phosphoproteins (Chakrabarty and Brattain, 1987). In Chinese hamster ovary cell lines, resistance to mitomycin appears to be associated with either or both of bioactivation and DNA excision repair (Dulhanty et al., 1989). A resistant human breast tumour cell line (MCF-7) produced less hydroxyl radicals and DNA cross-linking with mitomycin than a sensitive cell line (Dusre et al., 1990). A strain of L5178Y cells which showed increased sensitivity to mitomycin C contained much elevated levels of DT-diaphorase (Begleiter et al., 1989) and a resistant L1210 cell line had enhanced non-protein sulphydryl levels and reduced mitomycin uptake (Dorr et al., 1987).

16. TEROXIRONE

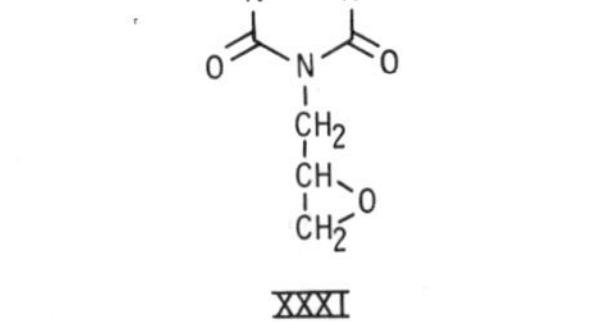

XXXI

The molecule of teroxirone (1,3,5-triazine-2,4,6 (^{1}H, ^{3}H, ^{5}H)trione-1,3,5-tris(oxiranylmethyl)-(α); Henkel compound) (XXXI) contains three alkylating epoxide groups (Budnowski, 1968). It is the more soluble of a pair of stereoisomers and has greater activity against the P-388 and L1210 animal leukaemias than its isomeric counterpart (Atassi et al., 1980). Phase I trials of different formulations of the drug have been carried out in Europe (Cavalli et al., 1981; Piccart et al., 1981) and in the U.S.A. (Rubin et al., 1983; Neidhart et al., 1984).

The characterization of teroxirone pharmacology has been carried out using an assay based on the HPLC of the derivative of teroxirone with diethyl dithiocarbamate (Ames et al., 1984). With epoxides this reagent produces adducts of high UV absorption and ready extractability (cf. dianhydrogalactitol above). Using this method teroxirone could be detected to a limit of 15 ng/mL in plasma. In rabbits infused with [^{14}C]-teroxirone there was rapid loss of parent drug ($t_{1/2} < 5$ min) from the plasma, but much slower loss of radioactivity. The urinary excretion of teroxirone in 24 hr was less than 1% of the dose, although 65% of the radioactivity was excreted in the same period. Similar results were obtained for teroxirone plasma levels ($t_{1/2}$ 1.4 min) and urinary excretion ($< 1\%$) in patients receiving rapid infusion of the drug. At doses below 140 mg/m^2 the detection of the drug in human plasma became inconsistent. In the Phase I trial of Piccart et al. (1981) limited pharmacokinetic data for teroxirone were obtained using a GC assay. The drug was cleared very rapidly from the plasma and concentrations of only ca. 1 μg/mL could be found after infusions of 2000 mg/m^2.

The rapid loss of the drug from plasma is not due to chemical hydrolysis because $< 10\%$ decomposition was found in 2 hr incubations in pH 7.4 buffers (Ames et al., 1984). Rapid decomposition occurs however when teroxirone is incubated with microsomes. As this is independent of NADPH concentrations and inhibited by cyclohexene oxide it appears to be caused by epoxide hydrase. No metabolic activity was found with lung homogenates or microsomes however.

The Phase I trials that have been carried out with teroxirone have shown that myelosuppression or local thrombophlebitis is the dose-limiting toxicity (Piccart et al., 1981; Rubin et al., 1983; Neidhart et al., 1984).

Many other epoxide analogues of teroxirone have more recently been synthesized and tested (Fischer et al., 1984a). The activity in animal tumours of 1,2,4-triglycidylurazole (XXXII) is high (Atassi et al., 1984; Fischer et al., 1984b) and this compound is also undergoing preclinical testing as a possible replacement for teroxirone. Its water solubility is higher (at 7%) than that of teroxirone (1%) and its therapeutically effective dose appears to be about half of that of teroxirone (Atassi et al., 1984). Triglycidylurazole may be determined by HPLC with a sensitivity in plasma of 250 ng/mL (Welsh et al., 1984). In mice the $t_{1/2}\alpha$ for plasma elimination of triglycidylurazole is 1.5 min and $t_{1/2}\beta$ 5 min.

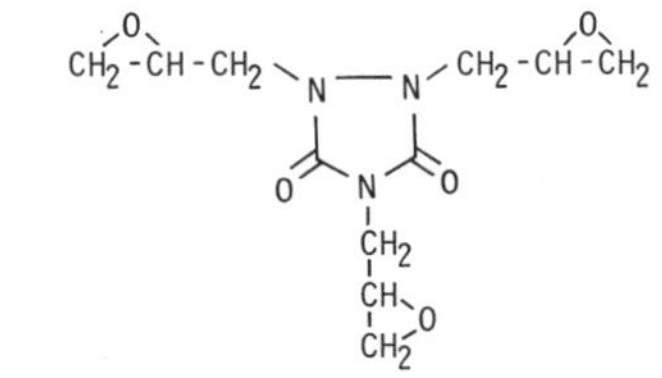

XXXII

17. CONCLUSION

It is apparent that alkylating agents have demonstrated significant effectiveness against human cancers. As indicated in Section 1 the main consideration in the development (past and future) of these agents is in methods of increasing their selectivity towards tumour cells. Progress over the 40 years since the introduction of nitrogen mustard is exemplified by the synthesis of spirohydantoin mustard for treatment of tumours in lipophilic areas and by the development of mitomycin C for use in hypoxic areas. A highly significant feature in the future development of alkylating agents in chemotherapy is the animal test system used for their screening. Previously these systems tended to be rather favourable for detecting alkylating ability per se in a new compound. As future alkylating agents will be designed with a particular tumour or tissue in mind it will clearly be necessary to select or create testing systems appropriate for the proposed drug's activity.

Further developments in increasing the selectivity of alkylating agents could depend either on increasing the transport of the drug to the tumour site (for example by coupling it with an antibody for a tumour-associated antigen, or with a hormone for hormonally sensitive tumours) or on promoting the chemical activation of the drug at the tumour site (e.g. by metabolism by a tumour-specific enzyme). Although toxicity to normal tissues will naturally decrease with an increase in the tumour-selectivity of the alkylating agents, further reductions are necessary and may be achievable with developments of chemical protecting agents, as exemplified by the use of Mesna® to minimize bladder toxicity from cyclophosphamide.

For currently used agents we are still faced with immediate and severe toxic effects in the treated patient and as the success of cancer treatment increases there may well be in the future a more significant incidence of later adverse consequences of chemotherapy, such as carcinogenesis. The success of future alkylating agent drugs will be totally dependent on the extent of both of these short- and long-term toxicities.

REFERENCES

Ackland, S. P., Choi, K. E., Ratain, M. J., Egorin, M. J., Williams, S. F., Sinkule, J. A. and Bitran, J. D. (1988) Human plasma pharmacokinetics of thio-TEPA following administration of high-dose thio-TEPA and cyclophosphamide. *J. clin. Oncol.* **6:** 1192–1196.

Adair, C. G,. Bridges, J. M. and Desai, Z. R. (1986) Can food affect the bioavailability of chlorambucil in patients with haematological malignancies? *Cancer Chemother. Pharmac.* **17:** 99–102.

Adair, C. G. and McElnay, J. C. (1986) Studies on the mechanism of gastrointestinal absorption of melphalan and chlorambucil. *Cancer Chemother. Pharmac.* **17:** 95–98.

Adair, C. G. and McElnay, J. D. (1987) The effect of dietary amino acids on the gastrointestinal absorption of melphalan and chlorambucil. *Cancer Chemother. Pharmac.* **19:** 343–346.

Adair, C. G., Burns, D. T., Crockard, A. D. and Harriott, M. (1985) Determination of chlorambucil in plasma using reversed-phase high-performance liquid chromatography. *J. Chromatog. Biomed. Appl.* **342:** 447–451.

Ahmed, A. E. and Hsu, T. F. (1981) Quantitative analysis of melphalan and its major hydrolysate in patients and animals by reversed-phase high-performance liquid chromatography. *J. Chromatog.* **222:** 453–460.

Ahmed, A. E., Hsu, T. F., El-Azhary, R. A., Moawad, H. and Costanzi, J. (1982a) Macromolecular interactions of [^{14}C-ring] melphalan in blood. *Biochem. Pharmac.* **31:** 1615–1619.

Ahmed, A. E., Hsu, T. F., El-Azhary, R. A., Moawad, H., Farrish, H. H. and Costanzi, J. (1982b) Tissue distribution and macromolecular interactions of [^{14}C-ring] melphalan in the rat. *Cancer Chemother. Pharmac.* **8:** 271–276.

Akhtar, M. H., Begleiter, A., Johnson, D., Lown, J. W., McLaughlin, L. and Sim, S.-K. (1975) Antitumour antibiotics. VI Correlation of covalent cross-linking of DNA by bifunctional aziridinoquinones with their antineoplastic activity. *Can. J. Chem.* **53:** 2891–2905.

Alberts, D., Chang, S. Y., Melnick, L., Himmelstein, K., Walson, P., Gross, J. and Salmon, S. (1977) Melphalan (M) disposition in man. *Proc. Am. Ass. Cancer Res.* **18:** 128.

Alberts, D. S., Chang, S. Y., Chen, H. G., Evans, T. L. and Moon, T. E. (1979a) Oral melphalan kinetics. *Clin. Pharmac. Ther.* **26:** 737–745.

Alberts, D. S., Chang, S. Y., Chen, H. G., Larcom, B. J., Jones, S. E. (1979b) Pharmacokinetics and metabolism of chlorambucil in man: a preliminary report. *Cancer Treat. Rev.* **6**(Suppl.): 9–17.

Alberts, D. S., Chang, S. Y., Chen, H. G., Moon, T. E., Evans, T. L., Furner, R. L., Himmelstein, K. and Gross, J. F. (1979c) Kinetics of intravenous melphalan. *Clin. Pharmac. Ther.* **26:** 73–80.

Alberts, D. S., Chang, S. Y., Chen, H. G., Larcom, B. J. and Evans, T. L. (1980a) Comparative pharmacokinetics of chlorambucil and melphalan in man. *Rec. Res. Cancer Res.* **74:** 124–131.

Alberts, D. S., Chen, H. G., Benz, D. and Mason, N. L. (1981) Effect of renal dysfunction in dogs on the disposition and marrow toxicity of melphalan. *Br. J. Cancer* **43:** 330–334.

Alberts, D. S., Chen, H. G., Chang, S. Y. and Peng, Y. M. (1980b) The disposition of intraperitoneal bleomycin, melphalan and vinblastine in cancer patients. *Rec. Res. Cancer Res.* **74:** 293–299.

Alexander, P. and Lett, J. T. (1960) The biological significance of the changes produced in the deoxyribonucleic acid of cells treated with radiomimetic alkylating agents. *Biochem. Pharmac.* **4:** 34–48.

Allen, E. and Seaman, W. (1955) Method of assay for ethyl-enimine derivatives. *Anal. Chem.* **27:** 540–543.

Ames, B. N., Durston, W. E., Yamasaki, E. and Lee, F. D. (1973) Carcinogens are mutagens: a simple test system combining liver homogenates for activation and bacteria for detection. *Proc. natn. Acad. Sci. U.S.A.* **70:** 2281–2285.

Ames, M. M., Kovach, J. S. and Rubin, J. (1984) Pharmacogical characterization of teroxirone, a tripoxide antitumour agent in rats, rabbits and humans. *Cancer Res.* **44:** 4151–4156.

Andersson, L., Edsmyr, F., Jöhnsson, G. and Könyves, I. (1977) Estramustine phosphate therapy in carcinoma of the prostate. *Rec. Res. Cancer Res.* **60:** 73–77.

Andersson, S. B., Gunnarsson, P. O., Nilsson, T. and Forshell, G. P. (1981) Metabolism of oestramustine phosphate (Estracyt) in patients with prostatic carcinoma. *Eur. J. Drug Metab. Pharmacokin.* **2:** 149–154.

Andrews, N. C., Weiss, A. J., Ansfield, F. J., Rochlin, D. B. and Mason, J. H. (1971) Phase I study of dibromodulcitol (NSC 1048OO). *Cancer Chemother. Rep.* **55:** 61–65.

Andrews, N. C., Weiss, A. J., Wilson, W. and Nealon, T. (1974) Phase II study of dibromodulcitol (NSC 104800). *Cancer Chemother. Rep.* **58:** 653–660.

ANDREWS, P. A., MURPHY, M. P. and HOWELL, S. B. (1986) Differential sensitization of human ovarian carcinoma and mouse L1210 cells to cisplatin and melphalan by glutathione depletion. *Molec. Pharmac.* **30:** 643–650.

ANON (1966) Qualitative and quantitative tests for melphalan. *J. Pharm. Sci.* **55:** 726–727.

APPELGREN, L. E., FORSGREN, B., GUSTAFSSON, J. A., POUSETTE, A. and HÖGBERG, B. (1978) Autoradiographic studies of ^{3}H-oestramustine in the rat ventral prostate. *Acta. Pharm. Toxic.* **43:** 368–374.

ARDIET, C., TRANCHARD, B., BIRON, P., REBATTU, P. and PHILIP, T. (1986) Pharmacokinetics of high dose intravenous melphalan in children and adults with forced diuresis. *Cancer Chemother. Pharmac.* **16:** 300–305.

ARONEY, R. S., KAPLAN, R. S., SALEMAN, M., MONTGOMERY, E. and WIERNIK, P. H. (1982) A Phase II trial of AZQ (NSC 182986) in patients with recurrent primary or metastatic brain tumours. *Proc. Am. Soc. clin. Oncol.* **1:** 24.

ATASSI, G., DUMONT, P. and VANHAELEN, C. (1984) Characterization of the activity of triglycidylurazol (TGU; NSC 332488): a new antineoplastic compound. *Eur. J. Cancer clin. Oncol.* **20:** 1187–1191.

ATASSI, G., SPREAFICO, F., DUMONT, P., NAYER, P. and KLASTERSKY, J. (1980a) Antitumoural effect in mice of a new triepoxyde derivation: 1,3,5-triglycidyl-*S*-triazinetrione (NSC 296934). *Eur. J. Cancer.* **16:** 1561–1567.

ATHANASIOU, K. and ARZIMANOGLOU, I. (1986) Mutagenicity and clastogenicity of the antineoplastic agents homo-aza-steroidal ester of *p*-bis(2-chloroethyl) aminophenyl acetic acid and chlorambucil. *Mutat. Res.* **175:** 165–169.

AUTRUP, H., THURLOW, B. J. and WARWICK, G. P. (1974) Activation by reductive cleavage of potentially cytotoxic azo compounds by human hepatocellular carcinoma. *Biochem. Pharmac.* **23:** 2341–2345.

AXELROD, A. R., BERMAN, L. and MURPHY, R. V. (1953) Clinical and hematologic effects of triethylene melamine. *Am. J. Med.* **15:** 684–694.

BALL, C. R. and DOUBLE, J. A. (1974) Enzyme activated anti-tumour agents. Conjugates of *p*-hydroxyaniline mustard as substrates for hydrolytic enzymes. *Biochem. Pharmac.* **23:** 3173–3177.

BALL, C. R., CONNORS, T. A., DOUBLE, J. A., USHAZY, V. and WHISSON, M. E. (1966) Comparison of nitrogen mustard-sensitive and resistant Yoshida sarcoma. *Int. J. Cancer* **1:** 319–327.

BANERJEE, A. and BENEDICT, W. F. (1979) Production of sister-chromatid exchanges by various cancer chemotherapeutic agents. *Cancer Res.* **39:** 797–799.

BANK, B. B., KANGANIS, D., LEIBES, L. F. and SILBER, R. (1989) Chlorambucil pharmacokinetics and DNA binding in chronic lymphocytic leukemia lymphocytes. *Cancer Res.* **49:** 554–559.

BARBHAIYA, R. H., PAPP, E. A., VAN HARKEN, D. R. and SMYTH, R. D. (1984) Pharmacokinetics of mitomycin C in dogs: application of a high-performance liquid chromatographic assay. *J. Pharm. Sci.* **73:** 1220–1223.

BARRANCO, S. C., TOWNSEND, C. M., WEINTRAUB, B., BEASLEY, E. G., MACLEAN, K. K., SHAEFFER, J., LIU, N. H. and SCHELLENBERG, K. (1990) Changes in glutathione content and resistance to anticancer agents in human stomach cancer cells induced by treatments with melphalan in vitro. *Cancer Res.* **50:** 3614–3618.

BASTHOLT, L., JOHANSSON, C.-J., PFEIFFER, P., SVENSSON, L., JOHANSSON, S. A., GUNNARSSON, P. O. and MOURIDSEN, H. (1991) A pharmacokinetic study of prednimustine as compared with prednisolone plus chlorambucil in cancer patients. *Cancer Chemother. Pharmac.* **28:** 205–210.

BATIST, G., TORRES-GARCIA, S., DEMUYS, J-M., GREENE, D., LEHNERT, S., ROCHON, M. and PANASCI, L. (1989) Enhanced DNA cross-link removal: the apparent mechanism of resistance in a clinically relevant melphalan-resistant human breast cancer cell line. *Molec. Pharmac.* **36:** 224–230.

BAXTER, M. A., CHAHWALA, S. B., HICKMAN, J. A. and SPURGIN, G. E. (1982) The effects of nitrogen mustard (HN2) on activities of the plasma membrane of PC6A mouse plasmacytoma cells. *Biochem. Pharmac.* **31:** 1773–1778.

BECHER, R. and PRESCHER, G. (1988) Induction of sister chromatid exchanges and chromosomal aberrations by busulfan in Philadelphia chromosome-positive chronic myeloid leukemia and normal bone marrow. *Cancer Res.* **48:** 3435–3439.

BEDFORD, P. and FOX, B. W. (1982) Repair of DNA interstrand crosslinks after busulphan. *Cancer Chemother. Pharmac.* **8:** 3–7.

BEDFORD, P. and FOX, B. W. (1983) DNA–DNA interstrand cross-linking by dimethanesulphonic acid esters. Correlation with cytotoxicity and antitumour activity in the Yoshida lymphosarcoma model and relationship to chain length. *Biochem. Pharmac.* **32:** 2297–2301.

BEGLEITER, A. and GOLDENBERG, G. J. (1979) Transport of melphalan by amino acid carriers in MCF-7 human breast cancer cells in vitro. *Proc. Am. Ass. Cancer Res.* **20:** 240.

BEGLEITER, A. and GOLDENBERG, G. J. (1983) Uptake and decomposition of chlorambucil by L5178Y lymphoblasts in vitro. *Biochem. Pharmac.* **32:** 535–539.

BEGLEITER, A., FROESE, E. K. and GOLDENBERG, G. J. (1980) A comparison of melphalan transport in human breast cancer cells and lymphocytes in vitro. *Cancer Lett.* **10:** 243–251.

BEGLEITER, A., GROVER, J. and GOLDENBERG, G. J. (1982) Mechanism of efflux of melphalan from L5178Y lymphoblasts in vitro. *Cancer Res.* **42:** 987–991.

BEGLEITER, A., LAM, H.-Y. P., GROVER, J., FROESE, E. K. and GOLDENBERG, G. J. (1979) Evidence for active transport of melphalan by two amino acid carriers in L5178Y lymphoblasts in vitro. *Cancer Res.* **39:** 353–359.

BEGLEITER, A., ROBOTHAM, E., LACEY, G. and LEITH, M. K. (1989) Increased sensitivity of quinone resistant cells to mitomycin C. *Cancer Lett.* **45:** 173–176.

BELEJ, M. A., TROETEL, W. M., WEISS, A. J., STAMBAUGH, J. E. and MANTHEI, R. W. (1972) The absorption and metabolism of dibromodulcitol in patients with advanced cancer. *Clin. Pharmac. Ther.* **13:** 563–572.

BELLAMY, W. T., DALTON, W. S., GLEASON, M. C., GROGAN, T. M. and TRENT, J. M. (1991) Development and characterization of a melphalan-resistant human multiple myeloma cell line. *Cancer Res.* **51:** 995–1002.

BENCKHUIJSEN, C., VAROSSIEAU, F. J., HART, A. A. M., WIEBERDINK, J. and NOORDHOEK, J. (1986) Pharmacokinetics of melphalan in isolated perfusion of the limbs. *J. Pharmac. exp. Ther.* **237:** 583–588.

BENCKHUYSEN, C., TER HART, H. G. J. and VAN DIJK, P. J. (1981) Enhanced cytostatic effectiveness of aniline mustard against 7,12-dimethylbenz[a]anthracene induced rat mammary tumours during regression in response to ovariectomy. *Cancer Treat. Rep.* **65:** 567–574.

BENEDICT, W. F., BAKER, M. S., HAROUN, L., CHOI, E. and AMES, B. N. (1977) Mutagenicity of cancer chemotherapeutic agents in the *Salmonella*/Microsome test. *Cancer Res.* **37:** 2209–2213.

BERENBAUM, M. C., TIMMIS, G. M. and BROWN, I. N. (1967) The relation between the physico-chemical properties and immunosuppression effects of an homologous series of sulphonic acid esters. *Immunology* **13:** 517–522.

BERGEL, F. and STOCK, J. A. (1953) Cytotoxic alpha amino acids and peptides. *Br. Emp. Cancer Camp. A. Rep.* **31:** 6–7.

BERGEL, F. and STOCK, J. A. (1954) Cyto-active amino-acid and peptide derivatives: Part I Substituted phenylalanines. *J. Chem. Soc.* 2409–2417.

BERGER, M. R., HABS, M. and SCHMAHL, D. (1986) Long term toxicology effects of prednimustine in comparison with chlorambucil, prednisolone and chlorambucil plus prednisolone in Sprague–Dawley rats. *Sem. Oncol.* **13** (Suppl. 1): 8–13.

BERGH, J., BJÖRK, P., WESTLIN, J.-E. and NILSSON, S. (1988) Expression of an oestramustine-binding associated protein in human lung cancer cell lines. *Cancer Res.* **48:** 4615–4619.

BERK, P. D., GOLDBERG, J. D., SILVERSTEIN, M. N., WEINFELD, A., DONOVAN, P. B., ELLIS, J. T., LANDAW, S. A., LASZLO, J., NAJEAN, Y., PISCIOTTA, A. V. and WASSERMAN, L. R. (1981) Increased incidence of acute leukemia in polycythemia vera associated with chlorambucil therapy. *New Engl. J. Med.* **304:** 441–447.

BERNIER, L. G., GAUDREAULT, R. C., PAGE, M. and JOLY, L. P. (1984a) Fluorescence determination of microconcentrations of chlorambucil after photoactivation. *J. Pharm. Sci.* **73:** 1157–1158.

BERNIER, L. G., PAGE, M., GAUDREAULT, R. C. and JOLY, L. P. (1984b) A chlorambucil-anti-CEA conjugate cytotoxic for human colon adenocarcinoma cells in vitro. *Br. J. Cancer* **49:** 245–246.

BEROZA, M. and BORKOVEC, A. B. (1964) The stability of Tepa and other aziridine chemosterilants. *J. med. Chem.* **7:** 44–49.

BETTERIDGE, R. F., BOSANQUET, A. G. and GILBY, E. D. (1990) Pharmacokinetics of 2,5-diaziridinyl-3,6-bis(2-hydroxyethylamino)-1,4-benzoquinone (BZQ, NSC 224070) during a Phase I clinical trial. *Eur. J. Cancer* **26:** 107–112.

BETTERIDGE, R. F., BOSANQUET, A. G., HUNT, P. and GILBY, E. D. (1988) Determination of diaziridinyl-3,6-bis(2-hydroxyethylamino)-1,4-benzoquinone in plasma by solid-phase extraction and high-performance liquid chromatography. *J. Chromatog. Biomed. Appl.* **432:** 352–357.

BIANCHI, M. S., LARRAMENDY, M. L. and BIANCHI, N. O. (1986) Mitomycin C-induced damage and repair in human and pig lymphocytes. *Mutat. Res.* **160:** 27–32.

BIBBY, M. C., MCDERMOTT, B. J., DOUBLE, J. A., PHILLIPS, R. M., LOADMAN, P. M. and BURGESS, L. (1987) Influence of the tissue distribution of thio-TEPA and its metabolite, TEPA, on the response of murine colon tumours. *Cancer Chemother. Pharmac.* **20:** 203–206.

BJÖRK, P., FORSGREN, B., GUSTAFSSON, J. A., POUSETTE, A. and HÖGBERG, B. (1982) Partial characterization and "quantitation" of a human prostatic oestramustine-binding protein. *Cancer Res.* **42:** 1935–1942.

BJORNSSON, T. D., SCHOLD, S. C., FRIEDMAN, H. S., SCHNEIDER, D. and FALLETTA, J. M. (1985) Pharmacokinetics of diaziquone after three different dosage regimens. *Cancer Treat. Rep.* **69:** 1383–1385.

BLACK, S. M., BEGGS, J. D., HAYES, J. D., BARTOSZEK, A., MURAMATSU, M., SAICAI, M. and WOLF, C. R. (1990) Expression of human glutathione*S*-transferase in *Saccharomyces cerevisiae* confers resistance to the anticancer drugs adriamycin and chlorambucil. *Biochem. J.* **268:** 309–315.

BLANZ, J., ROSENFELD, C., PROKSCH, B., EHNINGER, G. and ZELLER, K.-P. (1990) Quantitation of busulfan in plasma by high-performance liquid chromatography using postcolumn photolysis. *J. Chromatog. Biomed. Appl.* **532:** 429–437.

BLIGH, H. F. J., BARTOSZEK, A., ROBSON, C. N., HICKSON, I. D., KASPER, C. B., BEGGS, J. D. and WOLF, C. R. (1990) Activation of mitomycin C by NADPH: cytochrome P-450 reductase. *Cancer Res.* **50:** 7789–7792.

BLOSMANIS, R., WRIGHT, J. A. and GOLDENBERG, G. J. (1987) Sensitivity to melphalan as a function of transport activity and proliferative rate in BALB/c 3T3 fibroblasts. *Cancer Res.* **47:** 1273–1277.

BOCCARDO, F., DECENSI, A., GUARNERI, D., MARTORNANA, G., GILBERTI, C. and GIULIANI, L. (1988) Estramustine phosphate (estracyt) following androgens in man with refractory stage D2 prostate cancer. *Cancer Chemother. Pharmac.* **22:** 172–174.

BOLTON, M. G., COLVIN, O. M. and HILTON, J. (1991) Specificity of isozymes of murine hepatic glutathione-*S*-transferase for the conjugation of glutathione with L-phenylalanine mustard. *Cancer Res.* **51:** 2410–2415.

BOONE, I. U., ROGERS, B. S. and WILLIAMS, D. L. (1962) Toxicity, metabolism and tissue distribution of carbon-14 labelled *N,N',N''*-triethylenethiophosphoramide (thio-TEPA) in rats. *Toxic. appl. Pharmac.* **4:** 344–353.

Borowy-Borowski, H., Lipman, R., Chowdary, D. and Tomasz, M. (1990a) Duplex oligodeoxyribonucleotides cross-linked by mitomycin C at a single site: synthesis, properties and cross-link reversibility. *Biochemistry* **29:** 2992–2999.

Borowy-Borowski, H., Lipman, R. and Tomasz, M. (1990b) Recognition between mitomycin C and specific DNA sequences for cross-link formation. *Biochemistry* **29:** 2999–3006.

Bosanquet, A. G. (1985) Stability of melphalan solutions during preparation and storage. *J. Pharm. Sci.* **74:** 348–351.

Bosanquet, A. G. and Bird, M. C. (1988) Degradation of melphalan in vitro: rationale for the use of continuous exposure in chemosensitivity assays. *Cancer Chemother. Pharmac.* **21:** 211–215.

Bosanquet, A. G. and Clarke, H. E. (1986) Chlorambucil: stability of solutions during preparation and storage. *Cancer Chemother. Pharmac.* **18:** 176–179.

Bosanquet, A. G. and Gilby, E. D. (1982a) Measurement of plasma melphalan at therapeutic concentrations using isocratic high-performance liquid chromatography. *J. Chromatog.* **232:** 345–354.

Bosanquet, A. G. and Gilby, E. D. (1982b) Pharmacokinetics of oral and intravenous melphalan during routine treatment of multiple myeloma. *Eur. J. Cancer clin. Oncol.* **18:** 355–362.

Bosanquet, A. G. and Gilby, E. D. (1984) Comparison of the fed and fasting states on the absorption of melphalan in multiple myeloma. *Cancer Chemother. Pharmac.* **12:** 183–186.

Boyland, E., Staunton, M. D. and Williams, K. (1961) Experimental regional administration (perfusion and infusion) of chlorambucil (*p*-*N*,*N*-di(chloroethyl) aminophenyl butyric acid). *Br. J. Cancer* **15:** 498–510.

Brandt, L., Konyves, I. and Moller, T. R. (1975) Therapeutic effect of Leo 1031, an alkylating corticosteroid ester in lymphoproliferative disorders. I. Chronic lymphocytic leukaemia. *Acta Med. scand.* **197:** 317–322.

Briele, H. A., Djuric, M., Jung, D. T., Mortell, T., Patel, M. K., Das Gupta, T. K. (1985) Pharmacokinetics of melphalan in clinical isolation perfusion of the extremities. *Cancer Res.* **45:** 1885–1889.

Brookes, P. and Lawley, P. D. (1961a) The alkylation of guanosine and guanylic acid. *J. Chem. Soc.* pp. 3923–3928.

Brookes, P. and Lawley, P. D. (1961b) The reaction of mono- and di-functional alkylating agents with nucleic acids. *Biochem. J.* **80:** 496–503.

Brown, J. M. and Hirst, D. G. (1982) Effect of clinical levels of misonidazole on the response of tumour and normal tissues in the mouse to alkylating agents. *Br. J. Cancer* **45:** 700–708.

Brown, T. D., Ettinger, D. S. and Donehower, R. C. (1986) A Phase I trial of spirohydantoin mustard (NSC 172112) in patients with advanced cancer. *J. clin. Oncol.* **4:** 1270–1276.

Brox, L. W., Gowans, B. and Belch, A. (1980) L-phenylalanine mustard (melphalan) uptake and cross-linking in the RPMI 6410 human lymphoblastoid cell line. *Cancer Res.* **40:** 1169–1172.

Brox, L., Birkett, L. and Belch, A. (1979) Pharmacology of intravenous melphalan in patients with multiple myeloma. *Cancer Treat. Rev.* **6** (Suppl.): 27–32.

Bucci, L. R. and Meistrich, M. L. (1987) Effects of busulfan on murine spermatogenesis: cytotoxicity, sterility, sperm abnormalities and dominant lethal mutations. *Mutat. Res.* **176:** 259–268.

Buchanan, L. J. and Riches, A. C. (1987) Testosterone-induced DNA synthesis in cultured rat ventral prostate: effects of estracyt and its derivatives. *Br. J. Cancer* **55:** 47–51.

Budnowski, M. (1968) Preparation and properties of the diastereoisomeric 1,3,5-triglycidyl-*S*-triazinetriones. *Angew. Chem. Int. Ed. Engl.* **7:** 827–828.

Bukhari, A., Connors, T. A., Gilsenan, A. M., Ross, W. C. J., Tisdale, M. J., Warwick, G. P. and Wilman, D. E. V. (1973) Cytotoxic agents designed to be selective for liver cancer. *J. natn. Cancer Inst.* **50:** 243–247.

Bukhari, M. A., Everett, J. L. and Ross, W. C. J. (1972) Aryl-2-halogenoalkylamines-XXVI Glucuronic, sulphuric and phosphoric esters of p-di-2-chloroethylaminophenol. *Biochem. Pharmac.* **21:** 963–967.

Buller, A. L., Clapper, M. L. and Tew, K. D. (1987) Glutathione-*S*-transferase in nitrogen mustard resistant and sensitive cell lines. *Molec. Pharmac.* **31:** 575–578.

Butler, J., Hoey, B. M. and Lea, J. S. (1987) The reduction of anti-tumour diaziridinyl benzoquinones. *Biochim. biophys. Acta* **925:** 144–149.

Butler, J., Hoey, B. M. and Ward, T. H. (1989) The alkylation of DNA in vitro by 2,5-bis(2-hydroxyethylamino)-3,6-diaziridinyl-1,4-benzoquinone (BZQ)-I. *Biochem. Pharmac.* **38:** 923–927.

Byington, K. H., Bowe, C. C. and McKinsey, D. S. (1980) Biliary excretion of melphalan by control and anuric rats. *Biochem. Pharmac.* **29:** 2518–2520.

Catovsky, D. and Galton, D. A. G. (1971) Myelomonocytic leukaemia supervening on chronic lymphocytic leukakemia. *Lancet* **i:** 478–479.

Cavaliere, A., Pietropaoli, N., Alberti, P. F. and Vitali, R. (1990) Chlorambucil carcinogenesis in BALB/c mice. *Cancer Lett.* **55:** 115–120.

Cavalli, F., Kaplan, S., Varini, M. and Joss, R. (1981) Phase I trial of 1,3,5-triglycidyl-*S*-triazinetrione (TGT, NSC 296934). *Proc. Am. Ass. Cancer Res.* **22:** 191.

Ceccherini, I., Sbrana, I. and Loprieno, N. (1988) Kinetics of chromosomal aberrations and first mitosis division in human lymphocytes exposed to mitomycin C. *Mutat. Res.* **208:** 183–188.

Cera, C. and Crothers, D. M. (1989) Modulation of mitomycin cross-linking by DNA bending in the *Escherichia coli* CAP protein–DNA complex. *Biochemistry* **28:** 3908–3911.

Chakrabarty, S. and Brattain, M. G. (1987) Molecular comparisons of acquired and native mitomycin C resistance in human colon carcinoma cells. *Cancer Lett.* **37:** 267–276.

CHAN, K. K., BOLGER, M. B. and PANG, V. S. (1985) Statistical moment theory in chemical kinetics. *Anal. Chem.* **57:** 2145–2151.

CHAN, P. K. (1989) Cross-linkage of nucleoplasmin in tumour cells by nitrogen mustard. *Cancer Res.* **49:** 3271–3275.

CHANG, S. Y., ALBERTS, D. S., FARQUAR, D., MELNICK, L. R., WALSON, P. D. and SALMON, S. E. (1978b) Hydrolysis and protein binding of melphalan. *J. Pharm. Sci.* **67:** 682–684.

CHANG, S. Y., ALBERTS, D. S., MELNICK, L. R., WALSON, P. D. and SALMON, S. E. (1978a) High-pressure liquid chromatographic analysis of melphalan in plasma. *J. Pharm. Sci.* **67:** 679–682.

CHANG, S. Y., EVANS, T. L. and ALBERTS, D. S. (1979) The stability of melphalan in the presence of chloride ion. *J. Pharm. Pharmac.* **31:** 853–854.

CHANG, S. Y., EVANS, T. L., ALBERTS, D. S. and SIPES, I. G. (1978c) The stability of L-phenylalanine mustard in bile. *Life Sci.* **23:** 1697–1702.

CHANG, S. Y., LARCOM, B. J., ALBERTS, D. S., LARSEN, B., WALSON, P. D. and SIPES, I. G. (1980) Mass spectrometry of chlorambucil, its degradation products and its metabolite in biological samples. *J. Pharm. Sci.* **69:** 80–84.

CHAUBE, S., KURY, G. and MURPHY, M. L. (1967) Teratogenic effects of cyclophosphamide (NSC 26271) in the rat. *Cancer Chemother. Rep.* **51:** 363–376.

CHEN, T.-L., GROCHOW, L. B., HUROWITZ, L. A. and BRUNDRETT, R. B. (1988) Determination of busulfan in human plasma by gas chromatography with electron-capture detection. *J. Chromatog.* **425:** 303–309.

CHIPMAN, J. K., HIROM, P. C. and MILLBURN, P. (1980) Biliary excretion and enterohepatic circulation of aniline mustard metabolites in the rat and the rabbit. *Biochem. Pharmac.* **29:** 1299–1301.

CHIRIGOS, M. A. and MEAD, J. A. R. (1964) Experiments on determination of melphalan by fluorescence. Interaction with protein and various solutions. *Anal. Biochem.* **7:** 259–268.

CHIUTEN, D. F., ROZENCWEIG, M., VON HOFF, D. D. and MUGGIA, F. M. (1981) Clinical trials with the hexitol derivatives in the U.S. *Cancer* **47:** 442–451.

CHOI, K. E., RATAIN, M. J., WILLIAMS, S. F., GOLICK, J. A., BESCHORNER, J. C., FULLEM, L. J. and BITRAN, J. D. (1989) Plasma pharmacokinetics of high-dose oral melphalan in patients treated with trialkylator chemotherapy and autologous bone marrow reinfusion. *Cancer Res.* **49:** 1318–1321.

CHOI, K. E., SINKULE, J. A., CROM, W. R., THOMPSON, E. I. and EVANS, W. E. (1985) High-performance liquid chromatographic assay of mitomycin in biological fluids. *J. Chromatog.* **345:** 197–202.

CHOU, F., KHAN, A. H. and DRISCOLL, J. S. (1976) Potential central nervous system antitumour agents. Azindinylbenzoquinones. 2. *J. med. Chem.* **19:** 1302–1308.

CHUN, E. H. L., GONZALES, L., LEWIS, F. S., JONES, J. and RUTMAN, R. J. (1969) Differences in the in vivo alkylation and cross-linking of nitrogen mustard-sensitive and resistant lines of Lettre–Ehrlich ascite tumours. *Cancer Res.* **29:** 1184–1194.

CLAASSEN, E., KORTBEEK, H. and ARWERT, F. (1986) Effects of mitomycin C on the rate of DNA synthesis in normal and Fanconi anaemia cells. *Mutat. Res.* **165:** 15–19.

CLEMENT, J. J., GORDON, M. S., WODINSKY, I., CATANE, R. and JOHNSON, R. K. (1980) Enhancement of antitumour activity of alkylating agents by the radiation sensitizer misonidazole. *Cancer Res.* **40:** 4165–4170.

COHEN, B. E., EGORIN, M. J., KOHLHEPP, E. A., ALSNEL, J. and GUTIERREZ, P. L. (1986) Human plasma pharmacokinetics and urinary excretion of thio-TEPA and its metabolites. *Cancer Treat. Rep.* **70:** 859–864.

COHEN, C., VAN ARTSDALEN, E. R. and HARRIS, J. (1948) Reaction kinetics of aliphatic tertiary chloroethylamines in dilute aqueous solution. I. The cyclization process. *J. Am. Chem. Soc.* **70:** 281–285.

COHEN, N. A., EGORIN, M. J., SNYDER, S. W.. ASHAR, B., WIETHARN, B. E., PAN, S.-S., ROSS, D. D. and HILTON, J. (1991) Interaction of *N,N′,N″*-triethylenethiophosphoramide and *N,N′,N″*-triethylenephosphoramide with cellular DNA. *Cancer Res.* **51:** 4360–4366.

COHEN, R. J. and CROTHERS, D. M. (1970) Preparation and characterization of monodisperse cross-linked low molecular weight deoxyribonucleic acid. *Biochemistry* **9:** 2533–2539.

COHN, P. (1957) The distribution of radioactivity in tissues of the rat following the administration of a nitrogen mustard derivative. (*p*-di-(2-chloroethyl)amino-D,L-phenyl [β-^{14}C]alanine). *Br. J. Cancer* **11:** 258–267.

COLE, R. C., MYERS, T. J. and KATSKY, A. W. (1978) Pulmonary disease with chlorambucil therapy. *Cancer* **41:** 455–459.

COLEMAN, C. N., CARLSON, R. W., HALSEY, J., KOHLER, M., GRIBBLE, M., SIKIC, B. I. and JACOBS, C. (1988) Enhancement of the clinical activity of melphalan by the hypoxic cell sensitizer misonidazole. *Cancer Res.* **48:** 3528–3532.

COLEMAN, C. N., FRIEDMAN, M. K., JACOBS, C., HALSEY, J., IGNOFFO, R., LEIBEL, S., HIRST, V. K., GRIBBLE, M., CARTER, S. K. and PHILLIPS, T. L. (1983) Phase I trial of intravenous L-phenyl-alanine mustard plus the sensitizer misonidazole. *Cancer Res.* **43:** 5022–5025.

COLVIN, M. (1982) The alkylating agents. In: *Pharmacological Principles of Cancer Treatment*, pp. 276–308, CHABNER, B. (ed.) W. B. Saunders, Philadelphia.

CONKLIN, J. W., UPTON, A. C. and CHRISTENBERRY, K. W. (1965) Further observations on late somatic effects of radiomimetic chemicals and X-rays in mice. *Cancer Res.* **25:** 20–27.

CONNER, M. K., GUZZIE, P. J. and NEFT, R. E. (1989) Temporal SCE and cytotoxicity responses of murine cells following in vivo treatment with MNU or L-PAM. *Mutat. Res.* **224:** 135–142.

CONNORS, T. A. and WHISSON, M. E. (1966) Cure of mice bearing advanced plasma cell tumours with aniline mustard: the relationship between glucuronidase activity and tumour sensitivity. *Nature* **210:** 866–867.

CONNORS, T. A., FARMER, P. B., FOSTER, A. B., GILSENAN, A. M., JARMAN, M. and TISDALE, M. J. (1973a) Metabolism of aniline mustard [*N,N*-di-(2-chloroethyl)aniline]. *Biochem. Pharmac.* **22:** 1971–1980.

CONNORS, T. A., FOSTER, A. B., GILSENAN, A. M., JARMAN, M. and TISDALE, M. J. (1972) Chemical trapping of a reactive metabolite. The metabolism of the azomustard 2′-carboxy-4-di-(2-chloroethyl)amino-2-methylazobenzene. *Biochem. Pharmac.* **21:** 1309–1316.

CONNORS, T. A., GILSENAN, A. M., ROSS, W. C. J., BUKHARI, A., TISDALE, M. J. and WARWICK, G. P. (1973b) Agents designed specifically for the treatment of liver cancer. In: *Chemotherapy of Cancer Dissemination and Metastasis*, pp. 367–374, GARATTINI, S. and FRANCHI, G. (eds) Raven Press, New York.

CORNBLEET, M. A., MCELWAIN, T. J., KUMAR, P. J., FILSHIE, J., SELBY, P., CARTER, R. L., HEDLEY, D. W., CLARK, M. L. and MILLAR, J. L. (1983) Treatment of advanced malignant melanoma with high-dose melphalan and autologous bone marrow transplantation. *Br. J. Cancer* **48:** 329–334.

COSTA, G., ENGLE, R. L. JR and SCHILLING, A. (1973) Melphalan and prednisone: an effective combination for the treatment of multiple myeloma. *Am. J. Med.* **54:** 589–599.

CRAIG, A. W. and JACKSON, H. (1955) The metabolism of ^{32}P-labelled triethylenephosphoramide in relation to its anti-tumour activity. *Br. J. Pharmac.* **10:** 321–325.

CRAIG, A. W., FOX, B. W. and JACKSON, H. (1959) Metabolic studies of ^{32}P-labelled triethylene thiophosphoramide. *Biochem. Pharmac.* **3:** 42–50.

CRATHORN, A. R. and HUNTER, G. D. (1957) The effect of nitrogen mustards on the incorporation of amino acids into protein by *Staphylococcus aureus*. *Biochem. J.* **67:** 37–41.

CRESPI, C. L., SEIXAS, G. M. and PENMAN, B. W. (1987) The induction of aneuploidy by nitrogen mustard in a human lymphoblastoid cell line. *Mutat. Res.* **190:** 69–76.

CSETENYI, J., AFRA, D., KERPEL-FRONIUS, S., HORVATH, I. P., INSTITORIS, L. and ECKHARDT, S. (1983) The distribution of [^{3}H]-dibromodulcitol in the central nervous system of patients with brain tumour. *Eur. J. Cancer clin. Oncol.* **19:** 1389–1392.

CSETENYI, J., GATI, E., HEGEDUS, L., HORVATH, I. P. and HOLCZINGER, L. (1985) Rat liver-mediated degradation of dibromodulcitol. *Eur. J. Cancer clin. Oncol.* **21:** 881–885.

CURT, G. A., CONNORS, T. A., MURRAY-LYON, I. M. and TATTERSALL, M. N. H. (1977) The clinical pharmacology of a hepatoma-specific alkylating agent. *Biochem. Pharmac.* **26:** 1715–1718.

CURT, G. A., SCKILSKY, R., KELLY, J., KUFTA, C., SMITH, B., THOMAS, C. and YOUNG, R. C. (1982) Phase II study of aziridinyl benzoquinone (AZQ) in high grade gliomas. *Proc. Am. Soc. clin. Oncol.* **1:** 13.

CUZICK, J., ERSKINE, S., EDELMAN, D. and GALTON, D. A. G. (1987) A comparison of the incidence of the myelodysplastic syndrome and acute myeloid leukaemia following melphalan and cyclophosphamide treatment for myelomatosis. *Br. J. Cancer* **55:** 523–529.

CZEJKA, M. J., JÄGER, W. and SCHÜLLER, J. (1989) Mitomycin C determination using loop-column extraction: a rapid and sensitive high-performance liquid chromatographic assay for pharmacokinetic studies with Spherex starch particles. *J. Chromatog.* **497:** 336–341.

DALTON, J. T., GEUNS, E. R. and LAI-SIM AU, J. (1989) High-performance liquid chromatographic determination of mitomycin C in rat and human plasma and urine. *J. Chromatog.* **495:** 330–337.

DAVIS, T. P., PENG, Y., GOODMAN, G. E. AND ALBERTS, D. S. (1982) HPLC, MS and pharmacokinetics of melphalan, bisantrene and 13-cis retinoic acid. *J. Chrom. Sci.* **20:** 511–516.

DAVIS, W. and ROSS, W. C. J. (1963) The formation of epoxides from cytotoxic polyol methanesulphonates under physiological conditions. *Biochem. Pharmac.* **12:** 915–917.

DEAN, S. W., GIBSON, N. W. and TEW, K. D. (1986a) Selection of nitrogen mustard resistance in a rat tumour cell line results in loss of guanine-O^{6}-alkyl transferase activity. *Molec. Pharmac.* **30:** 77–80.

DEAN, S. W., JOHNSON, A. B. and TEW, K. D. (1986b) A comparative analysis of drug-induced DNA effects in a nitrogen mustard resistant cell line expressing sensitivity to nitrosoureas. *Biochem. Pharmac.* **35:** 1171–1176.

DEEN, D. F., HOSHINO, T., WILLIAMS, M. E., NOMURA, K. and BARTLE, P. M. (1979) Response on 9L tumour cells in vitro to spirohydantoin mustard. *Cancer Res.* **39:** 4336–4340.

DEMOL, N. J., LUSTHOF, K. J. and DECUYPER, J. (1988) DNA modifications by potential antitumour bisaziridinylquinones. *Biochem. Pharmac.* **37:** 1837–1838.

DEN HARTIGH, J., VAN OORT, W. J., BOCKEN, M. C. Y. M. and PINEDO, H. M. (1981) High-performance liquid chromatographic determination of the antitumour agent mitomycin C in human plasma. *Anal. Chim. Acta* **127:** 47.

DEN HARTIGH, J., MCVIE, J. G., VAN OORT, W. J. and PINEDO, H. M. (1983) Pharmacokinetics of mitomycin C in humans. *Cancer Res.* **43:** 5017–5021.

DIXON, R., BROOKS, M. and GILL, G. (1980) Estramustine phosphate: plasma concentrations of its metabolites following oral administration to man, rat and dog. *Res. Commun. Chem. Path. Pharmac.* **27:** 17–29.

DOPPLER, W., HOFMANN, J., MALY, K. and GRUNICKE, H. H. (1988) Protection of Ehrlich ascites tumour cells against the antiproliferative effect of mechlorethamine (nitrogen mustard) by 5-*N,N*-dimethylamiloride. *Cancer Res.* **48:** 2454–2457.

DOPPLER, W., HOFMANN, J., OBERHUBER, H., MALY, K. and GRUNICKE, H. (1985) Nitrogen mustard interference with potassium transport systems in Ehrlich ascites tumour cells. *J. Cancer Res. clin. Oncol.* **110:** 35–41.

DORR, R. T. (1987) Reduced thiol content in L1210 cells treated with BSO increases DNA cross linking by melphalan. *Biochem. biophys. Res. Commun.* **144:** 47–52.

DORR, R. T., LIDDIL, J. D., TRENT, J. M. and DALTON, W. S. (1987) Mitomycin C resistant L1210 leukemia cells: association with pleiotropic drug resistance. *Biochem. Pharmac.* **36:** 3115–3120.

DORR, R. T., SOBLE, M. and ALBERTS, D. S. (1988) Efficacy of sodium thiosulfate as a local antidote to mechlorethamine skin toxicity in the mouse. *Cancer Chemother. Pharmac.* **22:** 299–302.

DOSKOCIL, J. (1965) Reaction of deoxyribonucleic acid with triethylene melamine. *Cell. Czech. Chem. Commun.* **30:** 2434–2443.

DOUBLE, J. A. and WORKMAN, P. (1977) A new high-glucuronidase mouse tumour curable by aniline mustard therapy. *Cancer Treat. Rep.* **61:** 909–911.

DRISCOLL, J. S., DUDECK, L., CONGLETON, G. and GERAN, R. I. (1979) Potential CNS antitumour agents VI. Aziridinylbenzoquinones III. *J. Pharm. Sci.* **68:** 185–188.

DRISCOLL, J. S., HAZARD, G. F., WOOD, JR, H. B. and GOLDIN, A. (1974) Structure antitumour activity relationships among quinone derivations. *Cancer Chemother. Rep.* **4:** 1–362.

DUCORE, J. M. and MCNAMARA, L. (1986) Effect of α-difluoromethylornithine on L-phenylalanine mustard-induced cytotoxicity and DNA interstrand cross-linking in a human cell line in vitro. *Cancer Res.* **46:** 1068–1072.

DUCORE, J. M., ERICKSON, L. C., ZWELLING, L. A., LAURENT, G. and KOHN, K. W. (1982) Comparative studies of DNA cross-linking and cytotoxicity in Burkitt's lymphoma cell lines treated with *cis*-diammine dichloroplatinum (II) and L-phenylalanine mustard. *Cancer Res.* **42:** 897–902.

DULHANTY, A. M., LI, M. and WHITMORE, G. F. (1989) Isolation of Chinese hamster ovary cell mutants deficient in excision repair and mitomycin C bioactivation. *Cancer Res.* **49:** 117–122.

DULIK, D. M. and FENSELAU, C. (1987) Conversion of melphalan to 4-(glutathionyl)phenylalanine. A novel mechanism for conjugation by glutathione-*S*-transferases. *Drug. Metab. Disp.* **15:** 195–199.

DULIK, D. M., COLVIN, D. M. and FENSELAU, C. (1990) Characterization of glutathione conjugates of chlorambucil by fast atom bombardment and thermospray liquid chromatography/mass spectrometry. *Biomed. Environ. Mass Spec.* **19:** 248–252.

DULIK, D. M., FENSELAU, C. and HILTON, J. (1986) Characterization of melphalan-glutathione adducts whose formation is catalyzed by glutathione transferases. *Biochem. Pharmac.* **35:** 3405–3409.

DUNN, C. D. R. (1974) The chemical and biological properties of busulphan (myleran). *Exp. Hematol.* **2:** 101–117.

DUNN, C. D. R. and ELSON, L. A. (1970) The effect of a homologous series of dimethanesulphonoxy-alkanes on haemopoietic colony forming units in the rat. *Chem. Biol. Interact.* **2:** 273–280.

DUPERRAY, A., TRANQUI, L., ALIX, J.-L. and CORDONNIER, D. (1988) Effect of mitomycin C on prostacyclin synthesis by human endothelial cells. *Biochem. Pharmac.* **37:** 4753–4757.

DUSRE, L., COVEY, J. M., COLLINS, C. and SINHA, B. K. (1989) DNA damage, cytotoxicity and free radical formation by mitomycin C in human cells. *Chem.-Biol. Interact.* **71:** 63–78.

DUSRE, L., RAJAGOPALAN, S., ELIOT, H. M., COVEY, J. M. and SINHA, B. K. (1990) DNA interstrand cross-link and free radical formation in a human multidrug-resistant cell line from mitomycin C and its analogs. *Cancer Res.* **50:** 648–652.

DUVALL, L. R. (1961) Ross azo mustard. *Cancer Chemother. Rep.* **14:** 174–179.

EAGAN, R. T., AMES, M. M., POWIS, G. and KOVACH,J. S. (1982) Clinical and pharmacologic evaluation of split-dose intermittent therapy with dianhydrogalactitol. *Cancer Treat. Rep.* **66:** 283–287.

ECKHARDT, S., CSETENYI, J., HORVATH, I. P., KERPEL-FRONIUS, S., SZAMEL,I., INSTITORIS, L., SZLOVIK, F., PASZTOR, E. and AFRA, D. (1977) Uptake to labelled dianhydrogalactitol into human gliomas and nervous tissue. *Cancer Treat. Rep.* **61:** 841–847.

ECKHARDT, S., SELLEI, C., HORVATH, I. P. and INSTITORIS, L. (1963) Effect of 1,6-dibromo-1,6-dideoxy-D-mannitol on chronic granulocytic leukemia. *Cancer Chemother. Rep.* **33:** 57–61.

EGAN, C. M., JONES, C. R. and MCCLUSKEY, M. (1981) Method for the measurement of melphalan in biological samples by high performance liquid chromatography with fluorescence detection. *J. Chromatog. Biomed. Appl.* **224:** 338–342.

EGORIN, M. J. and SNYDER, S. W. (1990) Characterization of nonexchangeable radioactivity in L1210 cells incubated with [^{14}C]thio-TEPA: labelling of phosphatidylethanolamine. *Cancer Res.* **50:** 4044–4049.

EGORIN, M. J., COHEN, B. E., KOHLHEPP, E. A. and GUTIERREZ, P. L. (1985) Gas-liquid chromatographic analysis of *N,N′,N″*-triethylene thiophosphoramide and *N,N′,N″*-triethylene-phosphoramide in biological samples. *J. Chromatog.* **343:** 196–202.

EGORIN, M. J., SNYDER, S. W. and WIETHARN, B. E. (1990) Effects of ethanolamine and choline on thio-TEPA accumulation and cytotoxicity in L1210 cells. *Cancer Res.* **50:** 4322–4327.

EGORIN, M. J., SNYDER, S. W., PAN, S.-S and DALY, C. (1989) Cellular transport and accumulation of thio-TEPA in murine, human and avian cells. *Cancer Res.* **49:** 5611–5617.

EHLING, U. H. and NEUHÄUSER-KLAUS, A. (1989) Induction of specific-locus and dominant lethal mutations in male mice by chlormethine. *Mutat. Res.* **227:** 81–89.

EHLING, U. H. and NEUHÄUSER-KLAUS, A. (1991) Induction of specific-locus and dominant lethal mutations in male mice by busulfan. *Mutat. Res.* **249:** 285–292.

EHRSSON, H. and HASSAN, M. (1983) Determination of busulfan in plasma by GC-MS with selected-ion monitoring. *J. Pharm. Sci.* **72:** 1203–1205.

EHRSSON, H. and HASSAN, M. (1984) Binding of busulfan to plasma proteins and blood cells. *J. Pharm. Pharmac.* **36:** 694–696.

EHRSSON, H. and LÖNROTH, U. (1982) Degradation of melphalan in aqueous solutions—influence of human albumin binding. *J. Pharm. Sci.* **71:** 826–827.

EHRSSON, H., EKSBORG, S. and LINDFORS, A. (1986) Quantitative determination of melphalan in plasma by liquid chromatography after derivatization with *N*-acetylcysteine. *J. Chromatog. Biomed. Appl.* **380:** 222–228.

EHRSSON, H., EKSBORG, S., JSTERBORG, A., MELLSTEDT, H. and LINDFORS, A. (1989) Oral melphalan pharmacokinetics in relation to dose in patients with multiple myeloma. *Med. Oncol. Tumor Pharmac.* **6:** 151–154.

EHRSSON, H., EKSBORG, S., WALLIN, I. and NILSSON, S. O. (1980b) Degradation of chlorambucil in aqueous solution. *J. Pharm. Sci.* **69:** 1091–1094.

EHRSSON, H., EKSBORG, S., WALLIN, I., MÄRDE, Y. and JOANSSON, B. (1980a) Determination of chlorambucil in plasma by GLC with selected-ion monitoring. *J. Pharm. Sci.* **69:** 710–712.

EHRSSON, H., HASSAN, M., EHRNEBO, M. and BERAN, M. (1983a) Busulfan kinetics. *Clin. Pharmac. Ther.* **34:** 86–89.

EHRSSON, H., LÖNROTH, U., WALLIN, I., EHRNEBO, M. and NILSSON, S. O. (1981) Degradation of chlorambucil in aqueous solution—influence of human albumin binding. *J. Pharm. Pharmac.* **33:** 313–315.

EHRSSON, H., WALLIN, I., NILSSON, S. O. and JOHANSSON, B. (1983b) Pharmacokinetics of chlorambucil in man after administration of the free drug and its prednisolone ester. (Prednimustine, LRO 1031). *Eur. J. clin. Pharmac.* **24:** 251–253.

EHRSSON, H., WALLIN, I., SIMONSSON, B., HARTVIG, P. and ÖBERG, G. (1984) Effect of food on pharmacokinetics of chlorambucil and its main metabolite, phenylacetic acid mustard. *Eur. J. clin. Pharmac.* **27:** 111–114.

EINHORN, N. (1978) Acute leukemia after chemotherapy (melphalan). *Cancer* **41:** 444–447.

EINHORN, N., EKLUND, G. and LAMBERT, B. (1988) Solid tumours and chromosome aberrations as late side effects of melphalan therapy in ovarian carcinoma. *Acta Oncol.* **27:** 215–219.

EKSBERG, S., EHRSSON, H. and LINDFORS, A. (1983) Liquid chromatographic determination of mitomycin C in human plasma and urine. *J. Chromatog.* **274:** 263–270.

ELLIOTT, E. M. and LING, V. (1981) Selection and characterization of Chinese hamster ovary cell mutants resistant to melphalan. *Cancer Res.* **41:** 393–400.

ELSON, L. A. (1951) A study of the nutritional and other systemic factors influencing the response of host and tumour to carcinogenic and therapeutic agents, including both chemicals and ionising radiation. *Br. Emp. Cancer Camp. A. Rep.* **29:** 299–303.

ELSON, L. A. (1958) The effects of myleran (1,4-dimethane sulphonyloxybutane) and homologous compounds on the blood. *Biochem. Pharmac.* **1:** 39–47.

ELSON, L. A., JARMAN, M. and ROSS, W. C. J. (1968) Toxicity, haemotological effects and anti-tumour activity of epoxides derived from disubstituted hexitols. Mode of action of mannitol myleran and dibromomannitol. *Eur. J. Cancer* **4:** 617–625.

EPSTEIN, J., ROSENTHAL, R. W. and ESS, R. J. (1955) Use of β-(4-nitrobenzyl)pyridine as analytical reagent for ethylenimines and alkylating agents. *Anal. Chem.* **27:** 1435–1439.

EVANS, C. G., BODELL, W. J., TOKUDA, K., DOANE-SETLER, P. and SMITH, M. T. (1987) Glutathione and related enzymes in rat brain tumour cell resistance to 1,3-bis(2-chloroethyl)-1-nitrosourea and nitrogen mustard. *Cancer Res.* **47:** 2525–2530.

EVANS, T. L., CHANG, S. Y., ALBERTS, D. S., SIPES, I. G. and BRENDEL, K. (1982) In vitro degradation of L-phenylalanine mustard (L-PAM). *Cancer Chemother. Pharmac.* **8:** 175–178.

EVENAAR, A. H., WINS, E. H. R. and VAN PUTTEN, L. M. (1973) Cell killing effectiveness of an alkylating steroid (Leo 1031). *Eur. J. Cancer* **9:** 773–774.

EVERETT, J. L., ROBERTS, J. R. and ROSS, W. C. J. (1953) Aryl-2-halogenoalkylamines XII. Some carboxylic derivatives of *N,N*-di-2-chloroethylaniline. *J. Chem. Soc.* 2386–2392.

FARMER, P. B. and NEWELL, D. R. (1983) Alkylating Agents. In: *Pharmacokinetics of Anti-cancer Agents in Humans*, pp. 77–111, AMES, M. M., POWIS, G. and KOVACH, J. S. (eds) Elsevier, Amsterdam.

FARMER, P. B., FOSTER, A. B., JARMAN, M., NEWELL, D. R., ODDY, M. R. and KIBURIS, J. H. (1979) The metabolism of deuterated analogues of chlorambucil by the rat. *Chem. Biol. Interact.* **28:** 211–224.

FEIT, P. W. (1961) Stereoisomere 1,4-di-*O*-methansulfonyl-butan-1,2,3,4-tetrole. *Tetrahedron Lett.* **20:** 716–717.

FEIT, P. W. (1964) 1,4-Bis-methanesulfonates of the stereoisomeric butanetetraols and related compounds. *J. Med. Chem.* **7:** 14–17.

FENNELLY, J. F. (1979) Addisonian syndrome associated with treosulfan. *Lancet* **i:** 106.

FENNELLY, J.(1977) Treosulfan in the management of ovarian cancer. *Br. J. Obstet. Gynecol.* **84:** 300–303.

FERNO, M., BORG, A. and IDVALL, I. (1987a) Estramustine binding site in human breast cancer biopsy samples. Its relation to oestrogen and progesterone receptor levels, age and menopausal status. *Eur. J. Cancer clin. Oncol.* **23:** 1505–1510.

FERNO, M., BORG, A., INGVAR, C. and JONSSON, P. E. (1987b) Estrogen receptor and binding site for oestramustine in metastatic malignant melanoma. *Anticancer Res.* **7:** 741–744.

FISCHER, H., ZEIDLER, U., BUDNOWSKI, M., ATASSI, G., DUMONT, P., VENDITTI, J. and YODER, O. C. (1984a) Investigation of the antitumour activity of new epoxide derivatives. Part I. Triazinetrione derivatives. *Arzneim. Forsch.* **34:** 543–547.

FISCHER, H., MOELLER, H., BUDNOWSKI, M., ATASSI, G., DUMONT, P., VENDITTI, J. and YODER, O. C. (1984b)

Investigation of the antitumour activity of new epoxide derivatives. Part II. *N*-Glycidylated oxo-nitrogen heterocycles. *Arzneim. Forsch.* **34:** 663–668.

FISHER, B., SHERMAN, B., ROCKETTE, H., REDMOND, C., MARGOLESE, R. and FISHER, E. R. (1979) L-Phenylalanine mustard (L-PAM) in the management of premenopausal patients with preliminary breast cancer. *Cancer* **44:** 847–857.

FITZSIMMONS, W. E., GHALIE, R. and KAIZER, H. (1990) The effect of hepatic enzyme inducers on busulfan neurotoxicity and myelotoxicity. *Cancer Chemother. Pharmac.* **27:** 226–228.

FLORA, K. P., CRADDOCK, J. C. and KELLEY, J. A. (1982) The hydrolysis of spirohydantoin mustard. *J. Pharm. Sci.* **71:** 1206–1211.

FLORA, K. P., SMITH, S. L. and CRADDOCK, J. C. (1979) Application of a simple high-performance liquid chromatographic method for the determination of melphalan in the presence of its hydrolysis products. *J. Chromatog.* **177:** 91–97.

FOREMAN, W. W., MURRAY, A. and RONZIO, A. R. (1950) Micro-syntheses with tracer elements II Methyl bis(2-chloroethylamine hydrochloride (nitrogen mustard) and methyl bromide labelled with carbon-14. *J. Org. Chem.* **15:** 119–122.

FORSGREN, B., BJÖRK, P., CARLSTROM, K., GUSTAFSSON, J. A., POUSETTE, A. and HÖGBERG, B. (1979a) Purification and distribution of a major protein in rat prostate that binds oestramustine, a nitrogen mustard derivation of oestradiol-17. *Proc. natn. Acad. Sci. U.S.A.* **76:** 3149–3153.

FORSGREN, B., GUSTAFSSON, J. A., POUSETTE, A. and HÖGBERG, B. (1979b) Binding characteristics of a major protein in rat ventral prostate cytosol that interacts with oestramustine, a nitrogen mustard derivation of 17-oestradiol. *Cancer Res.* **39:** 5155–5164.

FORSHELL, G. P. and NILSSON, H. (1974) The distribution of radioactivity after administration of labelled oestramustine phosphate (Estracyt®), oestradiol-17 phosphate and oestradiol to rats. *Acta Pharm. Toxic.* **35 (Suppl. 1):** 28.

FORSHELL, G. P., MUNTZING, J., EK, A., LINDSTREDT, E. and DENCKER, H. (1976) The absorption, metabolism and excretion of Estracyt (NSC 89199) in patients with prostatic cancer. *Invest. Urol.* **14:** 128–131.

FRANKFURT, O. S., SECKINGER, D. and SUGARBAKER, E. V. (1990) Flow cytometric analysis of DNA damage and repair in the cells resistant to alkylating agents. *Cancer Res.* **50:** 4453–4457.

FRECKMAN, H. A., FRY, H. L., MENDEZ, F. L. and MAURER, E. R. (1964) Chlorambucil-prednisolone therapy for disseminated breast carcinoma. *J. Am. Med. Ass.* **189:** 23–26.

FREDHOLM, B., JENSEN, G., LINDSKOG, M. and MÜNTZING, J. (1974) Effects of oestramustine phosphate (Estracyt R) on growth of DMBA-induced mammary tumours in rats. *Acta Pharm. Toxic.* **35** (Suppl. 1): 28.

FRICK, H. C., TRETTER, P., TRETTER, W. and HYMAN, G. A. (1968) Disseminated carcinoma of the ovary treated by L-phenylalanine mustard. *Cancer* **21:** 508–513.

FRIDEN, B., WALLIN, M., DEINUM, J., PRASAD, V. and LUDUENA, R. (1987) Effect of oestramustine phosphate on the assembly of trypsin-treated microtubules and microtubules reconstituted from purified tubulin with either tau, MAP2, or the tubulin-binding fragment of MAP2. *Arch. Biochem. Biophys.* **257:** 123–130.

FRIEDMAN, H. S., SKAPEK, S. X., COLVIN, O. M., ELION, G. B., BLUM, M. R., SAVINA, P. M., HILTON, J., SCHOLD, S. C., KURTZBERG, J. and BIGNER, D. D. (1988) Melphalan transport, glutathione levels and glutathione-*S*-transferase activity in human medulloblastoma. *Cancer Res.* **48:** 5397–5402.

FRIEDMAN, O. M. and BOGER, E. (1961) Colorimetric estimation of nitrogen mustards in aqueous media. Hydrolytic behaviour of bis(beta-chloroethyl) amine, nor HN2. *Anal Chem.* **33:** 906–910.

FROESE, G., HANADE, J. F. and LINFORD, J. H. (1969) A comparison of the biologic activities and of the chemical properties of chlorambucil and trenimon. *Cancer Res.* **29:** 800–806.

FUJI, T. and NAKATSUKA, T. (1983) Potentiating effects of caffeine on teratogenicity of alkylating agents in mice. *Teratology* **28:** 29–33.

FUJITA, H. (1971) Comparative studies on the blood level, tissue distribution, excretion and inactivation of anticancer drugs. *Jap. J. clin. Oncol.* **1:** 151–162.

FUJIWARA, K., SAIKUSA, H., YASUNO, M. and KITAGAWA, T. (1982) Enzyme immunoassay for the quantification of mitomycin C using / galactosidase as a label. *Cancer Res.* **42:** 1487–1491.

FURNER, R. L. and BROWN, R. K. (1980) L-Phenylalanine mustard (L-PAM): the first 25 years. *Cancer Treat. Rep.* **64:** 559–574.

FURNER, R. L., BROWN, R. K. and DUNCAN, G. (1977a) Pharmacokinetics of the absorption, distribution and elimination of melphalan in the dog. *Cancer Treat. Rep.* **61:** 1637–1646.

FURNER, R. L., BROWN, R. K. and DUNCAN, G. (1977b) ^{14}C-L-phenylalanine mustard (^{14}C-L-PAM): studies on absorption, distribution, degradation and elimination in the dog. *Proc. Am. Ass. Cancer Res.* **18:** 41.

FURNER, R. L., MELLETT, L. B., BROWN, R. K. and DUNCAN, G. (1976) A method for the measurement of L-phenylalanine mustard in the mouse and dog by high-pressure liquid chromatogoraphy. *Drug Metab. Dispos.* **4:** 577–583.

GALTON, D. A. G. (1953) Myleran in chronic myeloid leukaemia. Results of treatment. *Lancet* **i:** 208–213.

GAMCSIK, M. P., HAMILL, T. G. and COLVIN, M. (1990) NMR studies of the conjugation of mechlorethamine with glutathione. *J. med. Chem.* **33:** 1009–1014.

GANDARA, D. R., GEORGE, C. B., RIES, C. A., KORETZ, M. M. and LEWIS, J. P. (1987) Treatment of refractory chronic lymphocytic leukemia with prednimustine: a Phase II study using strict response criteria. *Cancer Chemother. Pharmac.* **19:** 165–168.

GATI, E. and SOMFAI-RELLE, S. (1982) Effect of phenobarbital on the toxicity and antitumour activity of dibromodulcitol and dianhydrogalactitol. *Arzneim. Forsch.* **32:** 149–151.

GAUSS, W. (1958) Uber die Umsetzung einiger Alkoxy-*p*-benzochinone mit Ähylenimin. *Chem. Ber.* **91:** 2216–2222.

GAVER, R. C., DEEB, G., PITTMAN, K. A., ISSELL, B. F., MITTELMAN, A. and SMYTH, R. D. (1983) Disposition of orally administered ^{14}C-prednimustine in cancer patients. *Cancer Chemother. Pharmac.* **11:** 139–143.

GELEZIUNAS, R., MCQUILLAN, A., MALAPETSA, A., HUTCHINSON, M., KOPRIVA, D., WAINBERG, M. A., HISCOTT, J., BRAMSON, J. and PANASCI, L. (1991) Increased DNA synthesis and repair-enzyme expression in lymphocytes from patients with chronic lymphocytic leukemia resistant to nitrogen mustards. *J. natn. Cancer Inst.* **83:** 557–564.

GELLHORN, A., KLIGERMAN, M. M. and JAFFE, I. (1952) Triethylenemelamine in clinical cancer chemotherapy. *Am. J. Med.* **13:** 428–431.

GERA, S., MUSCH, E., OSTERHELD, H. K. O. and LOOS, U. (1989) Relevance of the hydrolysis and protein binding of melphalan to the treatment of multiple myeloma. *Cancer Chemother. Pharmac.* **23:** 76–80.

GERAN, R. I., CONGLETON, G. F., DUDECK, L. E., ABBOTT, B. J. and GARGUS, J. L. (1974) A mouse ependymoblastoma as an experimental model for screening potential antineoplastic drugs. *Cancer Chemother. Rep.* **4:** 53–87.

GHOSE, T., NORNELL, S. T., GUCLU, A., CAMERON, D., BODURTH, A. and MCDONALD, A. S. (1972) Immunochemotherapy of cancer with chlorambucil-carrying antibody. *Br. Med. J.* **3:** 495–499.

GILMAN, A. and PHILIPS, F. S. (1946) The biological actions and therapeutic applications of the chloroethyl amines and sulfides. *Science* **103:** 409–415.

GODENECHE, D., MADELMONT, J. C., SAUVEZIE, B. and BILLAUD, A. (1975) Etude de la cinetique d'absorption, de distribution et d'elimination de l'acide *N,N*-dichloro-2,ethyl,*p*-amino-phenyl-4-butyrique (chloraminophene) marque au ^{14}C chez le rat. *Biochem. Pharmac.* **24:** 1303–1308.

GOLDACRE, R. J., LOVELESS, A. and ROSS, W. C. J. (1949) Mode of production of chromosome abnormalities by the nitrogen mustards. *Nature* **163:** 667–669.

GOLDENBERG, G. J. (1974) Drug-induced stimulation of nitrogen mustard and choline transport and other systems in L5178Y lymphoblasts in vitro. *Cancer Res.* **34:** 2511–2516.

GOLDENBERG, G. J. (1976) Drug-induced stimulation of transport of hydrolyzed nitrogen mustard and choline by normal and leukemic cells in vitro. *Cancer Res.* **36:** 978–981.

GOLDENBERG, G. J. and FROESE, E. K. (1985) Antagonism of the cytocidal activity and uptake of melphalan by tamoxifen in human breast cancer cells in vitro. *Biochem. Pharmac.* **34:** 763–770.

GOLDENBERG, G. J. and SINHA, B. K. (1973a) Protection of L5178Y lymphoblasts by choline and ethanolamine against cytocidal effect of nitrogen mustard in vitro. *Cancer Res.* **33:** 1253–1257.

GOLDENBERG, G. J. and SINHA, B. K. (1973b) Nitrogen mustard sensitivity and choline transport in Walker 256 carcinsarcoma cells in vitro. *Cancer Res.* **33:** 2584–2587.

GOLDENBERG, G. J., LAM, H.-Y. P. and BEGLEITER, A. (1979) Active carrier-mediated transport of melphalan by two separate amino acid transport systems in LPC-1 plasmacytoma cells in vitro. *J. biol. Chem.* **254:** 1057–1064.

GOLDENBERG, G. J., LEE, M., LAM, H.-Y. P. and BEGLEITER, A. (1977) Evidence for carrier-mediated transport of melphalan by L5178Y lymphoblasts in vitro. *Cancer Res.* **37:** 755–760.

GOLDENBERG, G. J., LYONS, R. M., LEPP, J. A. and VANSTONE, C. L. (1971a) Sensitivity to nitrogen mustard as a function of transport activity and proliferative rate in L5178Y lymphoblasts. *Cancer Res.* **31:** 1616–1619.

GOLDENBERG, G. J., VANSTONE, C. L., ISRAELS, L. G., ILSE, D. and BIHLER, I. (1970) Evidence for a transport carrier of nitrogen mustard in nitrogen mustard-sensitive and resistant L5178Y lymphoblasts. *Cancer Res.* **30:** 2285–2291.

GOLDENBERG, G. J., VANSTONE,C. L. and BIHLER, I. (1971b) Transport of nitrogen mustard on the transport-carrier for choline in L5178Y lymphoblasts. *Science* **172:** 1148–1149.

GOLDENTHAL, E. I., NADKARNI, M. V. and SMITH, P. K. (1958) The excretion of radioactivity following administration of tri-^{14}C-ethylenimine-*S*-triazine in normal mice. *J. Pharmac. exp. Ther.* **122:** 431–441.

GOLDSTEIN, L. S. (1987) Dominant lethal mutations induced in mouse spermatogonia by mechlorethamine, procarbazine and vincristine admintered in 2-drug and 3-drug combinations. *Mutat. Res.* **191:** 171–176.

GORAS, J. T., KNIGHT, J. B., IWAMOTO, R. H. and LIM, P. (1970) Gas–liquid chromatographic determination of melphalan. *J. Pharm. Sci.* **59:** 561–563.

GORMLEY, P. E., WOOD, J. H. and POPLECK, D. G. (1981) Ability of a new antitumour drug, AZQ, to penetrate into CSF. *Pharmacology* **22:** 196–198.

GOUYETTE, A., HARTMANN, O. and PICO, J.-L. (1986) Pharmacokinetics of high-dose melphalan in children and adults. *Cancer Chemother. Pharmac.* **16:** 184–189.

GREEN, J. A., VISTICA, D. T., YOUNG, R. C., HAMILTON, T. C., ROGAN, A. M. and OZOLS, R. F. (1984) Potentiation of melphalan cytotoxicity in human ovarian cancer cell lines by glutathione depletion. *Cancer Res.* **44:** 5427–5431.

GREENE, M. H., HARRIS, E. L., GERSHENSON, D. M., MALKASIAN, G. D., MELTON, L. J., DEMBO, A. J., BENNETT, J. M., MOLONEY, W. C. and BOICE, J. D. (1986) Melphalan may be a more potent leukemogen than cyclophosphamide. *Ann. intern. Med.* **105:** 360–367.

GREIG, N. H., DALY, E. M. SWEENEY, D. J. and RAPOPORT, S. I. (1990a) Pharmacokinetics of chlorambucil-tertiary butyl ester, a lipophilic chlorambucil derivative that achieves and maintains high concentrations in brain. *Cancer Chemother. Pharmac.* **25:** 320–325.

GREIG, N. H., GENKA, S., DALY, E. M., SWEENEY, D. J. and RAPOPORT, S. I. (1990b) Physicochemical and pharmacokinetic parameters of seven lipophilic chlorambucil esters designed for brain penetration. *Cancer Chemother. Pharmac.* **25:** 311–319.

GREIG, N. H., MOMMA, S., SWEENEY, D. J., SMITH, Q. R. and RAPOPORT, S. I. (1987) Facilitated transport of melphalan at the rat blood–brain barrier by the large neutral amino acid carrier system. *Cancer Res.* **47:** 1571–1576.

GREIG, N. H., STAHLE, P. L., SHETTY, H. V., GENKA, S., JOHN, V., SONCRANT, T. T. and RAPOPORT, S. I. (1990c) High-performance liquid chromatographic analysis of chlorambucil tert-butyl ester and its active metabolites chlorambucil and phenylacetic mustard in plasma and tissue. *J. Chromatog. Biomed. Appl.* **534:** 279–286.

GREIG, N. H., SWEENEY, D. J. and RAPOPORT, S. I. (1988) Comparative brain and plasma pharmacokinetics and anticancer activities of chlorambucil and melphalan in the rat. *Cancer Chemother. Pharmac.* **21:** 1–8.

GRIFFIN, J. P., NEWMAN, R. A., MCCORMACK, J. J. and KRAKOFF, I. H. (1982) Clinical and clinical pharmacologic studies of aziridinylbenzoquinone. *Cancer Treat. Rep.* **66:** 1321–1325.

GROCHOW, L. B., GROSSMAN, S., GARRETT, S., MURRAY, K., TRUMP, D. and COLVIN, M. (1982) Pharmacokinetics of intraventricular thio-TEPA (TT) in patients with meningeal carcinomatosis. *Proc. Am. Soc. clin. Oncol.* **1:** 19.

GROCHOW, L. B., JONES, R. J., BRUNDRETT, R. B., BRAINE, H. G., CHEN, T.-L., SARAL, R., SANTOS, G. W. and COLVIN, O. M. (1989) Pharmacokinetics of busulfan: correlation with veno-occlusive disease in patients undergoing bone marrow transplantation. *Cancer Chemother. Pharmac.* **25:** 55–61.

GRUENEBERG, D. A., OJWANG, J. O., BENASUTTI, M., HARTMAN, S. and LOECHLER, E. L. (1991) Construction of a human shuttle vector containing a single nitrogen mustard interstrand DNA–DNA cross-link at a unique plasmid location. *Cancer Res.* **51** 2268–2272.

GRUNICKE, H., DOPPLER, W., FINCH, S. A. E., GREINERT, R., GRÜNEWALD, K., HOFMANN, J., MALY, K., STIER, A., SCHEIDL, F. and THOMAS, J. K. (1985) Effects of nitrogen mustard on potassium transport systems and membrane structure of Ehrlich ascites tumour cells. *Adv. Eng. Reg.* **23:** 277–290.

GRUNICKE, H., PUTZER, H., SCHEIDL, F., WOLFF-SCREINER, E. and GRUNEWALD, K. (1982) Inhibition of tumour growth by alkylation of the plasma membrane. *Biosci. Rep.* **2:** 601–604.

GULATI, D. K., WOJCIECHOWSKI, J. P. and KAUR, P. (1990) Comparison of single-, double- or triple-exposure protocols for the rodent bone marrow/peripheral blood micronucleus assay using 4-aminobiphenyl and treosulphan. *Mutat. Res.* **234:** 135–139.

GUNNARSSON, P. O., ANDERSON, S.-B. and JOHANSSON, S.-A. (1983) The hydrolysis of oestramustine phosphate; in vitro studies. *Eur. J. Drug Metab. Pharmac.* **8:** 395–402.

GUNNARSSON, P. O., JOHANSSON, S.-Å. and SVENSSON, L. (1984) Cholesterol ester formation by transesterification of chlorambucil: a novel pathway in drug metabolism. *Xenobiotica* **14:** 569–574.

GUNNARSSON, P.-O., FORSHELL, G. P., FRITJOFSSON, A. and NORLEN, B. J. (1981) Plasma concentrations of oestramustine phosphate and its major metabolites in patients with prostatic carcinoma treated with different doses of oestramustine phosphate (Estracyt®). *Scand. J. Urol. Nephrol.* **15:** 201–205.

GUPTA, V., SINGH, S. V., AHMAD, H., MEDH, R. D. and AWASTHI, Y. C. (1989) Glutathione and glutathione-S-transferases in a human plasma cell line resistant to melphalan. *Biochem. Pharmac.* **38:** 1993–2000.

GUTIERREZ, P. I., FRIEDMAN, R. D. and BACHUR, N. R. (1982) Biochemical activation of AZQ [3,6-diaziridinyl-2,5-bis(carboethoxyamino)-1,4-benzoquinone] to its free radical species. *Cancer Treat. Rep.* **66:** 339–342.

GUTIERREZ, P. L., NAYAR, M. S. B., NARDINO, R. and CALLERY, P. S. (1987) The chemical reduction of diaziquone: products and free radical intermediates. *Chem.-Biol. Interact.* **64:** 23–37.

HACES, A., DRISCOLL, J. S., ROTH, J. S., HEIDEMAN, R. L. and KELLEY, J. A. (1986) Spiromustine analogs. Relationships between structure, plasma stability and antitumour activity. *J. Pharmac. Sci.* **75:** 313–316.

HADDOW, A. and TIMMIS, G. M. (1953) Myleran in chronic myeloid leukaemia. Chemical constitution and biological action. *Lancet* **i:** 207–208.

HAGEN, B. and NILSEN, O. G. (1987) The binding of thio-TEPA in human serum and to isolated serum protein fractions. *Cancer Chemother. Pharmac.* **20:** 319–323.

HAGEN, B., NEVERDAL, G., WALSTAD, R. A. and NILSEN, O. G. (1990) Long-term pharmacokinetics of thio-TEPA, TEPA and total alkylating activity following i. v. bolus administration of thio-TEPA in ovarian cancer patients. *Cancer Chemother. Pharmac.* **25:** 257–262.

HAGEN, B., WALSETH, F., WALSTAD, R. A. and IVERSEN, T. (1985) Gas chromatographic assay of triethylenethiophosphoramide in serum and urine. *J. Chromatog.* **345:** 173–177.

HAGEN, B., WALSETH, F., WASTAD, R. A., IVERSEN, T. and NILSEN, O. G. (1987) Single and repeated dose pharmacokinetics of thio-TEPA in patients treated for ovarian carcinoma. *Cancer Chemother. Pharmac.* **19:** 143–148.

HAGEN, B., WALSTAD, R. A. and NILSEN, O. G. (1988) Pharmacokinetics of thio-TEPA at two different doses. *Cancer Chemother. Pharmac.* **22:** 356–358.

HALL, A., ROBSON, C. N., HICKSON, I. D., HARRIS, A. L., PROCTOR, S. J. and CATTAN, A. R. (1989) Possible role of inhibition of glutathione-*S*-transferase in the partial reversal of chlorambucil resistance by indomethacin in a Chinese hamster ovary cell line. *Cancer Res.* **49:** 6265–6268.

HAMANA, K., KAWADA, K., SUGIOKA, K., NAKANO, M., TERO-KUBOTA, S. and IKEGAMI, Y. (1985) DNA strand scission by enzymatically reduced mitomycin C: evidence for participation of the hydroxyl radical in the DNA damage. *Biochem. Int.* **10:** 301–309.

HAMILTON, T. C., WINKER, M. A., LOWIE, K. G., BATIST, G., BEHRENS, B. C., TSURUO, T., GROTZINGER, K. R., MCKOY, W. M., YOUNG, R. C. and OZOLS, R. F. (1985) Augmentation of adriamycin, melphalan and cisplatin cytotoxicity in drug-resistant and sensitive human ovarian carcinoma cell lines by buthionine sulfoximine mediated glutathione depletion. *Biochem. Pharmac.* **34:** 2583–2586.

HAMPEL, K. E., KOBER, B., RÖSCH, D., GERHARTZ, H. and MEINIG, K.-H. (1966) The action of cytostatic agents on the chromosomes of human leukocytes in vitro. *Blood* **27:** 816–823.

HANBY, W. E., HARTLEY, G. S., POWELL, E. O. and RYDON, H. N. (1947) The chemistry of 2-chloroalkylamines Part II. Reactions of tertiary 2-chloroalkylamines in water. *J. Chem. Soc.* pp. 519–527.

HANDA, K. and SATO, S. (1975) Generation of free radicals of quinone group-containing anti-cancer chemicals in NADPH-microsome system as evidenced by initiation of sulfite oxidation. *Gann* **66:** 43–47.

HANSSON, J., BERHANE, K., CASTRO, V. M., JUNGNELIUS, U., MANNERVIK, B. and RINGBORG, W. (1991) Sensitization of human melanoma cells to the cytotoxic effect of melphalan by the glutathione transferase inhibitor ethacrynic acid. *Cancer Res.* **51:** 94–98.

HANSSON, J., EDGREN, M., EHRSSON, H., RINGBORG, U. and NILSSON, B. (1988) Effect of D,L-buthionine-*S,R*-sulfoximine on cytotoxicity and DNA cross-linking induced by bifunctional DNA-reactive cytostatic drugs in human melanoma cells. *Cancer Res.* **48:** 19–26.

HANSSON, J., LEWENSOHN, R., RINGBORG, W. and NILSSON, B. (1987) Formation and removal of DNA cross-links induced by melphalan and nitrogen mustard in relation to drug-induced cytotoxicity in human melanoma cells. *Cancer Res.* **47:** 2631–2637.

HARRAP, K. R. and HILL, B. T. (1970) The selectivity of action of alkylating agents and drug resistance III. The uptake and degradation of alkylating drugs by Yoshida ascites sarcoma cells in vitro. *Biochem. Pharmac.* **19:** 209–217.

HARRAP, K. R., RICHES, P. G., GILBY, E. D., SELLWOOD, S. M., WILKINSON, R. and KONYVES, I. (1977) Studies on the toxicity and antitumour activity of prednimustine, a prednisolone ester of chlorambucil. *Eur. J. Cancer* **13:** 873–881.

HART, R. D., PERLOFF, M. and HOLLAND, J. F. (1981) One-day VATH (Vinblastine, adriamycin, thio-TEPA and halotestin) therapy for advanced breast cancer refractory to chemotherapy. *Cancer* **48:** 1522–1527.

HARTLEY, J. A., FORROW, S. M. and SOUHAMI, R. L. (1990) Effect of ionic strength and cationic DNA affinity binders on the DNA sequence selective alkylation of guanine-N7-positions by nitrogen mustard. *Biochemistry* **29:** 2985–2991.

HARTLEY-ASP, B. (1984) Estramustine induced mitotic arrest in two human prostatic carcinoma cell-lines DU 145 and PC 3. *Prostate* **5:** 93–100.

HARTLEY-ASP, B. (1986) The antitumour effects of prednimustine in vitro and in vivo. *Sem. Oncol.* **13** (Suppl. 1): 3–7.

HARTLEY-ASP, B. and GUNNARSSON, P.-O. (1982a) Cytotoxicity and mode of action of oestramustine, the dephosphorylated metabolite of estracyt R and its components in the human prostatic carcinoma cell line DU 145. *Proc. Am. Ass. Cancer Res.* **23:** 168.

HARTLEY-ASP, B. and GUNNARSSON, P.-O. (1982b) Growth and cell survival following treatment with oestramustine, nor-nitrogen mustard, oestradiol and testosterone of a human prostatic cancer cell line (DU 145). *J. Urol.* **127:** 818–822.

HARTLEY-ASP, B. and KRUSE, E. (1986) Nuclear protein matrix as a target for oestramustine-induced cell death. *Prostate* **9:** 387–395.

HARTLEY-ASP, B., GUNNARSSON, P. O. and LILJEKVIST, J. (1986) Cytotoxicity and metabolism of prednimustine, chlorambucil and prednisolone in a Chinese hamster cell line. *Cancer Chemother. Pharmac.* **16:** 85–90.

HASHIMOTO, Y. and SHUDO, K. (1985) Chemical modification of DNA with mutacarcinogens. III. Reductive alkylation of DNA with mitomycin C. *Environ. Health Perspec.* **62:** 219–222.

HASHIMOTO, Y., SHUDO, K. and OKAMOTO, T. (1983) Modification of deoxyribonucleic acid with reductive activated mitomycin C. Structures of modified nucleotides. *Chem. Pharm. Bull.* **31:** 861–869.

HASSAN, M. and EHRSSON, H. (1983) Gas chromatographic determination of busulfan in plasma with electron-capture detection. *J. Chromatog.* **277:** 374–380.

HASSAN, M. and EHRSSON, H. (1986) Metabolism of ^{14}C-busulfan in isolated perfused rat liver. Proc. 10th European Drug Metabolism Workshop, Guildford, U.K. 6–11 July, 1986, p. 93.

HASSAN, M. and EHRSSON, H. (1987a) Metabolism of ^{14}C-busulfan in isolated perfused rat liver. *Eur. J. Drug Metab. Pharmac.* **12:** 71–76.

HASSAN, M. and EHRSSON, H. (1987b) Urinary metabolites of busulfan in the rat. *Drug Metab. Disp.* **15:** 399–402.

HASSAN, M., ÖBERG, G., BEKASSY, A. N., ASCHAN, J., EHRSSON, H., LJUNGMAN, P., LONNERHOLM, G., SMEDMYR, B., TAUBE, A., WALLIN, I. and SIMONSSON, B. (1991) Pharmacokinetics of high-dose busulphan in relation to age and chronopharmacology. *Cancer Chemother. Pharmac.* **28:** 130–134.

HASSAN, M., ÖBERG, G., EHRSSON, H., EHRNEBO, M., WALLIN, I., SMEDMYR, B., TÖTTERMAN, T., EKSBORG, S. and SIMONSSON, B. (1989) Pharmacokinetic and metabolic studies of high-dose busulphan in adults. *Eur. J. clin. Pharmac.* **36:** 525–530.

HASSAN, M., EHRSSON, H., WALLIN, I. and EKSBORG, S. (1988) Pharmacokinetic and metabolic studies of busulfan in rat plasma and brain. *Eur. J. Drug Metab. Pharmac.* **13:** 301–305.

HATA, T., SANO, Y., SUGAWARA, R., MATSUMAE, A., KANAMORI, K., SHIMNA, T. and HOSHI, T. (1956) Mitomycin, a new antibiotic from *Streptomyces*. I. *J. Antibiotics* **9:** 141–146.

HEDLEY, D. W., MCELWAIN, T. J., MILLAR, J. L. and GORDON, M. Y. (1978) Acceleration of bone-marrow recovery by pre-treatment with cyclophosphamide in patients receiving high-dose melphalan. *Lancet* **ii:** 966–967.

HEIDEMAN, R. L., COLE, D. E., BALIS, F., SATO, J., REAMAN, G. H., PACKER, R. J., SINGHER, L. J., ETTINGER, L. J., GILLESPIE, A., SAM, J. and POPLACK, D. G. (1989) Phase I and pharmacokinetic evaluation of thio-TEPA in the cerebrospinal fluid and plasma of pediatric patients: evidence for dose-dependent plasma clearance of thio-TEPA. *Cancer Res.* **49:** 736–741.

HEIDEMAN, R. L., KELLEY, J. A., PACKER, R. J., REAMAN, G. H., ROTH, J. S., BALIS, F., ETTINGER, L. J., DOHERTY, K. M., JEFFRIES, S. L. and POPLACK, D. G. (1988) A pediatric Phase I and pharmacokinetic study of spirohydantoin mustard. *Cancer Res.* **48:** 2292–2295.

HELLIGER, W., HOFMANN, J., MALY, K., DOPPLER, W., HERMANN, B.-J., HOCK, W., PUSCHENDORF, B. and GRUNICKE, H. (1988) Differential sensitivity of histone acetylation in nitrogen-mustard sensitive and resistant cells. Relation to drug uptake, formation and repair of DNA-interstrand cross-links. *Eur. J. Cancer clin. Oncol.* **24:** 1861–1868.

HENDRY, J. A., HOMER, R. F., ROSE, F. L. and WALPOLE, A. L. (1951) Cytotoxic agents: III Derivatives of ethyleneimine. *Br. J. Pharmac.* **6:** 357–410.

HENNER, W. D., FURLONG, E. A., FLAHERTY, M. D., SHEA, T. C. and PETERS, W. P. (1987) Measurement of busulfan in plasma by high-performance liquid chromatography. *J. Chromatog.* **416:** 426–432.

HENNER, W. D., FURLONG, E. A., KELLEY, S. L. and ROSOWSKY, A. (1985) Assay for mitolactol and its bifunctional alkylating metabolites in plasma. *J. Pharmac. Sci.* **74:** 983–986.

HENRIKSSON, R., BJERMER, L., VON SCHOULTZ, E. and GRANKVIST, K. (1990) The effect of oestramustine on microtubuli is different from the direct action via oxygen radicals on DNA and cell membrane. *Anticancer Res.* **10:** 303–310.

HESTON, W. E. (1949) Induction of pulmonary tumours in strain A mice with methylbis(chloroethyl)amine hydrochloride. *J. natn. Cancer Inst.* **10:** 125–130.

HESTON, W. E. (1950) Carcinogenic action of the mustards. *J. natn. Cancer Inst.* **11:** 415–423.

HILL, B. T. (1972) Studies on the transport and cellular distribution of chlorambucil in the Yoshida ascites sarcoma. *Biochem. Pharmac.* **21:** 495–502.

HILL, B. T. (1975) Differential effects of cytotoxic concentrations of chlorambucil on drug-resistant and drug-sensitive cell lines of the Yoshida ascites sarcoma in culture. *Eur. J. Cancer* **11:** 9–16.

HILL, B. T. and HARRAP, K. R. (1972) The uptake and utilization of chlorambucil by lymphocytes from patients with chronic lymphocytic leukaemia. *Br. J. Cancer* **26:** 439–443.

HILL, B. T. and RICHES, P. G. (1971) The absorption, distribution and excretion of ^{3}H-chlorambucil in rats bearing the Yoshida ascites sarcoma. *Br. J. Cancer* **25:** 831–837.

HILL, B. T., JARMAN, M. and HARRAP, K. R. (1971) Selectivity of action of alkylating agents and drug resistance. 4. Synthesis of tritium-labelled chlorambucil and a study of its cellular uptake by drug-sensitive and drug-resistant strains of the Yoshida ascites sarcoma in vitro. *J. med. Chem.* **14:** 614–618.

HILTON, J., SESSIONS, R. H. and WALKER, M. D. (1977) Cross-linking of DNA in rat brain tumour and bone marrow by spirohydantoin mustard (SHM). *Proc. Am. Ass. Cancer Res.* **18:** 112.

HINCHLIFFE, M., NCNALLY, N. J. and STRATFORD, M. R. L. (1983) The effect of radiosensitizers on the pharmacokinetics of melphalan and cyclophosphamide in the mouse. *Br. J. Cancer* **48:** 375–383.

HOBAN, P. R., WALTON, M. I., ROBSON, C. N., GODDEN, J., STRATFORD, I. J., WORKMAN, P., HARRIS, A. L. and HICKSON, I. D. (1990) Decreased NADPH: cytochrome P-450 reductase activity and impaired drug activation in a mammalian cell line resistant to mitomycin C under aerobic but not hypoxic conditions. *Cancer Res.* **50:** 4692–4697.

HOEY, B. M., BUTLER, J. and SWALLOW, A. J. (1988) Reductive activation of mitomycin C. *Biochemistry* **27:** 2608–2614.

HOFMANN, J., DOPPLER, W., JAKOB, A., MALY, K., POSCH, L., UBERALL, F. and GRUNICKE, H. H. (1988) Enhancement of the antiproliferative effect of *cis*-diamminedichloroplatinum (II) and nitrogen mustard by inhibitors of protein kinase C. *Int. J. Cancer* **42:** 382–388.

HOLCENBERG, J., ANDERSON, T., RITCH, P., SKIBBA, J., HOWSER, D., RING, B. and ADAMS, S. (1983) Intraperitoneal chemotherapy with melphalan plus glutaminase. *Cancer Res.* **43:** 1381–1388.

HORNEMANN, U., HO, Y. K., MACKEY, J. K. and SRIVASTAVA, S. C. (1976) Studies on the mode of action of the mitomycin antibiotics. Reversible conversion of mitomycin C into sodium 7-aminomitosane-9a-sulphonate. *J. Am. Chem. Soc.* **98:** 7069–7074.

HORNEMANN, U., KELLER, P. J. and KOZLOWSKI, J. F. (1979) Formation of 1-ethylxanthyl-2,7-diaminomitosene and 1,10-diethylxanthyl-2,7-diaminodecarbamoyl mitosene in aqueous solution upon reduction–reoxidation of mitomycin C in the presence of potassium ethylxanthate. *J. Am. Chem. Soc.* **101:** 7121–7124.

HORSMAN, M. R., EVANS, J. W. and BROWN, J. M. (1984) Enhancement of melphalan-induced tumour cell killing by misonidazole: an interaction of competing mechanisms. *Br. J. Cancer* **50:** 305–316.

HORVATH, I. P., CSETENYI, J., KERPEL-FRONIUS, S., HINDY, I. and ECKHARDT, S. (1979) Metabolism and pharmacokinetics of dibromodulcitol (DBD, NSC-104800) in man. I. Metabolites of DBD. *Eur. J. Cancer* **15:** 337–344.

HORVATH, I. P., CSETENYI, J., KERPEL-FRONIUS, S., INSTITORIS, L., HEGEDUS, L. and ECKHARDT, S. (1982a)

Metabolism and pharmacokinetics of dibromodulcitol (DBD, NSC-104800) in man. II. Pharmacokinetics of DBD. *Eur. J. Cancer clin. Oncol.* **18:** 1211–1219.

HORVATH, I. P., CSETENYI, J., KERPEL-FRONIUS, S., HELEDUS, L., KANYAR, B. and ECKHARDT, S. (1986) Pharmacokinetics and metabolism of dianhydrogalactitol DAG in patients: a comparison with the human disposition of dibromodulcitol DBD. *Eur. J. Cancer clin. Oncol.* **22:** 163–171.

HORVATH, I. P., SOMFAI-RELLE, S., HEGEDUS, L. and JARMAN, M. (1982b) Toxicity, antitumour and haematological effects of 1,2-anhydro-6-bromo-galactitol and D-mannitol: a comparison with the related dibromo- and dianhydro-derivatives. *Eur. J. Cancer clin. Oncol.* **18:** 573–577.

HOWELL, S. B., PFEIFLE, C. E. and OLSHEN, R. A. (1984) Intraperitoneal chemotherapy with melphalan. *Ann. intern. Med.* **101:** 14–18.

HU, E. and HOWELL, S. B. (1983) Pharmacokinetics of intra-arterial mitomycin C in humans. *Cancer Res.* **43:** 4474–4477.

HUDSON, R. F., TIMMIS, G. M. and MARSHALL, R. D. (1959) A physico-chemical investigation into the biological action of myleran and related sulphonic acid esters. *Biochem. Pharmac.* **1:** 48–59.

I.A.R.C. (1975a) *Monograph on the Evaluation of Carcinogenic Risk of Chemicals to Man, Vol.* 9. *Some aziridines* N-, S- and O-mustards and selenium, pp. 85–94, I.A.R.C., Lyon.

I.A.R.C. (1975b) *Monograph on the Evaluation of Carcinogenic risk of Chemicals to Man, Vol.* 9. *Some aziridines* N-, S- and O-mustards and selenium, pp. 193–207, I.A.R.C., Lyon.

I.A.R.C. (1979) *Evaluation of Carcinogenic Risk of Chemicals to Humans*, p. 37, I.A.R.C., Lyon.

I.A.R.C. (1981) *Monographs on the evaluation of the carcinogenic risk of chemicals to humans. Vol.* 26. *Some antineoplastic and immunosuppressive agents*, pp. 115–136, I.A.R.C., Lyon.

I.A.R.C. (1982a) *Monographs on the evaluation of the carcinogenic risk of chemicals to humans* pp. 170–172, I.A.R.C., Lyon

I.A.R.C. (1982b) *Monographs on the evaluation of the carcinogenic risk of chemicals to humans.* pp. 68–71, I.A.R.C., Lyon.

INABA, M. (1973) Mechanism of resistance of Yoshida sarcoma to nitrogen mustard. III. Mechanism of supressed transport of nitrogen mustard. *Int. J. Cancer* **11:** 231–236.

INABA, M. and SAKURAI, Y. (1971) Mechanism of resistance of Yoshida sarcoma to nitrogen mustard. *Int. J. Cancer* **7:** 430–435.

INABA, M. and SAKURAI, Y. (1977) Role of DNA repair in natural resistance of rat ascites hepatomas to nitogen mustard. *Gann* **68:** 15–19.

INSTITORIS, E. and FOX, B. W. (1978) The interaction of dianhydrogalactitol with DNA in cultured Yoshida sarcoma cells. *Chem.-Biol. Interact.* **22:** 99–107.

INSTITORIS, E. and TAMAS, J. (1980) Alkylation by 1,2:5,6-dianhydrogalactitol of deoxyribonucleic acid and guanosine. *Biochem. J.* **185:** 659–666.

INSTITORIS, L. (1981) In vivo study on alkylation site in DNA by the bifunctional dianhydrogalactitol. *Chem.-Biol. Interact.* **35:** 207–216.

INSTITORIS, L., DZURILLAY, E. and PETHES, G. (1973) Comparative studies on the in vivo distribution pattern of dibromodulcitol and diepoxydulcitol. *Z. Krebsforsch.* **79:** 49–59.

ISRAELS, L. G. and RITZMANN, S. E.(1960) Laboratory and clinical studies on a new azo-mustard, 4-di-2″-chloroethylamino-2-methylazo-benzene-2-carboxylic acid (CB 1414) *Acta Un. Int. Contra. Cancrum.* **16:** 665–672.

IYENGAR, B. S., DORR, R. T., SHIPP, N. G. and REMERS, W. A. (1990) Alkylation of DNA by C-10 of 2,7-diaminomitosene. *J. med. Chem.* **33:** 253–257.

IYER, V. N. and SZYBALSKI, W. (1963) A molecular mechanism of mitomycin action: linking of complementary DNA strands. *Proc. natn. Acad. Sci. U.S.A.* **50:** 355–362.

IYER, V. N. and SZYBALSKI, W. (1964) Mitomycins and porfiromycin: chemical mechanism of activation and cross-linking of DNA. *Science* **145:** 55–58.

JÖHNSSON, G., HÖGBERG, B. and NILSSON, T. (1977) Treatment of advanced prostatic cancer with oestramustine phosphate (Estracyt R). *Scand. J. Urol. Nephrol.* **11:** 231–238.

JÖNSSON, P.-E., INGVAR, C., FERNO, M., HAFSTRÖM, L. and RUDENSTAM, C.-M. (1988) Phase II study of oestramustine phosphate (Estracyt®) in patients with metastatic melanoma. *Eur. J. Cancer clin. Oncol.* **24:** 413–415.

JAKHAMMER, T., OLSSON, A. and SVENSSON, L. (1977) Mass fragmentographic determination of prednimustine and chlorambucil in plasma. *Acta Pharm. Suec.* **14:** 485–496.

JENEY, A., CONNORS, T. A. and JONES, M. (1978) The toxicity of merophan after pretreatment with subtoxic dose. *Acta Phys. Hung.* **33:** 89–94.

JOHNSSON, J. E., TROPE, C., MATTSSON, W., GRUNDSELL, H., ASPEGREN, K. and KONYVES, I. (1979) Phase II study of Leo 1031 (Prednimustine) in advanced ovarian carcinoma. *Cancer Treat. Rep.* **63:** 421–424.

JOHNSTON, J. B., ISRAELS, L. G., GOLDENBERG, G. J., ANHALT, C. D., VERBURG, L., MOWAT, M. R. A. and BEGLEITER, A. (1990) Glutathione-*S*-transferase activity, sulphydryl levels and DNA cross-linking activity with chlorambucil in chronic lymphocytic leukemia. *J. natn. Cancer Inst.* **82:** 776–779.

JOSTES, R. F., WILLIAMS, M. E. and DEEN, D. F. (1985) The effect of treatment with single and split doses of spirohydantoin mustard on the growth delay of 9L rat brain tumour multicellular spheroids. *Eur. J. Cancer clin. Oncol.* **21:** 975–979.

KÖNYVES, I., NORDENSKJÖLD, B., FORSHELL, G. P., DE SCHRYVER, A. and WESTERBERG-LARSSON, H. (1975)

Preliminary clinical and absorption studies with prednimustine in patients with mammary carcinoma. *Eur. J. Cancer* **11:** 841–844.

KADOHAMA, N., KIRDANI, R. Y., MADAJEWICZ, S., MURPHY, G. P. and SANDBERG, A. A. (1979) Estramustine. Metabolic pattern and possible mechanisms for its action in prostate cancer. *N.Y. State J. Med.* **79:** 1005–1009.

KADOHAMA, N., KIRDANI, R. Y., MURPHY, G. P. and SANDBERG, A. A. (1978) Estramustine phosphate: metabolic aspects related to its action in prostatic cancer. *J. Urol.* **119:** 235–239.

KALLAMA, S. and HEMMINKI, K. (1986) Stabilities of 7-alkylguanosines and 7-deoxyguanosines formed by phosphoramide mustard and nitrogen mustard. *Chem-Biol. Interact.* **57:** 85–96.

KALYANARAMAN, B., PEREZ-REYES, E. and MASON, R. P. (1980) Spin-trapping and direct electron spin resonance investigations of the redox mechanism of quinone anticancer drugs. *Biochim. biophys. Acta* **630:** 119–130.

KANJE, M., DEINUM, J., WALLIN, M., EKSTRÖM, P., EDSTRÖM, A. and HARTLEY-ASP, B. (1985) Effect of oestramustine phosphate on the assembly of isolated bovine brain micro-tubules and fast axonal transport in the frog sciatic nerve. *Cancer Rep.* **45:** 2234–2239.

KAPLAN, D. J. and TOMASZ, M. (1982) Altered physicochemical properties of the deoxyribonucleic acid-mitomycin C complex. Evidence for a conformational change in deoxyribonucleic acid. *Biochemistry* **21:** 3006–3013.

KARCHMER, R. K., AMARE,M., LARSEN, W. E., MALLOUK, A. G. and CALDWELL, G. G. (1974) Alkylating agents as leukaemogens in multiple myeloma. *Cancer* **33:** 1103–1107.

KATO, S., YAMASHITA, K., KIM, T., TAJIRI, T., ONDA, M. and SATO, S. (1988) Modification of DNA by mitomycin C in cancer patients detected by ^{32}P-postlabeling analysis. *Mutat. Res.* **202:** 85–91.

KAZEMIFARD, A. G. and MORGAN, D. J. (1990) Determination of busulfan in plasma by high performance liquid chromatography. *J. Chromatog. Biomed. Appl.* **528:** 274–276.

KELLEY, J. A. and CHONG, E. D. S. (1981) Reverse phase HPLC determination of AZQ in biological fluids. *J. Liq. Chromatog.* **4:** 1855–1867.

KELLEY, S. L., PETERS, W. P., ANDERSEN, J., FURLONG, E. A., FREI, E. and HENNER, W. D. (1986) Pharmacokinetics of dibromodulcitol in humans: a phase I study. *J. clin. Oncol.* **4:** 753–761.

KELLIE, S. J. and KINGSTON, J. E. (1987) Ovarian failure after high-dose melphalan in adolescents. *Lancet* **i:** 1425.

KENNEDY, K. A. and SARTORELLI, A. C. (1979) Metabolic activation of mitomycin C by isolated liver nuclei and microsomes. *Fed. Proc.* **38:** 443.

KENNEDY, K. A., MCGURL, J. D., LEONDARIDIS, L. and ALABASKER, O. (1985a) pH dependence of mitomycin C-induced cross-linking activity in EMT6 tumour cells. *Cancer Res.* **45:** 3541–3547.

KENNEDY, K. A., MIMNAUGH, E. G., TRUSH, M. A. and SINHA, B. K. (1985b) Effects of glutathione and ethyl xanthate on mitomycin C activation by isolated rat hepatic or EMT6 mouse mammary tumour nuclei. *Cancer Res.* **45:** 4071–4076.

KENNEDY, K. A., ROCKWELL, S. and SARTORELLI, A. C. (1980) Preferential activation of mitomycin C to cytotoxic metabolites by hypoxic tumour cells. *Cancer Res.* **40:** 2356–2360.

KENNEDY, K. A., SLIGAR, S. G., POLOMSKI, L. and SARTORELLI, A. C. (1982) Metabolic activation of mitomycin C by liver microsomes and nuclei. *Biochem. Pharmac.* **31:** 2011–2016.

KESSEL, D. and THOMPSON, P. (1986) Photosensitization of leukaemia L1210 cells with diaziquone. *Cancer Res.* **46:** 5587–5588.

KESSEL, D., MYERS, M. and WODINSKY, I. (1969) Accumulation of two alkylating agents, nitrogen mustard and busulfan, by murine leukemia cells in vitro. *Biochem. Pharmac.* **18:** 1229–1234.

KEYES, S. R., FRACASSO, P. M., HEIMBROOK, D. C., ROCKWELL, S., SLIGAR, S. G. and SARTORELLI, A. C. (1984) Role of NADPH: Cytochrome C reductase and DT-diaphorase in the bio-transformation of mitomycin C. *Cancer Res.* **44:** 5638–5643.

KEYES, S. R., ROCKWELL, S. and SARTORELLI, A. C. (1985) Enhancement of mitomycin C cytotoxicity to hypoxic tumour cells by dicoumarol in vivo and in vitro. *Cancer Res.* **45:** 213–216.

KHAN, A. H. and DRISCOLL, J. S. (1976) Potential central nervous system antitumour agents. Aziridinylbenzoquinones I. *J. Med. Chem.* **19:** 313–317.

KIMURA, T., STERNSON, L. A. and HIGUCHI, T. (1976) Gas-chromatographic analysis for 1,2:5,6-dianhydrogalactitol, an anti-neoplastic agent, in plasma. *Clin. Chem.* **22:** 1639–1643.

KING, C. L., HITTELMAN, W. N. and LOO, T. L. (1984a) Induction of DNA strand breaks and cross-links by 2,5-diaziridinyl-3,6-bis(carboethoxyamino)-1,4-benzoquinone in Chinese hamster ovary cells. *Cancer Res.* **44:** 5634–5637.

KING, C. L., WONG, S.-K. and LOO, T. L. (1984b) Alkylation of DNA by the new anticancer agent 3,6-diaziridinyl-2,5-bis(carboethoxyamino)-1,4-benzoquinone (AZQ). *Eur. J. Cancer clin. Oncol.* **20:** 261–264.

KIRDANI, R. Y., MÜNTZING, J., VARKARAKIS, M. J., MURPHY, G. P. and SANDBERG, A. A. (1974) Studies on the antiprostatic action of estracyt, a nitrogen mustard of oestradiol. *Cancer Res.* **34:** 1031–1037.

KIRDANI, R. Y., MITTELMAN, A., MURPHY, G. P. and SANDBERG, A. A. (1975) Studies on phenolic steroids in human subjects. XIV. Fate of a nitrogen mustard of oestradiol-17. *J. clin. Endocr. Metab.* **41:** 305–318.

KIRDANI, R. Y., MURPHY, G. P. and SANDBERG, A. A. (1977) Studies on a nitrogen mustard of oestradiol in dogs and rats. *Proc. Soc. exp. Biol. Med.* **155:** 94–98.

KIRDANI, R. Y., MURPHY, G. P. and SANDBERG, A. A. (1978) Some metabolic aspects of a nitrogen mustard of prednisolone. *Oncology* **35:** 47–53.

KITAMURA, S. and TATSUMI, K. (1983) Azoreductase activity of liver aldehyde oxidase. *Chem. Pharm. Bull.* **31:** 3334–3337.

KLAMERTH, O. L. and KAPUN, M. (1971) The influence of trenimon upon deoxyribonucleic acid in vitro. *Eur. J. Biochem.* **21:** 199–203.

KLATT, O., GRIFFIN, A. C. and STEHLIN, J. S. (1960) Method for determination of phenylalanine mustard and related alkylating agents in blood. *Proc. Soc. exp. Biol. Med.* **104:** 629–631.

KLIGERMAN, A. D., EREXSON, G. L., WILMER, J. L. and SCHOLD, S. C. (1987) Sister chromatid exchange induction in patients with anaplastic gliomas undergoing treatment with radiation plus diaziquone or 1,3-bis(2-chloroethyl)-1-nitrosourea. *Cancer Res.* **47:** 631–635.

KOBAYASHI, T., BLASBERG, R. G., PATLAK, C. S. and FENSTERMACHER, J. D. (1979) Spirohydantoin mustard (NSC 172112) penetration of brain and systemic organs. *Proc. Am. Ass. Cancer Res.* **20:** 104.

KODAMA, M. (1967) The interaction of mitomycin C with deoxyribonucleic acid in vitro. *J. Biochem.* (*Tokyo*) **61:** 162–167.

KOHN, K. W. (1979) DNA as a target in cancer chemotherapy. Measurement of macromolecular DNA damage produced in mammalian cells by anticancer agents and carcinogens. *Meth. Cancer Res.* **16:** 291–345.

KOHN, K. W., HARTLEY, J. A. and MATTES, W. B. (1987) Mechanisms of DNA sequence selective alkylation of guanine-N7 positions by nitrogen mustards. *Nucleic Acids Res.* **15:** 10531–10549.

KOHN, K. W., HARTLEY, J. A. and MATTES, W. B. (1988) Mechanisms of DNA sequence selective alkylations of guanine-N7 positions by nitrogen mustards. *Biochem. Pharmac.* **37:** 1799–1800.

KONO, A., HARA, Y., EGUCHI, S. and TANAKA, M. (1979) Determination of mitomycin C in biomedical specimens by high performance liquid chromatography. *J. Chromatog.* **164:** 404–406.

KORBITZ, B. C. and REIQUAM, C. W. (1969) *Clin. Med.* **76:** 16–22.

KOZLOV, N. E. and BERNSHTEIN, V. N. (1968) Qualitative and quantitative analysis of drugs of the bis(2-chloroethyl) group. *Aktual. Vop. Farm.* 61–65.

KRAMER, R. A., GREENE, K., AHMAD, S. and VISTICA, D. T. (1987) Chemosensitization of L-phenylalanine mustard by the thiol-modulating agent buthionine sulfoximine. *Cancer Res.* **47:** 1593–1597.

KRUSE, E. and HARTLEY-ASP, B. (1989a) A time study on the uptake of oestramustine into prostatic tumour 1013L cells in vitro. *Biochem. Pharmac.* **38:** 702–704.

KRUSE, E. and HARTLEY-ASP, B. (1989b) The effect of oestramustine, nor-nitrogen mustard and tauromustine on macromolecular labelling in the human prostatic tumour cell line 1013L. *Pharmac. Toxic.* **64:** 9–13.

KRUSE, E., JOHANSSON, S.-A., HARTLEY-ASP, B. and GUNNARSSON, P. O. (1988) Distribution and metabolism of oestramustine in HeLa cells and the human prostatic tumour cell line 1013L. *Biochem. Pharmac.* **37:** 3161–3167.

KULKARNI, S. S., LEVENTON, G. S., HUYNH, L., CHOW, H., DICKE, K. A. and ZANDER, A. R. (1985) Effect of pretreatment with cyclophosphamide on high dose toxicity of melphalan in mice. *Cancer Res.* **45:** 5431–5435.

KUNZ, B. A. and MIS, J. R. A. (1989) Mutational specificities of 1,3-bis(2-chloroethyl)-1-nitrosourea and nitrogen mustard in the SUP4-O gene of *Saccharomyces cerevisiae*. *Cancer Res.* **49:** 279–283.

KYLE, R. A., PIERRE, R. V. and BAYRD, E. D. (1975) Multiple myeloma and acute leukemia associated with alkylating agents. *Arch. intern. Med.* **135:** 185–192.

LAMBERT, B., HOLMBERG, K. and EINHORN, N. (1986) Chromosome damage and second malignancy in patients treated with melphalan. *I.A.R.C. Sci. Publ.* **78:** 147–160.

LAMBERT, B., RINGBORG, U., LINDBLAD, A. and STEN, M. (1981) Sister-chromatid exchange in peripheral lymphocytes of human subjects: the effect of cigarette smoking and anticancer chemotherapy. *Mutat. Res.* **85:** 235.

LARIONOV, L. F., SHKODINSKAJA, E. N., TROOSHEIKINA, N. I., KHOKHLOV, A. S., VASINA, O. S. and NOVIKOVA, M. A. (1955) Studies on the anti-tumour activity of *p*-di-(2-chloroethyl) aminophenylalanine (Sarcolysine). *Lancet* **ii:** 169–171.

LAW, I. P. and BLOM, J. (1977) Second malignancies in patients with multiple myeloma. *Oncology* **34:** 20–24.

LAWLEY, P. D. and BROOKES, P. (1867) Interstrand cross-linking of DNA by difunctional alkylating agents. *J. molec. Biol.* **25:** 143–160.

LAZARUS, H. M., REED, M. D., SPITZER, T. R., RABAA, M. S. and BLUMER, J. L. (1987) High dose iv thio-TEPA and cryopreserved autologous bone marrow transplantation for therapy of refractory cancer. *Cancer Treat. Rep.* **71:** 689–695.

LEA, J. S., GARNER, H. J., BUTLER, J., HOEY, B. M. and WARD, T. H. (1988) The lack of correlation between toxicity and free radical formation of two diaziridinyl benzoquinones. *Biochem. Pharmac.* **37:** 2023–2025.

LEE, F. Y. F. and WORKMAN, P. (1986) Altered pharmacokinetics in the mechanism of chemosensitization: effects of nitroimidazoles and other chemical modifiers on the pharmacokinetics, antitumour activity and acute toxicity of selected nitrogen mustards. *Cancer Chemother. Pharmac.* **17:** 30–37.

LEE, F. Y. F., COE, P. and WORKMAN, P. (1986) Pharmacokinetic basis for the comparative antitumour activity and toxicity of chlorambucil, phenylacetic mustard and $\beta\beta$-difluorochlorambucil (CB 7103) in mice. *Cancer Chemother. Pharmac.* **17:** 21–29.

LEFF, P. and BARDSLEY, W. G. (1979) Pharmacokinetics of chlorambucil in ovarian carcinoma using a new HPLC assay. *Biochem. Pharmac.* **28:** 1289–1292.

LEISTENSCHNEIDER, W. and NAGEL, R. (1980) Estracyt therapy of advances prostatic cancer with special reference to control of therapy with cytology and DNA cytophotometry. *Eur. Urol.* **6:** 111–115.

LEONARD, R. C. F., SMART, G. E., LIVINGSTONE, J. R. B., CORNBLEET, M. A., KERR, G. R., FLETCHER, S., WEBB, J. N. and SMYTH, J. F. (1989) Randomised trial comparing prednimustine with combination chemotherapy in advanced ovarian carcinoma. *Cancer Chemother. Pharmac.* **23:** 105–110.

LEVIN, V. A. (1980) Relationship of octanol/water partition coefficient and molecular weight to rat brain capillary permeability. *J. med. Chem.* **23:** 682–684.

LEVIN, V. A. and WHEELER, K. T. (1982) Chemotherapeutic approaches to brain tumours. Experimental observations with dianhydrogalactitol and dibromodulcitol. *Cancer Chemother. Pharmac.* **8:** 125–131.

LEVIN, V. A., FREEMAN-DOVE, M. A. and MAROTEN, C. E. (1976) Dianhydrogalactitol (NSC 132313): Pharmacokinetics in normal and tumour-bearing rat brain and antitumour activity against three intracerebral rodent tumours. *J. natn. Cancer Inst.* **56:** 535–539.

LEWIS, C., LAWSON, N., RANKIN, E. M., MORRISON, G., MACLEAN, A. B., CORDINER, J., CASSIDY, J., KERR, D. J. and KAYE, S. B. (1990) Phase I and pharmacokinetic study of intraperitoneal thioTEPA in patients with ovarian cancer. *Cancer Chemother. Pharmac.* **26:** 283–287.

LIAO, J. T. F., COLLINS, W. T., HILES, R. A., KARCHER, R. V. and FRICK, S. (1983) Phase II report of Task 1: intravenous lethality and toxicity studies in CD2F1 mice and Sprague–Dawley rats and toxicity study in beagle dogs of spirohydantoin mustard (NSC 172112). *Chem. Abs.* **99:** 47611.

LINFORD, J. H. (1961) Some interactions of nitrogen mustards with constituents of human blood serum. *Biochem. Pharmac.* **8:** 343–357.

LINFORD, J. H. (1962) The recovery of free chlorambucil from solution in blood serum. *Biochem. Pharmac.* **11:** 693–706.

LINFORD, J. H. (1963) The influence of pH on the reactivity of chlorambucil. *Biochem. Pharmac.* **12:** 317–324.

LINFORD, J. H. (1973) 2,3,5-Tris-ethylenimino-1,4-benzo quinone (Trenimon). Some chemical and biological properties. *Chem.-Biol. Interactions* **6:** 149–168.

LINFORD, J. H., FROESE, A. and ISRAELS, L. G. (1963) Interaction of chlorambucil with cell surfaces. *Nature* **197:** 1068–1070.

LINFORD, J. H., HRYNIUK, W. and ISRAELS, L. G. (1969) Adsorption to human red blood cells of chlorambucil and other biological alkylating agents. *Biochem. Pharmac.* **18:** 2723–2735.

LIPMAN, R., WEAVER, J. and TOMASZ, M. (1978) Electrostatic complexes of mitomycin C with nucleic acids and polyanions. *Biochim. biophys. Acta* **521:** 779–791.

LIPSETT, M. N. and WEISSBACK, A. (1965) The site of alkylation of nucleic acids by mitomycin. *Biochemistry* **4:** 206–211.

LOEB, V. (1964) Dihydroxybusulfan (NSC 39069) in chronic myelocytic leukaemia and miscellaneous malignant neoplasms. *Cancer Chemother. Rep.* **42:** 39–43.

LOHMAR, F., MUSCH, E., VON UNRUH, G. E. and MUHLENBRUCH, B. J. (1989) Gas chromatographic assay for chlorambucil and phenylacetic mustard in plasma. *J. Chromatog. Biomed. Appl.* **495:** 281–287.

LOKICH, J. J., EGORIN, M. J., COHEN, B. E., BERN, M. M., ZIPOLI, T. E. and MOORE, C. (1989) A Phase I study of thio-TEPA administered by short-term and protracted continuous infusion. *Cancer* **63:** 46–50.

LOWN, J. W., BEGLEITER, A., JOHNSON, D. and MORGAN, A. R. (1976) Studies related to antitumour antibiotics. Part V. Reactions of mitomycin C with DNA examined by ethidium fluorescence assay. *Can. J. Biochem.* **54:** 110–119.

LU, K., SAVARAJ, N., YAP, B. S., BEDIKIAN, A. Y., FENN, L., BENJAMIN, R. S. and LEO, T. L. (1983) Clinical pharmacology of 2,5′-diaziridinyl-3,6-biscarboethoxyamino-1,4-benzoquinone (AZQ). *Eur. J. Cancer clin. Oncol.* **19:** 603–606.

LUSTHOF, K. J., DEMOL, N. J., JANSSEN, L. H. M., VERBOOM, W. and REINHOUDT, D. N. (1989) DNA alkylation and formation of DNA interstrand cross-links by potential antitumour 2,5-bis(1-aziridinyl)-1,4-benzoquinones. *Chem.-Biol. Interact.* **70:** 249–262.

LUSTHOF, K. J., DEMOL, N. J., JANSSEN, L. H. M., PRINS, B., VERBOOM, W. and REINHOUDT, D. N. (1990a) Interactions between potential anti-tumour 2,5-bis(1-aziridinyl)-1,4-benzoquinone derivatives and glutathione: reductive activation, conjugation and DNA damage. *Anti-Cancer Drug Design* **5:** 283–290.

LUSTHOF, K. J., RICHTER, W., DEMOL, N. J., JANSSEN, L. H. M., VERBOOM, W. and REINHOUDT, D. N. (1990b) Reductive activation of potential antitumour bis(aziridinyl)benzoquinones by xanthine oxidase: competition between oxygen reduction and quinone reduction. *Arch. Biochem. Biophys.* **277:** 137–142.

LYONS, R. M. and GOLDENBERG, G. J. (1972) Active transport of nitrogen mustard and choline by normal and leukemic human lymphoid cells. *Cancer Res.* **32:** 1679–1685.

M. V., GOLDENTHAL, E. I. and SMITH, P. K. (1954) The distribution of radioactivity following administration of triethylenimino-*S*-triazine-^{14}C in tumour-bearing and control mice. *Cancer Res.* **14:** 559–562.

MACKICHAN, J. J. and BECHTER, T. P. (1990) Quantitation of busulfan in plasma by high-performance liquid chromatography. *J. Chromatog. Biomed. Appl.* **532:** 424–428.

MADAJEWICZ, S., CATANE, R., MITTELMAN, A., WAJSMAN, Z. and MURPHY, G. P. (1980) Chemotherapy of advanced, hormonally resistant prostatic carcinoma. *Oncology* **37:** 53–56.

MAMURIS, Z., GERBAULT-SEUREAU, M., PRIEUR, M., POUILLART, P., DUTRILLAUX, B. and AURIAS, A. (1989) Chromosomal aberrations in lymphocytes of patients treated with melphalan. *Int. J. Cancer.* **43:** 80–86.

MARCHAND, D. H., REMMEL, R. P. and ABDEL-MONEM (1988) Biliary excretion of a glutathione conjugate of busulfan and 1,4-diiodobutane in the rat. *Drug Metab. Dispos.* **16:** 85–90.

MAREEL, M. M., STORME, G. A., DRAGONETTI, C. H., DE BRUYNE, G. K., HARTLEY-ASP, B., SEGERS, J. L. and RABAEY, M. L. (1988) Antiinvasive activity of oestramustine on malignant MO_4 mouse cells and on DU-145 human prostate carcinoma cells in vitro. *Cancer Res.* **48:** 1842–1849.

MARSHALL, R. S., ERLICHMAN, C. and RAUTH, A. M. (1985) A bioassay to measure cytotoxicity of plasma from patients treated with mitomycin C. *Cancer Res.* **45:** 5939–5943.

MARSHALL, R. S., PATERSON, M. C. and RAUTH, A. M. (1991) Studies on the mechanism of resistance to mitomycin C and porfiromycin in a human cell strain derived from a cancer-prone individual. *Biochem. Pharmac.* **41:** 1351–1360.

MARTIN, A. D., BEER, R. W. G., BOSANQUET, A. G. and GILBY, E. D. (1982) The effect of alkylating agents and other drugs on the accumulation of melphalan by murine L1210 leukaemia cells in vitro. *Biochem. Pharmac.* **31:** 2727–2732.

MASTERS, J. R. W., MCDERMOTT, B. J., JENKINS, W. E. A., FENWICK, E., SHAH, P. J. R., MUNDY, A. R., LOADMAN, P. M. and BIBBY, M. C. (1990) ThioTEPA pharmacokinetics during intravesical chemotherapy and the influence of Tween 80. *Cancer Chemother. Pharmac.* **25:** 267–273.

MATAGNE, R. (1967) Activity of L-threitol-1,4-bismethane sulphonate on early chromosomes in relation to chemical transformation during treatment. *Mutat. Res.* **4:** 621–630.

MATHESON, D., BRUSICK, D. and CARRANO, R. (1978) Comparison of the relative mutagenic activity for eight antineoplastic drugs in the Ames *Salmonella*/microsome and TK + mouse lymphoma assays. *Drug Chem. Toxic.* **1:** 277–304.

MATSUMOTO, I. and LARK, K. G. (1963) Altered DNA isolated from cells treated with mitomycin C. *Exp. Cell Res.* **32:** 192–196.

MATTES, W. B., HARTLEY, J. A. and KOHN, K. W. (1986) DNA sequence selectivity of guanine-N7 alkylation by nitrogen mustards. *Nucleic Acids Res.* **14:** 2971–2987.

MAUGER, A. B. and ROSS, W. C. J. (1962) Aryl-2-halogeno-alkylamines-XX. The preparation and properties of some di-2-chloroethyl-aminoaryl substituted hydantoins and related amino acids. *Biochem. Pharmac.* **11:** 847–858.

MCDERMOTT, B. J., DOUBLE, J. A. and BIBBY, M. C. (1985) Gas chromatographic analysis of triethylenethiophosphoramide and triethylenephosphoramide in biological specimens. *J. Chromatog.* **338:** 335–345.

MCELWAIN, T. J., HEDLEY, D. W., BURTON, G., CLINK, H. M., GORDON, M. Y., JARMAN, M., JUTTNER, C. A., MILLAR, J. K., MILSTED, R. A. V., PRENTICE, G., SMITH, I. E., SPENCE, D. and WOODS, M. (1979) Marrow autotransplantation accelerates haematological recovery in patients with malignant melanoma treated with high-dose melphalan. *Br. J. Cancer* **40:** 72–80.

MCLEAN, A., NEWELL, D. and BAKER, G. (1976) The metabolism of chlorambucil. *Biochem. Pharmac.* **25:** 2331–2335.

MCLEAN, A., NEWELL, D., BAKER, G. and CONNORS, T. A. (1980) The metabolism of chlorambucil. *Biochem. Pharmac.* **29:** 2039–2047.

MCLEAN, A., WOODS, R. L., CATOVSKY, D. and FARMER, P. (1979) Pharmacokinetics and metabolism of chlorambucil in patients with malignant disease. *Cancer Treat. Rev.* **6 Suppl:** 33–42.

MCNALLY, N. J. (1982) Enhancement of Chemotherapy Agents. In: *Chemical Modifications: Radiation and Cytotoxic Drugs*, pp. 593–598, SUTHERLAND, R. M. (ed.) Pergamon Press, New York.

MEEKS, R. G. (1983) Preclinical single dose lethality of spiro-hydantoin mustard (NSC 172112) in CD2F1 mice. *Chem. Abs.* **99:** 16186 V.

MEEKS, R. G. and FRICK, S. (1983) Preclinical intravenous lethality and toxicity studies of spirohydantoin mustard (NSC 172112) in CS2F1 mice, Sprague-Dawley rats and beagle dogs. *Chem. Abs.* **99:** 250a.

MELLETT, L. B. and WOODS, L. A. (1960a) The fluorometric estimation of mechlorethamine (mustargen) and its biological disposition in the dog. *Cancer Res.* **20:** 518–523.

MELLETT, L. B. and WOODS, L. A. (1960b) The comparative physiological disposition of thioTEPA and TEPA in the dog. *Cancer Res.* **20:** 524–532.

MELLETT, L. B., HODGSON, P. E. and WOODS, L. A. (1962) Absorption and fate of C^{14}-labelled *N,N′,N″*-triethylene-thiophosphoramide (thioTEPA) in humans and dogs. *J. Lab. clin. Med.* **60:** 818–825.

MERCADO, C. M. and TOMASZ, M. (1977) Circular dichroism of mitomycin–DNA complexes. Evidence for a conformational change in DNA. *Biochemistry* **16:** 2040–2046.

MERKER, P. C., WODINSKY, I. and GERAN, R. I. (1975) Review of selected experimental brain tumour models used in chemotherapy experiments. *Cancer Chemother. Rep.* **59:** 729–736.

MIKKELSEN, R. B., ASHER, C. and HICKS, T. (1985) Extracellular pH, transmembrane distribution and cytotoxicity of chlorambucil. *Biochem. Pharmac.* **34:** 2531–2534.

MILLAR, B. C., MAITLAND, J. A., MILLAR, J. L. and BELL, J. B. G. (1989) Melphalan transport into human malignant lymphoid cells differs from the murine equivalent in vitro. *Br. J. Cancer* **59:** 710–713.

MILLAR, J. L. and MCELWAIN, T. J. (1978) Combinations of cytotoxic agents that have less than expected toxicity on normal tissues in mice. *Antibiot. Chemother.* **23:** 271–282.

MILLAR, J. L., HUDSPITH, B. N. and BLACKETT, N. M. (1975) Reduced lethality in mice receiving a combined dose of cyclophosphamide and busulphan. *Br. J. Cancer* **32:** 193–198.

MILLAR, J. L., HUDSPITH, B. N., MCELWAIN, T. J. and PHELPS, T. A. (1978) Effect of high-dose melphalan on marrow and intestinal epithelium in mice pretreated with cyclophosphamide. *Br. J. Cancer* **38:** 137–142.

MILNER, A. L., KLATT, O., YOUNG, S. E. and STEHLIN, J. S. (1965) The biochemical mechanism of action of

L-phenylalanine mustard. I. Distribution of L-phenylalanine mustard-^{3}H in tumour-bearing rats. *Cancer Res.* **25:** 259–264.

MINOR, D. R., ALLEN, R. E., ALBERTS, D., PENG, Y., TARDELL, G. and HUTCHINSON, J. (1985) A clinical and pharmacokinetic study of isolated limb perfusion with heat and melphalan for melanoma. *Cancer* **55:** 2638–2644.

MISCHLER, N. E., EARHARDT, R. H., CARR, B. and TORMEY, D. C. (1979) Dibromodulcitol. *Cancer Treat. Rev.* **6:** 191–204.

MITCHELL, M. P. and WALKER, I. G. (1972) Studies on the cytotoxicity of myleran and dimethyl myleran. *Can. J. Biochem.* **50:** 1074–1081.

MITOMA, C., ONODERA, T., TAKEGOSHI, T. and THOMAS, D. W. (1977) Metabolic disposition of chlorambucil in rats. *Xenobiotica* **7:** 205–220.

MITTELMAN, A., CATANE, R. and MURPHY, G. P. (1977) New steroidal alkylating agents in advanced stage D carcinoma of the prostate. *Cancer Treat. Rep.* **61:** 307–310.

MIZUNO, M., YOSHINO, H., HASHIDA, M. and SEZAKI, H. (1987) Decreased transport of D-glucose and L-alanine across brush-border membrane vesicles from small intestine of rats treated with mitomycin C. *Biochim. biophys. Acta* **902:** 93–100.

MOLLER, T. R., BRANDT, L., KONYVES, I. and LINDBERG, L. G. (1975) Therapeutic effect of Leo 1031, an alkylating cortico-steroid ester in lymphoproliferative disorders. II. Lymphocytic lymphoma. *Acta Med. Scand.* **197:** 323–327.

MOORE, H. W. (1977) Bioactivation as a model for drug design. Bioreductive alkylation. *Science* **197:** 527–532.

MOSSOBA, M. M. and GUTIERREZ, P. L. (1985) Diaziquone as a potential agent for photoirradiation therapy: formation of the semiquinone and hydroxyl radicals by visible light. *Biochem. biophys. Res. Commun.* **132:** 445–452.

MOSSOBA, M. M., ALIZADEH, M. and GUTIERREZ, P. L. (1985) Mechanism for the reductive activation of diaziquone. *J. Pharm. Sci.* **74:** 1249–1254.

MOURIDSEN, H. T., KEISTENSNEN, D., HALSKOV NIELSEN, J. and DOMBERNOWSKY, P. (1980) Phase II trial of prednimustine L-1031, (NSC 134087) in advanced breast cancer. *Cancer* **46:** 253–255.

MOY, B. C. and TEW, K. D. (1986) Differences in the nuclear matrix phosphoproteins and of a wild-type and nitrogen mustard-resistant rat breast carcinoma cell line. *Cancer Res.* **46:** 4672–4676.

MULCAHY, R. T., GIPP, J. J., UBLACKER, G. A. and MCCLELLAND, R. A. (1990) Enhancement of melphalan (L-PAM) toxicity by reductive metabolites of 1-methyl-2-nitroimidazole, a model nitroimidazole chemosensitizing agent. *Biochem. Pharmac.* **40:** 2671–2676.

MUNGER, D., STERNSON, L. A. and PATTON, T. F. (1978) Studies on the distribution of dianhydrogalactitol into the central nervous system of the rat. *Cancer Treat. Rep.* **62:** 409–412.

MUNGER, D., STERNSON, L. A., REPTA, A. J. and HIGUCHI, T. (1977) High-performance liquid chromatographic analysis of dianhydrogalactitol in plasma by derivatization with diethyldithiocarbamate. *J. Chromatog.* **143:** 375–382.

MURPHY, M. L., DEL MORO, A. and LACON, C. (1958) The comparative effects of five polyfunctional alkylating agents on the rat fetus, with additional notes on the chick embryo. *Ann. NY Acad. Sci.* **68:** 762–782.

MURRAY, D. and MEYN, R. E. (1983) Enhancement of the DNA cross-linking activity of melphalan by misonidazole in vivo. *Br. J. Cancer* **47:** 195–203.

MURRAY, D. and MEYN, R. E. (1986) Cell cycle-dependent cytotoxicity of alkylating agents: determination of nitrogen mustard-induced DNA cross-links and their repair in Chinese hamster ovary cells synchronized by centrifugal elutriation. *Cancer Res.* **46:** 2324–2329.

MURRAY-LYON, I. M., TATTERSALL, M. H. B., THOMAS, H., SHERLOCK, S., COCHRANE, M., WILLIAMS, R. and READ, A. E. (1978). CB 10-252 in the treatment of primary hepatocellular carcinoma. *Med. Chir. Dig.* **7:** 425–426.

MUSSER, S. M., PAN, S.-S. and CALLERY, P. S. (1989) Liquid chromatography thermospray mass spectrometry of DNA adducts formed with mitomycin C, porfiromycin and thio-TEPA. *J. Chromatog.* **474:** 197–207.

NADKARNI, M. V., GOLDENTHAL, E. I. and SMITH, P. K. (1957) The distribution of radioactivity following administration of triethylenephosphoramide-^{32}P in tumour-bearing and control mice. *Cancer Res.* **17:** 97–101.

NADKARNI, M. V., TRAMS, E. G. and SMITH P. K. (1961) Excretion and distribution studies with radioisotope labelled alkylating drugs in cancer patients. *Cancer* **14:** 953–956.

NADKARNI, M. V., TRAMS, E. G. and SMITH, P. K. (1956) Observations on the rapid disappearance of radioactivity from blood after intravenous triethylene melamine ^{14}C. *Proc. Am. Ass. Cancer Res.* **2:** 136.

NADKARNI, M. V., TRAMS, E. G. and SMITH, P. K. (1959) Preliminary studies on the distribution and fate of TEM, TEPA and Myleran in the human. *Cancer Res.* **19:** 713–718.

NAGAO, T. and FUJIKAWA, K. (1990) Genotoxic potency in mouse spermatogonial cells of triethylenemelamine, mitomycin C, ethylnitrosourea, procarbazine and propyl methanesulfonate as measured by F_1 congenital defects. *Mutat. Res.* **229:** 123–128.

NAGOURNEY, R. A., MESSENGER, J. C., KERN, D. H. and WEISENTHAL, L. M. (1990) Enhancement of anthracycline and alkylation cytotoxicity by ethacrynic acid in primary cultures of human tissues. *Cancer Chemother. Pharmac.* **26:** 318–322.

NATH, J., KRISHNA, G., PETERSEN, M. and ONG, T. (1988) Sister-chromatid exchanges induced by triethylenemelamine: in vivo and in vivo/in vitro studies in mouse and Chinese hamster bone marrow and spleen cells. *Mutat. Res.* **206:** 73–82.

NATIONAL BLADDER CANCER COLLABORATIVE GROUP (1977) The role of intravesical thio-TEPA in the management of superficial bladder cancer. *Cancer Res.* **37:** 2916–2917.

NEFT, R. E., SCHOL, H. M. and CASCIANO, D. A. (1989) Triethylene melamine-induced sister-chromatid exchange in murine lymphocytes exposed in vivo. *Mutat. Res.* **222:** 323–328.

NEIDHART, J. A., DEROCHER, D., GREVER, M. R., KRAUT, E. H. and MALSPEIS, L. (1984) Phase I trial of teroxirone. *Cancer Treat. Rep.* **68:** 1115–1119.

NEWELL, D. R., CALVERT, A. H., HARRAP, K. R. and MCELWAIN, T. J. (1983a) Studies on the pharmacokinetics of chlorambucil and prednimustine in man. *Br. J. clin. Pharmac.* **15:** 253–258.

NEWELL, D. R., CALVERT, A. H., HARRAP, K. R. and MCELWAIN, T. J. (1983b) The clinical pharmacology of chlorambucil and prednimustine. *Br. J. clin. Pharmac.* **16:** 762–763.

NEWELL, D. R., HART, L. I. and HARRAP, K. R. (1979) Estimation of chlorambucil, phenyl acetic mustard and prednimustine in human plasma by high-performance liquid chromatography. *J. Chromatog. Biomed. Appl.* **164:** 114–119.

NEWELL, D. R., SHEPHERD, C. R. and HARRAP, K. R. (1981) The pharmacokinetics of prednimustine and chlorambucil in the rat. *Cancer Chemother. Pharmac.* **6:** 85–91.

NG, S. and WAXMAN, D. J. (1990) Biotransformation of *N,N',N''*-triethylenethiophosphoramide: oxidative desulfuration to yield *N,N',N''*-triethylenephosphoramide associated with suicide inactivation of a phenobarbital-inducible hepatic P-450 monooxygenase. *Cancer Res.* **50:** 464–471.

NG, S. and WAXMAN, D. J. (1991) *N,N',N''*-Triethylenethiophosphoramide (Thio-TEPA) oxygenation by constitutive hepatic P450 enzymes and modulation of drug metabolism and clearance in vivo by P450-inducing agents. *Cancer Res.* **51:** 2340–2345.

NGUYEN, B., BISWAL, S. and GUTIERREZ, P. L. (1988) The influence of diaziquone free radicals on the in vitro activity of diaziquone. *Xenobiotica* **18:** 593–602.

NIESSEN, W. M. A., BERGERS, P. J. M., TJADEN, U. R. and VAN DER GREEF, J. (1988) Phase-system switching as an on-line sample pretreatment in the bioanalysis of mitomycin C using supercritical fluid chromatography. *J. Chromatog.* **454:** 243–251.

NINANE, J., BAURAIN, R., DE SELYS, A., TROUET, A. and CORNU, G. (1985) High dose melphalan in children with advanced malignant disease. *Cancer Chemother. Pharmac.* **15:** 263–267.

NISSEN-MEYER, R. and HOST, H. (1960) A comparison between the hematological side effects of cyclophosphamide and nitrogen mustard. *Cancer Chemother. Rep.* **9:** 51–55.

NORPOTH, K., ADDICKS, H. W. and WITTING, U. (1973) Quantitative determination of alkylating cytostatics on the thin layer chromatography (TLC) plate with 4-pyridinecarboxaldehyde 2-benzothiazolylhydrazone. *Arzneim-Forsch.* **23:** 1529–1535.

O'DWYER, P. J., LACRETA, F., ENGSTROM, P. F., PETER, R., TARTAGLIA, L., COLE, D., LITWIN, S., DE VITO, J., POPLACK, D., DELAP, R. J. and COMIS, R. L. (1991) Phase I/pharmacokinetic reevaluation of thioTEPA. *Cancer Res.* **51:** 3171–3176.

OBE, G. and BECK, B. (1979) Trenimon: biochemical, physiological and genetic effects on cells and organisms. *Mutat. Res.* **65:** 21–70.

OBERC-GREENWOOD, M. A., SMITH, B. H., COOKE, C., ELLIS, J. R., KORNBLITH, P. L. and MCKEEVER, P. E. (1983) Mitochondrial toxicity of 2,5-diaziridinyl-3,6-bis(carboethoxyamino)-1, 4-benzoquinone. *J. natn. Cancer Inst.* **71:** 723–733.

OBRECHT, P., WOENCKHAUS, J. W. and FUSENIG, N. E. (1967) Die Verteilung von Tris-aethylenimino benzochinon (Trenimon[R]) in organismus der Ratte. *Eur. J. Cancer* **3:** 29–36.

OGAWA, M., BERGSAGEL, D. E. and MCCULLOCH, E. A. (1973) Studies of nitrogen mustard transport by mouse myeloma and hemopoietic precursor cells. *Cancer Res.* **33:** 3172–3175.

OJWANG, J. O., GRUENEBERG, D. A. and LOECHIER, E. L. (1989) Synthesis of a duplex oligonucleotide containing a nitrogen mustard interstrand DNA–DNA cross-link. *Cancer Res.* **49:** 6529–6537.

OPPITZ, M. M., MUSCH, E., MALEK, M., RÜB, H. P., VON UNRUH, G. E., LOOS, U. and MÜHLENBRUCH, B. (1989) Studies on the pharmacokinetics of chlorambucil and prednimustine in patients using a new high-performance liquid chromatographic assay. *Cancer Chemother. Pharmac.* **23:** 208–212.

OSTERBORG, A., EHRSSON, H., EKSBORG, S., WALLIN, I. and MELLSTEDT, H. (1989) Pharmacokinetics of oral melphalan in relation to renal function in multiple myeloma patients. *Eur. J. Cancer clin. Oncol.* **25:** 899–903.

OSTERHELD, H. K. O., MUSCH, E., VON UNRUH, G. E., LOOS, U., RAUSCHECKER, H. and MÜHLENBRUCH, B. J. (1988) A sensitive high-performance liquid chromatographic assay for melphalan and its hydrolysis products in blood and plasma. *Cancer Chemother. Pharmac.* **21:** 156–162.

ÖTVÖS, L. and ELEKES, I. (1975) Stereochemistry of the reactions of biopolymers. III. Steric hindrance in the reaction of DNA with bifunctional alkylating agents. Definition of τ and μ substituents. *Tetrahedron Lett.* **29:** 2477–2480.

OWEN, W. R. and STEWART, P. J. (1979) Kinetics and mechanism of chlorambucil hydrolysis. *J. Pharm. Sci.* **68:** 992–996.

OZOLS, R. F., LOWIE, K. G., PLOWMAN, J., BEHRENS, B. C., FINE, R. L., DYKES, D. and HAMILTON, T. C. (1987) Enhanced melphalan cytotoxicity in human ovarian cancer in vitro and in tumour-bearing nude mice by buthionine sulfoximine depletion of glutathione. *Biochem. Pharmac.* **36:** 147–153.

PACHECO, D. Y., STRATTON, N. K. and GIBSON, N. W. (1989) Comparison of the mechanism of action of busulfan with hepsulfan, a new anti-leukemic agent in the L1210 cell line. *Cancer Res.* **49:** 5108–5110.

PALLANTE, S. L., PENSELAU, C., MENNEL, R. G., BRUNDRETT, R. B., APPLER, M., ROSENSHEIN, N. B. and COLVIN, M. (1980) Quantitation by gas chromatography—chemical ionization—mass spectrometry of phenylalanine mustard in plasma of patients. *Cancer Res.* **40:** 2268–2272.

PALMER, R. G., DORE, C. and DENMAN, A. M. (1985) Chlorambucil-induced chromosome damage to human lymphocytes. *Lancet* **ii:** 1438–1439.

PAN, S.-S., ANDREWS, P. A., GLOVER, C. J. and BACHUR, N. R. (1984) Reductive activation of mitomycin C and mytomycin C metabolites catalysed by NADPH-cytochrome P-450 reductase and xanthine oxidase. *J. biol. Chem.* **259:** 959–966.

PAN, S.-S., IRACKI, T. and BACHUR, N. R. (1986) DNA alkylation by enzyme-activated mitomycin C. *Molec. Pharmac.* **29:** 622–628.

PANASCI, L., HENDERSON, D., TORRES-GARCIA, S. J., SKALSKI, V., CAPLAN, S. and HUTCHINSON, M. (1988) Transport, metabolism and DNA interaction of melphalan in lymphocytes from patients with chronic lymphocytic leukemia. *Cancer Res.* **48:** 1972–1976.

PANASCI, L., MCQUILLAN, A., COHEN, J. and ZACKON, I. (1990) The effect of prolonged incubations and heat denaturation on melphalan-induced DNA cross-links as measured by the ethidium bromide fluorescence assay. *Cancer Lett.* **50:** 129–132.

PARSONS, P. G., CARTER, F. B., MORRISON, L. and REGIUS M. (1981) Mechanism of melphalan resistance developed in vitro in human melanoma cells. *Cancer Res.* **41:** 1525–1534.

PATRICK, J. B., WILLIAMS, R. P., MEYER, W. E., FULMAR, W., COSULICH, D. B., BROSCHARD, R. W. and WEBB, J. S. (1964) Aziridinomitosenes: a new class of antibiotics related to the mitomycins. *J. Am. Chem. Soc.* **86:** 1889–1890.

PAVELIC, J., ZGRADIC, I. and PAVELIC, K. (1991) Presence of oestrogen receptors on target cells and antiproliferative activity of oestramustine phosphate: positive correlation for human tumours in vitro. *J. Cancer Res. clin. Oncol.* **117:** 244–248.

PAZDUR, R., REDMAN, B. G., CORBETT, T., PHILLIPS, M. and BAKER, L. H. (1987) Phase I trial of spiromustine (NSC 172112) and evaluation of toxicity and schedule in a murine model. *Cancer Res.* **47:** 4213–4217.

PEDERSEN-BJERGAARD, J., MORKHANSEN, M., GEISLER, C. H. and NISSEN, N. I. (1980a) Clinical trial of prednimustine, Leo 1031 (NSC 134087) in patients with non-Hodgkin lymphomata and chronic lymphocytic leukaemia previously treated with steroids and alkylating agents. *Acta. Med. scand.* **207:** 215–220.

PEDERSEN-BJERGAARD, J., NISSEN, N. I., SØRENSEN, H. M., HOU-JENSEN, K., LARSEN, M. S., ERNST, P., ERSBØL, J., KNUDTZON, S. and ROSE, C. (1980b) Acute non-lymphocytic leukemia in patients with ovarian carcinoma following long-term treatment with treosulfan (dihydroxybusulfan) *Cancer* **45:** 19–29.

PEDERSEN-BJERGAARD, J., SØRENSEN, H. M., HOU-JENSEN, K. and ERSBØL, J. (1979) Acute non-lymphocytic leukemic (ANLL) in patients with ovarian cancer following long term treatment with treosulfan (= dihydroxybusulfan). *Proc. Am. Ass. Cancer Res.* **20:** 287.

PENG, C. T. (1957) Distribution and metabolite fate of S^{35}-labelled myleran (busulfan) in normal and tumour bearing rats. *J. Pharmac. exp. Ther.* **120:** 229–238.

PENG, G. W., MARQUEZ, V. E. and DRISCOLL, J. S. (1975) Potential central nervous system antitumour agents. Hydantoin derivatives. *J. med. Chem.* **18:** 846–849.

PERTICONE, P. and LAMBERT, B. (1986) Effects of liquid holding by L-ethionine on the SCE frequency induced by nitrogen mustard in human lymphocyte cultures. *Mutat. Res.* **175:** 171–177.

PETERS, W. P., HENNER, W. D., GROCHOW, L. B., OLSEN, G., EDWARDS, S., STANBUCK, H., STUART, A., GOCKERMAN, J., MOORE, J., BAST, R. C., SEIGLER, H. F. and COLVIN, O. M. (1987) Clinical and pharmacologic effects of high dose single agent busulfan with autologous bone marrow support in the treatment of solid tumours. *Cancer Res.* **47:** 6402–6406.

PETERSON, C., FORSGREN, B. and HOGBERG, B. (1983) Subcellular localization of oestramustine in rat ventral prostate following intravenous injection. *Acta Physiol. scand.* **Suppl. 515:** 55–63.

PHILIPS, F. S., SCHWARTZ, H. S. and STERNBERG, S. S. (1960) Pharmacology of mitomycin C. I. Toxicity and pathological effects. *Cancer Res.* **20:** 1354–1361.

PICCART, M., ROZENCWEIG, M., DODION, P., CUMPS, E., CRESPEIGNE, N., MAKAROFF, O., ATASSI, G., KISNER, D. and KENIS, Y. (1981) Phase I clinical trial with alpha 1,3,5-triglycidyl-*S*-triazinetrione (NSC 296934). *Eur. J. Cancer clin. Oncol.* **17:** 1263–1266.

PIEPER, R. O. and ERICKSON, L. C. (1990) DNA adenine adducts induced by nitrogen mustards and their role in transcription termination in vitro. *Carcinogenesis* **11:** 1739–1746.

PLOWMAN, J. and ADAMSON, R. H. (1979) The disposition of spirohydantoin mustard (NSC 172112) in rats and dogs. *Xenobiotica* **9:** 379–391.

PLOWMAN, J., LAKINGS, D. B., OWENS, E. S. and ADAMSON, R. H. (1977) Initial studies on the penetration of spirohydantoin mustard into the cerebrospinal fluid of dogs. *Pharmacology* **15:** 359–366.

POLITI, P. M., RAJAGOPALAN, S. and SINHA, B. K. (1989) Free-radical formation by mitomycin C and its novel analogs in cardiac microsomes and the perfused rat heart. *Biochim. biophys. Acta* **992:** 341–348.

POUSETTE, A., BJORK, P. and CARLSTROM, K. (1987) Hormonal regulation of an oestramustine-binding protein in the submaxillary gland of the rat. *J. Steroid Biochem.* **26:** 31–34.

PRADOS, M., RODRIGUEZ, L., SEAGER, M., SILVER, P. and LEVIN, V. (1987) Phase II study of spirohydantoin mustard for the treatment of recurrent malignant gliomas. *Cancer Treat. Rep.* **71:** 1105–1106.

PRESANT, C. A. and CARR, D. (1980) Amphotericin B (Fungizone®) enhancement of nitrogen mustard uptake by human tumour cells. *Biochem. biophys. Res. Commun.* **93:** 1067–1073.

PRICE, C. C. (1975) Chemistry of alkylation. In: *Handbook of Experimental Pharmacology*, Vol. 38, pp. 1–5, SARTORELLI, A. C. and JOHNS, D. G. (eds). Springer, Berlin.

PRICER, W. E. and WEISSBACH, A. (1965) Enzymatic utilization and degradation of DNA treated with mitomycin C or ultraviolet light. *Biochemistry* **4:** 200–206.

PRINS, B., KOSTER, A. S., VERBOOM, W. and REINHOUDT, D. N. (1989) Microsomal superoxide anion production and NADPH-oxidation in a series of 22 aziridinylbenzoquinones. *Biochem. Pharmac.* **38:** 3753–3757.

PRIOR, J. and WHITE, I. (1978) Addisonian syndrome associated with treosulfan. *Lancet* **ii:** 1207–1208.

PRITSOS, C. A. and SARTORELLI, A. C. (1986) Generation of reactive oxygen radicals through bioactivation of mitomycin antibiotics. *Cancer Res.* **46:** 3528–3532.

PRITSOS, C. A., CONSTANTINIDES, P. P., TRITTON, T. R., HEIMBROOK, D. C. and SARTORELLI, A. C. (1985) Use of high-performance liquid chromatography to detect hydroxyl and superoxide radicals generated from mitomycin C. *Anal. Biochem.* **150:** 294–299.

PYATIGORSKAYA, T. L., ZHILKOVA, O. Y., SHELKOVSKY, V. S., ARKHANGELOVA, N. M., GRIZODUS, A. I. and SUKHODUB, L. F. (1987) Hydrolysis of 1,1′,1″phosphinothioylidinetrisaziridine (Thiotepa) in aqueous solution. *Biomed. Environ. Mass Spec.* **14:** 143–148.

RAINE, D. N. (1962) Estimation of thio-TEPA in urine. *J. Pharm. Pharmac.* **14:** 614–615.

RANDHAWA, V. S., STEWART, F. A., DENEKAMP, J. and STRATFORD, M. R. L. (1985) Factors influencing the chemosensitization of melphalan by misonidazole. *Br. J. Cancer* **51:** 219–228.

RANKIN, E. M., HARVEY, C., KNIGHT, R. K. and RUBENS, R. D. (1987) Phase II trial of prednimustine as first-line chemotherapy in patients with advanced breast cancer. *Cancer Treat. Rep.* **701:** 1107–1108.

RAUTH, A. M., MOHINDRA, J. K. and TANNOCK, I. F. (1983) Activity of mitomycin C for aerobic and hypoxic cells in vitro and in vivo. *Cancer Res.* **43:** 4154–4158.

RAVINDRANATHAN, M. P., PAUL, V. J. and KURIAKOSE, E. T. (1972) Cataract after busulphan treatment. *Br. med. J.* 1: 218–219.

REDDY, M. V. and RANDERATH, K. (1987) ^{32}P-Analysis of DNA adducts in somatic and reproductive tissues of rats treated with the anticancer antibiotic, mitomycin C. *Mutat. Res.* **179:** 75–88.

REDWOOD, W. R. and COLVIN, M. (1980) Transport of melphalan by sensitive and resistant L1210 cells. *Cancer Res.* **40:** 1144–1149.

REECE, P. A., DALE, B. M., MORRIS, R. G., KOKASEK, D., GEE, D., ROGERSON, S. and SAGE, R. E. (1987) Effect of L-leucine on oral melphalan kinetics in patients. *Cancer Chemother. Pharmac.* **20:** 256–258.

REECE, P. A., HILL, H. S., GREEN, R. M., MORRIS, R. G., DALE, B. M., KOTASEK, D. and SAGE, R. E. (1988) Renal clearance and protein binding of melphalan in patients with cancer. *Cancer Chemother. Pharmac.* **22:** 348–352.

REECE, P. A., KOTASEK, D., MORRIS, R. G., DALE, B. M. and SAGE, R. E. (1986) The effect of food on oral melphalan absorption. *Cancer Chemother. Pharmac.* **16:** 194–197.

REEVES, B. R. and MARGOLES, C. (1974) Preferential location of chlorambucil-induced breakage in the chromosomes of normal human lymphocytes. *Mutat. Res.* **26:** 205–208.

REEVES, B. R., CASEY, G., HARRIS, H. and DINNING, W. J. (1985) Long-term cytogenetic follow-up study of patients with uveitis treated with chlorambucil. *Carcinogenesis* **6:** 1615–1619.

REICH, S. D. (1979) Clinical pharmacology of mitomycin C. In: *Mitomycin C: Current status and new developments*, p. 243, CARTER, S. K., CROOKE, S. T. (eds) Academic Press, London.

REIMER, R. R., HOOVER, R., FRAUMENI, J. F. and YOUNG, R. C. (1977) Acute leukemia after alkylating therapy of ovarian cancer. *New Engl. J. Med.* **297:** 177–181.

REYNOLDS, J. E. F. (ED) (1982) *Martindale The Extra Pharmacopoeia*, 28th edn, pp. 221–222, Pharmaceutical Press.

RICHES, P. G. and HARRAP, K. R. (1973) Some effects of chlorambucil on the chromatin of Yoshida ascites sarcoma cells. *Cancer Res.* **33:** 389–393.

RICHES, P. G. and HARRAP, K. R. (1975) The binding of [^{3}H]-chlorambucil to nuclear proteins of the Yoshida ascites sarcoma. *Chem.-Biol. Interact.* **11:** 291–299.

RICHTER, P., CALAMERA, J. C., MORGENFELD, M. C., KIERSZENBAUM, A. L., LAVIERI, J. C. and MANCINI, R. E. (1970) Effect of chlorambucil on spermatogenesis in the human with malignant lymphoma. *Cancer* **25:** 1026–1030.

RINCHIK, E. M., BANGHAM, J. W., HUNSICKER, P. R., CACHEIRO, N. L. A., KWON, B. S., JACKSON, I. J. and RUSSELL, L. B. (1990) Genetic and molecular analysis of chlorambucil-induced germ-line mutations in the mouse. *Proc. natn. Acad. Sci. U.S.A.* **87:** 1416–1420.

RITTER, C., RUTMAN, R. J. and PROOD, C. (1989) In vitro inhibition of nitrogen mustard efficacy by postincubation of treated cells in serum protein. *Cancer Biochem. Biophys.* **10:** 299–302.

ROBERT, J., BARBIER, P., MANASTER, J. and JACOBS, E. (1968) Hepatotoxicity of cytostatic drugs evaluated by liver-function tests and appearance of jaundice. *Digestion* **1:** 229–232.

ROBERTS, J. J. and WARWICK, G. P. (1961) The mode of action of alkylating agents. III. The formation of 3-hydroxytetra-hydrothiophene-1:1-dioxide from 1:4-dimethanesulphonyl-oxybutane (myleran), *S*-β-L-alanyltetrahydrothiophenium mesylate, tetrahydrothiophene and tetrahydrothiophene-1:1-dioxide in the rat, rabbit and mouse. *Biochem. Pharmac.* **6:** 217–227.

ROBINSON, R. and WATT, J. S. (1934) Some derivatives of 3-ethylpyridine and 2:3-furano (2′:3′)pyridine. *J. Chem. Soc.* 1536–1543.

ROBSON, C. N., ALEXANDER, J., HARRIS, A. L. and HICKSON, I. D. (1986) Isolation and characterization of a Chinese hamster ovary cell line resistant to bifunctional nitrogen mustards. *Cancer Res.* **46:** 6290–6294.

ROBSON, C. N., LEWIS, A. D., WOLF, C. R., HAYES, J. D., HALL, A., PROCTOR, S. J., HARRIS, A. L. and HICKSON, I. D. (1987) Reduced levels of drug-induced DNA cross-linking in nitrogen mustard-resistant Chinese hamster ovary cells expressing elevated glutathione*S*-transferase activity. *Cancer Res.* **47:** 6022–6027.

ROCKWELL, S., KEYES, S. R. and SARTORELLI, A. C. (1988) Modulation of the cytotoxicity of mitomycin C to EMT6 mouse mammary tumour cells by dicoumarol in vitro. *Cancer Res.* **48:** 5471–5474.

ROCKWELL, S., KEYES, S. R. and SARTORELLI, A. C. (1989) Modulation of the antineoplastic efficacy of mitomycin C by dicoumarol in vivo. *Cancer Chemother. Pharmac.* **24:** 349–353.

ROE, F. J. C. and SALAMAN, M. H. (1955) Further studies on incomplete carcinogenesis: triethylenemelamine (TEM), 1,2-benzanthracene and β-propiolactone as initiators of skin tumour formation in the mouse. *Br. J. Cancer* **9:** 177–203.

ROSE, L. M., JAMES, R. H., DUNCAN, S. and STRUCK, R. F. (1982) High-performance liquid chromatographic determination of spirohydantoin mustard in a clinically acceptable formulation of fat emulsion. *J. Chromatog.* **246:** 152–156.

ROSENBLUM, I. and STEIN, A. A. (1963) Preferential distribution of diphenylhydantoin in primary brain tumours. *Biochem. Pharmac.* **12:** 1453–1454.

ROSS, W. C. J. (1949) Aryl-2-halogenoalkylamines. Part I. *J. Chem. Soc.* pp. 183–191.

ROSS, W. C. J. (1975a) The conjugation of chlorambucil with humanβ-globulin. *Chem.-Biol. Interact.* **10:** 169–172.

ROSS, W. C. J. (1975b) The conjugation of chlorambucil with humanβ-globulin: confirmation that the drug is bound in an active form. *Chem.-Biol. Interact.* **11:** 139–143.

ROSS, W. C. J. and WARWICK, G. P. (1955) Reduction of cytotoxic azo compounds by hydrazine and by the xanthine oxidase-xanthine system. *Nature* **176:** 298–299.

ROSS, W. C. J. and WARWICK, G. P. (1956a) Aryl-2-halogeno-alkylamines. Part XVI. The preparation of derivatives of 4-[di-(2-choroalkyl)amino] azobenzenes. *J. Chem. Soc.* 1364–1369.

ROSS, W. C. J. and WARWICK, G. P. (1956b) Aryl-2-halogeno-alkylamines. Part XVIII. The rates of reduction of substituted 4-di-(2-chloroethyl) aminoazobenzenes by stannous chloride, hydrazine and the xanthine oxidase-xanthine system. *J. Chem. Soc.* 724–1732.

ROSS, W. E., EWIG, R. A. G. and KOHN, K. W. (1978) Differences between melphalan and nitrogen mustard in the formation and removal of DNA cross-links. *Cancer Res.* **38:** 1502–1506.

ROTH, E. F., ARNONE, A., BOOKCHIN, R. M. and NAGEL, R. L. (1981) Chemical modification of human hemoglobin by antisickling concentrations of nitrogen mustard. *Blood* **58:** 300–308.

RUBIN, J., KOVACK, J. S., MOERTEL, C. G., AMES, M., CREAGEN, E. T. and O'CONNELL, M. J. (1983) Phase I study of Henkel (HKL) compound on single day and daily for five day schedules. *Proc. Am. Soc. clin. Oncol.* **2:** 23.

RUHLAND, A., FLEER, R. and BRENDEL, L. M. (1978) Genetic activity of chemicals in yeast: DNA alterations and mutations induced by alkylating anti-cancer agents. *Mutat. Res.* **58:** 241–250.

RUNDLES, R. W. and BARTON, W. B.(1952) Triethylene melamine in the treatment of neoplastic disease. *J. Hematol.* **7:** 483–507.

RUTMAN, R. J., AVADHANI, N. G. and RITTER, C. (1977) Activation in vitro of nitrogen mustard by liposomal transport. *Biochem. Pharmac.* **26:** 85–88.

RUTMAN, R. J., CHUN, E. H. L. and JONES, J. (1969) Observations on the mechanism of the alkylation reaction between nitrogen mustard and DNA. *Biochim. biophys. Acta* **174:** 663–673.

RUTMAN, R. J., CHUN, E. H. L. and LEWIS, F. S. (1968) Permeability difference as a source of resistance to alkylating agents in Ehrlich tumour cells. *Biochem. biophys. Res. Commun.* **32:** 650–657.

SALAMAN. M. H. and ROE, F. J. C. (1956) Further tests for tumour-initiating activity: *N,N*-di-(2-chloroethyl)-*p*-aminophenylbutyric acid (CB 1348) as an initiator of skin tumour formation in the mouse. *Br. J. Cancer* **10:** 363–378.

SANO, A., MATSUTANI, S. and TAKITANI, S. (1988) High-performance liquid chromatography of the anti-tumour agent triethylenethiophosphoramide and its metabolite triethylenephosphoramide with sodium sulphide, taurine and *o*-phthalaldehyde as pre-column fluorescent derivatization reagents. *J. Chromatog.* **458:** 295–301.

SANO, Y., HOSHINO, T., BJERKVIG, R. and DEEN, D. F. (1983) The relative resistance of non-cycling cells in 9L multicellular spheroids to spirohydantoin mustard. *Eur. J. Cancer clin. Oncol.* **19:** 1451–1456.

SARNA, G. P., CHAMPLIN, R. and GALE, R. P. (1982) Phase I study of high-dose mitomycin with autologous bone marrow support. *Cancer Treat. Rep.* **66:** 277–281.

SARTORELLI, A. C. (1986) The role of mitomycin antibiotics in the chemotherapy of solid tumours. *Biochem. Pharmac.* **35:** 67–69.

SATO, S., INUI, N., IKEDA, Y. and HIRAGA, Y. (1989) A comparison of intraperitoneal injection and oral gavage in the micronucleus test with mitomycin C in mice. *Mutat. Res.* **223:** 387–390.

SCHILSKY, R. L., KELLEY, J. A., IHDE, D. C., HOWSER, D. M., CORDES, R. S. and YOUNG R. C. (1981) Phase I trial and pharmacokinetics of aziridinylbenzoquinone (NSC 182986) in humans. *Cancer Res.* **42:** 1582–1586.

SCHLAGER, J. J. and POWIS, G. (1988) Mitomycin C is not metabolized by but is an inhibitor of human kidney NAD(P)H: (quinone-acceptor) oxidoreductase. *Cancer Chemother. Pharmac.* **22:** 126–130.

SCHMÄHL, D. and OSSWALD, H. (1970) Experimentelle Untersuchungen über carcinogene Wirkungen von Krebs-Chemotherapeutica und Immunosuppressiva. *Arzneim. Forsch.* **20:** 1461–1467.

SCHMÄHL, D., HABS, M., LORENZ, M. and WAGNER, I. (1982) Occurrence of second tumours in man after anticancer drug treatment. *Cancer Treat. Rev.* **9:** 167–194.

SCHMALBACH, T. K. and BORCH, R. F. (1989) Myeloprotective effect of diethyldithiocarbamate treatment following 1,3-bis(2-chloroethyl)-1-nitrosourea, adriamycin, or mitomycin C in mice. *Cancer Res.* **49:** 2574–2577.

SCHMIDT, H. and LISS, E. (1978) Different uptake of two alkylating substances by ascites tumour cells. *Arzneim. Forsch.* **28:** 2150–2152.

SCHMIDT, L. H., FRANKLIN, R., SULLIVAN, R. and FLOWERS, A. (1965) Comparative pharmacology of alkylating agents. *Cancer Chemother. Rep.* **2:** 1–1528.

SCHWARTZ, H. S. (1962) Pharmacogy of mitomycin C: II. In vitro metabolism by rat liver. *J. Pharmac. exp. Ther.* **136:** 250–258.

SCHWARTZ, H. S. and PHILIPS, F. S. (1961) Pharmacogy of mitomycin C. II. Renal excretion and metabolism by tissue homogenates. *J. Pharmac. exp. Ther.* **133:** 335–342.

SCHWARTZ, H. S., SODERGREN, J. E. and PHILIPS, F. S.(1963) Mitomycin C: chemical and biological studies on alkylation. *Science* **142:** 1181–1183.

SELBY, P. J., LOPES, N., MUNDY, J., CROFTS, M., MILLAR, J. L. and MCELWAIN, T. J. (1987) Cyclophosphamide priming reduces intestinal damage in man following high dose melphalan chemotherapy. *Br. J. Cancer* **55:** 531–533.

SELLEI, C., ECKHARDT, S., HORVATH, I. P., KRALOVANSZKY, J. and INSTITORIS, L. (1969) Clinical and pharmacologic experience with dibromodulcitol (NSC 104800), a new antitumour agent. *Cancer Chemother. Rep.* **53:** 377–384.

SHARPE, H. B. A. (1971) Observations on the effect of therapy with nitrogen mustard or a derivative on chromosomes of human peripheral blood lymphocytes. *Cell Tissue Kinet.* **4:** 501–504.

SHELBY, M. D., GULATI, D. K., TICE, R. R. and WOJCIECHOWSKI, J. P. (1989) Results of tests for micronuclei and chromosomal aberrations in mouse bone marrow cells with the human carcinogens 4-aminobiphenyl, treosulphan and melphalan. *Env. Molec. Mutagen.* **13:** 339–342.

SHEPHERD, K. M. and SAGE, R. E. (1986) DNA binding by adriamycin, melphalan, *cis*-dichlorodiammine platinum (II) and nornitrogen mustard assessed by restriction enzyme block. *Res. Commun. Chem. Path. Pharm.* **54:** 367–378.

SHIBA, S., TERAWAKI, A., TAGUCHI, T. and KAWAMATA, J. (1959) Selective inhibition of formation of deoxyribonucleic acid in *Escherichia coli* by mitomycin C. *Nature* **183:** 1056–105.

SHIMKIN, M. B. (1954) Pulmonary tumour induction in mice with chemical agents used in the clinical management of lymphomas. *Cancer* **7:** 410–413.

SHIMKIN, M. B., WEISBURGER, J. H., WEISBURGER, E. K., GUBAREFF, N. K. and SUNTZEFF, V. (1966) Bioassay of 29 alkylating chemicals by the pulmonary tumour response in strain A mice. *J. natn. Cancer Inst.* **36:** 915–935.

SHIRAISHI, T., NIO, Y., OHGAKI, K. and TOBE, T. (1989) The inhibitory effect of a conjugate of human immunoglobulin G and melphalan K18, on DNA synthesis of human tumour cells. *Anticancer Res.* **9:** 599–604.

SHOEMAKER, D. D., O'DWYER, P. J., MARSONI, S., PLOWMAN, J., DAVIGNON, J. P. and DAVIS, R. D. (1983) Spriomustine: a new agent entering clinical trials. *Invest. New Drugs* **1:** 303–308.

SHOTTON, D., LYNCHBURG, V. and MONIE, I. W. (1963) Possible teratogenic effect of chlorambucil on a human fetus. *J. Am. Med. Ass.* **186:** 74–75.

SIEGEL, D., GIBSON, N. W., PREUSCH, P. C. and ROSS, D. (1990a) Metabolism of mitomycin C by DT-diaphorase: role in mitomycin C-induced DNA damage and cytotoxicity in human colon carcinoma cells. *Cancer Res.* **50:** 7483–7489.

SIEGEL, D., GIBSON, N. W., PREUSCH, P. C. and ROSS, D. (1990b) Metabolism of diaziquone by NAD(P)H: (quinone acceptor) oxidoreductase (DT-diaphorase): role in diaziquone-induced DNA damage and cytotoxicity in human colon carcinoma cells. *Cancer Res.* **50:** 7293–7300.

SILBER, R., POTMESI, M. and BANK, B. B. (1989) Studies on drug resistance in chronic lymphocytic leukemia. *Adv. Enzym. Reg.* **29:** 267–276.

SILVA, J. M. and O'BRIEN, P. J. (1989) Diaziquone-induced cytotoxicity in isolated rat hepatocytes. *Cancer Res.* **49:** 5550–5554.

SKAPEK, S. X., COLVIN, O. M., GRIFFITH, O. W., ELION, G. B., BIGNER, D. D. and FRIEDMAN, H. S. (1988) Enhanced melphalan cytotoxicity following buthionine sulfoximine-mediated glutathione depletion in a human medulloblastoma xenograft in athymic mice. *Cancer Res.* **48:** 2764–2767.

SKAPEK, S. X., VAN DELLEN, A. F., MCMAHON, D. P., POSTELS, D. G., GRIFFITH, O. W., BIGNER, D. D. and FRIEDMAN, H. S. (1991) Melphalan-induced toxicity in nude mice following pretreatment with buthionine sulfoximine. *Cancer Chemother. Pharmac.* **28:** 15–21.

SKIPPER, H. E., BENNETT, L. L. and LANGHAM, W. H. (1951) Overall tracer studies with C^{14}-labelled nitrogen mustard in normal and leukemic mice. *Cancer* **4:** 1025–1027.

SKURAI, Y. and ITO, K. (1960) Paper chromatographic detection of nitrogen mustard. *Chem. Pharm. Bull.* **8:** 655–656.

SMYTH, M. J., PIETERSZ, G. A. and MCKENZIE, I. F. C. (1986b) Potentiation of the in vitro cytotoxicity of chlorambucil by monoclonal antibodies. *J. Immun.* **137:** 3361–3366.

SMYTH, M. J., PIETERSZ, G. A. and MCKENZIE, I. F. C. (1987) Selective enhancement of antitumour activity of *N*-acetyl melphalan upon conjugation to monoclonal antibodies. *Cancer Res.* **47:** 62–69.

SMYTH, M. J., PIETERSZ, G. A., CLASSON, B. J. and MCKENZIE, I. F. C. (1986a) Specific targeting of chlorambucil to tumours with the use of monoclonal antibodies. *J. natn. Cancer Inst.* **76:** 503–510.

SOMFAI-RELLE, S., SUZUKAKE, K., VISTICA, B. P. and VISTICA D. T. (1984) Reduction in cellular glutathione by buthionine sulfoximine and sensitization of murine tumour cells resistant to L-phenylalanine mustard. *Biochem. Pharmac.* **33:** 485–490.

SOSTMAN, H. D., MATTHAY, R. A. and PUTMAN, C. E. (1977) Cytotoxic drug-induced lung disease. *Am. J. Med.* **62:** 608–615.

SPIEGEL, J. F., EGORIN, M. J., COLLINS, J. M., KAPLAN, R. and BACHUR, N. R. (1982) The murine metabolism and disposition of aziridinylbenzoquinone (AZQ) (NSC 182986). *Proc. Am. Ass. Cancer Res.* **23:** 177.

STEARNS, M. E. and TEW, K. D. (1985) Antimicrotubule effects of oestramustine, an antiprostatic tumour drug. *Cancer Res.* **45:** 3891–3897.

STEARNS, M. E. and TEW, K. D. (1988) Estramustine binds MAP-2 to inhibit microtubule assembly in vitro. *J. Cell Sci.* **89:** 331–342.

STEARNS, M. E., JENKINS, D. P. and TEW, K. D. (1985) Dansylated oestramustine, a fluorescent probe for studies of oestramustine uptake and identification of intracellular targets. *Proc. natn. Acad. Sci. U.S.A.* **82:** 8483–8487.

STEARNS, M. E., WANG, M. and SOUSA, O. (1991) Evidence that estramustine binds MAP-1A to inhibit type IV collagenase secretion. *J. Cell Sci.* **98:** 55–63.

STEARNS, M. E., WANG, M., TEW, K. D. and BINDER, L. I. (1988) Estramustine binds a MAP-1-like protein to inhibit microtubule assembly in vitro and disrupt microtubule organization in DU 145 cells. *J. Cell Biol.* **107:** 2647–2656.

STEEGE, J. F. and CALDWELL, D. S. (1980) Renal agenesis after first trimester exposure to chlorambucil. *South. Med. J.* **73:** 1414–1415.

STEIGBIGEL, R. T., KIM, H., POTOLSKY, A. (1974) Acute myeloproliferative disorder following long-term chlorambucil therapy. *Arch. Intern. Med.* **134:** 728–731.

STONER, G. D., SHIMKIN, M. B., KNIAZEFF, A. J., WEISBURGER, J. H., WEISBURGER, E. K. and GORI, G. B. (1973) Tests for carcinogenicity of food additives and chemotherapeutic agents by the pulmonary tumour response in strain A mice. *Cancer Res.* **33:** 3069–3085.

STOTT, H., FOX, W., GIRLING, D. J., STEPHENS, R. J. and GALTON, D. A. G. (1977) Acute leukaemia after busulphan. *Br. Med. J.* **ii:** 1513–1517.

SULING, W. J., STRUCK, R. F., WOOLLEY, C. W. and SHANNON, W. M. (1983) Metabolism of spirohydantoin mustard in the mouse. Isolation of an alkylating, mutagenic metabolite. *Biochem. Pharmac.* **32:** 523–527.

SUZUKAKE, K., PETRO, B. J. and VISTICA, D. T. (1982) Reduction in glutathione content of L-Pam resistant L1210 cells confers drug sensitivity. *Biochem. Pharmac.* **31:** 121–124.

SUZUKAKE, K., VISTICA, B. P. and VISTICA, D. T. (1983) Dechlorination of L-phenylalanine mustard by sensitive and resistant tumour cells and its relationship to intracellular glutathione content. *Biochem. Pharmac.* **32:** 165–167.

SVILAND, L., ROBINSON, A., PROCTOR, S. J. and BATEMAN, D. N. (1987) Interaction of cimetidine with oral melphalan. *Cancer Chemother. Pharmac.* **20:** 173–175.

SWEENEY, D. J., GREIG, N. H. and RAPOPORT, S. I. (1985) High-performance liquid chromatographic analysis of melphalan in plasma, brain and peripheral tissue by O-phthalaldehyde derivatization and fluorescence detection. *J. Chromatog.* **339:** 434–439.

SYKES, M. P., KARNOFSKY, D. A., PHILIPS, F. S. and BURCHENAL, J. H. (1953) Clinical studies on triethylene phosphoramides and diethylene phosphoramide compounds with nitrogen mustard like activity. *Cancer* **6:** 142–148.

SZIKLAI, I. L., AFRA, D., ORDOGH, M., INSTITORIS, L., KERPEL-FRONIUS, S. and SZABO, E. (1990) The distribution of bromine content of dibromodulcitol in the central nervous system of patients with malignant gliomas. *Eur. J. Cancer* **26:** 79–82.

TAHA, I. A.-K., AHMAD, R. A.-J. and ROGERS, H. J. (1981) Melphalan estimation by quantitative thin-layer chromatography. Observations on melphalan hydrolysis in vitro and pharmacokinetics in rabbits. *Cancer Chemother. Pharmac.* **5:** 181–184.

TAHA, I. A.-K., AHMAD, R. A.-J., GRAY, H., ROBERTS, C. I. and ROGERS, H. J. (1982) Plasma melphalan and prednisolone concentrations during oral therapy for multiple myeloma. *Cancer Chemother. Pharmac.* **9:** 57–60.

TAHA, I. A.-K., AHMAD, R. A.-J., ROGERS, D. W., PRITCHARD, J. and ROGERS, H. J. (1983) Pharmacokinetics of melphalan in children following high-dose intravenous injection. *Cancer Chemother. Pharmac.* **10:** 212–216.

TAN, C., HANCOCK, C., MILLER, L., CAPARROS, B. and LEYLAND-JONES, B. (1982) Phase I study of aziridinylbenzoquinone (AZQ, NSC 183986) in children with cancer. *Proc. Am. Ass. Cancer Res.* **23:** 120.

TAN, K. B., MATTERN, M. R., BOYCE, R. A. and SCHEIN, P. S. (1987) Elevated DNA topoisomerase II activity in nitrogen mustard-resistant human cells. *Proc. natn. Acad. Sci. U.S.A.* **84:** 7668–7671.

TAN, K. B., PER, S. R., BOYCE, R. A., MIRABELLI, C. K. and CROOKE, S. T. (1988) Altered expression and transcription of the topoisomerase II gene in nitrogen mustard-resistant human cells. *Biochem. Pharmac.* **37:** 4413–4416.

TANIMURA, T. (1968) Relation of dosage and time of administration to teratogenic effects of thioTEPA in mice. *Okajima. Folia Anat. Jap.* **44:** 203–253.

TATTERSALL, M. H. N., JARMAN, M., NEWLANDS, E. S., HOLYHEAD, L., MILSTEAD, R. A. V. and WEINBERG, A. (1978) Pharmacokinetics of melphalan following oral or intravenous administration in patients with malignant disease. *Eur. J. Cancer* **14:** 507–513.

TAYLOR, Y. C., EVANS, J. W. and BROWN, J. M. (1983) Mechanism of sensitization of Chinese hamster ovary cells to melphalan by hypoxic treatment with misonidazole. *Cancer Res.* **43:** 3175–3181.

TEICHER, B. A., CRAWFORD, J. M., HOLDEN, S. A. and CATHCART, K. N. S. (1987a) Effects of various oxygenation conditions on the enhancement by Fluosol-DA of melphalan antitumour activity. *Cancer Res.* **47:** 5036–5041.

TEICHER, B. A., HOLDEN, S. A. and JACOBS, J. L. (1987b) Approaches to defining the mechanism of enhancement by Fluosol-DA 20% with carbogen of melphalan antitumour activity. *Cancer Res.* **47:** 513–518.

TEICHER, B. A., HOLDEN, S. A. and ROSE, C. M. (1985) Differential enhancement of melphalan cytotoxicity in tumour and normal tissue by Fluosol-DA® and oxygen breathing. *Int. J. Cancer* **36:** 585–589.

TEICHER, B. A., WAXMAN, D. J., HOLDEN, S. A., WANG, Y., CLARKE, L., SOTOMAYOR, E. A., JONES, S. M. and FREI, E. (1989) Evidence for enzymatic activation and oxygen involvement in cytotoxicity and antitumour activity of *N,N,N''*-triethylenethiophosphoramide. *Cancer Res.* **49:** 4996–5001.

TENG, S. P., WOODSON, S. A. and CROTHERS, D. M. (1989) DNA sequence specificity of mitomycin cross-linking. *Biochemistry* **28:** 3901–3907.

TERRANOVA, A. C. (1969) Automated procedure for the determination of the aziridine moieties of *N,N'*-tetramethylene bis(1-aziridinecarboxamide) and other compounds containing aziridine. *J. Agric. Food Chem.* **17:** 1047–1051.

TEW, K. D. and STEARNS, M. E. (1987) Hormone-independent, non-alkylating mechanism of cytotoxicity for estramustine. *Urol. Res.* **15:** 155–160.

TEW, K. D. and STEARNS, M. E. (1989) Estramustine—a nitrogen mustard/steroid with antimicrotubule activity. *Pharmac. Ther.* **43:** 299–319.

TEW, K. D. and TAYLOR, D. M. (1978) Tissue distribution and nucleic acid binding of chlorambucil-^{3}H in tumour-bearing rats. *Experientia* **34:** 1215–1216.

TEW, K. D., BOMBER, A. M. and HOFFMAN, S. J. (1988) Ethacrynic acid and piriprost as enhancers of cytotoxicity in drug resistant and sensitive cell lines. *Cancer Res.* **48:** 3622–3625.

TEW, K. D., WOODWORTH, A. and STEARNS, M. E. (1986) Relationship of glutathione depletion and inhibition of glutathione-*S*-transferase activity to the antimitotic properties of estramustine. *Cancer Treat. Rep.* **70:** 715–720.

THORPE, P. E. and ROSS, W. C. J. (1982) The preparation and cytotoxic properties of antibody-toxin conjugates. *Immun. Rev.* **62:** 119–158.

TILBY, M. J., LAWLEY, P. D. and FARMER, P. B. (1990) Alkylation of DNA by melphalan in relation to immunoassay of melphalan-DNA adducts: characterization of mono-alkylated and cross-linked products from reaction of melphalan with dGMP and GMP. *Chem.-Biol. Interact.* **73:** 183–194.

TILBY, M. J., STYLES, J. M. and DEAN, C. J. (1987) Immunological detection of DNA damage caused by melphalan using monoclonal antibodies. *Cancer Res.* **47:** 1542–1546.

TIMMIS, G. M. (1950) Reported in *Br. Emp. Cancer Camp. Ann. Rep.* **28:** 58.

TINSLEY, P. W., O'DWYER, P. J. and LA CRETA, F. P. (1989) High-performance liquid chromatographic analysis of *N,N',N''*-triethylenethiophosphoramide in human plasma. *J. Chromatog.* **495:** 318–323.

TISDALE, M. J. and PHILLIPS, B. J. (1978) Cyclic nucleotide metabolism in Walker carcinoma cells resistant to alkylating agents. *Biochem. Pharmac.* **27:** 947–952.

TJADEN, U. R., DE BRUIJN, E. A., VAN DER HOEVEN, R. A. M., JOL, C., VAN DER GREEF, J. and LINGEMAN, H. (1987) Automated analysis of mitomycin C in body fluids by high-performance liquid chromatography with on-line sample pre-treatment. *J. Chromatog.* **420:** 53–62.

TJADEN, U. R., LANGENBERG, J. P., ENSING, K. and VAN BENNEKOM, W. P. (1982) Determination of mitomycin C in plasma, serum and urine by high-performance liquid chromatography with ultra-violet and electrochemical detection. *J. Chromatog.* **232:** 355–367.

TJANDRA, J. J., PIETERSZ, G. A., TEH, J. G., CUTHERBERTSON, A. M., SULLIVAN, J. R., PENFOLD, C. and MCKENZIE, I. F. C. (1989) Phase I clinical trial of drug-monoclonal antibody conjugates in patients with advanced colorectal carcinoma: a preliminary report. *Surgery* **106:** 533–545.

TOCH, R. (1953) Clinical studies on the carcinolytic action of triethylenephosphoramide. *Cancer* **6:** 135–141.

TOKUDA, K. and BODELL, W. J. (1987) Cytotoxicity and sister chromatid exchange in 9L cells treated with monofunctional and bifunctional nitrogen mustards. *Carcinogenesis* **8:** 1697–1701.

TOMASZ, M. (1976) H^2O^2 generation during the redox cycle of mitomycin C and DNA-bound mitomycin C. *Chem.-Biol. Interactions* **13:** 89–97.

TOMASZ, M. and LIPMAN, R. (1979) Alkylation reactions of mitomycin C at acid pH. *J. Am. Chem. Soc.* **101:** 6063–6067.

TOMASZ, M. and LIPMAN, R. (1981) Reductive metabolism and alkylating activity of mitomycin C induced by rat liver microsomes. *Biochemistry* **20:** 5056–5061.

TOMASZ, M., (1970) Novel assay of 7-alkylation of guanine residues in DNA. Application to nitrogen mustard, triethylenemelamine and mitomycin C. *Biochim. Biophys. Acta* **213:** 288–295.

TOMASZ, M., CHAWLA, A. K. and LIPMAN, R. (1988) Mechanism of monofunctional and bifunctional alkylation of DNA by mitomycin C. *Biochemistry* **27:** 3182–3187.

TOMASZ, M., CHOWDARY, D., LIPMAN, R., SHIMOTAKAHARA, S., VEIRO, D., WALKER, V. and VERDINE, G. L. (1986a) Reaction of DNA with chemically or enzymatically activated mitomycin C: Isolation and structure of the major covalent adduct. *Proc. natn Acad. Sci. U.S.A.* **83:** 6702–6706.

TOMASZ, M., LIPMAN, R., CHOWDARY, D., PAWLAK, J., VERDINE G. L. and NAKANISHI, K. (1987a) Isolation and structure of a covalent cross-link adduct between mitomycin C and DNA. *Science* **235:** 1204–1208.

TOMASZ, M., LIPMAN, R., LEE, M. S., VERDINE, G. L. and NAKANISHI, K. (1987b) Reaction of acid-activated mitomycin C with calf thymus DNA and model guanines: elucidation of the base-catalyzed degradation of N7-alkylguanine nucleosides. *Biochemistry* **26:** 2010–2027.

TOMASZ, M., LIPMAN, R., SNYDER, J. K. and NAKANISHI, K.(1983) Full structure of a mitomycin C dinucleoside phosphate adduct. Use of a differential FT-IR spectroscopy in microscale structural studies. *J. Am. Chem. Soc.* **105:** 2059–2063.

TOMASZ, M., LIPMAN, R., VERDINE, G. L. and NAKANISHI, K. (1986b) Reassignment of the guanine-binding mode of reduced mitomycin C. *Biochemistry* **25:** 4337–4344.

TOMASZ, M., MERCADO, C. M., OLSON, J. and CHATTERJIE, N. (1974) The mode of interaction of mitomycin C with deoxyribonucleic acid and other polynucleotides in vitro. *Biochemistry* **13:** 4878–4887.

TONG, W. P. and LUDLUM, D. B. (1980) Cross-linking of DNA by busulfan. Formation of diguanyl derivatives. *Biochim. biophys. Acta* **608:** 174–181.

TORRES-GARCIA, S. J., COUSINEAU, L., CAPLAN, S. and PANASCI, L. (1989) Correlation of resistance to nitrogen mustards in chronic lymphocytic leukemia with enhanced removal of melphalan-induced DNA cross-links. *Biochem. Pharmac.* **38:** 3122–3123.

TORRES-GARCIA, S., MCQUILLAN, A. and PANASCI, L. (1988) Correlation between the cytotoxicity of melphalan and DNA cross-links as detected by the ethidium bromide fluorescence assay in the F_1 variant of B_{16} melanoma cells. *Biochem. Pharmac.* **37:** 3189–3192.

TRAMS, E. G. and KLOPP, C. T. (1955) Distribution of radiocarbon in liver choline, creatine and methionine after the injection of methyl-C^{14} bis(β-chloroethyl) amine. *Cancer Res.* **15:** 617–619.

TRAMS, E. G. and NADKARNI, M. V. (1956) Studies on the *N*-dealkylation of nitrogen mustard and triethylene melamine by liver homogenates. *Cancer Res.* **16:** 1069–1075.

TRAMS, E. G., NADKARNI, M. V., DEQUATTRO, V., MAENGWYN-DAVIES, G. D. and SMITH, P. K.(1959) Dimethanesulphonoxybutane (Myleran). Preliminary studies on distribution and metabolic fate in the rat. *Biochem. Pharmac.* **2:** 7–16.

TRITSCH, G. L., SHUKLA, S. K., MITTELMAN, A. and MURPHY, G. P. (1974) Estracyt (NSC 89199) as a substrate for phosphatases in human serum. *Invest. Urol.* **12:** 38–39.

TWENTYMAN, P. R. and WORKMAN, P. (1983a) Chemosensitization by lipophilic nitroimidazoles. *Br. J. Cancer* **48:** 17–26.

TWENTYMAN, P. R. and WORKMAN, P. (1983b) An investigation of the possibility of chemosensitization by clinically achievable concentrations of misonidazole. *Br. J. Cancer* **47:** 187–194.

UNDERBERG, W. J. M. and LINGEMAN, H. (1983) Aspects of the chemical stability of mitomycin and porfinomycin in acidic solution. *J. Pharm. Sci.* **72:** 549–553.

VALERIOTE, F. and GRATES, H. E. (1989) Potentiation of nitrogen mustard cytotoxicity by disulfiram, diethyldithiocarbamic acid and diethylamine in mice. *Cancer Res.* **49:** 6658–6661.

VAN HAZEL, G. A. and KOVACH, J. S. (1982) Pharmacokinetics of mitomycin C in rabbit and human. *Cancer Chemother. Pharmac.* **8:** 189–192.

VAN MAELE-FABRY, G. and PICARD, J. J. (1987) Evaluation of the embryotoxic potential of ten chemicals in the whole mouse embryo culture. *Teratology* **36:** 95–106.

VASSAL, G., DEROUSSENT, A., HARTMANN, O., CHALLINE, D., BENHAMOU, E., ALTEAU-CONNES, D., BRUGIÈRES, L., KALIFA, C., GOUYETTE, A. and LEMERLE, J. (1990) Dose-dependent neurotoxicity of high-dose busulfan in children: a clinical and pharmacological study. *Cancer Res.* **50:** 6203–6207.

VASSAL, G., GOUYETTE, A., HARTMANN, O., PICO, J. L. and LEMERLE, J. (1989) Pharmacokinetics of high-dose busulfan in children. *Cancer Chemother. Pharmac.* **24:** 386–390.

VASSAL, G., RE, M. and GOUYETTE, A. (1988) Gas chromatographic-mass spectrometric assay for busulfan in biological fluids using a deuterated internal standard. *J. Chromatog. Biomed. Appl.* **428:** 357–361.

VERLY, W. G. and BRAKIER, L. (1969) The lethal action of monofunctional and bifunctional alkylating agents on T7 coliphage. *Biochim. biophys. Acta* **174:** 674–685.

VERWEIJ, J., DEN HARTIGH, J., STUURMAN, M., DE VRIES, J. and PINEDO, H. M. (1987a) Relationship between clinical parameters and pharmacokinetics of mitomycin C. *J. Cancer Res. clin. Oncol.* **113:** 91–94.

VERWEIJ, J., VAN ZANTEN, T., SOUREN, T., GOLDING, R. and PINEDO, H. M. (1987b) Prospective study on the dose relationship of mitomycin C-induced interstitial pneumonitis. *Cancer* **60:** 756–761.

VERWEY, J., DE VRIES, J. and PINEDO, H. M. (1987) Mitomycin C-induced renal toxicity, a dose-dependent side effect? *Eur. J. Cancer clin. Oncol.* **23:** 195–199.

VIDRA, I., SIMON, K., INSTITORIS, L., CSÖREGH, I. and CZUGLER, M. (1982) The chemical transformation products of 1,6-dibromo 1,6-dideoxygalactitol and 1,2:5,6-dianhydro-galactitol in aqueous solution. *Carbohyd. Res.* **111:** 41–57.

VISTICA, D. T. (1979) Cytotoxicity as an indicator for transport mechanism. Evidence that melphalan is transported by two leucine-preferring carrier systems in the L1210 murine leukaemia cell. *Biochem. biophys. Acta* **550:** 309–317.

VISTICA, D. T. and RABINOWITZ, M. (1979) Concentration uptake of melphalan, a cancer chemotherapeutic agent which is transported by the leucine-preferring carrier system. *Biochem. biophys. Res. Commun.* **86:** 929–932.

VISTICA, D. T., RABON, A. and RABINOWITZ, M. (1978a) Interference with melphalan transport and therapy in the L1210 murine leukemia system, its significance and prevention. *Proc. Am. Ass. Cancer Res.* **20:** 44.

VISTICA, D. T., RABON, A. and RABINOWITZ, M. (1978b) Enhancement of melphalan therapy with glutaminase: asparaginase. *Res. Commun. Chem. Path. Pharmac.* **22:** 83–92.

VISTICA, D. T., RABON, A. and RABINOWITZ, M. (1979a) Amino acid conferred protection against melphalan interference with melphalan therapy by L-leucine, a competitive substrate for transport. *Cancer Lett.* **6:** 7–13.

VISTICA, D. T., RABON, R. and RABINOWITZ, M. (1979b) Cytotoxicities of the L and D isomers of phenylalanine mustard in L1210 cells. *Biochem. Pharmac.* **28:** 3221–3225.

VISTICA, D. T., TOAL, J. N. and RABINOWITZ, M. (1978d) Amino-acid conferred protection against melphalan: interference with leucine protection of melphalan cytotoxicity by the basic amino acids in cultured murine L1210 leukaemia cells. *Molec. Pharmac.* **14:** 1136–1142.

VISTICA, D. T., TOAL, J. N. and RABINOWITZ, M. (1978c) Amino-acid conferred protection against melphalan—Characterization of melphalan transport and correlation of uptake with cytotoxicity in cultured L1210 murine leukaemia cells. *Biochem. Pharmac.* **27:** 2865–2870.

VISTICA, D. T., TOAL, J. N. and RABINOWITZ, M. (1976) Amino-acid conferred resistance to melphalan. I. Structure–activity relationship in cultured murine L1210 leukemia cells. *Cancer Treat. Rep.* **60:** 1363–1367.

VODOPICK, H., HAMILTON, H. E., JACKSON, H. L., PENG, C. T. and SHEETS, R. F. (1969) Metabolic fate of tritiated busulfan in man. *J. Lab. clin. Med.* **73:** 266–276.

VON SCHOULTZ, E., GUNNARSSON, P.-O. and HENRICKSSON, R. (1989) Uptake, metabolism and antiproliferative effect of estramustine phosphate in human glioma cell lines. *Anticancer Res.* **9:** 1713–1716.

VON SCHOULTZ, E., LUNDBLAD, D., BERGH, J., GRANKVIST, K. and HENRICKSSON, R. (1988) Estramustine binding protein and anti-proliferative effect of estramustine in human glioma cell lines. *Br. J. Cancer* **58:** 326–329.

VROMANS, R. M., VAN DE STRAAT, R., GROENEVELD, M. and VERMEULEN, P. E. (1990) One-electron reduction of mitomycin C rat liver: role of cytochrome P-450 and NADPH-cytochrome P-450 reductase. *Xenobiotica* **20:** 967–978.

WAKAKI, S., MARUMO, H., TOMIOKA, K., SHIMIZU, G., KATO, E., KAMADA, H., KUDO, S. and FUJIMOTO, Y. (1958) Isolation of new fractions of antitumour mitomycins. *Antibiot. Chemother.* **8:** 228–240.

WALLIN, M., DEINUM, J. and FRIDEN, B. (1985) Interaction of oestramustine phosphate with microtubule-associated proteins. *FEBS Letters* **179:** 289–293.

WALLIN, M., DEINUM, J. and HARTLEY-ASP, B. (1986) Estramustine phosphate inhibits microtubule assembly by binding to the microtubule-associated proteins. *Ann. NY Acad. Sci.* **466:** 423–425.

WALPOLE, A. L. (1958) Carcinogenic action of alkylating agents. *Ann. NY Acad. Sci.* **68:** 750–761.

WANG, M. and STEARNS, M. E. (1988) Blocking of collagenase secretion by estramustine during in vitro tumour cell invasion. *Cancer Res.* **48:** 6262–6271.

WANG, M., TEW, K. D. and STEARNS, M. E. (1987) Immunofluorescent studies of the anti-microtubule effects of the anti-cancer drug estramustine. *Anticancer Res.* **7:** 1165–1172.

WANG, P., BENNETT, R. A. O. and POVIRK, L. F. (1990) Melphalan-induced mutagenesis in an SV40-based shuttle vector: predominance of A. T
T. A transversions. *Cancer Res.* **50:** 7527–7531.

WEBB, J. S., COSULICH, D. B., MOWAT, J. H., PATRICK, J. B., BROSCHARD, R. W., MEYER, W. E., WILLIAMS, R. P., WOLF, C. F., FULMOR, W., PIDACKS, C. and LANCASTER, J. E. (1962) The structures of mitomycins A, B and C and porfiromycin — Part 1. *J. Am. Chem. Soc.* **84:** 3185–3187.

WEISBACH, A. and LISIO, A. (1965) Alkylation of nucleic acids by mitomycin C and porfiromycin. *Biochemistry* **4:** 196–200.

WEISBURGER, J. H., GRISWOLD, D. P., PREJEAN, J. D., CASEY, A. E., WOOD, H. B. and WEISBURGER, E. K. (1975) The carcinogenic properties of some of the principal drugs used in clinical cancer chemotherapy. *Rec. Res. Cancer Res.* **52:** 1–17.

WELSH, J., STUART, J. F. B., SETANOIANS, A., BLACKIE, R. G. G., BILLIAERT, P., HALBERT, G. and CALMAN, K. C. (1984) The analysis and animal pharmacokinetics of 1,2,4-tri-glycidyl urazol using a high-pressure liquid chromatographic technique. *Cancer Chemother. Pharmac.* **12:** 198–200.

WELSH, J., STUART, J. F. B., SOUKOP, M., CUNNINGHAM, D., BLACKIE, R., SANGSTER, G. and CALMAN, K. C. (1982) The pharmacokinetics of oral and i.v. treosulfan. *Br. J. Cancer* **46:** 467.

WHEELER, G. P. and SKIPPER, H. E. (1957) Studies with mustards. III. In vivo fixation of ^{14}C from nitrogen mustard ^{14}CH^{3} in nucleic acid fractions of animal tissues. *Arch. Biochem. Biophys.* **72:** 465–475.

WHISSON, M. E. and CONNORS, T. A. (1965a) Drug-induced regression of large plasma cell tumours. *Nature* **205:** 406.

WHISSON, M. E. and CONNORS, T. A. (1965b) Cure of mice bearing advanced plasma cell tumours with aniline mustard. *Nature* **206:** 689–691.

WHITE, I. N. H., SUZANGER, M., MATTOCKS, A. R., BAILEY, E., FARMER, P. B. and CONNORS, T. A. (1989)

Reduction of nitromin to nitrogen mustard: unscheduled DNA synthesis in aerobic or anaerobic rat hepatocytes, JB1, BL8 and Walker carcinoma cell lines. *Carcinogenesis* **10:** 2113–2118.

WILCOCK, C. and HICKMAN, J. A. (1988) Characterization of a $Na^+/K^+/Cl^-$ cotransporter in alkylating agent-sensitive L1210 murine leukemia cells. *Biochim. biophys. Acta* **946:** 359–367.

WILCOCK, C., CHAHWALA, S. B. and HICKMAN, J. A. (1988) Selective inhibition of bis(2-chloroethyl)methylamine (nitrogen mustard) of the $Na^+/K^+/Cl^-$ cotransporter of murine L1210 leukemia cells. *Biochim. biophys. Acta* **946:** 368–378.

WILKINSON, R., GUNNARSSON, P. O., FORSHELL, G. P., RENSHAW, J. and HARRAP, K. R. (1978) The hydrolysis of prednimustine by enzymes from normal and tumour tissues. In: *Advances in Tumor Prevention, Detection and Characterization*, pp. 260–273, DAVIS, W. and HARRAP, K. R. (eds) Excerpta Medica, Amsterdam.

WILLIAMSON, C. E., KIRBY, J. G., MILLER, J. I., SASS, S., KRAMER, S. P., SEIGMAN, A. M. and WITTEN, B. (1966) Enzyme alterable alkylating agents. IX. The enzymatic transformation of some nitrogen mustards in the presence of carbon dioxide: implications in respiration. *Cancer Res.* **26:** 323–330.

WOLPERT, M. K. and RUDDON, R. W. (1969) A study on the mechanism of resistance to nitrogen mustard (HN2) in Ehrlich ascites tumour cells: comparison of uptake of HN2-^{14}C into sensitive and resistant cells. *Cancer Res.* **29:** 873–879.

WOODHOUSE, K. W., HAMILTON, P., LENNARD, A. and RAWLINS, M. D. (1983) The pharmacokinetics of melphalan in patients with multiple meyloma: an intravenous/oral study using a conventional dose regimen. *Eur. J. clin. Pharmac.* **24:** 283–285.

WORKMAN, P. (1978) Inhibition of human prostatic tumour acid phosphatase by *N,N-p*-di-2-chloroethylaminophenol, *N,N-p*-di-2-chloroethylaminophenyl phosphate and other difunctional nitrogen mustards. *Chem.-Biol. Interact.* **20:** 103–112.

WORKMAN, P. and DOUBLE, J. A. (1978) Enzyme activated anti-tumour agents. IV. Comparative kinetics of *N,N-p*-di-2-chloroethylaminophenyl phosphate hydrolysis catalysed by phosphatases of normal and neoplastic tissues. *Biochem. Pharmac.* **27** :199–202.

WORKMAN, P., BALL, C. R. and DOUBLE, J. A. (1976a) Enzyme activated anti-tumour agents. II. The role of alkaline phosphatase in the release of *p*-hydroxyaniline mustard from its phosphate in cells in culture. *Biochem. Pharmac.* **25:** 1139–1144.

WORKMAN, P., DOUBLE, J. A. and WILMAN, D. E. V. (1976b) Enzyme activated anti-tumour agents. III. Hydrolysis of conjugates of *p*-hydroxyaniline mustard in aqueous solution. *Biochem. Pharmac.* **25:** 2347–2350.

WORKMAN, P., OPPITZ, M., DONALDSON, J. and LEE, F. Y. F. (1987) High-performance liquid chromatography of chlorambucil analogs. *J. Chromatog.* **422:** 315–321.

WRIGHT, J. C., GOLOMB, F. M. and GUMPORT, S. L. (1958) Summary of results with triethylenethiophosphoramide. *Ann NY Acad. Sci.* **68:** 937–966.

WRIGHT, J. C., PRIGOT, A., WRIGHT, L. T. and ARONS, I. (1952) Further observations on the use of triethylene melamine in neoplastic diseases. *Arch. Intern. Med.* **89:** 387–404.

YERUSHALMI, A. and YAGIL, C. (1980) The interaction of chromatin with alkylating agents. The monofunctional action of bis (2-chloroethyl)methylamine. *Eur. J. Biochem.* **103:** 237–246.

YOUNG, C. W., YAGODA, A., BITTAR, E. S., SMITH, S. W., GRABSTALD, H. and WHITMORE, W.(1976) Therapeutic trial of aniline mustard in patients with advanced cancer. *Cancer* **38:** 1887–1895.

ZACKHEIM, H. S. and SMUCKLER, E. A.(1980) Tumorigenic effect of topical mechlorethamine, BCNU and CCNU in mice. *Experientia* **36:** 1211–1212.

ZAKARIA, M. and BROWN, P. R. (1982) Rapid assay for plasma chlorambucil and phenyl acetic mustard using reversed-phase liquid chromatography. *J. Chromatog. Biomed. Appl.* **230:** 381–389.

ZEIGER, E. and PAGANO, D. A. (1989) Mutagenicity of the human carcinogen treosulphan in *Salmonella. Environ. Molec. Mutagen.* **13:** 343–346.

ZIMBER, A., PERK, K. and LIVNAT, I. (1988) Priming with low doses of methyl-CCNU reduce the toxicity of high doses of methyl-CCNU and melphalan and increase the lifespan of mice implanted with Lewis lung carcinoma. *Br. J. Cancer* **57:** 266–270.

ZWELLING, L. A., MICHAELS, S., SCHWARTZ, H., DOBSON, P. P. and KOHN, K. W. (1981) DNA cross-linking as an indicator of sensitivity and resistance of mouse L1210 leukemia to *cis*-diamminedichloroplatinum (II) and L-phenylalanine mustard. *Cancer Res.* **41:** 640–649.

Garth Powis, editor.
(1994) *Anticancer Drugs: Reactive Metabolism and Drug Interactions*,
Pergamon Press Ltd, pp. 79–156
Printed in the United Kingdom

CHAPTER 2

METABOLISM AND PHARMACOKINETIC BEHAVIOR OF CYCLOPHOSPHAMIDE AND RELATED OXAZAPHOSPHORINES

N. E. SLADEK

Department of Pharmacology, University of Minnesota, 3-249 Millard Hall, 435 Delaware Street S.E., Minneapolis, MN 55455, U.S.A.

1. INTRODUCTION

Synthesis of the first clinically useful oxazaphosphorine, viz. 2-bis[(2-chloroethyl)amino]tetrahydro-2H-1,3,2-oxazaphosphorine 2-oxide was reported more than three decades ago (Arnold and Bourseaux, 1958). In the intervening years, this agent, which goes by the nonproprietary name of cyclophosphamide, has enjoyed widespread use as an antineoplastic and immunosuppressive drug. Other oxazaphosphorines (Fig. 1) are also emerging as potentially useful therapeutic agents. Thus, cyclophosphamide and some of its congeners are of demonstrated clinical utility in the treatment of (1) various lymphoproliferative and myeloproliferative disorders (Calabresi and Chabner, 1990; American Medical Association, 1992), (2) certain solid malignancies (Calabresi and Chabner, 1990; American Medical Association, 1992) and (3) various clinical maladies whose etiology includes an autoimmune component (Fauci et al., 1971; Mukherjee, 1971; Gonsette et al., 1977; Marmont et al., 1979; McCarty and Carrera, 1982; Hauser et al., 1983; Horslev-Peterson et al., 1983; Balow et al., 1984; Myers, 1987; Calabresi and Chabner, 1990; De Vita et al., 1991; American Medical Association, 1992). Most of the disorders for which therapy with oxazaphosphorines is of proven clinical value are listed in Table 1.

Cyclophosphamide has also proven to be of value in transplantation protocols where it is used at high doses as an immunosuppressant to 'condition' recipients and as a tumor-ablative agent (Starzl et al., 1971; Thomas et al., 1975; Champlin and Gale, 1984; Phillips and Connors, 1987; Kennedy et al., 1991). In addition, analogs of 'activated cyclophosphamide', e.g. 4-hydroperoxycyclophosphamide and mafosfamide, may be of value for *regional* chemotherapy of cancer (Arndt et al., 1987; Phillips et al., 1992). Moreover, these agents have already been shown to be of value when used ex vivo for the purpose of purging autologous bone marrow of neoplastic cells prior to transplantation (Sharkis et al., 1980; Kluin-Nelemans et al., 1984; Manna et al., 1986; Yeager et al., 1986; Santos et al., 1989; Sindermann et al., 1989; Jones and Santos, 1990; Rizzoli and Mangoni, 1990; Gorin et al., 1991; Kennedy et al., 1991). Ex vivo purging of allogenic bone marrow for the purpose of minimizing graft-versus-host disease has been suggested (Shand, 1978; Korbling et al., 1982; Kohn and Sladek, 1988).

Recent investigations have shown cyclophosphamide to be of potential synergistic therapeutic value in the treatment of certain cancers when combined with interleukin 2 (IL-2) and ex vivo IL-2-expanded allogeneic lymphokine-activated (LAK) cells or ex vivo IL-2-expanded tumor-infiltrating lymphocytes (TIL). As an added benefit, cyclophosphamide reduces the toxicity effected by IL-2 administration, at least in animal models. The basis for cyclophosphamide's synergistic action in these protocols has not been established. In the case of allogeneic LAK cells, which are not T-cells, it may be acting by suppressing the host immune system thus permitting the survival of the donor allogeneic LAK cells. TIL cells are T-cells and thus may be inhibited by T-suppressor cells and other suppressor factors, e.g. those associated with B-cells, macrophages and tumor cells. Cyclophosphamide may potentiate the antitumor action of TIL by inhibiting T-suppressor cell

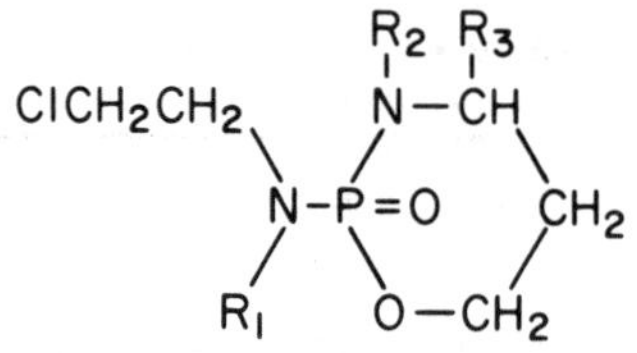

OXAZAPHOSPHORINE	R_1	R_2	R_3
CYCLOPHOSPHAMIDE			H–
4-HYDROPEROXYCYCLOPHOSPHAMIDE	$ClCH_2CH_2$–	H–	HOO–
MAFOSFAMIDE			^-O_3S–CH_2CH_2–S–
IFOSFAMIDE	H–	$ClCH_2CH_2$–	H–
4-HYDROPEROXYIFOSFAMIDE			HOO–
TROFOSFAMIDE	$ClCH_2CH_2$–	$ClCH_2CH_2$–	H–

FIG. 1. Chemical structures of several oxazaphosphorines.

TABLE 1. *Disorders for which the Oxazaphosphorines are of Demonstrated Clinical Value*

Myeloproliferative and lymphoproliferative disorders
- (1) Leukemias
  - (a) Chronic lymphocytic leukemia
  - (b) Chronic granulocytic leukemia (ineffective in acute blastic crises)
  - (c) Acute myelogenous and monocytic leukemia
  - (d) Acute lymphoblastic leukemia in children
- (2) Malignant lymphomas
  - (a) Hodgkin's disease
  - (b) Burkitt's lymphoma
  - (c) Follicular lymphoma
  - (d) Lymphocytic lymphosarcoma
  - (e) Reticulum cell sarcoma
  - (f) Lymphoblastic lymphosarcoma
- (3) Multiple myeloma
- (4) Mycosis fungoides

Solid malignancies
- (1) Neuroblastoma
- (2) Wilms' tumor
- (3) Retinoblastoma
- (4) Adenocarcinoma of the ovary
- (5) Rhabdomyosarcoma
- (6) Carcinomas of the lung, breast and cervix

Disorders with an autoimmune component
- (1) Rheumatoid arthritis
- (2) Multiple sclerosis
- (3) Wegener's granulamatosis
- (4) Systemic lupus erythematosus
- (5) Proliferative glomerulonephritis
- (6) Autoallergic ocular disease

TABLE 2. *Current and Potential Uses of the Oxazaphosphorines where the Uneconomic Species is of Lymphoid Lineage*

	Use		Uneconomic species
In vivo	Lymphoproliferative disorders*		Malignant lymphoid cells
	Immunosuppression	Pretransplant conditioning	Non-malignant lymphoid cells
		Autoimmune disorders	
	Immunoaugmentation		T-suppressor cells
Ex vivo	Marrow transplantation	Autologous	Malignant lymphoid cells†
		Allogenic	GVHD-producing T-lymphocytes

*The oxazaphosphorines are also of value in the treatment of certain myeloproliferative disorders and solid malignancies.
†More frequently, this modality has been used to treat myeloproliferative disorders.

and/or other suppressor factor production.* In any event, 'adoptive immunotherapy', as the above-described approaches have been termed, shows promise as a therapeutic strategy in the treatment of certain neoplasms (Rosenberg, 1984; Rosenberg et al., 1986, 1988; Awwad and North, 1988; Papa et al., 1988; Lafreniere et al., 1989). The immunoaugmenting action of the oxazaphosphorines, manifested when these agents are given alone at low doses (Hilgard et al., 1985; Mokyr and Dray, 1987; Berd and Mastrangelo, 1988; Awwad and North, 1989; Reissman et al., 1989), may also have clinical potential.

Intriguing, too, is the recent observation (Simard and Jolicoeur, 1991) suggesting that the oxazaphosphorines may be of therapeutic benefit when used to treat certain acquired immunodeficiency syndromes.

Noteworthy is that, in those cases where the oxazaphosphorines have demonstrated or suspected therapeutic value, the target cell, i.e. the uneconomic species, is often of lymphoid lineage (Table 2).

The oxazaphosphorines are believed to be of therapeutic value in each of these clinical settings

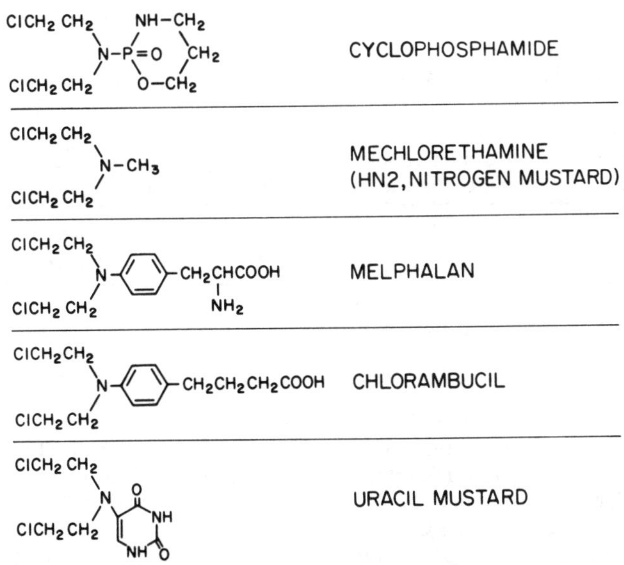

FIG. 2. Chemical structures of cyclophosphamide and several other clinically useful bifunctional nitrogen mustards. Note that common to all of these agents is the bis-(2-chloroethyl)-amine moiety.

*Selective inhibition of T-suppressor cells by 'activated cyclophosphamide' analogs thus facilitating the ex vivo activation and expansion of tumor-reactive lymphocytes has also been proposed (Inge et al., 1992).

TABLE 3. *Therapeutic Indices of Cyclophosphamide and Chlorambucil in Rats Bearing the Walker 256 Carcinoma*

Drug	ED_{50}, mg/kg*	TD_{50}, mg/kg†	TI‡
Cyclophosphamide	0.7	19	27
Chlorambucil	0.8	3	4

*Dose that inhibited the intramuscular growth of the Walker 256 carcinosarcoma 50%; values were obtained as described by Sladek (1972a).

†Dose that depressed the peripheral blood leukocyte count to 50% of control values when the count was made three days after the administration of the drug; values were obtained as described by Sladek (1972a).

‡Therapeutic index: TD_{50}/ED_{50}.

because of their ability to cross-link the DNA of target cells thus rendering them nonviable (see Sections 5 and 6). There are a number of other drugs that are toxic to such cells. Some, e.g. melphalan, chlorambucil, uracil mustard and mechlorethamine (Fig. 2), even effect their cytotoxic action by an identical mechanism (Calabresi and Chabner, 1990). Of them all, however, the oxazaphosphorines are often considered to be the most clinically useful. The question is why?

The answer is relatively straightforward. When employing cytotoxic drugs, the underlying strategy is always to injure the uneconomic species without injuring the economic species. Thus, the goal is to spare critical normal cells, e.g. pluripotent hematopoietic cells, while poisoning cancer cells when the drugs are used as antineoplastic agents, and various, relatively differentiated, cells of the immune system when immunomodulation is the therapeutic goal. It follows that the drug that does this best is the one that will be the most useful clinically. Relative to other currently available nitrogen mustards, indeed, most other cytotoxic agents, the oxazaphosphorines very often do it best. The point is clearly illustrated by the experiments presented in Tables 3 and 4. Cyclophosphamide exhibited, by far, the greater margin of safety when in vivo therapeutic indices were determined for it and another nitrogen mustard, viz. chlorambucil (Table 3). Thus, the two agents were approximately equipotent with regard to their antitumor activity but chlorambucil was much more potent with regard to toxicity towards normal cells. Similarly, cyclophosphamide exhibited the greatest margin of safety when ex vivo therapeutic indices were determined for it and three other cross-linking agents, two of which, viz. mechlorethamine and melphalan, are also nitrogen mustards (Table 4). Bone marrow toxicity is often the major dose-limiting factor in the chemotherapy of neoplastic diseases. The results of the foregoing experiments are as expected then,

TABLE 4. *Ex Vivo Therapeutic Indices of Mafosfamide (Cyclophosphamide) and Several Other Cross-linking Agents*

	EC_{50}, μM*			TI‡	
Drug	L1210	P388	TC_{50}, μM†	L1210	P388
Cyclophosphamide§	10	1	87	8.7	87
Mechlorethamine	0.16	0.08	0.13	0.8	2
Melphalan	0.80	0.21	2.2	2.8	10
Cisplatin	35	1.5	26	0.7	17

*Drug concentration that inhibited the ex vivo growth of mouse L1210 or P388 cells by 50%; values were obtained as described by Sladek et al. (1985).

†Drug concentration that inhibited the ex vivo growth of mouse CFU-GEMM by 50%; values were obtained as described by Kohn et al. (1987b).

‡Therapeutic index: TC_{50}/EC_{50}.

§The test drug was actually mafosfamide. As described in detail later in this chapter, cyclophosphamide per se is without cytotoxic activity. CFU-GEMM and L1210 and P388 cells are unable to activate it because they lack the enzyme that catalyzes the activation. Mafosfamide is often used in place of cyclophosphamide in in vitro and ex vivo experiments, as it was here, because it gives rise to the same metabolites as does cyclophosphamide without the necessity of enzymatic participation.

given the knowledge that cyclophosphamide is relatively hematopoietic stem cell-sparing (Fried et al., 1977; Sensenbrenner et al., 1979; Neidhart et al., 1990). Colvin and Hilton (1981) demonstrated cyclophosphamide's relatively favorable margin of safety in another way. They found that when cyclophosphamide was given to L1210 tumor-bearing mice, more DNA was cross-linked in the L1210 leukemic cells than in the bone marrow cells obtained from these animals. This was in contrast to the results obtained with phosphoramide mustard; it produced similar degrees of DNA cross-linking in the leukemia and bone marrow cells.

The question then becomes, what is the biological basis for oxazaphosphorine-specific selectivity, that is, the selectivity above and beyond that exhibited by other nitrogen mustards?

In view of the existing, as well as the additional potential, therapeutic importance of the oxazaphosphorines, the search for the answer to this question has been, and remains, compelling; many laboratories have pursued it. Since cyclophosphamide itself is therapeutically inactive, i.e. it is a prodrug, much of the investigative effort has been directed toward identifying metabolites of cyclophosphamide, characterizing the reactions that give rise to their formation, identifying the catalysts of these reactions, and evaluating the cytotoxic potential of the identified metabolites. This knowledge was deemed to be particularly important early on for at least four reasons: the cytotoxic action of cyclophosphamide had to be due to one or more of its metabolites, the untoward effects of cyclophosphamide were very likely produced by one or more of its metabolites, the basis for cyclophosphamide's relatively favorable therapeutic index was very likely related to its metabolism, and there was great potential for modulating, whether favorably or unfavorably in terms of the therapeutic outcome, its metabolism.

This review attempts to summarize the results of these investigations; particular emphasis is placed on the metabolism of cyclophosphamide and other oxazaphosphorines as it relates to the therapeutic efficacy of these agents. The reader is advised that a symposium held in London, England and published in *Cancer Treatment Reports* (Cox et al., 1976a) and reviews authored by Hill (1975), Brock and Hohorst (1977), Friedman et al. (1979), Colvin and Hilton (1981), Stec (1982), Zon (1982), Brock (1983, 1986, 1989), Hengst and Kempf (1984), Sladek (1987, 1988) and Brock et al. (1988) provide excellent earlier summaries of oxazaphosphorine chemistry and pharmacology.

2. RATIONALE FOR SYNTHESIS

Formulation of the rationale that ultimately led to the synthesis of cyclophosphamide and other oxazaphosphorines was by Seligman and coworkers (Seligman et al., 1949; Rutenburg et al., 1954; Friedman and Seligman, 1954). Known at the time was that mechlorethamine and certain other rather chemically simple bis-(2-chloroethyl)-amines, i.e. bifunctional nitrogen mustards, were highly toxic to cells by virtue of their ability to readily form highly reactive carbonium ions (Fig. 3). Unfortunately, these compounds exhibited only minimal selectivity, i.e. they were approximately equitoxic to normal and neoplastic cells. It was also known that decreasing the basicity of the nitrogen atom of bis-(2-chloroethyl)-amine would markedly retard, if not completely prevent, carbonium ion formation, and that the basicity of the nitrogen atom could be decreased by the placement of an electron-withdrawing group on it. Finally, it had been reported that a number of malignant epithelial tumors had, relative to normal tissues, high levels of phosphoroamidase activity (Gomori, 1948). Phosphoroamidases catalyze the hydrolysis of nitrogen-phosphorous bonds. Hence, the idea was to conjugate bis-(2-chloroethyl)-amine with a suitable electron-withdrawing substituted phosphoryl group thus producing a 'transport' or 'latent' form of the drug, i.e. a prodrug. The prodrug would be activated when the bis-(2-chloroethyl)-amine residue was separated from the phosphoryl residue as a consequence of phosphoroamidase-catalyzed hydrolysis (Fig. 4). Selectivity would be achieved because of the purported relatively greater phosphoroamidase activity in tumor tissue.

Despite a substantial effort (Rutenburg et al., 1954; Friedman and Seligman, 1954), Seligman's laboratory never did synthesize a clinically useful agent.* However, another laboratory met with

*Ironically, they did synthesize phosphoramide mustard (Friedman and Seligman, 1954), a metabolite of cyclophosphamide now recognized as ultimately effecting its cytotoxic action (see Sections 3 and 6).

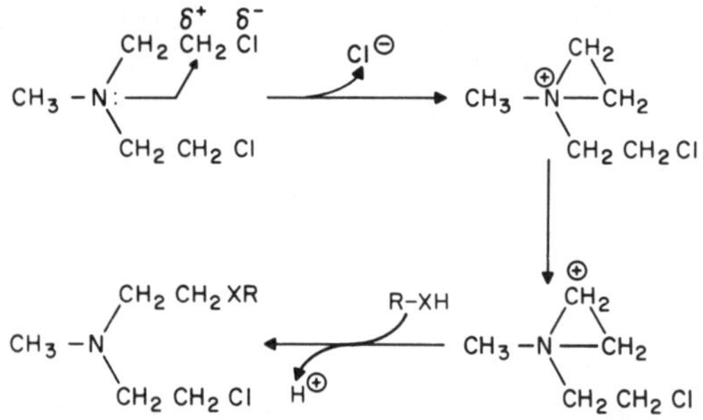

FIG. 3. Mechanism by which nitrogen mustards form covalent bonds with nucleophilic residues. Initially, one of the chloroethyl side chains undergoes a first-order (Sn1) intramolecular cyclization, releasing chloride ion to form a highly reactive ethylenimmonium intermediate. The latter, in turn, yields an electrophilic (electron deficient) carbonium ion that can react with a large number of nucleophilic (electron rich) residues by a second-order (Sn2) nucleophilic substitution reaction. Nucleophilic residues (X) include, but are not limited to, amino, hydroxyl, sulfhydryl and imidazole groups of proteins and nucleic acids. The second chloroethyl side chain can then undergo the same sequence of events.

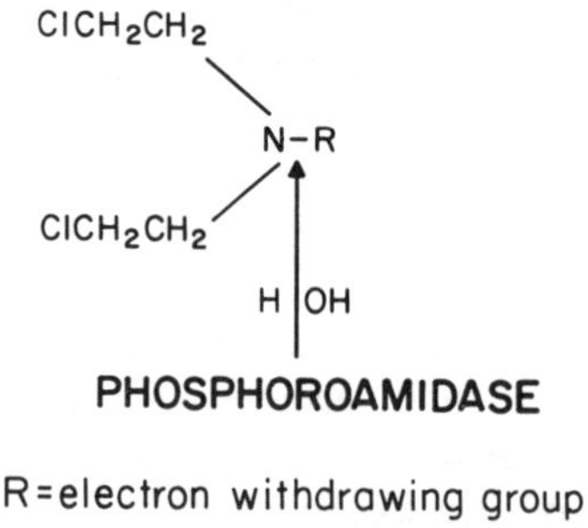

FIG. 4. Rationale for the synthesis of cyclophosphamide and like compounds. Conjugation of an electron-withdrawing group (R) with bis-(2-chloroethyl)-amine yields nitrogen mustards that are relatively inactive. Substituted phosphoryls are electron-withdrawing; they were to be conjugated to bis-(2-chloroethyl)-amine via a nitrogen-phosphorus bond to produce a prodrug. Phosphoroamidase cleaves such bonds. Cleavage of the prodrug by phosphoroamidase was to yield the active metabolite, viz. bis-(2-chloroethyl)-amine. Selectivity was to be achieved because of the purportedly relatively greater phosphoroamidase activity in tumor tissue.

more success. Embracing the concept outlined above, Arnold and coworkers (Arnold and Bourseaux, 1958; Arnold et al., 1961) synthesized many hundreds of phosphorous-containing compounds; one of these was cyclophosphamide, a prodrug that was quickly shown to be relatively selectively toxic to tumor cells growing in rodents and later, to certain human neoplasms. Almost from the beginning, however, it was recognized that activation of cyclophosphamide was not by target tumor cells, as had been intended according to the original rationale for its synthesis, since tumor cells sensitive to the drug in vivo were not sensitive to it in vitro (Arnold et al., 1958). Thus, vigorous pursuit of an understanding of its metabolism followed and continues to the present day.

3. METABOLISM OF CYCLOPHOSPHAMIDE AND OTHER OXAZAPHOSPHORINES

A somewhat abridged scheme of the current understanding of cyclophosphamide activation is presented in Fig. 5.

Cyclophosphamide, itself without cytotoxic activity, is first hydroxylated to yield 4-hydroxycyclophosphamide which exists in equilibrium with its ring-opened tautomer, aldophosphamide. The tautomers are, themselves, also without cytotoxic activity. They serve as transport forms for acrolein and phosphoramide mustard, each of which is cytotoxic; the latter effects the bulk of cyclophosphamide's therapeutic action.

Hydroxylation to the 4-hydroxy intermediate is catalyzed primarily, if not exclusively, by the mixed-function oxidases present in the endoplasmic reticulum of liver. The subsequent ring-opening of 4-hydroxycyclophosphamide to aldophosphamide is subject to general-acid catalysis although the presence of a general-acid catalyst is not an absolute requirement for the reaction to take place, since water-catalyzed ring-opening proceeds quite readily (Borch and Millard, 1987). β-Elimination of acrolein from aldophosphamide to yield phosphoramide mustard is catalyzed by bases; albumin, exonucleases and other, as yet unidentified, enzymes may also catalyze this reaction.

Only the salient features of cyclophosphamide bioactivation are presented in Fig. 5. Additional, though not all, aspects of cyclophosphamide metabolism are presented in Figs 6 and 7. Thus, the transport forms of cyclophosphamide are not simply 4-hydroxycyclophosphamide and aldophosphamide, but rather *cis-* and *trans*-4-hydroxycyclophosphamide, iminocyclophosphamide, aldophosphamide and aldophosphamide hydrate (Borch and Getman, 1984; Borch et al., 1984; Zon et al., 1984; Borch and Millard, 1987) (Fig. 6). Iminocyclophosphamide is present only transiently

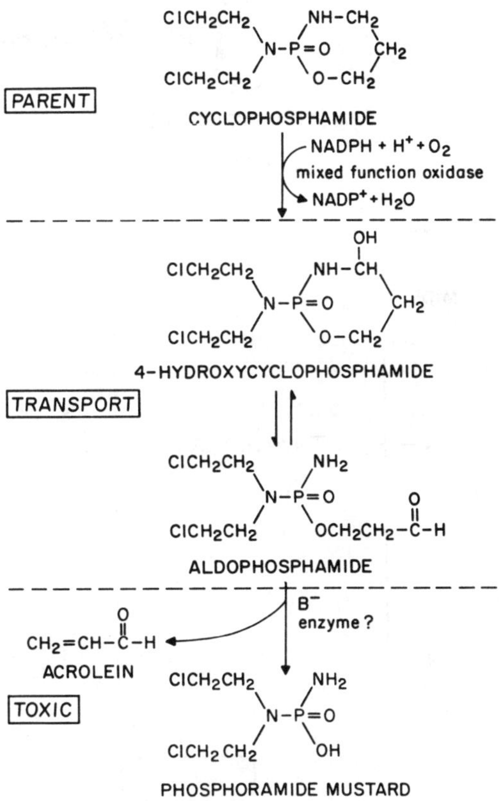

FIG. 5. Activation of cyclophosphamide: an abridged scheme.

(Fenselau et al., 1982; Borch and Getman, 1984; Kwon et al., 1987a,b; Boyd et al., 1987); approximate relative amounts of the transport forms at pseudoequilibrium are given in Table 5.

The transport forms of cyclophosphamide may be converted to metabolites other than phosphoramide mustard and acrolein (Fig. 7). Thus, the transport forms may conjugate with various sulfhydryls, e.g. glutathione, to form the 4-thiocyclophosphamide adduct (Draeger et al., 1976; Hohorst et al., 1976; Peter et al., 1976; Voelcker et al., 1976; Brock and Hohorst, 1977; Peter

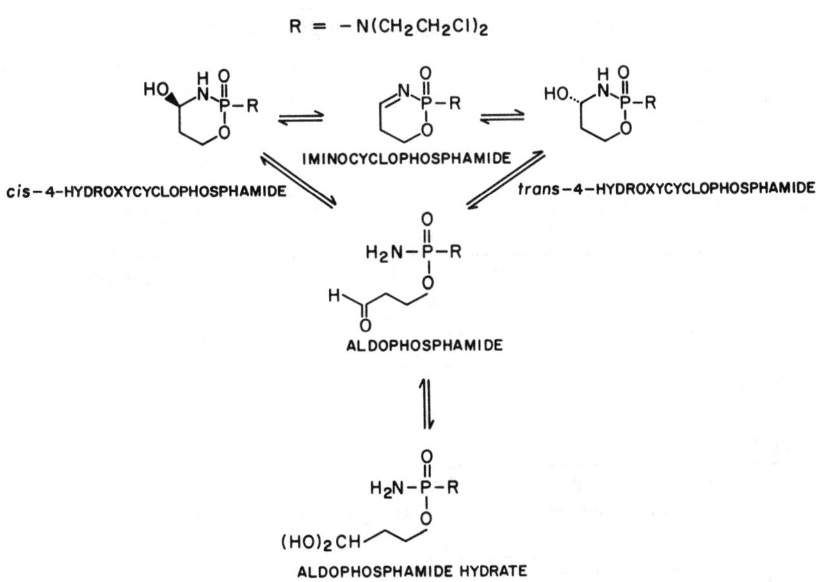

FIG. 6. Transport forms of cyclophosphamide.

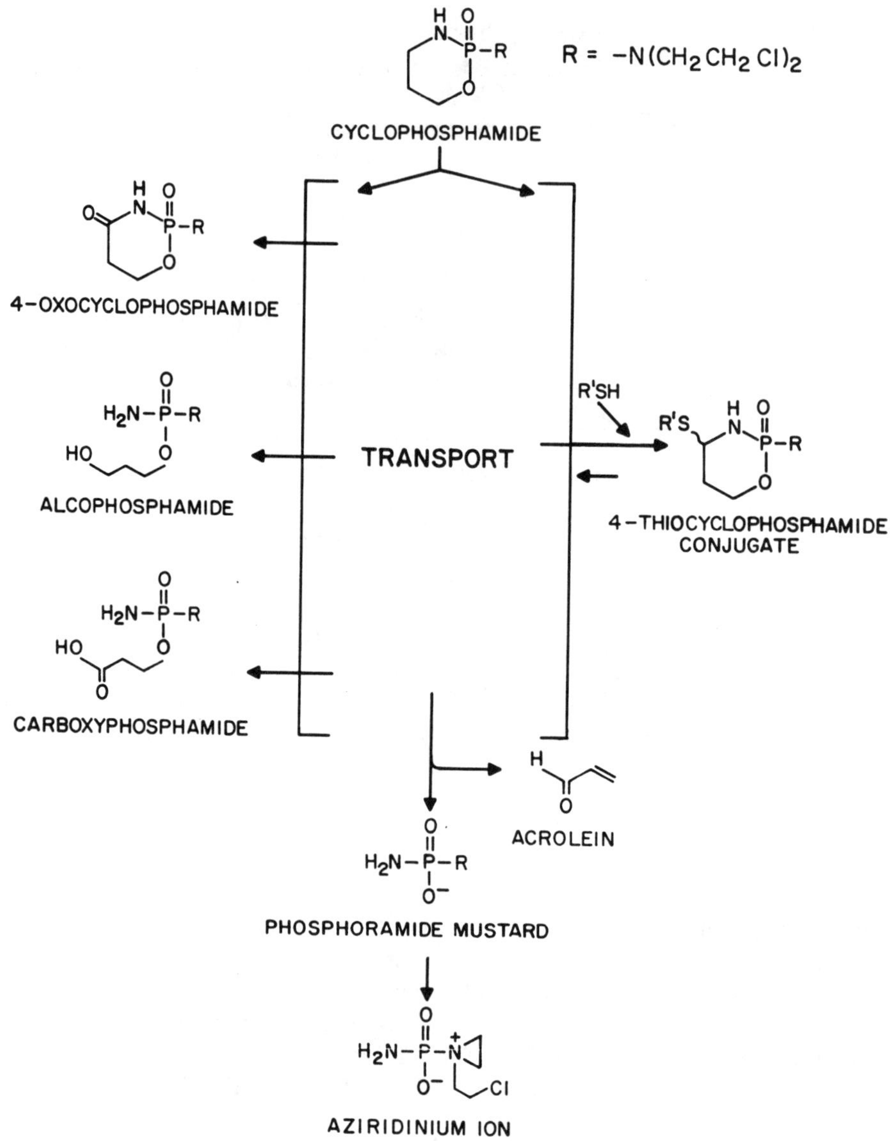

FIG. 7. Metabolism of cyclophosphamide.

TABLE 5. *Approximate Relative Amounts of the Transport Forms of Cyclophosphamide at Pseudoequilibrium in Aqueous Solutions*

Transport form	Borch et al., 1984*	Borch and Millard, 1987†	Zon et al., 1984‡
cis-4-Hydroxycyclophosphamide	13.8	9.6	14.3
trans-4-Hydroxycyclophosphamide	6.8	6.6	7.5
Iminocyclophosphamide	§	§	§
Aldophosphamide	1.0	1.0	1.0
Aldophosphamide hydrate	3.5	2.8	2.3

*Phosphate or cacodylate buffer, 0.1 M, pH 7.0; 25°C.

†Acetate (pH 4.3–5.3), cacodylate (pH 5.4–7.3), citrate (pH 5.0–6.3) or phosphate (pH 5.3–7.0) buffer, 0.1 M; 37°C.

‡2,6-Dimethylpyridine buffer, 1.0 M, pH 7.4; 37°C.

§None detectable.

and Hohorst, 1979; Brock, 1983; Zon et al., 1984; Kwon et al., 1987a; Lee, 1991). This reaction is readily reversible and proceeds without benefit of enzyme involvement. Conjugation of the transport forms with glutathione to form the 4-thiocyclophosphamide metabolite may also be catalyzed by an enzyme, viz. glutathione-*S*-transferase (Pallante et al., 1986).

Irreversible conjugation of glutathione with the mustard moieties of phosphoramide mustard and those of the oxazaphosphorines that give rise to it is also thought to occur and, at least in part, may be catalyzed by some members of a family of enzymes collectively known as glutathione-*S*-transferases (Yuan et al., 1990, 1991), though this notion has been disputed (Seitz et al., 1989). Mammalian cytosolic glutathione-*S*-transferases have been divided into three major classes, viz. alpha (basic), mu (neutral) and pi (acidic) (Mannervik et al., 1985; Boyer, 1989). A fourth class is membrane-bound (Morgenstern et al., 1982, 1984; Boyer, 1989; Clapper and Tew, 1989a). All are relatively substrate nonspecific and some are known to catalyze the conjugation of glutathione to a number of nitrogen mustards (Colvin and Hilton, 1988; Colvin et al., 1988; Clapper and Tew, 1989b).

The most abundant urinary metabolite of cyclophosphamide is usually carboxyphosphamide (see Sections 3.1 and 4). Enzyme-catalyzed oxidation of aldophosphamide gives rise to this metabolite (see Section 3.3).

Minor urinary metabolites of cyclophosphamide include 4-oxocyclophosphamide (Hohorst et al., 1971; Bakke et al., 1971, 1972; Struck et al., 1975; Milsted and Jarman, 1982; Hadidi and Idle, 1988; Hadidi et al., 1988; Anthony et al., 1990; Boddy et al., 1992; Tasso et al., 1992) and alcophosphamide (Bakke et al., 1972; Connors et al., 1974; Struck et al., 1975; Domeyer and Sladek, 1980b; Hong and Chan, 1987; Hong et al., 1991). 4-Oxocyclophosphamide may be the product of a reaction, viz. oxidation of 4-hydroxycyclophosphamide, catalyzed by aldehyde oxidase (Hohorst et al., 1971). Aldehyde oxidase is a molybdenum-containing enzyme that catalyzes the oxidation of a wide range of aldehydes and *N*-heterocyclic compounds (Johns, 1967; Beedham, 1985; Beedham et al., 1987). Alternatively, carboxyphosphamide may spontaneously cyclize to form 4-oxocyclophosphamide (Hill et al., 1972). Several enzymes are able to catalyze the reduction of aldophosphamide to alcophosphamide (see Section 3.4). A schematic showing direct conversion of cyclophosphamide to alcophosphamide has also been published (Struck et al., 1987) but the reviewer is unaware of any evidence that substantiates that notion.

A variety of other metabolites have also been identified (Torkelson et al., 1974; Hill, 1975; Cox et al., 1976a; Friedman et al., 1979; Gurtoo et al., 1985; Hadidi and Idle, 1988; Hadidi et al., 1988; Boddy et al., 1992; Tasso et al., 1992) but have been excluded here for the sake of simplicity. Amongst these is bis-(2-chloroethyl)-amine. Originally thought to be, perhaps, the penultimate cytotoxic metabolite of cyclophosphamide (Brock and Hohorst, 1967), subsequent experimentation revealed that it is not particularly cytotoxic at physiological pH (see Section 6). The source of bis-(2-chloroethyl)-amine was at first inferred, and then shown, to be phosphoramide mustard (Struck, 1974; Struck et al., 1975; Colvin et al., 1976; Suling et al., 1978; Chan et al., 1985; Watson et al., 1986; Hemminki et al., 1987; Hong and Chan, 1991). The reaction is shown in Fig. 8. Phosphoramide mustard can give rise to bis-(2-chloroethyl)-amine without benefit of enzymatic intervention, as well as by an enzyme-mediated reaction (Levins and Rogers, 1965; Watson et al., 1986; Hong and Chan, 1991). The operative enzyme may be a phosphoroamidase (Grillo et al., 1978; Hong and Chan, 1991). The high levels of bis-(2-chloroethyl)-amine that are sometimes reported to be present in the systemic circulation and/or urine of animals and humans given cyclophosphamide may be largely artifactual in that the bis-(2-chloroethyl)-amine that is measured is probably largely the product of carboxyphosphamide decomposition during sample collection, storage and preparation (Jardine et al., 1978; Ludeman et al., 1992). Following its formation, bis-(2-chloroethyl)-amine quickly gives rise, without benefit of enzymatic intervention, to 3-(2-chloroethyl)-1,3-oxazolidine-2-one (Struck et al., 1975; Chan et al., 1985, 1986; Hong and Chan, 1991; Hong et al., 1991).

3.1. Oxidation of Cyclophosphamide to 4-Hydroxycyclophosphamide/Aldophosphamide

Foley et al. (1961) were the first to demonstrate hepatic enzyme involvement in the activation of cyclophosphamide. They found cyclophosphamide to be without cytotoxic activity when added

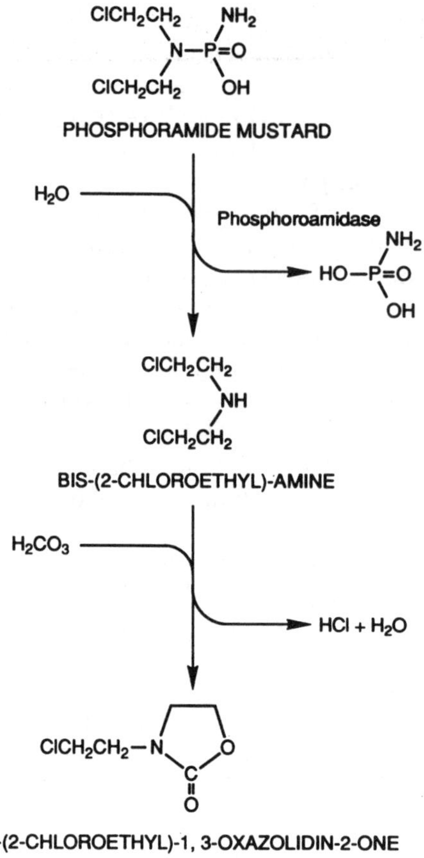

FIG. 8. Metabolism of phosphoramide mustard.

directly to cultured mammalian cells even when those cells were derived from tumors sensitive to cyclophosphamide in vivo. However, incubation of cyclophosphamide with liver homogenates gave rise to a substance (or substances) that inhibited the growth of these cells.

Catalysis by microsomal mixed-function oxidases was strongly suspected when it was observed that, of various hepatic subcellular fractions, microsomes were most active in activating cyclophosphamide and that the reaction required NADPH and O_2; moreover, pretreatment with SKF 525A, a known inhibitor of these enzymes, inhibited cyclophosphamide metabolism, and pretreatment with phenobarbital, a known inducer of microsomal mixed-function oxidase activity, stimulated its metabolism (Brock and Hohorst, 1963, 1967; Brock, 1967).

Subsequently, several laboratories contributed extensively to conclusively establishing and characterizing hepatic microsomal mixed-function oxidase-catalyzed oxidation of cyclophosphamide (Cohen and Jao, 1970; Connors et al., 1970, 1972; Sladek, 1971, 1972a,b; Short and Gibson, 1971; Hill et al., 1972). K_m values are between 0.5 and 1.5 mM when total enzyme activity present in hepatic microsomes obtained from rodents is evaluated; the pH optimum is about 7.4 (Sladek, 1971). Binding of cyclophosphamide to microsomal hemoprotein, viz. cytochrome P450, generates a Type I difference spectrum (Sladek, 1971).

There are a number of mixed-function oxidases (cytochrome P450s) present in hepatic microsomes and other mammalian tissues (Burke and Orrenius, 1979; Gram, 1980; Guengerich, 1989; Patel, 1990; Ryan and Levin, 1990; Nebert et al., 1991). The absolute abundance of each in any given tissue varies and is influenced by age, sex, diet, etc. Predictably, these enzymes are not equally proficient in catalyzing the bioactivation of cyclophosphamide (Table 6); indeed, some appear to be essentially incapable of catalyzing the reaction (Clarke and Waxman, 1989; LeBlanc and Waxman, 1989; Doehmer et al., 1990). Most proficient in catalyzing it in rat liver is the phenobarbital-inducible enzyme, P450 IIB1, and in livers obtained from rats treated with phenobarbital, this enzyme catalyzes the bulk of cyclophosphamide bioactivation; the apparent K_m

TABLE 6. *Rat P450 Enzyme-catalyzed Oxidation of Cyclophosphamide to 4-Hydroxycyclophosphamide*

P450*	CYP†	pmol/min/nmol P450‡
IIB1	*2B1*	26,100
IIC11	*2C11*	2,720
IIB2	*2B2*	610
IIA2	*2A2*	500
IIC6	*2C6*	260
IA1	*1A1*	160
IIC12	*2C12*	140
IIA1	*2A1*	110
IIC13	*2C13*	90
IIIA1	*3A1*	40
IA2	*1A2*	20

*Trivial name of gene product.

†Gene symbol according to Nebert et al. (1991).

‡Reconstituted enzyme systems consisting of the purified P450 enzyme of interest, NADPH P450 reductase, and dilauroyl-phosphatidylcholine were used to quantify catalytic activity. The substrate (cyclophosphamide) concentration was 0.5 mM.

Reprinted from Clarke and Waxman (1989), with permission of the authors and the copyright holder, American Association for Cancer Research, Philadelphia.

value is 162 μM (Clarke and Waxman, 1989). However, other enzymes in rat liver, viz. P450s IIC6 and IIC11, also catalyze the reaction and account for the bulk of hepatic enzyme-catalyzed bioactivation when liver is obtained from untreated adult male rats, i.e. constitutively, P450s IIC6 and IIC11 are present in much greater abundance than is P450 IIB1 (Clarke and Waxman, 1989). Cytochrome P450s IIC11 and IIC6 are male-specific and phenobarbital-inducible, respectively.

Less is known about the enzymes that catalyze the oxidation of cyclophosphamide in humans. P450 enzymes exhibiting structural similarity to rat P450s IIC6 (Meehan et al., 1988) and IIC11 (Yasumori et al., 1987) have been identified in humans. Whether these and/or others are the enzymes that catalyze the bulk of cyclophosphamide oxidation in human liver remains to be determined. Induction by barbiturates and phenytoins of P450-catalyzed oxidation of cyclophosphamide has been demonstrated in humans (Mellet et al., 1969; Cohen et al., 1971; Jao et al., 1972; Bagley et al., 1973; Sladek et al., 1980, 1984a; Egorin et al., 1982) but the identity of the relevant P450(s) that is (are) induced by these agents is unknown. Numerous other xenobiotics are known to induce one or more of the various cytochrome P450s (Okey, 1990).

Oxidation of cyclophosphamide is ordinarily catalyzed largely, if not exclusively, by mixed-function oxidases present in the endoplasmic reticulum of liver. However, mixed-function oxidases, including those that catalyze the oxidation of cyclophosphamide, are also found in other tissues. For example, P450 IIB1 is constitutively expressed in rat lung where it is also inducible by phenobarbital and although not detected in adrenal, kidney or small intestine obtained from untreated rats, this enzyme was clearly expressed in these organs when they were obtained from phenobarbital-treated rats (Christou et al., 1987). The expectation is that these enzymes are likely to be present in neoplastic cells that are derived from such tissues/organs and that the relevant enzymes may even be expressed in neoplastic cells that are derived from normal cells that do not ordinarily express them. Indeed, constitutive expression and phenobarbital inducibility of P450 IIB1 has been observed in carcinogen-induced liver nodules (Schwarz et al., 1987) and the former was observed in neoplastic lesions in kidney (Tsuda et al., 1987).

Assuming that rat cytochrome P450-catalyzed cyclophosphamide metabolism is not totally unlike that in humans, the foregoing observations suggest that cyclophosphamide may be subject to activation within some *target* tissues as well and that the rate at which this occurs can be modulated; the therapeutic significance of the latter is obvious.

Very recently, Smith and Kehrer (1991) and Kanekal and Kehrer (1993) obtained evidence

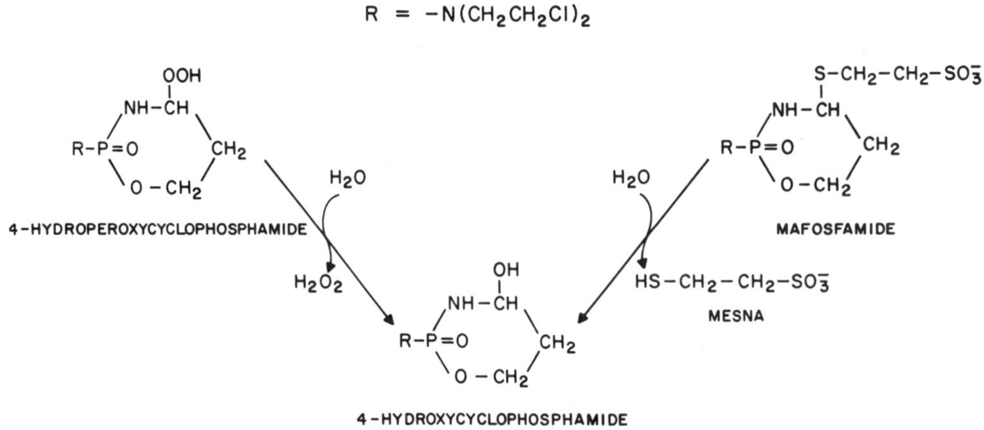

FIG. 9. Mafosfamide and 4-hydroperoxycyclophosphamide (perfosfamide): relatively stable oxazaphosphorines that, under physiological conditions, readily give rise to 4-hydroxycyclophosphamide without benefit of enzymatic involvement.

suggesting that bioactivation of cyclophosphamide can also occur via a mixed-function oxidase-independent pathway, at least in some tissues, e.g. lung. Suspected is hydroperoxide-dependent oxidation (cooxidation) of cyclophosphamide catalyzed by prostaglandin H synthetase.

The identity of the metabolite resulting from hepatic microsomal mixed-function oxidase-catalyzed oxidation of cyclophosphamide was not immediately apparent. Identification of carboxyphosphamide as the most abundant cyclophosphamide metabolite in the urine of sheep (Bakke et al., 1971, 1972), dogs (Struck et al., 1971) and humans (Struck et al., 1971) provided an important clue as did the fact that other urinary metabolites included 4-oxocyclophosphamide and one that yielded β-hydroxypropionamide on hydrolysis.* The presence of these metabolites suggested to Struck et al. (1971), Hohorst et al. (1971) and Takamizawa et al. (1972) that the oxidative step occurs on carbon 4 of cyclophosphamide, that is, that the initial metabolite of hepatic microsomal mixed-function oxidase-catalyzed oxidation of cyclophosphamide was 4-hydroxycyclophosphamide, that, in solution, 4-hydroxycyclophosphamide would give rise to its acyclic tautomer now known by the trivial name, aldophosphamide, and that these tautomers were intermediates in the generation of carboxyphosphamide (and 4-oxocyclophosphamide). Such a scheme had been considered earlier by Norpoth and coworkers (Norpoth, 1969; Norpoth et al., 1970) but, after investigating the possibility, these investigators rejected it. Ultimately, isolation and chemical and pharmacological characterization of the relevant (derivatized) metabolites, viz. 4-hydroxycyclophosphamide and aldophosphamide, and the observation that, under appropriate conditions, they gave rise to carboxyphosphamide, established the correctness of the proposed route (Hill et al., 1972; Sladek, 1973a,b; Connors et al., 1974; Struck, 1974, 1976; Völker et al., 1974; Takamizawa et al., 1975; Myles et al., 1977; Fenselau et al., 1977).

4-Hydroxycyclophosphamide can also be generated from mafosfamide and 4-hydroperoxycyclophosphamide (Fig. 9). Such conversion occurs fairly rapidly under physiological conditions and without benefit of enzymatic involvement (van der Steen et al., 1973; Völker et al., 1974; Low et al., 1982; Borch and Getman, 1984; Niemeyer et al., 1984, 1989; Kwon et al., 1987a). Thus, 4-hydroxycyclophosphamide, 4-hydroperoxycyclophosphamide and mafosfamide are, in most respects, essentially pharmacologically equivalent (Takamizawa et al., 1975; Von Hoff, 1984; Sladek et al., 1985). This equivalence and the relatively greater chemical stability of mafosfamide and 4-hydroperoxycyclophosphamide, as compared to that of 4-hydroxycyclophosphamide, make the former useful in investigations and applications where it is desired to examine the effects of, or utilize, 4-hydroxycyclophosphamide, i.e. to by-pass enzyme-catalyzed cyclophosphamide hydroxylation to 4-hydroxycyclophosphamide.

Similarly, aldophosphamide (aldoifosfamide) can be generated from an acid-labile acetalglycoside of 2,3-dideoxy-D-erythro-2-hexenopyranose and aldophosphamide (Tietze et al., 1989, 1990)

*The most abundant urinary metabolite in rabbits is 4-oxocyclophosphamide (Anthony et al., 1990).

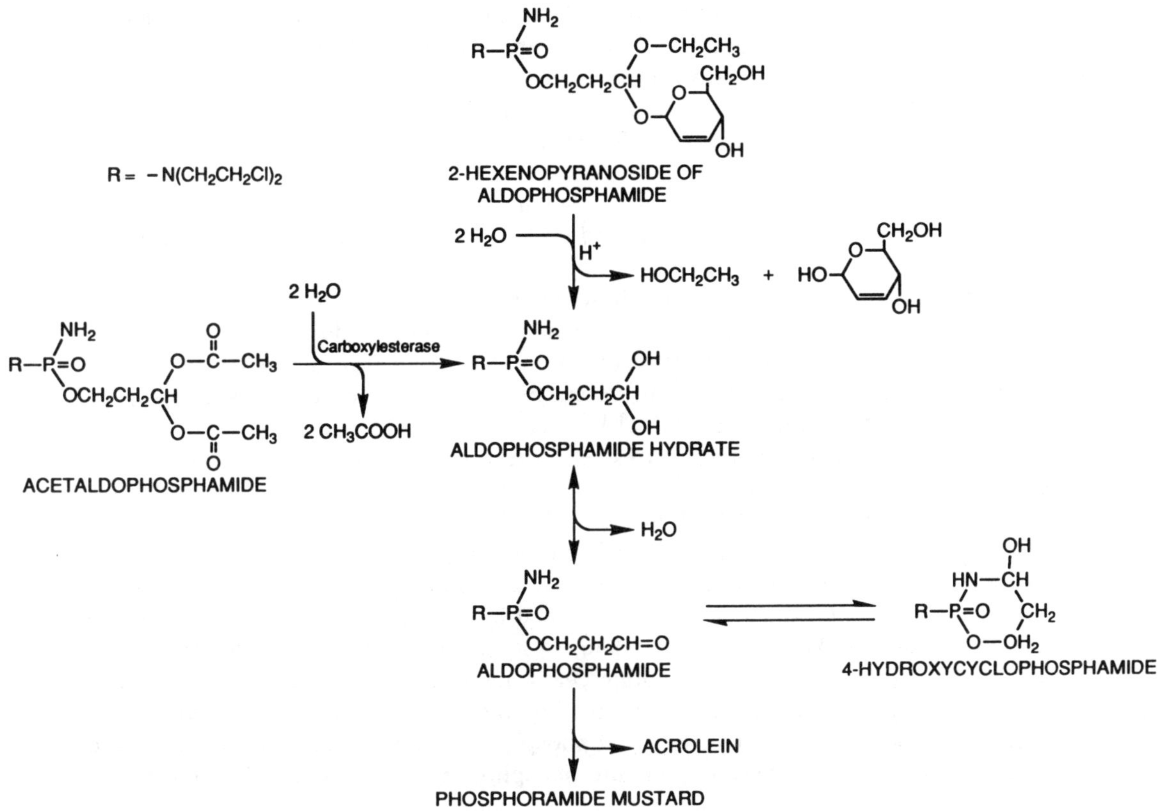

FIG. 10. Metabolism of acetaldophosphamide and a 2-hexenopyranoside of aldophosphamide.

(Fig. 10). Alternatively, it can be generated from acetaldophosphamide (acetaldoifosfamide) but, in this case, the participation of a carboxylesterase (carboxyl ester hydrolase) is required; these enzymes are ubiquitous in mammalian tissue (Beran et al., 1988; Andersson et al., 1990; Wang and Farquhar, 1991) (Fig. 10).

3.2. β-Elimination of Acrolein from Aldophosphamide to Generate Phosphoramide Mustard

Although he did not pursue this possibility either, Norpoth (1969) was also the first to propose that cyclophosphamide could ultimately give rise to phosphoramide mustard. Alarcon and Meienhofer's (1971) observation that acrolein was formed when cyclophosphamide was incubated with liver microsomes, together with the knowledge that the initial metabolite of hepatic microsomal mixed-function oxidase-catalyzed oxidation of cyclophosphamide was 4-hydroxycyclophosphamide in equilibrium with its acyclic tautomer aldophosphamide, led Colvin et al. (1973) and Connors et al. (1974) to suggest the formation of phosphoramide mustard as a consequence of the β-elimination of acrolein from aldophosphamide. Each group isolated phosphoramide mustard after incubating cyclophosphamide with the relevant rodent hepatic subcellular fraction to buttress this notion. Similarly, Völker et al. (1974) reported that 4-hydroxycyclophosphamide 'spontaneously' decomposed to phosphoramide mustard when incubated at 37°C in phosphate buffer, pH 7.0. Ultimate proof was the isolation of phosphoramide mustard from biological fluids of mice (Struck et al., 1975) and humans (Fenselau et al., 1975) given cyclophosphamide.

β-Elimination of acrolein from aldophosphamide to yield phosphoramide mustard is catalyzed by various bases, e.g. hydroxyl ion, carbonate ion and dianionic phosphate (Low et al., 1982, 1983; Borch et al., 1984). Kinetically, conversion is first-order with respect to the oxazaphosphorine as well as with respect to the catalytic base. The mechanism is apparently one of general base catalysis (Low et al., 1983; Borch and Millard, 1987). Catalytic constants of 2710, 3.09, 0.194 and 0.000006 $min^{-1}M^{-1}$ were obtained for hydroxyl ion-, carbonate ion-, dianionic phosphate- and water-catalyzed, respectively, conversion of aldophosphamide to phosphoramide mustard and acrolein at 37°C (Low et al., 1983). Energy of activation was approximately 20 kcal/mol when dianionic phosphate was used as the catalyst (Low et al., 1983).

Conversion of 4-hydroxycyclophosphamide/aldophosphamide to phosphoramide mustard and acrolein may also be catalyzed by enzymes (Voelcker et al., 1981; Wagner and Heydrich, 1982; Bielicki et al., 1983, 1984; Hohorst et al., 1983, 1986; Sladek et al., 1984b; Kwon et al., 1987a,c; Hong et al., 1991). Catalytic activity of apparent enzyme origin was found in serum, lymphocytes, lymphatic tissues (spleen and thymus), kidneys and testicles; it was not found in liver, muscle, heart, brain or erythrocytes.

Albumin appears to be the catalytic species present in serum (Wagner and Heydrich, 1982; Kwon et al., 1987c). As enzymes go, however, its catalytic activity is very modest; the catalytic constants of human and bovine albumin are, respectively, 285 and 83 $min^{-1}M^{-1}$ at 37°C. Possible is that aldophosphamide binds to a specific site on the enzyme and that the binding site is adjacent to an enzyme residue that functions as a general base catalyst.

The identity of the enzyme(s) catalyzing this reaction in other tissues has not been established but 3′,5′-exonucleases, especially those associated with DNA polymerase, are suspected (Voelcker et al., 1981; Bielicki et al., 1983, 1984; Hohorst et al., 1983, 1986). Macromolecules that contain both of these catalytic activities may have the capacity to add, in the presence of a DNA template, nucleotides to the 3′-OH terminus of a polynucleotide chain (polymerase) and proof-read and, if necessary, correct (excision by the exonuclease followed by the addition of the correct nucleotide) the product. According to Hohorst et al. (1986), 4-hydroxycyclophosphamide structurally resembles the 3′-OH terminus of a polynucleotide chain, i.e. it is a pseudodinucleotide. Their view is that 4-hydroxycyclophosphamide therefore readily binds to the polymerase portion of the macromolecule and that, because 4-hydroxycyclophosphamide is recognized as an aberration, the exonuclease portion comes into play to generate phosphoramide mustard and acrolein.

3.3. OXIDATION OF ALDOPHOSPHAMIDE TO CARBOXYPHOSPHAMIDE

Oxidation of aldophosphamide to carboxyphosphamide is catalyzed largely by NAD(P)-linked aldehyde dehydrogenases (Fig. 11). Hill et al. (1972) were the first to demonstrate that an aldehyde dehydrogenase catalyzed the formation of carboxyphosphamide from a metabolite, presumed to be aldophosphamide, of cyclophosphamide. They used a commercial preparation of yeast aldehyde dehydrogenase to make this point.

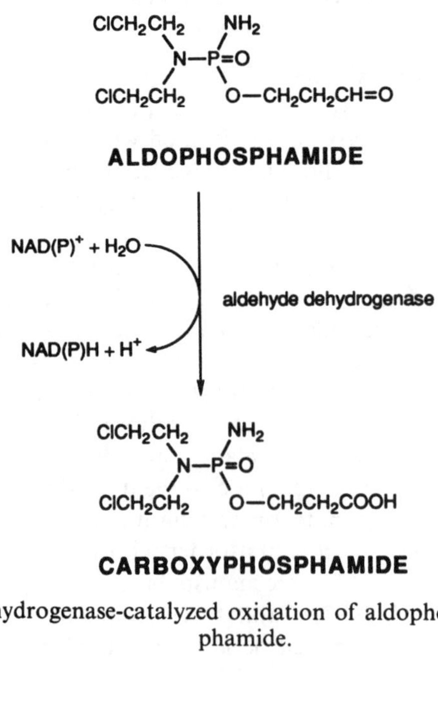

FIG. 11. Aldehyde dehydrogenase-catalyzed oxidation of aldophosphamide to carboxyphosphamide.

TABLE 7. *Mouse NAD-linked Aldehyde Dehydrogenase-catalyzed Oxidation of Aldophosphamide*: K_m *Values**

AHD-	K_m, μM
1a	2,530
1b	1,540
2	16
3	†
4	284
5a	170
5b	147
6	‡
7a	†
7b	†
8a	16
8b	38
9	101
10	121
11	1,200§
12a	354
12b	532
12c	336
13	117

*Data from Manthey (1988), Sladek et al. (1989) and Manthey et al. (1990).

†Aldophosphamide is not a substrate for this enzyme.

‡Aldophosphamide is a substrate for this enzyme, but the K_m value was not determined.

§Nucleotide co-factor was NADP.

TABLE 8. *Human NAD-linked Aldehyde Dehydrogenase-catalyzed Oxidation of Aldophosphamide*: K_m *Values*

Enzyme	K_m, μM
ALDH-1	52
ALDH-2	1,193
ALDH-3 (stomach)	‡
ALDH-3 (breast)	640
ALDH-4†	‡
ALDH-5	‡
Succinic semialdehyde dehydrogenase	560
Betaine aldehyde dehydrogenase	‡
γ-Aminobutyraldehyde dehydrogenase	§

*Data from Sladek et al. (1990), Dockham et al. (1992) and Sreerama and Sladek (1992).

†Also known as glutamic-γ-semialdehyde dehydrogenase.

‡Aldophosphamide is not a substrate for this enzyme.

§Whether aldophosphamide is a substrate for this enzyme remains to be determined.

There are a number of aldehyde dehydrogenases present in mammalian tissues. Not all of them catalyze the oxidation of aldophosphamide to carboxyphosphamide. Thus, of the 13 aldehyde dehydrogenases identified in mouse tissues, 11 catalyze this reaction (Table 7). One, viz. AHD-2, the most abundant aldehyde dehydrogenase in mouse liver cytosol, accounts for the bulk (> 80%) of the total hepatic activity when the aldophosphamide concentration is pharmacological. It and AHD-8 exhibit the most favorable K_m values.

There are at least eight 'aldehyde dehydrogenases', viz. ALDHs 1–5 and succinic semialdehyde, betaine aldehyde and γ-aminobutyraldehyde, dehydrogenase, present in human tissues (Kurys et al., 1989; Yin et al., 1989; Goedde and Agarwal, 1990). Variants of ALDHs 1 and 2 have been found in some people (Yoshida et al., 1989; Goedde and Agarwal, 1990). Tissue-specific isoforms of ALDH-3 may also be present (Sreerama and Sladek, 1991, 1992). Of the eight human 'aldehyde dehydrogenases' thus far examined in our laboratory, four, viz. ALDH-1, ALDH-2, breast ALDH-3 and succinic semialdehyde dehydrogenase, were found to catalyze the detoxification of cyclophosphamide (Table 8). ALDH-1, the most abundant aldehyde dehydrogenase in human liver cytosol, seems to be the most important. It exhibits the most favorable K_m value and accounts for more than 80% of the total hepatic activity when the aldophosphamide concentration is pharmacological.

One or more of the relevant aldehyde dehydrogenases is (are) present in most normal tissues/organs/cells including pluripotent and multipotent hematopoietic progenitor cells, stomach and intestine mucosal cells and erythrocytes (Cox et al., 1975b; Domeyer and Sladek, 1980b, 1981; Kohn and Sladek, 1985, 1987; Kohn et al., 1987a,b; Jones et al., 1987; Colvin et al., 1988; Manthey, 1988; Manthey and Sladek, 1988, 1989; Sahovic et al., 1988; Russo and Hilton, 1988; Russo et al., 1989; Sladek et al., 1989, 1990; Goedde and Agarwal, 1990; Kastan et al., 1990; Manthey et al., 1990; Dockham et al., 1992). On the other hand, tumor cells often contain very little of, or even totally lack, the relevant aldehyde dehydrogenase activity (see Section 9.3) although relatively large amounts of it were present in oxazaphosphorine-resistant mouse L1210 and P388 lymphocytic leukemia cells (Hilton, 1984a,b; Sladek and Landkamer, 1985; Kohn et al., 1987a; Manthey, 1988;

Colvin and Hilton, 1988; Colvin et al., 1988; Russo and Hilton, 1988; Russo et al., 1989; Sladek et al., 1989; Radin et al., 1991), in rat hepatoma cell lines (Lin and Lindahl, 1987) and in a metastatic Wilms tumor nodule taken from liver (Manthey, 1988).

Aldehyde dehydrogenases also catalyze the metabolism of ethanol (acetaldehyde) and thus have been studied extensively. Of particular relevance to the subject at hand is that (1) the majority of the aldehyde dehydrogenases catalyze the oxidation of many endo- and xenobiotic aldehydes, (2) each aldehyde dehydrogenase exhibits a unique, albeit usually broad, substrate specificity, (3) the specific aldehyde dehydrogenase complement varies with each tissue and some aldehyde dehydrogenases are tissue specific and (4) specific aldehyde dehydrogenase complement is subject to genetic variability (Mather and Holmes, 1984; Sladek et al., 1989; Ehrig et al., 1990; Goedde and Agarwal, 1990).

Hill et al. (1972) reported that purified rabbit liver aldehyde oxidase could also catalyze the formation of carboxyphosphamide from a metabolite, presumably aldophosphamide, of cyclophosphamide. Although both may be operative, aldehyde dehydrogenase rather than aldehyde oxidase is thought to be the predominating enzyme activity in vivo since (1) experiments in which surrogate aldehydes such as butyraldehyde and benzaldehyde were used as substrates showed that, whereas dehydrogenase activity is virtually ubiquitous, oxidase activity is confined to the soluble fraction of liver and only a few other tissues and that dehydrogenase activity far exceeds oxidase activity in those tissues and subcellular fractions where both activities are found and (2) oxidation of aldophosphamide to carboxyphosphamide by a rodent hepatic soluble fraction could not be demonstrated in the absence of NAD even when incubation conditions were made optimal for the expression of aldehyde oxidase activity (Domeyer and Sladek, 1980b).

Consistent with this notion are the observations that known inhibitors of aldehyde dehydrogenase activity, e.g. disulfiram and cyanamide, inhibited the conversion of aldophosphamide to carboxyphosphamide in vivo and potentiated the antitumor, leukopenic and lethal action of cyclophosphamide (Donelli et al., 1976; Cox et al., 1976b; Domeyer and Sladek, 1981; Habs et al., 1981; Hacker et al., 1982), as would be expected if a dehydrogenase was operative and catalyzed a detoxifying reaction (see Section 6).

In disagreement with the foregoing contention are the reports that disulfiram and other inhibitors of aldehyde dehydrogenases did not potentiate the antitumor action of cyclophosphamide in some in vivo models (Montgomery and Struck, 1973; Cox et al., 1976b; Domeyer, 1977). Moreover, in at least one in vivo rodent tumor model, pyridoxal, an inhibitor of the oxidase but not of the dehydrogenases, also potentiated the antitumor action of cyclophosphamide (Hill et al., 1972).

3.4. Reduction of Aldophosphamide to Alcophosphamide

Potentially, any of several alcohol dehydrogenases (Vallee and Bazzone, 1983; Burnell and Bosron, 1989; Ehrig et al., 1990; Yasunami et al., 1991) and pyridine nucleotide-dependent aldo-keto reductases (Felsted and Bachur, 1980; Wermuth, 1985; Ohta et al., 1991) may catalyze the reduction of aldophosphamide to alcophosphamide (Fig. 12) since these enzymes, like the aldehyde dehydrogenases, catalyze the biotransformation of many carbonyls. Thus far, the reaction has been shown to be catalyzed by horse liver alcohol dehydrogenase (Domeyer and Sladek, 1980b) and by a human alcohol dehydrogenase, aldehyde reductase, aldose reductase and an unidentified aldo-keto reductase (Parekh and Sladek, 1993). K_m values for the human enzymes were 1.1, 1.6, 0.15 and ca. 0.10 mM, respectively, suggesting that, of the enzymes studied thus far, aldose reductase and the unidentified aldo-keto reductase are most likely to catalyze the reduction of aldophosphamide in vivo.

Alcohol dehydrogenases, as the name indicates, also catalyze the oxidation of alcohols to aldehydes; whether they, and/or other enzymes, catalyze the reverse reaction, i.e. the oxidation of alcophosphamide to aldophosphamide, is not known. However, Hong and Chan (1987) found phosphoramide mustard to be the major circulating and urinary metabolite in rats given alcophosphamide i.v. As pointed out by these investigators, one way in which phosphoramide mustard could be generated from alcophosphamide would be if the latter was first oxidized to aldophosphamide, i.e. aldophosphamide served as an intermediate in the overall conversion. They also pointed out that phosphoramide mustard may be formed directly via *O*-dealkylation of

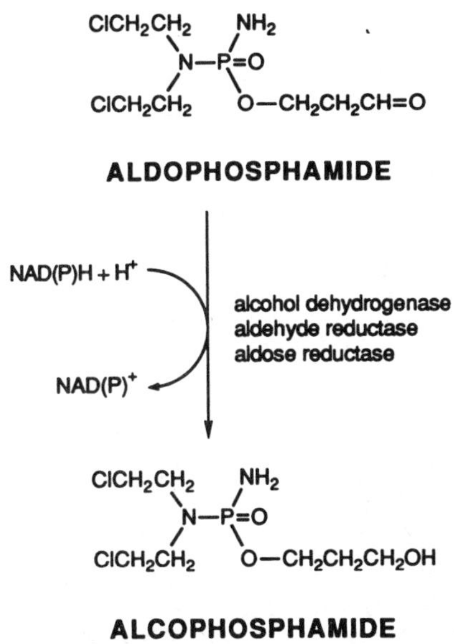

FIG. 12. Enzyme-catalyzed reduction of aldophosphamide to alcophosphamide. The reaction is shown as being irreversible in all cases but this has not been established.

alcophosphamide. *O*-Dealkylation of alcophosphamide to phosphoramide mustard in extracellular fluids seems more likely given that alcophosphamide exhibits only weak antitumor activity (see Section 6), that phosphoramide mustard generated outside of the target cell is not very toxic to it (see Sections 6 and 7), that enzymes that are likely to catalyze the oxidation of alcophosphamide to aldophosphamide are likely to be found only within cells, and that enzymes (esterases) that may catalyze the hydrolysis (*O*-dealkylation) of alcophosphamide to phosphoramide mustard are often found outside of cells.

3.5. Additional Aspects of Oxazaphosphorine Metabolism

Cyclophosphamide contains a chiral center at the phosphorous atom. However, in humans, stereoselective metabolism is minimal and of no apparent therapeutic consequence (Jarman et al., 1979; Farmer, 1988; Holm et al., 1990). Thus, continued clinical use of the racemic mixture, rather than switching to one of the enatiomers, seems warranted.

Cyclophosphamide analogs that are of demonstrated clinical utility or show promise in preclinical models include ifosfamide and trofosfamide. The metabolism of these oxazaphosphorines, particularly that of ifosfamide, has also been studied though not nearly as exhaustively (Allen and Creaven, 1972; Hill et al., 1973; Cox et al., 1976a; Low et al., 1983; Brade et al., 1985; Farmer, 1988; Zalupski and Baker, 1988; Kwon and Borch, 1989; Masurel et al., 1990; Ruzicka and Ruenitz, 1992). Essentially, metabolism of these analogs is identical to that of cyclophosphamide (Fig. 13).

4. PHARMACOKINETICS

Absorption, distribution and excretion of cyclophosphamide per se has been intensely investigated in both animals and humans, especially the latter. Grochow and Colvin (1980, 1983) reviewed and summarized much of the early information dealing with the clinical pharmacokinetics of this agent. More recent reviews of this subject have been authored by Sladek (1988) and Moore (1991). It is clear that interpatient variability is substantial. Much less is known about the pharmacokinetics of the clinically important circulating metabolites of cyclophosphamide, viz. 4-hydroxycyclophosphamide/aldophosphamide and, to a lesser extent, phosphoramide mustard (see Section 7).

Cyclophosphamide is given both parenterally and orally. The apparent systemic availability of cyclophosphamide per se after oral administration is somewhat short of total largely because of first-pass hepatic metabolism (bioactivation) to 4-hydroxycyclophosphamide/aldophosphamide; in

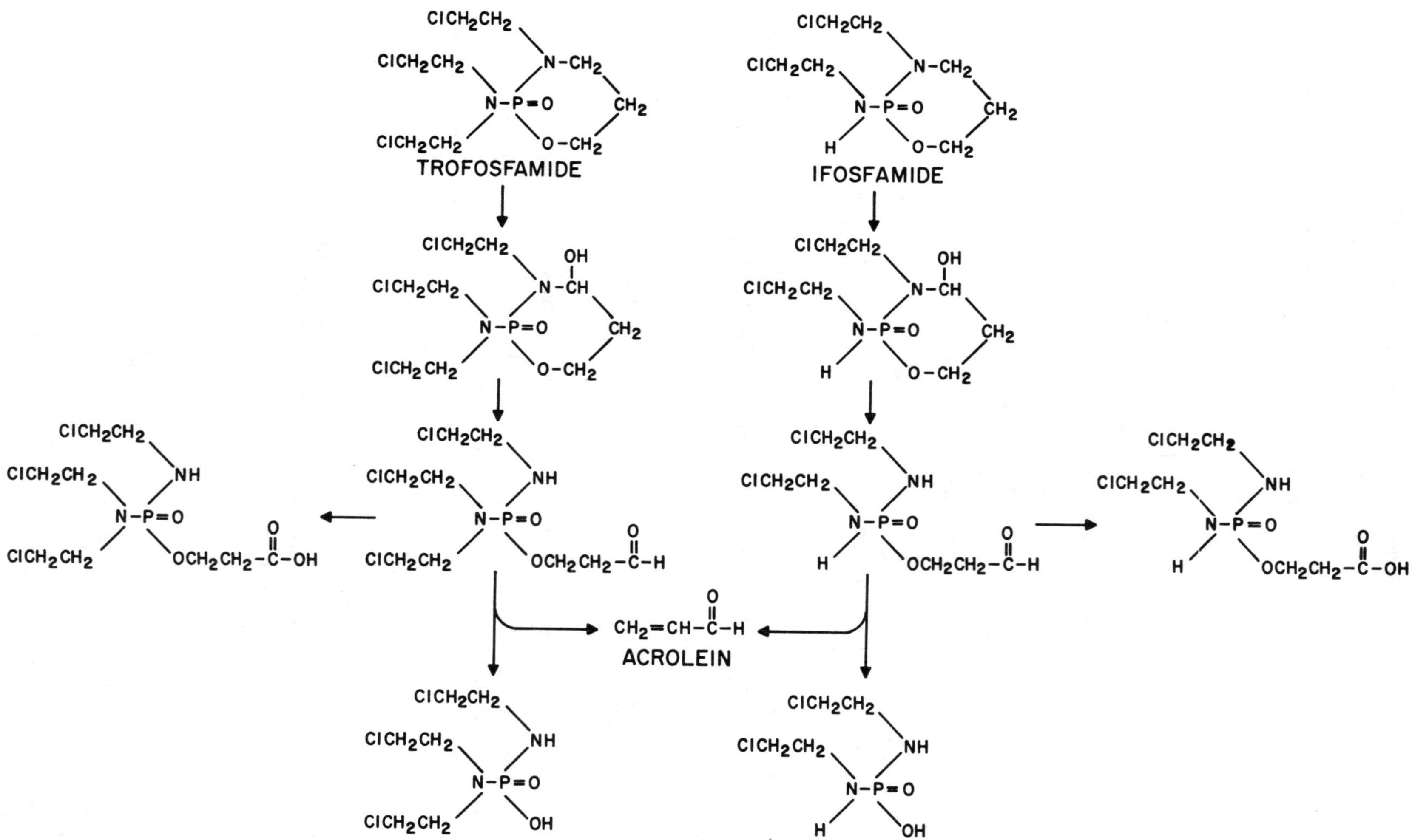

FIG. 13. Metabolism of trofosfamide and ifosfamide.

TABLE 9. *Apparent Volume of Distribution of Cyclophosphamide in Humans*

V_d, L/kg		
Mean	Range	Reference
0.64	—	Bagley et al., 1973
0.57	—	Mouridsen et al., 1974
0.58	0.48–0.77	Faber et al., 1974
0.52	0.47–0.58	Faber et al., 1975
0.71	0.58–0.77	Juma et al., 1979a
0.70	—	Juma et al., 1979b
0.78	0.31–2.49	Bramwell et al., 1979
1.12	0.49–1.90	D'Incalci et al., 1979a
0.68	0.51–0.83	Sladek et al., 1980
0.81	0.49–1.47	Edwards et al., 1980
0.74	0.50–1.00	Juma et al., 1980
0.58	0.29–0.86	Ritschel et al., 1981
0.68	0.58–0.77	Juma et al., 1981
0.64	0.52–0.74	Juma and Ogada, 1983
0.61	0.47–0.97	Juma et al., 1984
0.52	0.24–1.08	Powis et al., 1987
0.49	0.19–0.79	Tasso et al., 1992

TABLE 10. *Serum Protein Binding of Cyclophosphamide in Humans*

Binding, %	Reference
0	Linford, 1961
13	Bagley et al., 1973
24	Jardine et al., 1978
36	Jarman et al., 1979
13	Juma et al., 1979b
20	Edwards et al., 1980

fact, the true bioavailability of the parent compound is very nearly total (D'Incalci et al., 1979a; Juma et al., 1979a; Wagner and Fenneberg, 1984; Struck et al., 1987; De Bruijn et al., 1988). The drug also readily enters the circulation following inhalation or dermal application (Hirst et al., 1984; Sessink et al., 1991). The distribution volume is approximately 0.67 L/kg in humans (Table 9). This value is consistent with distribution of the drug in total body water. Such distribution is as expected since cyclophosphamide is a relatively small, unionized molecule that does not bind substantially to serum proteins (Table 10), nor is it known to be sequestered by any tissue.

Total body clearance of the parent compound in humans occurs at a mean rate of about 95 mL/min (range: 26–220 mL/min) but, on average, only about 11% of total body clearance is effected by the kidney (Table 11). This is because removal of cyclophosphamide from the body is primarily by hepatic metabolism, on average, only about 13% of it is excreted unchanged in the urine (range: 2–86%) (Table 12), and excretion in the feces or by the lungs is insignificant (Cohen

TABLE 11. *Clearance of Cyclophosphamide in Humans*

Cl_R, mL/min*		Cl_T, mL/min†		
Mean	Range	Mean	Range	Reference
10.7	5.2–15.9	—	—	Cohen et al., 1971
5.6	1.1–11.2	67	48–86	Juma et al., 1979a
6.1	1.2–11.2	80	43–200	Bramwell et al., 1979
7.4	2.9–16.5	81	43–160	Edwards et al., 1980
—	—	69	36–96	Juma et al., 1980
—	—	118	—	Wagner et al., 1980a
17.6	10.1–35.5	—	—	Wagner et al., 1980b
—	—	89	35–154	Ritschel et al., 1981
—	—	67	54–82	Juma et al., 1981
18.3	8.0–67.0	—	—	Wilkinson et al., 1983
—	—	103	—	Tchekmedyian et al., 1986
—	—	70	26–167	Powis et al., 1987
—	—	102	65–172	De Bruijn et al., 1988
—	—	119	65–175	Lartigue-Mattei et al., 1988
—	—	93	56–133	Moore et al., 1988
—	—	124	53–198	Alberts et al., 1991
—	—	146	72–220	Ayash et al., 1991
8.5	6.8–9.7	—	—	Tasso et al., 1992

*Renal clearance.
†Total body clearance.

TABLE 12. *Fraction of Administered Cyclophosphamide Excreted Unchanged in the Urine of Humans*

Fraction Excreted Unchanged		
Mean	Range	Reference
0.11	0.07–0.14	DeVita and Adamson, 1970
0.21	0.07–0.36	DeVita and Adamson, 1970
0.14	—	Cohen et al., 1971
0.11	0.03–0.19	Bagley et al., 1973
0.11	0.04–0.21	Mouridsen et al., 1974
0.10	0.04–0.15	Faber et al., 1974
0.11	0.06–0.19	Mouridsen et al., 1976
0.20	0.16–0.25	Jardine et al., 1978
0.07	0.02–0.12	Juma et al., 1979a
0.05	0.04–0.08	Jarman et al., 1979
0.14	0.04–0.26	Sladek et al., 1980
0.17	—	Wagner et al., 1980a
0.17	0.09–0.33	Wagner et al., 1980b
0.12	0.05–0.24	Milsted and Jarman, 1982
0.09	—	Tchekmedyian et al., 1986
0.14	0.06–0.23	Schuler et al., 1987
0.13	0.03–0.31	Hadidi et al., 1988
0.14	—	Bailey et al., 1991
0.14	0.01–0.32	Fasola et al., 1991
0.03	0.00–0.06	Boddy et al., 1992
0.32	0.05–0.86	Tasso et al., 1992

et al., 1971; Bagley et al., 1973). Although little of it appears in the feces, cyclophosphamide concentrations in the bile approach those in the plasma (Dooley et al., 1982) indicating that it undergoes extensive enterohepatic recirculation. The excretion of cyclophosphamide in human milk contraindicates its administration to nursing mothers (Wiernik and Duncan, 1971; Duncan et al., 1973).

Given a total body clearance of 95 mL/min, a volume of distribution of 0.67 L/kg and a body weight of 70 kg, a plasma elimination half-life value of about 6 hr can be expected for cyclophosphamide in adult humans. In fact, plasma elimination half-life values for cyclophosphamide vary considerably in adult humans (range: 108–1272 min) but the mean value is about 6–7 hr (Table 13). Plasma elimination half-life values are considerably shorter in mature mice (6–25 min), rats (29–93 min), dogs (32 min) and monkeys (48 min) (Mellett and El Dareer quoted in De Vita and Adamson, 1970; Voelcker and Haeglsperger, 1982; Sladek et al., 1984b; Hong et al., 1991).

The rate at which cyclophosphamide is removed from the body appears to be relatively slower in obese patients (Powis et al., 1987). This may reflect a relatively slower rate of hepatic mixed-function oxidase-catalyzed metabolism of cyclophosphamide in these individual which, in turn, may reflect relatively lower levels of the relevant P450(s); evidence for this notion has been summarized by Powis et al. (1987).

Children and young adults apparently metabolize cyclophosphamide somewhat faster than do adults; the mean plasma elimination half-life value in this population is about 4–5 hr (range: 129–516 min) (Table 14). Activity of hepatic microsomal mixed-function oxidases is known to be greater in children than in adults (Garrettson and Dayton, 1970; Alvares et al., 1975; Done et al., 1977; Vesell, 1977) although the reverse is true in animals, i.e. mixed-function oxidase activity increases with maturation in animals.

The transport forms of cyclophosphamide, i.e. 4-hydroxycyclophosphamide and aldophosphamide (see Section 7), do not ionize and, in the rat, appear to distribute in a volume, viz. 936 mL/kg, greater than total body water (Hong et al., 1991). The ultimate cytotoxic form of cyclophosphamide, i.e. phosphoramide mustard (see Section 6), distributes into a considerably smaller volume when placed into the circulation; values of 339 and 440 mL/kg were obtained in rats (Sladek et al., 1984b; Genka et al., 1990). Phosphoramide mustard is largely ionized at physiological pH (Engle et al., 1989, 1982) and, moreover, binds to both rat (20–60%) and human

TABLE 13. *Plasma (Whole Blood, Serum) Elimination Half-life of Cyclophosphamide after Intravenous Administration to Adult (≥ 19 years of age) Humans*

$t_{1/2}$, min		
Mean	Range	Reference
452	198–750	DeVita and Adamson, 1970
437	234–678	Cohen et al., 1971
414	234–552	Bagley et al., 1973
416	174–623	Mouridsen et al., 1974
443	267–607	Faber et al., 1974
435	226–566	Faber et al., 1975
313	189–496	Mouridsen et al., 1976
440	306–641	D'Incalci et al., 1979a
479	358–742	Juma et al., 1979a
493	—	Juma et al., 1979b
448	222–960	Bramwell et al., 1979
447	—	Jarman et al., 1979
474	210–960	Edwards et al., 1980
332	108–725	Ottolenghi et al., 1980
533	382–607	Juma et al., 1980
257	—	Wagner et al., 1980a
255	—	Wagner et al., 1980b
372	—	Fuks et al., 1981
352	312–378	Ritschel et al., 1981
462	—	Riggs et al., 1981
493	358–743	Juma et al., 1981
654	642–660	Wilkinson et al., 1983
306	—	Graham et al., 1983
455	342–597	Juma and Ogada, 1983
437	410–480	Sladek et al., 1984a
318	—	Tchekmedyian et al., 1986
457	152–984	Powis et al., 1987
507	390–654	Schuler et al., 1987
427	240–756	De Bruijn et al., 1988
428	—	Erlichman et al., 1988
282	218–401	Lartigue-Mattei et al., 1988
296	197–377	Moore et al., 1988
513	140–1272	Egorin et al., 1989
376	258–540	Alberts et al., 1991
366	—	Bailey et al., 1991
279	120–444	Schuler et al., 1991

TABLE 14. *Plasma (Whole Blood) Elimination Half-life of Cyclophosphamide after Intravenous administration to Children and Juveniles (≤ 18 years of Age)*

$t_{1/2}$, min		
Mean	Range	Reference
279	180–390	DeVita and Adamson, 1970
272	145–390	Sladek et al., 1980
250	208–297	Juma et al., 1984
210	150–260	Sladek et al., 1984a
383	312–516	Schuler et al., 1987
303	264–342	Schuler et al., 1991
238	129–489	Tasso et al., 1992

(39%) plasma proteins (Jardine et al., 1978; Voelcker et al., 1978; Genka et al., 1990).* Penetration into cerebrospinal fluid and brain tissue by 4-hydroxycyclophosphamide/aldophosphamide and by phosphoramide mustard is poor at best (Suling et al., 1978; Egorin et al., 1982; Arndt et al., 1988;

*4-Hydroxycyclophosphamide/aldophosphamide may also bind to specific sites on plasma proteins; carboxyphosphamide and 4-oxocyclophosphamide do not (Voelcker et al., 1978).

TABLE 15. *Apparent Plasma Elimination Half-lives of Cyclophosphamide, 4-Hydroxycyclophosphamide/Aldophosphamide, and Phosphoramide Mustard after Parenteral Administration of Cyclophosphamide*

	Apparent $t_{1/2}$, min						
	Cyclophosphamide		HA*		PM†		
Species	Mean	Range	Mean	Range	Mean	Range	Reference
Mice	6	—	16	—	—	—	Voelcker and Haeglsperger, 1982
Mice	—	—	17	—	29	—	Powers and Sladek, 1983
Rats	37	—	37	—	—	—	Sladek et al., 1982
Rats	—	—	30	—	55	—	Powers and Sladek, 1983
Rats	29	—	34	—	55	—	Sladek et al., 1984b
Humans‡	533	382–607	—	—	521	334–756	Juma et al., 1980
Humans‡	493	358–743	—	—	500	346–620	Juma et al., 1981
Humans§	88	45–150	118	70–190	182	75–320	Sladek et al., 1984a
Humans§	176	129–255	—	—	116	67–184	Tasso et al., 1992

*4-Hydroxycyclophosphamide/aldophosphamide.
†Phosphoramide mustard.
‡ $\geq$ 19 years of age.
§ $\leq$ 18 years of age.

Genka et al., 1990). Actual total body clearance values of 16 and 81 mL/min/kg have been reported for phosphoramide mustard and 4-hydroxycyclophosphamide/aldophosphamide, respectively, in adult rats (Genka et al., 1990; Hong et al., 1991).

The apparent plasma elimination half-life values for 4-hydroxycyclophosphamide/aldophosphamide and phosphoramide mustard in humans (and animals) given cyclophosphamide have also been determined (Table 15). Typical results in a patient given cyclophosphamide, 50 mg/kg, by i.v. infusion are shown in Fig. 14. Elimination of not only the parent compound, but also the two metabolites, is approximately first-order. Maximum plasma concentrations of 4-hydroxycyclophosphamide/aldophosphamide and phosphoramide mustard were about 6–16% and 9–18%, respect-

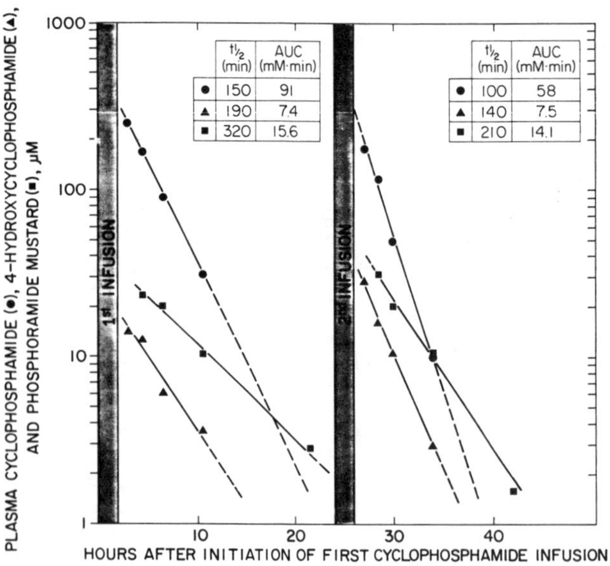

FIG. 14. Plasma concentrations of cyclophosphamide, 4-hydroxycyclophosphamide/aldophosphamide and phosphoramide mustard in a 6-year-old male patient (18.5 kg) given cyclophosphamide, 50 mg/kg, by i.v. infusion over a 1- to 2-hr period on each of two successive days. Reprinted from Sladek et al. (1984a).

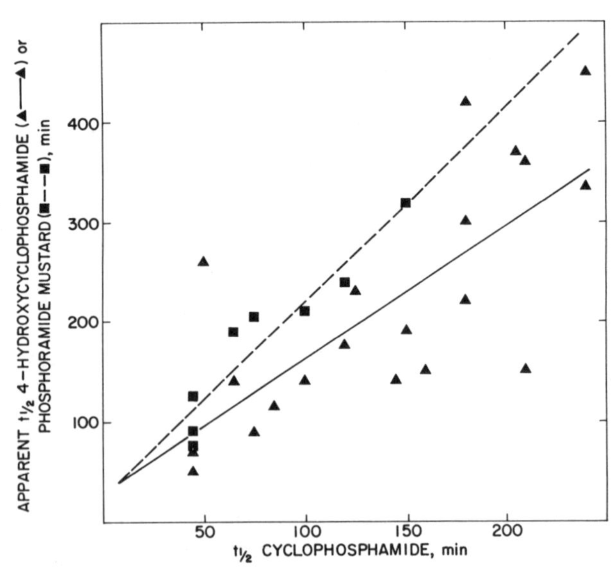

FIG. 15. Apparent plasma half-lives of 4-hydroxycyclophosphamide/aldophosphamide and phosphoramide mustard as a function of the respective plasma half-lives of cyclophosphamide. Cyclophosphamide, 50–60 mg/kg, was given by i.v. infusion over a 1- to 2-hr period to children and young adults (< 19 years of age). Modified from Sladek et al. (1984a).

TABLE 16. *Area under the Plasma (Whole Blood, Serum) Concentration vs Time Curve (AUC) Normalized for Dose for 4-Hydroxycyclophosphamide/Aldophosphamide and Phosphoramide Mustard in Patients (Rodents) Given Cyclophosphamide*

Species	Cyclophosphamide (mg/kg)	AUC/dose, mM·min/mg/kg		Reference
		HA*	PM†	
Mice	100	0.05	—	Voelcker and Haeglsperger, 1982
	65	0.04	0.02	Powers and Sladek, 1983
Rats	50	0.04	—	Sladek et al., 1982
	50	0.03	0.05	Powers and Sladek, 1983
	50	0.03	0.05	Sladek et al., 1984b
	20	0.05	—	Hong et al., 1991
Humans	6.4–12.5	—	0.38 (0.20–0.60)‡	Juma et al., 1980
	10	0.06	—	Wagner et al., 1980a
	10–20	0.06 (0.02–0.09)	—	Wagner et al., 1980b
	20	0.05	—	Wagner et al., 1981
	50–60	0.10 (0.05–0.15)	0.29 (0.24–0.36)	Sladek et al., 1984a
	50–60	0.03 (0.02–0.05)	—	Ehninger et al., 1985
	50–60	0.02 (0.00–0.04)	—	Schuler et al., 1987
	50–60	—	0.23 (0.15–0.33)	Moore et al., 1988
	50–60	0.02 (0.00–0.04)	—	Schuler et al., 1991

*4-Hydroxycyclophosphamide/aldophosphamide.
†Phosphoramide mustard.
‡Parenthesis: range.

ively, those of cyclophosphamide (Sladek et al., 1984a). Apparent plasma elimination half-life values for 4-hydroxycyclophosphamide/aldophosphamide and phosphoramide mustard increased approximately linearly with an increase in plasma half-life values for the parent compound; the slopes of these relationships were 1.35 and 1.97, respectively (Fig. 15). These observations and a comparison in male rats of the actual plasma half-life values for 4-hydroxycyclophosphamide/aldophosphamide (14 min)* and phosphoramide mustard (14 min) with the actual plasma half-life value obtained for cyclophosphamide (29 min) and the apparent plasma half-life values obtained for 4-hydroxycyclophosphamide/aldophosphamide (34 min) and phosphoramide mustard (55 min) following intraperitoneal cyclophosphamide administration (Sladek et al., 1984b),† strongly indicate that the major determinant with regard to the apparent plasma half-life of 4-hydroxycyclophosphamide/aldophosphamide is its rate of formation whereas in the case of phosphoramide mustard, an additional determinant, perhaps efflux from the cell, is operative.

As expected, plasma (blood) AUC values for 4-hydroxycyclophosphamide/aldophosphamide increase approximately linearly with an increase in the amount of cyclophosphamide administered (Wagner et al., 1980b; Sladek et al., 1984b). AUC values, obtained for 4-hydroxycyclophos-

*A nearly identical value, viz. 15 min, was recently reported by Genka et al. (1990).

†More recently, Hong et al. (1991) gave cyclophosphamide intravenously to somewhat older rats and obtained similar values, viz. actual mean plasma half-life values of 58 and 8 min for cyclophosphamide and 4-hydroxycyclophosphamide/aldophosphamide, respectively, and an apparent mean plasma half-life value of 55 min for 4-hydroxycyclophosphamide/aldophosphamide. They did not determine the actual plasma half-life value for phosphoramide mustard nor did they report the apparent mean plasma half-life for this metabolite following cyclophosphamide administration. However, following cyclophosphamide administration, the apparent plasma half-life value for phosphoramide mustard was about 2-fold greater than that for 4-hydroxycyclophosphamide/aldophosphamide in the representative experiment that was reported. Moreover, the apparent plasma half-life value for phosphoramide mustard was about 3-fold greater than that for 4-hydroxycyclophosphamide/aldophosphamide when the latter was given to male rats.

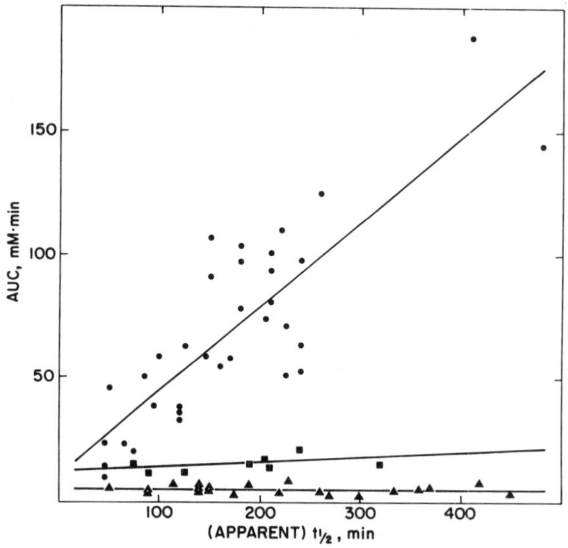

FIG. 16. Plasma AUC values for cyclophosphamide (●), 4-hydroxycyclophosphamide/aldophosphamide (▲) and phosphoramide mustard (■) as a function of their respective apparent (4-hydroxycyclophosphamide/aldophosphamide, phosphoramide mustard) or actual (cyclophosphamide) half-lives. Cyclophosphamide, 50–60 mg/kg, was given by i.v. infusion over a 1- to 2-hr period to children and young adults (< 19 years of age). Modified from Sladek et al. (1984a).

phamide/aldophosphamide and phosphoramide mustard following the administration of cyclophosphamide to humans or rodents and normalized for dose, are given in Table 16.* The disparity between the values obtained in humans and rodents for phosphoramide mustard suggests that a much greater fraction of the total dose is converted to phosphoramide mustard, or that elimination of phosphoramide mustard is much slower, in humans. Species variability in the rate at which serum albumin-catalyzed formation of phosphoramide mustard from aldophosphamide occurs has been reported and may be relevant in this regard (Kwon et al., 1987c). Although there is currently no supportive evidence, another possibility is that there are species differences in the binding of phosphoramide mustard to serum proteins.

Also as expected, at a given dose, AUC values for cyclophosphamide increase approximately linearly with an increase in its plasma half-life (Sladek et al., 1984a,b; Alberts et al., 1991) (Fig. 16). However, AUC values for 4-hydroxycyclophosphamide/aldophosphamide and phosphoramide mustard remain essentially constant with an increase in their respective apparent plasma half-life values (Sladek et al., 1984a,b) (Fig. 16). Since the apparent plasma half-lives of the metabolites increase as the plasma half-life of cyclophosphamide increases, it follows that the AUC values for 4-hydroxycyclophosphamide/aldophosphamide and phosphoramide mustard remain essentially constant as the plasma half-life of cyclophosphamide increases (Fig. 17). Others (Bagley et al., 1973; Juma et al., 1980; Wagner et al., 1980a,b; Moore et al., 1988; Lind et al., 1989; Alberts et al., 1991) have provided data consistent with these observations and/or have reached the same conclusion.†

*At variance with the observations reported in Table 16 for humans are those of Struck et al. (1987) and Alberts et al. (1991). They found that AUC values for 4-hydroxycyclophosphamide/aldophosphamide and phosphoramide mustard were nearly identical.

†One laboratory has reported data which is inconsistent with this notion (Ehninger et al., 1985; Schuler et al., 1987, 1991). These investigators noted that the plasma half-life of cyclophosphamide decreased when high doses of it were administered to patients on consecutive days and that associated with this decrease was an increase in the AUC value for 4-hydroxycyclophosphamide/aldophosphamide. The reason for the apparent discrepancy is not clear. Relative to those reported by Sladek et al. (1984a), values for both the peak concentrations and AUCs for 4-hydroxycyclophosphamide/aldophosphamide were very low, e.g. the mean day-1 AUC value, viz. 630 μM·min, reported by Schuler et al. (1987) was only about one-ninth the mean day-1 AUC value, viz. 5517 μM·min, reported by Sladek et al. (1984a), despite the fact that the dose and schedule (50–60 mg/kg daily), route of administration (i.v. infusion) and assay protocol were essentially identical. There were at least three, perhaps significant, differences in the experimental protocols. The Schuler patients were given

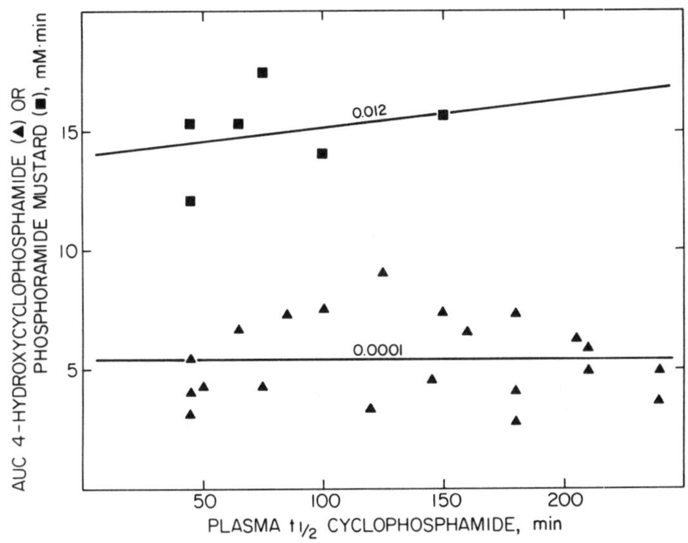

FIG. 17. Plasma AUC values for 4-hydroxycyclophosphamide/aldophosphamide and phosphoramide mustard as a function of the respective plasma half-life values for cyclophosphamide. Cyclophosphamide, 50–60 mg/kg, was given by i.v. infusion over a 1- to 2-hr period to children and young adults (< 19 years of age). The number associated with each line is the slope of that line. Data from Sladek et al. (1984a).

Such observations have also been made in animal experiments (Sladek et al., 1984b) and are as expected (Jao et al., 1972; Bagley et al., 1973; Sladek, 1972a,b; Goldstein et al., 1974) given the following scenario. Thus, assuming first-order kinetics, if the *only* change is to alter the rate at which the parent compound is converted to its metabolite, and if the parent compound is eliminated from the body primarily by metabolism, i.e. only a small fraction of it is eliminated by excretion so that regardless of the rate at which the parent compound is converted to its metabolite, ultimately almost all of it is, AUC values for the metabolite must remain constant as illustrated in Fig. 18.

Cyclophosphamide metabolites are ultimately eliminated primarily by renal mechanisms. Thus, in humans given radiolabeled cyclophosphamide, 62% (range: 41–82%) of the injected radioactivity was recovered in the urine within 48 hr and a small amount of additional radiolabeled material could be collected at later time points; recovery of radiolabel from stool and expired air was less than 4% (Bagley et al., 1973). Similar observations have been reported by others (De Vita and Adamson, 1970; Struck et al., 1971; Jao et al., 1972; Mouridsen et al., 1974; Wagner et al., 1980b; Hadidi and Idle, 1988; Hadidi et al., 1988; Tasso et al., 1992). The major urinary metabolites are carboxyphosphamide and, perhaps, phosphoramide mustard (see Section 3.1 and Table 17). The observations of Wagner et al. (1980b) further support the notion that phosphoramide mustard is a major urinary metabolite of cyclophosphamide. Minor urinary metabolites include 4-oxocyclophosphamide, alcophosphamide, bis-(2-chloroethyl)-amine and 4-hydroxycyclophosphamide/aldophosphamide (see Section 3.1 and Table 17). Less than 4% of the dose is excreted as 4-hydroxycyclophosphamide/aldophosphamide (Wagner et al., 1980b, 1981; Sladek et al., 1982). Intriguing, in view of the important role that aldehyde dehydrogenases play in oxazaphospharine metabolism/potency (see Sections 3.3 and 9.3), is the report that whereas in 6 of 14 patients, the mean percent of the administered dose excreted in the urine as carboxyphosphamide was 6.7%, in 4 of the 14 it was $\leq$ 0.1% (Hadidi et al., 1988). Others (Milsted and Jarman, 1982; Boddy et al., 1992; Tasso et al., 1992) also noted substantial interindividual variation in this regard. The long length of the urine collection period, the interindividual variation in urine pH (e.g.

Footnote continued
mesna; those of Sladek were not. Schuler and coworkers determined whole blood concentrations; Sladek and coworkers determined plasma concentrations. Finally, AUC values reported by Schuler and coworkers may be somewhat underestimated because they measured blood levels for only the first eight hours after the start of cyclophosphamide infusion.

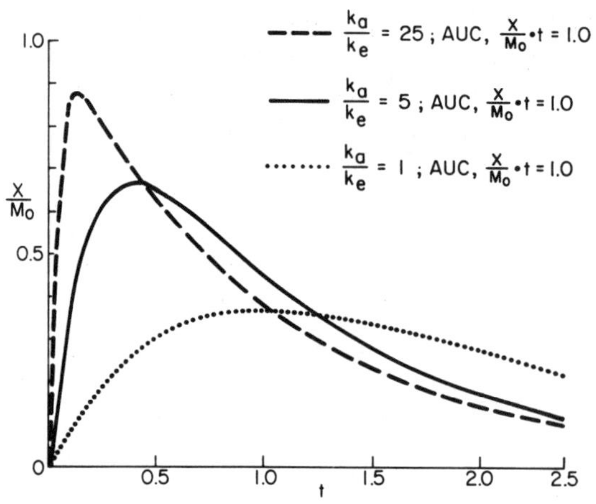

For $k_a = k_e : \frac{X}{M_o} = k_e t \left[e^{-k_e t} \right]$

For $k_a \neq k_e : \frac{X}{M_o} = \frac{k_a}{(k_e - k_a)} \left[e^{-k_a t} - e^{-k_e t} \right]$

Where:
M_o = *amount of drug introduced*
X = *amount of activated drug present at time t*
k_a = *rate constant of activation*
k_e = *rate constant of elimination*
t = *time*

FIG. 18. Predicted plasma concentrations and AUC values for the active metabolite of a prodrug, assuming that first-order kinetics describe its rate of formation (k_a) as well as its rate of removal (k_e) whether by excretion and/or further metabolism. Shown is the amount of metabolite (X) in the body as a fraction of the total amount of prodrug (M_o) placed into the body at time zero. The family of curves was generated by successively increasing k_a by 5-fold while keeping k_e constant. Only the first part of the relationship between X/M_o and t is shown here; the entire relationship was taken into account when AUC values were calculated. AUC values are expressed as (X/M_o) (t). Modified from Goldstein et al. (1974).

some drugs acidify the urine whereas others alkalinize it, and a largely vegetarian diet tends to yield an alkaline urine as opposed to the acid urine that is formed when the diet is rich in animal protein), and the instability of carboxyphosphamide in aqueous solution at physiological temperature and acid pH (Jardine, 1978; Ludeman et al., 1992) should be kept in mind when interpreting these observations.

Since clearance of cyclophosphamide and the therapeutically significant circulating metabolite,

TABLE 17. *Urinary Excretion of Carboxyphosphamide, 4-Oxycyclophosphamide and Phosphoramide Mustard in Humans Given Cyclophosphamide*

Percent of administered dose excreted in urine as						
Carboxyphosphamide*		4-Oxocyclophosphamide		Phosphoramide Mustard		
Mean	Range	Mean	Range	Mean	Range	Reference
≥15.0	—	≤2.0	—	—	—	Struck et al., 1971
—	—	—	—	1.9	1.2–2.8	Jardine et al., 1978
6.2	4.8–8.1	1.2	0.6–1.8	—	—	Jarman et al., 1979
≤10.1	≤3.8–≤15.9	—	—	—	—	Wagner et al., 1980b
12.1	3.2–33.9	1.1	0.8–1.5	—	—	Milsted and Jarman, 1982
3.1	0.1–10.1	1.0	0.4–3.9	18.5	2.7–52.9	Hadidi et al., 1988
1.9	0.0–13.6	0.4	0.0–2.1	3.3	0.1–10.9	Boddy et al., 1992
11.3	0.0–22.3	0.5	0.0–1.9	10.1	0.7–23.4	Tasso et al., 1992

*As pointed out by Jarman et al. (1979), the values for carboxyphosphamide may be somewhat underestimated because of its marked instability in aqueous solution at physiological temperature (Jardine et al., 1978); urinary pH may also be a factor (Ludeman *et al.*, 1992).

viz. 4-hydroxycyclophosphamide/aldophosphamide (see Section 7), is primarily by nonrenal mechanisms, impaired renal function would be expected to not affect the pharmacokinetic behavior of the parent compound or the metabolite and thus not to alter the therapeutic and toxic effects of cyclophosphamide. These expectations have been largely realized (Bramwell et al., 1979; Edwards et al., 1980; Wagner et al., 1980a; Juma et al., 1981). As expected, hemodialysis removes much of the parent compound as well as the metabolite (Bending and Finch, 1978; Milsted and Jarman, 1978; Wagner et al., 1980a; Wang et al., 1981). These subjects are discussed more fully in earlier reviews (Grochow and Colvin, 1980, 1983; Moore, 1991).

The absorption, distribution and excretion of ifosfamide per se has also been investigated (Creaven et al., 1974; Allen and Creaven, 1975a,b; Allen et al., 1976; Norpoth, 1976; Nelson et al., 1977; McNeil and Morgan, 1981; Wagner et al., 1981; Colvin, 1982; Klein et al., 1983; Piazza et al., 1984; Brade et al., 1985; Cerny et al., 1986; Wagner and Drings, 1986; Zalupski and Baker, 1988; Engineer et al., 1989; Lind et al., 1989). The metabolic transformations which ifosfamide undergoes are qualitatively the same as those which cyclophosphamide undergoes (Figs 5 and 13). However, the relative rates at which these transformations occur differ, resulting in a somewhat different overall pharmacokinetic picture. Thus, hydroxylation of ifosfamide occurs at a substantially slower rate, at least at higher doses, resulting in a longer plasma half-life. Moreover, as a consequence, another pathway, viz. dechloroethylation, becomes quantitatively important; dechloroethylation is ordinarily insignificant in the case of cyclophosphamide. It appears to be catalyzed by (a) phenobarbital-inducible cytochrome P450(s) (Ruzicka and Ruenitz, 1992). Since this pathway produces therapeutically inactive metabolites, the net result is that a smaller proportion of ifosfamide, as compared to cyclophosphamide, is converted to therapeutically active metabolites.

5. MECHANISM OF CYTOTOXIC ACTION

Like other bifunctional alkylating agents of the nitrogen mustard type, cyclophosphamide and other oxazaphosphorines are thought to effect their cytotoxic action primarily by cross-linking the two strands of DNA although ring cleavage and depurination may also be important (Calabresi and Chabner, 1990). Consistent with this notion is that interstrand DNA cross-linking was observed in neoplastic and, to a lesser extent, normal bone marrow, cells following the administration of cyclophosphamide to rodents (Colvin and Hilton, 1981; Hilton, 1984b; DeNeve et al., 1989; Wang et al., 1993); additional evidence for this contention is cited in the next section. The end result is cell cycle arrest in G_2M (D'Incalci et al., 1983; Uckun et al., 1985; Little and Mirkes, 1992). The oxazaphosphorines are cell-cycle nonspecific, i.e. they act on cells regardless of what stage of the cell cycle they are in, but as cells traverse the cell cycle from G_1 through S to G_2M their sensitivity to the oxazaphosphorines progressively decreases (Lee et al., 1992).

While interstrand DNA cross-linking is generally accepted as the primary mechanism by which the oxazaphosphorines effect their cytotoxic action, there is at least one dissenting view. Thus, Hohorst's laboratory is of the currently minority opinion that these agents act by alkylating DNA polymerase and/or primer/template DNA, either of which leads to inhibition of DNA polymerase activity (Bielicki et al., 1983, 1984; Hohorst et al., 1983, 1986). According to these investigators, DNA polymerase and template/primer DNA are particularly susceptible to attack because of their spatial proximity to the exonuclease which, in their view (see Section 3.2), catalyzes the release of the cytotoxic species, viz. phosphoramide mustard (see Section 6), from 4-hydroxycyclophosphamide.

Perhaps relevant to a discussion of oxazaphosphorine mechanism of action are the observations that, in vivo, tumor cells resistant to cyclophosphamide are not always cross-resistant to ifosfamide (Brock, 1979; Morgan et al., 1981; Antman et al., 1985; Brade et al., 1986; Pratt et al., 1987). Similarly, tumor cells resistant to 4-hydroperoxycyclophosphamide were not always fully cross-resistant to 4-hydroperoxyifosfamide in ex vivo experiments (Teicher et al., 1986), and failure to see parallel changes in sensitivity of cultured tumor cells to the ultimate cytotoxic metabolites of cyclophosphamide and ifosfamide, viz. phosphoramide mustard and ifosfamide mustard, respectively (see Section 6), has also been reported (Sladek et al., 1985).

Metabolism of cyclophosphamide and ifosfamide is thought to be qualitatively identical (see

Section 3.5) and both are thought to effect their cytotoxic action by cross-linking the two strands of DNA. However, they do differ structurally. In the case of cyclophosphamide and all clinically useful nitrogen mustards except ifosfamide, the 2-chloroethyl groups are attached to the same nitrogen atom (Fig. 2). In the case of ifosfamide, one of the 2-chloroethyl groups is attached to the extracyclic nitrogen atom and the other is attached to the nitrogen atom of the oxazaphosphorine ring. Moreover, the two nitrogen atoms are separated by a phosphorus atom (Fig. 1). It is tempting to speculate that while both cyclophosphamide and ifosfamide effect their cytotoxic action by cross-linking DNA, the spacial aspects of the interstrand DNA cross-links effected by these agents differ to the extent that enzymes operative in the repair of cyclophosphamide cross-linked DNA are incapable, or less capable, of repairing ifosfamide cross-linked DNA. According to this scenario, tumor cells resistant to cyclophosphamide and other bis-(2-chloroethyl) nitrogen mustards because of high repair capacity would still be sensitive to ifosfamide. Specificity of a repair enzyme, e.g. O^6-alkyl guanine alkyltransferase, for only a particular adduct/conformation is not without precedence (Gibson et al., 1985; D'Incalci et al., 1988; Hausheer et al., 1989).

6. PHOSPHORAMIDE MUSTARD—THE CYTOTOXIC METABOLITE

Since cyclophosphamide per se is without alkylating or cytotoxic activity, it follows that its cytotoxic action must be effected by one of its metabolites. Obvious contenders include 4-hydroxycyclophosphamide/aldophosphamide, 4-thiocyclophosphamide conjugates, carboxyphosphamide, 4-oxocyclophosphamide, alcophosphamide, acrolein and phosphoramide mustard. The following observations and considerations indicate that, of these, phosphoramide mustard, or more accurately, the aziridinium ion thereof, is, in fact, the metabolite that ultimately effects the bulk of cyclophosphamide's therapeutic action, most probably by cross-linking the two strands of DNA (see Section 5 and Fig. 19).

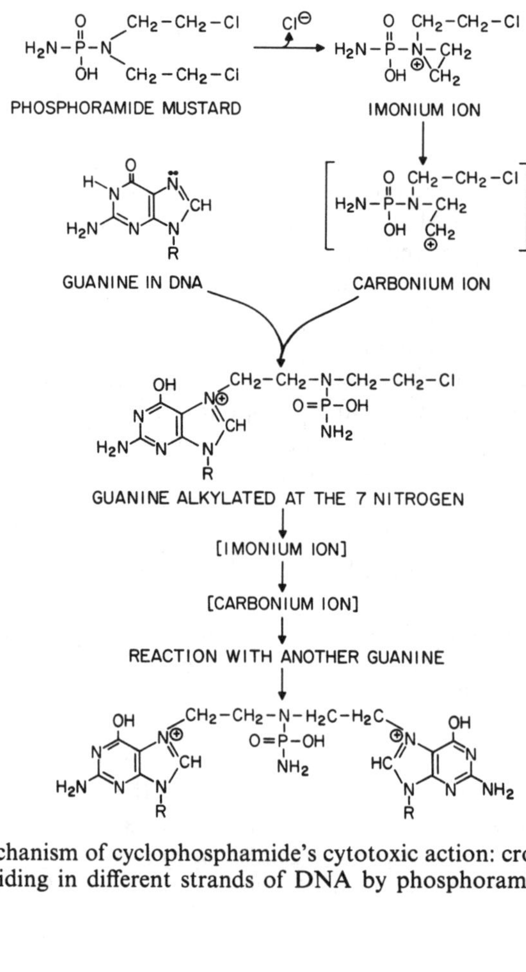

FIG. 19. Primary mechanism of cyclophosphamide's cytotoxic action: cross-linking of guanine residues residing in different strands of DNA by phosphoramide mustard.

Acrolein is highly cytotoxic to cultured tumor cells (Connors et al., 1974; Sladek et al., 1985; Blomgren and Hallström, 1991) and inactivates *Escherichia coli* DNA polymerase I (Bielicki et al., 1984). However, it can be ruled out as a possiblity for several reasons. Firstly, an analog of cyclophosphamide in which the bis-(2-chloroethyl)-amine group has been replaced by diethylamine, viz. dechlorocyclophosphamide, readily produces acrolein on microsomal metabolism (Alarcon et al., 1972) but lacks antitumor activity (Arnold et al., 1961). It, of course, cannot give rise to a bifunctional alkylating metabolite such as phosphoramide mustard. Secondly, 4-hydroperoxycyclophosphamide and an analog thereof in which the bis-(2-chloroethyl)-amine group has again been replaced by diethylamine, viz. 4-hydroperoxy-dechlorocyclophosphamide, spontaneously produce, at approximately the same rates, acrolein at physiological pH and temperature but only 4-hydroperoxycyclophosphamide gives rise to a bifunctional alkylating metabolite, viz. phosphoramide mustard, decreases the viability of mouse L1210 leukemia cells (Wrabetz et al., 1980), is toxic to human MLS ovarian cancer cells at low concentrations (Lee, 1991), or inactivates *E. coli* polymerase I (Bielicki et al., 1984). Thirdly, phenylketophosphamide, an analog of aldophosphamide that gives rise to phosphoramide mustard but that cannot give rise to acrolein, exhibits antitumor activity (Ludeman et al., 1986a,b). Finally, acrolein produces single-strand DNA breaks but not interstrand DNA cross-links (Erickson et al., 1980; Cairney et al., 1984).*

4-Hydroxycyclophosphamide/aldophosphamide and surrogates thereof, e.g. 4-hydroperoxycyclophosphamide and several 4-thiocyclophosphamide conjugates, are highly cytotoxic to tumor cells ex vivo and in vivo (Struck et al., 1975; Hohorst et al., 1976; Peter et al., 1976; Brock and Hohorst, 1977; Sladek, 1977a,b,c; Peter and Hohorst, 1979; Erickson et al., 1980; Sladek et al., 1985). Moreover, DNA cross-linking is observed after exposure of cultured tumor cells to these agents (Erickson et al., 1980; Ramonas et al., 1981; Hilton, 1984a,b; Cairney et al., 1984) and *E. coli* DNA polymerase I (which also contains 3′,5′-exonuclease activity) is inactivated when it is incubated with them (Bielicki et al., 1984; Hohorst et al., 1986). However, 4-hydroxycyclophosphamide/aldophosphamide can also be ruled out as a possibility because, per se, it is not an alkylating species at physiological pH and temperature (Struck et al., 1975; Draeger et al., 1976; Hohorst et al., 1976).

Carboxyphosphamide and 4-oxocyclophosphamide are also not alkylating species (Hohorst et al., 1971, 1976; Brock and Hohorst, 1977) nor do they or alcophosphamide exhibit significant cytotoxic activity ex vivo or in vivo (Norpoth et al., 1970; Hohorst et al., 1971; Struck et al., 1971; Sladek, 1973b; Connors et al., 1974; Friedman et al., 1976; Montgomery and Struck, 1976). Thus, these metabolites can be ruled out as well.

That leaves phosphoramide mustard. Although usually not as potent as 4-hydroxycyclophosphamide/aldophosphamide or surrogates thereof, it is cytotoxic to tumor cells ex vivo and in vivo (Maddock et al., 1966; Struck et al., 1975; Hohorst et al., 1976; Friedman et al., 1976; Brock and Hohorst, 1977; Sladek, 1977b,c; Erickson et al., 1980; Sladek et al., 1985) and it is an alkylating species at physiological pH and temperature (Struck et al., 1975; Colvin et al., 1976; Hohorst et al., 1976; Brock and Hohorst, 1977). Interstrand DNA cross-links are found after exposure of cultured tumor cells to phosphoramide mustard (Surya et al., 1978; Erickson et al., 1980; Ramonas et al., 1981; Hilton, 1984a; Cairney et al., 1984) and the time course of DNA cross-linking appearance in general, as well as interstrand DNA cross-links specifically, is similar to that obtained when these cells are exposed to 4-hydroxycyclophosphamide/aldophosphamide or surrogates thereof (Erickson et al., 1980; Ramonas et al., 1981; Hilton, 1984a; Cairney et al., 1984). Alkylation of target molecules, e.g. the N-7 position of guanosine, by phosphoramide mustard proceeds directly via an aziridinium intermediate rather than after cleavage to bis-(2-

*There is evidence, however, to suggest that acrolein mediates the immunoenhancing effects of low-dose cyclophosphamide (Kawabata and White, 1988).

chloroethyl)-amine† or other metabolites (Colvin et al., 1976; Mehta et al., 1980; Vu et al., 1981; Chetsanga et al., 1982; Kallama and Hemminki, 1984; Hemminki, 1985; Benson et al., 1988). A cross-linked dimer, viz. *N,N*-bis[2(5′-phospho-7-guanosinyl)-ethyl]phosphorodiamidic acid, has been isolated following the incubation of phosphoramide mustard and guanosine 5′-monophosphate (Vu et al., 1981). The instability of phosphoramide mustard-guanosine adducts, potentially leading to ring cleavage and/or depurination, has been repeatedly reported (Mehta et al., 1980; Vu et al., 1981; Chetsanga et al., 1982; Kallama and Hemminki, 1984; Hemminki, 1985). Finally, phosphoramide mustard inactivates *E. coli* DNA polymerase I (Bielicki et al., 1984).

The apparent discrepancy between the belief that phosphoramide mustard is the ultimate cytotoxic species and the observations that the cytotoxic potency of 4-hydroxycyclophosphamide/aldophosphamide is usually much greater than is that of phosphoramide mustard can be explained by the knowledge that phosphoramide mustard, because it is largely ionized at physiological pH (see Section 4), does not get into cells as readily as does 4-hydroxycyclophosphamide/aldophosphamide (Lenssen and Hohorst, 1979; Boyd et al., 1986; Sonawat et al., 1990). An extension of this line of thought is that, unless extracellular phosphoramide mustard concentrations greatly exceed those of 4-hydroxycyclophosphamide/aldophosphamide, the bulk of cyclophosphamide's therapeutic action must be due to the phosphoramide mustard released from 4-hydroxycyclophosphamide/aldophosphamide after the latter enters the target cell (see Section 7).

That phosphoramide mustard, and not 4-hydroxycyclophosphamide/aldophosphamide, a 4-thiocyclophosphamide conjugate, carboxyphosphamide, 4-oxocyclophosphamide, or alcophosphamide, should be the cytotoxic species is as expected from chemical considerations (Friedman, 1967; Colvin et al., 1976; Friedman et al., 1979; Brock, 1983).

Cytotoxic activity of the nitrogen mustards is directly related to their ability to covalently react (alkylate) with nucleophiles, i.e. to the reactivity of the 2-chloroethyl-amine functions. Reactivity is directly related to the basicity of the nitrogen atom of the 2-chloroethylamine. Basicity is decreased by attaching electrophilic (electron-withdrawing) functions to the amino nitrogen and increased by attaching nucleophilic (electron-donating) functions.

Esterified phosphates are electrophiles. Thus, cyclophosphamide and cyclophosphamide metabolites containing an intact phosphorous ester bond (esters of phosphoramide mustard), e.g. 4-hydroxycyclophosphamide/aldophosphamide, 4-thiocyclophosphamide conjugates, carboxyphosphamide, 4-oxocyclophosphamide and alcophosphamide, are expected to be without alkylating and cytotoxic activity; they are.

Unesterified phosphates are also ordinarily electrophiles. However, the unesterified hydroxyl group of phosphoramide mustard (pK_a 4.75) is dissociated at physiological pH and thus bears a negative charge (Engle et al., 1979, 1982). This charge is distributed over the entire molecule, enhancing the basicities of the phosphoramide nitrogens. Hence, the tertiary (mustard) nitrogen is sufficiently nucleophilic to allow aziridinium ion formation and subsequent alkylation.

†Bis-(2-chloroethyl)-amine has also been considered to be the metabolite that effects the cytotoxic actions of cyclophosphamide. It is cytotoxic to tumor cells ex vivo and in vivo (Sladek, 1973b; Struck et al., 1975; Friedman et al., 1976; Sladek, 1977b,c; Brock and Hohorst, 1977; Sladek et al., 1985) although it usually is not as potent as 4-hydroxycyclophosphamide/aldophosphamide or surrogates thereof. However, there is little or no evidence indicating that significant amounts of bis-(2-chloroethyl)-amine are generated and accumulated in vivo following cyclophosphamide administration. Accumulation would not be expected because, at physiological pH and bicarbonate concentrations, bis-(2-chloroethyl)-amine quickly gives rise, without benefit of enzymatic intervention, to 3-(2-chloroethyl)-1,3-oxazolidine-2-one (see Section 3); the latter is devoid of cytotoxic activity or potential. Moreover, bis-(2-chloroethyl)-amine is, relative to phosphoramide mustard, a weak alkylating agent (Struck et al., 1975; Colvin et al., 1976; Hohorst et al., 1976; Brock and Hohorst, 1977) at physiological pH and temperature. This is as expected for chemical reasons (Colvin et al., 1976; Friedman et al., 1979). Upon intramolecular cyclization, bis-(2-chloroethyl)-amine does give rise to the corresponding aziridinium ion but, at physiological pH, the aziridinium ion of bis-(2-chloroethyl)-amine is quickly converted to chloroethylaziridine (Friedman and Boger, 1961). Chloroethylaziridine is a neutral species and hence relatively stable, i.e. per se it is essentially without alkylating activity. In contrast, the tetra-substituted aziridinium cation of phosphoramide mustard cannot similarly form a neutral species; thus, all of it is available for reaction. Finally bis-(2-chloroethyl)-amine does not effect interstrand DNA cross-links; rather, it effects DNA–protein cross-links (Hilton, 1984a) and the time course of cross-link appearance following exposure of cultured tumor cells to bis-(2-chloroethyl)-amine differs from that obtained when such cells are exposed to 4-hydroxycyclophosphamide/aldophosphamide or surrogates thereof (Hilton, 1984a).

Theoretical considerations predict that the most favorable DNA sequence for phosphoramide mustard-effected interstrand cross-linking is 5′-GC-3′ and that thymine methyl groups adjacent to guanine will inhibit phosphoramide mustard-effected cross-linking (Hausheer et al., 1989). Intriguing is the notion that acquired resistance to phosphoramide mustard may be the consequence of methylation of an adjacent cytosine, or replacement of the usual adjacent base with thymine, in a critical and otherwise sensitive (to phosphoramide mustard-effected cross-linking) area of the genome (Hausheer et al., 1989).

Although acrolein does not effect the cytotoxic action of cyclophosphamide, it may serve to augment the cytotoxic action of the metabolite, viz. phosphoramide mustard, that does (Crook et al., 1986; Lee, 1991). The basis for this notion are the observations that (1) sensitivity to 4-hydroxycyclophosphamide/aldophosphamide (phosphoramide mustard) and a surrogate thereof, viz. 4-hydroperoxycyclophosphamide, increases as the cellular concentration of glutathione decreases (Crook et al., 1986; McGown and Fox, 1986; Chresta et al., 1990; Peters et al., 1990, 1991; Lee, 1991; Lee et al., 1991) and (2) acrolein irreversibly conjugates with glutathione thus effectively removing it from the cell (Crook et al., 1986; Lee, 1991). Possible mechanisms by which glutathione may protect cells against the cytotoxic action of cyclophosphamide are discussed elsewhere in this chapter.

Intermediates analogous to phosphoramide mustard are thought to be the therapeutically important cytotoxic metabolites of other oxazaphosphorines.

7. 4-HYDROXYCYCLOPHOSPHAMIDE/ALDOPHOSPHAMIDE—THE SIGNIFICANT CIRCULATING METABOLITE AND THE ONE RESPONSIBLE FOR CYCLOPHOSPHAMIDE-SPECIFIC SELECTIVITY

While it was generally agreed early on that phosphoramide mustard is the active cytotoxic species, the identity of the pharmacologically important, circulating (transport) form of cyclophosphamide (and other oxazaphosphorines) was, until relatively recently, the subject of considerable controversy. Some (Montgomery and Struck, 1973; Struck et al., 1975, 1979, 1983; Friedman et al., 1976; Hipkens et al., 1981) had favored phosphoramide mustard itself. Our laboratory (Domeyer and Sladek, 1980a; Powers and Sladek, 1983; Sladek et al., 1984a, 1985) and several others (Connors et al., 1974; Brock, 1976; Brock and Hohorst, 1977; Hilton, 1984b) had favored 4-hydroxycyclophosphamide/ aldophosphamide.

The identity of the pharmacologically important circulating form of cyclophosphamide is of substantial consequence because of an important ramification. Thus, if it is phosphoramide mustard, the cytotoxic action would be effected by phosphoramide mustard generated outside of target cells and the basis for oxazaphosphorine-specific selectivity would have to reside solely with this metabolite. On the other hand, if it is 4-hydroxycyclophosphamide/aldophosphamide, the cytotoxic action of cyclophosphamide would be effected by phosphoramide mustard generated from 4-hydroxycyclophosphamide/aldophosphamide within target cells and the basis for oxazaphosphorine-specific selectivity could reside with either 4-hydroxycyclophosphamide/aldophosphamide and/or phosphoramide mustard.

Since cell-kill by any DNA cross-linking agent will be directly proportional to the cytotoxic potency of that agent, the amount of that agent to which the cells are exposed and the length of time that the cells are exposed to that amount of agent, it follows that the individual contribution of circulating 4-hydroxycyclophosphamide/aldophosphamide and phosphoramide mustard to the cytotoxic effect of cyclophosphamide will depend on their relative potency and AUC values.

Substantial amounts of both 4-hydroxycyclophosphamide/aldophosphamide and phosphoramide mustard are found in the plasma of rodents and humans given cyclophosphamide. Plasma AUC values for 4-hydroxycyclophosphamide/aldophosphamide and phosphoramide mustard in mice, rats and humans given cyclophosphamide are presented in Table 18. In humans and rats, AUC values for phosphoramide mustard exceed those for 4-hydroxycyclophosphamide/aldophosphamide though not by a lot; the opposite is the case in mice.

The sensitivities of several mouse and human, normal and cultured tumor, cells to 4-hydroxycyclophosphamide/aldophosphamide and phosphoramide mustard are presented in columns 6 and

TABLE 18. *Plasma AUC Values for 4-Hydroxycyclophosphamide/Aldophosphamide and Phosphoramide Mustard in Mice, Rats and Humans given Cyclophosphamide*

Species	Cyclophosphamide (mg/kg)	AUC, mM·min		
		HA*	PM†	PM/HA‡
Mice	65	2.3	1.5	0.7
Rats	50	1.5	2.5	1.7
Humans	50–60	5.4	15.4	2.9§

*4-Hydroxycyclophosphamide/aldophosphamide.

†Phosphoramide mustard.

‡Since AUC values for 4-hydroxycyclophosphamide/aldophosphamide and phosphoramide mustard increase approximately linearly with an increase in the amount of cyclophosphamide administered (see Section 4), it follows that the relative amount of the two metabolites will be independent of the dose of cyclophosphamide. Since AUC values for 4-hydroxycyclophosphamide/aldophosphamide and phosphoramide mustard are independent of the rate at which cyclophosphamide is converted to 4-hydroxycyclophosphamide/aldophosphamide (see Section 4), it follows also that the relative amount of the two metabolites will be independent of this parameter.

§Others have reported ratios that are near unity (Struck et al., 1987; Alberts et al., 1991).

Data from Powers and Sladek (1983) and Sladek et al. (1984a,b).

7, respectively, of Table 19. With the exception of an oxazaphosphorine-resistant tumor cell line, viz. L1210/OAP*, all cells are more sensitive to 4-hydroxycyclophosphamide/aldophosphamide. Other cultured tumor cells have also been observed to be more sensitive to 4-hydroxycyclophosphamide/aldophosphamide than to phosphoramide mustard. For example, rat W256 (Powers and Sladek, 1983), rat Yoshida sarcoma (Brock, 1976), human malignant melanoma G3361 (N. E. Sladek, unpublished observations), human breast adenocarcinoma MCF-7 (N. E. Sladek, unpublished observations), human Burkitt's lymphoma Namalwa (N. E. Sladek, unpublished observations), human small cell lung cancer N417 (Ruckdeschel et al., 1987) and human Eagle KB (Struck et al., 1975), cells are approximately 20X, 25X, 18X, 16X, 15X, > 10X and 5X, respectively, more sensitive to 4-hydroxycyclophosphamide/aldophosphamide.

Having determined the cytotoxic potency and AUC values for these agents, the percent of total cell-kill hypothetically due to either circulating 4-hydroxycyclophosphamide/aldophosphamide or phosphoramide mustard can be estimated for each cell type by the two relationships that follow:

$$\%\mathrm{TCK}_{\mathrm{HA}} = \frac{(100)([\mathrm{AUC/LC}]_{\mathrm{HA}}/[\mathrm{AUC/LC}]_{\mathrm{PM}})}{1 + ([\mathrm{AUC/LC}]_{\mathrm{HA}}/[\mathrm{AUC/LC}]_{\mathrm{PM}})}$$

$$\%\mathrm{TCK}_{\mathrm{PM}} = 100 - \%\mathrm{TCK}_{\mathrm{HA}}$$

In these relationships,% $\mathrm{TCK}_{\mathrm{HA}}$ is the percent of the total cell-kill due to circulating 4-hydroxycyclophosphamide/aldophosphamide,% $\mathrm{TCK}_{\mathrm{PM}}$ is the percent of total cell-kill due to circulating phosphoramide mustard, AUC is the area under the plasma concentration curve for each of the two metabolites under consideration, and LC is the potency of each of these metabolites. LC is expressed as the concentration of drug required to kill a certain fraction e.g. 50 or 99%, of the target cell population ex vivo when exposure to the drug is for an exact amount of time, e.g. 30 min. For the relationship to have meaning, the amount of cell-kill must be determined during a time period in which cell survival decreases in an approximately log-linear manner during the period of drug exposure.

When the AUC and potency values presented in Tables 18 and 19, respectively, are substituted into the above relationship, the percent of total cell-kill hypothetically effected by circulating

*L1210/CPA cells are resistant specifically to 4-hydroxycyclophosphamide/aldophosphamide and other oxazaphosphorines, i.e. they are not resistant to non-oxazaphosphorines such as phosphoramide mustard. Indeed, they are collaterally sensitive to the latter (Sladek et al., 1985).

TABLE 19. *Percent of Total Cell-Kill Hypothetically Due to Circulating 4-Hydroxycyclophosphamide/Aldophosphamide and Phosphoramide Mustard*

Species	Cell: Name	Cell: Origin	Cell: Type		LC_{50}, μM*: HA‡	LC_{50}, μM*: PM§	% Cell-kill†: HA	% Cell-kill†: PM
Mouse	P388/0	Static suspension culture	Malignant	Lymphoid	1.0	16	96	4
Mouse	L1210/0	Static suspension culture	Malignant	Lymphoid	10	56	90	10
Mouse	P388/CLA	Static suspension culture	Resistant malignant	Lymphoid	9.5	40	87	13
Mouse	L1210/OAP	Static suspension culture	Resistant malignant	Lymphoid	102	49	42	58
Mouse	B-Cells (LPS)	Spleens from healthy donors	Non-malignant	Lymphoid	7.6	295	98	2
Mouse	T-Cells (PHA)	Spleens from healthy donors	Non-malignant	Lymphoid	16	262	96	4
Mouse	T-Cells (ConA)	Spleens from healthy donors	Non-malignant	Lymphoid	17	312	97	3
Mouse	T_h (Clone 176–24)	Cultured clones obtained from spleens of healthy donors	Non-malignant	Lymphoid	7.5	219	98	2
Mouse	T_c (Clone 193–7)	Cultured clones obtained from spleens of healthy donors	Non-malignant	Lymphoid	6.5	344	99	1
Mouse	BFU-E	Bone marrow from healthy donors	Non-malignant	Erythroid progenitors	32	148	88	12
Mouse	CFU-E	Bone marrow from healthy donors	Non-malignant	Erythroid progenitors	9	41	88	12
Mouse	CFU-GM	Bone marrow from healthy donors	Non-malignant	Myeloid progenitors	71	180	80	20
Mouse	CFU-Mk	Bone marrow from healthy donors	Non-malignant	Megakaryocytoid progenitors	63	123	75	25
Mouse	CFU-GEMM	Bone marrow from healthy donors	Non-malignant	Multipotent progenitors	87	98	63	37
Mouse	CFU-S	Bone marrow from healthy donors	Non-malignant	Pluripotent progenitors	78	140	73	27
Human	HPB-Null	ALL	Malignant	Pre-B blast	2.5	48	87	13
Human	Molt-4	ALL	Malignant	T blast II	7.7	112	84	16
Human	Raji	Burkitt's lymphoma	Malignant	B blast I	16	316	87	13
Human	U-937	Histiocytic lymphoma	Malignant	Monoblast	10	262	90	10
Human	KG-1	AML	Malignant	Pre-myeloid blast	21	141	70	30
Human	K-562	CML	Malignant	Pre-erythroid blast	34	222	70	30
Human	BFU-E	Bone marrow from healthy donors	Non-malignant	Erythroid progenitors	20	135	70	30
Human	CFU-GM	Bone marrow from healthy donors	Non-malignant	Myeloid progenitors	20	174	75	25
Human	CFU-Mk	Bone marrow from healthy donors	Non-malignant	Megakaryocytoid progenitors	16	115	72	28
Human	CFU-Mix	Bone marrow from healthy donors	Non-malignant	Multipoint progenitors	18	130	72	28

*Concentration of drug needed to kill 50% of cells. Mafosfamide was used as a surrogate for 4-hydroxycyclophosphamide/aldophosphamide. Drug exposure was for 30 min. Data from Smith and Sladek (1985); Sladek et al. (1985); Kohn et al. (1987a,b); and N. E. Sladek, F. R. Kohn, P. C. Smith and G. L. Landkamer, unpublished observations.

†Calculated as described in the text from LC_{50} and AUC values presented in this table and in Table 18, respectively. The calculated percent of total cell-kill hypothetically effected by circulating 4-hydroxycyclophosphamide/aldophosphamide values in humans are even greater when AUC values for 4-hydroxycyclophosphamide/aldophosphamide and phosphoramide mustard obtained by others (Struck et al., 1987; Alberts et al., 1991) are used to make this calculation.

‡4-hydroxycyclophosphamide/aldophosphamide.

§Phosphoramide mustard.

4-hydroxycyclophosphamide/aldophosphamide always, with one expection, viz. the value for L1210/OAP cells, exceeds 60% and frequently exceeds 80% (Table 19, column 8). Thus, it seems clear that, in the vast majority of cases, 4-hydroxycyclophosphamide/aldophosphamide will be the circulating metabolite of major importance although circulating phosphoramide mustard is not entirely without significance in many cases especially with regard to bone marrow toxicity. Occasionally, as for example when tumor cells become resistant specifically to oxazaphosphorines, phosphoramide mustard could be the circulating metabolite of major importance. However, this possibility may be largely academic, i.e. it is not likely to be of clinical significance, because cyclophosphamide would most probably not be used in such a case since to use it would be akin to giving phosphoramide mustard, a drug with a very poor therapeutic index, i.e. a very poor margin of safety (see below).

Supportive of the notion that 4-hydroxycyclophosphamide/aldophosphamide is usually the circulating metabolite of major importance are several additional observations. All of the cytotoxic activity (towards cultured rat W256 tumor cells) found in the plasma of cyclophosphamide-treated rats could be accounted for by the 4-hydroxycyclophosphamide/aldophosphamide found there; conversely, only a very small amount of the cytotoxic activity could be accounted for by the phosphoramide mustard present (Powers and Sladek, 1983). In vivo, antibody-forming cells in mice were much more sensitive to cyclophosphamide than they were to phosphoramide mustard, indicating that a precursor, viz. 4-hydroxycyclophosphamide/aldophosphamide, of the latter was the significant circulating agent (Sensenbrenner et al., 1979; Colvin and Hilton, 1981). Thiosulfate, a strong nucleophile that does not readily enter into cells, prevented the cytotoxic action of phosphoramide mustard against cultured tumor cells but not that of 4-hydroxycyclophosphamide/aldophosphamide (Powers and Sladek, 1978; Powers, 1981); it did not prevent the cytotoxic action of plasma taken from cyclophosphamide-treated rats against cultured tumor cells (N. E. Sladek, unpublished observations). There are examples of cyclophosphamide-resistant tumor cell lines that are fully cross-resistant to other oxazaphosphorines, e.g. 4-hydroxycyclophosphamide/aldophosphamide, but that remain fully, or at least partially, sensitive to non-oxazaphosphorine nitrogen mustards, e.g. phosphoramide mustard (Wampler et al., 1978; Gerhartz et al., 1979; Schmid et al., 1980; Struck et al., 1983; Schabel et al., 1983; Hilton, 1984b; Sladek et al., 1985; Koelling et al., 1990). Perhaps most persuasive is recognition that the basis for cyclophosphamide-specific selectivity resides with 4-hydroxycyclophosphamide/aldophosphamide (see below). As discussed earlier, the basis for cyclophosphamide-specific selectivity can only reside with this metabolite if it is the pharmacologically important circulating metabolite, i.e. it cannot reside with 4-hydroxycyclophosphamide/aldophosphamide if phosphoramide mustard is the circulating metabolite of importance.

That 4-hydroxycyclophosphamide/aldophosphamide, and not phosphoramide mustard, is the pharmacologically dominant circulating metabolite is indeed fortunate because examination of the LC_{50} data presented in Table 19 indicates that, as compared to phosphoramide mustard, 4-hydroxycyclophosphamide/aldophosphamide is likely to exhibit the more favorable margin of safety in both mice and humans. For example, if mouse L1210/0 tumor cells are viewed as the uneconomic species and mouse CFU-S are viewed as the economic species, the 'therapeutic indices' are 7.8 (78/10) and 2.5 (140/56) for 4-hydroxycyclophosphamide/aldophosphamide and phosphoramide mustard, respectively. A similar conclusion is arrived at if mouse T-cells are viewed as the uneconomic species and mouse CFU-S are viewed as the economic species as would be the case if immunomodulation was the therapeutic goal. While not as dramatic in all cases, the same holds in humans. Thus, if HPB-Null tumor cells are viewed as the uneconomic species and CFU-Mix are viewed as the economic species, the 'therapeutic indices' are 7.2 (18/2.5) for 4-hydroxycyclophosphamide/aldophosphamide and 2.7 (130/48) for phosphoramide mustard.

Given that 4-hydroxycyclophosphamide/aldophosphamide is the circulating metabolite of major pharmacological importance, consideration of the foregoing strongly suggests that the basis for cyclophosphamide-specific selectivity resides with this metabolite. Several additional observations can be cited to support this contention. Except in those, currently hypothetical, cases where cyclophosphamide is used to treat tumors that contain a relevant cytochrome P450, the basis for cyclophosphamide-specific selectivity cannot reside with the parent compound as was originally intended since it, per se, is without cytotoxic activity and is converted to 4-hydroxycyclophos-

TABLE 20. *Therapeutic Indices of Cyclophosphamide, Its Metabolites and Mechlorethamine in Rats Bearing the Yoshida Sarcoma*

Drugs	ED_{50}, mg/kg*	LD_{50}, mg/kg†	TI‡
Cyclophosphamide	1.25	220	176
4-hydroperoxycyclophosphamide	1.25	97.5	78
4-hydroxycyclophosphamide/aldophosphamide	1.25	150	120
4-Oxocyclophosphamide	>800	>800	—
Carboxyphosphamide	200	~800	~4
Phosphoramide mustard	20	61	3.1
Acrolein	>2.15	7.3	<3.4
Bis-(2-chloroethyl)-amine	40	100	2.5
Mechlorethamine	0.25	1.1	4.4

*Dose that effected a 'cure' in 50% of the rats.
†Dose that was lethal to 50% of the rats.
‡Therapeutic index: LD_{50}/ED_{50}.
Reprinted from Brock (1976), with permission of the author.

phamide/aldophosphamide largely as a consequence of hepatic (nontarget cell) enzyme activity. It cannot reside with phosphoramide mustard since (1) therapeutic indices (determined in an in vivo model as described in Table 3) of 26 and 17 were obtained when cyclophosphamide and phosphoramide mustard, respectively, were given to rats bearing the Walker 256 carcinoma (Powers, 1981) and (2) more DNA was cross-linked in L1210 leukemic cells than in bone marrow cells when cyclophosphamide was given to L1210 tumor-bearing mice but not when phosphoramide mustard was given (Colvin and Hilton, 1981). In fact, the experiments of Brock (1976) clearly point to 4-hydroxycyclophosphamide/aldophosphamide, at least in those cases where cyclophosphamide is likely to exhibit some therapeutic utility. He reported that, in rats bearing the Yoshida ascites sarcoma, the therapeutic index of 4-hydroxycyclophosphamide/aldophosphamide approached that of cyclophosphamide whereas that of phosphoramide mustard, acrolein, bis-(2-chloroethyl)-amine, 4-oxocyclophosphamide and carboxyphosphamide did not (Table 20).

One observation is seemingly at odds, however, with the conclusions that 4-hydroxycyclophosphamide/aldophosphamide is usually the circulating metabolite of major importance and thus, that cyclophosphamide-specific selectivity resides with 4-hydroxycyclophosphamide/aldophosphamide. Decreasing the plasma AUC value for 4-hydroxycyclophosphamide/aldophosphamide by administering phenobarbital, an inducer of hepatic NAD-linked aldehyde dehydrogenase activity, did not alter the therapeutic response to cyclophosphamide in two strains of mice (Hipkens et al., 1981). However, only one dose of cyclophosphamide, 150 mg/kg, was used and the first determination of the plasma concentration of 4-hydroxycyclophosphamide/aldophosphamide was made at 10 min after cyclophosphamide injection in one strain and at 15 min in the other. It is possible that 150 mg/kg of cyclophosphamide is much more than is needed to give the maximum therapeutic response and/or that the peak of the 4-hydroxycyclophosphamide/aldophosphamide concentration was missed in the phenobarbital-treated mice. Alternatively, the tumor cells (mouse L1210, mouse Gardner lymphosarcoma) used to measure the therapeutic response may have been substantially more sensitive to phosphoramide mustard than to 4-hydroxycyclophosphamide/aldophosphamide but, if so, they would seem to be, overall, the exception to the rule.

The reader should also be aware that one group of investigators holds views that differ from the conclusions reached herein. Hohorst and coworkers (1986) contend that the circulating metabolite of major pharmacological importance is neither 4-hydroxycyclophosphamide/aldophosphamide nor phosphoramide mustard but rather 4-(SR)-sulfidocyclophosphamide where the SR moiety can be either a low molecular weight thiol or a thiol group of a protein. They further contend that oxazaphosphorine-specific selectivity resides not with 4-hydroxycyclophosphamide/aldophosphamide or phosphoramide mustard but rather with 4-(SR)-sulfidocyclophosphamide. It is not clear what the cellular basis for the selectivity supposedly exhibited by this agent might be and the evidence in support of these contentions is minimal. Moreover, were they correct, 4-(SR)-sulfidocyclophosphamides would be expected to exhibit therapeutic indices as good as, or even better than, those exhibited by either cyclophosphamide or 4-hydroxycyclophosphamide/aldophosphamide; this is not the case (Peter and Hohorst, 1979; Hirano et al., 1980; Ramonas et al., 1981).

8. ACROLEIN—THE METABOLITE THAT INDUCES HEMORRHAGIC CYSTITIS

The clinical usefulness of cyclophosphamide (as well as of ifosfamide) is frequently limited by its urotoxic effects in the form of a hemorrhagic cystitis (Stillwell and Benson, 1988; Levine and Richie, 1989). There is good evidence that acrolein, released from 4-hydroxycyclophosphamide/aldophosphamide (or comparable intermediates in the case of ifosfamide and trofosfamide) in newly-formed urine, is the metabolite responsible for oxazaphosphorine-induced hemorrhagic cystitis.

It was shown early on (Philips et al., 1961; Bellin et al., 1974) that probably the consequence of bladder damage was a local action of cyclophosphamide metabolites present in the urine. Phosphoramide mustard and bis-(β-chloroethyl)-amine were quickly eliminated as candidate toxicants because, relative to cyclophosphamide, they were essentially without bladder toxicity when given in approximately equimolar doses to rats (Philips et al., 1961; Maddock et al., 1966; Cox, 1979; Brock et al., 1981). Moreover, cyclophosphamide, phosphoramide mustard and bis-(β-chloroethyl)-amine were relatively non-toxic to the bladder when instilled directly into it (Brock et al., 1979, 1981; Sladek et al., 1982). Subsequently, several observations led to the presently held view that acrolein, released in the newly-formed urine from 4-hydroxycyclophosphamide/aldophosphamide, is the primary causative urotoxic agent. Thus, direct instillation of 4-hydroxycyclophosphamide/aldophosphamide or acrolein into rat bladder induced toxicity to that organ; the urotoxic potency of acrolein was about 5–10 times that of 4-hydroxycyclophosphamide/aldophosphamide (Brock et al., 1979, 1981; Sladek et al., 1982). Urotoxicity was not induced by an analog of cyclophosphamide, 5,5-dimethylcyclophosphamide, which is hydroxylated in vivo in position 4 of the oxazaphosphorine ring but which cannot give rise to acrolein (Brock et al., 1979, 1981; Cox, 1979). Urotoxicity was induced by another analog of cyclophosphamide, dechlorocyclophosphamide, in which the bis-(β-chloroethyl)-amine group has been replaced by diethylamine (Brock et al., 1979, 1981; Cox, 1979). Dechlorocyclophosphamide is not an alkylating agent nor does it give rise to one; however, it readily produces acrolein on microsomal metabolism (Alarcon et al., 1972). Direct installation of 4-hydroxy-dechlorocyclophosphamide into rat bladder also induced toxicity in that organ (Brock et al., 1981). Following i.p. administration of cyclophosphamide to rats, about 3.5% of the dose was excreted in the urine as 4-hydroxycyclophosphamide/aldophosphamide. This amount of 4-hydroxycyclophosphamide/aldophosphamide, upon conversion to acrolein, was found to be sufficient to account for the urotoxic effects of cyclophosphamide (Sladek et al., 1982).

Acrolein may be generated from 4-hydroxycyclophosphamide/aldophosphamide both before and after urine formation. It is likely that only the acrolein generated in newly-formed urine contributes to the urotoxic action of cyclophosphamide. This is because acrolein is highly reactive and thus has a relatively short biological half-life, especially in an environment where there are numerous macro-, and other, molecules, e.g. proteins, with which to react; urine is comparatively free of such molecules.

Oxazaphosphorines also frequently induce alopecia and their potential as defleecing agents has been explored (Dolnick et al., 1969). Other antitumor agents, viz. adriamycin and vincristine, also cause hair loss but this untoward effect is usually not seen when other alkylating agents, including phosphoramide mustard (Nathanson et al., 1967; Feil and Lamoureux, 1974), are given. Thus, it is tempting to speculate that acrolein is the causative metabolite with regard to oxazaphosphorine-induced alopecia as well. However, Feil and Lamoureux (1974) have explored the structure–function requirements for depilation and found that at least two chloroethyl groups and the intact ring structure are required.

Cyclophosphamide also induces other untoward effects, e.g. ovarian, pulmonary and cardiac toxicities. Phosphoramide mustard appears to be responsible for ovarian toxicity (Plowchalk and Mattison, 1991) but, otherwise, the responsible metabolite(s) is(are) not known. The subject has been reviewed (Fraiser et al., 1991). Finally, cyclophosphamide is a potent teratogen. The teratogenic action of this agent appears to be mediated by phosphoramide mustard (Mirkes et al., 1981; Mirkes, 1985; Slott and Hales, 1988; Hales, 1989; Hales et al., 1989).

9. POSSIBLE CELLULAR DETERMINANTS OF OXAZAPHOSPHORINE-SPECIFIC SELECTIVITY

Substantial effort has been put into the identification of the operative, cellular determinant(s) of oxazaphosphorine-specific selectivity. By definition, those events that would influence sensitivity to all cross-linking agents or even all nitrogen mustards, e.g. various DNA repair mechanisms, cannot account for this selectivity. That is not to say that these determinants of cellular sensitivity to cross-linkings agents are not operative, only that they cannot account for the oxazaphosphorine-*specific* selectivity.

Given that 4-hydroxycyclophosphamide/aldophosphamide is the pharmacologically important circulating metabolite, that the cytotoxic action of cyclophosphamide is effected largely by phosphoramide mustard released from 4-hydroxycyclophosphamide/aldophosphamide within cells, and that the cytotoxic selectivity of cyclophosphamide resides with 4-hydroxycyclophosphamide/aldophosphamide, oxazaphosphorine-specific selectivity must, in some way, be accounted for by the micro-pharmacokinetic behavior of 4-hydroxycyclophosphamide/aldophosphamide, i.e. the way that this metabolite is handled by cells. Several scenarios can be envisaged: differentially greater uptake and/or trapping by the sensitive species, differentially greater activation by the sensitive species and differentially greater inactivation by the insensitive species. While all may be operative, and operating in concert, only the latter has been clearly demonstrated to be so.

9.1. Differentially Greater Uptake and/or Trapping by the Sensitive Species

The passage of a drug through the plasma membrane into the cell interior can be a passive, viz. filtration or passive diffusion, or an active, i.e. one that involves the active participation of membrane components, process. Active processes include pinocytosis and carrier-mediated transport.

Little is known about the permeation of 4-hydroxycyclophosphamide/aldophosphamide into cells. At a minimum, passive diffusion would be expected since 4-hydroxycyclophosphamide/aldophosphamide is a neutral species. Additionally, carrier-mediated transport may be operative (Redwood et al., 1982). Supporting this notion, although of no apparent pharmacological significance per se, is the observation that cyclophosphamide itself gains entry into cells, at least in part, by a carrier-mediated process (Goldenberg et al., 1974).

Incubation of 4-hydroxycyclophosphamide/aldophosphamide with thiols has been shown to give rise to 4-thiocyclophosphamide conjugates (Peter et al., 1976; Voelcker et al., 1976; Draeger and Hohorst, 1976; Draeger et al., 1976; Hohorst et al., 1976; Brock and Hohorst, 1977; Peter and Hohorst, 1979; Zon et al., 1984; Kwon et al., 1987a). These conjugates are, themselves, incapable of alkylation (or exerting a cytotoxic action) but they do retain the potential to do so since the conjugating reactions are readily and fully reversible. Conjugation may be with the thiol group of a small molecule or a macromolecule. 'Trapping' of, in effect, a latent cytotoxic agent within the cell would occur if the conjugate was ionized and/or if it was of sufficient size. Intracellular formation of 4-thiocyclophosphamide conjugates and retardation of 4-hydroxycyclophosphamide/aldophosphamide efflux from cells have been reported (Draeger and Hohorst, 1976; Sonawat et al., 1990). Alternatively, differentially greater uptake by the sensitive species of a conjugated thiol generated extracellularly could be operative.

There is, however, currently no evidence that differential uptake or efflux of 4-hydroxycyclophosphamide/aldophosphamide accounts for all or any part of oxazaphosphorine-specific selectivity.

9.2. DIFFERENTIALLY GREATER ACTIVATION BY THE SENSITIVE SPECIES

According to this scenario, conversion of aldophosphamide to phosphoramide mustard would occur more readily in the sensitive species.*

Since conversion of aldophosphamide to phosphoramide mustard can be the result of 'spontaneous', general base-catalyzed-β-elimination of acrolein from the former, it follows that the rate at which aldophosphamide is converted to phosphoramide mustard will increase as the (intracellular) general base concentration increases and vice versa. Moreover, since general base concentration increases as the pH of the environment increases, it follows also that the rate at which 4-hydroxycyclophosphamide/aldophosphamide is converted to phosphoramide mustard will increase as intracellular pH increases and vice versa.

Candidate intracellular general base catalysts of the reaction under consideration include carbonate and inorganic and organic phosphates (Low et al., 1982, 1983). Intracellular phosphate levels apparently may vary according to cell type. Values of about 10 and 20 mM have been reported for hepatocytes and Ehrlich ascites cells, respectively (Coe and Lee, 1969); presumably, most of the phosphate is present in the organic state (Simonsen and Cornelius, 1978). Many tumor cells exhibit greater glycolysis relative to that observed in normal cells (Warburg, 1930; Racker, 1972); it is conceivable that intracellular levels of inorganic and organic phosphates are elevated in these cells (Marx, 1981; Vaupel et al., 1989). Differences in intracellular pH between normal and tumor cells might also be expected if the metabolic activity of normal and tumor cells differs; differences in pH have been reported (Poole et al., 1964; Schloerb et al., 1965; Poole, 1967; Poole and Butler, 1969; Waddell and Bates, 1969; Racker, 1972; Vaupel et al., 1989). However, changes in intracellular pH compatible with survival are not likely to be of sufficient magnitude to substantially affect the rate at which 4-hydroxycyclophosphamide/aldophosphamide is converted to phosphoramide mustard (Low et al., 1982, 1983). Indeed, intracellular pH, as opposed to extracellular pH, appears to be regulated within a narrow range (Vaugel et al., 1989). Moreover, the rate at which aldophosphamide is converted to phosphoramide mustard is not likely to be the only relevant event influenced by intracellular pH (see Section 10.2); thus, the net effect of differences in intracellular pH on cellular sensitivity to the oxazaphosphorines is difficult to predict. There are, at present, no known examples of differential rates of base-catalyzed activation accounting for the differential sensitivity that cells exhibit towards cyclophosphamide and other oxazaphosphorines.

Conversion of 4-hydroxycyclophosphamide/aldophosphamide, and perhaps thiol conjugates thereof, to phosphoramide mustard may also be catalyzed by enzymes (see Section 3.2). Again, however, there is, at this time, no conclusive evidence that the differential sensitivity that cells exhibit towards cyclophosphamide and other oxazaphosphorines can be accounted for, in part or totally, by differential rates of enzyme-catalyzed activation although noteworthy may be that relatively greater amounts of activating activity were found in cells and tissues, viz. lymphocytes and lymphatic tissues (spleen and thymus), that are relatively sensitive to oxazaphosphorines (Voelecker et al., 1981; Bielicki et al., 1983; Hohorst et al., 1986).

9.3. DIFFERENTIALLY GREATER INACTIVATION BY THE INSENSITIVE SPECIES

Since irreversible detoxification of cyclophosphamide occurs when 4-hydroxycyclophosphamide/aldophosphamide is oxidized to carboxyphosphamide, and since several aldehyde dehydrogenases are capable of catalyzing this reaction, it follows that the amount of the relevant aldehyde dehydrogenases in a cell will play a major role in determining the sensitivity of that cell to cyclophosphamide and other oxazaphosphorines, and that the relative amounts of these enzymes in the economic and uneconomic species could be a major factor with regard to the ultimate margin of safety exhibited by these agents. First offered 20 years ago as a possible explanation for the relatively favorable therapeutic index exhibited by cyclophosphamide (Sladek, 1973b; Domeyer and Sladek, 1974; Conners et al., 1974), this notion is now an established fact; supportive evidence follows.

*Another, albeit remote, possibility is that conversion of cyclophosphamide to 4-hydroxycyclophosphamide could occur more readily in the sensitive species. The possibility can be viewed as being remote because, to date, the presence of a relevant cytochrome P450 in human neoplasms sensitive to cyclophosphamide has yet to be demonstrated.

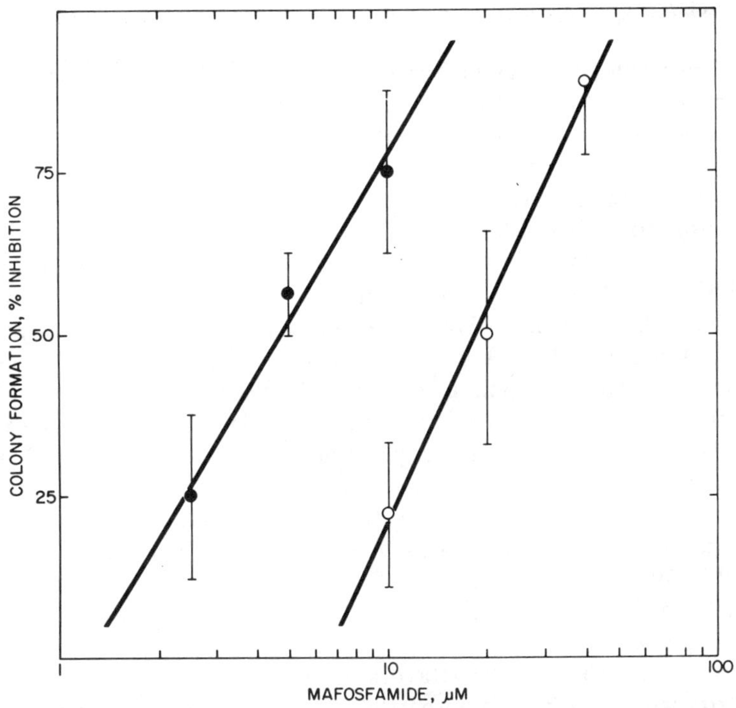

FIG. 20. Ex vivo sensitivity of human multipotent hematopoietic progenitor cells to 4-hydroxy-cyclophosphamide/aldophosphamide in the presence of an aldehyde dehydrogenase inhibitor, viz. disulfiram. Nonadherent, light density mononuclear bone marrow cells were incubated for 60 min at 37°C in the presence (●) and absence (○) of 10 μM disulfiram. Vehicle or mafosfamide was then added and incubation was continued at 37°C for an additional 30 min. Following incubation, the cells were harvested, resuspended in drug-free medium and assayed for viable multipotent hematopoietic progenitor cells (CFU-Mix assay). Points, mean and range of values obtained in duplicate plates. Modified from Kohn et al. (1987a).

Most (ordinarily sensitive to alkylating agents) critical normal cells, e.g. pluripotent and multipotent hematopoietic progenitor cells, contain significant amounts of the relevant aldehyde dehydrogenase activity, which is not too surprising since aldehyde dehydrogenase activity (measured with acetaldehyde, indole-3-acetaldehyde, butyraldehyde or benzaldehyde utilized as substrates) has been found in nearly every nonmalignant tissue (see Section 3.3). Inclusion of an inhibitor of aldehyde dehydrogenase during drug exposure increases the sensitivity of these cells to the cytotoxic action of the oxazaphosphorines (Fig. 20). On the other hand, tumor cells often contain very little of, or even totally lack, the relevant aldehyde dehydrogenases. Included are oxazaphosphorine-sensitive L1210 and P388 leukemia cells (Hilton, 1984a,b; Sladek and Landkamer, 1985; Kohn et al., 1987a; Manthey and Sladek, 1989), Walker 256 carcinosarcoma cells (Cox et al., 1975b, 1976b), 14 different human tumor cell lines of lymphoid or myeloid origin (Kohn et al., 1987a; N. E. Sladek, unpublished observations), two other human cell lines (breast adenocarcinoma MCF-7 and melanoma G-3361) (N. E. Sladek, unpublished observations), and 112 primary human tumor samples (B-ALL, T-ALL, CLL, HCL, AML, CML and NHL) obtained from oxazaphosphorine-naive patients (N. E. Sladek and F. Uckun, unpublished observations). Indirect evidence (test substrates were butyraldehyde and benzaldehyde) suggests that Novikoff rat hepatoma cells and mouse MC-79 and MBE sarcoma cells also lack a relevant enzyme (Domeyer and Sladek, 1980b).

An approximately inverse correlation was observed between aldehyde dehydrogenase activity and the sensitivity of several rodent tumor cell lines, several human leukemia cell lines and leukemic cells derived from marrow aspirates of several patients, to 'activated' cyclophosphamide (4-hydroxy-cyclophosphamide/aldophosphamide); disulfiram, a known inhibitor of aldehyde dehydrogenases, potentiated the cytotoxic action of 'activated' cyclophosphamide against those cells with relatively high amounts of aldehyde dehydrogenase activity (Hilton and Colvin, 1984; Colvin and Hilton, 1988).

4-Methylcyclophosphamide and phenylketophosphamide exhibit a lower therapeutic index than does cyclophosphamide (Cox et al., 1975a, 1976b; Ludeman et al., 1986b). 4-Methylcyclophosphamide, like cyclophosphamide, is first converted to a 4-hydroxy metabolite which then undergoes ring-opening and gives rise to phosphoramide mustard. Phenylketophosphamide is an analog of aldophosphamide in which the aldehyde moiety has been replaced with a phenylketone group; it, too, gives rise to phosphoramide mustard. However, metabolites corresponding to carboxyphosphamide cannot be formed from either of these agents because phenylketophosphamide and the ring-opened metabolite of 4-methylcyclophosphamide are not aldehydes and therefore not substrates for aldehyde dehydrogenases. Thus, aldehyde dehydrogenases cannot play a role in any selective toxicity that 4-methylcyclophosphamide and phenylketophosphamide might exhibit. All else being the same then, cyclophosphamide, 4-methylcyclophosphamide and phenylketophosphamide should exhibit the same therapeutic index if aldehyde dehydrogenases are not important determinants with regard to the selective toxicity exhibited by cyclophosphamide; if these enzymes are important determinants, the therapeutic index exhibited by cyclophosphamide should exceed, as was the case, that exhibited by 4-methylcyclophosphamide and phenylketophosphamide.

Finally, the therapeutic index of cyclophosphamide is lowered when an inhibitor of aldehyde dehydrogenases is also given (Cox et al., 1976b). This would be as expected if differentially greater inactivation by aldehyde dehydrogenases in the economic species accounted for a part of the favorable therapeutic index.

Thus, the conclusion that the relatively favorable margin of safety exhibited by cyclophosphamide and other oxazaphosphorines is, in part or even totally, due to aldehyde dehydrogenases as these enzymes favorably affect differences in the balance between the formation of cytotoxic metabolites and conversion to inactive metabolites in neoplastic and critical normal cells such as hematopoietic stem cells is inescapable.

There are other pathways by which cells *could* detoxify cyclophosphamide and thus, potentially, there may be additional determinants of cellular sensitivity to the oxazaphosphorines, some of which are likely to be oxazaphosphorine-specific.

Irreversible detoxification occurs when 4-oxocyclophosphamide or bis-(2-chloroethyl)-amine/3-(2-chloroethyl)-1,3-oxazolidin-2-one are generated from 4-hydroxycyclophosphamide and phosphoramide mustard, respectively (see Sections 3 and 6). It follows that the amount of the enzymes, viz. aldehyde oxidase and, putatively, phosphoroamidase, respectively, that catalyze the formation of these metabolites in relevant tissues/cells would also play a role in determining cellular sensitivity to cyclophosphamide and other oxazaphosphorines. However, beyond the foregoing, nothing further can be said about this subject at the present time.

Detoxification occurs when aldophosphamide is reduced to alcophosphamide. However, this reaction, and thus detoxification, is apparently reversible (see Section 3.4) and it is not clear at this time whether the enzymes that catalyze this reaction play a role in determining cellular sensitivity to cyclophosphamide and other oxazaphosphorines.

Reversible detoxification also occurs when 4-hydroxycyclophosphamide or aldophosphamide is joined with glutathione to form the corresponding 4-thiocyclophosphamide conjugate. Irreversible detoxification occurs when the mustard moiety of phosphoramide mustard is joined with glutathione. These reactions may be catalyzed by one or more of the glutathione-*S*-transferases but also proceed without benefit of enzymatic involvement (see Section 3). Thus, intracellular glutathione and/or, perhaps, relevant glutathione-*S*-transferases may also be operative determinants of cellular sensitivity to the oxazaphosphorines.

Reversible detoxification resulting from the conjugation of 4-hydroxycyclophosphamide or aldophosphamide with glutathione to form the corresponding 4-thiocyclophosphamide adduct would almost certainly be oxazaphosphorine-specific but it is not at all certain that such an occurrence would decrease the cytotoxic potential of the oxazaphosphorines. Reversible 'removal' of 4-hydroxycyclophosphamide/aldophosphamide by glutathione would serve to decrease the rate at which the former was converted to phosphoramide mustard. However, given that the cell-kill effected by phosphoramide mustard is directly proportional to the product of its concentration and exposure time, such a decrease would not be of any therapeutic consequence if, as is likely to be the case, the total amount of phosphoramide mustard that is ultimately generated, and thus the product of phosphoramide mustard concentration and exposure time, remained essentially unaltered.

Irreversible detoxification resulting from glutathione-*S*-transferase-catalyzed conjugation of phosphoramide mustard with glutathione may or may not be oxazaphosphorine-specific, but conjugation of the sort described proceeding without benefit of enzyme involvement would almost certainly not be oxazaphosphorine-specific, i.e. it would likely extend to all nitrogen mustards, if not to all cytotoxic agents, that kill cells after forming highly reactive electrophiles.

Supporting the notion that one or more of the glutathione-*S*-transferases are operative determinants of cellular sensitivity to the oxazaphosphorines are the observations that pan-glutathione-*S*-transferase activity (quantified with a surrogate substrate, viz. 1-chloro-2,4-dinitrobenzene) is often elevated in tumor cells that acquire resistance to the oxazaphosphorines (McGown and Fox, 1986; Colvin and Hilton, 1988). However, in at least one investigation, pan-glutathione-*S*-transferase activity and cellular sensitivity to the oxazaphosphorines were not inversely related (Sladek, 1993). Thus, while catalysis of glutathione conjugation with either the mustard moiety of phosphoramide mustard, or with 4-hydroxycyclophosphamide or aldophosphamide to generate the corresponding 4-thiocyclophosphamide conjugate, by a *specific* glutathione-*S*-transferase cannot be ruled out as an operative determinant of cellular sensitivity to the oxazaphosphorines, this possibility seems unlikely. Even more remote is the possibility that oxazaphosphorine-*specific* sensitivity is determined by one or more of the glutathione-*S*-transferases since associated with increased pan-glutathione-*S*-transferase activity was a decreased sensitivity to both 'activated' cyclophosphamide (4-hydroxycyclophosphamide/aldophosphamide) and phosphoramide mustard (McGown and Fox, 1986; Colvin and Hilton, 1988).

Several laboratories have shown that cellular sensitivity to the oxazaphosphorines is increased when the cellular glutathione concentration is decreased and vice versa (Crook et al., 1986; McGown and Fox, 1986; Chresta et al., 1990; Peters et al., 1990, 1991; Lee, 1991; Lee et al., 1991; Richardson and Siemann, 1992). These observations support, but do not prove, the notion that glutathione is an operative determinant of cellular sensitivity to the oxazaphosphorines. If glutathione is indeed an operative determinant of cellular sensitivity to the oxazaphosphorines, identification of the specific mechanism by which it does so is not possible at this time because of the many possibilities (see above and below and Sections 3 and 9.1) and because of the many conflicting observations. For example, with regard to the latter point, in one of the aforementioned investigations the inverse relationship was oxazaphosphorine-*specific* (Crook et al., 1986), i.e. cellular sensitivity to the cytotoxic action of 'activated' cyclophosphamide varied inversely with cellular glutathione concentration, whereas cellular sensitivity to the cytotoxic action of phosphoramide mustard was essentially unaffected when the cellular concentration of glutathione was lowered, but in another investigation (McGown and Fox, 1986) it was not, i.e. associated with an increase in gluathione levels was a decrease in cellular sensitivity to both 'activated' cyclophosphamide and phosphoramide mustard.

With regard to possible mechanisms, there is yet at least one more way by which glutathione could, in theory, act as a cellular determinant of sensitivity to (specifically) the oxazaphosphorines in some cells, viz. those in which relevant aldehyde dehydrogenases are present. Glutathione readily conjugates with acrolein (see Section 6). In vitro at least, acrolein is a potent inhibitor of some aldehyde dehydrogenases (Ferencz-Biro and Pietruszko, 1984; Nagasawa et al., 1984; Mitchell and Petersen, 1988). Thus, as is observed experimentally (see above), an increase in intracellular glutathione concentration would decrease the cytotoxic potency of the oxazaphosphorines (and vice versa) in those cells where a relevant aldehyde dehydrogenase was operative. This is because more of the aldophosphamide would be converted to carboxyphosphamide, thus less of it would be available for conversion to phosphoramide mustard. Changes in cellular sensitivity to the oxazaphosphorines due to this mechanism could be tempered somewhat since the glutathione–acrolein adduct is a good substrate for some aldehyde dehydrogenases (Mitchell and Petersen, 1989; Manthey, 1988) and thus could inhibit aldehyde dehydrogenase-catalyzed detoxification of aldophosphamide.

Mechanisms other than bioinactivation may also be operative. Perhaps noteworthy in this regard is that glutathione may facilitate the repair of cross-linked DNA (Perez et al., 1990; Mistry and Harrap, 1991). Such a mechanism is not likely to be oxazaphosphorine-specific.

10. MODULATION OF CYCLOPHOSPHAMIDE METABOLISM AND THE THERAPEUTIC CONSEQUENCES

Since (a) cyclophosphamide is known to undergo extensive metabolism, (b) the therapeutic and untoward effects of drugs are often influenced by the rate at which they are metabolized and (c) the rate at which drugs are metabolized may be influenced by numerous external and internal 'environmental' factors, as well as by the inclusion of other drugs in the therapeutic regimen, the question arises as to whether the therapeutic and/or untoward effects of cyclophosphamide will be substantially different from the 'usual' in patients whose 'environmental state' differs from the 'norm', or in patients who have received, or are receiving, various other drugs. The following sections describe principles and observations which allow some insight as to the answer to this question. Modulation of each of the relevant reactions of cyclophosphamide metabolism (and the therapeutic and toxic responses thereof) are considered separately to facilitate the presentation of this material.

10.1. OXIDATION OF CYCLOPHOSPHAMIDE TO 4-HYDROXYCYCLOPHOSPHAMIDE/ALDOPHOSPHAMIDE

Since total body clearance of cyclophosphamide is about 95 mL/min (see Section 4), clearance is primarily by hepatic metabolism (see Section 4) and hepatic blood flow in humans is about 1500 mL/min (Altman and Dittmer, 1971), cyclophosphamide clearance will be sensitive to changes in relevant hepatic enzyme levels (hepatic function) but not to changes in hepatic blood flow. However, for reasons discussed below, changes in the rate at which cyclophosphamide is cleared from the body, that is, the rate at which hepatic enzymes catalyze its oxidation to 4-hydroxycyclophosphamide, should not affect the magnitude of its therapeutic action nor should they affect its therapeutic index.

The activity of the hepatic microsomal mixed-function oxidase system which catalyzes the oxidation of cyclophosphamide to 4-hydroxycyclophosphamide/aldophosphamide is often influenced by the introduction of other xeno- and endobiotics (Conney, 1967; Mannering, 1968; Vesell, 1977; Pelkonen and Nebert, 1982; Okey, 1990). Literally hundreds of xenobiotics, e.g. phenobarbital, are known to induce hepatic microsomal mixed-function oxidase activity, and competitive inhibition is often observed because this enzyme system is not very specific with regard to the xeno- and endobiotics that it will accept as substrates; moreover, depression of enzyme activity by xeno- and endobiotics is also not uncommon. Thus, the potential for drug interactions at this level is very high.

Demonstrated inducers of cyclophosphamide hydroxylation in rodents and/or humans include barbiturates and phenytoin (Rauen and Kramer, 1964; Brock, 1967; Mellett et al., 1969; Cohen and Jao, 1970; Cohen et al., 1971; Jao et al., 1972; Sladek, 1972a; Bagley et al., 1973; Donelli et al., 1976, 1977; Alberts et al., 1978; Sladek et al., 1980, 1984a,b; Egorin et al., 1982). Moreover, as judged by plasma half-life values, cyclophosphamide appears to induce its own metabolism in humans (Table 21), though not in animals; indeed, hepatic microsomal mixed-function oxidase activity is frequently decreased after the administration of cyclophosphamide to the latter (Tardiff and DuBois, 1969; Donelli et al., 1970, 1973, 1976; Donelli and Garattini, 1971; Sladek, 1972a; Gurtoo et al., 1976). Ifosfamide also appears to induce its own metabolism in humans (Table 22).

An explanation for the species difference is yet to be substantiated. Administration of cyclophosphamide (or cisplatin) to adult male rats is known to increase the cellular concentration (synthesis) of some cytochrome P450s, e.g. IIA1, decrease that of others, e.g. IIC11, and not change that of still others, e.g. IIC6; the net effect is to decrease the rate of hepatic cytochrome P450-catalyzed oxidation of cyclophosphamide to 4-hydroxycyclophosphamide/aldophosphamide (LeBlanc and Waxman, 1990; LeBlanc et al., 1992). It may be that, because of quantitative and qualitative species differences in cytochrome P450 composition, the net effect of such cyclophosphamide-induced changes in humans is to increase the rate at which this reaction occurs in liver. Increased enzyme activity can also be due to the activation of existing enzyme; drug-meditated

TABLE 21. *Cyclophosphamide-induced Decreases in Cyclophosphamide Plasma Half-life Values in Humans*

	$t_{1/2}$ (min) on day*					
Daily dose, mg/kg	1	2	3	4	other	Reference
9–10	376				229†	Bagley et al., 1973
1–2	440				292‡	D'Incalci et al., 1979a,b
60	207	125				Sladek et al., 1980
53–56	267			127		Sladek et al., 1980
50	306	222	174	156		Graham et al., 1983
50–60	208	126				Sladek et al., 1984a
60	282	180				Ehninger et al., 1985
50	438			260		Ehninger et al., 1985
60	365	281				Schuler et al., 1987
50	539	420		260		Schuler et al., 1987
≤10	401	292	262	231		Lartigue-Mattei et al., 1988
50–60	296	176				Moore et al., 1988
60	301	173				Schuler et al., 1991
50	258	155		132		Schuler et al., 1991

*$t_{1/2}$s were determined on the day of cyclophosphamide administration indicated.
†Average of $t_{1/2}$s determined on days three and five of cyclophosphamide administration.
‡$t_{1/2}$s determined 6–13 months after the initiation of daily cyclophosphamide administration.

activation of existing cytochrome P450 enzymes is not without precedence (Benford et al., 1981). Phosphorylation of an enzyme can cause its inactivation. More to the point, phosphorylation of cytochrome P450s IIB1 and IIB2 by protein kinase A inactivates these enzymes (Oesch-Bartlomowicz et al., 1990). Perhaps, as opposed to the case in rodents, the homolog(s) of cytochrome P450s IIB1 and/or IIB2, or some other relevant cytochrome P450, is(are) ordinarily constitutively present in human liver but is(are) fully phosphorylated and thus in an inactive state; given the foregoing, cyclophosphamide could activate the enzyme by promoting its(their) dephosphorylation, or more likely, could appear to activate it(them) by preventing its(their) inactivation (phosphorylation). The hypothesis is presented in Fig. 21. Alteration (regulation) of enzyme activity in this way, as opposed to increased enzyme synthesis, would probably be more rapid, occurring in a matter of perhaps hours rather than days. In this regard, it may be of relevance that, in humans, measurable 'induction' occurs within 24 hr (Tables 21 and 22), and that the putative induction is apparently short-lived since plasma half-life values for cyclophosphamide do not decrease when the time interval between repeated cyclophosphamide administration and, thus, cyclophosphamide plasma half-life determinations, is ≥ 2–3 days (Mouridsen et al., 1974; Sladek et al., 1980; Wilkinson et al., 1983; Powis et al., 1987; Lartigue-Mattei et al., 1988).

Agents demonstrated to inhibit/depress the catalysis of cyclophosphamide hydroxylation include morphine, thioacetamide, cobalt chloride, SKF 525A, metyrapone, quinine, progesterone, 7,8-benzoflavone, deoxycorticosterone, estradiol-17β, chloramphenicol, allopurinol and prednisolone (Brock and Hohorst, 1963; Dixon, 1968; Hart and Adamson, 1969; Sladek, 1972a,b; Bagley et al., 1973; Faber et al., 1974, 1975). Of particular relevance, cytochrome P450-catalyzed oxidation of cyclophosphamide to 4-hydroxycyclophosphamide was significantly compromised in male rats given cisplatin (Clarke and Waxman, 1989; LaBlanc et al., 1992).

Numerous other internal and external environmental factors, e.g. disease status, age, diet, circadian and seasonal variations, and stress, can also markedly influence the basal level of hepatic microsomal mixed-function oxidase activity (Vesell, 1977). For example, it is generally depressed

TABLE 22. *Ifosfamide-induced Decreases in Ifosfamide Plasma Half-life Values in Humans*

	$t_{1/2}$ (min) on day*					
Daily dose, g/m^2	1	2	3	4	5	Reference
1.2–2.0	324–348				186–204	Engineer et al., 1989
1.5	347	225	231	208	208	Lind et al., 1989

*$t_{1/2}$s were determined on the day of cyclophosphamide administration indicated.

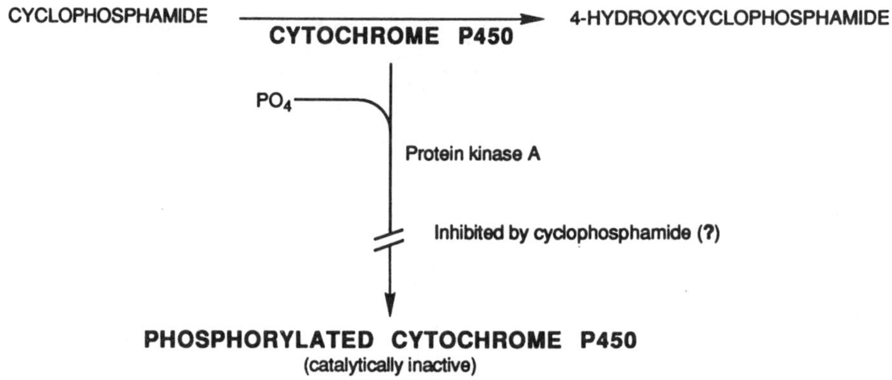

FIG. 21. Regulation of selected cytochrome P450 catalytic activity: a hypothesis. Established is that some, but not all, cytochrome P450s catalyze the oxidation of cyclophosphamide to 4-hydroxycyclophosphamide and that protein kinase A catalyzes the phosphorylation and thus, inactivation, of at least some of the relevant enzymes. Remaining to be determined is whether cyclophosphamide and/or one of its metabolites inhibits protein kinase A-catalyzed inactivation of relevant cytochrome P450s and if so, how. One possibility would be direct inactivation of protein kinase A. There are others. For example, protein kinase A is a cAMP-dependent enzyme. Thus, inactivation of relevant cytochrome P450s catalyzed by protein kinase A would presumably decrease as the intracellular concentration of cAMP decreases.

in tumor-bearing animals (Kato, 1977; Sladek et al., 1978; Garattini et al., 1988). However, little is known about the relative activity of this enzyme system in cancer patients and cancer-free 'normal' human subjects. Hepner and co-workers (Hepner and Vesell,1975; Hepner et al., 1976) reported that it was depressed, as judged by the aminopyrine breath test, in patients with malignant disease that included metastatic involvement of the liver. Higuchi et al. (1978, 1980), utilizing antipyrine half-life as an indicator, reported depressed hepatic drug metabolizing activity in patients with disseminated gastric carcinoma. On the other hand, antipyrine half-lives in patients with localized gastric carcinoma (Higuchi et al., 1978, 1980) or lung cancer (Tschanz et al., 1977) were only slightly (and not significantly) longer relative to those in control subjects. As another example, mature laboratory animals generally exhibit greater hepatic microsomal mixed-function oxidase activity than do immature animals (Short et al., 1976; Neims et al., 1976) although the opposite appears to be the case in man (see Section 4). The plasma half-life of cyclophosphamide in children is substantially lower than that ordinarily found in adults thus strongly indicating that hepatic microsomal mixed-function oxidase-catalyzed oxidation of cyclophosphamide occurs at a faster rate in the former (see Section 4).

It seems clear from the foregoing considerations then, that the rate at which cyclophosphamide is oxidized to 4-hydroxycyclophosphamide/aldophosphamide is highly subject to modulation. Perhaps reflecting such modulation is the substantial variability in the plasma half-life of cyclophosphamide in humans (see Section 4); since less than 20% of the parent compound is usually excreted as such (see Section 4) and very little, if any, of the parent compound is directly converted to metabolites other than 4-hydroxycyclophosphamide/aldophosphamide, the observed variability must largely reflect differences in the rate at which cyclophosphamide is converted to 4-hydroxy-cyclophosphamide/aldophosphamide.

The question is whether variability in the rate at which cyclophosphamide is oxidized to 4-hydroxycyclophosphamide/aldophosphamide is accompanied by variability in the therapeutic and (systemic) untoward responses to cyclophosphamide. The expectation is that it will not, given that the rate at which cyclophosphamide is converted to 4-hydroxycyclophosphamide/aldophosphamide by nontarget tissue, e.g. liver, is the *only* change effected and that most of the cyclophosphamide is ultimately converted to this metabolite. This is because (1) the AUC value for the relevant circulating metabolite, viz. 4-hydroxycyclophosphamide/aldophosphamide, is not expected to change in the face of increases or decreases in the rate at which a given dose of cyclophosphamide is converted to this metabolite (see Section 4) and (2) the cytotoxic effects of

TABLE 23. *Cell-kill by 4-Hydroxycyclophosphamide/Aldophosphamide as a Function of the Drug Concentration and Exposure Time*

Mafosfamide*, μM	Exposure time, min	Product, min × μM	Surviving fraction†
9	60	540	0.06 ± 0.01
18	30	540	0.05 ± 0.01
36	15	540	0.05 ± 0.01

*Mafosfamide was used as a surrogate for 4-hydroxycyclophosphamide/aldophosphamide.

†Mouse L1210 cells were exposed to different concentrations of mafosfamide for various exposure times such that the product of the two was constant. They were then cultured in suspension and surviving fractions were determined as described by Sladek et al. (1985). Values represent the mean ± S.E. of measurements on duplicate cultures.

N. E. Sladek (unpublished observations).

cyclophosphamide are directly proportional to AUC values for 4-hydroxycyclophosphamide/aldophosphamide (Jusko, 1971) (Table 23).

Experimentation has borne out the prediction, at least in one model system (Table 24). Thus, the administration of phenobarbital (known to induce hepatic microsomal mixed-function oxidase-catalyzed oxidation of cyclophosphamide to 4-hydroxycyclophosphamide/aldophosphamide, see above) decreased the plasma half-life of cyclophosphamide, did not change the AUC value obtained for 4-hydroxycyclophosphamide/aldophosphamide or phosphoramide mustard, and did not change the dose of cyclophosphamide required to inhibit the intramuscular growth of Walker 256 carcinosarcoma by 50%. Moreover, pretreatment with phenobarbital did not elicit a significant quantitative change in an untoward response, viz. leukopenia, to cyclophosphamide (Sladek, 1972a). Thus, the therapeutic index of cyclophosphamide also was not changed. The expected results were also obtained in female rats and following the administration of cobalt chloride, metyrapone, or relatively low doses of SKF 525A to male rats, i.e. when hepatic microsomal mixed-function oxidase activity was comparatively low (female rats) or depressed/inhibited as a consequence of drug administration (Sladek, 1972a,b). Similarly, phenobarbital or SKF 525A pretreatment did not alter the antitumor (leukemia L1210) efficacy of cyclophosphamide in mice (Hart and Adamson, 1969).

There is also a clinical example validating the prediction (Alberts et al., 1991). Thus, while the plasma AUC and half-life values for cyclophosphamide were increased when ranitidine was given with it, AUC values for 4-hydroxycyclophosphamide/aldophosphamide and phosphoramide mustard remained unchanged and there was no increase in cyclophosphamide-induced leukopenia or granulocytopenia.

Some observations seemingly challenge the view that increasing or decreasing the rate at which cyclophosphamide is oxidized to 4-hydroxycyclophosphamide/aldophosphamide in nontarget cells does not alter the therapeutic and/or untoward response(s) to cyclophosphamide.

The dose of cyclophosphamide required to inhibit the intramuscular growth of Walker 256 carcinosarcoma by 50% was substantially increased when rats were pretreated with 3-methylcholanthrene (Sladek, 1972a) or relatively high doses of SKF 525A (Sladek, 1972b). 3-Methylcholanthrene depresses, and SKF 525A inhibits, rat hepatic microsomal mixed-function

TABLE 24. *Therapeutic Efficacy of Cyclophosphamide as a Function of Its Rate of Hydroxylation in Control and Phenobarbital-treated Male Rats*

Parameter	Control	Phenobarbital
Cyclophosphamide: plasma half-life, min*	29	6
Cyclophosphamide: % of dose excreted in urine†	8.5	0.5
4-Hydroxycyclophosphamide/aldophosphamide: AUC, mM·min*	1.6	1.5
Phosphoramide Mustard: AUC, mM·min*	2.6	2.6
Cyclophosphamide: ED_{50}, mg/kg‡	0.69	0.73

*Data from Sladek et al. (1984b).

†N. E. Sladek (unpublished observations).

‡Dose of cyclophosphamide that inhibited the intramuscular growth of the Walker 256 carcinosarcoma 50%. Data from Sladek (1972a).

oxidase-catalyzed oxidation of cyclophosphamide to 4-hydroxycyclophosphamide/aldophosphamide. AUC values for 4-hydroxycyclophosphamide/aldophosphamide, and thus the therapeutic response to cyclophosphamide, should not be altered by these changes (see Section 4). However, AUC values are decreased after 3-methylcholanthrene administration (N. E. Sladek, unpublished observations). Perhaps 3-methylcholanthrene also induces aldehyde dehydrogenase-catalyzed oxidation of 4-hydroxycyclophosphamide/aldophosphamide to carboxyphosphamide, thus violating one of the conditions of the original construct. 3-Methylcholanthrene is known to induce hepatic aldehyde dehydrogenase-catalyzed oxidation of various aldehydes, e.g. acetaldehyde, in rats (Deitrich et al., 1978; Nakanishi et al., 1979; Marselos et al., 1979; Törrönen et al., 1981). Accurate AUC values for 4-hydroxycyclophosphamide/aldophosphamide are difficult to obtain when animals are pretreated with high doses of SKF 525A prior to the administration of cyclophosphamide. This is because plasma levels of 4-hydroxycyclophosphamide/aldophosphamide in such animals are very low at all time points making accurate measurement difficult. However, the AUC values are almost certainly decreased in these animals since the urinary excretion of the parent compound is substantially increased (N. E. Sladek, unpublished observations). Thus, an explanation for the unexpected response obtained when animals were pretreated with a relatively high dose of SKF 525A may be that the AUC value for 4-hydroxycyclophosphamide/aldophosphamide was significantly decreased because the rate at which cyclophosphamide was converted to 4-hydroxycyclophosphamide/aldophosphamide was depressed to such an extent that significantly greater amounts of the parent compound were excreted, thus again violating one of the conditions of the original construct. Additional factors may have been operative since increased excretion of the parent compound, at best, only partially accounted for the decreased antitumor effect of cyclophosphamide in these animals.

Pretreatment of rabbits with cimetidine, a histamine-H_2 antagonist known to impair hepatic drug metabolism, increased cyclophosphamide's plasma half-life as well as the AUC value for 4-hydroxycyclophosphamide/aldophosphamide (Anthony et al., 1990), and pretreatment of DBA/2 mice with cimetidine increased the antileukemic activity of cyclophosphamide as well as its toxicity to pluripotent bone marrow stem cells (Dorr and Alberts, 1982; Dorr et al., 1986). AUC values for 4-hydroxycyclophosphamide/aldophosphamide were not determined in the latter studies but it was shown that the AUC value for total alkylating metabolites in the plasma was increased. Also, pretreatment of DBA/2 mice with phenobarbital, known to induce hepatic microsomal mixed-function oxidase activity, reduced the antileukemic activity of cyclophosphamide although toxicity to pluripotent bone marrow stem cells remained unaltered (Alberts and van Daalen Wetters, 1976). Again AUC values for 4-hydroxycyclophosphamide/aldophosphamide were not determined but it was shown that the AUC value for total alkylating metabolites in the plasma was decreased; subsequently, Hipkens et al. (1981) reported that AUC values for 4-hydroxycyclophosphamide/aldophosphamide were indeed decreased when DBA/2 mice were pretreated with phenobarbital. Reconciliation of these observations with the conclusion presented in the first paragraph of this section is again not easy. Since the AUC values were altered, it is obvious that one of the conditions of the original construct must again have been violated. Which was violated is not so obvious. It may be that, at least in the case of the phenobarbital experiments, an explanation similar to the one offered in the case of 3-methylcholanthrene is viable, i.e. that phenobarbital induced aldehyde dehydrogenase-catalyzed oxidation of 4-hydroxycyclophosphamide/aldophosphamide to carboxyphosphamide. Phenobarbital is a demonstrated inducer of aldehyde dehydrogenase activity in a number of mouse strains (Redmond and Cohen, 1971; Deitrich et al., 1972; Smolen et al., 1980; Hipkens et al., 1981; Timms and Holmes, 1981) as well as in certain rat strains (Deitrich, 1971; Deitrich et al., 1972, 1975, 1978; Koivula and Koivusalo, 1975b; Petersen et al., 1977; Marselos et al., 1979; Nakanishi et al., 1979; Dunn et al., 1989; Vasiliou and Marselos, 1989). However, it may not induce a relevant aldehyde dehydrogenase in DBA/2 mice since it did not induce liver cytosolic aldehyde dehydrogenase-catalyzed oxidation of acetaldehyde to acetic acid in these animals (Hipkens et al., 1981) although it did induce the mitochondrial enzyme that catalyzes the oxidation of propanal (Smolen et al., 1980).

Alternatively, it may be that cimetidine inhibited the cytochrome P450(s) that catalyze(s) the conversion of cyclophosphamide to didechlorodihydroxycyclophosphamide (Struck et al., 1984; Gurtoo et al., 1985) and/or (di)dechloroethylcyclophosphamide plus chloroacetaldehyde (Ruzicka and Ruenitz, 1992). Assuming that the cytochrome P450(s) that catalyze these reactions are different from those that catalyze the oxidation of cyclophosphamide to 4-hydroxycyclophosphamide/aldophosphamide and that the latter are relatively insensitive to inhibition by cimetidine, and knowing that didechlorodihydroxycyclophosphamide, (di)dechloroethylcyclophosphamide and chloroacetaldehyde are all essentially without relevant cytotoxic activity and do not give rise to metabolites that are cytotoxic, treatment with cimetidine would be expected, and as was the case, to increase (1) AUC values for 4-hydroxycyclophosphamide/aldophosphamide, (2) antileukemic activity and (3) toxicity, *if* catalysis of the detoxifying reactions was ordinarily a quantitatively important event—available evidence indicates that it is not. Similarly, phenobarbital may, at least in some species, differentially induce the cytochrome P450(s) that catalyze(s) the irreversible detoxification of cyclophosphamide referred to above. In that case, treatment with phenobarbital would be expected, and as was the case, to decrease (1) AUC values for 4-hydroxycyclophosphamide/aldophosphamide and (2) antileukemic activity.

Interferon and poly I:C decreased the rate at which cyclophosphamide was oxidized to 4-hydroxycyclophosphamide in mice; associated with the decreased rate was decreased lethality and antitumor activity (Ishikawa et al., 1991). Again, AUC values for 4-hydroxycyclophosphamide/aldophosphamide were not determined but the AUC value for total alkylating metabolites in the plasma appeared to be unaltered or even slightly increased. As before, a plausible explanation for the inconsistency in these observations is not readily apparent.

There is also some question as to whether the cytotoxic effects of cyclophosphamide are indeed directly proportional to plasma AUC values for 4-hydroxycyclophosphamide/aldophosphamide. Thus, Hipkens et al. (1981) reported that, in control and phenobarbital-pretreated mice given cyclophosphamide, an apparent 11-fold difference in AUC values for 4-hydroxycyclophosphamide/aldophosphamide was not accompanied by any difference in the antileukemic potency of the parent compound, and Voelcker and Haeglsperger (1982) reported that somewhat greater antitumor activity was obtained when 4-hydroxycyclophosphamide/aldophosphamide concentrations were high over a short period of time as opposed to low over a long period of time.

Finally, increasing or decreasing the rate at which ifosfamide is C-4 hydroxylated may well be accompanied by corresponding changes in AUC values for the hydroxylated metabolite and thus in the therapeutic and untoward responses to ifosfamide. This is because ifosfamide, in contrast to cyclophosphamide, appears to have two quantitatively important fates, viz. hydroxylation and dechloroethylation; the latter pathway produces only therapeutically inactive metabolites. Alterations in the relative rates at which these reactions occur would result in changes in the AUC values for the hydroxylated metabolite and thus the cytotoxic and untoward responses to ifosfamide.

Relevant cytochrome P450s may also be present (and subject to modulation) in certain neoplastic cells, perhaps including some against which cyclophosphamide is used as a therapeutic agent. In that event, cyclophosphamide would be activated within target cells and modulation of enzyme activity *would* alter the cytotoxic potency of this agent against such cells in an entirely predictable manner. The point is nicely illustrated by the experiment of Doehmer et al. (1990) (Table 25).

TABLE 25. *Activation of Oxazaphosphorines by Genetically Engineered V79 Chinese Hamster Cells**

		IC_{90}, mM		
Cell line	Cytochrome P450	Cyclophosphamide	Ifosfamide	Ifosfamide mustard
V79	None	>2.0	>2.0	0.013
SD1	IIB1	1.2	2.0	0.013

*Data from Doehmer et al. (1990). The cytotoxic activity of cyclophosphamide and ifosfamide was quantified in V79 cells and in V79 cells genetically engineered to express active cytochrome P450 IIB1 (SD1).

10.2. β-ELIMINATION OF ACROLEIN FROM ALDOPHOSPHAMIDE TO GENERATE PHOSPHORAMIDE MUSTARD

4-Hydroxycyclophosphamide/aldophosphamide is a neutral species and readily enters cells where some of it is converted to phosphoramide mustard; phosphoramide mustard is largely ionized at physiological pH and consequently has great difficulty passing through cell membranes (see Sections 4 and 6). Thus, most cells are more sensitive to 4-hydroxycyclophosphamide/aldophosphamide than they are to phosphoramide mustard (see Section 7). Moreover, 4-hydroxycyclophosphamide almost always exhibits a more favorable therapeutic index than does phosphoramide mustard (see Section 7). Therefore, the expectation is that, almost always, the cytotoxic action of cyclophosphamide will increase or decrease, and that the therapeutic index of this agent will improve or worsen, as the rate at which 4-hydroxycyclophosphamide/aldophosphamide is converted to phosphoramide mustard in the extracellular space and non-target cells decreases or increases, respectively.

Phosphoramide mustard itself is a cytotoxic metabolite whereas 4-hydroxycyclophosphamide/aldophosphamide is not (see Section 6). Therefore, the cytotoxic action of cyclophosphamide against a given cell population will increase or decrease directly as the rate at which 4-hydroxycyclophosphamide/aldophosphamide is converted to phosphoramide mustard within these cells, whether uneconomic, e.g. neoplastic, or economic, e.g. normal, increases or decreases. If the rate is increased or decreased only in uneconomic cells, the therapeutic index will improve or worsen, respectively (Table 26). Just the opposite will be the case if the rate is altered only in critical economic cells, i.e. the therapeutic index will worsen or improve as the rate is increased or decreased, respectively. No change in the therapeutic index will be obtained if there is no selectivity with regard to the change in rate.

Conversion of 4-hydroxycyclophosphamide/aldophosphamide to phosphoramide mustard is catalyzed by general bases and perhaps enzymatically, (see Section 3.2).

Given that enzymic catalysis of this reaction does indeed occur in vivo, it is likely that the rate at which it occurs is subject to the influence of numerous external and internal 'environmental' factors, as well as to the inclusion of other drugs in the therapeutic regimen, i.e. those factors and drugs that affect the catalytic activity of the enzyme(s) in question. However, these factors and drugs cannot be identified at this time because the relevant enzyme(s) has(have) not yet been conclusively identified (see Section 3.2). Interesting, because of the potential ramifications, is the report (Kwon et al., 1987c) that albumin catalyzes the conversion of aldophosphamide to phosphoramide mustard.

It is known with certainty, however, that the reaction is catalyzed by general bases, e.g. dianionic phosphate and carbonate (see Section 3.2). In vivo, these bases originate from the conjugate acid-base pairs that serve to buffer extracellular and intracellular body fluids. At a given pH, catalytic activity varies directly with the concentration of the conjugate acid-base pairs (Fig. 22); at a given concentration of such conjugates, it varies directly with the pH since, according to the

TABLE 26. *Effects of Altering the Rate at which Aldophosphamide is Converted to Phosphoramide Mustard on the Therapeutic and Untoward Responses to, and Therapeutic Index of, Cyclophosphamide*

Site*	Rate	Effect of change in rate on: Therapeutic response	Untoward response†	Therapeutic index
Neoplastic cells	↑	↑	—	↑
	↓	↓	—	↓
Critical normal cells	↑	—	↑	↓
	↓	—	↓	↑
Neoplastic and critical normal cells	↑	↑	↑	—
	↓	↓	↓	—

*Site of change in rate.

†Systemic untoward responses caused by phosphoramide mustard generated within critical normal cells.

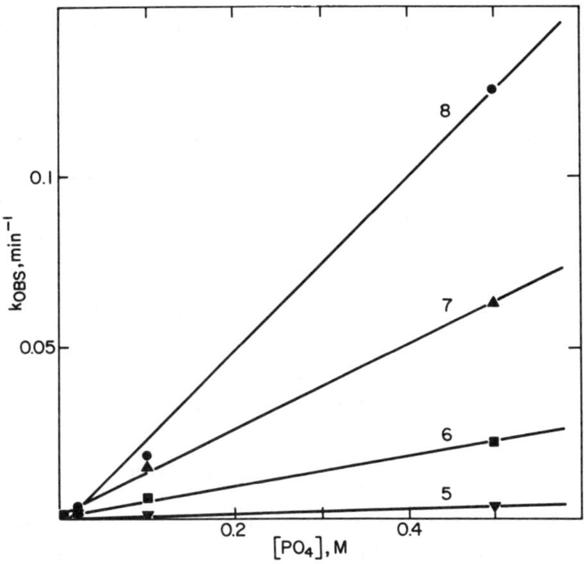

FIG. 22. Rate of acrolein and phosphoramide mustard release from 4-hydroxycyclophosphamide/aldophosphamide as a function of pH and phosphate buffer concentration. The number identifying each curve refers to the pH of the medium. Modified from Low et al. (1982).

Henderson–Hasselbalch relationship, the fraction of a conjugate acid-base pair that is present as the base varies directly with the pH.

Modulation of extra- and/or intracellular conjugate acid-base pair concentrations and/or pH by 'environmental' factors, e.g. carbon dioxide tension, nutrients, e.g. glucose infusion, and drugs (chemicals), e.g. iodoacetate, has been demonstrated (Poole et al., 1964; Schloerb et al., 1965; Poole, 1967; Waddell and Bates, 1969; Poole and Butler, 1969; Simonsen and Cornelius, 1978; Harguindey et al., 1979; Jähde and Rajewsky, 1982; Osinsky et al., 1987). That such modulation is sufficient to significantly, from the viewpoint of therapeutic or untoward responses, alter the rate at which 4-hydroxycyclophosphamide/aldophosphamide is systemically converted to phosphoramide mustard remains to be demonstrated. However, if the urinary bladder is viewed as a cell, albeit a rather large one, the principle has been demonstrated in an extrasystemic model (Table 27). The other metabolite released from 4-hydroxycyclophosphamide/aldophosphamide, when it gives rise to phosphoramide mustard, is acrolein. Oxazaphosphorine-induced bladder toxicity is effected by this metabolite after it is liberated in newly-formed urine (see Section 8). Bladder toxicity varied directly with pH and/or the phosphate buffer concentration when 4-hydroxycyclophosphamide/aldophosphamide was dissolved in phosphate-buffered aqueous solutions and placed into the

TABLE 27. *Bladder Toxicity Effected by 4-Hydroxycyclophosphamide/Aldophosphamide**

pH	PO_4, mM	HPO_4^{2-}, mM†	Increase in bladder weight, mg
6	4	0.4	14
6	40	4	28
8	4	4	29
8	40	40	70

*Female rats were anesthetized, their bladders were catheterized, and 4-hydroperoxycyclophosphamide (used as a surrogate for 4-hydroxycyclophosphamide/aldophosphamide) was infused in 0.2 mL of a phosphate buffer. One hour later, infusates were removed, bladders were flushed with a normal saline solution, and catheters were removed. Bladder wet weights were determined 48 hr after infusion. 4-Hydroperoxycyclophosphamide was omitted from the infusate to obtain control bladder weights, ca. 100 mg. Data from Sladek et al. (1982).

†Approximation based on a pK_a of 7.

bladder lumen. These experiments also call attention to the fact that the urotoxic potential of cyclophosphamide will be influenced by all of those factors that alter urinary pH and conjugate acid-base pair concentrations. Included are drugs, e.g. certain diuretics and acidifying and alkalinizing agents, hormonal status, disease status, diet, age and chronorhythmic variability.

As mentioned earlier, the rate at which aldophosphamide is converted to phosphoramide mustard is not likely to be the only relevant event influenced by intracellular pH. For example, the stability and reactivity of phosphoramide mustard and its aziridinium ion is also pH-dependent (Engle et al., 1979; Zon, 1982). Thus, the net effect of a change in intracellular pH on cellular sensitivity to the oxazaphosphorines is difficult to predict. Instructive in this regard may be the observations of Jähde and coworkers (1989a,b, 1991); they report that cellular sensitivity to mafosfamide, 4-hydroperoxycyclophosphamide, bis-(2-chloroethyl)-amine, mechlorethamine, melphalan and chlorambucil *increases* as the intracellular pH decreases. Curiously, a decrease in intracellular pH did not increase cellular sensitivity to 4-hydroperoxyifosfamide.

10.3. Oxidation of Aldophosphamide to Carboxyphosphamide

Carboxyphosphamide and aldophosphamide are, themselves, each without cytotoxic activity. However, carboxyphosphamide does not give rise to a cytotoxic metabolite in vivo whereas aldophosphamide does. Therefore, the cytotoxic action of cyclophosphamide increases or decreases when catalysis of this reaction is by cells, e.g. hepatocytes, other than target uneconomic cells, e.g. neoplastic cells, or critical economic cells, e.g. pluripotent bone marrow stem cells, and is decreased or increased, respectively. In essence, increasing or decreasing the rate at which 4-hydroxycyclophosphamide/aldophosphamide is oxidized to carboxyphosphamide is not unlike decreasing or increasing the amount of cyclophosphamide given since the ultimate effect is to simply decrease or increase the amount of circulating 4-hydroxycyclophosphamide/aldophosphamide available for uptake by neoplastic or critical normal cells. The therapeutic index remains unchanged in this scenario.

The cytotoxic action of cyclophosphamide against a given cell population, whether uneconomic or economic, will increase or decrease, respectively, as the rate at which 4-hydroxycyclophosphamide/aldophosphamide is converted to carboxyphosphamide in these cells decreases or increases (Table 28). If the rate is increased or decreased only in uneconomic cells, the therapeutic index will worsen or improve, respectively. Just the opposite will be the case if the rate is altered in critical economic cells, i.e. the therapeutic index will improve or worsen as the rate is increased or decreased, respectively. No change in the therapeutic index will be obtained if oxidation occurs in both uneconomic and critical economic cells and there is no selectivity with regard to the change in rate.

For the most part, oxidation of aldophosphamide to carboxyphosphamide is catalyzed by aldehyde dehydrogenases (see Section 3.3).

Aldehyde dehydrogenase-catalyzed oxidation of acetaldehyde, propionaldehyde and benzal-

Table 28. *Effects of Altering the Rate at which Aldophosphamide is Converted to Carboxyphosphamide on the Therapeutic and Untoward Responses to, and Therapeutic Index of, Cyclophosphamide*

		Effect of change in rate on:		
Site*	Rate	Therapeutic response	Untoward response†	Therapeutic index
Neoplastic cells	↑	↓	—	↓
	↓	↑	—	↑
Critical normal cells	↑	—	↓	↑
	↓	—	↑	↓
Neoplastic and critical normal cells	↑	↓	↓	—
	↓	↑	↑	—

*Site of change in rate.

†Systematic untoward responses caused by phosphoramide mustard generated within critical normal cells.

dehyde by rodent liver fractions is known to be induced by several agents. Included are phenobarbital, a sedative hypnotic (Deitrich, 1971; Redmond and Cohen, 1971; Deitrich et al., 1972, 1975, 1978; Koivula and Koivusalo, 1975b; Petersen et al., 1977; Marselos et al., 1979; Nakanishi et al., 1979; Smolen et al., 1980; Hipkens et al., 1981; Timms and Holmes, 1981; Dunn et al., 1989; Vasiliou and Marselos, 1989); clofibrate, a hypolipidemic agent (Kramar and Kremser, 1984; Panchenko et al., 1985); tetrachlorodibenzo-*p*-dioxin (TCDD), the notorious contaminant of Agent Orange (Petersen et al., 1977; Deitrich et al., 1978 Dunn et al., 1988); the insecticides mirex and DDT (Deitrich et al., 1978); polychlorinated biphenyls and β-naphthoflavone (Deitrich et al., 1978); 3-methylcholanthrene, 3,4-benzpyrene and other carcinogenic hydrocarbons (Deitrich et al., 1975, 1978; Marselos et al., 1979; Törrönen et al., 1981; Lin et al., 1984; Vasiliou and Marselos, 1989); and 2-acetylaminofluorene, yet another carcinogen (Lindahl, 1982). Although not directly demonstrated in these studies, at least some of the induced aldehyde dehydrogenases almost certainly significantly participate in the oxidation of aldophosphamide to carboxyphosphamide. For example, phenobarbital induces the major cytosolic aldehyde dehydrogenase in rat liver; the mouse and human homologs of this enzyme are known to catalyze this reaction with good proficiency (see Section 3.3). Induction is restricted to certain tissues, the identity of which varies with the inducer (Deitrich et al., 1972; Marselos et al., 1979; Vasiliou and Marselos, 1989), and is subject to genetic influence (Deitrich, 1971; Deitrich et al., 1972, 1978; Vasiliou and Marselos, 1989). Not known or, at best, uncertain, is whether any of these agents induce the activity of the relevant aldehyde dehydrogenases in humans, and, if they do, whether they induce the relevant enzyme activity in either uneconomic cells and/or critical economic cells. Nevertheless, the potential for clinically relevant drug interactions is obvious.

Normal human hematopoietic progenitor cells that have been incubated with certain cytokines, viz. TGF-beta 3 or IL-1 and TNF-alpha, are less sensitive to the cytotoxic action of 4-hydroperoxycyclophosphamide than are hematopoietic progenitor cells that have not (Moreb et al., 1989a,b, 1990, 1992; Lemoli et al., 1992; Zucali et al., 1992). Germane to the present discussion is the evidence, albeit less than conclusive, indicating that the loss of sensitivity to 4-hydroperoxycyclophosphamide exhibited by normal hematopoietic progenitor cells preincubated with IL-1 plus TNF-alpha is, at least in part, the consequence of cytokine-induced relevant aldehyde dehydrogenase activity (Moreb et al., 1992). Noteworthy, especially from the viewpoint of a potentially useful clinical strategy, are the reports that similar treatment of lymphoma and leukemia cells did not result in a loss of sensitivity to 4-hydroperoxycyclophosphamide, presumably because a relevant aldehyde dehydrogenase was not induced in these cells (Moreb et al., 1989a,b, 1990; Lemoli et al., 1992).

Other compounds are known to inhibit/depress the activity of one or more, but not necessarily all, of the hepatic aldehyde dehydrogenases. Best studied are the so-called 'alcohol deterrents', viz. disulfiram and cyanamide (Fig. 23). These agents have been shown to inhibit/depress rat hepatic aldehyde dehydrogenase-catalyzed oxidation of 4-hydroxycyclophosphamide/aldophosphamide to

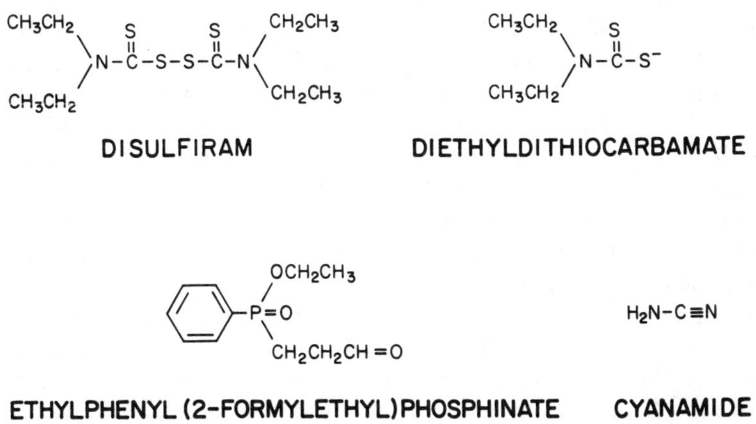

FIG. 23. Structural formulae of several known and suspected inhibitors of NAD-linked aldehyde dehydrogenases.

TABLE 29. *NAD-linked Aldehyde Dehydrogenase Catalysis of the Oxidation of Aldophosphamide to Carboxyphosphamide by Soluble and Particulate Fractions Obtained from Mouse Liver and Oxazaphosphorine-Sensitive and -Resistant L1210 cells*

	V_{max}, nmol/min/mg protein	
Source	Soluble	Particulate
Mouse liver	36	5
L1210/0*	0	0
L1210/OAP†	40	0

*Oxazaphosphorine-sensitive.
†Oxazaphosphorine-resistant.
Reprinted from Manthey and Sladek (1986), with permission of the copyright holder, Williams and Wilkins, Co., Baltimore.

carboxyphosphamide (Domeyer and Sladek, 1980b, 1981). The expectation would be that treatment of cells containing relevant aldehyde dehydrogenases with these agents will increase their sensitivity to the oxazaphosphorines. This expectation has been realized experimentally. Mouse L1210/OAP cells contain a relevant aldehyde dehydrogenase (Table 29). So do mouse P388/CLA cells. In each of these cell lines, the relevant aldehyde dehydrogenase has been identified as AHD-2 (Colvin et al., 1988; Russo and Hilton, 1988; Russo et al., 1989; Mirkes et al., 1990; C. L. Manthey and N. E. Sladek, unpublished observations). The sensitivity of cultured L1210/OPA and P388/CLA cells to the oxazaphosphorines was dramatically increased when cells were treated with cyanamide prior to exposure to the oxazaphosphorines (Fig. 24). Treatment with disulfiram or diethyldithiocarbamate, a metabolite of disulfiram, also sensitized these cells to the oxazaphosphorines (Sladek and Landkamer, 1985), as did treatment with ethylphenyl(2-formylethyl)phosphinate, a suspected inhibitor of aldehyde dehydrogenase activity (Fig. 25). None of these agents increased the sensitivity of cultured L1210/0 or P388/0 cells to the oxazaphosphorines (Sladek and Landkamer, 1985). L1210/0 cells lack a relevant aldehyde dehydrogenase (Table 29) and, as compared to L1210/OAP cells, are much more sensitive to the oxazaphosphorines (Sladek et al., 1985). P388/0 cells also lack a relevant aldehyde dehydrogenase (C. L. Manthey and N. E. Sladek, unpublished observations) and, as compared to P388/CLA cells, are much more sensitive to the oxazaphosphorines (Sladek et al., 1985). Similar observations have been reported by others (Hilton, 1984a,b; Colvin et al., 1988; Russo and Hilton, 1988; Russo et al., 1989).

The effect of disulfiram and cyanamide pretreatment on the antitumor action of cyclophosphamide has also been studied in tumor-bearing rodents. Even though some of the neoplastic lines used in these experiments may lack the relevant aldehyde dehydrogenases, the expectation would be that the antitumor activity of cyclophosphamide would be increased by the co-administration of either disulfiram or cyanamide since (1) rodent liver does contain at least some of the relevant aldehyde dehydrogenases (see Section 3.3), (2) at least some of the relevant hepatic aldehyde dehydrogenases are subject to inhibition by disulfiram and cyanamide and (3) inhibition of these enzymes would lead to an increased plasma AUC value for 4-hydroxycyclophosphamide/aldophosphamide. The results have not, however, always met the expectation. Thus, in two investigations (Donelli et al., 1976; Hacker et al., 1982), administration of disulfiram increased the antitumor action of cyclophosphamide, but in two others (Montgomery and Struck, 1973; Cox et al., 1976b) it did not. In yet another study, the antitumor action of cyclophosphamide was not increased by pretreatment with cyanamide (Domeyer, 1977).

On the other hand, potentiation of the untoward effects of cyclophosphamide by disulfiram and cyanamide has been more consistently observed. Thus, (1) cyclophosphamide-induced toxicity, as measured by peripheral blood leukocyte counts, was increased by both disulfiram (Hacker et al., 1982) and cyanamide (N. E. Sladek, unpublished observations) pretreatment, (2) mice treated with cyclophosphamide plus disulfiram exhibited a somewhat greater decrease in total marrow cellularity than did those treated with the oxazaphosphorine alone (Gamelli et al., 1986) and (3)

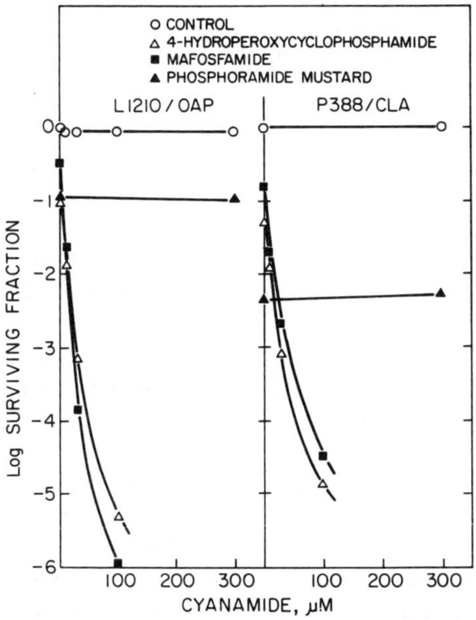

FIG. 24. Sensitivity of cultured oxazaphosphorine-resistant cells to 4-hydroxycyclophosphamide/aldophosphamide in the presence of an inhibitor of aldehyde dehydrogenase activity, viz. cyanamide. Tumor cells were incubated with vehicle or cyanamide for 60 min at 37°C. 4-Hydroperoxycyclophosphamide, mafosfamide, phosphoramide mustard, or vehicle was then added and incubation was continued at 37°C for an additional 30 min. Concentrations of cytotoxic agents were 35 (L1210/OAP) and 24 (P388/CLA) μM 4-hydroperoxycyclophosphamide; 43 (L1210/OAP) and 30 (P388/CLA) μM mafosfamide; and 90 (L1210/OAP) and 220 (P388/CLA) μM phosphoramide mustard. Cells were harvested at the end of the incubation period and subsequently resuspended and grown in a drug-free medium. Surviving fractions were determined by a back-extrapolation method. Each point represents the mean of measurements on duplicate cultures. Modified from Sladek and Landkamer (1985).

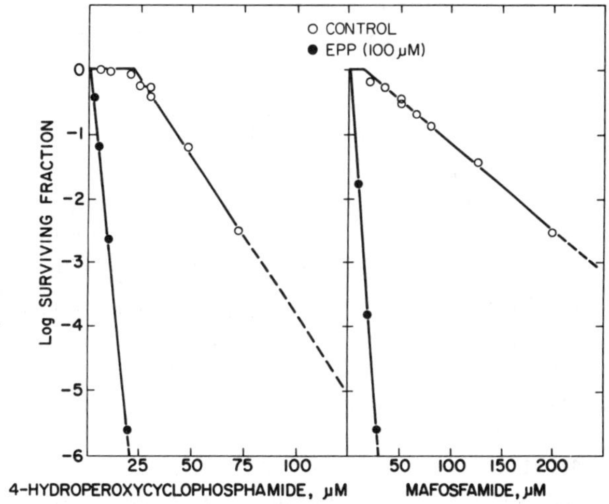

FIG. 25. Sensitivity of cultured oxazaphosphorine-resistant L1210/OAP cells to 4-hydroxycyclophosphamide/aldophosphamide in the presence of an inhibitor of aldehyde dehydrogenase activity, viz., ethylphenyl(2-formylethyl)phosphinate (EPP). L1210/OAP cells were incubated with vehicle or 100 μM EPP for 60 min at 37°C. 4-Hydroperoxycyclophosphamide or mafosfamide was then added and incubation was continued at 37°C for an additional 30 min. Cells were harvested at the end of the incubation period and subsequently resuspended and grown in drug-free medium. Surviving fractions were determined by a back-extrapolation method. Each point represents the mean of measurements on duplicate cultures. Modified from Sladek and Landkamer (1985).

potentiation of the lethal effects of cyclophosphamide by disulfiram has been reported by two laboratories (Cox et al., 1976b; Habs et al., 1981).

All in all, potentiation of cyclophosphamide's therapeutic and/or untoward effects in humans by disulfiram and cyanamide would seem to be a distinct possibility in view of their demonstrated clinical utility as alcohol deterrents.

Another agent known to inhibit aldehyde dehydrogenase activity is chloral hydrate. This drug is used clinically for sedative/hypnotic purposes. It is a potent inhibitor of some, but not all, rat, sheep and human hepatic aldehyde dehydrogenases (Crow et al., 1974; Koivula and Koivusalo, 1975a; Sidhu and Blair, 1975; Weiner et al., 1982). Of particular relevance, mouse AHD-2-catalyzed oxidation of aldophosphamide to carboxyphosphamide is highly sensitive to inhibition by chloral hydrate (Maki and Sladek, 1993) whereas mouse AHD-8-, AHD-12- and AHD-13-catalyzed oxidation of this substrate is not (Zhoo and Sladek, 1992; Maki and Sladek, 1993). Of even greater relevance, human ALDH-1-catalyzed oxidation of aldophosphamide to carboxyphosphamide is highly sensitive to inhibition by chloral hydrate whereas human ALDH-2- and SSDH-catalyzed oxidation of this substrate is not (Dockham et al., 1992).

Inclusion of chloral hydrate in the drug-exposure medium potentiated the cytotoxic action of mafosfamide against cultured L1210/OAP and P388/CLA cells; chloral hydrate did not potentiate the cytotoxic action of mafosfamide against cultured tumor cells lacking the relevant aldehyde dehydrogenase activity, viz. L1210/0 and P388/0 cells (Sladek et al., 1989; Maki and Sladek, 1993). Others (Donelli et al., 1976) reported that chloral hydrate potentiated the antitumor action of cyclophosphamide in vivo, viz. in mice bearing a mammary carcinoma or the Lewis lung carcinoma. Perhaps of most interest is that exposure to chloral hydrate ex vivo did not sensitize murine or human (one subject) pluripotent hematopoietic cells to mafosfamide (Sladek et al., 1989; Maki and Sladek, 1993).

These observations suggest the possibility of differentially potentiating the cytotoxic action of the oxazaphosphorines in a therapeutically favorable manner by selectively inhibiting the relevant aldehyde dehydrogenase activity in the uneconomic species. Of course, such a strategy would only be of value if the uneconomic species contained significant amounts of the relevant aldehyde dehydrogenase activity in the first place, as it might for example, at least in some instances, when an initially cyclophosphamide-sensitive tumor cell population becomes resistant to this agent.

Along the same vein, a cursory review of the medical literature reveals that, in addition to those already mentioned, there are at least 30 drugs in current clinical use that produce a disulfiram-like effect when taken prior to the ingestion of alcohol, i.e. nausea, vasodilation, pulsating headache, etc. Included are griseofulvin, chloramphenicol, furazolidone, quinacrine, isosorbide dinitrate, the hypoglycemic sulfonylureas chlorpropamide and tolbutamide, and the cephalosporin antibiotics that contain a methyltetrazolethiol side-chain, e.g. moxalactam, cefamandole and cefoperazone (Uri and Parks, 1983; Sladek et al., 1989). Disulfiram is believed to induce these symptoms by virtue of its ability to inhibit aldehyde dehydrogenases, thus preventing the oxidation of acetaldehyde, generated from ethanol, to acetic acid. Presumably, some or all of these drugs, many of which are used in cancer patients, also induce the disulfiram-like effect by inhibiting aldehyde dehydrogenases. This is almost certainly so in the case of the cephalosporin antibiotics (Yamanaka et al., 1983; Brien et al., 1985; Kitson, 1986). In pursuance of this line of thought, it has already been shown that at least some of these agents, e.g. chloramphenicol, isosorbide dinitrate and the cephalosporins that contain a methyltetrazolethiol side-chain, inhibit the aldehyde dehydrogenases that catalyze the oxidation of 4-hydroxycyclophosphamide/aldophosphamide to carboxyphosphamide (Sladek et al., 1989). It is not known whether they inhibit the relevant enzyme activity in all tissues; the potential for both favorable and unfavorable drug interactions, however, is obvious.

Activity of the relevant aldehyde dehydrogenases may also be depressed by the chronic ingestion of alcohol (Goedde and Agarwal, 1990) or by female sex steroids, as for example, during pregnancy or when taking birth control pills (Jeavons and Zeiner, 1984).

Although each of the relevant aldehyde dehydrogenases will accept only a certain spectrum of substrates, that spectrum is rather broad and there is considerable overlap (Manthey and Sladek, 1989; Sladek et al., 1989, 1990; Manthey et al., 1990; Dockham et al., 1992). Thus, it might be expected that substrates for the relevant aldehyde dehydrogenases will compete with 4-hydroxycyclophosphamide/aldophosphamide for the catalytic site and thus inhibit its oxidation. This expectation, too, has been realized. Thus, butyraldehyde inhibited the oxidation of 4-hydroxycyclophosphamide/aldophosphamide to carboxyphosphamide catalyzed by rat liver aldehyde dehydrogenase (Domeyer and Sladek, 1980b). It would also be expected that inclusion of such 'alternative substrates' in the drug exposure medium would potentiate the cytotoxic action of the oxazaphosphorines against cells containing the relevant aldehyde dehydrogenase activity. Acetaldehyde and benzaldehyde sensitized both L1210/OAP cells and CPU-GEMM to mafosfamide (Sladek, et al., 1989). Moreover, several phosphorylated acetals and aldehydes, including ethylphenyl(2-formylethyl)phosphinate, potentiated the antitumor activity of cyclophosphamide in vivo (Cates et al., 1980); these compounds are all potential substrates for, or inhibitors of, aldehyde dehydrogenase isozymes.

Cyclophosphamide is often only one of the antineoplastic agents included in the therapeutic regimen. It is not known whether other antineoplastic agents (or modalities) alter the relevant aldehyde dehydrogenase activity. At least one of these, viz. procarbazine, probably does. One of the metabolites of procarbazine is an aldehyde, viz. *n*-isopropyl-*p*-formylbenzamide (Weinkam and Shiba, 1978; Dunn et al., 1979). Acting as an alternative substrate, it markedly potentiated the cytotoxic action of mafosfamide against cultured L1210/OAP cells; it did not potentiate the cytotoxic action of this agent against cultured tumor cells lacking the relevant aldehyde dehydrogenase activity, viz. L1210/0 cells (Maki and Sladek, 1991).

The presence of a tumor often depresses the activity of various enzymes, e.g. hepatic microsomal mixed-function oxidases (see Section 10.1). However, a tumor burden, viz. Walker 256 carcinosarcoma or P388 lymphoma growing i.p., s.c. or i.m., did not alter the rate at which rodent hepatic aldehyde dehydrogenases catalyzed the oxidation of butyraldehyde to butyric acid (Domeyer and Sladek, 1980b).

The administration of cyclophosphamide also alters the activity of various enzymes. Thus, hepatic microsomal mixed-function oxidase activity is decreased and increased when rodents and humans, respectively, are given relatively large doses of cyclophosphamide (see Section 10.1). However, hepatic aldehyde dehydrogenase-catalyzed oxidation of butyraldehyde to butyric acid was not increased or decreased when rats were given cyclophosphamide, 200 mg/kg (Domeyer and Sladek, 1981).

Almost half of all Orientals and South American Indians lack the functional form of one of the major aldehyde dehydrogenases, viz. ALDH-2, present in the remainder of their countrymen, in most North American and Mexican Indians, and in all Caucasians and Blacks (Goedde and Agarwal, 1990). However, this is not likely to be of any significance with regard to the metabolic fate and therapeutic potential of cyclophosphamide since ALDH-2 appears to contribute little or nothing to cyclophosphamide detoxification (see Section 3.3).

ALDH-1 almost certainly does contribute significantly to the detoxification of cyclophosphamide (see Section 3.3). Variants of ALDH-1 that do not, or only poorly, catalyze the oxidation of acetaldehyde have been found, at the expense of ALDH-1, in both Orientals and Caucasians, though the frequency is almost surely much lower than 50% (Yoshida et al., 1983, 1989; Eckey et al., 1986). The expectation is that such variants would not, or would only poorly, catalyze the detoxification of cyclophosphamide. The inability to detoxify cyclophosphamide by this mechanism is likely to be therapeutically significant.

10.4. Reduction of Aldophosphamide to Alcophosphamide

Alcophosphamide per se is also without cytotoxic activity. The identity of all of the enzymes that catalyze the reduction of aldophosphamide to alcophosphamide is yet to be established. Candidates and those already identified include the alcohol dehydrogenases and the pyridine nucleotide-dependent aldo-keto reductases (see Section 3.4). A number of drugs inhibit one or more of these enzymes (Deis and Lester, 1979; Felsted and Bachur, 1980; Burnell and Bosron, 1989). Unlike carboxyphosphamide, alcophosphamide can give rise to a cytotoxic metabolite, viz. phosphoramide mustard, although it is not clear how, or where, this occurs (see Section 3.4). Thus, it is uncertain what the effects of increasing or decreasing the rate at which aldophosphamide is reduced to alcophosphamide would be on the therapeutic and untoward response to, and therapeutic index of, cyclophosphamide. The effects, if any, are likely to be minimal and in the same direction as when oxidation of aldophosphamide to carboxyphosphamide is modulated (Table 28).

10.5. Conjugation of 4-Hydroxycyclophosphamide/Aldophosphamide or Phosphoramide Mustard with Glutathione

The exact mechanism(s) by which glutathione and/or glutathione-*S*-transferases influence(s) cellular sensitivity to cyclophosphamide is(are) uncertain; indeed, it is not certain that glutathione and/or especially glutathione-*S*-transferases *are* determinants of cellular sensitivity to the oxazaphosphorines (see Section 9.3). Thus, it is somewhat premature to discuss the modulation of these unidentified mechanisms. None-the-less, a few introductory comments follow.

Reversible detoxification would occur if 4-hydroxycyclophosphamide/aldophosphamide is joined with glutathione to form the corresponding 4-thiocyclophosphamide conjugate in vivo. Irreversible detoxification would occur if the mustard moiety of phosphoramide mustard is joined with glutathione in vivo. There is evidence to suggest that either or both reactions may be catalyzed by one or more glutathione-*S*-transferases but both reactions can occur without benefit of enzymatic involvement (see Section 3).

Modulation of the reversible reaction may be without therapeutic or toxic consequence (see Section 9.3); if there are any consequences, they will be in the same direction as those effected by modulation of aldophosphamide oxidation to carboxyphosphamide (Table 28).

The therapeutic and toxic consequences of modulating the irreversible reaction will be identical to those effected by modulating the oxidation of aldophosphamide to carboxyphosphamide (Table 28).

A number of agents are known to modulate glutathione-*S*-transferase activity and cellular glutathione concentration (van Bladeren and van Ommen, 1991; Black and Wolf, 1991; Meister, 1991; O'Dwyer et al., 1992). For example, buthionine sulfoximine is known to lower cellular glutathione concentrations by inhibiting the biosynthesis of glutathione. Unfortunately, the use of this particular agent is not likely to be advantageous because, as might be expected, it enhances not only the antineoplastic action (see Section 9.3) but also the urotoxic and lethal effects of cyclophosphamide, at least in mice (Ishikawa et al., 1989).

10.6. Oxidation of 4-Hydroxycyclophosphamide to 4-Oxocyclophosphamide and Hydrolysis of Phosphoramide Mustard to Bis-(2-chloroethyl)-amine

4-Oxocyclophosphamide is without cytotoxic activity and it cannot give rise to a metabolite with such activity. Its formation may be from 4-hydroxycyclophosphamide in a reaction catalyzed by aldehyde oxidase (see Section 3). Little is known about modulation of aldehyde oxidase activity in vivo (Beedham, 1985) but in vitro inhibitors of the enzyme are known (Johns, 1967).

Relative to phosphoramide mustard, bis-(2-chloroethyl)-amine is only weakly cytotoxic; it does not give rise to a strongly cytotoxic metabolite. Irreversible hydrolysis of phosphoramide mustard to bis-(2-chloroethyl)-amine may be catalyzed by a phosphoroamidase but can occur without benefit of enzymatic involvement (see Section 3). There are no demonstrated modulators of this reaction and modulators of the putative phosphoroamidase activity have yet to be identified.

The effects of altering the rate at which aldophosphamide is oxidized to 4-oxocyclophosphamide, or at which phosphoramide mustard is hydrolyzed to bis-(2-chloroethyl)-amine, on the therapeutic and untoward responses to, and therapeutic index of, cyclophosphamide would be identical to those indicated in Table 28 for aldophosphamide conversion to carboxyphosphamide.

11. SOME IMPORTANT UNANSWERED QUESTIONS AND FUTURE DIRECTIONS

Despite the wealth of knowledge already accumulated with regard to the metabolism of the oxazaphosphorines and the important role that biotransformation plays in the therapeutic efficacy of these agents, the final chapter on this subject is yet to be written since several important questions have yet to be satisfactorily answered.

More information is needed about the tissue distribution, substrate specificity, sensitivity to inhibitors and inducibility, of the relevant aldehyde dehydrogenases. The contribution of erythrocyte ALDH-1 to the overall catalysis of aldophosphamide oxidation to carboxyphosphamide needs to be clarified. Not known is whether the therapeutic and toxic consequences of cyclophosphamide administration differ from the 'usual' in patients that express aldehyde dehydrogenase variants, especially those of ALDH-1. Suggesting that the ability to catalyze the oxidation of aldophosphamide to carboxyphosphamide varies considerably in patients, for whatever reason, are the reports that the fraction of the administered cyclophosphamide dose excreted in urine as carboxyphosphamide varies widely from patient to patient (Milsted and Jarman, 1982; Hadidi et al., 1988; Boddy et al., 1992; Tasso et al., 1992). Still to be clarified is the relative in vivo importance of enzyme-catalyzed (1) reduction of aldophosphamide to alcophosphamide, (2) oxidation of 4-hydroxycyclophosphamide to 4-oxocyclophosphamide and (3) hydrolysis of phosphoramide mustard to bis-(2-chloroethyl)-amine, and modulation thereof. Yet to be determined, also, is whether conversion of 4-hydroxycyclophosphamide/aldophosphamide to phosphoramide mustard is enzymatically mediated in vivo as has been suggested and whether enzyme-catalyzed oxidation of cyclophosphamide to 4-hydroxycyclophosphamide ever occurs in target tissue. Should enzymatic involvement be established, a whole new set of questions concerning the basis for oxazaphosphorine-specific selectivity, and potential modulation of such catalysis, would have to be addressed as well.

The relative importance of glutathione and/or glutathione-S-transferases as determinants of cellular sensitivity to the oxazaphosphorines and oxazaphosphorine-specific selectivity, also needs to be clarified. Questions concerning modulation would have to be addressed if either or both are important.

Rodent tumor cell populations that exhibit an acquired resistance to the oxazaphosphorines are often not cross-resistant to other cross-linking agents (Sladek, 1993). In at least two such instances, the phenotypic basis for the acquired resistance was increased detoxification due to increased levels of a relevant aldehyde dehydrogenase. More information is needed about the genotypic basis for the increased enzyme levels. Unfortunately, acquired resistance to the oxazaphosphorines also often occurs in humans. Whether it is occasionally/inevitably due to increased aldehyde dehydrogenase-catalyzed detoxification remains to be determined. Increased rates of detoxification catalyzed by relevant reductases, oxidases, etc., or decreased rates of activation catalyzed by relevant enzymes present in target cells, are some other possibilities. Knowledge of the foregoing could be therapeutically exploited in several ways. For example, the use of an agent that inhibits γ-glutamylcysteine synthetase, thus glutathione synthesis, e.g. buthionine sulfoximine; glutathione-S-transferase, e.g. indomethacin; or aldehyde dehydrogenase, e.g. disulfiram, cyanamide or chloral hydrate; to sensitize tumor cells that are otherwise insensitive to the oxazaphosphorines might be of value if the biochemical basis for the relative insensitivity is greater than normal glutathione levels, glutathione-S-transferase activity, or aldehyde dehydrogenase activity, respectively (Hilton, 1984a; Sladek and Landkamer, 1985; Crook et al., 1986; Russo and Hilton, 1988; Russo et al., 1989; Clapper and Tew, 1989b; Hall et al., 1989; Sladek et al., 1989; Chresta et al., 1990; Perez et al., 1990; Peters et al., 1990, 1991; Lee, 1991; Mistry and Harrap, 1991; Sladek, 1993). Of course, these strategies would be successful only if the target enzyme was not also as important in protecting critical normal cells from the cytotoxic action of the oxazaphosphorines.

Inasmuch as cancer prevention is still a goal that is far from being realized, organ/tissue transplantation is likely to become even more common in future years and, increasingly, newly emerging evidence suggests that the etiology of many of the so-called chronic disorders, e.g. rheumatoid arthritis, insulin-dependent diabetes, multiple sclerosis, myasthenia gravis, systemic lupus erythematosus, alopecia areata, etc., includes an autoimmune component, a more pragmatic question is how to translate the scientific community's hard-won existing understanding of oxazaphosphorine pharmacokinetics and pharmacodynamics into the design of new, even more useful, antineoplastic and/or immunosuppressive agents. A major drawback of the oxazaphosphorines is that they are carcinogenic. All DNA–DNA cross-linking agents probably are. Thus, pursuit of an 'improved cyclophosphamide' would not seem to be sagacious. However, advantage could be taken of the fact that some critical normal cell populations, e.g. pluripotent hematopoietic cells, contain the relevant aldehyde dehydrogenase activity, whereas some undesired cell populations, malignant or normal depending on the therapeutic goal, may not. Aldehydes or precursors thereof

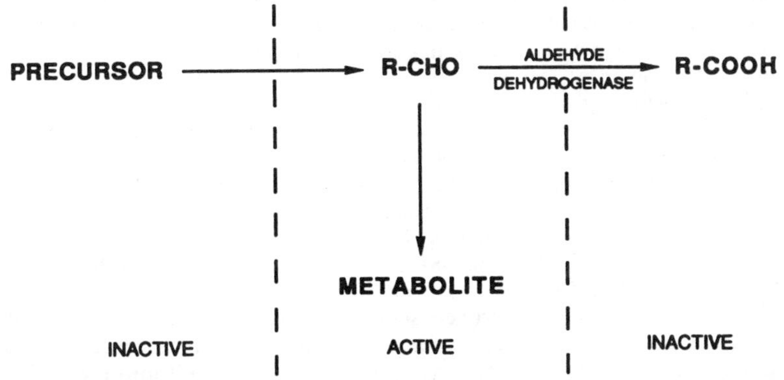

FIG. 26. The design of cytotoxic agents that are selectively toxic to the uneconomic species because of a differently greater relevant aldehyde dehydrogenase activity in the economic species: general considerations.

should be sought, which (1) as aldehydes or metabolites thereof (other than the corresponding acids) are cytotoxic and (2) as aldehydes, are substrates for relevant aldehyde dehydrogenases present in the economic species (Fig. 26). In this scenario, the oxidized products of aldehyde dehydrogenase catalysis, i.e., the corresponding acids, would be without cytotoxic activity. Cytotoxicity could be by any mechanism that does not lead to malignancy. Cytotoxic aldehydes are not unheard of (Perin et al., 1978; Schauenstein and Esterbauer, 1979; Canuto et al., 1985; Hauptlorenz et al., 1985).

N-(5,5-diacetoxypentyl)doxorubicin, a new, highly potent, analog of doxorubicin showing a great deal of early promise (Zwelling et al., 1991; Cherif and Farquhar, 1992), may very well be an agent that behaves in the proposed/desired manner (Fig. 27). Spermine dialdehyde, an immunosuppressive agent, may be another (Kazmi et al., 1992).

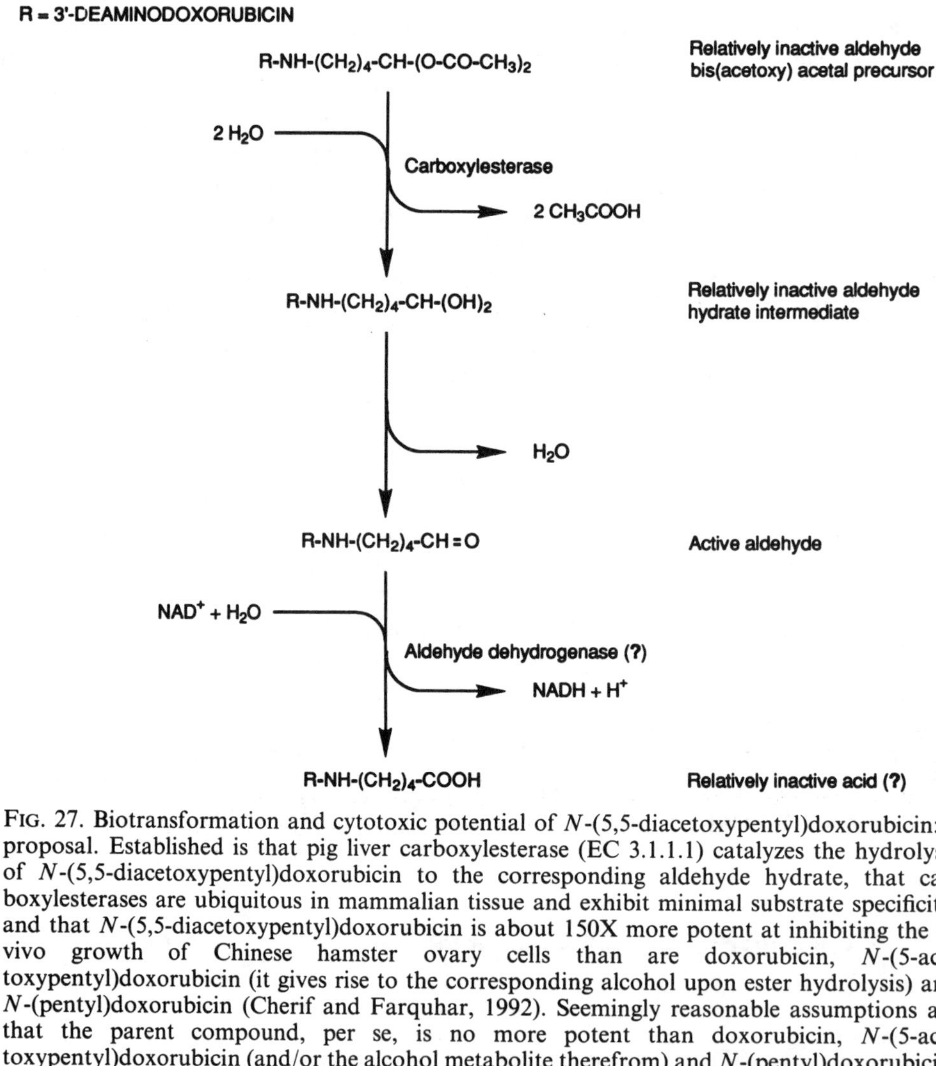

FIG. 27. Biotransformation and cytotoxic potential of *N*-(5,5-diacetoxypentyl)doxorubicin: a proposal. Established is that pig liver carboxylesterase (EC 3.1.1.1) catalyzes the hydrolysis of *N*-(5,5-diacetoxypentyl)doxorubicin to the corresponding aldehyde hydrate, that carboxylesterases are ubiquitous in mammalian tissue and exhibit minimal substrate specificity, and that *N*-(5,5-diacetoxypentyl)doxorubicin is about 150X more potent at inhibiting the ex vivo growth of Chinese hamster ovary cells than are doxorubicin, *N*-(5-acetoxypentyl)doxorubicin (it gives rise to the corresponding alcohol upon ester hydrolysis) and *N*-(pentyl)doxorubicin (Cherif and Farquhar, 1992). Seemingly reasonable assumptions are that the parent compound, per se, is no more potent than doxorubicin, *N*-(5-acetoxypentyl)doxorubicin (and/or the alcohol metabolite therefrom) and *N*-(pentyl)doxorubicin, and thus, that it is the aldehyde metabolite that effects the cytotoxic action that is observed. Remaining to be determined also is whether the aldehyde is a substrate for any of the aldehyde dehydrogenases that are present in the economic species and if so, whether the acid that is thus produced is relatively without cytotoxic activity. Both seem to be reasonable expectations since a number of the aldehyde dehydrogenases exhibit only minimal substrate specificity, and, relative to aldehydes, acids are not very chemically reactive; chemical reactivity is thought to be an absolute requirement for the increased potency and was built into the molecule with a specific rationale in mind (Cherif and Farquhar, 1992). Perhaps instructive is that *N*-(5-acetoxypentyl)doxorubicin (presumably the *alcohol* metabolite thereof) was much less potent than was *N*-(5,5-diacetoxypentyl)doxorubicin (presumably the *aldehyde* metabolite thereof).

Fruitful also, may be the design of agents that selectively (1) induce the activity of the relevant aldehyde dehydrogenases in the economic species or (2) inhibit/depress the activity of the relevant enzyme in the uneconomic species when it is present in this species. Finally, increasing the margin of safety of oxazaphosphorines by inserting a gene coding for a relevant aldehyde dehydrogenase into the economic species, e.g. autologous bone marrow, may be possible.

Acknowledgements—Investigations conducted by the author and reviewed herein were funded by USPHS Grants CA 21737, CA 26357, CA 70383 and GM 15477; ACS Grant CH-106; Bristol-Myers Squibb Company Grant 100-R220; and the University of Minnesota Bone Marrow Transplant Research Fund. Secretarial assistance was provided by Ms. Gina Valentini.

REFERENCES

ALARCON, R. A. and MEIENHOFER, J. (1971) Formation of the cytotoxic aldehyde acrolein during in vitro degradation of cyclophosphamide. *Nature New Biol.* **233:** 250–252.

ALARCON, R. A., MEIENHOFER, J. and ATHERTON, E. (1972) Isophosphamide as a new acrolein-producing antineoplastic isomer of cyclophosphamide. *Cancer Res.* **32:** 2519–2523.

ALBERTS, D. S. and VAN DAALEN WETTERS, T. (1976) The effect of phenobarbital on cyclophosphamide antitumor activity. *Cancer Res.* **36:** 2785–2789.

ALBERTS, D. S., PENG, Y. M., CHEN, H. S. and STRUCK, R. F. (1978) Effect of phenobarbital on plasma levels of cyclophosphamide and its metabolites in the mouse. *Br. J. Cancer* **38:** 316–324.

ALBERTS, D. S., MASON-LIDDIL, N., PLESIA, P. M., ROE, D. J., DORR, R. T., STRUCK, R. F. and PHILLIPS, J. G. (1991) Lack of ranitidine effects on cyclophosphamide bone marrow toxicity or metabolism: a placebo-controlled clinical trial. *J. natn. Cancer Inst.* **83:** 1739–1743.

ALLEN, L. M. and CREAVEN, P. J. (1972) In vitro activation of isophosphamide (NSC-109724), a new oxazaphosphorine, by rat liver microsomes. *Cancer Treat. Rep.* **56:** 603–610.

ALLEN, L. M. and CREAVEN, P. J. (1975a) Pharmacokinetics of ifosfamide. *Clin. Pharmac. Ther.* **17:** 492–498.

ALLEN, L. M. and CREAVEN, P. J. (1975b) Human pharmacokinetic model for isophosphamide (NSC-109724). *Cancer Chemother. Rep.* **59:** 877–882.

ALLEN, L. M., CREAVEN, P. J. and NELSON, R. L. (1976) Studies of the human pharmacokinetics of isophosphamide (NSC-109724). *Cancer Treat. Rep.* **60:** 451–458.

ALTMAN, P. L. and DITTMER, D. S. (EDS) (1971) *Respiration and Circulation.* Federation of American Societies for Experimental Biology, Bethesda.

ALVARES, A. P., KAPELNER, S., SASSA, S. and KAPPAS, A. (1975) Drug metabolism in normal children, lead-poisoned children, and normal adults. *Clin. Pharmac. Ther.* **17:** 179–183.

AMERICAN MEDICAL ASSOCIATION (1992) Oncolytic drugs. In: *Drug Evaluations Annual.* pp. 1843–1896, American Medical Association, Chicago.

ANDERSSON, B. S., WANG, Y.-Q., MCCREDIE, K. B. and FARQUHAR, D. (1990) Suitability of a new stable acetal analog of aldoifosphamide for purging leukemic cells from human bone marrow. *Leukemia* **4:** 435–440.

ANTHONY, L. B., LONG, Q.-C., STRUCK, R. F. and HANDE, K. R. (1990) The effect of cimetidine on cyclophosphamide metabolism in rabbits. *Cancer Chemother. Pharmac.* **27:** 125–130.

ANTMAN, K. H., MONTELLA, D., ROSENBAUM, C. and SCHWEN, M. (1985) Phase II trial of ifosfamide with mesna in previously treated metastatic sarcoma. *Cancer Treat. Rep.* **69:** 499–504.

ARNDT, C. A. S., COLVIN, O. M., BALIS, F. M., LESTER, C. M., JOHNSON, G. and POPLACK, D. G. (1987) Intrathecal administration of 4-hydroperoxycyclophosphamide in rhesus monkeys. *Cancer Res.* **47:** 5932–5934.

ARNDT, C. A. S., BALIS, F. M., LESTER-MCCULLY, C., COLVIN, O. M. and POPLACK, D. G. (1988) Cerebrospinal fluid penetration of active metabolites of cyclophosphamide and ifosfamide in rhesus monkeys. *Cancer Res.* **48:** 2113–2115.

ARNOLD, H. and BOURSEAUX, F. (1958) Synthese und abbau cytostatisch wirksamer cyclischer *N*-phosphamidester des bis-(β-chloräthyl)-amins. *Angew. Chem.* **70:** 539–544.

ARNOLD, H., BOURSEAUX, F. and BROCK, N. (1958) Chemotherapeutic action of a cyclic nitrogen mustard phosphamide ester (B 518-ASTA) in experimental tumors of the rat. *Nature* **181:** 931.

ARNOLD, H., BOURSEAUX, F. and BROCK, N. (1961) Über beziehungen zwischen chemischer konstitution und cancertoxischer wirkung in der reihe der phosphamidester de bis-(β-chorāthyl)-amins. *Arzneim.-Forsch. Drug Res.* **11:** 143–158.

AWWAD, M. and NORTH, R. J. (1988) Cyclophosphamide (Cy)-facilitated adoptive immunotherapy of a Cy-resistant tumor. Evidence that Cy permits the expression of adoptive T-cell mediated immunity by removing suppressor T cells rather than by reducing tumor burden. *Immunology* **65:** 87–92.

AWWAD, M. and NORTH, R. J. (1989) Cyclophosphamide-induced immunologically mediated regression of a cyclophosphamide-resistant murine tumor: a consequence of eliminating precursor $L3T4^+$ suppressor T-cells. *Cancer Res.* **49:** 1649–1654.

AYASH, L. J., WRIGHT, J. E., TRETYAKOV, O., GONIN, R., ELIAS, A., WHEELER, C., EDER, J. P., ROSOWSKY, A.,

ANTMAN, K. and FREI, E., III (1992) Cyclophosphamide pharmacokinetics: correlation with cardiac toxicity and tumor response. *J. clin. Oncol.* **10:** 995–1000.

BAGLEY, C. M., JR, BOSTICK, F. W. and DE VITA, V. T., JR (1973) Clinical pharmacology of cyclophosphamide. *Cancer Res.* **33:** 226–233.

BAILEY, H., MULCAHY, R. T., TUTSCH, K. D., ROZENTAL, J. M., ALBERTI, D., ARZOOMANIAN, R. Z., TOMBES, M. B., TRUMP, D. L. and WILDING, G. (1991) A phase I study of SR-2508 and cyclophosphamide administered by intravenous injection. *Cancer Res.* **51:** 1099–1104.

BAKKE, J. E., FEIL, V. J. and ZAYLSKIE, R. G. (1971) Characterization of the major sheep urinary metabolites of cyclophosphamide, a defleecing chemical. *J. Agric. Food Chem.* **19:** 788–790.

BAKKE, J. E., FEIL, V. J., FJELSTUL, C. E. and THACKER, E. J. (1972) Metabolism of cyclophosphamide by sheep. *J. Agric. Food Chem.* **20:** 384–388.

BALOW, J. E., AUSTIN, H. A., III, MUENZ, L. R., JOYCE, K. M., ANTONOVYCH, T. T., KLIPPEL, J. H., STEINBERG, A. D., PLOTZ, P. H. and DECKER, J. L. (1984) Effect of treatment on the evolution of renal abnormalities in lupus nephritis. *New Engl. J. Med.* **311:** 491–495.

BEEDHAM, C. (1985) Molybdenum hydroxylases as drug-metabolizing enzymes. *Drug Metab. Rev.* **16:** 119–156.

BEEDHAM, C., BRUCE, S. E., CRITCHLEY, D. J., AL-TAYIB, Y. and RANCE, D. J. (1987) Species variation in hepatic aldehyde oxidase activity. *Eur. J. Drug Metab. Pharmacokinet.* **12:** 307–310.

BELLIN, H. J., CHERRY, J. M. and KOSS, L. G. (1974) Effects of a single dose of cyclophosphamide. V. Protective effect of diversion of the urinary stream on dog bladder. *Lab. Invest.* **30:** 43–47.

BENDING, M. R. and FINCH, R. E. (1978) Haemodialysis during cyclophosphamide treatment. *Br. med. J.* **1:** 1145–1146.

BENFORD, D. J., BRIDGES, J. W., BOOBIS, A. R., KAHN, G. C., BRODIE, M. J. and DAVIES, D. S. (1981) The selective activation of cytochrome P-450 dependent microsomal hydroxylases in human and rat liver microsomes. *Biochem. Pharmac.* **30:** 1702–1703.

BENSON, A. J., MARTIN, C. N. and GARNER, R. C. (1988) *N*-(2-hydroxyethyl)-*N*-[2-(7-guanyl)ethyl]amine, the putative major DNA adduct of cyclophosphamide in vitro and in vivo in the rat. *Biochem. Pharmac.* **37:** 2979–2985.

BERAN, M., ANDERSSON, B. S., WANG, Y., MCCREDIE, K. B. and FARQUHAR, D. (1988) The effects of acetaldophosphamide, a novel stable aldophosphamide analog, on normal human and leukemic progenitor cells in vitro: implications for use in bone marrow purging. *Cancer Res.* **48:** 339–345.

BERD, D. and MASTRANGELO, M. J. (1988) Active immunotherapy of human melanoma exploiting the immunopotentiating effects of cyclophosphamide. *Cancer Invest.* **6:** 337–349.

BIELICKI, L., VOELCKER, G. and HOHORST, H. J. (1983) Enzymatic toxicogenation of 'activated' cyclophosphamide by 3′–5′ exonucleases. *J. Cancer Res. clin. Oncol.* **105:** 27–29.

BIELICKI, L., VOELCKER, G. and HOHORST, H. J. (1984) Activated cyclophosphamide: an enzyme-mechanism-based suicide inactivator of DNA polymerase/3′–5′ exonuclease. *J. Cancer Res. clin. Oncol.* **107:** 195–198.

BLACK, S. M. and WOLF, C. R. (1991) The role of glutathione-dependent enzymes in drug resistance. *Pharmac. Ther.* **51:** 139–154.

BLOMGREN, H. and HALLSTRÖM, M. (1991) Possible role of acrolein in 4-hydroperoxycyclophosphamide-induced cell damage in vitro. *Methods Find. exp. clin. Pharmac.* **13:** 11–14.

BODDY, A. V., FURTUN, Y., SARDAS, S., SARDAS, O. and IDLE, J. R. (1992) Individual variation in the activation and inactivation of metabolic pathways of cyclophosphamide. *J. natn. Cancer Inst.* **84:** 1744–1748.

BORCH, R. F. and GETMAN, K. M. (1984) Base-catalyzed hydrolysis of 4-hydroperoxycyclophosphamide: evidence for iminocyclophosphamide as an intermediate. *J. med. Chem.* **27:** 485–490.

BORCH, R. F. and MILLARD, J. A. (1987) The mechanism of activation of 4-hydroxycyclophosphamide. *J. med. Chem.* **30:** 427–431.

BORCH, R. F., HOYE, T. R. and SWANSON, T. A. (1984) In situ preparation and fate of *cis*-4-hydroxycyclophosphamide and aldophosphamide: ^{1}H and ^{31}P NMR evidence for equilibration of *cis*- and *trans*-4-hydroxycyclophosphamide with aldophosphamide and its hydrate in aqueous solution. *J. med. Chem.* **27:** 490–494.

BOYD, V. L., ROBBINS, J. D., EGAN, W. and LUDEMAN, S. M. (1986) ^{31}P Nuclear magnetic resonance spectroscopic observation of the intracellular transformations of oncostatic cyclophosphamide metabolites. *J. med. Chem.* **29:** 1206–1210.

BOYD, V. L., SUMMERS, M. F., LUDEMAN, S. M., EGAN, W., ZON, G. and REGAN, J. B. (1987) NMR spectroscopic studies of intermediary metabolites of cyclophosphamide. 2. Direct observation, characterization and reactivity studies of iminocyclophosphamide and related species. *J. med. Chem.* **30:** 366–374.

BOYER, T. D. (1989) The glutathione-*S*-transferases: an update. *Hepatology* **9:** 486–496.

BRADE, W. P., HERDRICH, K. and VARINI, M. (1985) Ifosfamide—pharmacology, safety and therapeutic potential. *Cancer Treat. Rev.* **12:** 1–47.

BRADE, W., SEEBER, S. and HERDRICH, K. (1986) Comparative activity of ifosfamide and cyclophosphamide. *Cancer Chemother. Pharmac.* **18:** S1–S9.

BRAMWELL, V., CALVERT, R. T., EDWARDS, G., SCARFFE, H. and CROWTHER, D. (1979) The disposition of cyclophosphamide in a group of myeloma patients. *Cancer Chemother. Pharmac.* **3:** 253–259.

BRIEN, J. F., TAM, G. S., CAMERON, R. J., STEENAART, N. A. E. and LOOMIS, C. W. (1985) A comparative study of the inhibition of hepatic aldehyde dehydrogenases in the rat by methyltetrazolethiol, calcium carbimide and disulfiram. *Can. J. Physiol. Pharmac.* **63:** 438–443.

BROCK, N. (1967) Pharmacologic characterization of cyclophosphamide (NSC-26271) and cyclophosphamide metabolites. *Cancer Chemother. Rep.* **51:** 315–325.

BROCK, N. (1976) Comparative pharmacologic study in vitro and in vivo with cyclophosphamide (NSC-26271), cyclophosphamide metabolites, and plain nitrogen mustard compounds. *Cancer Treat. Rep.* **60:** 301–307.

BROCK, N. (1979) The special position of ifosfamide in the series of cytostatically active oxazaphosphorines. *Adv. Med. Oncol. Res. Educ.* **5:** 39–47.

BROCK, N. (1983) Oxazaphosphorine cytostatics: structure–activity relationships, selectivity and metabolism, regional detoxification. In: *Structure–Activity Relationships of Anti-tumor Agents*, pp. 239–267, REINHOUDT, D. N., CONNORS, T. A., PINEDO, H. M. and VAN DE POLL, K. W. (eds) Martinus Nijhoff Publishers, Boston.

BROCK, N. (1986) Ideas and reality in the development of cancer chemotherapeutic agents, with particular reference to oxazaphosphorine cytostatics. *J. Cancer Res. clin. Oncol.* **111:** 1–12.

BROCK, N. (1989) Oxazaphosphorine cytostatics: past–present–future. *Cancer Res.* **49:** 1–7.

BROCK, N. and HOHORST, H. J. (1963) Über die aktivierung von cyclophosphamid in vivo und in vitro. *Arzneim.-Forsch. Drug Res.* **13:** 1021–1031.

BROCK, N. and HOHORST, H. J. (1967) Metabolism of cyclophosphamide. *Cancer* **20:** 900–904.

BROCK, N. and HOHORST, H. J. (1977) The problem of specificity and selectivity of alkylating cytostatics: studies on *N*-2-chloroethylamido-oxazaphosphorines. *Z. Krebsforsch. Klin. Onkol.* **88:** 185–215.

BROCK, N., STEKAR, J., POHL, J., NIEMEYER, U. and SCHEFFLER, G. (1979) Acrolein, the causative factor of urotoxic side-effects of cyclophosphamide, ifosfamide, trofosfamide and sufosfamide. *Arzneim.-Forsch. Drug Res.* **29:** 659–661.

BROCK, N., POHL, J. and STEKAR, J. (1981) Studies on the urotoxicity of oxazaphosphorine cytostatics and its prevention. Experimental studies on the urotoxicity of alkylating compounds. *Eur. J. Cancer* **17:** 595–607.

BROCK, N., HILGARD, P., PEUKERT, M., POHL, J. and SINDERMANN, H. (1988) Basis and new developments in the field of oxazaphosphorines. *Cancer Invest.* **6:** 513–532.

BURKE, M. D. and ORRENIUS, S. (1979) Isolation and comparison of endoplasmic reticulum membranes and their mixed function oxidase activities from mammalian extrahepatic tissues. *Pharmac. Ther.* **7:** 549–599.

BURNELL, J. C. and BOSRON, W. F. (1989) Genetic polymorphism of human liver alcohol dehydrogenase and kinetic properties of the isoenzymes. In: *Human Metabolism of Alcohol. Regulation, Enzymology and Metabolites of Ethanol*, pp. 65–75, CROW, K. E. and BATT, R. D. (eds) CRC Press, Boca Raton.

CAIRNEY, A. E. L., SLADEK, N. E. and WOODS, W. G. (1984) DNA crosslinking by 4-hydroperoxycyclophosphamide in sensitive and resistant mouse leukemia cells. *Proc. Am. Ass. Cancer Res.* **25:** 339.

CALABRESI, P. and CHABNER, B. A. (1990) Chemotherapy of neoplastic diseases. In: *The Pharmacological Basis of Therapeutics*, 8th edn, pp. 1202–1263, GILMAN, A. G., RALL, T. W., NIES, A. S. and TAYLOR, P. (eds) Pergamon Press, New York.

CANUTO, R. A., BIOCCA, M. E., MUZIO, G., GARCEA, R. and DIANZANI, M. U. (1985) The effect of various aldehydes on the respiration of rat liver and hepatoma AH-130 cells. *Cell Biochem. Func.* **3:** 3–8.

CATES, L. A., JONES, G. S., JR, GOOD, D. J., TSAI, H. Y.-L., LI, V.-S., CARON, N., TU, S.-C. and KIMBALL, A. P. (1980) Cyclophosphamide potentiation and aldehyde oxidase inhibition by phosphorylated aldehydes and acetals. *J. med. Chem.* **23:** 300–304.

CERNY, T., MARGISON, J. M., THATCHER, N. and WILKINSON, P. M. (1986) Bioavailability of ifosfamide in patients with bronchial carcinoma. *Cancer Chemother. Pharmac.* **18:** 261–264.

CHAMPLIN, R. E. and GALE, R. P. (1984) Role of bone marrow transplantation in the treatment of hematologic malignancies and solid tumors: critical review of syngeneic, autologous and allogeneic transplants. *Cancer Treat. Rep.* **68:** 145–161.

CHAN, K. K., WATSON, E. and HONG, S.-C. (1985) The application of stable isotopes in antineoplastic drug research. In: *Topics in Pharmacological Sciences*, pp. 249–267, BREIMER, D. D. and SPEISER, P. (eds) Elsevier Science Publishers B.V., Amsterdam.

CHAN, K. K., HONG, S.-K., WATSON, E. and DENG, S. K. (1986) Identification of new metabolites of phosphoramide and nor-nitrogen mustards and cyclophosphamide in rat urine using ion cluster techniques. *Biomed. Environ. Mass Spectrom.* **13:** 145–154.

CHERIF, A. and FARQUHAR, D. (1992) *N*-(5,5-diacetoxypent-1-yl)doxorubicin: A new intensely potent doxorubicin analog. *J. med. Chem.* **35:** 3208–3214.

CHETSANGA, C. J., POLIDORI G. and MAINWARING, M. (1982) Analysis and excision of ring-opened phosphoramide mustard-deoxyguanine adducts in DNA. *Cancer Res.* **42:** 2616–2621.

CHRESTA, C. M., CROOK, T. R. and SOUHAMI, R. L. (1990) Depletion of cellular glutathione by *N,N'*-bis(*trans*-4-hydroxycyclohexyl)-*N'*-nitrosourea as a determinant of sensitivity of K562 human leukemia cells to 4-hydroperoxycyclophosphamide. *Cancer Res.* **50:** 4067–4071.

CHRISTOU, M., WILSON, N. M. and JEFCOATE, C. R. (1987) Expression and function of three cytochrome P-450 isozymes in rat extrahepatic tissues. *Arch. Biochem. Biophys.* **258:** 519–534.

CLAPPER, M. L. and TEW, K. D. (1989a) Identification of a glutathione *S*-transferase associated with microsomes of tumor cells resistant to nitrogen mustards. *Biochem. Pharmac.* **38:** 1915–1921.

CLAPPER, M. L. and TEW, K. D. (1989b) Alkylating agent resistance. In: *Drug Resistance in Cancer Therapy*, pp. 125–150, OZOLS, R. F. (ed.) Kluwer Academic Publishers, Boston, Dordrecht and London.

CLARKE, L. and WAXMAN, D. J. (1989) Oxidative metabolism of cyclophosphamide: identification of the hepatic monooxygenase catalysts of drug activation. *Cancer Res.* **49:** 2344–2350.

COE, E. L. and LEE, I. Y. (1969) Phosphorylation of 2-D-deoxyglucose and associated inorganic phosphate uptake in ascites tumor cells. *Biochemistry* **8:** 685–693.

COHEN, J. L. and JAO, J. Y. (1970) Enzymatic basis of cyclophosphamide activation by hepatic microsomes of the rat. *J. Pharmac. exp. Ther.* **174:** 206–210.

COHEN, J. L., JAO, J. Y. and JUSKO, W. J. (1971) Pharmacokinetics of cyclophosphamide in man. *Br. J. Pharmac.* **43:** 677–680.

COLVIN, M. (1982) The comparative pharmacology of cyclophosphamide and ifosfamide. *Sem. Oncol.* **9** (Suppl. 1): 2–7.

COLVIN, M. and HILTON, J. (1981) Pharmacology of cyclophosphamide and metabolites. *Cancer Treat. Rep.* **65:** 89–95.

COLVIN, M. and HILTON, J. (1988) Cellular resistance to cyclophosphamide. In: *Mechanisms of Drug Resistance in Neoplastic Cells*, pp. 161–171, WOOLEY, P. V., III and TEW, K. D. (eds) Academic Press, New York.

COLVIN, M., PADGETT, C. A. and FENSELAU, C. (1973) A biologically active metabolite of cyclophosphamide. *Cancer Res.* **33:** 915–918.

COLVIN, M., BRUNDRETT, R. B., KAN, M. N. N., JARDINE, I. and FENSELAU, C. (1976) Alkylating properties of phosphoramide mustard. *Cancer Res.* **36:** 1121–1126.

COLVIN, M., RUSSO, J. E., HILTON, J., DULIK, D. M. and FENSELAU, C. (1988) Enzymatic mechanisms of resistance to alkylating agents in tumor cells and normal tissues. *Adv. Enzyme Regul.* **27:** 211–221.

CONNEY, A. H. (1967) Pharmacological implications of microsomal enzyme induction. *Pharmac. Rev.* **19:** 317–366.

CONNORS, T. A., GROVER, P. L. and MCLOUGHLIN, A. M. (1970) Microsomal activation of cyclophosphamide in vivo. *Biochem. Pharmac.* **19:** 1533–1535.

CONNORS, T. A., FOSTER, A. B., GILSENAN, A. M., JARMAN, M. and TISDALE, M. J. (1972) Observations on the metabolism of cyclophosphamide. *Biochem. Pharmac.* **21:** 1373–1376.

CONNORS, T. A., COX, P. J., FARMER, P. B., FOSTER, A. B. and JARMAN, M. (1974) Some studies of the active intermediates formed in the microsomal metabolism of cyclophosphamide and isophosphamide. *Biochem. Pharmac.* **23:** 115–129.

COX, P. J. (1979) Cyclophosphamide cystitis—identification of acrolein as the causative agent. *Biochem. Pharmac.* **28:** 2045–2049.

COX, P. J., FARMER, P. B. and JARMAN, M. (1975a) The microsomal metabolism of some analogues of cyclophosphamide: 4-methylcyclophosphamide and 6-methylcyclophosphamide. *Biochem. Pharmac.* **24:** 599–606.

COX, P. J., PHILLIPS, B. J. and THOMAS, P. (1975b) The enzymatic basis of the selective action of cyclophosphamide. *Cancer Res.* **35:** 3755–3761.

COX, P. J., FARMER, P. B. and JARMAN, M. (EDS) (1976a) Proceedings of the symposium on the metabolism and mechanism of action of cyclophosphamide. *Cancer Treat. Rep.* **60:** 299–525.

COX, P. J., PHILLIPS, B. J. and THOMAS, P. (1976b) Studies on the selective action of cyclophosphamide (NSC-26271): inactivation of the hydroxylated metabolite by tissue-soluble enzymes. *Cancer Treat. Rep.* **60:** 321–326.

CREAVEN, P. J., ALLEN, L. M., ALFORD, D. A. and COHEN, M. H. (1974) Clinical pharmacology of isophosphamide. *Clin. Pharmac. Ther.* **16:** 77–86.

CROOK, T. R., SOUHAMI, R. L., WHYMAN, G. D. and MCLEAN, A. E. M. (1986) Glutathione depletion as a determinant of sensitivity of human leukemia cells to cyclophosphamide. *Cancer Res.* **46:** 5035–5038.

CROW, K. E., KITSON, T. M., MACGIBBON, A. K. H. and BATT, R. D. (1974) Intracellular localization and properties of aldehyde dehydrogenase from sheep liver. *Biochim. biophys. Acta* **350:** 121–128.

DE BRUIJN, E. A., SLEE, P. H. TH. J., VAN OOSTEROM, A. T., LAMEIJER, D. W., ROOZENDAAL, K. J. and TJADEN, U. R. (1988) Pharmacokinetics of intravenous and oral cyclophosphamide in the presence of methoxtrexate and fluorouracil. *Pharm. Week. Sci. Ed.* **10:** 200–206.

DEIS, F. H. and LESTER, D. (1979) Biochemical pharmacology of pyrazoles. In: *Biochemistry and Pharmacology of Ethanol*, **2:** 303–323, MAJCHROWICZ, E. and NOBLE, E. (eds) Plenum Press, New York.

DEITRICH, R. A. (1971) Genetic aspects of increase in rat liver aldehyde dehydrogenase induced by phenobarbital. *Science* **173:** 334–336.

DEITRICH, R. A., COLLINS, A. C. and ERWIN, V. G. (1972) Genetic influence upon phenobarbital-induced increase in rat liver supernatant aldehyde dehydrogenase activity. *J. biol. Chem.* **247:** 7232–7236.

DEITRICH, R. A., TROXELL, P. A. and ERWIN, V. G. (1975) Characteristics of the induction of aldehyde dehydrogenase in rat liver. *Cancer Res.* **44:** 5219–5226.

DEITRICH, R. A., BLUDEAU, P., ROPER, M. and SCHMUCK, J. (1978) Induction of aldehyde dehydrogenase. *Biochem. Pharmac.* **27:** 2343–2347.

DENEVE, W., VALERIOTE, F., EDELSTEIN, M., EVERETT, C. and BISCHOFF, M. (1989) In vivo DNA cross-linking by cyclophosphamide: comparison of human chronic lymphatic leukemia cells with mouse L1210 leukemia and normal bone marrow cells. *Cancer Res.* **49:** 3452–3456.

DE VITA, V. T. and ADAMSON, R. H. (1970) The metabolism of ^{14}C-cyclophosphamide: comparative drug metabolism studies on African and American patients with lymphosarcoma and Burkitt's tumor. *Prog. Antimicrob. Anticancer Chemother.* **2:** 218–225.

DE VITA, S., NERI, R. and BOMBARDIERI, S. (1991) Cyclophosphamide pulses in the treatment of rheumatic diseases: an update. *Clin. exp. Rheumat.* **9:** 179–193.

D'INCALCI, M., BOLIS, G., FACCHINETTI, T., MANGIONI, C., MORASCA, L., MORAZZONI, P. and SALMONA, M. (1979a) Decreased half life of cyclophosphamide in patients under continual treatment. *Eur. J. Cancer* **15:** 7–10.

D'INCALCI, M., FACCHINETTI, T., BOLIS, G., MANGIONI, C. and MORASCA, L. (1979b) Pharmacokinetics of cyclophosphamide after prolonged low dose treatment in ovarian cancer patients. *Eur. J. Drug Metab. Pharmacokinet.* **4:** 83–85.

D'INCALCI, M., TORTI, L., DAMIA, G., ERBA, E., MORASCA, L. and GARATTINI, S. (1983) Ovarian reticular cell sarcoma of the mouse (M5076) made resistant to cyclophosphamide. *Cancer Res.* **43:** 5674–5680.

D'INCALCI, M., CITTI, L., TAVERNA, P. and CATAPANO, C. V. (1988) Importance of the DNA repair enzyme O^6-alkyl guanine alkyltransferase (AT) in cancer chemotherapy. *Cancer Treat. Rev.* **15:** 279–292.

DIXON, R. L. (1968) Effect of chloramphenicol on the metabolism and lethality of cyclophosphamide in rats. *Proc. Soc. exp. biol. Med.* **127:** 1151–1155.

DOCKHAM, P. A., LEE, M.-O. and SLADEK, N. E. (1992) Identification of human liver aldehyde dehydrogenases that catalyze the oxidation of aldophosphamide and retinaldehyde. *Biochem. Pharmac.* **43:** 2453–2469.

DOEHMER, J., SEIDEL, A., OESCH, F. and GLATT, H. R. (1990) Genetically engineered V79 Chinese hamster cells metabolically activate the cytostatic drugs cyclophosphamide and ifosfamide. *Environ. Health Perspect.* **88:** 63–65.

DOLNICK, E. H., LINDAHL, I. L., TERRILL, C. E. and REYNOLDS, P. J. (1969) Cyclophosphamide as a chemical 'defleecing' agent for sheep. *Nature* **221:** 467–468.

DOMEYER, B. E. (1977) Biotransformation of 'activated' cyclophosphamide. Ph.D. Thesis, University of Minnesota, Minneapolis.

DOMEYER, B. E. and SLADEK, N. E. (1974) Potential for in vivo inactivation of a cyclophosphamide metabolite (aldophosphamide) by tumor enzymes. *Fed. Proc.* **33:** 581.

DOMEYER, B. E. and SLADEK, N. E. (1980a) Kinetics of cyclophosphamide biotransformtion in vivo. *Cancer Res.* **40:** 174–180.

DOMEYER, B. E. and SLADEK, N. E. (1980b) Metabolism of 4-hydroxycyclophosphamide/aldophosphamide in vitro. *Biochem. Pharmac.* **29:** 2903–2912.

DOMEYER, B. E. and SLADEK, N. E. (1981) Inhibition by cyanamide of 4-hydroxycyclophosphamide/aldophosphamide oxidation to carboxyphosphamide. *Biochem. Pharmac.* **30:** 2065–2073.

DONE A. K., COHEN, S. N. and STREBEL, L. (1977) Pediatric clinical pharmacology and the 'therapeutic orphan'. *Ann. Rev. Pharmac. Toxic.* **17:** 561–573.

DONELLI, M. G. and GARATTINI, S. (1971) Drug metabolism after repeated treatments with cytotoxic agents. *Eur. J. Cancer* **7:** 361–364.

DONELLI, M. G., FRANCHI, G. and ROSSO, R. (1970) The effect of cytotoxic agents on drug metabolism. *Eur. J. Cancer* **6:** 125–126.

DONELLI, M. G., COLOMBO, T. and GARATTINI, S. (1973) Effect of cyclophosphamide on the activity and distribution of pentobarbital in rats. *Biochem. Pharmac.* **22:** 2609–2614.

DONELLI, M. G., BARTOSEK, I., GUAITANI, A., MARTINI, A., COLOMBO, T., PACCIARINI, M. A. and MODICA, R. (1976) Importance of pharmacokinetic studies on cyclophosphamide (NSC-26271) in understanding its cytotoxic effect. *Cancer Treat. Rep.* **60:** 395–401.

DONELLI, M. G., VECCHI A., BOSSI, A., COLOMBO, T., SIRONI, M., PANTAROTTO, C., GARATTINI, S. and SPREAFICO, F. (1977) Effect of phenobarbital on cyclophosphamide cytotoxic activity and pharmacokinetics in mice. *Tumori* **63:** 137–146.

DOOLEY, J. S., JAMES, C. A., ROGERS, H. J. and STUART-HARRIS, R. (1982) Biliary elimination of cyclophosphamide in man. *Cancer Chemother. Pharmac.* **9:** 26–29.

DORR, R. T. and ALBERTS, D. S. (1982) Cimetidine enhancement of cyclophosphamide antitumor activity. *Br. J. Cancer* **45:** 35–43.

DORR, R. T., SOBLE, M. J. and ALBERTS, D. S. (1986) Interaction of cimetidine but not ranitidine with cyclophosphamide in mice. *Cancer Res.* **46:** 1795–1799.

DRAEGER, U. and HOHORST, H. J. (1976) Permeation of cyclophosphamide (NSC-26271) metabolites into tumor cells. *Cancer Treat. Rep.* **60:** 423–427.

DRAEGER, U., PETER, G. and HOHORST, H. J. (1976) Deactivation of cyclophosphamide (NSC-26271) metabolites by sulfhydryl compounds. *Cancer Treat. Rep.* **60:** 355–359.

DUNCAN, J. H., COLVIN, O. M. and FENSELAU, C. (1973) Mass spectrometric study of the distribution of cyclophosphamide in humans. *Toxic. appl. Pharmac.* **24:** 317–323.

DUNN, D. L., LUBET, R. A. and PROUGH, R. A. (1979) Oxidative metabolism of *N*-isopropyl-α-(2-methylhydrazino)-*p*-toluamide hydrochloride (procarbazine) by rat liver microsomes. *Cancer Res.* **39:** 4555–4563.

DUNN, T. J., LINDAHL, R. and PITOT, H. C. (1988) Differential gene expression in response to 2,3,7,8-tetrachlorodibenzo-*p*-dioxin (TCDD). Noncoordinate regulation of a TCDD-induced aldehyde dehydrogenase and cytochrome P-450c in the rat. *J. biol. Chem.* **263:** 10878–10886.

DUNN, T. J., KOLESKE, A. J., LINDAHL, R. and PITOT, H. C. (1989) Phenobarbital-inducible aldehyde dehydrogenase in the rat. cDNA sequence and regulation of the mRNA by phenobarbital in responsive rats. *J. biol. Chem.* **264:** 13057–13065.

ECKEY, R., AGARWAL, D. P., SAHA, N. and GOEDDE, H. W. (1986) Detection and partial characterization of a variant form of cytosolic aldehyde dehydrogenase isozyme. *Human Gen.* **72:** 95–97.

EDWARDS, G., CALVERT, R. T., CROWTHER, D., BRAMWELL, V. and SCARFFE, H. (1980) Repeated investigations of cyclophosphamide disposition in myeloma patients receiving intermittent chemotherapy. *Br. J. clin. Pharmac.* **10:** 281–285.

EGORIN, M. J., KAPLAN, R. S., SALCMAN, M., AISNER, J., COLVIN, M., WIERNIK, P. H. and BACHUR, N. R. (1982) Cyclophosphamide plasma and cerebrospinal fluid kinetics with and without dimethyl sulfoxide. *Clin. Pharmac. Ther.* **32:** 122–128.

EGORIN, M. J., FORREST, A., BELANI, C. P., RATAIN, M. J., ABRAMS, J. S. and VAN ECHO, D. A. (1989) A limited sampling strategy for cyclophosphamide pharmacokinetics. *Cancer Res.* **49:** 3129–3133.

EHNINGER, G., SCHULER, U., WAGNER, T. and OSTENDORF, P. (1985) Cyclophosphamide pharmacokinetics and metabolism after repeated high dose administration in BMT. *Exp. Hemat.* **13:** 153.

EHRIG, T., BOSRON, W. F. and LI, T.-K. (1990) Alcohol and aldehyde dehydrogenase. *Alcohol Alcohol.* **25:** 105–116.

ENGINEER, M. S., AYELE, W., LEGHA, S. S. and NEWMAN, R. A. (1989) Clinical pharmacology of ifosfamide. *Proc. Am. Ass. Cancer Res.* **30:** 249.

ENGLE, T. W., ZON, G. and EGAN, W. (1979) ^{31}P NMR investigations of phosphoramide mustard: evaluation of pH control over the rate of intramolecular cyclization to an aziridinium ion and the hydrolysis of this reactive alkylator. *J. med. Chem.* **22:** 897–899.

ENGLE, T. W., ZON, G. and EGAN, W. (1982) ^{31}P NMR kinetic studies of the intra- and intermolecular alkylation chemistry of phosphoramide mustard and cognate *N*-phosphorylated derivatives of *N,N*-bis(2-chloroethyl)amine. *J. med. Chem.* **25:** 1347–1357.

ERICKSON, L. C., RAMONAS, L. M., ZAHARKO, D. S. and KOHN, K. W. (1980) Cytotoxicity and DNA cross-linking activity of 4-sulfidocyclophosphamides in mouse leukemia cells in vitro. *Cancer Res.* **40:** 4216–4220.

ERLICHMAN, C., SOLDIN, S. J., HARDY, R. W., THIESSEN, J. J., STURGEON, J. F. G., FINE, S. and BASKERVILLE, T. (1988) Disposition of cyclophosphamide on two consecutive cycles of treatment in patients with ovarian carcinoma. *Arzneim.-Forsch. Drug Res.* **38:** 839–842.

FABER, O. K., MOURIDSEN, H. T. and SKOVSTED, L. (1974) The biotransformation of cyclophosphamide in man: influence of prednisone. *Acta Pharmac. Toxic.* **35:** 195–200.

FABER, O. K., MOURIDSEN, H. T. and SKOVSTED, L. (1975) The effect of chloramphenicol and sulphaphenazole on the biotransformation of cyclophosphamide in man. *Br. J. clin. Pharmacol.* **2:** 281–285.

FARMER, P. B. (1988) Enantiomers of cyclophosphamide and iphosphamide. *Biochem. Pharmac.* **37:** 145–148.

FASOLA, G., GRECO, P. L., CALORI, E., ZILLI, M., VERLICCHI, F., MOTTA, M. R., RICCI, P., BACCARANI, M. and TURA, S. (1991) Pharmacokinetics of high-dose cyclophosphamide for bone marrow transplantation. *Haematologica* **76:** 120–125.

FAUCI, A. S., WOLFF S. M. and JOHNSON, J. S. (1971) Effect of cyclophosphamide upon the immune response in Wenener's granulomatosis. *New Engl. J. Med.* **285:** 1493–1496.

FEIL, V. J. and LAMOUREUX, C. H. (1974) Alopecia activity of cyclophosphamide metabolites and related compounds in sheep. *Cancer Res.* **34:** 2596–2598.

FELSTED, R. L. and BACHUR, N. R. (1980) Mammalian carbonyl reductases. *Drug Metab. Rev.* **11:** 1–60.

FENSELAU, C., KAN, M.-N. N., BILLETS, S. and COLVIN, M. (1975) Identification of phosphorodiamidic acid mustard as a human metabolite of cyclophosphamide. *Cancer Res.* **35:** 1453–1457.

FENSELAU, C., KAN, M.-N. N., RAO, S. S., MYLES, A., FRIEDMAN, O. M. and COLVIN, M. (1977) Identification of aldophosphamide as a metabolite of cyclophosphamide in vitro and in vivo in humans. *Cancer Res.* **37:** 2538–2543.

FENSELAU, C., LEHMAN, J. P., MYLES, A., BRANDT, J., YOST, G. S., FRIEDMAN, O. M. and COLVIN, O. M. (1982) Iminocyclophosphamide as a chemically reactive metabolite of cyclophosphamide. *Drug Met. Disp.* **10:** 636–640.

FERENCZ-BIRO, K. and PIETRUSZKO, R. (1984) Inhibition of human aldehyde dehydrogenase isozymes by propionaldehyde. *Alcohol. clin. Exp. Res.* **8:** 302–307.

FOLEY, G. E., FRIEDMAN, O. M. and DROLET, B. P. (1961) Studies on the mechanism of action of cytoxan—evidence of activation in vivo and in vitro. *Cancer Res.* **21:** 57–63.

FRAISER, L. H., KANEKAL, S. and KEHRER, J. P. (1991) Cyclophosphamide toxicity. Characterizing and avoiding the problem. *Drugs* **42:** 781–795.

FRIED, W., KEDO, A. and BARONE, J. (1977) Effects of cyclophosphamide and of busulfan on spleen colony-forming units and on hematopoietic stroma. *Cancer Res.* **37:** 1205–1209.

FRIEDMAN, O. M. (1967) Studies of some newer phosphoramide mustards. *Cancer Chemother. Rep.* **51:** 347–357.

FRIEDMAN, O. M. and BOGER, E. (1961) Colorimetric estimation of nitrogen mustards in aqueous media. Hydrolytic behavior of bis(beta-chloroethyl)-amine, norHN2. *Anal. Chem.* **3:** 906–910.

FRIEDMAN, O. M. and SELIGMAN, A. M. (1954) Preparation of *N*-phosphorylated derivatives of bis-β-chloroethylamine. *J. Am. Chem. Soc.* **76:** 655–658.

FRIEDMAN, O. M., WODINSKY, I. and MYLES, A. (1976) Cyclophosphamide (NSC-26271)-related phosphoramide mustards—recent advances and historical perspective. *Cancer Treat. Rep.* **60:** 337–346.

FRIEDMAN, O. M., MYLES, A. and COLVIN, M. (1979) Cyclophosphamide and related phosphoramide mustards. Current status and future prospects. *Adv. Cancer Chemother.* **1:** 143–204.

FUKS, J. Z., EGORIN, M. J., AISNER, J., OSTROW, S. S. KLEIN, M. E., BACHUR, N. R., COLVIN, M. and WIERNIK,

P. H. (1981) Cyclophosphamide and dimethylsulfoxide in the treatment of squamous carcinoma of the lung. Therapeutic efficacy, toxicity, and pharmacokinetics. *Cancer Chemother. Pharamac.* **6:** 117–120.

GAMELLI, R. L., ERSHLER, W. B., HACKER, M. P. and FOSTER, R. S. (1986) The effect of disulfiram on cyclophosphamide-mediated myeloid toxicity. *Cancer Chemother. Pharmac.* **16:** 153–155.

GARATTINI, S., GHEZZI, P. and D'INCALCI, M. (1988) Effects of cancer disease on the metabolism of anticancer agents. *Pharmac. Ther.* **37:** 57–65.

GARRETTSON, L. K. and DAYTON, P. G. (1970) Disappearance of phenobarbital and diphenylhydantoin from serum of children. *Clin. Pharmac. Ther.* **11:** 674–679.

GENKA, S., DEUTSCH, J., STAHLE, P. L., SHETTY, U. H., JOHN, V., ROBINSON, C., RAPOPORT, S. I. and GREIG, N. H. (1990) Brain and plasma pharmacokinetics and anticancer activities of cyclophosphamide and phosphoramide mustard in the rat. *Cancer Chemother. Pharmac.* **27:** 1–7.

GERHARTZ, H. H., LISS, E. and SCHMIDT, H. (1979) Cyclophosphamide-resistant Yoshida ascites tumor cells and their cross reistance to some alkylating agents. *J. Cancer Res. clin. Oncol.* **94:** 257–263.

GIBSON, N. W., ZLOTOGORSKI, C. and ERICKSON, L. C. (1985) Specific DNA repair mechanisms may protect some human tumor cells from DNA interstrand crosslinking by chloroethylnitrosoureas but not from crosslinking by other anti-tumor alkylating agents. *Carcinogenesis* **6:** 445–450.

GOEDDE, H. W. and AGARWAL, D. P. (1990) Pharmacogenetics of aldehyde dehydrogenase (ALDH). *Pharmac. Ther.* **45:** 345–371.

GOLDENBERG, G. J., LAND, H. B. and CORMACK, D. V. (1974) Mechanism of cyclophosphamide transport by L5178Y lymphoblasts in vitro. *Cancer Res.* **34:** 3274–3282.

GOLDSTEIN, A., ARONOW, L. and KALMAN, S. M. (1974) *Principles of Drug Action: The Basis of Pharmacology*, 2nd edn, pp. 333–338, John Wiley and Sons, New York.

GOMORI, G. (1948) Histochemical demonstration of sites of phosphamidase activity. *Proc. Soc. exp. biol. Med.* **69:** 407–409.

GONSETTE, R. E., DEMONTY, L. and DELMOTTE, P. (1977) Intensive immunosuppression with cyclophosphamide in multiple sclerosis. *J. Neurol.* **214:** 173–181.

GORIN, N. C., LABOPIN, M., MELONI, G., KORBLING, M., CARELLA, A., HERVE, P., BURNETT, A., RIZZOLI, V., ALESSANDRINO, E. P., BJORKSTRAND, B., FERRANT, A., LOWENBERG, B., COSER, P., SIMONSSON, B., HELBIG, W., BRUNET MAURI, S., VERDONCK, L. F., IRIONDO, A., POLLI, E., COLOMBAT, P., FRANKLIN, I. M., SOUILLET, G. and WILLEMZE, R. (1991) Autologous bone marrow transplantation for acute myeloblastic leukemia in Europe: further evidence of the role of marrow purging by mafosfamide. *Leukemia* **5:** 896–904.

GRAHAM, M. I., SHAW, I. C., SOUHAMI, R. L., SIDAU, B., HARPER, P. G. and MCLEAN, A. E. M. (1983) Decreased plasma half-life of cyclophosphamide during repeated high-dose administration. *Cancer Chemother. Pharmac.* **10:** 192–193.

GRAM, T. E. (1980) *Extrahepatic Metabolism of Drugs and Other Foreign Compounds*. SP Medical and Scientific Books, New York.

GRILLO, T. A. I., BAXTER-GRILLO, D. L. and ABEGUNDE, J. O. A. (1978) Light and electron histochemistry of phosphoamidase with ρ-chloranilidophosphonic acid and with cyclophosphamide (endoxan). *Histochemistry* **59:** 73–74.

GROCHOW, L. B. and COLVIN, M. (1980) Clinical pharmacokinetics of cyclophosphamide. *Clin. Pharmacokinet.* **4:** 380–394.

GROCHOW, L. B. and COLVIN, M. (1983) Clinical pharmacokinetics of cyclophosphamide. In: *Pharmacokinetics of Anticancer Agents in Humans*, pp. 135–154, AMES, M. M., POWIS, G. and KOVACH, J. S. (eds) Elsevier, Amsterdam.

GUENGERICH, F. P. (1989) Characterization of human microsomal cytochrome P-450 enzymes. *Ann. Rev. Pharmac. Toxic.* **29:** 241–264.

GURTOO, H. L., GESSNER, T. and CULLITON, P. (1976) Studies on the effects of cyclophosphamide, vincristine, and prednisone on some hepatic oxidations and conjugations. *Cancer Treat. Rep.* **60:** 1285–1294.

GURTOO, H. L., BANSAL, S. K., PAVELIC, Z. and STRUCK, R. F. (1985) Effects of the induction of hepatic microsomal metabolism on the toxicity of cyclophosphamide. *Br. J. Cancer* **51:** 67–75.

HABS, H., HABS, M. and SCHMÄHL, D. (1981) Influence of pretreatment with disulfiram on the acute toxicity of cyclophosphamide in male Sprague–Dawley rats. *Arzneim.-Forsch. Drug Res.* **31:** 530–531.

HACKER, M. P., ERSHLER, W. B., NEWMAN, R. A. and GAMELLI, R. L. (1982) Effect of disulfiram (tetraethylthiuram disulfide) and diethyldithiocarbamate on the bladder toxicity and antitumor activity of cyclophosphamide in mice. *Cancer Res.* **42:** 4490–4494.

HADIDI, A.-H. F. A. and IDLE, J. R. (1988) Combined thin-layer chromatography–photography–densitometry for the quantitation of cyclophosphamide and its four principal urinary metabolites. *J. Chromatogr.* **427:** 121–130.

HADIDI, A.-H. F. A., COULTER, C. E. A. and IDLE, J. R. (1988) Phenotypically deficient urinary elimination of carboxyphosphamide after cyclophosphamide administration to cancer patients. *Cancer Res.* **48:** 5167–5171.

HALES, B. F. (1989) Effects of phosphoramide mustard and acrolein, cytotoxic metabolites of cyclophosphamide, on mouse limb development in vitro. *Teratology* **40:** 11–20.

HALES, B. F., LUDEMAN, S. M. and BOYD, V. L. (1989) Embryotoxicity of phenyl ketone analogs of cyclophosphamide. *Teratology* **39:** 31–37.

HALL, A., ROBSON, C. N., HICKSON, I. D., HARRIS, A. L., PROCTOR, S. J. and CATTAN, A. R. (1989) Possible role of inhibition of glutathione *S*-transferase in the partial reversal of chlorambucil resistance by indomethacin in a Chinese hamster ovary cell line. *Cancer Res.* **49:** 6265–6268.

HARGUINDEY, S., HENDERSON, E. S. and NAEHER, C. (1979) Effects of systemic acidification of mice with sarcoma 180. *Cancer Res.* **39:** 4364–4371.

HART, L. G. and ADAMSON, R.H. (1969) Effect of microsomal enzyme modifiers on toxicity and therapeutic activity of cyclophosphamide in mice. *Arch. Int. Pharmacodyn. Ther.* **180:** 391–401.

HAUPTLORENZ, S., ESTERBAUER, H., MOLL, W., PUMPEL, R., SCHAUENSTEIN, E. and PUSCHENDORF, B. (1985) Effects of the lipid peroxidation product 4-hydroxynonenal and related aldehydes on proliferation and viability of cultured Ehrlich ascites tumor cells. *Biochem. Pharmac.* **34:** 3803–3809.

HAUSER, S. L., DAWSON, D. M., LEHRICH, J. R., BEAL, M. F., KEVY, S. V., PROPPER, R. D., MILLS, J. A. and WEINER, H. L. (1983) Intensive immunosuppression in progressive multiple sclerosis. A randomized, three-arm study of high-dose intravenous cyclophosphamide, plasma exchange, and ACTH. *New Engl. J. Med.* **308:** 173–180.

HAUSHEER, F. H., SINGH, U. C., SAXE, J. D. and COLVIN, O. M. (1989) Identification of local determinants of DNA interstrand crosslink formation by cyclophosphamide metabolites. *Anti-Cancer Drug Design* **4:** 281–294.

HEMMINKI, K. (1985) Binding of metabolites of cyclophosphamide to DNA in a rat liver microsomal system and in vivo in mice. *Cancer Res.* **45:** 4237–4243.

HEMMINKI, K., ALHONEN, A., LINKOLA, E. and HESSO, A. (1987) Kinetics of hydrolysis in vitro of nornitrogen mustard, a metabolite of phosphoramide mustard and cyclophosphamide. *Arch. Toxic.* **61:** 126–130.

HENGST, J. C. D. and KEMPF, R. A. (1984) Immunodulation by cyclophosphamide. *Clin. Immun. Allergy* **4:** 199–216.

HEPNER, G. W. and VESELL, E. S. (1975) Quantitative assessment of hepatic function by breath analysis after oral administration of [^{14}C]aminopyrine. *Ann. intern. Med.* **83:** 632–638.

HEPNER, G. W., UHLIN, S. R., LIPTON, A., HARVEY, H. A. and ROHRER, G. V. (1976) Abnormal aminopyrine metabolism in patients with hepatic neoplasm. *J. Am. Med. Ass.* **236:** 1587–1590.

HIGUCHI, T., NAKAMURA, T. and UCHINO, H. (1978) Microsomal enzymes in patients with gastric carcinoma as determined by plasma half-life of antipyrine. *Gann* **69:** 753–756.

HIGUCHI, T., NAKAMURA, T. and UCHINO, H. (1980) Antipyrine metabolism in cancer patients. *Cancer* **45:** 541–544.

HILGARD, P., POHL, J., STEKAR, J and VOEGELI, R. (1985) Oxazaphosphorines as biological response modifiers—experimental and clinical perspectives. *Cancer Treat. Rev.* **12:** 155–162.

HILL, D. L. (1975) *A Review of Cyclophosphamide.* Charles C. Thomas, Springfield, IL.

HILL, D. L., LASTER, W. R., JR and STRUCK, R. F. (1972) Enzymatic metabolism of cyclophosphamide and nicotine and production of a toxic cyclophosphamide metabolite. *Cancer Res.* **32:** 658–665.

HILL, D. L., LASTER, W. R., JR, KIRK, M. C., EL DAREER, S. and STRUCK, R. F. (1973) Metabolism of iphosphamide [2-(2-chloroethylamino)-3-(2-chloroethyl)tetrahydro-2H-1,3,2-oxazaphosphorine 2-oxide] and production of a toxic iphosphamide metabolite. *Cancer Res.* **33:** 1016–1022.

HILTON, J. (1984a) Deoxyribonucleic acid crosslinking by 4-hydroperoxycyclophosphamide in cyclophosphamide-sensitive and -resistant L1210 cells. *Biochem. Pharmac.* **33:** 1867–1872.

HILTON, J. (1984b) Role of aldehyde dehydrogenase in cyclophosphamide-resistant L1210 leukemia. *Cancer Res.* **44:** 5156–5160.

HILTON, J. and COLVIN, M. (1984) The role of aldehyde dehydrogenase activity in cyclophosphamide sensitivity of hematopoetic and leukemic cell populations. *Proc. Am. Ass. Cancer Res.* **25:** 339.

HIPKENS, J. H., STRUCK, R. F. and GURTOO, H. L. (1981) Role of aldehyde dehydrogenase in the metabolism-dependent biological activity of cyclophosphamide. *Cancer Res.* **41:** 3571–3583.

HIRANO, T., RINGSDORF, H. and ZAHARKO, D. S. (1980) Antitumor activity of monomeric and polymeric cyclophosphamide derivatives compared with in vitro hydrolysis. *Cancer Res.* **40:** 2263–2267.

HIRST, M., TSE, S., MILLS, D. G., LEVIN, L. and WHITE, D. F. (1984) Occupational exposure to cyclophosphamide. *Lancet* **i:** 186–188.

HOHORST, H. J., ZIEMANN, A. and BROCK, N. (1971) 4-Ketocyclophosphamide, a metabolite of cyclophosphamide. Formation, chemical and biological properties. *Arzneim-Forsch. Drug Res.* **21:** 1254–1257.

HOHORST, H. J., DRAEGER, U., PETER, G. and VOELCKER, G. (1976) The problem of oncostatic specificity of cyclophosphamide (NSC-26271): studies on reactions that control the alkylating and cytotoxic activity. *Cancer Treat. Rep.* **60:** 309–315.

HOHORST, H. J., BIELICKI, L. and VOELCKER, G. (1983) The mode of action of cyclophosphamide. In: *The Control of Tumor Growth and its Biological Bases*, pp. 445–451, DAVIS, W., MALTONI, C. and TANNEBERGER, S. (eds) Martinus Nijhoff Publishers, Boston.

HOHORST, H. J., BIELICKI, L. and VOELCKER, G. (1986) The enzymatic basis of cyclophosphamide specificity. In: *Advances in Enzyme Regulation*, **25:** 99–122, WEBER, G. (ed.) Pergamon Press, Oxford.

HOLM, K. A., KINDBERG, C. G., STOBAUGH, J. F., SLAVIK, M. and RILEY, C. M. (1990) Stereoselective pharmacokinetics and metabolism of the enantiomers of cyclophosphamide. *Biochem. Pharmac.* **39:** 1375–1384.

HONG, P. S. and CHAN, K. K. (1987) Identification and quantitation of alcophosphamide, a metabolite of cyclophosphamide, in the rat using chemical ionization mass spectrometry. *Biomed. Environ. Mass Spectrom.* **14:** 167–172.

HONG, P. S. and CHAN, K. K. (1991) Enzymatic detoxification of phosphoramide mustard by soluble fractions from rat organ tissues. *Drug Metab. Disp.* **19:** 568–573.

HONG, P. S., SRIGRITSANAPOL, A. and CHAN, K. K. (1991) Pharmacokinetics of 4-hydroxycyclophosphamide and metabolites in the rat. *Drug Metab. Disp.* **19:** 1–7.

HORSLEV-PETERSEN, K., BEYER, J. M. and HELIN, P. (1983) Intermittent cyclophosphamide in refractory rheumatoid arthritis. *Br. med. J.* **287:** 711–712.

INGE, T. H., HOOVER, S. K., FRANK, J. L., KAWABATA, T. T., BETHKE, K. P. and BEAR, H. D. (1992) Enhancement of cytotoxic T lymphocyte growth from spleens of P815-tumor-bearing host mice with mafosfamide. *Cancer Immun. Immunother.* **35:** 119–126.

ISHIKAWA, M., SASAKI, K.-I. and TAKAYANAGI, Y. (1989) Injurious effect of buthionine sulfoximine, an inhibitor of glutathione biosynthesis, on the lethality and urotoxicity of cyclophosphamide in mice. *Jap. J. Pharmac.* **51:** 146–149.

ISHIKAWA, M., SASAKI, K., TAKAYANAGI, Y. and SASAKI, K.-I. (1991) Perturbation of metabolism and disposition of cyclophosphamide by interferon and poly I:C, an interferon inducer, in mice. *Pharmac. Toxic.* **68:** 157–162.

JÄHDE, E. and RAJEWSKY, M. F. (1982) Tumor-selective modification of cellular microenvironment in vivo: effect of glucose infusion on the pH in normal and malignant rat tissues. *Cancer Res.* **42:** 1505–1512.

JÄHDE, E., GLÜSENKAMP, K.-H., KLÜNDER, I., HÜLSER, D. F., TIETZE, L.-T. and RAJEWSKY, M. F. (1989a) Hydrogen ion-mediated enhancement of cytotoxicity of bis-chloroethylating drugs in rat mammary carcinoma cells in vivo. *Cancer Res.* **49:** 2965–2972.

JÄHDE, E., GLÜSENKAMP, K.-H. and RAJEWSKY, M. F. (1989b) Increased drug cytotoxicity at reduced pH counteracts cyclophosphamide resistance in cultured rat mammary carcinoma cells. *Int. J. Cancer* **44:** 1082–1087.

JÄHDE, E., GLÜSENKAMP, K.-H. and RAJEWSKY, M. F. (1991) Nigericin enhances mafosfamide cytotoxicity at low extracellular pH. *Cancer Chemother. Pharmac.* **27:** 440–444.

JAO, J. Y., JUSKO, W. J. and COHEN, J. L. (1972) Phenobarbital effects on cyclophosphamide pharmacokinetics in man. *Cancer Res.* **32:** 2761–2764.

JARDINE, I., FENSELAU, C., APPLER, M., KAN, M. N., BRUNDRETT, R. B. and COLVIN, M. (1978) Quantiation by gas chromatography-chemical ionization mass spectrometry of cyclophosphamide, phosphoramide mustard, and nornitrogen mustard in the plasma and urine of patients receiving cyclophosphamide therapy. *Cancer Res.* **38:** 408–415.

JARMAN, M., MILSTED, R. A. V., SMYTH, J. F., KINAS, R. W., PANKIEWICZ, K. and STEC, W. J. (1979) Comparative metabolism of 2-[bis(2-chloroethyl)-amino]tetrahydro-2H-1,3,2-oxazaphosphorine-2-oxide (cyclophosphamide) and its enantiomers in humans. *Cancer Res.* **39:** 2762–2767.

JEAVONS, C. M. and ZEINER, A. R. (1984) Effects of elevated female sex steroids on ethanol and acetaldehyde metabolism in humans. *Alcohol. clin. Exp. Res.* **8:** 352–358.

JOHNS, D. G. (1967) Human liver aldehyde oxidase: differential inhibition of oxidation of charged and uncharged substrates. *J. clin. Invest.* **46:** 1492–1505.

JONES, R. J. and SANTOS, G. W. (1990) Autologous bone marrow transplantation with 4-hydroperoxycyclophosphamide purging. In: *Acute Myelogenous Leukemia: Progress and Controversies*, pp. 411–419, GALE, R. P. (ed.) Wiley-Liss, New York.

JONES, R. J., ZUEHLSDORF, M., ROWLEY, S. D., HILTON, J., SANTOS, G. W., SENSENBRENNER, L. L. and COLVIN, O. M. (1987) Variability in 4-hydroperoxycyclophosphamide activity during clinical purging for autologous bone marrow transplantation. *Blood* **70:** 1490–1494.

JUMA, F. and OGADA, T. (1983) Pharmacokinetics of cyclophosphamide in Kenyan Africans. *Br. J. clin. Pharmac.* **16:** 61–63.

JUMA, F. D., ROGERS, H. J. and TROUNCE, J. R. (1979a) Pharmacokinetics of cyclophosphamide and alkylating activity in man after intravenous and oral administration. *Br. J. clin. Pharmac.* **8:** 209–217.

JUMA, F. D., ROGERS, H. J. and TROUNCE, J. R. (1979b) The kinetics of salivary elimination of cyclophosphamide in man. *Br. J. clin. Pharmac.* **8:** 455–458.

JUMA, F. D., ROGERS, H. J. and TROUNCE, J. R. (1980) The pharmacokinetics of cyclophosphamide, phosphoramide mustard and nor-nitrogen mustard studied by gas chromatography in patients receiving cyclophosphamide therapy. *Br. J. clin. Pharmac.* **10:** 327–335.

JUMA, F. D., ROGERS, H. J. and TROUNCE, J. R. (1981) Effect of renal insufficiency on the pharmacokinetics of cyclophosphamide and some of its metabolites. *Eur. J. clin. Pharmac.* **19:** 443–451.

JUMA, F. D., KOECH, D. K., KASILI, E. G. and OGADA, T. (1984) Pharmacokinetics of cyclophosphamide in Kenyan African children with lymphoma. *Br. J. clin. Pharmac.* **18:** 106–107.

JUSKO, W. J. (1971) Pharmacodynamics of chemotherapeutic effects: dose–time–response relationships for phase-nonspecific agents. *J. Pharmaceut. Sci.* **60:** 892–895.

KALLAMA, S. and HEMMINKI, K. (1984) Alkylation of guanosine by phosphoramide mustard, chloromethine hydrochloride and chlorambucil. *Acta Pharmac. Toxicol.* **54:** 214–220.

KANEKAL, S. and KEHRER, J. P. (1993) Evidence for peroxidase-mediated metabolism of cyclophosphamide. *Drug Metab. Disp.* **21:** 37–42.

KASTAN, M. B., SCHLAFFER, E., RUSSO, J. E., COLVIN, O. M., CIVIN, C. I. and HILTON, J. (1990) Direct demonstration of elevated aldehyde dehydrogenase in human hematopoietic progenitor cells. *Blood* **75:** 1947–1950.

KATO, R. (1977) Drug metabolism under pathological and abnormal physiological states in animals and man. *Xenobiotica* **7:** 25–92.

KAWABATA, T. T. and WHITE, K. L., JR (1988) Enhancement of in vivo and in vitro murine immune responses by the cyclophosphamide metabolite acrolein. *Cancer Res.* **48:** 41–45.

KAZMI, S. M. I., LI, D., KOOP, K., CONANT, J. and LAU, C. Y. (1992) Role of aldehyde dehydrogenase in the biological activity of spermine dialdehyde, a novel immunosuppressive/purging agent. *Pharmac. Res.* **25:** 383–392.

KENNEDY, M. J., BEVERIDGE, R. A., ROWLEY, S. D., GORDON, G. B., ABELOFF, M. D. and DAVIDSON, N. E. (1991) High-dose chemotherapy with reinfusion of purged autologous bone marrow following dose-intense induction as initial therapy for metastatic breast cancer. *J. natn. Cancer Inst.* **83:** 920–926.

KITSON, T. (1986) The effect of 5,5′-dithiobis(1-methyltetrazole) on cytoplasmic aldehyde dehydrogenase and its implications for cephalosporin–alcohol reactions. *Alcohol. clin. exp. Res.* **10:** 27–32.

KLEIN, H. O., WICKRAMANAYAKE, P. D., COERPER, C., CHRISTIAN, E., POHL, J. and BROCK, N. (1983) High-dose ifosfamide and mesna as continuous infusion over five days—a phase I/II trial. *Cancer Treat. Rev.* **10**(Suppl. A): 167–173.

KLUIN-NELEMANS, H. C., LÖWENBERG, B., MARTENS, A. C. M. and HAGENBEEK, A. (1984) In vitro chemotherapy with ASTA-Z-7557: studies in rat and human acute myeloid leukemia. In: *Autologous Bone Marrow Transplantation and Solid Tumors*, pp. 33–39, MCVIE, J. G., DALESIO, O. and SMITH, I. E. (eds) Raven Press, New York.

KOELLING, T. M., YEAGER, A. M., HILTON, J., HAYNIE, D. T. and WILEY, J. M. (1990) Development and characterization of a cyclophosphamide-resistant subline of acute myeloid leukemia in the Lewis × Brown Norway hybrid rat. *Blood* **76:** 1209–1213.

KOHN, F. R. and SLADEK, N. E. (1985) Aldehyde dehydrogenase activity as the basis for the relative insensitivity of murine pluripotent hematopoietic stem cells to oxazaphosphorines. *Biochem. Pharmac.* **34:** 3465–3471.

KOHN, F. R. and SLADEK, N. E. (1987) Effects of aldehyde dehydrogenase inhibitors on the ex vivo sensitivity of murine late spleen colony-forming cells (day-12 CFU-S) and hematopoietic repopulating cells to mafosfamide (ASTA Z 7557). *Biochem. Pharmac.* **17:** 2805–2811.

KOHN, F. R. and SLADEK, N. E. (1988) Ex vivo treatment of murine splenocyte-supplemented bone marrow inocula with mafosfamide prior to allogeneic transplantation in an attempt to prevent lethal graft-versus-host disease without compromising engraftment. *Immunopharmac. Immunotoxic.* **10:** 387–398.

KOHN, F. R., LANDKAMER, G. J., MANTHEY, C. L., RAMSAY, N. K. C. and SLADEK, N. E. (1987a) Effect of aldehyde dehydrogenase inhibitors on the ex vivo sensitivity of human multipotent and committed hematopoietic progenitor cells and malignant blood cells to oxazaphosphorines. *Cancer Res.* **47:** 3180–3185.

KOHN, F. R., LANDKAMER, G. J. and SLADEK, N. E. (1987b) Effect of the aldehyde dehydrogenase inhibitor, cyanamide, on the ex vivo sensitivity of murine multipotent and committed hematopoietic progenitor cells to mafosfamide (ASTA Z 7557). *Immunopharmac. Immunotoxic.* **9:** 163–176.

KOIVULA, T. and KOIVUSALO, M. (1975a) Different forms of rat liver aldehyde dehydrogenase and their subcellular distribution. *Biochim. biophys. Acta* **397:** 9–23.

KOIVULA, T. and KOIVUSALO, M. (1975b) Partial purification and properties of a phenobarbital-induced aldehyde dehydrogenase of rat liver. *Biochim. biophys. Acta* **410:** 1–11.

KORBLING, M., HESS, A. D., TUTSCHKA, R. J., KAIZER, H., COLVIN, O. M. and SANTOS, G. W. (1982) 4-Hydroperoxycyclophosphamide: a model for eliminating residual human tumor cells and T-lymphocytes from bone marrow graft. *Br. J. Haemat.* **52:** 89–96.

KRAMAR, R. and KREMSER, K. (1984) Enhancement of aldehyde dehydrogenase activity in rat liver by clofibrate feeding. *Enzyme* **31:** 17–20.

KURYS, G., AMBROZIAK, W. and PIETRUSZKO, R. (1989) Human aldehyde dehydrogenase. Purification and characterization of a third isozyme with low K_m for γ-aminobutyraldehyde. *J. biol. Chem.* **264:** 4715–4721.

KWON, C. H. and BORCH, R. F. (1989) Effects of *N*-substitution on the activation mechanisms of 4-hydroxycyclophosphamide analogues. *J. med. Chem.* **32:** 1491–1496.

KWON, C. H., BORCH, R. F., ENGEL, J. and NIEMEYER, U. (1987a) Activation mechanisms of mafosfamide and role of thiols in cyclophosphamide metabolism. *J. med. Chem.* **30:** 395–399.

KWON, C. H., KIRK, M. C., STRUCK, R. F. and BORCH, R. F. (1987b) Spectroscopic detection of iminocyclophosphamide and its possible role in cyclophosphamide metabolism. *J. med. Chem.* **30:** 1110–1114.

KWON, C. H., MADDISON, K., LOCASTRO, L. and BORCH, R. F. (1987c) Accelerated decomposition of 4-hydroxycyclophosphamide by human serum albumin. *Cancer Res.* **47:** 1505–1508.

LAFRENIERE, R., BORKENHAGEN, K., BRYANT, L. D. and NG, E. (1989) Tumor-infiltrating lymphocytes cultured in recombinant interleukin-2: enhancement of growth, cytotoxicity, and phenotypic expression of cytotoxic T-cell antigens by cyclophosphamide given intravenously prior to tumor harvest. *J. biol. Response Modif.* **8:** 238–251.

LARTIGUE-MATTEI, C., CHABARD, J. L., TOUZET, C., CHOLLET, P., PLAGNE, R., PETIT, J. and BERGER, J. A. (1988) Pharmacokinetics of cyclophosphamide administered alone or in combination with vindesin or cisplatin in 5 patients with bronchial adenocarcinoma. *Biomed. Pharmacother.* **42:** 555–560.

LEBLANC, G. A. and WAXMAN, D. J. (1989) Interaction of anticancer drugs with hepatic monooxygenase enzymes. *Drug Metab. Rev.* **20:** 395–439.

LEBLANC, G. A. and WAXMAN, D. J. (1990) Mechanisms of cyclophosphamide action on hepatic P-450 expression. *Cancer Res.* **50:** 5720–5726.

LEBLANC, G. A., SUNDSETH, S. S., WEBER, G. F. and WAXMAN, D. J. (1992) Platinum anticancer drugs modulate P-450 mRNA levels and differentially alter hepatic drug and steroid hormone metabolism in male and female rats. *Cancer Res.* **52:** 540–547.

LEE, F. Y. F. (1991) Glutathione diminishes the anti-tumor activity of 4-hydroperoxycyclophosphamide by stabilising its spontaneous breakdown to alkylating metabolites. *Br. J. Cancer* **63:** 45–50.

LEE, F. Y. F., FLANNERY, D. J. and SIEMANN, D. W. (1991) Prediction of tumour sensitivity to 4-hydroperoxycyclophosphamide by a glutathione-targeted assay. *Br. J. Cancer* **63:** 217–222.

LEE, F. Y. F., FLANNERY, D. J. and SIEMANN, D. W. (1992) Modulation of the cell cycle-dependent cytotoxicity of adriamycin and 4-hydroperoxycyclophosphamide by novobiocin, an inhibitor of mammalian topoisomerase II. *Cancer Res.* **52:** 3515–3520.

LEMOLI, R. M., STRIFE, A., CLARKSON, B. D., HALEY, J. D. and GULATI, S. C. (1992) TGF-beta 3 protects normal human hematopoietic progenitor cells treated with 4-hydroperoxycyclophosphamide in vitro. *Exp. Hemat.* **20:** 1252–1256.

LENSSEN, U. and HOHORST, H. J., (1979) Zur frage der permeabilität von *N,N*-bis(2-chloräthyl)-phosphorsäurediamid in tumorzellen. *J. Cancer Res. clin. Oncol.* **93:** 161–164.

LEVINE, L. A. and RICHIE, J. P. (1989) Urological complications of cyclophosphamide. *J. Urol.* **141:** 1063–1069.

LEVINS, P. L. and ROGERS, W. I. (1965) Nuclear magnetic resonance study of stability of a salt of *N,N*-bis(2-chloroethyl)phosphorodiamidic acid (NSC-69945) in aqueous solution. *Cancer Chemother. Rep.* **44:** 15–17.

LIN, K.-H. and LINDAHL, R. (1987) Role of aldehyde dehydrogenase activity in cyclophosphamide metabolism in rat hepatoma cell lines. *Biochem. Pharmac.* **36:** 3305–3307.

LIN, K-H., WINTERS, A. L. and LINDAHL, R. (1984) Regulation of aldehyde dehydrogenase activity in five rat hepatoma cell lines. *Cancer Res.* **44:** 5219–5226.

LIND, M. J., MARGISON, J. M., CERNY, T., THATCHER, N. and WILKINSON, P. M. (1989) Comparative pharmacokinetics and alkylating activity of fractionated intravenous and oral ifosfamide in patients with bronchogenic carcinoma. *Cancer Res.* **49:** 753–757.

LINDAHL, R. (1982) Induction of aldehyde dehydrogenase during hepatocarcinogenesis. In: *Enzymology of Carbonyl Metabolism: Aldehyde Dehydrogenase and Aldo/Keto Reductase*, pp. 121–135, WEINER, H. and WERMUTH, B. (eds) Alan R. Liss, Inc., New York.

LINFORD, J. H. (1961) Some interactions of nitrogen mustards with constituents of human blood serum. *Biochem. Pharmac.* **8:** 343–357.

LITTLE, S. A. and MIRKES, P. E. (1992) Effects of 4-hydroperoxycyclophosphamide and 4-hydroperoxydechlorocyclophosphamide on the cell cycle of post implantation rat embryos. *Teratology* **45:** 163–173.

LOW, J. E., BORCH, R. F. and SLADEK, N. E. (1982) Conversion of 4-hydroperoxycyclophosphamide and 4-hydroxycyclophosphamide to phosphoramide mustard and acrolein mediated by bifunctional catalysts. *Cancer Res.* **42:** 830–837.

LOW, J. E., BORCH, R. F. and SLADEK, N. E. (1983) Further studies on the conversion of 4-hydroxyoxazaphosphorines to reactive mustards and acrolein in inorganic buffers. *Cancer Res.* **43:** 5815–5820.

LUDEMAN, S. M., BOYD, V. L., REGAN, J. B., GALLO, K. A., ZON, G. and ISHII, K. (1986a) Synthesis of reactive metabolite-analogues of cyclophosphamide for comparisons of NMR kinetic parameters and anticancer screening data. *Drugs exp. clin. Res.* **12:** 527–532.

LUDEMAN, S. M., BOYD, V. L., REGAN, J. B., GALLO, K. A., ZON, G. and ISHII, K. (1986b) Synthesis and antitumor activity of cyclophosphamide analogues. 4. Preparation, kinetic studies, and anticancer screening of 'phenylketophosphamide' and similar compounds related to the cyclophosphamide metabolite aldophosphamide. *J. med. Chem.* **29:** 716–727.

LUDEMAN, S. M., HO, C.-K., BOAL, J. H., SWEET, E. M. and CHANG, Y. H. (1992) Carboxyphosphamide: NMR studies of its stability and cell membrane permeability. *Drug Metab. Disp.* **20:** 337–338.

MADDOCK, C. L., HANDLER, A. H., FRIEDMAN, O. M., FOLEY, G. E. and FARBER, S. (1966) Primary evaluation of alkylating agent cyclohexylamine salt of *N,N*-bis(2-chloroethyl)phosphorodiamidic acid (NSC 69945; OMF-59) in experimental antitumor assay systems. *Cancer Chemother. Rep.* **50:** 629–638.

MAKI, P. A. and SLADEK, N. E. (1991) Potentiation of the cytotoxic action of mafosfamide by *N*-isopropyl-*p*-formylbenzamide, a metabolite of procarbazine. *Cancer Res.* **51:** 4170–4175.

MAKI, P. A. and SLADEK, N. E. (1993) Sensitivity of aldehyde dehydrogenases in murine tumor and hematopoietic progenitor cells to inhibition by chloral hydrate as determined by the ability of chloral hydrate to potentiate the cytotoxic action of mafosfamide. *Biochem. Pharmac.* **45:** 231–239.

MANNA, A., SPARAVENTI, G., PALAZZI, M. and PORCELLINI, A. (1986) In vitro active cyclophosphamide derivatives in cleansing procedures intended for autologous bone marrow transplantation. *Haematologica* **71:** 257–261.

MANNERING, G. J. (1968) Significance of stimulation and inhibition of drug metabolism in pharmacological testing. In: *Selected Pharmacological Testing Methods*, pp. 51–119, BURGER, A. (ed.) Marcel Dekker, Inc., New York.

MANNERVIK, B., ALIN, P., GUTHENBERG, C., JENSSON, H., TAHIR, M. K., WARHOLM, M. and JORNVALL, H. (1985) Identification of three classes of cytosolic glutathione transferase common to several mammalian species: correlations between structural data and enzymatic properties. *Proc. natn. Acad. Sci. U.S.A.* **82:** 7202–7206.

MANTHEY, C. L. (1988) Resolution and characterization of the aldehyde dehydrogenases important in cyclophosphamide metabolism. Ph.D. Thesis, University of Minnesota, Minneapolis.

MANTHEY, C. L. and SLADEK, N. E. (1986) Characterization of NAD-linked aldehyde dehydrogenase catalysis of the oxidation of aldophosphamide by mouse liver fractions. *Proc. Am. Ass. Cancer Res.* **27:** 421.

MANTHEY, C. L. and SLADEK, N. E. (1988) Kinetic characterization of the catalysis of 'activated' cyclophosphamide (4-hydroxycyclophosphamide/aldophosphamide) oxidation to carboxyphosphamide by mouse hepatic aldehyde dehydrogenases. *Biochem. Pharmac.* **37:** 2781–2790.

MANTHEY, C. L. and SLADEK, N. E. (1989) Aldehyde dehydrogenase-catalyzed bioinactivation of cyclophosphamide. *Prog. clin. Biol. Res.* **290:** 49–63.

MANTHEY, C. L., LANDKAMER, G. J. and SLADEK, N. E. (1990) Identification of the mouse aldehyde dehydrogenases important in aldophosphamide detoxification. *Cancer Res.* **50:** 4991–5002.

MARMONT, A. M., DAMASIO, E. E., GIORDANO, D., CERRI, R. and BANCHI, L. (1979) Some modern aspects of systemic lupus erythematosus with special reference to the treatment with cyclophosphamide of lupus nephropathy. *Adv. Inflam. Res.* **1:** 591–603.

MARSELOS, M., TORRONEN, R., KOIVULA, T. and KOIVUSALO, M. (1979) Comparison of phenobarbital- and carcinogen-induced aldehyde dehydrogenases in the rat. *Biochim. biophys. Acta* **583:** 110–118.

MARX, J. L. (1981) Tumor viruses and the kinase connection. *Science* **211:** 1336–1338.

MASUREL, D., HOUGHTON, P. J., YOUNG, C. L. and WAINER, I. W. (1990) Efficacy, toxicity, pharmacokinetics, and in vitro metabolism of the enantiomers of ifosfamide in mice. *Cancer Res.* **50:** 252–255.

MATHER, P. B. and HOLMES, R. S. (1984) Biochemical genetics of aldehyde dehydrogenase isozymes in the mouse: evidence for stomach- and testis-specific enzymes. *Biochem. Gen.* **22:** 981–995.

MCCARTY, D. J. and CARRERA, G. F. (1982) Intractable rheumatoid arthritis. Treatment with combined cyclophosphamide, azathioprine, and hydroxychloroquine. *J. Am. med. Ass.* **248:** 1718–1723.

MCGOWN, A. T. and FOX, B. W. (1986) A proposed mechanism of resistance to cyclophosphamide and phosphoramide mustard in a Yoshida cell line in vitro. *Cancer Chemother. Pharmac.* **17:** 223–226.

MCNEIL, N. O. and MORGAN, L. R., JR (1981) The bioavailability of oral and intravenous ifosfamide in the treatment of bronchogenic carcinoma. *Int. J. clin. Pharmac. Ther. Toxic.* **19:** 490–493.

MEEHAN, R. R., GOSDEN, J. R., ROUT, D., HASTIE, N. D., FRIEDBERG, T., ADESNIK, M., BUCKLAND, R., VAN HEYNINGEN, V., FLETCHER, J., SPURR, N. K., SWEENEY, J. and WOLF, C. R. (1988) Human cytochrome P-450 PB-1: a multigene family involved in mephenytoin and steroid oxidations that maps to chromosome 10. *Am. J. Human Gen.* **42:** 26–37.

MEHTA, J. R., PRZYBYLSKI, M. and LUDLUM, D. B. (1980) Alkylation of guanosine and deoxyguanosine by phosphoramide mustard. *Cancer Res.* **40:** 4183–4186.

MEISTER, A. (1991) Glutathione deficiency produced by inhibition of its synthesis, and its reversal; applications in research and therapy. *Pharmac. Ther.* **51:** 155–194.

MELLETT, L. B., EL DAREER, S. M., LUCE, J. K. and KREI, E. III (1969) Activation of cyclophosphamide metabolism in various species. *Pharmacologist* **11:** 273.

MILSTED, R. A. V. and JARMAN, M. (1978) Haemodialysis during cyclophosphamide treatment. *Br. med. J.* **1:** 820–821.

MILSTED, R. A. V. and JARMAN, M. (1982) Metabolism of high doses of cyclophosphamide. *Cancer Chemother. Pharmac.* **8:** 311–313.

MIRKES, P. E. (1985) Cyclophosphamide teratogenesis: a review. *Teratog. Carcinog. Mutagen.* **5:** 75–88.

MIRKES, P. E., FANTEL, A. G., GREENAWAY, J. C. and SHEPARD, T. H. (1981) Teratogenicity of cyclophosphamide metabolites: phosphoramide mustard, acrolein, and 4-ketocyclophosphamide in rat embryos cultured in vitro. *Toxic. appl. Pharmac.* **58:** 322–330.

MIRKES, P. E., ELLISON, A. and LITTLE, S. A. (1990) Role of aldehyde dehydrogenase in the detoxification of cyclophosphamide in rat embryos. *Adv. exp. med. Biol.* **284:** 85–90.

MISTRY, P. and HARRAP, K. R. (1991) Historical aspects of glutathione and cancer chemotherapy. *Pharmac. Ther.* **49:** 125–132.

MITCHELL, D. Y. and PETERSEN, D. R. (1988) Inhibition of rat liver aldehyde dehydrogenases by acrolein. *Drug Metab. Disp.* **16:** 37–42.

MITCHELL, D. Y. and PETERSEN, D. R. (1989) Metabolism of the glutathione-acrolein adduct, *S*-(2-aldehydoethyl)glutathione, by rat liver alcohol and aldehyde dehydrogenase. *J. Pharmac. exp. Ther.* **251:** 193–198.

MOKYR, M. B. and DRAY, S. (1987) Interplay between the toxic effects of anticancer drugs and host antitumor immunity in cancer therapy. *Cancer Invest.* **5:** 31–38.

MONTGOMERY, J. A. and STRUCK, R. F. (1973) The relationship of the metabolism of anticancer agents to their activity. *Prog. Drug Res.* **17:** 320–409.

MONTGOMERY, J. A. and STRUCK, R. F. (1976) Synthesis and structure–activity relationships of pre-activated analogs of cyclophosphamide (NSC-26271). *Cancer Treat. Rep.* **60:** 381–393.

MOORE, M. J. (1991) Clinical pharmacokinetics of cyclophosphamide. *Clin. Pharmacokinet.* **20:** 194–208.

MOORE, M. J., HARDY, R. W., THIESSEN, J. J., SOLDIN, S. J. and ERLICHMAN, C. (1988) Rapid development of enhanced clearance after high-dose cyclophosphamide. *Clin. Pharmac. Ther.* **44:** 622–628.

MOREB, J., ZUCALI, J. R., GROSS, M. A. and WEINER, R. S. (1989a) Protective effects of IL-1 on human hematopoietic progenitor cells treated in vitro with 4-hydroperoxycyclophosphamide. *J. Immun.* **142:** 1937–1942.

MOREB, J., ZUCALI, J. R., GROSS, M. A. and WEINER, R. S. (1989b) IL-1 protects human colony forming cells but not HL-60 and K562 leukemic cell lines from the toxic effects of 4-hydroperoxycyclophosphamide. In: *Autologous Bone Marrow Transplantation, Proceedings of the Fourth International Symposium*, pp. 637–643,

DICKE, K. A., SPITZER, G., JAGANNATH, S. and EVINGER HODGES, M. J. (eds) The University of Texas M.D. Anderson Cancer Center, Houston.

MOREB, J., ZUCALI, J. R. and RUETH, S. (1990) The effects of tumor necrosis factor-α on early human hematopoietic progenitor cells treated with 4-hydroperoxycyclophosphamide. *Blood* **76:** 681–689.

MOREB, J., ZUCALI, J. R., ZHANG, Y., COLVIN, O. M. and GROSS, M. A. (1992) Role of aldehyde dehydrogenase in the protection of hematopoietic progenitor cells from 4-hydroperoxycyclophosphamide by interleukin 1β and tumor necrosis factor. *Cancer Res.* **52:** 1770–1774.

MORGAN, L. R., POSEY, L. E., RAINEY, J., BICKERS, J., RYAN, D., VIAL, R. and HULL, E. W. (1981) Ifosfamide: a weekly dose fractionated schedule in bronchogenic carcinoma. *Cancer Treat. Rep.* **65:** 693–695.

MORGENSTERN, R., GUTHENBERG, C. and DEPIERRE, J. W. (1982) Microsomal glutathione-*S*-transferase. Purification, initial characterization and demonstration that it is not identical to the cytosolic glutathione-*S*-transferases A, B and C. *Eur. J. Biochem.* **128:** 243–248.

MORGENSTERN, R., LUNDQVIST, G., ANDERSSON, G., BALK, L. and DEPIERRE, J. W. (1984) The distribution of microsomal glutathione transferase among different organelles, different organs, and different organisms. *Biochem. Pharmac.* **33:** 3609–3614.

MOURIDSEN, H. T., FABER, O. and SKOVSTED, L. (1974) The biotransformation of cyclophosphamide in man: analysis of the variation in normal subjects. *Acta Pharmac. Toxic.* **35:** 98–106.

MOURIDSEN, H. T., FABER, O. and SKOVSTED, L. (1976) The metabolism of cyclophosphamide. Dose dependency and the effect of long-term treatment with cyclophosphamide. *Cancer* **37:** 665–670.

MUKHERJEE, A. P. (1971) Combined prednisolone, azathioprine, and cyclophosphamide treatment for persistent proliferative glomerulonephritis in adults. *Lancet* **ii:** 1350–1353.

MYERS, L. W. (1987) The use of cyclophosphamide to treat multiple sclerosis. *Clin. Neuropharmac.* **10:** 155–161.

MYLES, A., FENSELAU, C. and FRIEDMAN, O. M. (1977) Synthesis of aldophosphamide, a key cyclophosphamide metabolite. *Tetrahedron Lett.* **29:** 2475–2478.

NAGASAWA, H. T., ELBERLING, J. A. and DEMASTER, E. G. (1984) Latent inhibitors of aldehyde dehydrogenases as alcohol deterrent agents. *J. med. Chem.* **27:** 1335–1339.

NAKANISHI, S., SHIOHARA, E., TSUKADA, M., YAMAZAKI, H., NISHIGUCHI, K. and SALADIN, R. (1979) Genetic control of responsiveness of rat liver supernatant aldehyde dehydrogenase to phenobarbital and 3-methylcholanthrene. *Arch. Toxic.* **43:** 135–140.

NATHANSON, L., HALL, T. C., RUTENBERG, A. and SHADDUCK, R. K. (1967) Clinical toxicologic study of cyclohexylamine salt of *N,N*-bis(2-chloroethyl)phosphorodiamidic acid (NSC-69945; OMF-59). *Cancer Chemother. Rep.* **51:** 35–39.

NEBERT, D. W., NELSON, D. R., COON, M. J., ESTABROOK, R. W., FEYERSON, R., FUJII-KURIYAMA, Y., GONZALEZ, F. J., GUENGERICH, F. P., GUNSALUS, I. C., JOHNSON, E. F., LOPOR, J. C., SATO, R., WATERMAN, M. R. and WAXMAN, D. J. (1991) The P450 superfamily: update on new sequences, gene mapping, and recommended nomenclature. *DNA Cell Biol.* **10:** 1–14.

NEIDHART, J. A., KOHLER, W., STIDLEY, C., MANGALIK, A., PLAUCHE, A., ANDERSON, T., QUENZER, R. W. and RINEHART, J. J. (1990) Phase I study of repeated cycles of high-dose cyclophosphamide, etoposide, and cisplatin administered without bone marrow transplantation. *J. clin. Oncol.* **8:** 1728–1738.

NEIMS, A. H., WARNER, M., LOUGHNAN, P. M. and ARANDA, J. V. (1976) Developmental aspects of the hepatic cytochrome P450 monooxygenase system. *Ann. Rev. Pharmac. Toxic.* **16:** 427–445.

NELSON, R. L., ALLEN, L. M. and CREAVEN, P. J. (1977) Pharmacokinetics of divided-dose ifosfamide. *Clin. Pharmac. Ther.* **19:** 365–370.

NIEMEYER, U., ENGEL, J., SCHEFFLER, G., MOLGE, K., SAUERBIER, D. and WEIGERT, W. (1984) Chemical characterization of ASTA Z 7557 (INN mafosfamide, *cis*-4-sulfoethylthiocyclophosphamide), a stable derivative of 4-hydroxycyclophosphamide. *Invest. New Drugs* **2:** 133–139.

NIEMEYER, U., ENGEL, J., HILGARD, P., PEUKERT, M., POHL, J. and SINDERMANN, H. (1989) Mafosfamide—a derivative of 4-hydroxycyclophosphamide. *Prog. clin. Biochem. Med.* **9:** 35–60.

NORPOTH, K. (1969) Untersuchungen zur oxydativen umsetzung von Endoxan in vivo und in vitro. Münster, Habilitationsschrift, Fach Physiologische Chemi, Westfälischen Wilhelms-Universität.

NORPOTH, K. (1976) Studies on the metabolism of isophosphamide (NSC-109724) in man. *Cancer Treat. Rep.* **60:** 437–443.

NORPOTH, K., GOLOVINSKY, E. and RAUEN, H. M. (1970) Utersuchungen an hypothetischen metaboliten des 2-[bis(2-chloräthyl)amino]tetrahydro-2H-1,3,2-oxazaphosphorin-2-oxids (cyclophosphamide). *Hoppe-Seyler's Z. Physiol. Chem.* **351:** 377–383.

O'DWYER, P. J., HAMILTON, T. C., YOUNG, R. C. LACRETA, F. P., CARP, N., TEW, K. D., PADAVIC, K., COMIS, R. L. and OZOLS, R. F. (1992) Depletion of glutathione in normal and malignant human cells in vivo by buthionine sulfoximine: clinical and biochemical results. *J. natn. Cancer Inst.* **84:** 264–267.

OESCH-BARTLOMOWICZ, B., VOGEL, S., ARENS, H.-J. and OESCH, F. (1990) Modulation of the control of mutagenic metabolites derived from cyclophosphamide and ifosfamide by stimulation of protein kinase A. *Mutat. Res.* **232:** 305–312.

OHTA, M., TANIMOTO, T. and TANAKA, A. (1991) Localization, isolation and properties of three NADPH-dependent aldehyde reducing enzymes from dog kidney. *Biochim. biophys. Acta* **1078:** 395–403.

OKEY, A. B. (1990) Enzyme induction in the cytochrome P-450 system. *Pharmac. Ther.* **45:** 241–298.

OSINSKY, S., BUBNOVSKAJA, L. and SERGIENKO, T. (1987) Tumor pH under induced hyperglycemia and efficacy of chemotherapy. *Anticancer Res.* **7:** 199–202.

OTTOLENGHI, L., MORASCA, L., MARSONI, S., PIAZZA, E., SORESI, E., LIBRETTI, A. and GARATTINI, S. (1980) Plasma levels of cyclophosphamide in patients under polychemotherapeutic regimens. *Biomedicine* **32:** 123–127.

PALLANTE, S. L., LISEK, C. A., DULIK, D. M. and FENSELAU, C. (1986) Glutathione conjugates. Immobilized enzyme synthesis and characterization by fast atom bombardment mas spectrometry. *Drug Metab. Disp.* **14:** 313–318.

PANCHENKO, L. F., PIROZHKOV, S. V. and ANTONENKOV, V. D. (1985) Subcellular distribution and properties of a clofibrate-induced aldehyde dehydrogenase from rat liver. *Biochem. Pharmac.* **34:** 471–479.

PAPA, M. Z., YANG, J. C., VETTO, J. T., SHILONI, E., EISENTHAL, A. and ROSENBERG, S. A. (1988) Combined effects of chemotherapy and interleukin 2 in the therapy of mice with advanced pulmonary tumors. *Cancer Res.* **48:** 122–129.

PAREKH, H. K. and SLADEK, N. E. (1993) NADPH-dependent enzyme-catalyzed reduction of aldophosphamide, the pivotal metabolite of cyclophosphamide. *Proc. Am. Ass. Cancer Res.* **34:** 270.

PATEL, J. M. (1990) Metabolism and pulmonary toxicity of cyclophosphamide. *Pharmac. Ther.* **47:** 137–146.

PELKONEN, O. and NEBERT, D. W. (1982) Metabolism of polycyclic aromatic hydrocarbons: etiologic role in carcinogenesis. *Pharmac. Rev.* **34:** 189–222.

PEREZ, R. P., HAMILTON, T. C. and OZOLS, R. F. (1990) Resistance to alkylating agents and cisplatin: insights from ovarian carcinoma model systems. *Pharmac. Ther.* **48:** 19–27.

PERIN, A., SESSA, A. and CIARANFI, E. (1978) Carcinostatic effect of aliphatic aldehydes and aldehyde dehydrogenase activity in Ehrlich carcinoma, Sarcoma 180, and Yoshida AH 130 hepatoma. *Cancer Res.* **38:** 2180–2184.

PETER, G. and HOHORST, H. J. (1979) Synthesis and preliminary antitumor evaluation of 4-(SR)-sulfido-cyclophosphamides. *Cancer Chemother. Pharmac.* **3:** 181–188.

PETER, G., WAGNER, T. and HOHORST, H. J. (1976) Studies on 4-hydroperoxycyclophosphamide (NSC-181815): a simple preparation method and its application for the synthesis of a new class of 'activated' sulfur-containing cyclophosphamide (NSC-26271) derivatives. *Cancer Treat. Rep.* **60:** 429–435.

PETERS, R. H., BALLARD, K., OATIS, J. E., JOLLOW, D. J. and STUART, R. K. (1990) Cellular glutathione as a protective agent against 4-hydroperoxycyclophosphamide cytotoxicity in K-562 cells. *Cancer Chemother. Pharmac.* **26:** 397–402.

PETERS, R. H., JOLLOW, D. J. and STUART, R. K. (1991) Role of glutathione in the in vitro synergism between 4-hydroperoxycyclophosphamide and cisplatin in leukemia cell lines. *Cancer Res.* **51:** 2536–2541.

PETERSEN, D. R., COLLINS, A. C. and DEITRICH, R. A. (1977) Role of liver cytosolic aldehyde dehydrogenase isozymes in control of blood acetaldehyde concentrations. *J. Pharmac. exp. Ther.* **201:** 471–481.

PHILIPS, F. S., STERNBERG, S. S., CRONIN, A. P. and VIDAL, P. M. (1961) Cyclophosphamide and urinary bladder toxicity. *Cancer Res.* **21:** 1577–1589.

PHILLIPS, G. L. and CONNORS, J. M. (1987) Bone marrow transplantation for malignant lymphoma. In: *Progress in Bone Marrow Transplantation*, pp. 799–825, Gale, R. P. and Champlin, R. (eds) Alan R. Liss, New York.

PHILLIPS, P. C., THAN, T. T., CORK, L. C., HILTON, J., CARSON, B. S., COLVIN, O. M. and GROCHOW, L. B. (1992) Intrathecal 4-hydroperoxycyclophosphamide: neurotoxicity, cerebrospinal fluid pharmacokinetics, and antitumor activity in a rabbit model of VX2 leptomeningeal carcinomatosis. *Cancer Res.* **52:** 6168–6174.

PIAZZA, E., CATTANEO, M. T. and VARINI, M. (1984) Pharmacokinetic studies in lung cancer patients. *Cancer* **54:** 1187–1192.

PLOWCHALK, D. R. and MATTISON, D. R. (1991) Phosphoramide mustard is responsible for the ovarian toxicity of cyclophosphamide. *Toxic. appl. Pharmac.* **107:** 472–481.

POOLE, D. T. (1967) Intracellular pH of the Ehrlich ascites tumor cell as it is affected by sugar and sugar derivatives. *J. biol. Chem.* **242:** 3731–3736.

POOLE, D. T. and BUTLER, T.C. (1969) Effects of inhibitors of glycolysis on intracellular pH and on accumulation of glycolytic intermediates in the Ehrlich ascites tumor cell. *J. natn. Cancer Inst.* **42:** 1027–1033.

POOLE, D. T., BUTLER, T. C. and WADDELL, W. J. (1964) Intracellular pH of the Ehrlich ascites tumor cell. *J. natn. Cancer Inst.* **32:** 939–946.

POWERS, J. F. (1981) Circulating phosphoramide mustard and the pharmacologic action of cyclophosphamide. Ph.D. Thesis, University of Minnesota, Minneapolis.

POWERS, J. F. and SLADEK, N. E. (1978) Influence of thiosulfate on the cytotoxic action of cyclophosphamide metabolites. *Pharmacologist* **20:** 250.

POWERS, J. F. and SLADEK, N. E. (1983) Cytotoxic activity relative to 4-hydroxycyclophosphamide and phosphoramide mustard concentrations in the plasma of cyclophosphamide-treated rats. *Cancer Res.* **43:** 1101–1106.

POWIS, G., REECE, P., AHMANN, D. L. and INGLE, J. N. (1987) Effect of body weight on the pharmacokinetics of cyclophosphamide in breast cancer patients. *Cancer Chemother. Pharmac.* **20:** 219–222.

PRATT, C. B., HOROWITZ, M. E., MEYER, W. H., ETCUBANAS, E., THOMPSON, E. I., DOUGLASS, E. C., WILIMAS, J. A., HAYES, F. A. and GREEN, A. A. (1987) Phase II trial of ifosfamide in children with malignant solid tumors. *Cancer Treat. Rep.* **71:** 131–135.

RACKER, E. (1972) Bioenergetics and the problem of tumor growth. *Am. Sci.* **60:** 56–63.

RADIN, A. I., ZHAO, X.-L., WOO, T. H., COLVIN, O. M. and HILTON, J. (1991) Structure and expression of the cytosolic aldehyde dehydrogenase gene in cyclophosphamide-resistant murine leukemia L1210 cells. *Biochem. Pharmac.* **42:** 1933–1939.

Ramonas, L. M., Erickson, L. C., Klesse, W., Kohn, K. W. and Zaharko, D.S. (1981) Differential cytotoxicity and DNA cross-linking produced by polymeric and monomeric activated analogs of cyclophosphamide in mouse L1210 leukemia cells. *Molec. Pharmac.* **19:** 331–336.

Rauen, H. M. and Kramer, K. P. (1964) Der gesamtalkylantien-blutspiegel von ratten nach verabreichung von cyclophosphamid und acyclophosphamid. *Arzneim.-Forsch. Drug Res.* **14:** 1066–1067.

Redmond, G. and Cohen, G. (1971) Induction of liver acetaldehyde dehydrogenase: possible role in ethanol tolerance after exposure to barbiturates. *Science* **171:** 387–389.

Redwood, W. R., Hilton, J., Colvin, M. and Owens, A. H., Jr (1982) The cellular uptake of 4-hydroperoxycyclophosphamide. *Proc. Am. Ass. Cancer Res.* **23:** 169.

Reissmann, T., Voegeli, R., Pohl, J. and Hilgard, P. (1989) Augmentation of host antitumor immunity by low doses of cyclophosphamide and mafosfamide in two animal tumor models. *Cancer Immun. Immunother.* **28:** 179–184.

Richardson, M. E. and Siemann, D. W. (1992) Thiol manipulation as a means of overcoming drug resistance in a novel cyclophosphamide-induced resistant cell line. *Int. J. Radiation Oncol. Biol. Phys.* **22:** 781–784.

Riggs, C. E., Jr, Egorin, M. J., Fuks, J. Z., Schnaper, N., Duffey, P., Colvin, O. M., Aisner, J., Wiernik, P. H. and Bachur, N. R. (1981) Initial observations on the effects of Δ^9-tetrahydrocannabinol on the plasma pharmacokinetics of cyclophosphamide and doxorubicin. *J. clin. Pharmac.* **21:** 90S–98S.

Ritschel, W. A., Bykadi, G., Norman, E. J., Cluxton, R. J. and Denton, D. (1981) Salivary elimination of cyclophosphamide in man. *J. clin. Pharmac.* **21:** 461–465.

Rizzoli, V. and Mangoni, L. (1990) Pharmacological-mediated purging with mafosfamide in acute and chronic myeloid leukemias. *Prog. clin. Biol. Res.* **333:** 21–38.

Rosenberg, S. A. (1984) Adoptive immunotherapy of cancer: accomplishments and prospects. *Cancer Treat. Rep.* **68:** 233–255.

Rosenberg, S. A., Spiess, P. and Lafreniere, R. (1986) A new approach to the adoptive immunotherapy of cancer with tumor-infiltrating lymphocytes. *Science* **233:** 1318–1321.

Rosenberg, S. A., Packard, B. S., Aebersold, P. M., Solomon, D., Topalian, S. L., Toy, S. T., Simon, P., Lotze, M. T., Yang, J. C., Seipp, C. A., Simpson, C., Carter, C., Bock, S., Schwartzentruber, D., Wei, J. P. and White, D. E. (1988) Use of tumor-infiltrating lymphocytes and interleukin-2 in the immunotherapy of patients with metastatic melanoma. A preliminary report. *New Engl. J. Med.* **319:** 1676–1680.

Ruckdeschel, J. C., Carney, D. N., Oie, H. K., Russell, E. K. and Gazdar, A. F. (1987) In vitro chemosensitivity of human lung cancer cell lines. *Cancer Treat. Rep.* **71:** 697–704.

Russo, J. E. and Hilton, J. (1988) Characterization of cytosolic aldehyde dehydrogenase from cyclophosphamide resistant L1210 cells. *Cancer Res.* **48:** 2963–2968.

Russo, J. E., Hilton, J. and Colvin, O. M. (1989) The role of aldehyde dehydrogenase isozymes in cellular resistance to the alkylating agent cyclophosphamide. *Prog. clin. Biol. Res.* **290:** 65–79.

Rutenburg, A. M., Persky, L., Friedman, O. M. and Seligman, A. M. (1954) Toxicity in mice of new secondary nitrogen mustards. *J. Pharmac. exp. Ther.* **111:** 483–488.

Ruzicka, J. A. and Ruenitz, P. C. (1992) Cytochrome P-450-mediated *N*-dechloroethylation of cyclophosphamide and ifosfamide in the rat. *Drug Metab. Disp.* **20:** 770–772.

Ryan, D. E. and Levin, W. (1990) Purification and characterization of hepatic microsomal cytochrome P-450. *Pharmac. Ther.* **45:** 153–239.

Sahovic, E., Colvin, M., Hilton, J. and Ogawa, M. (1988) Role for aldehyde dehydrogenase in survival of progenitors for murine blast cell colonies after treatment with 4-hydroperoxycyclophosphamide in vitro. *Cancer Res.* **48:** 1223–1226.

Santos, G. W., Yeager, A. M. and Jones, R. J. (1989) Autologous bone marrow transplantation. *Ann. Rev. Med.* **40:** 99–112.

Schabel, F. M., Jr, Skipper, H. E., Trader, M. W., Laster, W. R., Jr, Griswold, D. P., Jr and Corbett, T. H. (1983) Establishment of cross-resistance profiles for new agents. *Cancer Treat. Rep.* **67:** 905–922.

Schauenstein, E. and Esterbauer, H. (1979) Formation and properties of reactive aldehydes. In: *Submolecular Biology in Cancer*, **67:** 225–244, Ciba Foundation Symposium London, 1978, Excerpta Medica, Amsterdam.

Schloerb, P. R., Blackburn, G. L., Grantham, J. J., Mallard, D. S. and Cage, G. K. (1965) Intracellular pH and buffering capacity of the Walker 256 carcinoma. *Surgery (St. Louis)* **58:** 5–11.

Schmid, F. A., Otter, G. M. and Stock, C. C. (1980) Resistance patterns of Walker carcinosarcoma 256 and other rodent tumors to cyclophosphamide and 1-phenylalanine mustard. *Cancer Res.* **40:** 830–833.

Schuler, U., Ehninger, G. and Wagner, T. (1987) Repeated high-dose cyclophosphamide administration in bone marrow transplantation: exposure to activated metabolites. *Cancer Chemother. Pharmac.* **20:** 248–252.

Schuler, U., Waidelich, P., Kolb, H., Wagner, T. and Ehninger, G. (1991) Pharmacokinetics and metabolism of cyclophosphamide administered after total body irradiation of bone marrow transplant recipients. *Eur. J. clin. Pharmac.* **40:** 521–523.

Schwarz, M., Peres, G., Buchmann, A., Friedberg, T., Waxman, D. J. and Kunz, W. (1987) Phenobarbital induction of cytochrome P-450 in normal and preneoplastic rat liver: comparison of enzyme and mRNA expression as detected by immunohistochemistry and in situ hybridization. *Carcinogenesis* **8:** 1355–1357.

SEITZ, D. E., WINTER, M. A. and PEARCE, H. L. (1989) Evaluation of the potential of glutathione-*S*-transferase to catalyze the reaction of phosphoramide mustard, cyclophosphamide or ifosfamide and N-acetylcysteine or glutathione. *Proc. Am. Ass. Cancer Res.* **30:** 497.

SELIGMAN, A. M., NACHLAS, M. M., MANHEIMER, L. H., FRIEDMAN, O. M. and WOLF, G. (1949) Development of new methods for the histochemical demonstration of hydrolytic intracellular enzymes in a program of cancer research. *Ann. Surg.* **130:** 333–341.

SENSENBRENNER, L. L., MARINI, J. J. and COLVIN, M. (1979) Comparative effects of cyclophosphamide, isophosphamide, 4-methylcyclophosphamide, and phosphoramide mustard on murine hematopoietic and immunocompetent cells. *J. natn. Cancer Inst.* **62:** 975–981.

SESSINK, P. J. M., VAN DEN BROEK, P. H. H. and BOS, R. P. (1991) Urinary cyclophosphamide excretion in rats after intrathecal, dermal, oral and intravenous administration of cyclophosphamide. *J. appl. Toxic.* **11:** 125–128.

SHAND, F. L. (1978) The capacity of microsomally-activated cyclophosphamide to induce immunosuppression in vivo. *Immunology* **35:** 1017–1025.

SHARKIS, S. J., SANTOS, G. W. and COLVIN, M. (1980) Elimination of acute myelogenous leukemic cells from marrow and tumor suspensions in the rat with 4-hydroperoxycyclophoshamide. *Blood* **55:** 521–523.

SHORT, C. R., KINDEN, D. A. and STITH, R. (1976) Fetal and neonatal development of the microsomal monooxygenase system. *Drug Metab. Rev.* **5:** 1–42.

SHORT, R. D. and GIBSON, J. E. (1971) Development of cyclophosphamide activation and its implications in perinatal toxicity to mice. *Toxic. appl. Pharmac.* **19:** 103–110.

SIDHU, R. S. and BLAIR, A. H. (1975) Human liver dehydrogenase. Kinetics of aldehyde oxidation. *J. biol. Chem.* **250:** 7899–7904.

SIMARD, C. and JOLICOEUR, P. (1991) The effect of anti-neoplastic drugs on murine acquired immunodeficiency syndrome. *Science* **251:** 305–308.

SIMONSEN, L. O. and CORNELIUS, F. (1978) Inorganic phosphate in Ehrlich ascites tumor cells and its distribution across the cell membrane. *Biochim. biophys. Acta* **511:** 213–223.

SINDERMANN, H., PEUKERT, M. and HILGARD, P. (1989) Bone marrow purging with mafosfamide—a critical survey. *Blut* **59:** 432–441.

SLADEK, N. E. (1971) Metabolism of cyclophosphamide by rat hepatic microsomes. *Cancer Res.* **31:** 901–908.

SLADEK, N. E. (1972a) Therapeutic efficacy of cyclophosphamide as a function of its metabolism. *Cancer Res.* **32:** 535–542.

SLADEK, N. E. (1972b) Therapeutic efficacy of cyclophosphamide as a function of inhibition of its metabolism. *Cancer Res.* **32:** 1848–1854.

SLADEK, N. E. (1973a) Evidence for an aldehyde possessing alkylating activity as the primary metabolite of cyclophosphamide. *Cancer Res.* **33:** 651–658.

SLADEK, N. E. (1973b) Bioassay and relative cytotoxic potency of cyclophosphamide metabolites generated in vitro and in vivo. *Cancer Res.* **33:** 1150–1159.

SLADEK, N. E. (1977a) Potentiation of the cytotoxic action of melphalan and 'activated' cyclophosphamide against tumor cells growing in vitro by centrophenoxine. *J. Pharmac. exp. Ther.* **200:** 17–24.

SLADEK, N. E. (1977b) Potentiation of antitumor drug action by centrophenoxine: specificity. *J. Pharmac. exp. Ther.* **201:** 518–526.

SLADEK, N. E. (1977c) Cytotoxic activity of alkylating agents in the presence of centrophenoxine and its hydrolysis products. *J. Pharmac. exp. Ther.* **203:** 630–639.

SLADEK, N. E. (1987) Oxazaphosphorines. In: *Metabolism and Actions of Anticancer Drugs*, pp. 48–90, POWIS, G. and PROUGH, R. (eds) Taylor and Francis, London.

SLADEK, N. E. (1988) Metabolism of oxazaphosphorines. *Pharmac. Ther.* **37:** 301–355.

SLADEK, N. E. (1993) Oxazaphosphorine-specific acquired cellular resistance. In: *Drug Resistance in Oncology*, pp. 375–411, TEICHER, B. A. (ed.) Marcel Dekker, New York.

SLADEK, N. E. and LANDKAMER, G. J. (1985) Restoration of sensitivity to oxazaphosphorines by inhibitors of aldehyde dehydrogenase activity in cultured oxazaphosphorine-resistant L1210 and cross-linking agent-resistant P388 cell lines. *Cancer Res.* **45:** 1549–1555.

SLADEK, N. E., DOMEYER, B. E., MERRIMAN, R. L. and BROPHY, G. T. (1978) Differential effects of Walker 256 carcinosarcoma cells growing subcutaneously, intramuscularly, or intraperitoneally on hepatic microsomal mixed-function oxygenase activity. *Drug Metab. Disp.* **6:** 412–417.

SLADEK, N. E., PRIEST, J., DOEDEN, D., MIROCHA, C. J., PATHRE, S. and KRIVIT, W. (1980) Plasma half-life and urinary excretion of cyclophosphamide in children. *Cancer Treat. Rep.* **64:** 1061–1066.

SLADEK, N. E., SMITH, P. C., BRATT, P. M., LOW, J. E., POWERS, J. F., BORCH, R. F. and COVENEY, J. R. (1982) Influence of diuretics on urinary general base catalytic activity and cyclophosphamide-induced bladder toxicity. *Cancer Treat. Rep.* **66:** 1889–1900.

SLADEK, N. E., DOEDEN, D., POWERS, J. F. and KRIVIT, W. (1984a) Plasma concentrations of 4-hydroxycyclophosphamide and phosphoramide mustard in patients repeatedly given high doses of cyclophosphamide in preparation for bone marrow transplantation. *Cancer Treat. Rep.* **68:** 1247–1254.

SLADEK, N. E., POWERS, J. F. and GRAGE, G. (1984b) Half-life of oxazaphosphorines in biological fluids. *Drug Metab. Disp.* **12:** 553–559.

SLADEK, N. E., LOW, J. E. and LANDKAMER, G. J. (1985) Collateral sensitivity to cross-linking agents exhibited by cultured L1210 cells resistant to oxazaphosphorines. *Cancer Res.* **45:** 625–629.

SLADEK, N. E., MANTHEY, C. L., MAKI, P. A., ZHANG, Z. and LANDKAMER, G. J. (1989) Xenobiotic oxidation catalyzed by aldehyde dehydrogenases. *Drug Metab. Rev.* **20:** 697–720.

SLADEK, N. E., DOCKHAM, P. A. and LEE, M.-O. (1990) Human and mouse hepatic aldehyde dehydrogenases important in the biotransformation of cyclophosphamide and the retinoids. *Adv. exp. med. Biol.* **284:** 97–104.

SLOTT, V. L. and HALES, B. F. (1988) Role of the 4-hydroxy intermediate in the in vitro embryotoxicity of cyclophosphamide and dechlorocyclophosphamide. *Toxic. Appl. Pharmac.* **92:** 170–178.

SMITH, P. C. and SLADEK, N. E. (1985) Sensitivity of murine B- and T-lymphocytes to oxazaphosphorine and non-oxazaphosphorine nitrogen mustards. *Biochem. Pharmac.* **34:** 3459–3463.

SMITH, R. D. and KEHRER, J. P. (1991) Cooxidation of cyclophosphamide as an alternative pathway for its bioactivation and lung toxicity. *Cancer Res.* **51:** 542–548.

SMOLEN, A., ATKINSON, N. and PETERSEN, D. R. (1980) The role of liver cytosolic aldehyde dehydrogenase in ethanol metabolism in DBA and C57B1 mice. In: *Alcohol and Aldehyde Metabolizing Systems-IV*, pp. 627–634, THURMAN, R. G. (ed.) Plenum Press, New York and London.

SONAWAT, H. M., LEIBFRITZ, D., ENGEL, J. and HILGARD, P. (1990) Biotransformation of mafosfamide in P388 mice leukemia cells: intracellular ^{31}P-NMR studies. *Biochim. biophys. Acta* **1052:** 36–41.

SREERAMA, L. and SLADEK, N. E. (1991) Apparently resistance-irrelevant elevated aldehyde dehydrogenase-3 activity in a breast adenocarcinoma cell line exhibiting oxazaphosphorine-specific acquired resistance. *Proc. Am. Ass. Cancer Res.* **32:** 352.

SREERAMA, L. and SLADEK, N. E. (1992) Identification of a novel class 3 aldehyde dehydrogenase over-expressed in a human breast adenocarcinoma cell line (MCF-7/OAP) exhibiting oxazaphosphorine-specific acquired resistance. *Proc. Am. Ass. Cancer Res.* **33:** 447.

STARZL, T. E., PUTNAM, C. W., HALGRIMSON, C. G., SCHROTER, G. T., MARTINEAU, G., LAUNOIS, B., CORMAN, J. L., PENN, I., BOOTH, A. S., JR, GROTH, C. G. and PORTER, K. A. (1971) Cyclophosphamide and whole organ transplantation in human beings. *Gynec. Obstetr.* **133:** 981–991.

STEC, W. J. (1982) Cyclophosphamide and its congeners. *J. Organophos. Chem.* **13:** 145–174.

STILLWELL, T. J. and BENSON, R. C. JR (1988) Cyclophosphamide-induced hemorrhagic cystitis. A review of 100 patients. *Cancer* **61:** 451–457.

STRUCK, R. F. (1974) Isolation and identification of a stabilized derivative of aldophosphamide, a major metabolite of cyclophosphamide. *Cancer Res.* **34:** 2933–2935.

STRUCK, R. F. (1976) Aldophosphamide: synthesis, characterization, and comparison with 'Hohorst's aldophosphamide'. *Cancer Treat. Rep.* **60:** 317–319.

STRUCK, R. F., KIRK, M. C., MELLETT, L. B., EL DAREER, S. and HILL, D. L. (1971) Urinary metabolites of the antitumor agent cyclophosphamide. *Molec. Pharmac.* **7:** 519–529.

STRUCK, R. F., KIRK, M. C., WITT, M. H. and LASTER, W. R., JR (1975) Isolation and mass spectral identification of blood metabolites of cyclophosphamide: evidence for phosphoramide mustard as the biologically active metabolite. *Biomed. Mass Spectrom.* **2:** 46–52.

STRUCK, R. F., TRADER, M. W., DYKES, D. J., CORBETT, T. H. and LASTER, W. R., JR (1979) Synthesis and antitumor evaluation of isophosphoramide mustard, the active metabolite of the clinical antitumor agent ifosfamide. In: *Current Chemotherapy and Infectious Disease. Proceedings of the Eleventh Congress of Chemotherapy*, pp. 1520–1522, NELSON, J. D. and GRASSI, C. (eds) American Society for Microbiology, Washington, D.C., Boston.

STRUCK, R. F., DYKES, D. J., CORBETT, T. H., SULING, W. J. and TRADER, M. W. (1983) Isophosphoramide mustard, a metabolite of ifosfamide with activity against murine tumors comparable to cyclophosphamide. *Br. J. Cancer* **47:** 15–26.

STRUCK, R. F., KARI, P., KALIN, J., MONTGOMERY, J. A., MARINELLO, A. J., LOVE, J., BANSAL, S. K. and GURTOO, H. L. (1984) Metabolism of cyclophosphamide by purified cytochrome P-450 from microsomes of phenobarbital-treated rats. *Biochem. biophys. Res. Commun.* **120:** 390–396.

STRUCK, R. F., ALBERTS, D. S., HORNE, K., PHILLIPS, J. G., PENG, Y.-M. and ROE, D. J. (1987) Plasma pharmacokinetics of cyclophosphamide and its cytotoxic metabolites after intravenous versus oral administration in a randomized, crossover trial. *Cancer Res.* **47:** 2723–2726.

SULING, W. J., STRUCK, R. F., WOOLLEY, C. W. and SHANNON, W. M. (1978) Comparative disposition of phosphoramide mustard and other cyclophosphamide metabolites in the mouse using the Salmonella/mutagenesis assay. *Cancer Treat. Rep.* **62:** 1321–1328.

SURYA, Y. A., ROSENFELD, J. M. and HILLCOAT, B. L. (1978) Cross-linking of DNA in L1210 cells and nuclei treated with cyclophosphamide and phosphoramide mustard. *Cancer Treat. Rep.* **62:** 23–29.

TAKAMIZAWA, A., TOCHINO, Y., HAMASHIMA, Y. and IWATA, T. (1972) Studies on cyclophosphamide metabolites and their related compounds. *Chem. Pharmac. Bull.* **20:** 1612–1616.

TAKAMIZAWA, A., MATSUMOTO, S., IWATA, T., TOCHINO, Y., KATAGIRI, K., YAMAGUCHI, K. and SHIRATORI, O. (1975) Studies on cyclophosphamide metabolites and their related compounds. Preparation of an active species of cyclophosphamide and related compounds. *J. med. Chem.* **18:** 376–383.

TARDIFF, R. G. and DUBOIS, K. P. (1969) Inhibition of hepatic microsomal enzymes by alkylating agents. *Arch. Int. Pharmacodyn. Ther.* **177:** 445–456.

TASSO, M. J., BODDY, A. V., PRICE, L., WYLLIE, R. A., PEARSON, A. D. J. and IDLE, J. R. (1992) Pharmacokinetics and metabolism of cyclophosphamide in paediatric patients. *Cancer Chemother. Pharmac.* **30:** 207–211.

TCHEKMEDYIAN, N. S., EGORIN, M. J., COHEN, B. E., KAPLAN, R. S., POPLIN, E. and AISNER, J. (1986) Phase I clinical and pharmacokinetic study of cyclophosphamide administered by five-day continuous intravenous infusion. *Cancer Chemother. Pharmac.* **18:** 33–38.

TEICHER, B. A., CUCCHI, C. A., LEE, J. B., FLATOW, J. L., ROSOWSKY, A. and FREI, E., III (1986) Alkylating agents: in vitro studies of cross-resistance patterns in human cell lines. *Cancer Res.* **46:** 4379–4383.

THOMAS, E. D., STORB, R., CLIFT, R. A., FEFER, A., JOHNSON, F. L., NEIMAN, P. E., LERNER, K. G., GLUCKSBERG, H. and BUCKNER, C. D. (1975) Bone-marrow transplantation. *New Engl. J. Med.* **292:** 832–843; 895–902.

TIETZE, L. F., NEUMANN, M., MÖLLERS, T., FISCHER, R., GLÜSENKAMP, K-H., RAJEWSKY, M. F. and JÄHDE, E. (1989) Proton-mediated liberation of aldophosphamide from a nontoxic prodrug: a strategy for tumor-selective activation of cytocidal drugs. *Cancer Res.* **49:** 4179–4184.

TIETZE, L. F., FISCHER, R., BELLER, M. and SEELE, R. (1990) Novel stable bioactivated cyclophosphamide derivatives for selective cancer chemotherapy, synthesis of aldophosphamide acetal-glycosides and their glycoconjugates. *Liebigs Ann. Chem.* 151–157.

TIMMS, G. P. and HOLMES, R. S. (1981) Genetics and ontogeny of aldehyde dehydrogenase isozymes in the mouse: evidence for a locus controlling the inducibility of the liver microsomal isozyme. *Biochem. Gen.* **19:** 1223–1236.

TORKELSON, A. R., LABUDDE, J. A. and WEIKEL, J. H., JR (1974) The metabolic fate of cyclophosphamide. *Drug Metab. Rev.* **3:** 131–165.

TÖRRÖNEN, R., NOUSIAINEN, U. and HÄNNINEN, O. (1981) Induction of aldehyde dehydrogenase by polycyclic aromatic hydrocarbons in rats. *Chemcio.-Biol. Interact.* **36:** 33–34.

TSCHANZ, C. HIGNITE, C. E., HUFFMAN, D. H. and AZARNOFF, D. L. (1977) Metabolic disposition of antipyrine in patients with lung cancer. *Cancer Res.* **37:** 3881–3886.

TSUDA, H., MOORE, M. A., ASAMOTO, M., INOUE, T., FUKUSHIMA, S., ITO, N., SATOH, K., AMELIZAD, Z. and OESCH, F. (1987) Immunohistochemically demonstrated altered expression of cytochrome P-450 molecular forms and epoxide hydrolase in *N*-ethyl-*N*-hydroxyethylnitrosamine-induced rat kidney and liver lesions. *Carcinogenesis* **8:** 711–717.

UCKUN, F. M., RAMAKRISHNAN, S. and HOUSTON, L. L. (1985) Increased efficiency in selective elimination of leukemia cells by a combination of a stable derivative of cyclophosphamide and a human B-cell-specific immunotoxin containing pokeweed antiviral protein. *Cancer Res.* **45:** 69–75.

URI, J. V. and PARKS, D. B. (1983) Disulfiram-like reaction to certain cephalosporins. *Ther. Drug Monit.* **5:** 219–224.

VALLEE, B. L. and BAZZONE, T. J. (1983) Isozymes of human liver alcohol dehydrogenase. *Curr. Top. Biol. med. Res.* **8:** 219–244.

VAN BLADEREN, P. J. and VAN OMMEN, B. (1991) The inhibition of glutathione *S*-transferases: mechanism, toxic consequences and therapeutic benefits. *Pharmac. Ther.* **51:** 35–46.

VAN DER STEEN, J., TIMMER, E. C., WESTRA, J. G. and BENCKHUYSEN, C. (1973) 4-Hydroperoxidation in the Fenton oxidation of the antitumor agent cyclophosphamide. *J. Am. Chem. Soc.* **95:** 7535–7536.

VASILIOU, V. and MARSELOS, M. (1989) Tissue distribution of inducible aldehyde dehydrogenase activity in the rat after treatment with phenobarbital or methylcholanthrene. *Pharmac. Toxic.* **64:** 39–42.

VAUPEL, P., KALLINOWSKI, F. and OKUNIEFF, P. (1989) Blood flow, oxygen and nutrient supply, and metabolic microenvironment of human tumors: a review. *Cancer Res.* **49:** 6449–6465.

VESELL, E. S. (1977) Genetic and environmental factors affecting drug disposition in man. *Clin. Pharmac. Ther.* **22:** 659–679.

VOELCKER, G. and HAEGLSPERGER, R. (1982) Die pharmakokinetik von cyclophosphamid und cyclophosphamid-metaboliten bei der maus und ihr einfluß auf die therapeutische wirkung von 'aktiviertem' cyclophosphamid (4-hydroxycyclophosphamid). *Arzneim.-Forsch. Drug Res.* **32:** 639–647.

VOELCKER, G., WAGNER, T. and HOHORST, H. J. (1976) Identification and pharmacokinetics of cyclophosphamide (NSC 26271) metabolites in vivo. *Cancer Treat. Rep.* **60:** 415–422.

VOELCKER, G., GIERA, H. P., JÄGER, L. and HOHORST, H. J. (1978) Zur binding von cyclophosphamid und cyclophosphamid-metaboliten an serum-albumin. *Z. Krebsforsch. Klin. Onkol.* **91:** 127–142.

VOELCKER, G., BIELICKI, L. and HOHORST, H. J. (1981) Evidence for enzymatic toxification of activated cyclophosphamide (4-hydroxycyclophosphamide). *J. Cancer Res. clin. Oncol.* **99:** A58–A59.

VÖLKER, G., DRÄGER, U., PETER, G. and HOHORST, H. J. (1974) Studien zum spontanzerfall von 4-hydroxycyclophosphamid und 4-hydroperoxycyclophosphamid mit hilfe der dünnschichtchromatographie. *Arzneim.-Forsch. Drug Res.* **24:** 1172–1176.

VON HOFF, D. D. (ED.) (1984) Proceedings of the Symposium on the New Oxazaphosphorine, ASTA Z 7557. *Invest. New Drugs. J. New Anticancer Agents* **2:** 131–262.

VU, V. T., FENSELAU, C. C. and COLVIN, O. M. (1981) Identification of three alkylated nucleotide adducts from the reaction of guanosine 5′-monophosphate with phosphoramide mustard. *J. Am. Chem. Soc.* **103:** 7362–7364.

WADDELL, W. J. and BATES, R. G. (1969) Intracellular pH. *Physiol. Rev.* **49:** 285–329.

WAGNER, T. and DRINGS, P. (1986) Pharmacokinetics and bioavailability of oral ifosfamide. *Arzneim.-Forsch. Drug Res.* **36:** 878–880.

WAGNER, T. and FENNEBERG, K. (1984) Bioavailability of cyclophosphamide from oral formulations. *Eur. J. clin. Pharmac.* **26:** 269–270.

WAGNER, T. and HEYDRICH, D. (1982) Wirkspiegel von cyclophosphamid und metaboliten im malignen pleuraergüssen bei intravenöser therapie. *Arzneim.-Forsch. Drug Res.* **5:** 566–568.

WAGNER, T., HEYDRICH, D., BARTELS, H. and HOHORST, H. J. (1980a) Einfluß von leberparenchymschäden, niereninsuffizienz und hämodialyse auf die pharmakokinetik von cyclophosphamid und seinen aktiviertem metaboliten. *Arzneim.-Forsch. Drug Res.* **30:** 1588–1592.

WAGNER, T., HEYDRICH, D., VOELCKER, G. and HOHORST, H. J. (1980b) Über blutspiegel und urin-ausscheidung von aktiviertem cyclophosphamid und seinen deaktivierungsprodukten beim menschen. *J. Cancer Res. clin. Oncol.* **96:** 79–92.

WAGNER, T., HEYDRICH, D., JORK, T., VOELCKER, G. and HOHORST, H. J. (1981) Comparative study on human pharmacokinetics of activated ifosfamide and cyclophosphamide by a modified fluorometric test. *J. Cancer Res. clin. Oncol.* **100:** 95–104.

WAMPLER, G. L., REGELSON, W. and BARDOS, T. J. (1978) Absence of cross-resistance to alkylating agents in cyclophosphamide-resistant L1210 leukemia. *Eur. J. Cancer* **14:** 977–982.

WANG, L. H., LEE, C. S., MAJESKE, B. L. and MARBURY, T. C. (1981) Clearance and recovery circulations in hemodialysis: application to plasma, red blood cell, and dialysate measurements for cyclophosphamide. *Clin. Pharmac. Ther.* **29:** 365–372.

WANG, Y. and FARQUHAR, D. (1991) Aldophosphamide acetal diacetate and structural analogs: synthesis and cytotoxicity studies. *J. med. Chem.* **34:** 197–203.

WANG, J.-Y., PROROK, G. and VAUGHAN, W. P. (1993) Cytotoxicity, DNA cross-linking, and DNA single-strand breaks induced by cyclophosphamide in a rat leukemia in vivo. *Cancer Chemother. Pharmac.* **31:** 381–386.

WARBURG, O. (1930) *The Metabolism of Tumors.* Constable, London.

WATSON, E., DEA, P. and CHAN, K. K. (1986) Kinetics of phosphoramide mustard hydrolysis in aqueous solution. *J. Pharmac. Sci.* **74:** 1283–1292.

WEINER, H., FREYTAG, S., FOX, J. M. and HU, J. H. J. (1982) Reversible inhibitors of aldehyde dehydrogenases. *Prog. clin. Biol. Res.* **114:** 91–102.

WEINKAM, R. J. and SHIBA, D. A. (1978) Metabolic activation of procarbazine. *Life Sci.* **22:** 937–946.

WERMUTH, B. (1985) Aldo-keto reductases. *Prog. clin. Biol. Res.* **174:** 209–230.

WIERNIK, P. H. and DUNCAN, J. H. (1971) Cyclophosphamide in human milk. *Lancet* **i:** 912.

WILKINSON, P. M., O'NEILL, P. A., THATCHER, N. and LUCAS, S. B. (1983) Pharmacokinetics of high-dose cyclophosphamide in patients with metastatic bronchogenic carcinoma. *Cancer Chemother. Pharmac.* **11:** 196–199.

WRABETZ, E., PETER, G. and HOHORST, H. J. (1980) Does acrolein contribute to the cytotoxicity of cyclophosphamide? *J. Cancer Res. clin. Oncol.* **98:** 119–126.

YAMANAKA, Y., YAMAMOTO, T. and EGASHIRA, T. (1983) Effects of cephem antibiotics on rat liver aldehyde dehydrogenases. *Jap. J. Pharmac.* **33:** 717–723.

YASUMORI, T., KAWANO, S., NAGATA, K., SHIMADA, M., YAMAZOE, Y. and KATO, R. (1987) Nucleotide sequence of a human liver cytochrome P-450 related to the rat male specific form. *J. Biochem. (Tokyo)* **102:** 1075–1082.

YASUNAMI, M., CHEN, C.-S. and YOSHIDA, A. (1991) A human alcohol dehydrogenase gene (ADH6) encoding an additional class of isozyme. *Proc. natn. Acad. Sci. U.S.A.* **88:** 7610–7614.

YEAGER, A. M., KAIZER, H., SANTOS, G. W., SARAL, R., COLVIN, O. M., STUART, R. K., BRAINE, H. G., BURKE, P. J., AMBINDER, R. F., BURNS, W. H., FULLER, D. J., DAVIS, J. M., KARP, J. E., MAY, W. S., ROWLEY, S. D., SENSENBRENNER, L. L., VOGELSANG, G. B. and WINGARD, J. R. (1986) Autologous bone marrow transplantation in patients with acute nonlymphocytic leukemia, using ex vivo marrow treatment with 4-hydroperoxycyclophosphamide. *New Engl. J. Med.* **315:** 141–147.

YIN, S.-J., LIAO, C.-S., WANG, S.-L., CHEN, Y.-J. and WU, C.-W. (1989) Kinetic evidence for human liver and stomach aldehyde dehydrogenase-3 representing a unique class of isozymes. *Biochem. Gen.* **27:** 321–331.

YOSHIDA, A., WANG, G. and DAVÉ, V. (1983) Determination of genotypes of human aldehyde dehydrogenase $ALDH_2$ locus. *Am. J. Human Gen.* **35:** 1107–1116.

YOSHIDA, A., DAVÉ, V., WARD, R. J. and PETERS, T. J. (1989) Cytosolic aldehyde dehydrogenase (ALDH1) variants found in alcohol flushers. *Ann. Human Gen.* **53:** 1–7.

YUAN, Z.-M., FENSELAU, C., DULIK, D. M., MARTIN, W., EMARY, W. B., BRUNDRETT, R. B., COLVIN, O. M. and COTTER, R. J. (1990) Laser desorption electron impact: application to a study of the mechanism of conjugation of glutathione and cyclophosphamide. *Anal. Chem.* **62:** 868–870.

YUAN, Z.-M., SMITH, P. B., BRUNDRETT, R. B., COLVIN, M. and FENSELAU, C. (1991) Glutathione conjugation with phosphoramide mustard and cyclophosphamide. A mechanistic study using tandem mass spectrometry. *Drug Metab. Disp.* **19:** 625–629.

ZALUPSKI, M. and BAKER, L. H. (1988) Ifosfamide. *J. natn. Cancer Inst.* **80:** 556–566.

ZHOO, N.-S. and SLADEK, N. E. (1992) Substrate specificity and other characteristics of a novel aldehyde dehydrogenase present in female DBA/2 mouse liver. *Drug Metab. Disp.* **20:** 134–136.

ZON, G. (1982) Cyclophosphamide analogues. *Prog. med. Chem.* **19:** 205–246.

ZON, G., LUDEMAN, S. M., BRANDT, J. A., BOYD, V. L., OZKAN, G., EGAN, W. and SHAO K.-L. (1984) NMR spectroscopic studies of intermediary metabolites of cyclophosphamide. A comprehensive kinetic analysis of the interconversion of *cis-* and *trans*-4-hydroxycyclophosphamide with aldophosphamide and the concomitant partitioning of aldophosphamide between irreversible fragmentation and reversible conjugation pathways. *J. med. Chem.* **27:** 466–485.

ZUCALI, J. R., MOREB, J. and BAIN, C. (1992) Protection of cells capable of reconstituting long-term bone marrow stromal cultures from 4-hydroperoxycyclophosphamide by interleukin 1 and tumor necrosis factor. *Exp. Hemat.* **20:** 969–973.

ZWELLING, L. A., ALTSCHULER, E., CHERIF, A. and FARQUHAR, D. (1991) *N*-(5,5-diacetoxypentyl)doxorubicin: a novel anthracycline producing DNA interstrand cross-linking and rapid endonucleolytic cleavage in human leukemia cells. *Cancer Res.* **51:** 6704–6707.

Garth Powis, editor.
(1994) *Anticancer Drugs: Reactive Metabolism and Drug Interactions*,
Pergamon Press Ltd, pp. 157–165
Printed in the United Kingdom

CHAPTER 3

METABOLISM OF TRIAZINE ANTICANCER AGENTS

M. D'Incalci
Istituto di Ricerche Farmacologiche "Mario Negri", Via Eritrea 62, 20157 Milan, Italy

1. INTRODUCTION

Triazine anticancer agents include the old alkylating agent triethylenimino-*S*-triazine (TEM) and methylmelamines (see structure in Fig. 1).

The activity of TEM is due to its alkylating moieties (i.e. aziridine rings) which bind to nucleophilic sites of nucleic acids and proteins. Its metabolism was investigated several years ago, and it was concluded that the drug is rapidly transformed to cyanuric acid, the major urinary metabolite (Nadkarni et al., 1985). Since no significant recent studies have been published on the metabolism of this compound, which is no longer used frequently by oncologists, this review article will deal only with the metabolism of hexamethylmelamine (HMM) and its derivatives.

Although these drugs have only a limited spectrum of activity, they are nevertheless among the effective available agents for some human malignancies (e.g. ovarian cancer) (Foster et al., 1986). Their mechanism of action is still unknown but metabolism is likely to be involved in the production of the active metabolites responsible for their effects. A further reason for reviewing the metabolism of methylmelamines is that metabolic studies have been the basis for the design of new analogs, one of which (trimelamol) is under clinical investigation at the moment.

2. STUDIES IN VITRO

HMM is metabolized by a series of oxidative *N*-demethylation steps occurring in liver and extrahepatically. The scheme of HMM metabolism is illustrated in Fig. 2.

2.1. Hepatic Metabolism

De Milo and Borkovec (1968), Worzalla et al. (1973) and Rutty and Connors (1977) first reported that HMM undergoes oxidative *N*-demethylation by hepatic microsomes (of rats or mice) with elimination of formaldehyde from methylol intermediates. Gescher et al. (1980) identified hydroxymethylpentamethylmelamine (HMPMM) as a major metabolite of HMM in incubation mixtures with fortified mouse liver 9000 × *g* or microsomal preparations. The HMPMM was identified either by HPLC or by GLC–MS after derivatization with a sililating reagent. HMPMM was also reported to be relatively stable: 29% of the initial HMPMM was recovered after 1-hr incubation at 37°C in buffered solution containing boiled microsomes (Gescher et al., 1980).

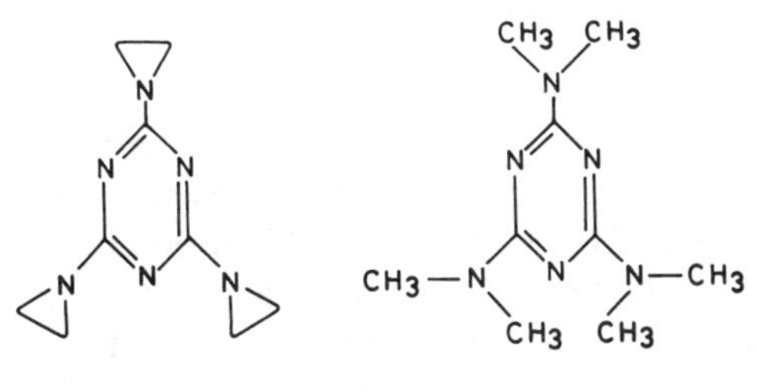

Fig. 1. Chemical structures of hexamethylmelamine (HMM) and triethylenmelamine (TEM).

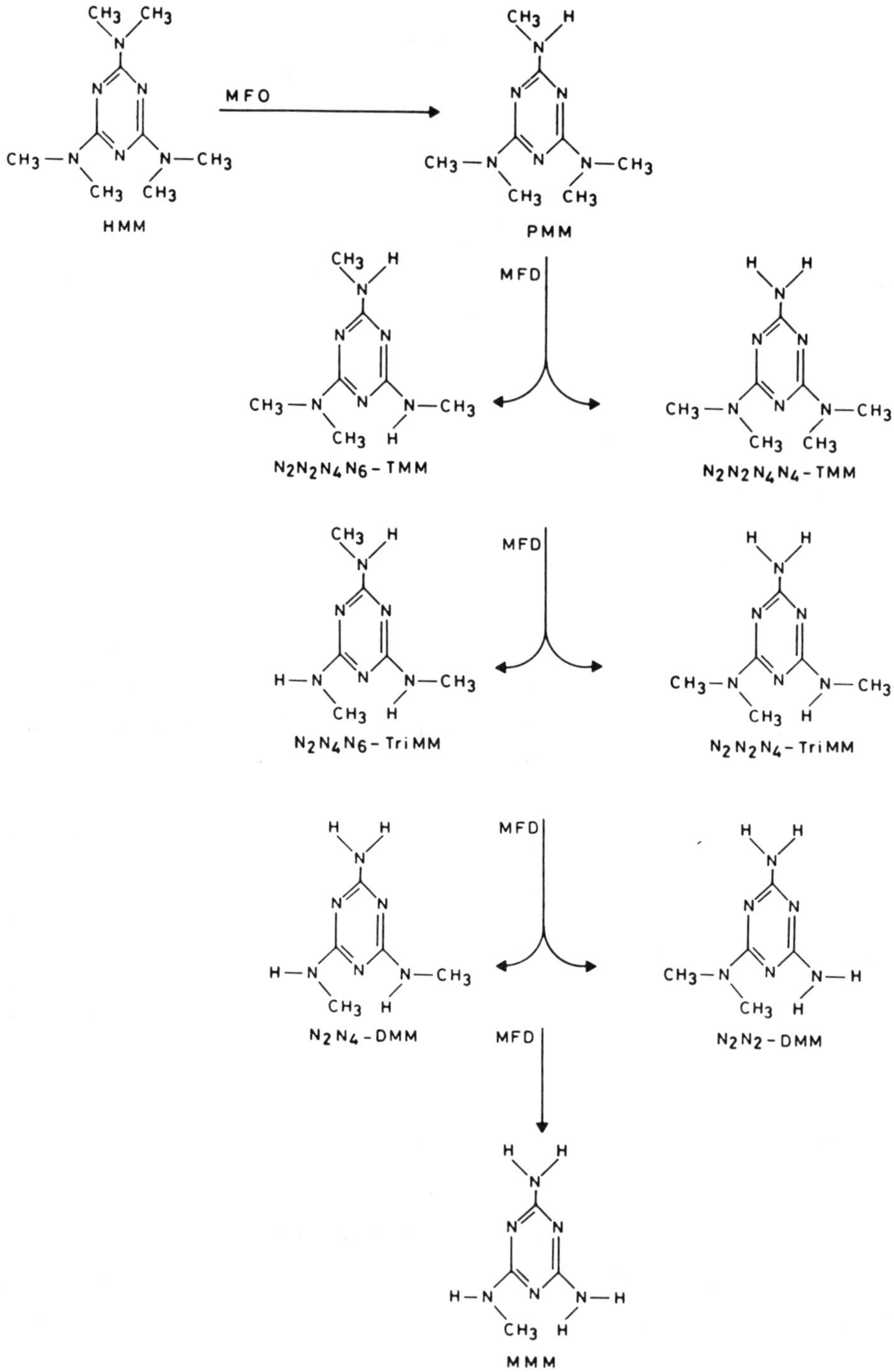

FIG. 2. Metabolism of HMM through the successive *N*-demethylation steps. MFO = mixed function oxygenase.

The other N-demethylated metabolites of HMM (i.e. pentamethylmelamine (PMM), tetramethylmelamines, trimethylmelamines, dimethylmelamines and monomethylmelamine) have also been identified and quantitated by HPLC or GLC–MS in different studies (Worzalla et al., 1974; D'Incalci et al., 1970; Ames et al., 1979; Hulshoff et al., 1980; Benvenuto et al., 1981).

Hydroxymethylmelamines, formed as intermediates of *N*-demethylation, are considered the active metabolites of HMM because of their ability to bind covalently to proteins and nucleic acids (Ames et al., 1983). In addition, they showed greater cytotoxic potency than HMM against murine (Rutty and Abel, 1980) or human (D'Incalci et al., 1980) cancer cell lines growing in vitro.

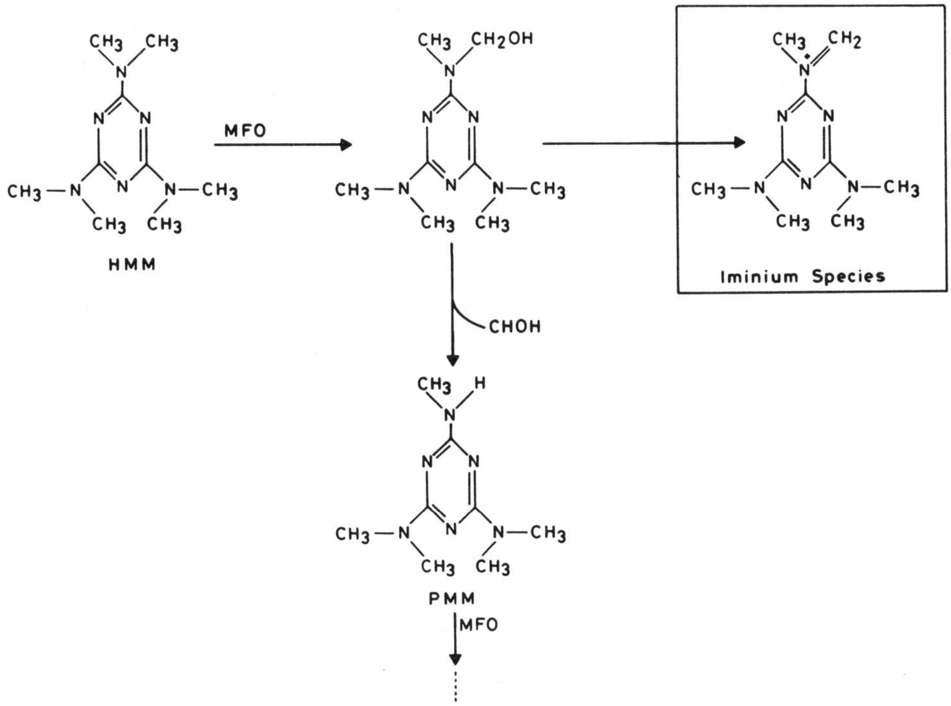

FIG. 3. Metabolic activation of HMM to chemical species likely to be responsible for its antitumoral activity.

Garattini et al. (1981) found that [ring-^{14}C]HMM was metabolized in vitro by mouse liver microsomes—in the presence of NADPH as a cofactor—to species able to bind proteins covalently. Ames et al. (1983) found that NADPH-dependent covalent binding of [methyl-^{14}C]HMM to rat microsomal proteins (probably mainly due to formaldehyde) was greater than that of [ring-^{14}C]HMM (probably due to hydroxymethylderivatives). NADPH-dependent covalent binding values of [ring-^{14}C]HMM and [methyl-^{14}C]HMM to calf thymus DNA, added to microsomal incubation mixtures, were approximately equal. They also found that the [ring-^{14}C]-labelled carbinolamine intermediate of HMM demethylation (HMPMM) covalently binds to microsomal proteins and, to a much greater extent, to calf thymus DNA. The covalent binding is explained by the formation of a reactive iminium species from HMPMM (see Fig. 3) able to react with nucleophiles.

2.2. Extrahepatic Metabolism

Borm et al. (1983, 1985) demonstrated intestinal oxidation of HMM and PMM by using rat intestinal microsomal or mitochondrial preparations, isolated intact mucosal cells and intestinal perfused segments. They found that both compounds were extensively metabolized by intestinal cells or extracts (the *N*-demethylation rates by microsomes and mitochondria were equivalent). For cellular systems, K_m and V_{max} were very similar for HMM and PMM. K_m was 53–65 μM and V_{max} 5.6–7.0 nmol/min/g intestine. Studies in everted intestinal perfused segments showed that HMM was metabolized approximately two times more than PMM, whereas PMM transport was three times greater than the transport of unchanged HMM. The intestinal metabolism of HMM, investigated by this technique, was found to predict events in vivo when the drug was administered intraduodenally.

Of great interest was the finding that some neoplastic cells are able to *N*-demethylate HMM or PMM, thus making plausible the idea that the antitumor activity of these drugs is partly due to activation in situ, with the formation of reactive intermediates (i.e. hydroxymethyl derivatives).

Begleiter et al. (1980) found that L5178Y lymphoblasts rapidly are able to convert HMM to PMM and other more polar metabolites. Garattini et al. (1981) showed that the microsomal fraction from the mouse ovarian reticular cell sarcoma M5076 was able to metabolize HMM with the formation of reactive products that bind macromolecules covalently. This binding was dependent on the presence of NADPH in the incubation mixture.

3. METABOLISM AND PHARMACOKINETICS IN DIFFERENT ANIMAL SPECIES

The majority of published studies refer to the mouse, which is the animal species most commonly used in experimental cancer chemotherapy. In our laboratories at the Mario Negri Institute, detailed studies have been made of C57BI female mice with M5076 ovarian reticular cell sarcoma (Broggini et al., 1981, 1982). After i.p. doses of 50 or 100 mg/kg HMM, peak plasma HMM levels were achieved in 45–60 min, corresponding to 1.4 ± 0.1 μg/ml and 3.4 ± 0.4 μg/ml, respectively. Then HMM concentrations declined monoexponentially with half-lives of about 44 and 49 min and AUC values (calculated experimentally up to 6 hr) of 129 and 393μg/ml $\times$ min.

After 50 or 100 mg/kg PMM i.p., plasma PMM peak levels of 2.0 ± 0.5 and 8.5 ± 0.8 μg/ml, respectively, were achieved in 30 min; the PMM plasma concentrations then dropped very rapidly with half-lives of 8 and 9 min. Table 1 illustrates the distribution of HMM or PMM after i.p. administration of each drug to M5076-bearing mice. Both compounds are distributed preferentially in fat tissue and lymph nodes. Concentrations of HMM or PMM were relatively high in spleen, liver and kidney but low in brain and tumor. Both HMM and PMM were extensively N-demethylated in mice, their major metabolites in plasma being $N_2N_2N_4N_6$ tetramethylmelamine and $N_2N_4N_6$ trimethylmelamine, but all the other N-demethylated products (see Fig. 2) were detectable too. Trimethyl and dimethylmelamines were the major urinary metabolites of HMM or PMM.

Hydroxymethylderivatives (e.g. HMPMM) were not detected in plasma or tissues of mice treated with HMM or PMM. However, their formation is indirectly suggested by other studies in which ^{14}C-HMM or ^{14}C-PMM were administered to M5076-bearing mice and in which it was possible to determine the radioactive species irreversibly bound to tissues macromolecules (Garattini et al., 1983, 1984). Significant covalent binding of radioactive metabolites was found in normal and neoplastic tissues. This was also reported by Morimoto et al. (1980) who investigated the amount of radioactivity bound to macromolecules in normal mice treated with [^{14}C-ring]HMM or [^{14}C-ring]PMM. Garattini's studies (Garattini et al., 1983, 1984) also gave some clues to the molecular species involved in the irreversible binding to DNA and thus possibly responsible for the antitumor activity. He found that after i.p. injection of [^{14}C-ring]-labelled PMM to M5076-bearing mice, covalent binding of radioactive species increased between 15 and 60 min, during which time the only metabolites that disappeared were PMM and $N_2N_2N_4N_6$ TMM. Thus, the reactive species for DNA binding should be sought in the metabolic step between PMM and $N_2N_2N_4N_6$ TMM, or possibly between $N_2N_2N_4N_6$ TMM and $N_2N_4N_6$ Tri MM. In fact the concentrations of

TABLE 1. *Distribution of HMM and PMM in M5076-bearing mice treated i.p. with 100 mg/kg HMM or PMM*

	HMM		PMM	
	Peak (tissue) / Peak (plasma)	AUC (tissue) / AUC (plasma)	Peak (tissue) / Peak (plasma)	AUC (tissue) / AUC (plasma)
Tumor	10	6	2	4
Liver	46	16	24	23
Spleen	81	25	60	61
Kidney	36	17	25	31
Heart	23	10	9	12
Brain	6	4	2	4
Adipose tissue	510	417	103	145
Lymph nodes	658	226	157	128
Small intestine	133	38	40	54

Figures represent the ratios of peak and AUC values in tissue and peak and AUC values in plasma. HMM and PMM were determined by a GLC method (D'Incalci et al., 1979). For further details see Broggini et al. (1981, 1982).

all other metabolites drop significantly between 1 and 8 hr during which time binding to DNA (or to other macromolecules) does not increase. That the more reactive metabolites of HMM or PMM are formed during the first *N*-demethylation steps is also suggested by other studies (Ames et al., 1983; Brindley et al., 1982; Ross et al., 1984; Cumber and Ross, 1977) and might explain why lower methylmelamines (e.g. tri-MMs) are not effective against tumors that are nevertheless susceptible to HMM or PMM (Ross et al., 1984; Lake et al., 1985). The presence of *N*-hydroxymethylmelamines as a metabolite of HMM or PMM in mice has been further demonstrated by Rutty et al. (1982) who quantitated in plasma the amount of formaldehyde released by *N*-hydroxymethylmelamines under the conditions of the Nash assay. Their study showed relatively high plasma concentrations of formaldehyde precursors in different strains of mice treated with i.v. doses of 90 mg/kg PMM. They also studied the formation of these metabolites in rodents and humans and found that plasma concentrations in hydroxymethylmelamines were much lower in rats than in mice and were undetectable in man. This led to the suggestions that the lower *N*-demethylation rate in man with lower *N*-hydroxymethylmelamine levels (the presumed active metabolites) was a great disadvantage, and could explain these drugs' scant activity in humans.

On the basis of this consideration, they synthesized trihydroxymethylmelamine (trimelamol), which should not require metabolic activation. This compound, which has shown activity in several rodent tumors, is under clinical investigation at the moment. Additional studies on the metabolism and pharmacokinetics of HMM and PMM have been made in rats and rabbits. In both these species, PMM disappears from plasma faster than HMM. Detailed studies of the elimination routes of these two drugs in rats (Colombo et al., 1982) showed that about 40% of HMM or PMM i.v. doses (25 mg/kg) were excreted in the urine as metabolites, more than 95% of which were N_2–N_4 dimethylmelamine and monomethylmelamine. Biliary excretion of HMM or PMM and their *N*-demethylated metabolites accounted for <2% of the administered dose. Only 0.3% was excreted with the feces, suggesting intestinal reabsorption or metabolism of a portion of the methylmelamines passing into the bile. Conjugates of methylmelamines with glucuronic acid or sulphate were found only in minute quantities in the urine or bile of rats treated with HMM or PMM. An additional conjugated product of PMM was also found after acid hydrolysis of bile or urines, but the chemical nature of this metabolite was not established.

A further interesting finding on the pharmacokinetics of PMM in the rat is the lower plasma drug clearance after high i.v. doses (50 mg/kg) (Colombo et al., 1981). Even though this dose-dependent kinetic pattern is likely to be due to saturation of metabolism, this point has not been investigated in detail.

The low bioavailability of HMM given orally to rabbits (Ames et al., 1979) or rats (Borm et al., 1985) is likely to be due mainly to a first-pass effect. Klippert et al. (1983) found that extensive gut wall metabolism was an important factor in the low HMM bioavailability after intraduodenal administration. HMM was not appreciably metabolized in the lung (Klippert et al., 1983).

4. METABOLISM AND PHARMACOKINETICS IN MAN

4.1. HMM

Because of its poor solubility in physiological solvents, HMM has been clinically used by the oral route. In different cancer patients receiving HMM p.o., plasma drug levels were very variable (D'Incalci et al., 1978) suggesting variable absorption and/or variable presystemic metabolism (in intestine and liver) as shown in other animal species. The variability of the levels of HMM and its metabolites was instead relatively low when the same patient was investigated repeatedly (see as an example Table 2). HMM distribution was investigated by determining the drug concentrations in surgical biopsies of 12 pelvic cancer patients receiving the drug before surgery (D'Incalci et al., 1982). The highest HMM concentrations were found in tissues such as omentum, or subcutaneous tissues that have a predominant lipidic component. HMM concentrations in the primary tumor were lower than in other tissues and were similar to those in plasma. HMM concentrations in metastases appeared to be higher than in the primary tumor, and, in metastases with a diameter <3 mm, drug levels were 2–10 times those of larger ones. Examples of tissue

TABLE 2. *Plasma Levels of HMM and Some of its Metabolites in an Ovarian Cancer Patient*

	AUC (μg × min/ml)		
	I° course	II° course	III° course
Hexamethylmelamine	184	153	121
Pentamethylmelamine	100	60	81
$N_2N_2N_4N_6$ Tetramethylmelamine	82	76	128
$N_2N_2N_4$ Trimethylmelamine	85	34	78
$N_2N_4N_6$ Trimethylmelamine	325	210	370

Pharmacokinetic studies were performed on the first oral dose (150 mg/m^2) of the 1st, 2nd and 3rd course. Each course consisted of 14 daily oral doses. The interval between two subsequent courses was 14 days. HMM and metabolites were determined by the method described by Hulshoff et al. (1980).

distribution in two ovarian cancer patients operated 8.5 and 9 hr after an oral dose of 135 mg/m^2 and 140 mg/m^2 HMM are illustrated in Fig. 4.

The concentration of HMM was determined in the cerebrospinal fluid in a 51-year-old cancer patient who had received an oral HMM dose of 130 mg/m^2 230 min earlier (D'Incalci et al., 1981b). Cerebrospinal fluid concentrations of HMM, PMM, TMM and Tri MM amounted to 6, 24, 47 and 100% respectively, of those in plasma. These differences were protein fractions of HMM, PMM and TMM, determined by equilibrium dialysis at 37°C, were in fact 6, 25 and 50%, respectively. The presence of ascites, the patient's age, the concomitant administration of adriamycin and cyclophosphamide, and obesity did not appear to influence the kinetics of HMM and metabolites (D'Incalci et al., 1981a). However, the influence of these factors could have been masked by the high interindividual variability of drug levels mainly due to the variable drug bioavailability.

The low and variable oral bioavailability of HMM has stimulated research for a parental formulation suitable for clinical use and clinical trials with a new i.v. injectable HMM preparation are in progress (Ames and Kovach, 1982).

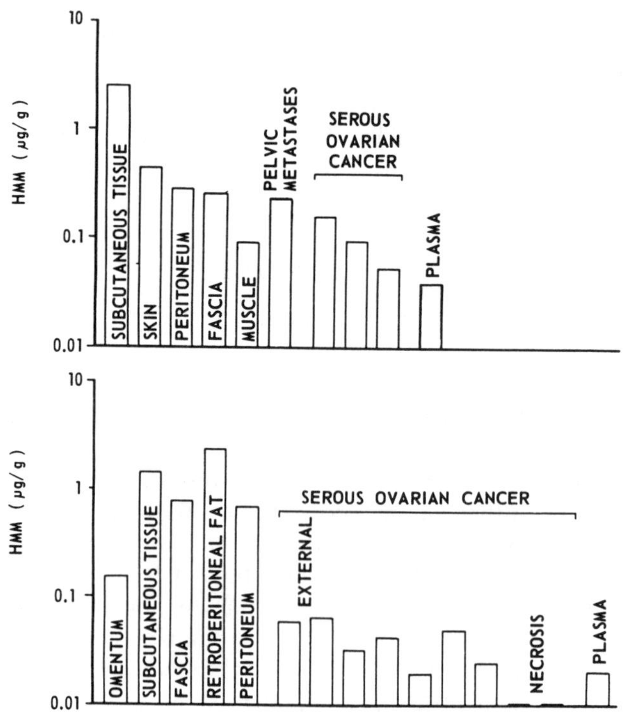

FIG. 4. HMM levels in surgical biopsies of two ovarian cancer patients obtained 8.5 hr (upper panel) and 9 hr (lower panel) after an oral dose of 135 mg/m^2 and 140 mg/m^2, respectively.

4.2. PMM

To overcome problems associated with the gastrointestinal toxicity and the variable oral bioavailability of HMM, it was proposed to investigate as an alternative its metabolite PMM which, being more water-soluble, could be given i.v. Several Phase I clinical trials with PMM have been conducted (Benvenuto et al., 1981; Ihde et al., 1981; Eagan et al., 1980; Goldberg et al., 1980; Van Echo et al., 1980; Ajani et al., 1982) and in some cases the drug pharmacokinetics were investigated in patients. All the results are in agreement about the rapid *N*-demethylation of PMM in humans.

Benvenuto et al. (1981) monitored PMM plasma levels in patients receiving PMM infusions at doses between 80 and 1500 mg/m^2. They did not find dose-dependent kinetics in patients ($n = 17$) with normal liver function whose PMM plasma clearance values were 180 L/hr. Plasma clearance was much reduced in patients with moderate ($n = 3$) or severe ($n = 3$) liver disease, to values of 17 and 15 L/hr, respectively. They found a relationship between the decrease in PMM clearance and drug neurotoxicity.

Ihde et al. (1981) investigated PMM pharmacokinetics in patients receiving i.v. doses between 80 and 1500 mg/m^2. They found peak levels were proportional to the doses, whereas plasma clearance values were dose-dependent. In cerebrospinal fluid obtained 40 min after PMM infusion the drug concentration was approximately 25% that in plasma.

The neurotoxicity of PMM in mice (Perego et al., 1984) or in man (Ihde et al., 1981; Eagan et al., 1980; Goldberg et al., 1980; Van Echo et al., 1980; Ajani et al., 1982) was an important drawback with this drug and explains why no further clinical investigations of its efficacy have been made.

5. DRUG INTERACTIONS

Not much work has been published on the interference of other drugs in the metabolism and pharmacokinetics of methylmelamines. In a recent study, we found that the HMM levels in plasma, liver and M5076 tumor were much lower when mice were pretreated with phenobarbital (PB) (Paolini and D'Incalci, 1986). The levels of all the *N*-demethylated metabolites except N_2N_4 dimethylmelamine were also lower. PB induction of HMM metabolism resulted in significant loss of antitumoral activity toward M5076 mouse reticular cell sarcoma and PC6 mouse plasmocytoma. This loss of HMM antitumor activity after PB pretreatment suggests that the time of exposure of tumor cells to the active metabolites (presumably the hydroxymethyl derivatives) is more important than the peak level which should actually be increased by metabolic induction. Cimetidine, which reportedly affects the microsomal metabolism of some drugs, had no effect on HMM metabolism and antitumor activity in mice (unpublished data).

6. CONCLUSIONS

In summary, this review article describes the available knowledge on the metabolism and pharmacokinetics of two methylmelamines, namely HMM and PMM. The relatively simple structure of methylmelamines, the specificity and sensitivity of the analytical assays probably due to different plasma protein binding of these compounds. The free plasma for determination of the parent compounds and any metabolic bioproducts and the availability of standards labelled in different positions have made these compounds particularly attractive as models for investigations of *N*-demethylation.

A first conclusive consideration is that HMM or PMM are good substrates for oxidative *N*-demethylation. The high stability of hydroxymethylmelamines, the intermediates of the *N*-demethylation reactions, suggests that they are responsible for the antitumor activity of methylmelamines. Their antitumor and cytotoxic activities may possibly be due to reactive iminium species, formed from hydroxymethylmelamines. Only the hydroxymethylmelamines formed during the first *N*-demethylations appear important in terms of covalent binding to DNA and protein and of antitumor activity, whereas central nervous system toxicity appears related to the formation of lower *N*-methylmelamines that cross the blood–brain barrier more efficiently. The dissociation between the mechanisms of toxicity and of antitumor activity makes it theoretically possible to counteract toxicity without losing the anticancer effects of the methylmelamines. Of reasonable interest is the fact that methylmelamines undergo an extrahepatic metabolism involving some tissues. Among these, the gastrointestinal tract can metabolize HMM or PMM very efficiently and this may partially explain the low bioavailability and gastrointestinal symptoms of HMM given orally.

HMM or PMM can also be transformed in tumor cells to species able to bind covalently to macromolecules. This finding requires further studies to assess the potential presence of enzymes in human tumors that can *N*-demethylate compounds for which this reaction represents metabolic activation. This knowledge could in fact be exploited to find more selective antitumoral agents. From the several pharmacokinetic studies conducted to date in different animal species, one can conclude that *N*-demethylation of methylmelamines varies widely; its efficiency decreases in mice, rats and humans, in that order.

Indeed, these interspecies differences may be relevant not only for methylmelamines, but for many other *N*-methyl-containing compounds for whose activity oxidative *N*-demethylation is crucial.

Acknowledgements—The generous contribution of the Italian Association for Cancer Research, Milan, Italy, is gratefully acknowledged. We wish to thank Ms Judy Baggott and Ms Antonella Palmiero for editorial assistance.

REFERENCES

AJANI, J. A., CABANILLAS, F. F. and BODEY, G. P. (1982) Phase I trial of pentamethylmelamine. *Cancer Treat. Rep.* **66:** 1227–1228.

AMES, M. M. and KOVACH, J. S. (1982) Parenteral formulation of hexamethylmelamine potentially suitable for use in man. *Cancer Treat. Rep.* **66:** 1579–1581.

AMES, M. M., POWIS, G., KOVACH, J. S. and EAGAN, R. T. (1979) Disposition and metabolism of pentamethylmelamine and hexamethylmelamine in rabbits and humans. *Cancer Res.* **39:** 5016–5021.

AMES, M. M., SANDERS, M. E. and TIEDE, W. S. (1983) Role of *N*-methylolpentamethylmelamine in the metabolic activation of hexamethylmelamine. *Cancer Res.* **43:** 500–504.

BEGLEITER, A., GROVER, J. and GOLDENBERG, G. J. (1980) Uptake and metabolism of hexamethylmelamine and pentamethylmelamine by L5178Y lymphoblasts in vitro. *Cancer Res.* **40:** 4489–4494.

BENVENUTO, J. A., STEWART, D. J., BENJAMIN, R. S. and LOO, T. L. (1981) Pharmacology of pentamethylmelamine in humans. *Cancer Res.* **41:** 566–569.

BORM, P., MINGELS, M.-J., HULSHOFF, A., FRANKHUYZEN-SIEREVOGEL, A. and NOORDHOEK, J. (1983) Rapid formation of *N*-hydroxymethylpentamethylmelamine by mitochondria from rat small intestinal epithelium. *Life Sci.* **33:** 2113–2119.

BORM, P. J. A., FRANKHUYZEN-SIEREVOGEL, A. C., WELLER, E. B. C. and NOORDHOEK, J. (1985) Absorption and metabolism of hexamethylmelamine and pentamethylmelamine in rat everted perfused gut segments: Correlation with in-vivo data. *J. Pharm. Pharmac.* **37:** 629–636.

BRINDLEY, C., GESCHER, A., LANGDON, S. P., BROGGINI, M., COLOMBO, T. and D'INCALCI, M. (1982) Studies of the mode of action of antitumour triazenes and triazines—III. Metabolism studies on hexamethylmelamine. *Biochem. Pharmac.* **31:** 625–631.

BROGGINI, M., COLOMBO, T., D'INCALCI, M., DONELLI, M. G., GESCHER, A. and GARATTINI, S. (1981) Pharmacokinetics of hexamethylmelamine and pentamethylmelamine in mice. *Cancer Treat. Rep.* **65:** 669–672.

BROGGINI, M., ROSSI, C., COLOMBO T. and D'INCALCI, M. (1982) Hexamethylmelamine and pentamethylmelamine tissue distribution in M5076/73A ovarian cancer-bearing mice. *Cancer Treat. Rep.* **66:** 127–133.

COLOMBO, T., TORTI, L. and D'INCALCI, M. (1981) Dose-dependent pharmacokinetics of PMM in the rat. *Cancer Chemother. Pharmac.* **5:** 201–203.

COLOMBO, T., BROGGINI, M., GESCHER, A. and D'INCALCI, M. (1982) Routes of elimination of hexamethylmelamine and pentamethylmelamine in the rat. *Xenobiotica* **12:** 315–321.

CUMBER, A. J. and ROSS, W. C. J. (1977) Analogues of hexamethylmelamine. The anti-neoplastic activity of derivatives with enhanced water solubility. *Chem.-Biol. Interact.* **17:** 349–357.

DEMILO, A. B. and BORKOVEC, A. B. (1968) Insect chemosterilants, VII. Oxidative degradation of hexamethylmelamine. *J. Med. Chem.* **11:** 961–963.

D'INCALCI, M., BOLIS, G., MANGIONI, C., MORASCA, L. and GARATTINI, S. (1978) Variable oral absorption of hexamethylmelamine in man. *Cancer Treat. Rep.* **62:** 2117–2119.

D'INCALCI, M., MORAZZONI, P. and PANTAROTTO, C. (1979) Gas chromatographic determination of hexamethylmelamine in mouse plasma. *Anal. Biochem.* **99:** 441–449.

D'INCALCI, M., ERBA, E., BALCONI, G., MORASCA, L. and GARATTINI, S. (1980) Time dependence of the in vitro cytotoxicity of hexamethylmelamine and its metabolites. *Br. J. Cancer* **41:** 630–635.

D'INCALCI, M., BEGGIOLIN, G., SESSA, C. and MANGIONI, C. (1981a) Influence of ascites on the pharmacokinetics of hexamethylmelamine and *N*-demethylated metabolites in ovarian cancer patients. *Eur. J. Cancer clin. Oncol.* **17:** 1331–1335.

D'INCALCI, M., SESSA, C., BEGGIOLIN, G. and MANGIONI, C. (1981b) Cerebrospinal fluid levels of hexamethylmelamine and *N*-demethylated metabolites. *Cancer Treat. Rep.* **65:** 350–351.

D'INCALCI, M., FARINA, P., SESSA, C., MANGIONI, C. and GARATTINI, S. (1982) Hexamethylmelamine distribution in patients with ovarian and other pelvic cancers. *Cancer Treat. Rep.* **66:** 231–235.

EAGAN, R. T., CREAGAN, E. T., RUBIN, J., O'CONNELL, M. J. and KOVACH, J. S. (1980) Early clinical trial of a 1-day intermittent schedule for pentamethylmelamine. *Cancer Treat. Rep.* **64:** 993–995.

FOSTER, B. J., CLAGETT-CARR, K., MARSONI, S., SIMON, R. and LEYLAND-JONES, B. (1986) Role of hexamethylmelamine in the treatment of ovarian cancer: Where is the needle in the haystack? *Cancer Treat. Rep.* **70:** 1003–1014.

GARATTINI, E., DONELLI, M. G., COLOMBO, T., PAESANI, R. and PANTAROTTO, C. (1981) In vivo and in vitro irreversible binding of hexamethylmelamine to liver and ovarian tumor macromolecules of mice. *Biochem. Pharmac.* **30:** 1151–1154.

GARATTINI, E., COLOMBO, T., DONELLI, M. G., CATALANI, P., BIANCHI, M., D'INCALCI, M. and PANTAROTTO, C. (1983) Distribution, metabolism, and irreversible binding of hexamethylmelamine in mice bearing ovarian carcinoma. *Cancer Chemother. Pharmac.* **11:** 51–55.

GARATTINI, E., BROGGINI, M., COCCIA, P., COLOMBO, T., ROSSI, C. and D'INCALCI, M. (1984) Biochemical studies on the ability of pentamethylmelamine to interact in vivo with DNA and proteins in a sensitive murine ovarian reticular cell sarcoma. *Biochem. Pharmac.* **33:** 2715–2722.

GESCHER, A., D'INCALCI, M., FANELLI, R. and FARINA, P. (1980) *N*-hydroxymethylpentamethylmelamine, a major in vitro metrabolite of hexamethylmelamine. *Life Sci.* **26:** 147–154.

GOLDBERG, R. S., GRIFFIN, J. P., MCSHERRY, J. W. and KRAKOFF, I. H. (1980) Phase I study of pentamethylmelamine. *Cancer Treat. Rep.* **64:** 1319–1322.

HULSHOFF, A., NEIJT, J. P., SMULDERS, C. F. A., VAN LOENEN, A. C. and PINEDO, H. M. (1980) Determination of hexamethylmelamine and metabolites in plasma or serum by gas–liquid chromatography with a nitrogen-sensitive detector. *J. Chromatogr.* **181:** 363–371.

IHDE, D. C., DUTCHER, J. S., YOUNG, R. C., CORDES, R. S., BARLOCK, A. L., HUBBARD, S. M., JONES, R. B. and BOYD, M. R. (1981) Phase I trial of pentamethylmelamine: A clinical and pharmacologic study. *Cancer Treat. Rep.* **65:** 755–762.

KLIPPERT, P. J. M., HULSHOFF, A., MINGELS, M.-J. J., HOFMAN, G. and NOORDHOEK, J. (1983) Low oral bioavailability of hexamethylmelamine in the rat due to simultaneous hepatic and intestinal metabolism. *Cancer Res.* **43:** 3160–3164.

LAKE, L. M., GRUNDEN, E. E. and JOHNSON, B. M. (1975) Toxicity and antitumor activity of hexamethylmelamine and its *N*-demethylated metabolites in mice with transplantable tumors. *Cancer Res.* **35:** 2858–2863.

MORIMOTO, M., GREEN, D., RAHMAN, A., GOLDIN, A. and SCHEIN, P. S. (1980) Comparative pharmacology of pentamethylmelamine and hexamethylmelamine in mice. *Cancer Res.* **40:** 2762–2767.

NADKARNI, M. V., GOLDENTHAL, E. I. and SMITH, P. K. (1985) The distribution of radioactivity following administration of triethylenimino-*S*-triazine-C^{14} in tumor-bearing and control mice. *Cancer Res.* **15:** 559–562.

PAOLINI, A. and D'INCALCI, M. (1986) Effect of phenobarbital pretreatment on the metabolism and antitumor activity of hexamethylmelamine. *Cancer Treat. Rep.* **70:** 513–516.

PEREGO, C., BROGGINI, M., GARATTINI, S., D'INCALCI, M., ACHILLI, G., LIPARTITI, M and PONZIO, F. (1984) Central side effects of pentamethylmelamine: Biochemical and behavioural studies. *Biochem. Pharmac.* **33:** 4011–4015.

ROSS, D., LANGDON, S. P., GESCHER, A. and STEVENS, M. F. G. (1984) Studies of the mode of action of antitumor triazenes and triazines. V. The correlation of the in vitro cytotoxicity and in vivo antitumour activity of hexamethylmelamine analogues with their metabolism. *Biochem. Pharmac.* **33:** 1131–1136.

RUTTY, C. J. and ABEL, G. (1980) In vitro cytotoxicity of the methylmelamines. *Chem.-Biol. Interact.* **29:** 235–246.

RUTTY, C. J. and CONNORS, T. A. (1977) In vitro studies with hexamethylmelamine. *Biochem. Pharmac.* **26:** 2385–2391.

RUTTY, C. J., NEWELL, D. R., MUINDI, J. R. F. and HARRAP, K. R. (1982) The comparative pharmacokinetics of pentamethylmelamine in man, rat, and mouse. *Cancer Chemother. Pharmac.* **8:** 105–111.

VAN ECHO, D. A., CHIUTEN, D. F., WHITACRE, M., AISNER, J., LICHTENFELD, J. L. and WIERNIK, P. H. (1980) Phase I trial of pentamethylmelamine in patients with previously treated malignancies. *Cancer Treat. Rep.* **64:** 1335–1339.

WORZALLA, J. F., JOHNSON, B. M., RAMIREZ, G. and BRYAN, G. T. (1973) *N*-demethylation of the antineoplastic agent hexamethylmelamine by rats and man. *Cancer Res.* **33:** 2810–2815.

WORZALLA, J. F., KAIMAN, B. D., JOHNSON, B. M., RAMIREZ, G. and BRYAN, G. T. (1974) Metabolism of hexamethylmelamine-ring-^{14}C in rats and man. *Cancer Res.* **34:** 2669–2674.

Garth Powis, editor.
(1994) *Anticancer Drugs: Reactive Metabolism and Drug Interactions*,
Pergamon Press Ltd, pp. 167–185
Printed in the United Kingdom

CHAPTER 4

THE METABOLISM OF TRIAZENE ANTITUMOR DRUGS

MICHAEL D. THREADGILL* AND ANDREAS GESCHER†

*School of Pharmacy and Pharmacology, University of Bath, Claverton Down, Bath BA2 7AY, U.K.
†Cancer Research Campaign Experimental Chemotherapy Group, Pharmaceutical Sciences Institute, Aston University, Aston Triangle, Birmingham B4 7ET, U.K.

1. INTRODUCTION

1-Aryl-3,3-dialkyltriazenes (1, Fig. 1) are carcinogens (Preussmann et al., 1969a; Druckrey, 1913) and the dimethyl analogues (1; R′, R″ CH_3) show potent antineoplastic activity against rodent tumors (Clarke et al., 1955; Burchenal et al., 1956). Use of these potently biologically active compounds has also been claimed for such diverse applications as herbicides (Mazza et al., 1974), reagents for the determination of heavy metals (Popescu and Danet, 1983) and agents to render grain unpalatable to pests (Adams and Wright, 1964). Structure–antitumor activity studies on 1-aryl-3,3-dialkyltriazenes have shown that at least one *N*-methyl group is necessary for activity and that substitution in the phenyl ring has little effect on activity against the TLX5 lymphoma in mice (Audette et al., 1973; Connors et al., 1976). However, quantitative structure–activity relationships (QSAR) established by Hatheway et al. (1978) and by Trinajstic et al. (1989) have indicated a good correlation between antitumor activity and the presence of electron-donating substituents on the phenyl ring but that partition coefficient (expressed as log *P*) has little effect. Various attempts have been made to attach the 3,3,-dimethyltriazen-1-yl-phenyl 'warhead' to 'delivery' moieties such as 2,4-diaminopyrimidines (Bliss et al., 1987) and peptides (Ionescu et al., 1981). 3-Acyl-1-(2-chloroethyl)-3-methyltriazenes have also been claimed to be useful antineoplastic agents (Michejda and Smith, 1989). During the last 25 years, the role of metabolism in the mechanisms of the carcinogenicity and cytotoxicity of aryldialkyltriazenes has been studied extensively. However, many important aspects of these mechanisms remain enigmatic. One heteroaryldimethyltriazene, 5-(3,3-dimethyltriazen-1-yl)imidazole-4-carboxamide (dacarbazine, DTIC; 2, Fig. 1), is of moderate clinical usefulness in the treatment of disseminated melanoma, cancer of the colon and Hodgkin's

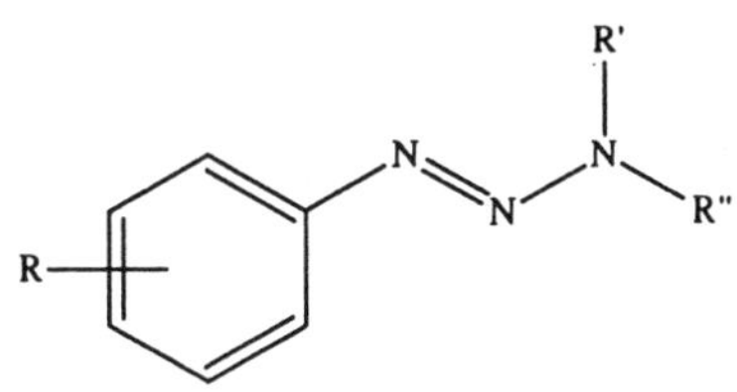

1

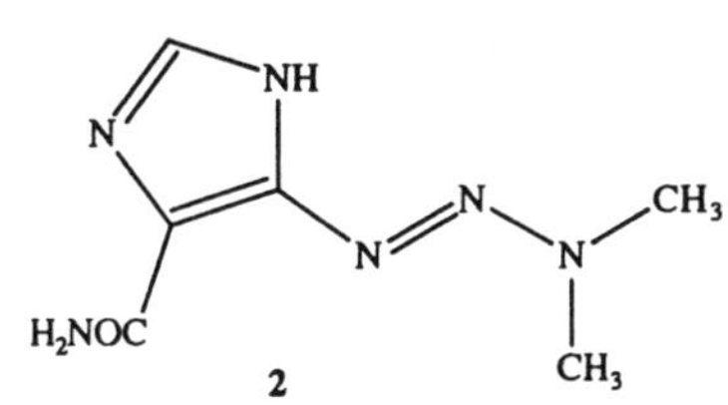

2

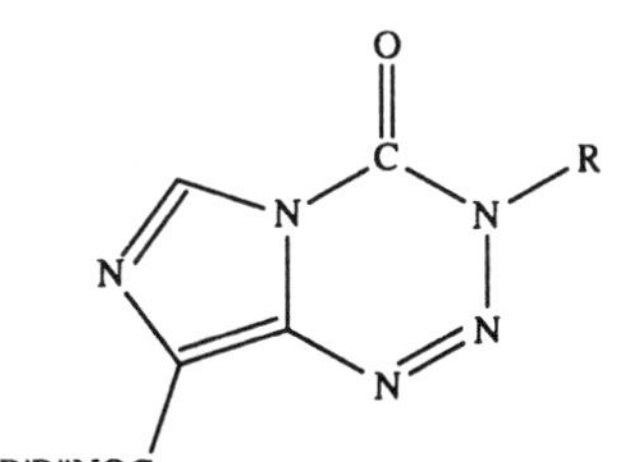

3: R = CH_2CH_2Cl; R',R" = H
4: R = CH_3; R',R" = H
5: R = CH_2CH_2Cl; R',R" = CH_3
6: R = CH_2CH_2Cl; R' = CH_3; R" = H

FIG. 1. Structures of arylalkyltriazenes (1), dacarbazine (2), mitozolomide (3), temozolomide (4) and analogues.

disease which is resistant to therapy with MOPP (a combination of mechlorethamine, vincristine, procarbazine and prednisone) (Loo et al., 1976; Spassova and Golovinsky, 1985). Some 1-aryl-3,3-dimethyltriazenes and 1-aryl-3-methyltriazenes also show strong antimetastatic activity which is probably mediated through xenogenization of the tumor cells, leading to attack by the immune system (Nardelli et al., 1984; Grill et al., 1987; Nifontov et al., 1988). Although DNA is generally taken to be the biochemical site of cytotoxic, carcinogenic and mutagenic action of triazenes, a correlation between inhibition of Ca^{2+}-activated ATPase and antimetastatic activity against the murine Lewis lung carcinoma has been noted (Nifontov et al., 1988). Curiously, most studies of the metabolism and mechanism of the antineoplastic action of dimethyltriazenes have been carried out using substituted phenyldimethyltriazenes rather than dacarbazine itself.

Recently, a number of cyclic arylmonoalkyltriazenes, the 3-alkyl-8-carbamoylimidazo[5,1-*d*]-1,2,3,5-tetrazin-4(3H)-ones (e.g. 3–6, Fig. 1) have been designed as potential therapeutic alternatives to dacarbazine (Stevens et al., 1984). They exhibit potent antineoplastic properties in rodents (Hickman et al., 1985; Fodstad et al., 1985). Mitozolomide (8-carbamoyl-3-(2-chloroethyl)-imidazo[5,1-*d*]-1,2,3,5-tetrazin-4(3H)-one; 3) underwent clinical trial and was found to cause severe prothromocytopenia as a clinically unacceptable, dose-limiting toxicity (Harding et al., 1988). Temozolomide (8-carbamoyl-3-methylimidazo[5,1-*d*]-1,2,3,5-tetrazin-1(3H)-one; 3) is currently under clinical evaluation.

The chemical properties and therapeutic aspects of the 1-aryl-3,3-dialkyltriazenes and the chemical properties of the imidazotetrazinones have been reviewed extensively (Kolar, 1984; Spassova and Golovinsky, 1985; Threadgill, 1990). Hence, this chapter is principally confined to aspects of their metabolism, together with appropriate biomimetic chemistry.

In aqueous solution at physiological or mildly basic pH, 1-aryl-3,3-dialkyltriazenes are moderately stable. In contrast, acidic environments cause rapid reversal of the usual synthetic reaction (Gescher et al., 1981), giving the arenediazonium salt (7, Fig. 2) and the protonated secondary amine (8). This degradation yields potently electrophilic species and therefore this pathway could be considered to be the source of biologically reactive entities. However, no firm evidence has been put forward to support the contention that this reaction occurs at a significant rate under physiological conditions.

The oxidative metabolism of 1-aryl-3,3-dialkyltriazenes by hepatic microsomes in vitro was first reported in 1967 (Druckrey et al., 1967) and this study and subsequent investigations (e.g. Preussmann et al., 1969b; Kolar and Schlesiger, 1976a; Kolar and Wildschütte, 1982) have left little

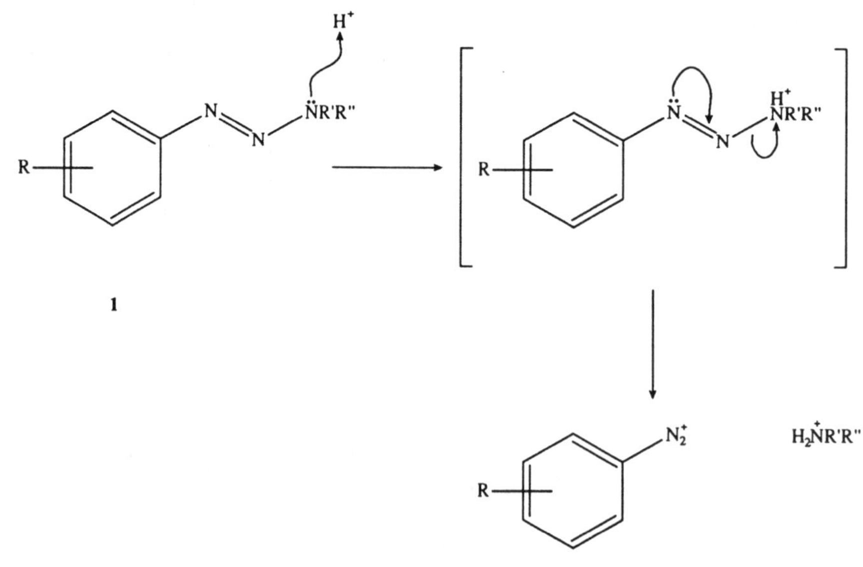

1

7 8

FIG. 2. Mechanism of acid-catalyzed decomposition of aryldialkyltriazenes by reversal of the general synthetic pathway.

doubt that oxidative *N*-dealkylation is a metabolic pathway essential for the biological properties of these compounds.

2. OXIDATIVE METABOLISM OF 1-ARYL-3,3-DIALKYLTRIAZENES AT THE ALKYL GROUPS

In the study by Preussmann et al. (1969b), 3,3-dimethyl-1-phenyltriazene (9, Fig. 3) was incubated with rat liver microsomes and NADPH. Formaldehyde was reported to be a metabolite and the authors suggested that the other product of this oxidation was 3-methyl-1-phenyltriazene (11, Fig. 3). Monoalkyltriazenes such as this are powerful directly-acting alkylating agents (13, Fig. 4) and are known to be carcinogens (Vaughan and Stevens, 1978). They react spontaneously with nucleophiles, giving the corresponding arylamine (14), molecular nitrogen and the alkylated nucleophile (15). It can be assumed that it is this reaction mechanism which is operative in biological alkylations involving monoalkyltriazenes rather than a reaction which has been claimed to involve the 'methyl carbonium ion' (16), as the latter is very unlikely to occur in aqueous biological media, although the methyl diazonium ion has been put forward as the ultimate mutagen derived from 3-acyl-1,3-dimethyltriazenes in *Salmonella* (Smith et al., 1986). Deuterium labelling studies have shown that diazoalkanes (17) are unlikely to be involved as intermediates in these alkylations (Lown and Singh, 1981). There is good evidence that the reaction between monomethyltriazenes and bionucleophiles such as nucleic acids can occur in vivo (Preussmann et al., 1969b; Kleihues et al., 1979; Margison et al., 1979). Therefore, the oxidative metabolic pathway (Fig. 3) has been postulated to be responsible for the generation of the ultimate cytotoxin which is responsible for the carcinogenicity and, possibly, the antitumor activity of aryldialkyltriazenes.

Many of the studies of the metabolism of aryldialkyltriazenes conducted in the wake of the original report by Preussmann et al. (1969b) used colorimetric determination of the aldehyde generated by hydroxylation of the *N*-alkyl group mediated by cytochromes *P*450 enzymes and subsequent hydrolysis/elimination. In that study, some 20–80% of the alkyl groups were oxidized to aldehydes, depending on the chemical nature of the alkyl moieties (on the basis that complete

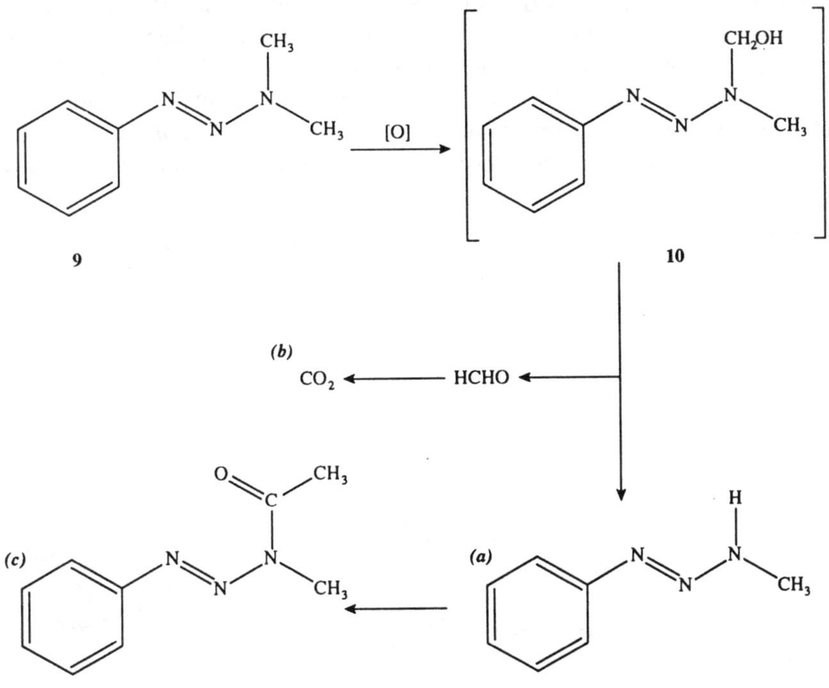

9 10 12 11

FIG. 3. Metabolism of 3,3-dimethyl-1-phenyltriazene (9) by rodent hepatic microsomes in vitro. (a) Preussmann and von Hodenberg, 1969. (b) Kleihues et al., 1976. (c) Pool, 1979b.

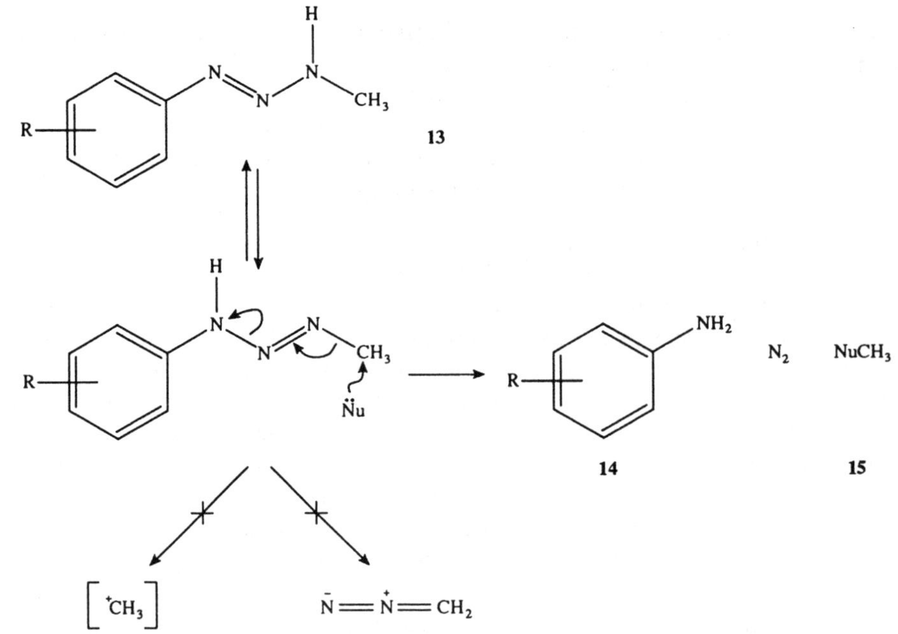

16 17

FIG. 4. Postulated mechanisms of methylation by monomethyltriazenes. Nu = H_2O, nucleophilic sites on DNA, proteins, etc.

removal of one of the two alkyl groups equals 100%). A later study showed that incubation of four (haloaryl)dimethyltriazenes and the unsubstituted 3,3-dimethyl-1-phenyltriazene with microsomes led to the loss of between 35 and 122% of the methyl groups as formaldehyde (calculated on the above basis) (Pool, 1979a). These results imply some oxidation of the second methyl group. 3,3-Dimethyl-1-phenyltriazene yielded the lowest and 1-(2,4,6-trichlorophenyl)3,3-dimethyltriazene (18, Fig. 5) gave the highest extent of oxidation at N-CH_3 (Pool, 1979a), although Kolar and Habs (1984) have reported that the presence of halogen substituents on the benzene ring decreases the extent of this metabolism. There have been several other studies on the effect of the nature of the (substituted)aryl group on the extent of metabolism at the N-CH_3 groups of aryldimethyltriazenes; some of these studies give conflicting results and conclusions (Preussmann et al., 1969b; Audette et al., 1973; Giraldi et al., 1975). Inhibition of this metabolism by metabolic products has been

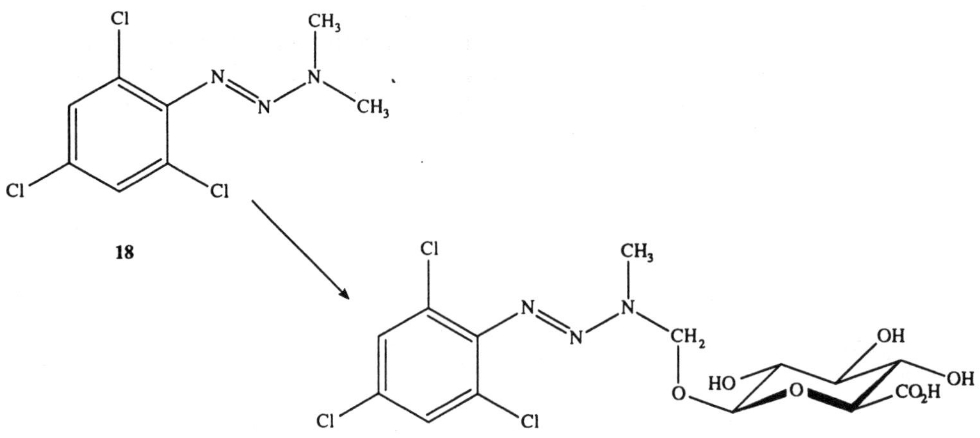

19

FIG. 5. Metabolic oxidation/conjugation of 3,3-dimethyl-1-(2,4,6-trichlorophenyl)triazene (18) in the mouse.

noted (Giraldi et al., 1975). The ultimate fate of some 40% of the radioactivity administered as 3,3-di[^{14}C]methyl-1-phenyltriazene to rats was reported to be exhalation as $^{14}CO_2$ by Kleihues et al. (1976). These workers and Hradec and Kolar (1985) also observed the formation of 7-[^{14}C]methylguanine and other methylated DNA and RNA bases. *N*-Hydroxy-*N*-methyltriazenes appear not to be substrates for oxidative metabolism (Preussmann et al., 1969b).

Work by Stevens et al. (1979) using chemical biomimetic oxidation of related triazenes in which the two alkyl groups are part of a heteroalicyclic ring has shown facile oxidation to nitrogen, although the chemical products were devoid of antitumor activity. The Udenfriend system has been used as a chemical model for the oxidative metabolism of 1-aryl-3,3-dimethyltriazenes to reactive methylating agents (Matrka et al., 1988).

Unambiguous and direct identification of a monoalkyltriazene as a metabolite of a 1-aryl-3,3-dimethyltriazene was first reported by Farina et al. (1982); 1-(4-acetylphenyl)-3-methyltriazene (21, Fig. 6), together with 4-aminoacetophenone (22), was found as a metabolite of 1-(4-acetylphenyl)-3,3-dimethyltriazene (20) both in the plasma of mice in vivo and in 9000 × *g* fractions of mouse liver homogenate in vitro. A more indirect observation of a monomethyltriazene as a metabolite of a dimethyltriazene has been made in that one of the metabolites found in incubations of rodent hepatic microsomes with 3,3-dimethyl-1-phenyltriazene was 3-acetyl-3-methyl-1-phenyltriazene (12, Fig. 3) (Pool, 1979b). Presumably, the formation of this *N*-acyltriazene involves the monomethyltriazene (11) as a metabolic intermediate which is subsequently acetylated.

The immediate metabolic precursors of 1-aryl-3-methyltriazenes, the 1-aryl-3-(hydroxymethyl)-3-methyltriazenes (26, Fig. 7A), have been synthesized (Gescher et al., 1978; Juillard et al., 1980). However, such carbinolamines have not yet been identified unambiguously as metabolites of aryldimethyltriazenes. At first sight, it is difficult to envisage how such compounds could be more selectively cytotoxic than their decomposition products, the monomethyltriazenes. Certain *N*-(hydroxymethyl)amines and *N*-(hydroxymethyl)amides related to *N*-(hydroxymethyl)-*N*-methyltriazenes have the ability to form, or can be in equilibrium with, electrophilic, potentially toxic imines or iminium ions, either themselves or after conjugation; the chemical features which predispose *N*-(hydroxymethyl) compounds to undergo such reactions under physiological conditions have been reviewed (Overton et al., 1985). Such an elimination reaction (Fig. 7A) could, on paper, be a mechanism by which hydroxymethyltriazenes exert toxicity in a manner different from that which renders monomethyltriazenes cytotoxic (Hemens et al., 1984; Soloway et al., 1983). However, a chemical and kinetic study of the reactions of 3-(hydroxymethyl)-3-methyl-1-(pyridin-3-yl)triazene with amine bases to give 3-methyl-1-(pyridin-3-yl)triazene as the sole product (Cheng et al., 1985) and the failure of the treatment of 1-aryl-3-(hydroxymethyl)-3-methyltriazenes with sodium cyanoborohydride, an iminium trapping agent, to yield 3,3-dimethyltriazenes (M. D. Threadgill, unpublished results) suggest that this is not an electrophilic reaction pathway open to *N*-(hydroxymethyl)triazenes under physiological conditions. Nevertheless, it has been shown that a reactive iminium is formed during chemical reactions of acetate and benzoate esters of *N*-(hydroxymethyl)triazenes (28 and 29, respectively, Fig. 7B) with nucleophiles. Presumably the enhanced leaving-group ability of the carboxylate leads to this increased electrophilicity (Hemens et al., 1984; Hemens and Vaughan, 1986; Iley et al., 1987a), although Vaughan et al. (1987) postulate a direct non-ionic S_N2 reaction of 28 with azide ion to give a new type of prodrug of monomethyltriazenes, which does not require oxidative metabolism. However, such acylation of a *N*-(hydroxymethyl)triazene has yet to be shown in biochemical experiments. Methyleneiminium triazenes are also formed during reactions of *N*-(hydroxymethyl)triazenes with nucleophiles under acidic conditions (Iley et al., 1987b, 1988).

The rather unstable nature of *N*-(hydroxymethyl)-*N*-methyltriazenes (Vaughan et al., 1984) has been claimed to mitigate against their role as the ultimate antineoplastic species derived from dimethyltriazenes. Nevertheless, the possibility that they are important as precursors of monomethyltriazenes with a transport function cannot be excluded, particularly if they are stabilized as the corresponding glucuronide acetate conjugate. It is pertinent in this context to note that Kolar and Carubelli (1979) identified 1-{[3-methyl-1-(2,4,6-trichlorophenyl)triazen-1-1]methyl}-β-D-glucuronic acid (19, Fig. 5) as a metabolite in the urine of mice which had received 3,3-dimethyl-1-(2,4,6-trichlorophenyl)triazene (18) and the authors suggested that this conjugate may, indeed, carry the monomethyltriazene to the target tissue. Metabolic conjugation of triazenes

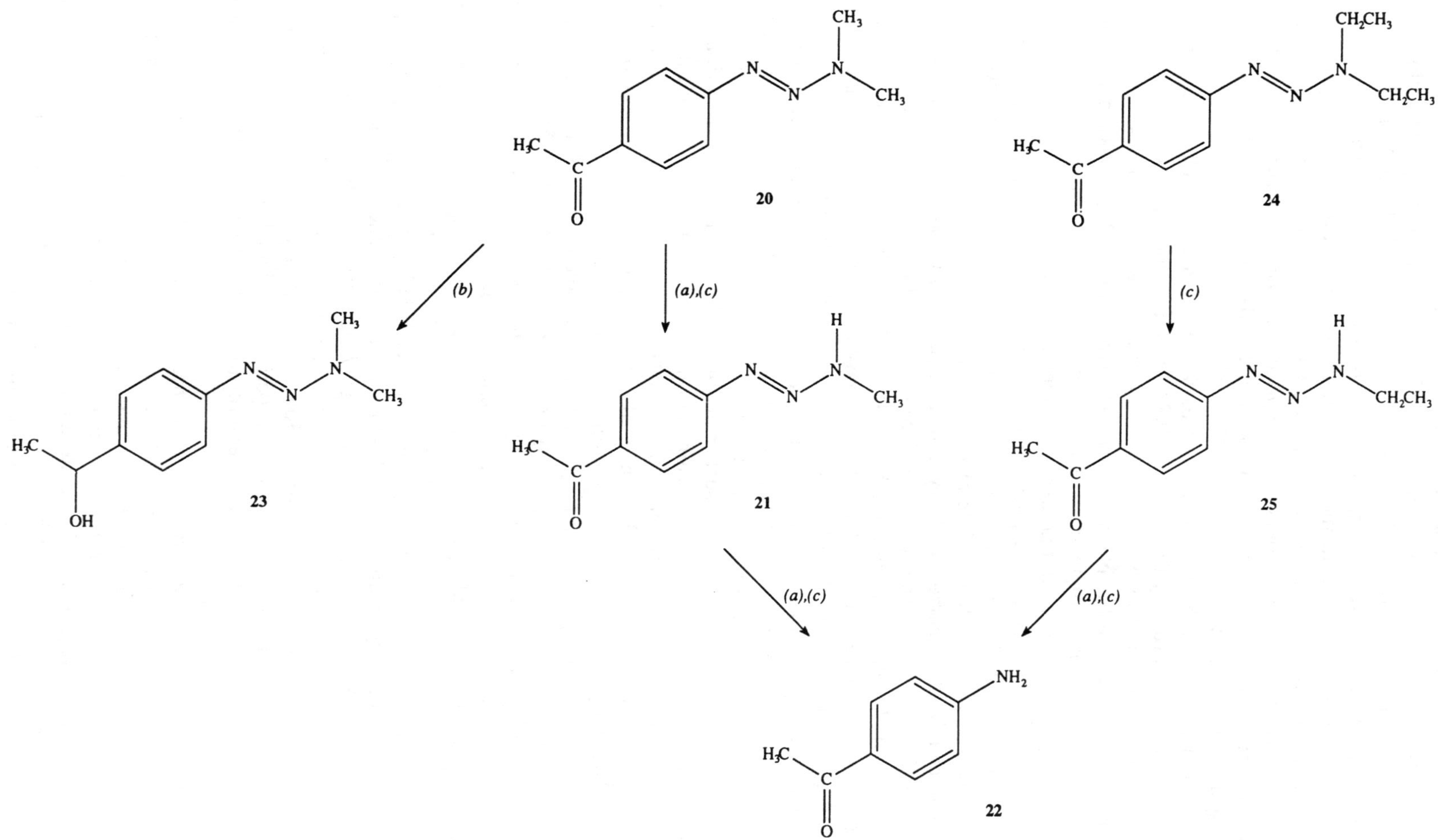

FIG. 6. Oxidative and reductive metabolic pathways demonstrated for 1-(4-acetylphenyl)triazenes (16) and (24). (a) Farina et al., 1982. (b) Farina et al., 1983. (c) Farina et al., 1986.

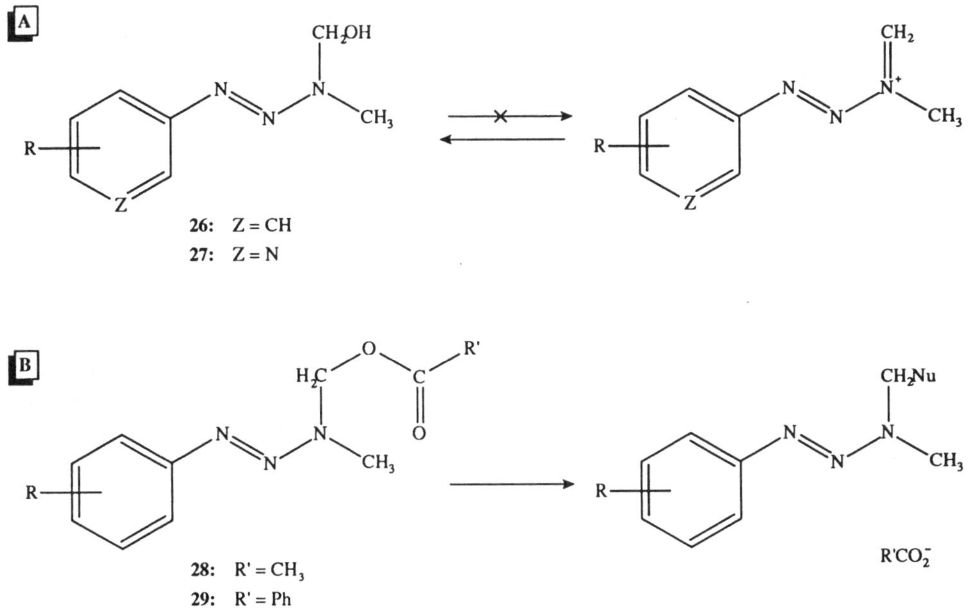

FIG. 7. (A) Electrophilic iminium ions from *N*-(hydroxymethyl)triazenes. (B) Electrophilic reactivity of *N*-(acyloxymethyl)triazenes.

to glutathione and to sulfate has yet to be reported, although a putative glutathione conjugate has been synthesized chemically (Iley et al., 1988).

Monomethyltriazenes and 3-(hydroxymethyl)-3-methyltriazenes generated as metabolites of dimethyltriazenes could be considered as substrates for further metabolism. Indeed, aniline is a metabolite of 3,3-dimethyl-1-phenyltriazene in vitro in amounts equimolar to the amount of formaldehyde formed (Druckrey et al., 1967; Preussmann et al., 1969b) and Toren et al. (1984) have detected methanol formed metabolically from 1-aryl-3-methyltriazenes and from a 1-aryl-3-(hydroxymethyl)-3-methyltriazene. When further oxidative metabolism is considered, it should be noted that analogous *N*-(hydroxymethyl)benzamides are subject to further metabolic oxidation at the methylene group yielding the corresponding *N*-(hydroxymethyl)benzamide which is excreted by the mouse in the urine (Ross et al., 1983). *N*-(Hydroxymethyl)triazenes, however, have not yet been reported to undergo this metabolic oxidation to afford the corresponding *N*-formyltriazenes which are highiy reactive entities (Ignasiak et al., 1975; Threadgill and Gledhill, 1986; Butler et al., 1987), although *N*-formyltriazenes are the principal products of oxidation of *N*-methyltriazenes and *N*-hydroxymethyltriazenes by a chemical model for cytochromes P450 (Iley and Ruecroft, 1988). Some evidence for a second biological oxidation has been obtained in experiments in which the fate of 1-(4-acetylphenyl)3-methyltriazene (21, Fig. 6) in suspensions of murine hepatocytes was investigated (Farina et al., 1983). The monomethyltriazene was consumed in this medium at a rate significantly more rapid than in suspensions of nonviable cells. The chemical nature of the products of this metabolic reaction are completely unknown.

Metabolic oxidation at the nitrogen atoms of the triazene group of an arylmonoalkyltriazene has been observed only once, in that 3-(4-carboxy-3-fluorophenyl)-1-methyltriazene-1-oxide was revealed by ^{19}F NMR spectroscopy to be a urinary metabolite of the corresponding dimethyltriazene, 3-fluoro-4-(3,3-dimethyltriazen-1-yl)benzoic acid (Vaughan and Wilman, 1991).

3. METABOLISM REMOTE FROM THE TRIAZENE MOIETY

1-Aryl-3,3-dimethyltriazenes undergo metabolism also at sites remote from the triazene moiety, i.e. in the aryl part of the molecule or involving transformation of functional groups attached thereto. Kolar and Schlesiger (1976b) reported indirect evidence for such metabolites in that the major urinary metabolite derived from 3,3-dimethyl-1-phenyltriazene in rats was found to be 4-aminophenol (30) with smaller amounts of the 3-amino and 2-amino isomers (31 and 32, respectively, Fig. 8). These authors also proposed ring-hydroxylated triazenes as metabolites of this substrate but only after chemical coupling with 1-(ethylamino)naphthalene to give the azo dyes 1-(ethylamino)-4(4-hydroxybenzeneazo)naphthalene (35) and 1-(ethylamino)-4-(2-hydroxybenzeneazo)naphthalene (36). This derivatization involves the loss of N^3 of the triazene (with its attached groups) and thus the urinary triazenes 33 and 34 may have been 3,3-dimethyl, 3-methyl or even 3-(hydroxymethyl)-3-methyl compounds. A more direct example of metabolism remote from the triazene moiety with confirmed retention of the N^3 substituents is that the ketone carbonyl group of 1-(4-acetylphenyl)-3,3-dimethyltriazene (20) was reduced by preparations of murine hepatic tissue in vitro to give 1-[4-(1-hydroxyethyl)phenyl]-3,3-dimethyltriazene (29, Fig. 6). Interestingly, this material retained an antitumor activity similar to that of the parent drug (Farina et al., 1983). The principal urinary metabolites of the experimental drug, 4-(3,3-dimethyl-1-triazenyl)benzoic acid (1; R = 4-CO_2H) have been found to be the glucuronide and glycine conjugates of the parent dimethyltriazene; the corresponding monomethyltriazene and its derivatives were not observed (Benfenati et al., 1989).

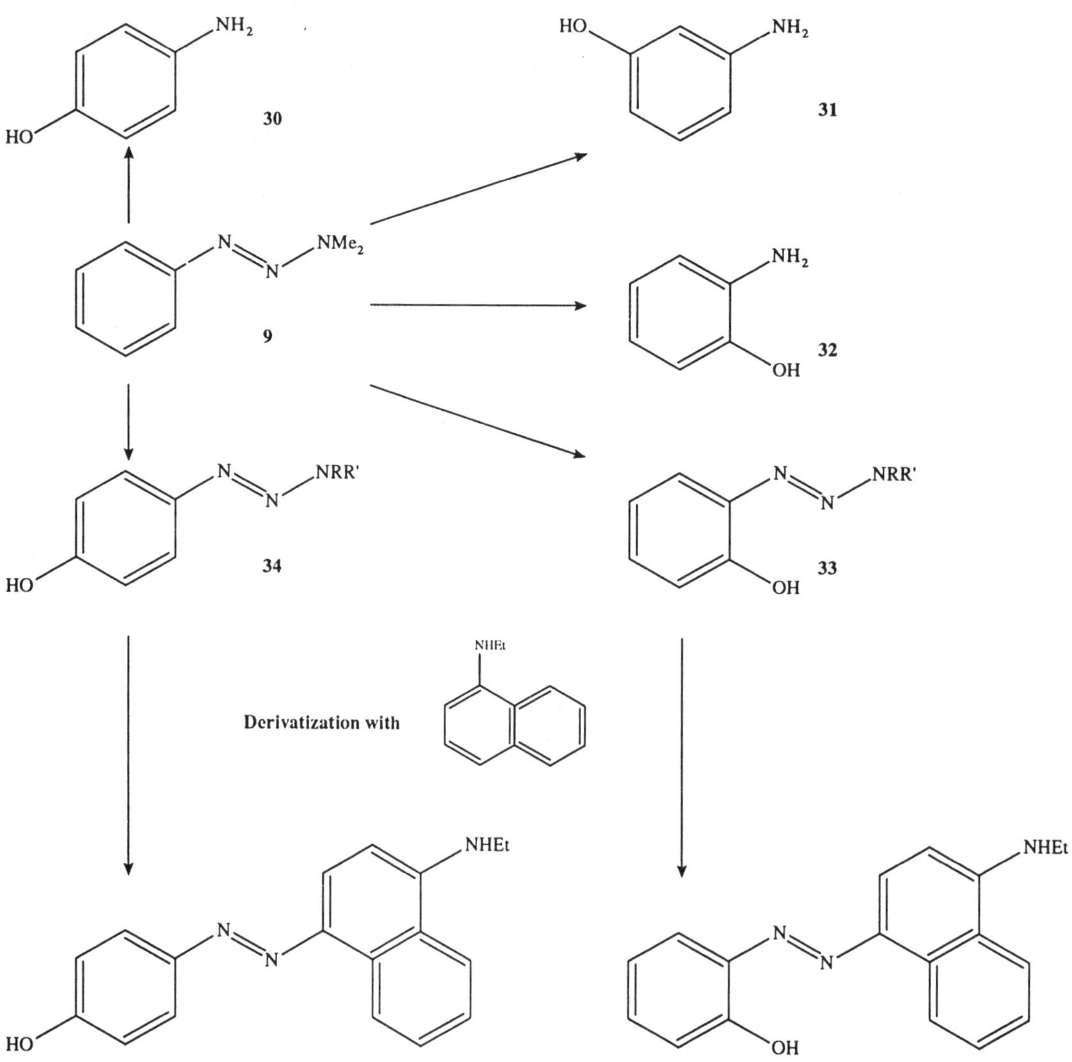

FIG. 8. Aryl-hydroxylated metabolites of 3,3-dimethyl-1-phenyltriazene (9) in the mouse. R = CH_3; R′ = H, CH_2OH, CH_3.

4. METABOLIC FATE OF 1-(IMIDAZOL-5-YL)-3-ALKYLTRIAZENES

The major urinary metabolite of dacarbazine (2) in man is 5-aminoimidazole-4-carboxamide (AIC: 39, Fig. 9) (Householder and Loo, 1969; Skibba et al., 1970a,b; Breithaupt et al., 1982). AIC has also been identified as a product of metabolism of dacarbazine in vitro in incubations with mouse liver microsomes (Hill, 1975) and with human and animal tumor tissue (Gerulath and Loo, 1972; Mizuno and Humphrey, 1972). From the mechanistic point of view, it is difficult to envisage how AIC could be formed by a metabolic pathway other than one implicating the intermediate formation of 5-(3-methyltriazen-1-yl)imidazole-4-carboxamide (MTIC: 38), followed by the tautomerism noted by Hooper and Vaughan (1981), amongst others, and subsequent hydrolysis. Many workers have reported that metabolism is required for the antitumor activity of dacarbazine to be manifest (Skibba et al., 1969a,b; Skibba and Bryan, 1971; Preussmann et al., 1969a). 5-[3-(Hydroxymethyl)-3-methyltriazen-1-yl]imidazole-4-carboxamide (HMTIC: 37, Fig. 9), the metabolic precursor of MTIC, has been characterized as a urinary metabolite of dacarbazine in rats (Kolar et al., 1980). Surprisingly, this hydroxymethyl compound was reported to be more stable than MTIC in polar solvents. This observation led to the suggestion that HMTIC may act as a transport form for MTIC, the postulated ultimate cytotoxic species derived from dacarbazine. After the manner of 3-methyl-1-phenyltriazene, MTIC decomposes spontaneously in aqueous media to form AIC (39) and was capable of alkylating biological nucleophiles such as DNA (Mizuno and Decker, 1976). The pharmacokinetic studies published so far on dacarbazine (Householder and Loo, 1971; Loo et al., 1968, 1976; Skibba et al., 1969a,b; Breithaupt et al., 1982) have not provided information on concentrations in plasma or tissue of metabolically generated HMTIC or MTIC. Therefore, the pharmacokinetic data available on dacarbazine is of limited value in helping to relate the efficacy or toxicity of this drug to the concentrations of cytotoxic or biologically inactive metabolites in body fluids and tissues. The major shortcoming of most of the pharmacokinetic data reported in the literature is the analytical procedure employed, a colorimetric method which determines the total amount of compounds with intact triazene linkages and therefore does not discriminate between dacarbazine, HMTIC and MTIC. The plasma elimination half-life of such species after

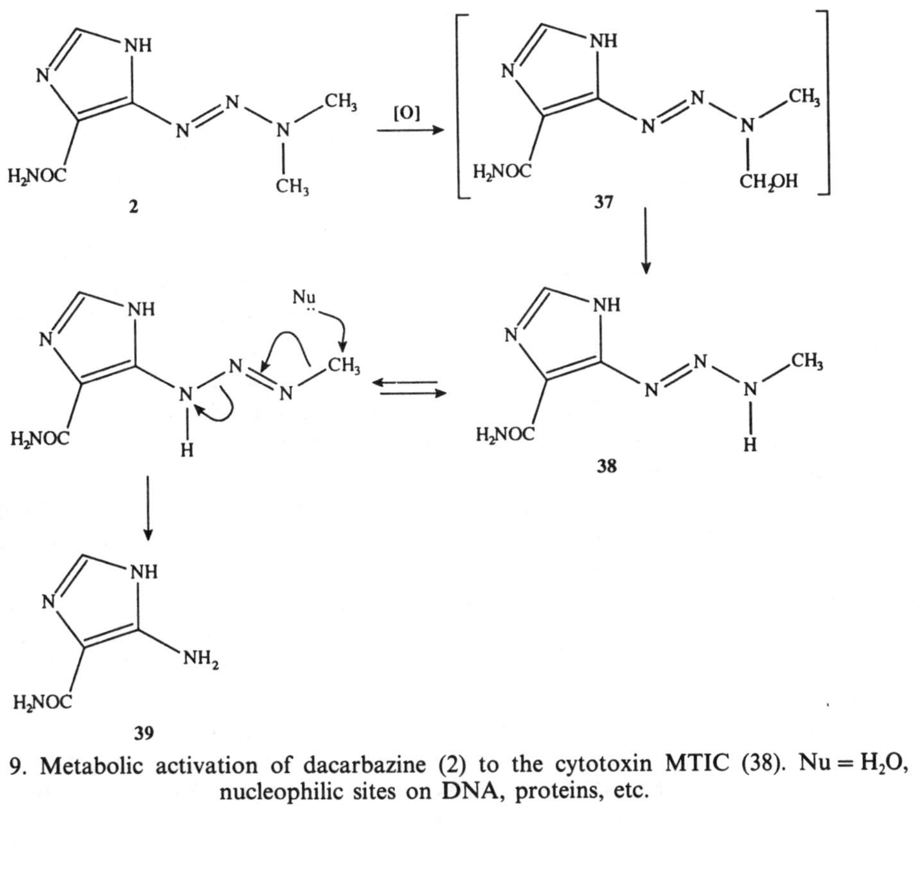

39

FIG. 9. Metabolic activation of dacarbazine (2) to the cytotoxin MTIC (38). Nu = H_2O, nucleophilic sites on DNA, proteins, etc.

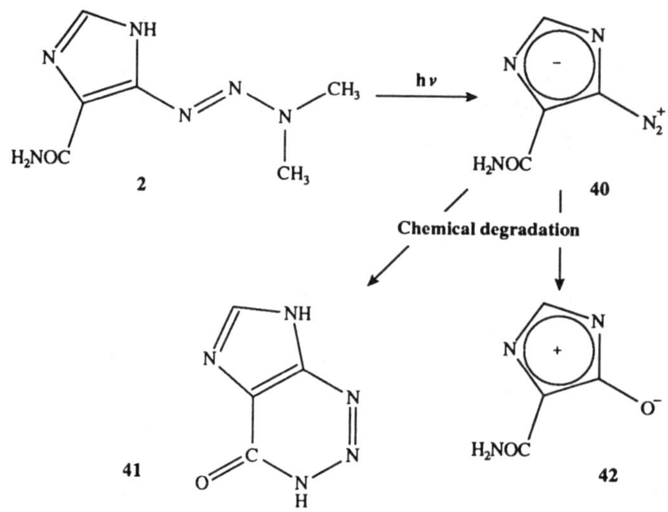

FIG. 10. Photodecomposition and subsequent chemical degradation of dacarbazine (2).

i.v. administration of dacarbazine to patients was 35 min (Loo et al., 1968). Measurement of plasma concentrations of dacarbazine using a HPLC method yielded a biphasic elimination profile with a terminal half-life of 41.4 min (Breithaupt et al., 1982). In this study, the plasma decay of metabolically generated AIC was monoexponential with a half-life of 43–116 min. The urinary recovery was 46–52% for dacarbazine and 9–18% for AIC. These pharmacokinetic data are in broad agreement with those obtained earlier with inferior analytical methods (Householder and Loo, 1969, 1971; Loo et al., 1968; Skibba et al., 1969a,b).

Dacarbazine is photolabile and reverts in light to its synthetic precursor 5-diazoimidazole-4-carboxamide (40, Fig. 10) (Horton and Stevens, 1981). This diazo compound and its decomposition products, 2-azahypoxanthine (41) and 4-carbamoylimidazolium-5-olate (42) have not been found as metabolites of dacarbazine in vivo, although the former has been implicated in the antibacterial action of the parent drug (Saunders and Schultz, 1972).

5. METABOLISM OF THE IMIDAZOTETRAZINONES

The metabolic fate of the imidazotetrazinones remains to be elucidated fully. Unlike the open chain dacarbazine which does not decompose under simulated physiological conditions, the cyclic mitozolomide (3) undergoes rapid hydrolytic ring-opening to give 5-[3-(2-chloroethyl)triazen-1-yl]imidazole-4-carboxamide (MCTIC: 44, Fig. 11) (Stevens et al., 1984) which may well be the ultimate antineoplastic metabolite of the parent drug (Horgan and Tisdale, 1984). MCTIC is an exceedingly short-lived compound with a $t_{1/2}$ of only 5.5 min at pH 7.5 (Horgan, 1985). Interestingly, this is the same compound as would be speculated to be formed by metabolic oxidative dealkylation of 5-[3,3-bis(2-chloroethyl)triazen-1-yl]imidazole-4-carboxamide (45), a dialkyltriazene with activity against tumors in the brain (Shealy et al., 1968; Levin et al., 1975). The great reactivity of 3-(2-chloroethyl)triazenes (46, Fig. 12) is thought to be due to their facile cyclization to 1,2,3-triazolines (48) or 1,2,3-triazolium salts (49) (Abraham et al., 1969; Lown and Singh, 1981). There is evidence to suggest that metabolism is an important determinant of the rate of deactivation of mitozolomide. Workman and Lee (1984) have shown that pretreatment of mice with phenobarbital reduces the activity of mitozolomide against the KHT sarcoma. In accordance with this finding, the area of the plasma-concentration-of-mitozolomide vs. time curve, determined in mice which had been pretreated with phenobarbital, was also significantly smaller than that in control mice (Brindley et al., 1986).

Hydrolytic ring-opening of temozolomide (4), the methyl analog of mitozolomide, should yield MTIC (38, Fig. 13). In order to test the hypotheses that temozolomide degrades to MTIC in physiological solutions and that MTIC mediates, or contributes to, the cytotoxicity of temozolo-

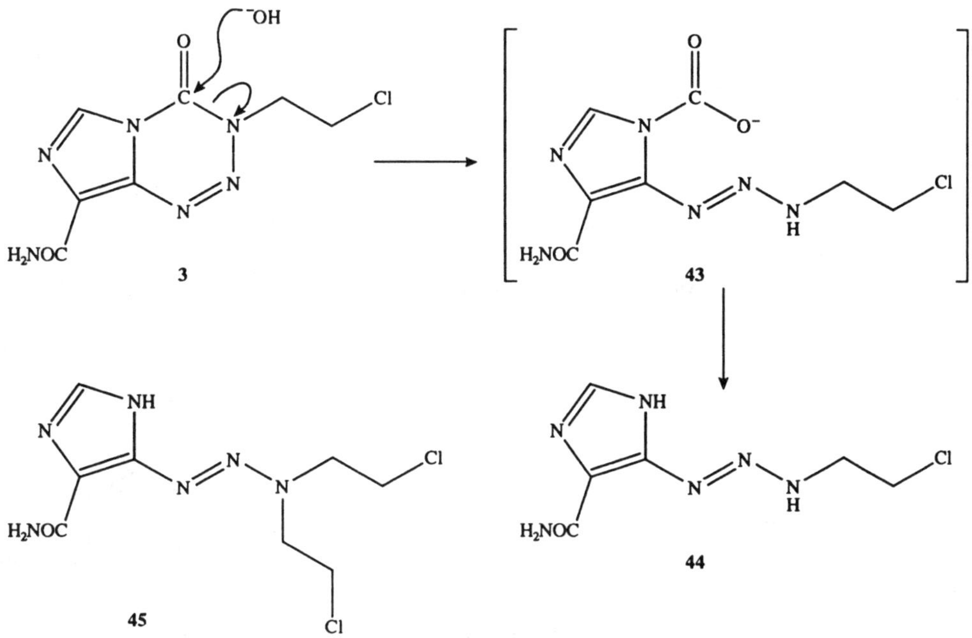

FIG. 11. Non-enzymic hydrolytic ring-opening of mitozolomide (3) to the active metabonate MCTIC (44).

mide, the drug was incubated with TLX5 cells. MTIC was detected by HPLC within 1 hr in the presence or absence of murine liver microsomes (Tsang et al., 1991). In contrast, when dacarbazine was incubated under the same conditions, MTIC was found only when microsomes were present. MTIC is also present in the urine of mice that have received temozolomide (Tsang et al., 1991). When temozolomide was incubated with preparation of murine liver, the drug was not metabolized at a measurable rate except for its chemical degradation to MTIC (Tsang et al., 1990). Contrastingly, the analogous 3-methylbenzo-1,2,3-triazin-4-one (52) was metabolically demethy-

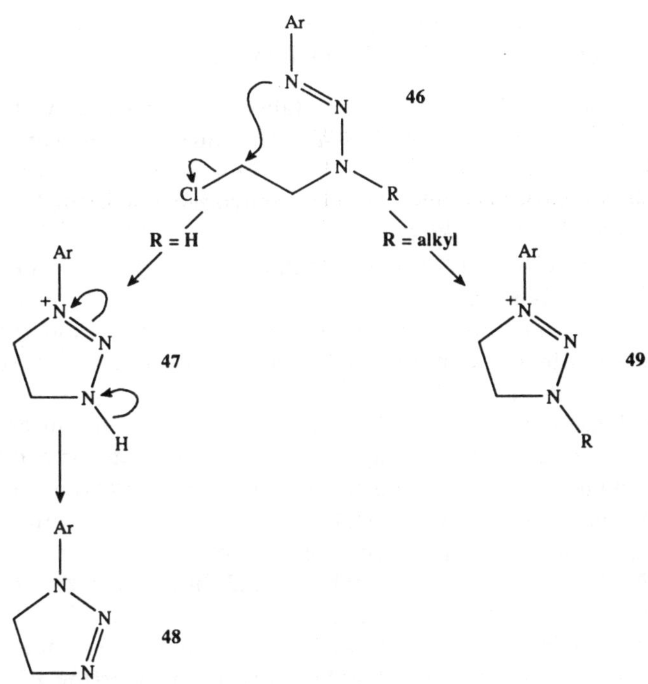

FIG. 12. Mechanism of cyclization degradation of *N*-(2-chloroethyl)triazenes.

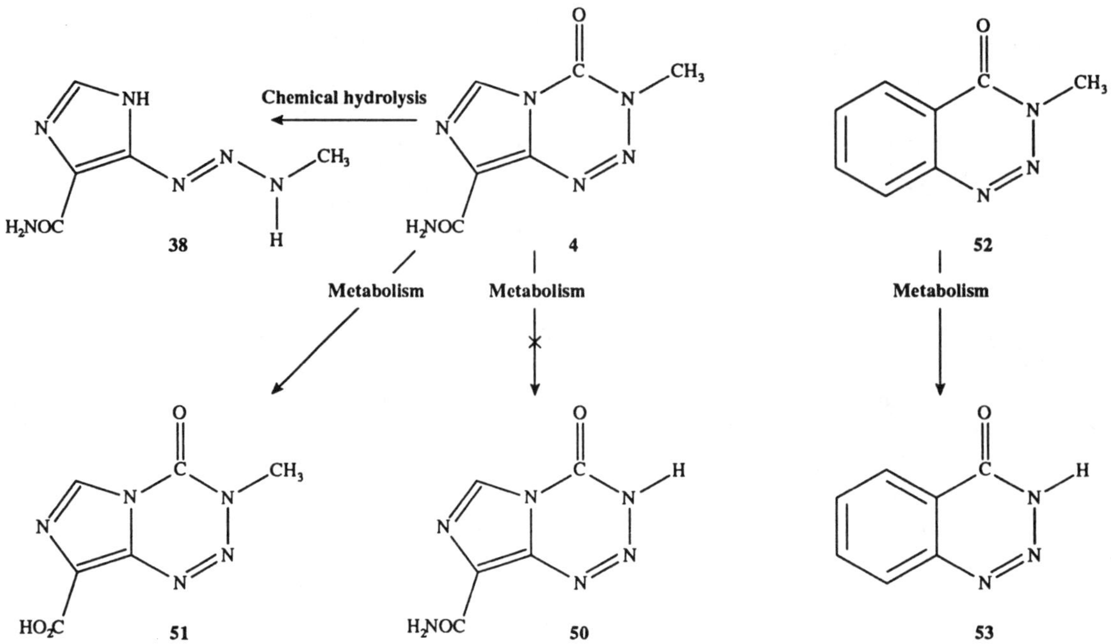

FIG. 13. Metabolic fate of temozolomide (4) in comparison with that of its non-antineoplastic analogue (52).

lated to give the benzotriazinone (53, Fig. 13). The major route of excretion of temozolomide in mice is via the kidneys. An acidic metabolite of temozolomide, probably a conjugate, was found in the urine of mice but its identity has not yet been established unambiguously. Another metabolite, the corresponding 8-carboxylic acid (51), has been found in the urine of human patients but not of mice. Unlike the unknown conjugate, this carboxylic acid was cytotoxic towards TLX5 lymphoma cells in vitro (Tsang et al., 1990).

6. THE ROLE OF METABOLISM IN THE MECHANISM OF ANTITUMOR ACTIVITY OF TRIAZENES

Many crucial mechanistic details that link the metabolism of triazenes with their antineoplastic activity remain obscure. Answers to the following three questions appear to be pivotal in the elucidation of this link:

(1) How can the aggressively reactive monomethyltriazene generated by metabolism of a dimethyltriazene cause selective cytotoxicity?

(2) Is the metabolic route which leads to the antineoplastic species identical with that which generates the carcinogenic metabolite?

(3) Are differences in the metabolism between dimethyltriazenes and other dialkyltriazenes responsible for the marked difference in antineoplastic activity observed in some murine tumors (Connors et al., 1976; Gescher et al., 1981)?

Even though the evidence for the involvement of metabolism in the mechanism of antitumor activity of dimethyltriazenes is overwhelming, the possibility that some dimethyltriazenes are themselves cytotoxic, under certain circumstances, without metabolic activation cannot be dismissed. Dacarbazine has been used in local therapy in patients with advanced malignant melanoma and soft tissue sarcoma of the extremities and regression of tumors has been observed (Aigner et al., 1983). Furthermore, 1-(4-carboxyphenyl)-3,3-dimethyltriazene (1; R 4-CO_2H, Fig. 1) did not undergo marked oxidative demethylation in vitro (Sava et al., 1982), yet it possessed antimetastatic properties in mice bearing the Lewis lung carcinoma (Giraldi et al., 1981). This drug also increased the survival of mice bearing the TLX5 lymphoma or the P388 leukemia without exerting marked cytotoxicity (Sava et al., 1982).

Some doubt has been cast on the contention that an electrophile as indiscriminate and non-selective as a monomethyltriazene could account for the antineoplastic activity of dimethyltriazenes (Gescher et al., 1981). This doubt was based on experiments in which the cytotoxicity of a monomethyltriazene was tested in a bioassay against a mouse TLX5 lymphoma cell line which had acquired resistance to dimethyltriazenes in vivo. The monomethyltriazene was found to be non-selectively toxic to both the sensitive and resistant lines, whereas incubation of the dimethyltriazene with a liver homogenate produced metabolites which were more toxic to the sensitive than to the resistant lymphoma cells (Gescher et al., 1981). However, cytotoxic metabolites of dimethyltriazenes, which are more selective than the monomethyltriazenes, have yet to be isolated or characterized. *N*-(Hydroxymethyl)triazenes were found to be equally as cytotoxic as their decomposition products, the monomethyltriazenes (Vaughan et al., 1984; Kohlsmith et al., 1984). Consequently, it has been suggested by some workers that the *N*-(hydroxymethyl) compounds may be the ultimate or proximate cytotoxic metabolites of dimethyltriazenes (Vaughan et al., 1984). The third question posed above has been addressed in a recent comparison of the antitumor activities and toxicities of 1-(4-acetylphenyl)-3,3-dimethyltriazene (20, Fig. 6) and 1-(4-acetylphenyl)3,3-diethyltriazene (24, Fig. 6) (Farina et al., 1986). The diethyltriazene was inactive against three murine tumors which were highly sensitive to the dimethyltriazene. However, the diethyltriazene was much more toxic to the host than was the dimethyl analogue. Both compounds were rapidly metabolized in vivo and in vitro and the monoalkyltriazenes (21 and 25, respectively) and 4-aminoacetophenone (22) were identified as metabolites of the parent compounds. However, the extent to which the drugs were *N*-dealkylated differed markedly. The amount of monoethyltriazene generated was only one third of the amount of monomethyl derivative found (Farina et al., 1986). This result suggests that the difference in activities between different dialkyltriazenes may indeed be due to differences in metabolism. A QSAR study has shown good correlation between antitumor activity and the presence of electron-donating substituents on the benzene ring of 3,3-dimethyl-1-(substituted)phenyltriazenes (Hatheway et al., 1978); this same chemical parameter also correlates with the extent of metabolic activation by hydroxylation at N-CH_3 by cytochromes P450 (Venger et al., 1979; Shusterman et al., 1989a,b). However, based upon studies involving induction of a cytochromes P450 by pretreatment with phenobarbital, Sava et al. (1988) raised some doubt about the role of metabolic activation in the antitumor activities and antimetastatic activities of 1-aryl-3,3-dimethyltriazenes against the Lewis lung carcinoma in the mouse. There has been one suggestion that arenediazonium metabonates of 1-aryl-3,3-dialkyltriazenes are responsible for their antitumor activity (Nifontov et al., 1984) but this conclusion is at variance with the vast majority of the literature.

On the basis of a preliminary pharmacokinetic study of dacarbazine and its metabolite MTIC in rodents and in human patients, Rutty (1983) suggested that the relative lack of antitumor activity of dacarbazine in man compared to rodents may be related to differences in the rate of hydroxylation at the *N*-methyl group; this hydroxylation is slow in man and fast in mice. It is, however, interesting to note that murine Sarcoma 180 cells themselves are capable of metabolizing dacarbazine (Mizuno and Humphrey, 1972).

Temozolomide is hydrolyzed chemically to its active metabonate MTIC, whereas this reactive electrophile is formed only after oxidative metabolism of dacarbazine. Thus, temozolomide may provide a pharmacokinetic advantage over dacarbazine in the clinical situation in the generation of the cytotoxic monomethyltriazene. A large number of analogues of mitozolomide and temozolomide have been synthesized with the aim of clarifying which chemical features of the imidazotetrazinone are essential for expression of their cytotoxic and antineoplastic properties. In analogues with a carboxamide at position 8, an NH appears to be required for maximal cytotoxicity in vitro. The dimethylcarboxamide 5 (Fig. 1) is markedly less cytotoxic in vitro than is mitozolomide (3) or the monomethylcarboxamide 6 (Horspool et al., 1989); nevertheless, the antitumor activity of the three agents in mice bearing the TLX5 lymphoma was very similar (Hickman et al., 1985; Lunt et al., 1987). The chemical stabilities of the three compounds are also similar. Incubation of 5 with marine hepatic microsomes led to increased cytotoxicity and to formation of the monomethyl analogue 6 (Horspool et al., 1989), suggesting that the latter causes or contributes to the antitumor effect of 5 in vivo. Interestingly, it has been demonstrated that $>89\%$ of the dose (10 mg kg^{-1}) of the administered dimethylcarboxamide is metabolized via the monomethylcarboxamide in the mouse.

7. THE ROLE OF METABOLISM IN THE MECHANISMS OF TOXICITY, MUTAGENICITY AND CARCINOGENICITY OF TRIAZENES

1-Aryl-3-methyltriazenes are direct-acting mutagens in the Ames assay (Malaveilie et al., 1982). The mutagenic activities of 1-aryl-3,3-dimethyltriazenes in *Drosophila melanogaster* have been reported to correlate with parameters on nucleophilicity which also correlate well with the extent of oxidative metabolic demethylation by cytochromes P450 (Vogel, 1989). Inhibition of cytochromes P450 causes a decrease in mutagenicity of 1-(2,4,6-trichlorophenyl)-3,3-dimethyltriazene (18) in this species, whereas inhibition of monoamine oxidase and of flavin monooxygenases caused increases in mutagenicity, suggesting again that metabolism by cytochromes P450 is required for mutagenic activity of this aryldimethyltriazene (Zijlstra and Vogel, 1988). In contrast, analogous studies with enzyme inhibitors indicated that the metabolism of dacarbazine (2) to the mutagenic derivative was mediated by flavin monooxygenases. It has been demonstrated that, for a wide range of aryldialkyltriazenes and heteroaryldimethyltriazenes (including dacarbazine), mutagenicity was manifest towards *Salmonella* in the Ames test after incubation with a rodent S9 microsomal preparation. In these QSAR studies, mutagenicity was found to correlate with the hydrophobicity (expressed as log P) and with parameters of electron density; extent of metabolism by cytochromes P450 also correlates with these parameters in a similar way (Venger et al., 1979; Hopfinger and Potenzone, 1982; Shusterman et al., 1989a,b). A strong relationship between toxicity to rats (expressed as LD_{50}) and these parameters has also been determined (Hansch et al., 1978).

Examples of benzenediazonium compounds, which are putative chemical breakdown products and metabolites of 3,3-dimethyl- or 3-methyl-triazenes, have been noted to be moderately carcinogenic in mice (Toth et al., 1989) and mutagens (Malaveille et al., 1982).

Kohn et al. (1988) have reported that the urine of patients who bave received dacarbazine (2) contains metabolites that are mutagenic to *Escherichia coli.*

8. CONCLUSIONS

It has been shown in very many studies that the principal metabolic process undergone by 1-aryl-3,3-dimethyltriazenes is oxidative hydroxylation at *N*-methyl group, with subsequent breakdown to the corresponding monomethyltriazene. It is also abundantly clear that this is a necessary metabolic step for the expression of beneficial antineoplastic activity of such triazenes, including the clinically used drug dacarbazine. Unfortunately, the molecular parameters which predispose these open-chain triazenes to metabolic activation as antitumor agents are effectively the same as those correlating with activation as mutagens, carcinogens and general toxins; oxidative metabolic activiation also requires that patients have competent hepatic function. Hence, one can only be pessimistic about the prospects of design of new dimethyltriazenes for therapeutic applications. Generation of the reactive and cytotoxic monomethyltriazenes non-enzymically from pro-drugs such as temozolomide may well constitute the way forward in the design of new compounds of this class for the effective treatment of cancers.

REFERENCES

ABRAHAM, D. J., RUTHERFORD, J. S. and ROSENSTEIN, R. D. (1969) Single crystal studies of chemotherapeutic agents. The structure of 1-(2-chloroethyl)-3(5)-(carbamoylimidazole-4-yl)-Δ^2-1,2,3-triazolinium chloride. *J. med. Chem.* **12:** 189–190.

ADAMS, F. H. and WRIGHT, D. P. (1964) Method of protecting plants and organic matter with substituted triazenes. U.S. Patent 3162571.

AIGNER, K., HILD, P., BREITHAUPT, H., HUNDEIKER, M., SCHWEMMLE, K., HENNEKING, K., ILLING, L. L., MERKER, G., PAUL, E., BRODKORB, J. and JUNGBLUTH, A. (1983) Isolated extremity perfusion with DTIC. An experimental and clinical study. *Anticancer Res.* **3:** 87–94.

AUDETTE, R. S. C., CONNORS, T. A., MANDEL, H. K., MERAI, K. and ROSS, W. C. J. (1973) Studies on the mechanism of action of the tumour inhibitory triazenes. *Biochem. Pharmac.* **22:** 1855–1864.

BENFENATI, E., FARINA, P., COLOMBO, T., DE BELLIS, G., CAPPODIFERRO, M. V. and D'INCALCI, M. (1989) Metabolism and pharmacokinetics of *p*-(3,3-dimethyl-1-triazeno)benzoic acid in M5076 sarcoma-bearing mice. *Cancer Chemother. Pharmac.* **24:** 354–358.

BLISS, E. A., GRIFFIN, R. J. and STEVENS, M. F. G. (1987) Structural studies on bioactive compounds. Part 5. A novel role for the azido group in lipophilic 2,4-diaminopyrimidine dihydrofolate reductase inhibitors. *J. Chem. Soc., Perkin Trans. 1* 2217–2228.

BREITHAUPT, H., DAMMANN, A. and AIGNER, K. (1982) Pharmacokinetics of dacarbazine (DTIC) and its metabolite 5-aminoimidazole-4-carboxamide (AIC) following different dose schedules. *Cancer Chemother. Pharmac.* **9:** 103–109.

BRINDLEY, C. J., ANTONIW, P. and NEWLANDS, E. S. (1986) Plasma and tissue decomposition of mitozolomide in mice. *Br. J. Cancer* **53:** 91–97.

BURCHENAL, J. H., DAGG, M. K., BEYER, M. and STOCK, C. C. (1956) Triazenes as antitumor agents. *Proc. Soc. exp. Biol. Med.* **91:** 398–403.

BUTLER, R. N., O'SHEA, P. D. and BURKE, L. A. (1987) Conjugated *N*-isocyanides; a reassessment and a correction of claimed stable conjugated *N*-isocyanides. Stable *N*-formyltriazenes; a confirmation. *J. Chem. Soc., Chem. Commun.* 1210–1212.

CHENG, S. C., FERNADES, L., ILEY, J. and ROSA, E. (1985) Triazene drug metabolites: base catalysed formation of *N*-alkyltriazenes from *N*-hydroxymethyl-*N*-methyltriazenes. *Tetrahedron Lett.* **26:** 1557–1560.

CLARKE, D. A., BARCLAY, R. K., STOCK, C. C. RONDESTVEDT, C. S., MULLER, A., PAGLIARO, A., O'LOUGHLIN, I. and HAGAN, P. (1955) Triazenes as inhibitors of mouse sarcoma 180. *Proc. Soc. exp. Biol. Med.* **90:** 484–489.

CONNORS, T. A., GODDARD, P. M., MERAI, K., ROSS, W. C. J. and WILLMAN, D. E. V. (1976) Tumour inhibitory triazenes: Structural requirements for an active metabolite. *Biochem. Pharmac.* **25:** 241–246.

DRUCKREY, H. (1973) Specific carcinogenic and teratogenic effects of 'indirect' alkylating methyl and ethyl compounds and their dependency on stages of oncogenic developments. *Xenobiotica* **3:** 271–303.

DRUCKREY, H., IVANKOVIC, S. and PREUSSMANN, R. (1967) Neurotropische carcinogene Wirkung von Phenyldimethyltriazen an Ratten. *Naturwissenschaften* **54:** 171.

FARINA, P., GESCHER, A., HICKMAN, J. A., HORTON, J. K., D'INCALCI, M., ROSS, D., STEVENS, M. F. G. and TORTI, L. C. (1982) Studies on the mode of action of antitumour triazenes and triazines. IV. The metabolism of 1-(4-acetylphenyl)-3,3-dimethyltriazene. *Biochem. Pharmac.* **31:** 1887–1892.

FARINA, P., BENFENATI, E., REGINATO, R., TORTI, L., D'INCALCI, M., THREADGILL, M. D. and GESCHER, A. (1983) Metabolism of the anticancer agent 1-(4-acetylphenyl)-3,3-dimethyltriazene. *Biomed. Mass Spectrom.* **10:** 485–488.

FARINA, P., TORTI, L., URSO, R., HORTON, J. K., GESCHER, A. and D'INCALCI, M. (1986) Comparison of metabolism and activity of an aryldimethyltriazene and an aryldiethyltriazene. *Biochem. Pharmac.* **35:** 209–215.

FODSTAD, O., AAMDAL, S., PIHL, A. and BOYD, M. R. (1985) Activity of mitozolomide (NSC 353451), a new imidazotetrazine, against xenografts from human melanomas, sarcomas, and lung and colon carcinomas. *Cancer Res.* **45:** 1778–1786.

GERULATH, A. H. and LOO, T. L. (1972) Mechanism of action of 5-(3,3-dimethyl-1-triazeno)imidazole-4-carboxamide in mammalian cells in culture. *Biochem. Pharmac.* **21:** 2335–2343.

GESCHER, A, HICKMAN, I. A., SIMMONDS, R. J., STEVENS, M. F. G. and VAUGHAN, K. (1978) α-Hydroxylated derivatives of antitumour dimethyltriazenes. *Tetrahedron Lett.* 5041–5044.

GESCHER, A., HICKMAN, J. A., SIMMONDS, R. J., STEVENS, M. F. G. and VAUGHAN, K. (1981) Studies on the mode of action of antitumour triazenes and triazines. II. Investigation of the selective toxicity of 1-aryl-3,3-dimethyltriazenes. *Biochem. Pharmac.* **30:** 89–93.

GIRALDI, T., NISI, C. and SAVA, G. (1975) Investigation on the oxidative *N*-demethylation of aryl triazenes in vitro. *Biochem. Pharmac.* **24:** 1793–1797.

GIRALDI, T., SAVA, G., CUMAN, R., NISI, C. and LASSIANI, L. (1981) Selectivity of the antimetastatic and cytotoxic effects of 1-*p*-(3,3-dimethyl-1-triazeno)benzoic acid potassium salt, (±)-1,2-di(3,5-dioxopiperazin-1-yl)propane and cyclophosphamide in mice bearing Lewis lung carcinoma. *Cancer Res.* **41:** 2524-2528.

GRILL, V., MALLARDI, F., ZORZET, S., PERISSIN, L. and GIRALDI, T. (1987) Morphological analysis of metastatic potential and antimetastatic drug effects in mice bearing two lines of Lewis lung carcinoma. *Clin. exp. Metastasis* **5:** 233–244.

HANSCH, C., HATHEWAY, G. J., QUINN, F. R. and GREENBERG, N. (1978) Antitumor 1-(X-aryl)-3,3- dialkyltriazenes. 2. On the role of correlation analysis in decision-making in drug modification. Toxicity quantitative structure-activity relationships of 1-(X-phenyl)3,3-dialkyltriazenes in mice. *J. med. Chem.* **21:** 574–577.

HARDING, M., NORTHCOTT, D., SMYTHE, J., STUART, N. S. A., GREEN, J. A. and NEWLANDS, E. (1988) Phase II evaluation of mitozolomide in ovarian cancer. *Br. J. Cancer* **57:** 113–114.

HATHEWAY, G. J., HANSCH, C., KIM, K. H., MILSTEIN, S. R., SCHMIDT, C. L., SMITH, R. N. and QUINN, F. R. (1978) Antitumor 1-(X-aryl)-3,3-dialkyltriazenes. 1. Quantitative structure-activity relationships vs. L1210 leukemia in mice. *J. med. Chem.* **21:** 563–574.

HEMENS, C. M. and VAUGHAN, K. (1986) Kinetic study of the solvolysis reactions of 1-aryl-3-acetoxymethyl-3-alkyltriazenes: evidence for iminium ion intermediates and the S_N1 mechanism. *J. Chem. Soc., Perkin Trans. 2* 11–15.

HEMENS, C. M., MANNING, H. W., VAUGHAN, K., LAFRANCE, R. J. and TANG, Y. (1984) Open chain nitrogen compounds. Part V. Hydroxymethyltriazenes: synthesis of some new alkyl homologues of the antitumour 3-methyl-3-hydroxymethyltriazenes and preparation of the derived acetoxymethyl, benzoyloxymethyl and methoxymethyltriazenes. *Can. J. Chem.* **62:** 741–748.

HICKMAN, J. A., STEVENS, M. F. G., GIBSON, N. W., LANGDON, S. P., FIZAMES, C., LAVALLE, F., ATASSI, G., LUNT, E. and TILSON, R. M. (1985) Experimental antitumour activity against murine tumour model systems of 8-carbamoyl-3-(2-chloroethyl)imidazo[5,1-*d*]-1,2,3,5-tetrazin-4(3H)-one (mitozolomide), a novel broad spectrum agent. *Cancer Res.* **45:** 3008–3013.

HILL, D. L. (1975) Microsomal metabolism of triazenylimidazoles. *Cancer Res.* **35:** 3106–3110.

HOOPER, D. L. and VAUGHAN, K. (1981) ^{13}C and ^{1}H Nuclear magnetic resonance study of solvent effects on tautomerism in 1-aryl-3-methyltriazenes. *J. Chem. Soc., Perkin Trans. 2* 1161–1165.

HOPFINGER, A. J. and POTENZONE, R. (1982) Ames test and antitumor activity of 1-(X-phenyl)-3,3- dimethyltriazenes. Quantitative structure-activity studies based on molecular shape analysis. *Molec. Pharmac.* **21:** 187–195.

HORGAN, C. M. T. (1985) Studies on mitozolomide (CCRG 81010), a new antineoplastic agent, PhD thesis, Aston University.

HORGAN, C. M. T. and TISDALE, M. J. (1984) Antitumour imidazotetrazines. IV. An investigation into the mechanism of antitumour activity of a novel and potent antitumour agent, mitozolomide. *Biochem. Pharmac.* **33:** 2185–2192.

HORSPOOL, K. R., QUARTERMAN, C. P., SLACK, J. A., GESCHER, A., STEVENS, M. F. G. and LUNT, E. (1989) Metabolism and murine pharmacokinetics of the 8-(N,N-dimethylcarboxamide) analogue of the experimental antitumor drug mitozolomide (N5C353451). *Cancer Res.* **49:** 5023–5026.

HORTON, J. K. and STEVENS, M. F. G. (1981) A new light on the photodecomposition of DTIC. *Biochem. Pharmac.* **33:** 808–811.

HOUSEHOLDER, G. E. and LOO, T. L. (1969) Elevated urinary excretion of 4-aminoimidazole-5-carboxamide in patients after i.v. injection of 4-(3,3-dimethyl-1-triazeno)imidazole-5-carboxamide. *Life Sci.* **8:** 533–536.

HOUSEHOLDER, G. E. and LOO, T. L. (1971) Disposition of 5-(3,3-dimethyl-1-triazeno)imidazole-4-carboxamide, a new antitumor agent *J. Pharmac. exp. Ther.* **179:** 386–395.

HRADEC, J. and KOLAR, G. F. (1985) Microsome-mediated alkylation of rat liver initiator tRNA by 3,3-dimethyl-1-phenyltriazene and its ring-chlorinated derivatives. *Carcinogenesis* **6:** 995–998.

IGNASIAK, T., SUSKO, J. and IGNASIAK, B. (1975) Structure of aromatic diazo cyanides; synthesis of diazoisocyanides. *J. Chem. Soc., Perkin Trans. 1* 2122–2129.

ILEY, J. and RUECROFT, G. (1988) Trinzene drug metabolites. Part 7. A biomimetic synthesis of *N*-alkyl-*N*-formyl triazenes. *J. Chem. Res., Synop.* 24–25.

ILEY, J., MOREIRA, R. and ROSA, E. (1987a) Triazene drug metabolites. Part 4. Kinetics and mechanism of the decomposition of 1-aryl-3-(benzoyloxymethyl)-3-methyltriazenes in mixed aqueous-organic solvents. *J. Chem. Soc., Perkin Trans. 1* 1503–1508.

ILEY, J., ROSA, E. and FERNANDES, L. (1987b) Triazene drug metabolites. Part 5. A simple direct synthesis of 3-(alkoxymethyl)- and 3-[(alkylthio)methyl]-1-aryl-3-alkyltriazenes from 1-aryl-3-(hydroxymethyl)-3-alkyltriazenes. *J. Chem. Res., Synop.* 264–265.

ILEY, J., MOREIRA, R., RUECROFT, G. and ROSA, E. (1988) Synthesis of *S*-cysteinyl, *S*-(*N*-acetylcysteinyl) and *S*-glutathionyl conjugates of *N*-hydroxymethyltriazenes. *Tetrahedron Lett.* **29:** 2707–2710.

IONESCU, D., NEAGU, V., DOBRE, V. and NICULESCU-DUVAZ, I. (1981) Potential anticancer agents. XXII. Pharmacological properties of some new triazene derivatives. *Neoplasma* **28:** 19–26.

JUILLARD, M., VERNIN, G. and METZGER, J. (1980) Triazenes; III. A convenient synthesis of triazenes with potential antitumour activity. *Synthesis* 116–117.

KLEIHUES, G. P., KOLAR, G. F. and MARGISON, G. P. (1976) Interaction of the carcinogen 3,3-dimethyl-1-phenyltriazene with nucleic acids of various rat tissues and the effect of a protein-free diet. *Cancer Res.* **36:** 2189–2193.

KLEIHUES, G. P., COOPER, H. K., BUECHELER, J., KOLAR, G. F. and DIESSNER, H. (1979) Mechanism of perinatal tumor induction by neuro-oncogenic alkylnitrosoureas and dialkyltriazenes. *Natn. Cancer Inst. Monograph* **51:** 227–231.

KOHLSMITH, D. J., VAUGHAN, K. and LUNER, S. J. (1984) Triazene metabolism. III. In vitro cytotoxicity towards M21 cells and in vivo antitumor activity of the proposed metabolites of the antitumor 1-aryl-3,3-dimethyltriazenes. *Can. J. Physiol. Pharmac.* **62:** 396–402.

KOHN, A., DONCHIN, M., JACOBS, J. Y., HORN, Y., GIBOR, Y., FISH, F., RIESENFELD, G., KIRENBERG, F. and LAMPERT, I. (1988) Detection of genotoxic substances in cancer patients receiving antineoplastic drugs. *Ann. N.Y. Acad. Sci.* **534:** 776–791.

KOLAR, G. F. (1984) Triazenes. In: *Chemical Carcinogens*, Vol. 2, pp. 869–914, American Chemical Society Monograph 182, American Chemical Society, Washington.

KOLAR, G. F. and CARUBELLI, R. (1979) Urinary metabolites of 1-(2,4,6-trichlorophenyl)-3,3-dimethyltriazene with an intact diazoamino structure. *Cancer Lett.* **7:** 209–214.

KOLAR, G. F. and HABS, H. (1984) Comparative metabolism and carcinogenicity of ring-halogenated 3,3-dimethyl-1-phenyltriazenes. *J. Cancer Res. clin. Oncol.* **108:** 71–75.

KOLAR, G. F. and SCHLESIGER, J. (1976a) Metabolism of the tumour-inhibitory 3,3-dimethyl-1-phenyltriazene and its 4-chlorophenyl analog. In: *Chemotherapy*, Vol. 8, pp. 91–96, HELLMAN, K. and CONNORS, T. A. (eds) Plenum Publishing Corp., New York.

KOLAR, G. F. and SCHLESIGER, J. (1976b) Urinary metabolites of 3,3-dimethyl-1-phenyltriazene. *Chem.-Biol. Interact.* **14:** 310–311.

KOLAR, G. F. and WILDSCHÜTTE, M. (1982) Metabolic activation of triazene cytostatics. In: *Biological Reactive*

Intermediates—II, Part B, pp. 1285–1296, SNYDER, R., PARKE, D. V., KOCSIS, J. J., JOLLOW, D. J., GIBSON, C. G. and WITMER, C. M. (eds) Plenum Publishing Corp., New York.

KOLAR, G. F., MAURER, M. and WILDSCHÜTTE, M. (1980) 5-(3-Hydroxymethyl-3-methyltriazeno)imidazole-4-carboxamide (DIC, DTIC, NSC 45388). *Cancer Lett.* **10:** 241–253.

LEVIN, V. A., CRAFTS, D., WILSON, C. B., KABRA, P., HANSCH, C., BOLDREY, E., ENOT, I. and NEELY, M. (1975) Relationship of lipophilicity to activity against intracerebral murine glioma 26 and preliminary phase II clinical trial of 5-3,3-bis(2-chloroethyl)1-triazenoimidazole-4-carboxamide (NSC-82196) in primary and secondary brain tumors. *Cancer Chemother. Rep.* **59:** 327–331.

LOO, T. L., LUCE, J. K., JARDINE, J. H. and FREI, E. (1968) Pharmacologic studies of the antitumor agent 5-(3,3-dimethyl-1-triazeno)imidazole-4-carboxamide. *Cancer Res.* **28:** 2448–2353.

LOO, T. L., HOUSEHOLDER, G. E., GERULATH, A. H., SAUNDERS, P. H. and FARQUHAR, D. L. (1976) Mechanism of action and pharmacology studies with DTIC (NSC 45388). *Cancer Treat. Rep.* **60:** 149–152.

LOWN, J. W. and SINGH, R. (1981) Synthesis of 3-(2-haloethyl)aryltriazenes and study of their reactions in aqueous solution. *Can. J. Chem.* **59:** 1347–1356.

LUNT, E., NEWTON, C. G., SMITH, C., STEVENS, G. P., STEVENS, M. F. G., STRAW, C. G., WARREN, R. J. A., FIZAMES, C., LAVELLE, F., LANGDON, S. P. and VICKERS, L. M. (1987) Antitumor imidazotetrazines. 14. Synthesis and antitumor activity of 6- and 8-substituted imidazo[5,1-*d*]-1,2,3,5-tetrazonones and 8-substituted pyrazolo[5,1-*d*]-1,2,3,5-tetrazinones. *J. med. Chem.* **30:** 357–366.

MALAVEILLE, C., BRUN, G., KOLAR, G. and BARTSCH, H. (1982) Mutagenic and alkylating activities of 3-methyl-1-phenyltriazenes and their possible role as carcinogenic metabolites of the parent dimethyl compounds. *Cancer Res.* **42:** 1446–1453.

MARGISON, G. P., LIKHACHEV, A. J. and KOLAR, G. F. (1979) *In vivo* alkylation of foetal, maternal and normal rat tissue nucleic acids by 3-methyl-1-phenyltriazene. *Chem.-Biol. Interact.* **25:** 345–353.

MATRKA, M., PÍPALOVÁ, J., BURES, D. and KRAMPERA, F. (1988) Chemické modely biotransformace IV. Studium karcinostatik odvozených od 1-fenyl-3,3-dimetyltriazenu. *Cesk. Farm.* **37:** 112–116.

MAZZA, M., PAGANI, G., CALDERARA, G. and VICARINI, L. (1974) Sull'attivita fitotossica di derivati triazenici. *Farmaco Ed. Sci.* **29:** 58–72.

MICHEJDA, C. J. and SMITH, R. H. (1989) 1-(2-Chloroethyl)-3-acyl-3-alkyltriazenes as neoplasm inhibitors. PCT Int. Appl. WO 89 09,207. *Chem. Abstr.* **112:** 157702.

MIZUNO, N. S. and DECKER, R. W. (1976) Alterations of DNA by 5-(3,3-dimethyl-1-triazeno)imidazole-4-carboxamide, NSC 407347. *Biochem. Pharmac.* **25:** 2643–2647.

MIZUNO, N. S. and HUMPHREY, E. W. (1972) Metabolism of 5-(3,3-dimethyl-1-triazeno)imidazole-4-carboxamide (NSC 43588) in human and tumor tissue. *Cancer Chemother. Rep.* **56:** 465–172.

NARDELLI, B., CONTESSA, A. R., ROMANI, L., SAVA, G., NISI, C. and FIORETTI, M. C. (1984) Immunogenic changes of murine lymphoma cells following in vitro treatment with aryl triazene derivatives. *Cancer Immun. Immunother.* **16:** 157–161.

NIFONTOV, V. I., BEL'SKAYA, N. P., CHERNOV, V. A., ERSHOVA, Y. A., VALIDUDA, G. I., DARIENKO, E. P., NIKIFOROVA, S. V. and PAKHOMOVA, E. Y. (1984) Reactivity and mechanism of the antitumor action of triazenes. *Khim.-Farm. Zh.* **18:** 1037–1041.

NIFONTOV, V. I., TAT'YANENKO, L. V., CHERNOV, V. A., BEL'SKAYA, N. P., SOKOLOVA, N. M., SHCHERBAKOVA, T. S. and ERSHOVA, Y. A. (1988) Reactivity and mechanism of the antitumor action of triazenes. III. Calcium ATPase as a possible triazene chemotherapy target. *Khim.-Farm. Zh.* **22:** 522–525.

OVERTON, M., HICKMAN, J. A., THREADGILL, M. D., VAUGHAN, K. and GESCHER, A. (1985) The generation of potentially toxic, reactive iminium ions from the oxidative metabolism of xenobiotic *N*-alkyl compounds. *Biochem. Pharmac.* **34:** 2055–2061.

POOL, B. L. (1979a) Microsomal mediated metabolism of dialkylaryltriazenes. I. Demethylation of ring-halogenated 3,3-dimethyltriazenes. *J. Cancer Res. clin. Oncol.* **93:** 215–220.

POOL, B. L. (1979b) Microsomal mediated metabolism of dialkylaryltriazenes. II. Isolation and identification of metabolites of 3,3-dimethyl-1-phenyltriazene. *J. Cancer Res. clin. Oncol.* **93:** 221–231.

POPESCU, M. and DANET, A. (1983) Mercury (II) complexes of phenyl-alpha-pyridyltriazene and *p*-nitrophenyl-alpha-pyridyltriazene; properties and analytic application in a spectrophotometric method. *Revue Roumaine de Chimie* **28:** 65–74.

PREUSSMANN, R., DRUCKREY, H., IVANKOVIC, S. and VON HODENBERG, A. (1969a) Chemical structure and carcinogenicity of aliphatic hydrazo-, azo- and azoxy compounds and of triazenes, potential in vivo alkylating agents. *Ann. N.Y. Acad. Sci.* **163:** 697–714.

PREUSSMANN, R., VON HODENBERG, A. and HENGY, H. (1969b) Mechanism of carcinogenesis of 1-aryl-3,3-dimethyltriazenes. Enzymatic dealkylation by rat liver microsomal fraction in vitro. *Biochem. Pharmac.* **18:** 1–13.

ROSS, D., FARMER, P. B., GESCHER, A., HICKMAN, J. A. and THREADGILL, M. D. (1983) The formation and metabolism of *N*-hydroxymethyl compounds-III. The metabolic conversion of *N*-methyl and *N*,*N*-dimethylbenzamides to *N*-hydroxymethyl compounds. *Biochem. Pharmac.* **32:** 1773–1781.

RUTTY, C. J. (1983) The species dependent pharmacokinetics of DTIC. *Br. J. Cancer* **48:** 140.

SAUNDERS, P. P. and SCHULTZ, G. A. (1972) Role of 4-diazoimidazole-5-carboxamide in the action of the antitumour agent DTIC in *Bacillus subtilis*. *Biochem. Pharmac.* **21:** 2065–2076.

SAVA, G., GIRALDI, T., LASSIANI, L. and NISI, C. (1982) Metabolism and mechanism of the antileukemic action of isomeric aryldimethyltriazenes. *Cancer Treat. Rep.* **66:** 1751–1755.

SAVA, G., ZORZET, S., PERISSIN, L., GIRALDI, T. and LASSIANI, L. (1988) Effects of an inducer and an inhibitor of hepatic metabolism on the antitumor action of triazenes. *Cancer Chemother. Pharmac.* **21:** 241–245.

SHEALY, Y. F., KRAUTH, C. A. and HOLUMN, L. B. (1968) Synthesis and properties of the antineoplastic agent 5(4)-(3,3-bis-(2-chloroethyl)-1-triazeno)imidazole-4(5)-carboxamide. *J. Pharm. Sci.* **57:** 83–86.

SHUSTERMAN, A. J., DEBNATH, A. K., HANSCH, C., HORN, G. W., FRONCZEK, F. R., GREENE, A. C. and WATKINS, S. F. (1989a) Mutagenicity of dimethyl heteroaromatic triazenes in the Ames test: the role of hydrophobicity and electronic effects. *Molec. Pharmac.* **36:** 939–944.

SHUSTERMAN, A. J., JOHNSON, A. S. and HANSCH, C., (1989b) Correlation of mutagenicity of 1,1-dimethyl-3-(X-phenyl)triazenes with molecular orbital energies and hydrophobicity. *Int. J. Quantum Chem.* **36:** 19–33.

SKIBBA, J. L. and BRYAN, G. T. (1971) Methylation of nucleic acids and urinary excretion of ^{14}C-labelled 7-methylguanine by rats and man after administration of 4(5)-(3,3bis-(2-chloroethyl)-1-triazeno)imidazole-5(4)-carboxamide. *Toxic. appl. Pharmac.* **18:** 707–719.

SKIBBA, J. L., RAMIREZ, G., BEAL, D. D. and BRYAN, G. T. (1969a) Preliminary clinical trial and the physiological disposition of 4(5)-(3,3-bis-(2-chloroethyl)1-triazeno)imidazole-5(4)-carboxamide in man. *Cancer Res.* **29:** 1944–1951.

SKIBBA, J. L., RAMIREZ, G., BEAL, D. D., JOHNSON, R. O. and BRYAN, G. T. (1969b) Metabolism of 4(5)-(3,3-bis-(2-chloroethyl)-1-triazeno)imidazole-5(4)-carboxamide (NSC 445388, DIC) in vivo and in vitro. *Proc. Am. Ass. Cancer Res.* **10:** 83.

SKIBBA, J. L., RAMIREZ, G., BEAL, D. D. and BRYAN, G. T. (1970a) *N*-Demethylation of the antineoplastic agent 4(5)-(3,3-bis-(2-chloroethyl)-1-triazeno)imidazole-5(4)-carboxamide by rats and man. *Cancer Res.* **30:** 147–150.

SKIBBA, J. L., RAMIREZ, G., BEAL, D. D. and BRYAN, G. T. (1970b) Metabolism of 4(5)-(3,3-bis-(2-chloroethyl)-1-triazeno)imidazole-5(4)-carboxamide to 4(5)-aminoimidazole-5(4)-carboxamide in man. *Biochem. Pharmac.* **19:** 2043–2051.

SMITH, R. H., MEHL, A. F., HICKS, A., DENLINGER, C. L., KRATZ, L., ANDREWS, A. W. and MICHEJDA, C. A. (1986) 1,3-Dimethyl-3-acyltriazenes: synthesis and chemistry of a novel class of biological methylating agents. *J. Org. Chem.* **51:** 3751–3757.

SOLOWAY, A. H., BRUMBAUGH, R. J. and WITTIAK, D. T. (1983) Carbinolamines and related structures—potential alkylating metabolites of clinically active anticancer drugs. *J. Theor. Biol.* **102:** 361–373.

SPASSOVA, M. K. and GOLOVINSKY, E. V. (1985) Pharmacobiochemistry of arylalkyltriazenes and their application in cancer chemotherapy. *Pharmac. Ther.* **27:** 333–352.

STEVENS, M. F. G., GESCHER, A. and TURNBULL, C. P. (1979) Antitumour activity, biomimetic oxidation and metabolism of heteroalicyclic triazenes. *Biochem. Pharmac.* **25:** 769–776.

STEVENS, M. F. G., HICKMAN, J. A., STONE, R., GIBSON, N. W., LUNT, E., NEWTON, C. G. and BAIG, G. U. (1984) Antitumour imidazotetrazines. I. Synthesis and chemistry of 8-carbamoyl-3-(2-chloroethyl)imidazo[5,1-*d*]-1,2,3,5-tetrazin-4-(3H)-one, a novel broad spectrum antitumour agent. *J. med. Chem.* **27:** 196–201.

THREADGILL, M. D. (1990) The chemistry of azolotetrazinones. In: *Chemistry of Antitumour Agents*, pp. 187–201, WILMAN, D. E. V. (ed.) Blackie, Glasgow.

THREADGILL, M. D. and GLEDHILL, A. P. (1986) Selective reactions in the triazene series. 2. Protodediazoniation of arenediazonium salts with formamide. *J. Chem. Soc., Perkin Trans. 1* 873–876.

TOREN, P. C., PLAKUNOV, I., PEYTON, A. L., COOPER, C. S. and WEINKAM, R. J. (1984) Quantitation of methanol formed in cell culture cytocoxicity assays and as a metabolite in microsome suspensions. *J. Chromatogr.* **305:** 171–177.

TOTH, B., TAYLOR, B., MATTSON, B. and GANNETT, P. (1989) Tumor induction by 4-(methyl)benzenediazonium sulfate in mice. *In Vivo* **3:** 17–22.

TRINAJSTIC, N., NICOLIC, S. and CARTER, S. (1989) QSAR: theory and application. *Kem. Ind.* **38:** 469–488.

TSANG, L. L. H., GESCHER, A., SLACK, J. A. and FARMER, P. B. (1990) Characterisation of urinary metabolites of temozolomide in humans and mice and evaluation of their cytotoxicity. *Cancer Chemother. Pharmac.* **26:** 429–436.

TSANG, L. L. H., QUARTERMAN, C. P., GESCHER, A. and SLACK, J. A. (1991) Comparison of the cytotoxicity in vitro of temozolomide and dacarbazine, prodrugs of 5-(3-methyltriazen-1-yl)imidazo-4-carboxamide (MTIC). *Cancer Chemother. Pharmac.* **27:** 342–346.

VAUGHAN, K. and STEVENS, M. F. G. (1978) Monoalkyltriazenes. *Chem. Soc. Rev.* **7:** 377–397.

VAUGHAN, K. and WILMAN, D. E. V. (1991) 1-Aryl-3,3-dimethyltriazene 3-oxides: evidence for a new hypothesis regarding the metabolism of antitumour 1-aryl-3,3-dimethyltriazenes. *J. Chem. Res. Synop.* 294–295.

VAUGHAN, K., TANG, Y., LLANOS, G., HORTON, J. K., SIMMONDS, R. J., HICKMAN, J. A. and STEVENS, M. F. G. (1984) Studies of the mode of action of antitumor triazenes and triazines. 6. 1-Aryl-3-(hydroxymethyl)-3-methyltriazenes: synthesis, chemistry and antitumor properties. *J. med. Chem.* **27:** 357–363.

VAUGHAN, K., NICHOLAS, K. U. K., SINGER, R. D., ROY, M. and GIBSON, N. W. (1987) Triazene metabolism. VI. 3-Azidomethyl-3-alkyl-1-aryltriazenes, a new class of antitumour triazene with potential prodrug applications. *Anticancer Drug Design* **2:** 279–287.

VENGER, B. H., HANSCH, C., HATHEWAY, G. J. and AMREIN, Y. U. (1979) Ames test of 1-(X-phenyl)-3,3-dialkyltriazenes: a quantitative structure–activity study. *J. med. Chem.* **22:** 473–476.

VOGEL, E. W. (1989) Nucleophilic selectivity of carcinogens as a determinant of enhanced mutational response in excision repair-defective strains in *Drosophila*: effects of 30 carcinogens. *Carcinogenesis* **10:** 2093–2106.

WORKMAN, P. and LEE, F. Y. F. (1984) Experimental antitumour activity and mechanism of action of the novel anticancer agent CCRG 81010. *Br. J. Cancer* **50:** 251.

ZIJLSTRA, J. A., and VOGEL, E. W. (1988) Influence of inhibition of the metabolic action on the mutagenicity of some nitrosamines, triazenes, hydrazines and seniciphylline in *Drosophila melanogaster*. *Mutat. Res.* **202:** 251–267.

Garth Powis, editor.
(1994) *Anticancer Drugs: Reactive Metabolism and Drug Interactions*,
Pergamon Press Ltd, pp. 187–207
Printed in the United Kingdom

CHAPTER 5

THE METABOLISM AND MODE OF ACTION OF 2-CHLOROETHYLNITROSOUREAS

DONALD J. REED

Department of Biochemistry and Biophysics, Oregon State University, Corvallis, OR 97331, U.S.A.

1. HISTORICAL BACKGROUND

After the initial observation by Greene and Greenberg (1960) (for a review see Ludlum, 1990) that 1-methyl-3-nitro-1-nitrosoguanidine increased the life-span of mice implanted intraperitoneally with leukemia L1210 cells, investigators at the Southern Research Institute observed that 1-methyl-1-nitrosourea was an even more effective agent against L1210 cells (Johnston et al., 1963). Subsequently, the Cancer Chemotherapy National Service Center screening program provided resources for the synthesis and testing of hundreds of *N*-nitrosoureas and their development as antitumor drugs. The congeners of major importance are those containing a 2-chloroethyl moiety on the nitrogen atom attached to the nitroso group. Three drugs emerged and underwent testing: 1,3-bis(2-chloroethyl)-1-nitrosourea (BCNU); 1-(2-chloroethyl)-3-cyclohexyl-1-nitrosourea (CCNU); and 1-(2-chloroethyl)-3-(*trans*-4-methylcyclohexyl)-1-nitrosourea (methyl CCNU). Because of the ability of these lipophilic drugs to cross the blood–brain barrier and to be effective against solid tumors (including brain tumors), as well as leukemias, great interest developed in their clinical efficacy. A large body of literature exists from nearly 30 years of study of these and of other nitrosoureas. The National Cancer Institute considers nitrosoureas to be one of the most important classes of antitumor agents developed by the Cancer Chemotherapy Program (Carter et al., 1972). The structures of many of the 2-chloroethylnitrosoureas (CENUs) are shown in Table 1.

2. CHEMICAL PROPERTIES AND ANALYTICAL PROCEDURES

Many CENUs have been synthesized and the variety of congeners is indicated in Table 1. Prominent infrared absorption bands in the carbonyl-stretching region (1620–1750 cm^{-1}) characterize the nitrosoureas. Nitrosation of urea functions was found to cause consistently a shift toward higher wave numbers in the carbonyl region (Johnston et al., 1963). Nitroso isomer identification has been established by proton magnetic resonance spectroscopy by demonstrating a spectral symmetry of the $ClCH_2CH_2N(NO)$ group (A_2B_2 system) (Johnston et al., 1966; Machinami et al., 1975). Mass spectra fragmentation patterns have been shown to be very useful in establishing nitroso isomer identification (May et al., 1975, 1979). UV absorbance at about 230 nm provides a means of detection and quantitation of nitrosoureas. Quantitation of nitrosoureas in biological extracts by HPLC at nanomole levels is made possible with sensitive UV flow detectors (May et al., 1975, 1979). An elegant analytical method based on stable isotope dilution analysis and mass spectrometry has been described for BCNU (Weinkam et al., 1978). Pharmacokinetic profiles have been established utilizing techniques that take into account the rapid clearance of most chloroethylnitrosoureas which is related to their chemical reactivity and tissue distribution. Various assays for CENUs are based on the use of radiolabeled compounds (Levin et al., 1978; Freed et al., 1982) mass spectrometric techniques (Smith et al., 1981, 1983; Smith and Cheung, 1982), normal or reverse-phase HPLC (Caddy et al., 1982; Yeager et al., 1984; Labarre et al., 1987; Polacek et al., 1988; Gordon et al., 1989; Bartosek et al., 1991).

Decomposition of CENUs in aqueous solution is spontaneous and dependent on pH, buffer and temperature (Figs 1 and 2). Typical decomposition rates afford a range of half-lives from 46 min for chlorozotocin (Montgomery, 1976) to 70 min for methyl CCNU (Reed et al., 1975). Isocyanate formation during nitrosourea degradation was established in early studies (Garrett et al., 1965). Alkylating species were observed indirectly with the nitrobenzylpyridine assay method (Wheeler and Chumley, 1967). Vinyl carbonium ions were suggested as the alkylating species from BCNU (Montgomery et al., 1967). However, Reed and co-workers (1975) examined in detail the decomposition of CCNU and methyl CCNU at pH 7–4 in phosphate buffer and found the major alkylating species to be capable of 2-chloroethylation. 2-Chloroethanol is a major decomposition product with small amounts of acetaldehyde, vinyl chloride and ethylene. At the same time, Colvin et al. (1974) concluded that BCNU decomposition produced primarily a chloroethylcarbonium ion intermediate as the alkylating species. Dependence on pH was later noted for the difference in degradation products, with low pH producing acetaldehyde, whereas neutral pH produces greatly enhanced quantities of 2-chloroethanol (Montgomery et al., 1975).

Recent studies illustrate the complexity of the degradation events of the CENUs. Lown and

TABLE 1. *Nitrosoureas and Certain of their Metabolites*

Code	*Compound*	R – = NH – C(=O) – N(NO) – CH_2 – CH_2 – Cl
BCNU NSC 409962	1,3–Bis(2–chloroethyl)–1–nitrosourea	R – CH_2–CH_2–Cl
CCNU NSC 79037	1–(2–Chloroethyl)–3–cyclohexyl–1–nitrosourea	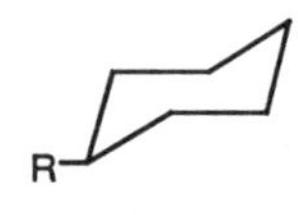
trans–2–hydroxy CCNU NSC 253947	1–(2–Chloroethyl)–3–*trans*–2–hydroxycyclohexyl)–1–nitrosourea	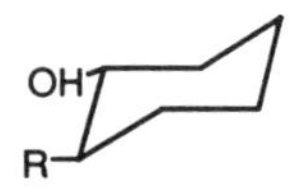
Me CCNU NSC 95441	1–(2–Chloroethyl)–3–(*trans*–4–methylcyclohexyl)–1–nitrosourea	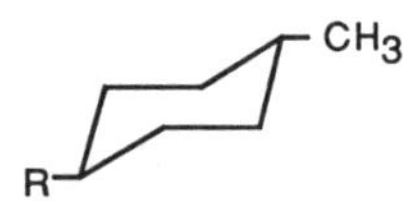
Chlorozotocin NSC 178248	1–(2–Chloroethyl)–3–(D–2–gluco-pyranosyl)–1–nitrosourea	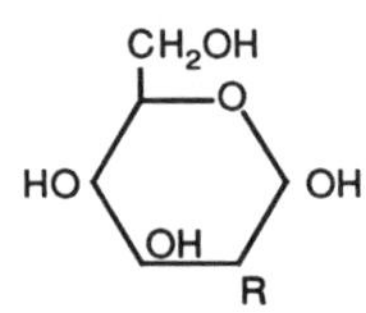
cis–Acid NSC 153174	1–(2–Chloroethyl)–3–(4–*cis*–carboxycyclohexyl)–1–nitrosourea	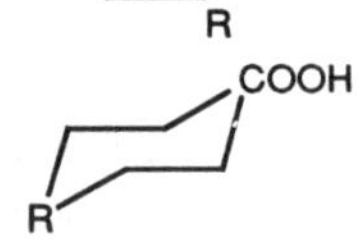
MCNU	1–(2–Chloroethyl)–3–(methyl–α–D–glucopyranose–6–yl)–1–nitrosourea	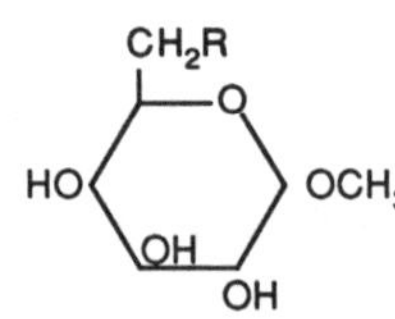
TA–077	1–(2–Chloroethyl)–3–isobutyl–3–(β–maltosyl)–1–nitrosourea	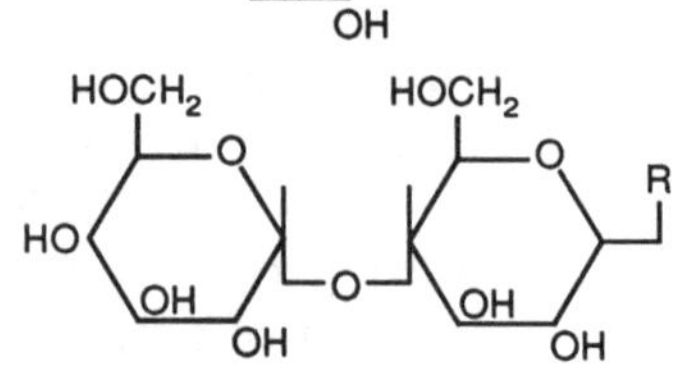
GANU NSC D 254157	1–(2–Chloroethyl)–3–(β–D–glucopyranosyl)–1–nitrosourea	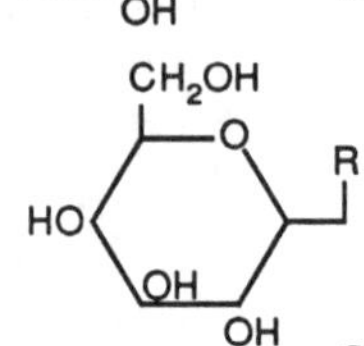

Continued opposite.

TABLE 1. (*Continued*)

Code	Compound	$R- = NH-C(=O)-N(NO)-CH_2-CH_2-Cl$
ACNU	1–(2–Chloroethyl)–3–(4–amino–2–methylpyrimidine–5–yl) methyl–1–nitrosourea	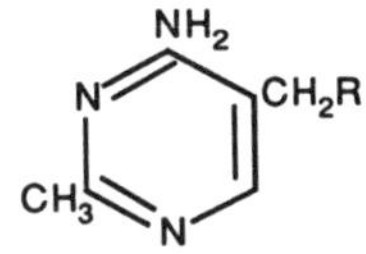
HECNU NSC 294895	1–(2–Chloroethyl)–3–(2–hydroxy-ethyl)–1–nitrosourea	$R-CH_2-CH_2OH$
CNCC 1.C.1.G.1325	*N,N′*–Bis[*N*–(2-chloroethyl)–*N*–nitrosocarbonyl]cystamine	$S-CH_2-CH_2-R$ / $S-CH_2-CH_2-R$
RPCNU 1.C.1.G.1163	1–(2–Chloroethyl)–3–(2,3,4–triacetyl–1–ribopyranosyl)–1–nitrosourea	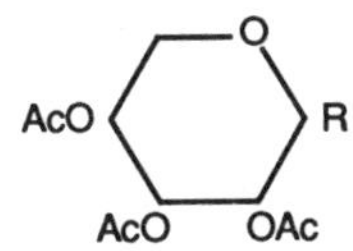
RFCNU 1.C.1.G.1105	1–(2–Chloroethyl)–3–[2,3–isopropylidene 5–(nitro–4–benzoyl)–1–ribofuranosyl]–1–nitrosourea	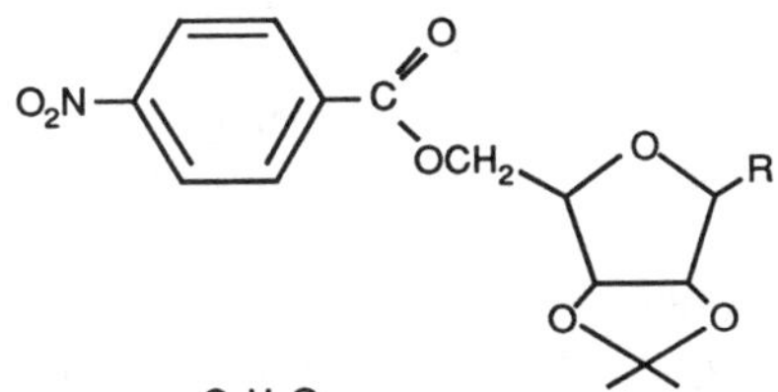
Fotemustine	Diethyl–1–[3–(2–chloroethyl)–3–nitrosoureido]ethyl phosphonate	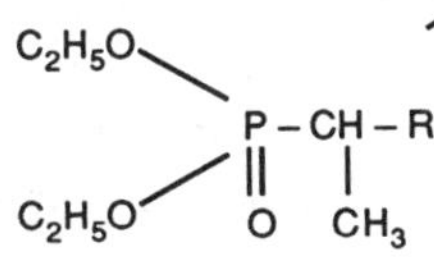

Code	Compound	*R = Bisnitrosourea*
BCyNU NSC -80590	1,3–Bis(cyclohexyl)–1–nitrosourea	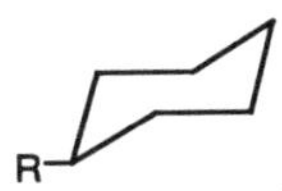
trans–4–Hydroxy BCyNU NSC -305715	1,3–Bis(*trans*–4–hydroxycyclo-hexyl)–1–nitrosourea	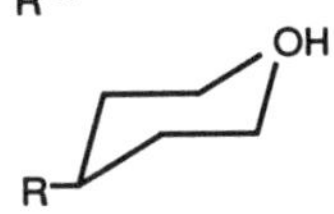
cis–4–Carboxyl BCyNU NSC -305716	1,3–Bis(*cis*–4–carboxylcyclo-hexyl)–1–nitrosourea	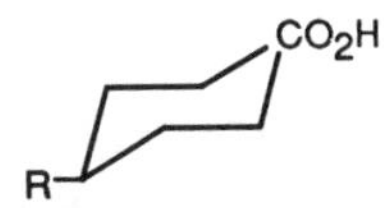

Chauhan (1981) described the synthesis of three 2-(alkylimino)-3-nitrosooxazolidines that correspond to degradation intermediates of BCNU, CCNU and methyl CCNU (Fig. 3). These intermediates are proposed to be formed via a minor pathway of degradation, yet may account in part for the 2-hydroxyethylated nucleoside products reported by other workers. The appropriateness of chloride ion as a leaving group for CENUs has been discussed in terms of an effective chemical compromise in reactivity. Although oxidative dechlorination by cytochrome P450 enzymes to yield imidazolidinone formation from 1-(2-chloroethyl)-3-(4-amino-2-methylpyrimidine-5-yl)methyl-1-nitrosourea (ACNU) is now documented (Nishigaki et al., 1985a), chloride leaving group ability is low enough to not favor competing pathways of nitrosourea degradation involving oxadiazoline, imino-*N*-nitrosooxazolidinones, or hybrid migrations which can limit 2-chloroethyl alkylations. Yet after chloroethylation, labilization of the chloride and production of interstrand crosslinks can occur (see Ludlum, 1990 for a review). It appears that the probability of crosslinking events is maximized with chloroethylation compared to other haloethylation

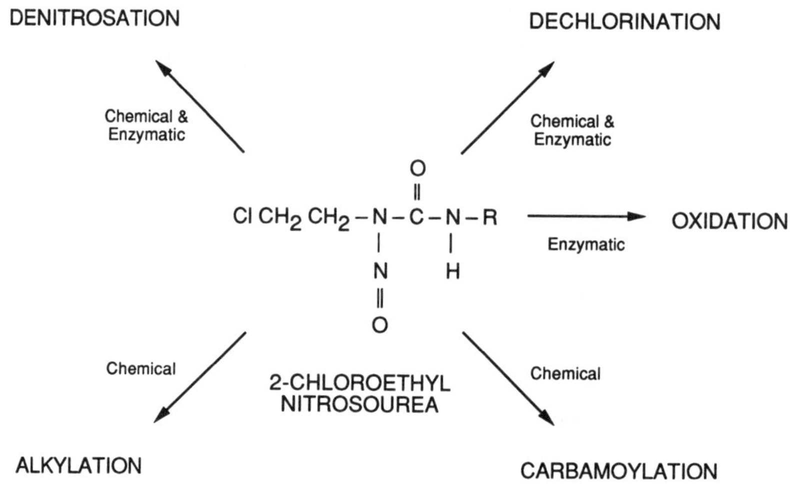

FIG. 1. Routes of chemical and metabolic degradation of 2-chloroethylnitrosoureas.

(Kohn, 1977). Interestingly, the 3-([1]H-decafluorocyclohexyl) analog of CCNU (FCCNU) rapidly converts to the corresponding 1-([1]H-decafluorocyclohexyl)-3-nitrosoimidazolidin-2-one by chloride being a leaving group (Foster et al., 1980). CCNU did not form a detectable quantity of the imidazolidine derivative, which suggests that a decafluorocyclohexyl moiety enhances the nucleophilicity of the *N*-3 nitrogen atom to facilitate the cyclization and the loss of chloride ion (Foster et al., 1980).

Brundrett (1980) has found evidence for the intermediacy of 4,5-dihydro-1,2,3-oxadiazole in BCNU decomposition. Formation of ethylene glycol as a degradation product of BCNU was noted. He concluded that its formation is best explained by an oxadiazole intermediate. Again this intermediate is thought to play only a minor role in the decomposition of BCNU at physiological pH and to have little or no antitumor activity (Brundrett, 1980).

Efforts to utilize CENUs for the treatment of solid tumors have led to the development of CENUs that could undergo preferential bioreductive activation in hypoxic tumors. Two of these

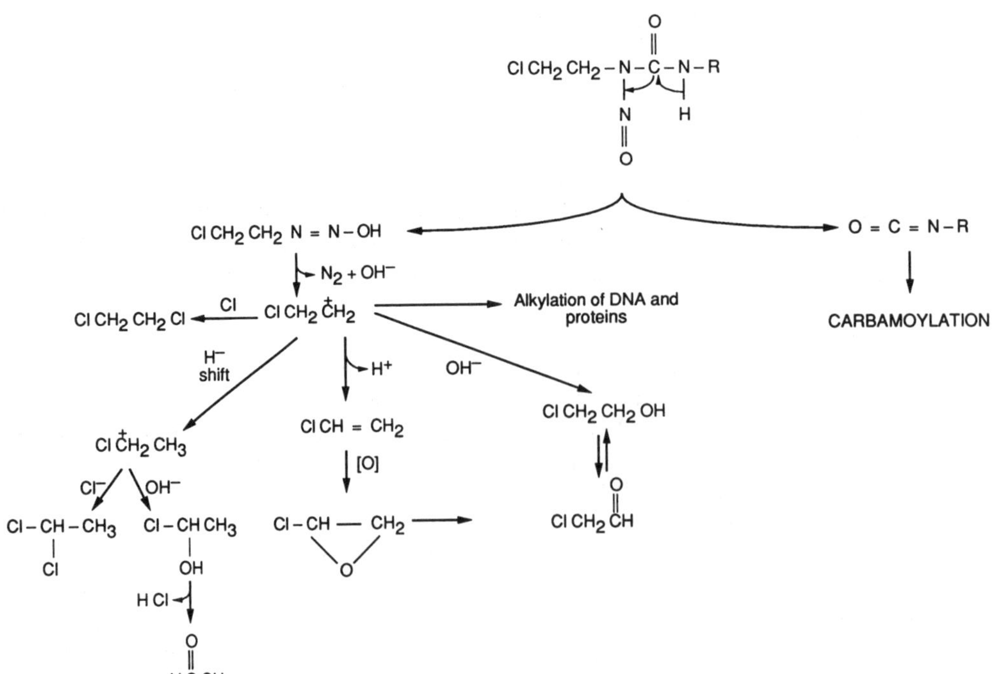

FIG. 2. Routes of chemical degradation of 2-chloroethylnitrosoureas.

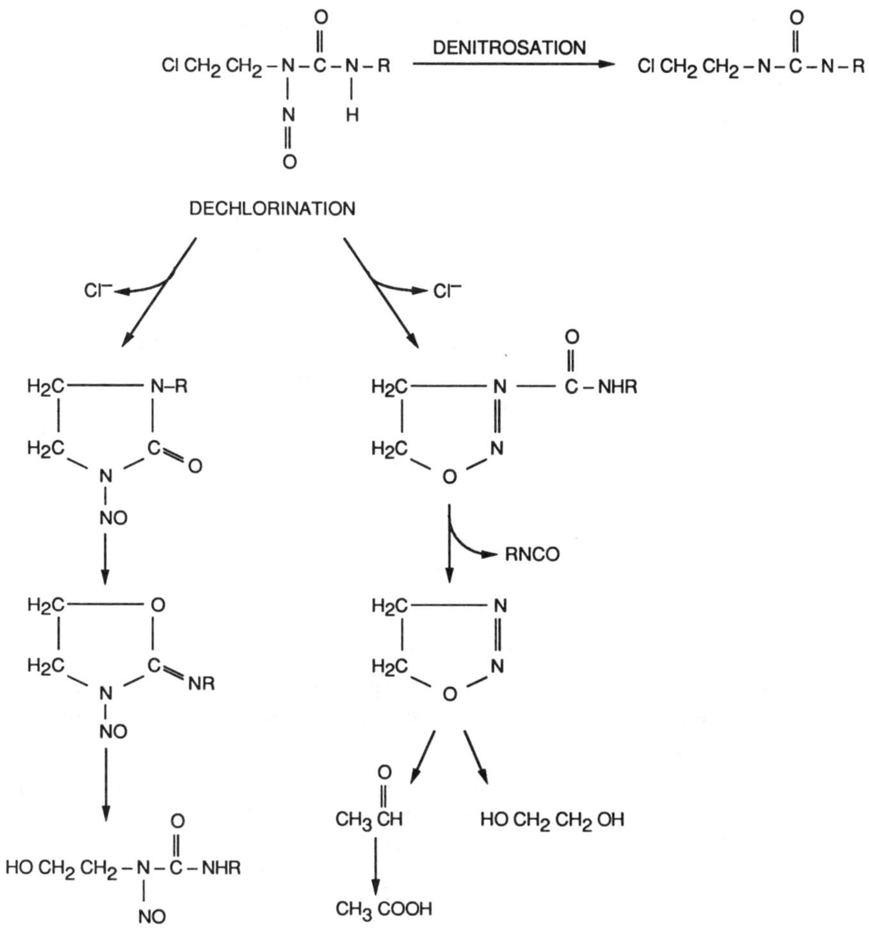

FIG. 3. The activation of 2-chloroethylnitrosoureas by denitrosation and dechlorination.

agents are 3,3′-bis-[*N*-(2-chloroethyl)-*N*-nitrosocarbamoyl]propyl disulfide (Lown et al., 1980) and a mixture of dinitrosated derivatives of *N,N*′-bis-[*N*-(2-chloroethyl)-*N*-carbamoyl]cystamine [CNCC-(D)] which contains a mixture of three dinitrosated isomers [CNCC-(C), (S), and (M)] (Imbach et al., 1981).

N-Me *cis*-CCNU, which is a nitrosourea that is incapable of the facile decomposition that characterizes the clinically useful nitrosoureas, has latent activity against an experimental solid tumor (Johnston et al., 1984b). Prior studies had suggested activation via enzymatic demethylation of fully substituted congeners as the basis for the latent activity. An important property of *N*-Me *cis*-CCNU is solubility in cold phosphate buffer with a half life at pH 7–4 of 4–2 hr (Johnston et al., 1984b).

Other new analogs of CENUs that are water-soluble, such as 1-(2-chloroethyl)-1-nitroso-3-(2-hydroxyethyl)urea (HECNU), are more effective antitumor agents in most model systems than are the clinically used compounds such as BCNU or chlorozotocin, according to preclinical studies. In this regard, HECNU was less toxic and less carcinogenic, and these differences were supported by its carbamoylating and alkylating potential, a glutathione reductase inhibition that did not parallel either its antitumor effectiveness or its chronic toxicity or carcinogenic potential (Eisenbrand, 1984). Thus HECNU and other CENUs with higher antitumor activity in preclinical trials also display a higher potential for DNA–DNA interstrand, crosslink in vivo (Eisenbrand, 1984). Several CENU analogs of 2′-deoxyuridine and 2′-deoxy-5-fluorouridine have been synthesized and tested for antitumor activity (Lin et al., 1986). 3′-CTNU was found to be three times more potent than BCNU in the inhibition of L1210 leukemia cells in culture. Possibly of greater interest—pyrimidine deoxyribonucleosides such as thymidine, 2′-deoxyuridine and 2′-deoxycytidine specifically prevent the inhibitory effects of the thymidine CENU, 3′-CTNU, which produced 'cures' in animal tests (Lin et al., 1986), and 3′-CdUNU and 3′-CFdUNU, which produced 90% and 60% 'cures' (survival > 60 days), respectively, where administered to mice bearing L1210 cells (Lin et al., 1986).

Weinkam and Dolan (1983) have compared the physical, chemical and kinetic parameters of five different CENUs in terms of the toxic effects on the growth of cultured P388 cells. They concluded that since the CENUs tested have the same activity at the cellular level, the difference in activity in vivo may be explained by differences in biodistribution (Weinkam and Dolan, 1983).

Because alterations of the 'carrier' moiety of CENUs affect both their physical and chemical properties, a major effort has been expended on nitrosourea derivatives containing a glucose carrier. TA-077 [1-(2-chloroethyl)-3-isobutyl-3-(β-maltosyl)-1-nitrosourea] is disubstituted at the *N*-3 position and upon activation does not produce an isocyanate moiety for carbamoylation. Evidence of toxicity of TA-077 in BDF1 mice indicates that it is a suitable drug for consecutive administration, in part because of the lack of toxicity associated with carbamoylation reactions (Fujimoto and Ogawa, 1985).

Fotemustine (diethyl-1-[3-(2-chloroethyl)-3-nitrosoureido]ethylphosphonate; S10036) has been synthesized and evaluated as a new CENU to achieve improved penetration of the cell membrane and better passage through the blood–brain barrier than other CENUs (Foster and Pardee, 1969; Montgomery and Mayo, 1974; Reed, 1984).

Interesting additions to the CENUs are the spin-labelled nitrosourea, 1-(2-chloroethyl)-3-(1-oxyl-2,2,6,6-tetramethylpiperidinyl)-1-nitrosourea (SL-CNU), and several of its analogs (Sosnovsky and Li, 1985). At equal molar doses, or at doses of equal toxicity level, SL-CNU was found to bc more active than CCNU.

The anticancer activity of several *N*-(2-fluoroethyl)-*N*-nitrosoureas has been determined, and a dihydroxycyclohexyl derivative was found to be the most effective (Johnston et al., 1984a).

A main feature of the CENUs is that the chemistry of the nitrosoureas is complex and new degradation products and metabolites continue to bc identified. New pathways illustrate the steps that may occur in the formation of these degradation and metabolic products. Some products are very reactive intermediates that appear to be essential for the biological effects of the nitrosoureas by mechanisms that remain poorly understood.

3. METABOLISM

The short half-lives of the nitrosoureas in buffer at physiological pH and in vivo as plasma half-lives led to an initial assumption that these drugs would have little opportunity to undergo metabolism in vivo (for a review see Reed, 1981). Not only was this assumption erroneous, but it is now generally accepted that the biological activity of CCNU is expressed through its oxidation metabolites; these are formed by an extremely rapid monohydroxylation of the cyclohexyl ring by cytochrome P450-dependent enzymes (Fig. 1). Evidence is accumulating to suggest that in vivo denitrosation and oxidative dechlorination are also important to the pharmacodynamics of certain nitrosoureas (Figs 1 and 3).

The therapeutic efficacies of the CENUs appear to involve their spontaneous chemical decomposition to yield electrophilic species that alkylate cellular macromolecules. The isocyanates may either carbamoylate macromolecules or undergo intramolecular carbamoylation to form cyclic urethanes. Alternative pathways of decomposition account for the diversity of products which are highly dependent upon the structure of individual CENUs.

4. ANIMAL STUDIES

4.1. Cytochrome P450 Monooxygenase-Dependent Hydroxylation

During the past 20 years cytochrome P450-dependent enzymes have been established as the major enzymes responsible for the biotransformation of lipophilic drugs. Lipophilic nitrosoureas, including CCNU and methyl CCNU, undergo cytochrome P450-dependent monooxygenation at cyclohexyl ring carbon atoms. Methyl CCNU is also hydroxylated in the 2-chloroethyl side-chain. Cytochrome P450 present in rat liver microsomes prepared from liver of phenobarbital-induced rats catalyses rapid monooxygenation of CCNU to yield five hydroxy CCNU metabolites (May et al., 1974, 1975; Hilton and Walker, 1975; Reed and May, 1975, 1977; Reed, 1981). Within 2 min after i.v. administration of CCNU to rats, a majority of the CCNU in the liver is metabolized and hydroxy CCNU metabolites are detectable in all organs examined (Reed and May, 1977). Methyl CCNU displays a slower rate of monooxygenation than CCNU and has a more complex metabolic pattern than CCNU (May et al., 1979). The presence of a *trans*-4-methyl group decreases the rate of monooxygenation of methyl CCNU 25% compared to CCNU (May et al., 1979). The methyl group is hydroxylated to some extent and a small amount of *trans*-4-hydroxy-*cis*-4-methyl CCNU formation occurs, possibly via a free-radical intermediate which facilitates some methyl group 'flip' (Potter and Reed, 1980).

Efforts have been made towards metabolism-directed design of new nitrosourea congeners. An attempt was made to direct the metabolic formation of specific hydroxy CCNU metabolites with specific deuterium labelling of the cyclohexyl ring (Farmer et al., 1978). Whereas a metabolic shift is achieved, the fraction of the metabolite desired, *trans*-2-hydroxy CCNU, remains too small compared to total metabolite formation for a noticeable change in therapeutic effect. More recently, cytochrome P450-dependent formation of alkylating metabolites of MeCCNU and CCNU have been observed with rat liver microsomes (Kramer, 1989). The alkylating metabolites were bound covalently to microsomal protein and DNA. In contrast, carbamoylation reactions were not affected significantly by microsomal metabolism of either CCNU or MeCCNU (Kramer, 1989).

Fluorinated congeners of CCNU have been synthesized and tested, in the hope that such congeners would be more effective antitumor agents than CCNU due to possible blocking of ring hydroxylation and changes in physicochemical characteristics (Foster et al., 1980). FCCNU was found to be more toxic and possess less antitumor activity than CCNU. This congener favors chemical decomposition via a 3-nitroso imidazolidin-2-one intermediate. A mixture of this intermediate and a 1-(nonafluorocyclohexyl) derivative appears to be responsible for the observed toxicity of FCCNU (Foster et al., 1980).

5. NITROSOUREA DENITROSATION

The lack of antitumor activity of methylurea as well as other ureas demonstrates the requirement for the *N*-nitroso moiety (Skipper et al., 1961). Chemically, the nitroso moiety of methyl CCNU can be quantitatively removed with the formation of methyl CCNU by hydrogenation in ethanol in the presence of 5% rhodium in charcoal at 25°C and 1 atm. (May et al., 1979) (Fig. 1). Biologically, BCNU undergoes denitrosation, which is catalyzed by liver microsomes in the presence of NADPH (Hill et al., 1975). Recent evidence has demonstrated that nitric oxide is formed as a product of denitrosation under anaerobic conditions (Potter and Reed, 1981) (Fig. 3). Cytochrome P450 can form a nitroso complex during denitrosation of CCNU with an absorption maximum at 445 nm (Reed and May, 1977). Certain nitrosoureas can undergo denitrosation in vivo with loss of antitumor activity, especially after induction of the liver endoplasmic reticulum with phenobarbital. Phenobarbital pretreatment of rats bearing intracerebral 9L tumors eliminates the antitumor activity of BCNU and decreases the efficacy of 1-(2-chloroethyl)-3-(2,6-dioxo-3-piperidyl)-1-nitrosourea (PCNU) and CCNU (Levin et al., 1979). Decreased systemic toxicity to the host rats is observed, which agrees with a microsomal-catalyzed rate of BCNU disappearance that doubles by phenobarbital pretreatment (Levin et al., 1979).

Denitrosation is a factor which may have importance in the design and efficacy of new nitrosourea drugs. Every nitrosourea examined so far can undergo anaerobic denitrosation catalyzed by liver microsomes in the presence of NADPH (Potter and Reed, 1981). The rates of denitrosation reveal a sufficient variation between the nitrosoureas tested to indicate that a low denitrosation rate may modify the therapeutic index of a congener. For example, a novel CENU, 1-(2-chloroethyl)-3-[2-(dimethylaminosulphonyl)ethyl]1-nitrosourea, tauromustine (TCNU), undergoes both demethylation and denitrosation. The rates of these reactions can be increased 10-fold for demethylation and six-fold for denitrosation by the induction of the cytochrome P450 system with phenobarbital pretreatment of rats (Seidegard et al., 1990).

6. OXIDATIVE DECHLORINATION

Recently it was stated that the major inactivation pathway of the CENUs was that of oxidative dechlorination (Figs 1 and 3) (Lemoine et al., 1991). The evidence for this pathway is on the basis of metabolites identified from in vitro incubations of ACNU with liver microsomes and cytosol. The degradation ACNU in vitro includes the spontaneous formation in phosphate buffer, pH 7.4, of an intramolecular cyclized product, 3,4-dihydro-7-methylpyrimido-[4,5-d]pyrimidin-2(1H)-one, with simultaneous liberation of the alkylating moiety. ACNU incubated with rat liver preparations yielded three metabolites; a denitrosated product and a product of oxidative dechlorination, 1-[(4-amino-2-methyl-5-pyrimidinyl)methyl]-5-hydroxy-3-nitroso-2-imidazolidinone (API). API, which also gave a denitrosation product, was formed by catalysis with microsomal enzymes which were induced by phenobarbital pretreatment, inhibited with SKF-525A, and carbon monoxide and dependent on NADPH and oxygen. Thus, it is assumed that oxidative dechlorination of ACNU is catalyzed by the microsomal mixed function oxidase presumably to form a reactive intermediate on the carbon that had been chlorinated. The nature of the metabolites and enzymes indicates that at least two enzymatic steps are involved which cause an oxidative dechlorination to API and a denitrosation process to yield 1-[(4-amino-2-methyl-5-pyrimidinyl)methyl 1-3-(2-chloroethyl)urea. The denitrosated product of the oxidative dechlorination was the remaining metabolite (Nishigaki et al., 1985a). Evidence for the formation of a reactive intermediate during oxidative dechlorination comes from the conversion of CCNU and MeCCNU by rat liver microsomes to metabolites that are trapped with semicarbazide to limit the extent of microsomal protein covalent labeling (Kramer, 1989). Cyclization to form the imidazolidinone ring could be via condensation between the newly formed reactive intermediate and the N1 nitrogen (Fig. 4). A similar intermediate has been proposed in the cytochrome P450 catalysis of the oxidative dechlorination of 1,2-dichloroethane to form 2-chloroethanol (Guengerich et al., 1980). Assuming that oxidative dechlorination could give the equivalent of an aliphatic carbonium ion, the fate of such a reactive intermediate would be extremely dependent on the nucleophiles in its presence to compete with the internal cyclization reaction to give the observed imidazolidinone product.

The major urinary metabolites of ACNU have been identified following intravenous administration of [^{14}C]ACNU into rats (Nishigaki et al., 1985b). An imidazolidinone compound, 1-[(4-amino-2-methyl-5-pyrimidinyl)methyl]-5-hydroxy-2-imidazolidinone, was the main metabolite with one of the other major metabolites being a nitrosated compound of the main metabolite, i.e. 1-[(4-amino-2-methyl-5-pyrimidinyl)methyl 1-5-hydroxy-3-nitroso-2-imidazolidinone. These metabolites indicate that oxidative dechlorination is the major pathway for ACNU metabolism in vivo and that denitrosation is another main pathway for inactivation of ACNU with loss of cytotoxicity. Also observed was the denitrosated parent urea and a cyclized pyrimidopyrimidine (Nishigaki et al., 1985b). Fotemustine metabolism includes the formation of an oxidative dechlorination product (Ings et al., 1990).

In a study of the CNS toxicity and cerebrospinal fluid (CSF) pharmacokinetics of intraventric-

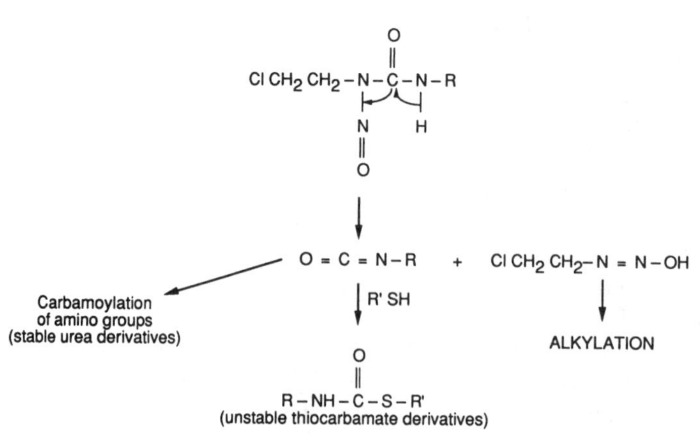

FIG. 4. The route of chemical degradation of 2-chloroethylnitrosoureas leading to carbamoylating products.

ularly administered ACNU in beagles, it was concluded that the disappearance of ACNU from CSF was due to hydrolytic decomposition with a half-time for CSF elimination of 18 min (Levin et al., 1985). Treatment of meningeal neoplasia may be limited since CSF elimination of ACNU is rapid compared to its equilibration time from ventricle to spinal-cerebral convexity-subarachnoid space (Levin et al., 1985).

7. CNCC METABOLISM

CNCC metabolism in rats displays a first-pass metabolism to yield four main metabolites (Godeneche et al., 1985). These metabolites arise from the bioreduction of the disulfide bridge of CNCC followed by *S*-methylation and oxidation to sulfinyl and sulfonyl derivatives. In vitro studies (Godeneche et al., 1986) have shown that a cytosolic thioreductase, a microsomal and cytosolic *S*-methyltransferase and a microsomal oxidase catalyze very rapid enzymatic reactions, which explains the non-detectable reduction products. An equally rapid metabolic sequence appears to cause a loss of the nitroso groups. All metabolic intermediates that retain both the nitroso group and the 2-chloroethyl moiety are potentially active antitumor agents.

8. HUMAN STUDIES

Clinical pharmacology of the CENUs has been reviewed (Levin, 1981). Unfortunately, the clinical relevance of analogs other than BCNU has not been assessed in terms of their pharmacokinetics and very little human metabolic data has been reported.

Human brain tumors have been examined for the pharmacokinetics of positron-labelled BCNU with positron emission tomography, and the results compared to those of normal brain (Diksic et al., 1984). Distribution of radioactivity in brain and plasma indicates a different rate of BCNU decomposition in the tumor than in normal brain, and the clearance of total radioactivity from the tumor is significantly slower than from the contralateral brain and plasma (Diksic et al., 1984).

9. RELATIONSHIP BETWEEN METABOLISM AND BIOLOGICAL ACTIVITY

Many nitrosoureas are remarkable in their ability to achieve complete cures of various tumors in test animals. Except for one factor, these drugs undoubtedly would be equally impressive in achieving cures of many neoplasms in humans. This factor, toxicity to normal cells as well as malignant cells, is extremely severe with the nitrosoureas. A wide range of toxicities is exhibited when nitrosoureas are administered to either test animals or humans. These include bone marrow suppression (myelosuppression or myelotoxicity), alopecia (loss of hair), interference with spermatogenesis, and of particular importance to patients, nausea and vomiting. Since rapidly proliferating cells or tissue have growth characteristics similar to tumor cells, they are the most susceptible to these cytotoxic effects. Alteration of genetic material is expressed not only by cytotoxicity, but also by the ability of the nitrosoureas to be mutagenic and somewhat carcinogenic. These effects have been reviewed (Ludlum, 1977, 1990). Cytotoxicity is so severe with the CENUs that cancer cell kill plays a greater role than transformation of normal cells to malignancy and tumor formation.

Non-enzymic degradation of CENUs, which may be protein-mediated under certain conditions (Weinkam et al., 1980), is responsible for the generation of a common but penultimate alkylating intermediate, 2-chloroethyldiazene hydroxide (Figs 1 and 2). This hypothetical intermediate (also known as a diazo-hydroxide) is very unstable and yet appears to have an important role in the selective alkylation events of DNA. This role has been discussed in detail for the corresponding diazene hydroxides derived from degradation of methyl and ethylnitrosourea (Jensen, 1978; Jensen and Reed, 1978). Formation of either 2-chloroethanol or 1-bromo-2-chloroethane in the presence of bromide ion during CCNU degradation is strong evidence for an intermediate capable of *t*-chloroethylation of biological molecules (Reed et al., 1975). Evidence against a classical S_N1 reaction mechanism for BCNU alkylation has been reported by Brundrett (Brundrett et al., 1976) from studies with deuterated BCNU. They proposed that a reaction which has a 2-chloroethylcarbonium ion intermediate would yield products predominantly from rearranged 1-chloro-ethylcarbonium ion and cyclic chloronium ions. The major product, 2-chloroethanol, was mostly unrearranged (90%) (Brundrett et al., 1976). Since S_N2 reactions of the diazene hydroxide are of low activation energy, little selectivity is proposed for the concerted loss of N_2 and alkylation of either sulphur, oxygen or nitrogen atoms (Brundrett et al., 1976). Differences in oxygen atom alkylation by ethyl- and methylnitrosoureas would suggest that alkylation site affinity for the diazene hydroxide cannot be ruled out entirely (Jensen and Reed, 1978).

9.1. ALKYLATION

Ludlum and co-workers have studied extensively alkylation modifications of DNA and RNA bases by nitrosoureas. Properties of these derivatives are reviewed (Ludlum and Tong, 1981). The modified bases have been categorized into two classes: those derived from a single substitution at a nucleophilic site and those involving a two-step modification. The haloethyl, hydroxyethyl, and aminoethyl modified bases are placed in the first group (Ludlum and Tong, 1981). The formation of diguanylethane represents a DNA crosslinking event which probably is intrastrand in nature but interstrand crosslinking cannot be ruled out at this time (Tong and Ludlum, 1981). Some of the unique cytotoxic properties of the nitrosoureas may relate to interstrand DNA crosslinking processes. The alkylation bifunctionality of the 2-haloethylnitrosoureas was established by Ludlum and coworkers (1975) when they isolated 3,*N*-4-ethanocytosine from the reaction of BCNU with polycytidylic acid. These findings were followed with reactions of CENUs with purified DNA by physical studies Kohn (1977) and Lown and coworkers (1978). Haloethylation was first demonstrated by Tong and Ludlum (1978) who isolated 2-fluroethylcytidine from the reaction of *N,N'*-bis(2-fluoroethyl)-*N*-nitrosourea with cytidine. 2-Haloethylnitrosoureas form the crosslinked structure 1-(3-cytosinyl),2-(1-guanyl)ethane in DNA. Following the synthesis of this crosslink by the reaction of O^6-(2-fluoroethyl)guanosine with deoxycytidine, a proposed mechanism involves an initial attack on the O-6 position of guanine, followed by a rearrangement and subsequent reaction with cytosine (MacFarland et al., 1990).

A new DNA adduct that may have relevance to either the therapeutic or carcinogenic actions of the CENUs is the N2,3-ethanoguanine isolated from CCNU-treated DNA (Habraken et al., 1990). This adduct is closely related to an etheno adduct formed by 2-chloroacetaldehyde a metabolite of the carcinogen, vinyl chloride and the CENUs.

Since we are able to describe some of these events chemically, we can more fully assess their impact on loss of cellular function, including cellular repair processes. New direct evidence now exists for the nature of DNA crosslinking by 2-haloethylnitrosoureas. Studies on DNA crosslinking have been reviewed (Kohn et al., 1981; Ludlum, 1990). Efforts to quantitate alkylation of DNA in intact cells and bone marrow have led workers to conclude that differences in DNA alkylation may relate to difference of bone marrow toxicity of nitrosoureas (Green et al., 1981). These workers conclude that decreased myelotoxicity of an individual nitrosourea compared to other nitrosoureas may relate more to localization of DNA modification within chromatin than alteration of rate and extent of DNA repair. In this regard, Tew (1981) has observed that within the nuclear matrix there exist transcriptionally active regions to chromatin that are preferentially modified by nitrosoureas. Briscoe et al. (1990) have examined the base sequence specificity of BCNU, CCNU, and methyl CCNU. Base sequence was found to have an effect upon alkylation of guanine by CENUs. A different effect was observed upon the *N*-7 position than on the O-6 position of guanine. Alkylation at the *N*-7 position of guanine was highly base sequence dependent; up to 50-fold.

The presence of specific modified bases in the DNA of sensitive compared to resistant cells after exposure to 2-haloethylnitrosoureas has been examined for direct evidence for the importance of specific DNA modifications. Cultured human glial cells that are resistant had a higher level of O^6-alkylguanine-DNA alkyltransferase and are several-fold more resistant to the 2-haloethylnitrosoureas than the sensitive line. As expected, the resistant cells have less 1-(3-deoxycytidyl)-2-(1-deoxyguanosinyl)ethane crosslinking than the sensitive cell line. In addition, however, there appears to be much reduced or absent 7-guanines in DNA of the resistant cell line compared to the sensitive cell (Bodell et al., 1988). Thus, the enzymatic removal and repair of DNA modifications caused by the 2-haloethylnitrosoureas have been utilized to establish the importance of DNA repair in preventing cytotoxicity. Habraken et al. (1991) have examined the release of N^2,3-ethanoguanine from haloethylnitrosourea-treated DNA by *Escherichia coli* 3-methyladenine DNA glycosylase II. Polyamines have been shown to interact with DNA to modulate chloroethylnitrosourea-induced DNA damage (Srivenugopal and AliOsman, 1990). These workers concluded that the interaction is not only a function of the charge on the polyamine molecule but also of the chemical structure of the polyamine. Other proteins shown to undergo alkylation of reactive thiolate anions include the enzymes O^6-alkylguanine-DNA alkyl-transferase (Meer et al., 1989), thioredoxin reductase, glutathione reductase, and ribonucleotide reductase (Schallreuter et al., 1990).

10. CARBAMOYLATION

Carbamoylation events can occur after nitrosourea degradation to yield an organic isocyanate and a diazene hydroxide (Fig. 4). As mentioned previously, the organic moiety of the isocyanate may contain a functional group such as a hydroxyl group leading to a possible intramolecular carbamoylation reaction to form a cyclic urethane. Extensive in vitro intramolecular carbamoylation is known to occur with chlorozotocin (Johnston et al., 1975) but whether exclusive intramolecular carbamoylation takes precedence in vivo over intermolecular carbamoylation is not known. The extent of intermolecular carbamoylation in vitro has been assayed by the carbamoylation of [^{14}C]lysine and quantitation of products by chromatography (Wheeler et al., 1974) (Fig. 4). This assay has been utilized extensively on the basis that the isocyanate would attack in a random manner any amino, hydroxyl or thiol functional group. Thus, classification of nitrosoureas based on their comparative carbamoylation of lysine in vitro has been utilized extensively to rank them on their in vivo or intracellular carbamoylating ability. Other assays of carbamoylation include the measurement of the extent of carbamoylation of the amino group of 5′-amino-5′-deoxythymidine (Brubaker et al., 1986), the thiol group of glutathione (Stahl et al., 1987), and intracellular esterases (Dive et al., 1988). Such comparisons are not an adequate estimate of protein modifications by the 2-chloroethylnitrosourea-derived organic isocyanates because some of the isocyanates are excellent pseudo substrates which are capable of irreversible inactivation of specific enzymes at their catalytic site.

A detailed review has focused on the effects of CENU carbamoylation of tumor metabolism (Lea, 1987). The author recognizes the major challenge in assessing the contribution of carbamoylation vs alkylation of the activities of the CENUs. However, carbamoylation appears to have a significant effect on tumors by inhibition of DNA repair and can have selective inhibitory effects on metabolite uptake and macromolecular synthesis in neoplastic tissues (Lea, 1987).

Originally, Brown and Wold (1973a,b) found that butyl isocyanate and octyl isocyanate were active-site-directed inactivators of elastase and chymotrypsin, respectively. Babson and Reed (1978) observed that active-site-specific inactivation of chymotrypsin occurred by cyclohexyl isocyanate released during degradation of CCNU. A 70-fold excess of lysine over chymotrypsin concentration is necessary to detect any effect on the stoichiometric inactivation of chymotrypsin (Babson and Reed, 1978). Subsequently, Frischer and Ahmad (1977) observed that only glutathione reductase out of 19 erythrocyte enzymes assayed is inactivated in vivo during chemotherapy of patients with BCNU. Further studies by Babson and Reed (1978) have shown that inactivation of glutathione reductase occurs only when the enzyme is in a reduced state (i.e. NADPH reduction) and two thiol groups are present at the active site. The inactivation of catalytic activity appears to occur as a thiocarbamate adduct forms between the isocyanate and possibly the distal thiol group at the active site (Babson and Reed, 1978). These findings have been extended to a detailed study of the inactivation of lipoamide dehydrogenase by BCNU-derived 2-chloroethyl isocyanate (Lohrer and Krauth-Siegel, 1990).

The importance of these observations is that certain enzymes and proteins have either a catalytic or functional site at a region of hydrophobicity that is capable of high-affinity binding of organic isocyanate with R groups of proper size and character. Thus a very high probability exists for a successful collision between a particular isocyanate and protein functional group. Active-site-directed interactions of this type take precedence over undirected reactions between other functional groups lacking the associated hydrophobic region for initial binding of the R group of the isocyanate. Such pockets or crevices in proteins have a very important role in the overall specificity and affinity of enzymes and other proteins (i.e. receptor proteins) for substrates and/or pseudo substrates. The ability of cyclohexyl isocyanate to prevent stoichiometrically the polymerization of brain tubulin is another example of highly specific irreversible binding of isocyanate to a protein (Brodie et al., 1980).

Very extensive use has been made of the BCNU inactivation of glutathione reductase in cells to examine the role of the glutathione redox cycle in protection against oxidative stress. For a review that describes this technique see Reed (1985). A very interesting finding is the selective activation in tumor cells of human heat shock gene transcription by chloroethylnitrosoureas mediated by isocyanate-induced damage and activation of heat shock transcription factor (Kroes et al., 1991). Activation of a subset of the human genes, HSP90 and HSP70 is strongly dependent on new protein synthesis and has little effect on other stress genes or on expression of the c-*fos*, c-*myc*, or beta-actin genes.

Additional evidence for the importance of the varying hydrophobic nature of the isocyanates released from CENUs is provided by a study of the calcium-dependent carbamoylation of calmodulin at Lys-75 by CCNU, methyl CCNU, and related derivatives such as hydroxylated metabolites (Mann and Vanaman, 1988). They found up to a 25-fold difference in concentration of CENU required for calmodulin modification. In addition, they concluded that Lys-75 is not essential for the function of calmodulin but is in a region of the molecule involved in interaction with phosphodiesterase and the binding of certain hydrophobic calmodulin antagonists.

11. ALKYLATION VS CARBAMOYLATION EFFECTS

Much of the effort on development of new nitrosoureas has been directed towards decreasing the dose-limiting bone marrow suppression. Chlorozotocin is an example of a drug which was designed to maintain therapeutic efficacy while attempting to minimize host toxicity (Anderson et al., 1975). The next section of this chapter will provide some views as to why chlorozotocin does not achieve this goal to the extent desired.

A comparison of chemical structure of carbamoylating groups suggests that for the CENUs, bifunctional alkylation is essential for antiglioma activity and that myelosuppression is at least partly correlated with carbamoylation (Ali-Osman et al., 1985). However, structural entities in the carbamoylating isocyanate, rather than a quantitative degree of carbamoylation, may be important in the degree of potential myelotoxicity (Ali-Osman et al., 1985).

A comparative study has been conducted to determine the relative organ-related toxicity of two CENUs, BCNU and HECNU, which possess different carbamoylating potential (Stahl and Eisenbrand, 1991). The findings indicate that bone marrow toxicity of CENUs primarily results from alkylation and not from carbamoylation. However, other organ-related toxic effects, such as lung toxicity, are probably a result of carbamoylating reactions of BCNU.

Thiols potentiate the interstrand crosslinking of DNA by CNCC-(C) as well as other CCNUs, which is explained by nucleophilic attack at the carbonyl group and subsequent stereoelectronically controlled decomposition of the tetrahedral intermediate (Lown et al., 1985). The reduced cytotoxic potential of CNCC-(S) has been described as an interaction between GSH and the drug, thereby protecting other more critical nucleophilic targets within the nucleus (Lown et al., 1985). It has been suggested that the decreased cytotoxic potential of CNCC-(S) is in agreement with a prolongation in the half-life of production of alkylating carbonium species and the lack of capacity to crosslink macromolecules (Farhi et al., 1984).

Four plasma metabolites of CNCC have been synthesized and evaluated for their antitumor activity. The metabolites are *N*′-(2-chloroethyl)-*N*-[2-(methylsulphinyl)ethyl]- and *N*′-(2-chloroethyl)-*N*-[2-(methylsulphonyl)ethyl]-*N*- or *N*′-nitrosoureas (Madelmont et al., 1985). Two of the four metabolites exhibited a greater antitumor activity than CNCC.

Specificity in ACNU and CCNU binding to the nucleosomal DNA of murine bone marrow and L1210 cells is in contrast to chlorozotocin and GANU binding preferentially to the linker DNA of bone marrow, but not tumor, cell chromatin (Dean et al., 1985). Differences in DNA linker length does not appear to be the basis for these quantitative differences in the tissue-specific toxicity of these CENUs which contain sugar moieties (Dean et al., 1985).

An in-depth investigation of resistance to DNA crosslinking agents in 9L cell lines with different sensitivities to CENUs has revealed that cellular resistance to CENUs is highly specific (Bodell et al., 1985b). DNA repair processes may mediate cellular resistance to CENUs, since the mechanism of resistance does not allow cross-resistance with other DNA crosslinking agents. Thus other crosslinking agents will not be cross-resistant unless they form alkylation products that are affected by repair processes which mediate resistance to CENUs (Bodell et al., 1985b).

Repair of DNA interstrand crosslink precursors, which is mediated by O^6-alkylguanine-DNA alkyltransferase activity, may be an important determinant of MeCCNU cytotoxicity. Evidence for this correlation comes from measurement of the extent of tumor regression and the level of O^6-methyl-guanine-DNA methyltransferase activity in tumor extracts of six different human rhabdomyosarcoma lines grown in immune-deprived female CBA/CaJ mice after treatment with MeCCNU (Brent et al., 1985). The level of this repair enzyme may be a clinically useful prediction of sensitivity of human tumor cells to the CENUs (Brent et al., 1985).

The induction of sister-chromatid exchanges (SCEs) in 9L rat brain tumor cells is 143-fold greater with ACNU than with 1-ethyl-1-nitrosourea (ENU) (Bodell et al., 1985a). Since on an equimolar basis ^{14}C labelling for [^{14}C]ACNU was about 3- to 2-fold higher than for [^{14}C]ENU, after correction for this difference the induction difference may be about 45-fold. The increased induction of SCEs caused by ACNU is thought to be a result of the formation of DNA interstrand crosslinks (Bodell et al., 1985a). Potentiation of BCNU-induced cytotoxicity in 9L cells by pretreatment with 6-thioguanine may result from increased formation of DNA crosslinks derived from the formation of S^6-(2-chloroethyl)-6-thioguanine in cellular DNA (Bodell et al., 1985c).

The levels of induction of SCEs and the cytotoxicity of ENU, MNU, ACNU and BCNU have been compared (Brent, 1984). The CENUs are 200-fold more cytotoxic and induce SCEs with 45-fold greater efficiency than ECU and MNU, which are not capable of crosslinking. It is suggested that crosslinking is probably the most important molecular event that leads to cell death and induction by SCEs.

A relationship may exist between the repair of O^6-substituted guanine derivatives and cellular resistance to CENUs in human tumor cells. Resistance of 9L-2, HU-188, and HU-253-2 cells to SCE induction and cytotoxicity by CENUs correlates to their increased capacity to remove O^6-(2-chloroethyl)guanine in DNA. O^6-Methylguanine-DNA methyltransferase removes a chloroethylation product that forms DNA crosslinks (Robins et al., 1983; Brent, 1984). Resistant cell lines have a higher cellular level of O^6-methylguanine-DNA methyl transferase, increased repair of O^6-methylguanine, and 50% fewer DNA interstrand crosslinks formed than do sensitive cells treated with the same concentration of CENU (Bodell et al., 1985d).

A major difference between 2-chloroethyl-(methylsulphonyl)methane sulphonate (ClEtSoSo) and the CENUs is that the CENUs, during chemical degradation, yield 2-hydroxyethyl intermediates and 7-hydroxyethyl hydroxylation products, whereas ClEtSoSo causes only chloroethylated products such as 7-chloroethylguanine (Gibson et al., 1986). Such a difference is thought to be important in the overall biological effects of these agents. In this regard, three chloroethylating antitumor agents have been compared for their DNA sequence selectivities of guanine-N'-alkylation. *Cis*-2-OH CCNU, ClEtSoSo, and mitozolomide alkylation of pBR322 DNA, followed by use of the Maxam and Gilbert sequencing technique to determine the alkylation of runs of three or more guanines in the DNA showed differences in the degree of alkylation of specific guanine bases (Hartley et al., 1986). ClEtSoSo alkylated all guanines to the same extent, while *cis*-2-OH CCNU preferentially alkylated the middle guanines as did mitozolomide, but not as intensely as *cis*-2-OH CCNU. Both 7-chloroethylation and 7-hydroxyethylation were similarly enhanced by the presence of adjacent guanines when *cis*-2-OH CCNU was the alkylator. The results imply that the alkylating intermediates, 2-chloroethyldiazohydroxide and 2-hydroxyethyldiazohydroxide react preferentially with the middle guanines because of the enhanced electronegativity created by the presence of neighboring guanines. The cationic character of these diazo intermediates is thought to be greater than with the other two alkylating agents.

It is suggested that CCNU has carbamoylating activity that is associated with inhibition of RNA processing and with the degree of chemopotentiation achieved with misonidazole (MISO) (Hill et al., 1984a). Also, such chemopotentiation by MISO does not appear to occur equally in all cell subpopulations derived from solid KHT sarcomas, and therefore some specificity of enhanced cell killing exists (Hill et al., 1984b). No loss in tumor cell sensitization was found with fractionation of CCNU treatment during chemopotentiation in vivo with KHT sarcoma, with and without MISO (Hill and Siemann, 1984). The combination of MISO with repeated low-dose treatment of CCNU results in a therapeutic gain (Hill and Siemann, 1984). The variable response to BCNU of human glioma cells, sorted according to DNA content, suggests a problem imposed by heterogeneity with regard to chemosensitivity even within a single tumor (Kobayashi et al., 1984).

Crosslinking mediated by X-rays has been proposed as the mechanism through which cell kill is increased by combination with BCNU that also induces DNA interstrand crosslinking (Tofilon et al., 1984).

A comparison of the alkylation of bone marrow DNA by chlorozotocin and CCNU indicates a quantitative equivalent level of DNA alkylation (Byrne et al., 1984). However, the bone marrow sparing effects of chlorozotocin may exist because in contrast to CCNU, chlorozotocin predominantly alkylates the transcriptionally inactive regions of chromatin. The lethal damage of CENUs alkylation in human bone marrow may be principally expressed in transcriptionally active regions of chromatin (Byrne et al., 1984).

The differential bone marrow toxicity exhibited by CENUs does not appear to be a carbamoylation-mediated difference in the rate and extent of DNA–DNA interstrand crosslink removal (Bedford and Eisenbrand, 1984). In the repair of DNA damage in the bone marrow of rats, the kinetics of crosslink removal was identical for chlorozotocin and BCNU (Bedford and Eisenbrand, 1984). These results are in agreement with studies on effects of carbamoylation on cell survival and DNA repair in normal human embryo cells (IMR-90). Carbamoylation may inhibit nucleotide excision repair that is not involved in the repair process of O^6-methylguanine-DNA methyltransferase (Sariban et al., 1984).

Evidence for in vivo carbamoylation of proteins by nitrosoureas includes not only organ and tissue distribution of radiolabel following administration of nitrosoureas radiolabelled in the isocyanate precursor moiety, but also the nature of the urinary metabolites. Kohlhepp et al. (1981) observed that major urinary metabolites of CCNU have molecular weights of 629, 413, 329 and 243 and they represent 5, 20, 2 and 5%, respectively, of total excreted ^{14}C following administration of ^{14}C ring-labelled CCNU. They concluded that the higher molecular weight metabolites are conjugates of peptides derived from active site-directed inactivation of specific enzymes. Lysine does not contribute significantly to the composition of the urinary metabolites. Major amino acids present in the peptides were cysteine, serine, glutamic acid, alanine, glycine and aspartic acid (Kohlhepp et al., 1981).

One must conclude that selective alkylation and carbamoylation events that modify macromolecules are both important in correlation of structure–activity relationships and that in vitro assays are unable to measure the selectivity of such specific macromolecular modifications in vivo.

12. ORGAN TOXICITY

12.1. NEPHROTOXICITY

Renal toxicity has been observed in patients after chemotherapy with MeCCNU (Weiss et al., 1983). Such toxicity is characterized as being cumulative dose dependent (> 1400 mg/m^2), delayed in onset (> 12 months), and often fatal (Kramer et al., 1986). Other CENUs cause renal failure, including CCNU (Weiss and Poster, 1982; Ellis et al., 1985) and chlorozotocin (Moriconi et al., 1985).

A model for CENU nephrotoxicity is based on a single, sublethal dose of MeCCNU or chlorozotocin to the Fischer 344 (F344) rat that produces chronic and progressive changes in renal function (Kramer et al., 1986). At equimolar doses chlorozotocin is a much more potent nephrotoxicant even though it causes much less carbamoylation on cellular macromolecules. Karyomegaly by MeCCNU and chlorozotocin was taken as evidence that both CENUs may have their toxic effects by virtue of extensive alkylation of renal DNA (Kramer et al., 1986).

12.2. Lung Toxicity

Lung damage caused by BCNU is characterized by fibrosing alveolitis and interstitial pneumonitis that can lead to pulmonary fibrosis, restrictive pulmonary failure, and death (Weiss et al., 1981; Muggia et al., 1983; Smith and Boyd, 1984a,b). Initial injury may occur in endothelial cells, causing changes in pulmonary and serum angiotensin, converting enzyme activity (Smith and Boyd, 1984a). Preferential destruction of lung glutathione reductase by BCNU precedes the development of severe lung injury (Smith and Boyd, 1984b).

BCNU has been shown to accentuate acute lung damage in mice with pre-existing lung damage that was produced by the administration of butylated hydroxytoluene (Kehrer and Klein-Szanto, 1985). A single dose of BCNU alone had a minimal toxic effect on lung tissue, whereas high doses of BCNU administered one day after butylated hydroxytoluene were related to the ability of BCNU to inhibit pulmonary glutathione reductase activity and the increased DNA synthesis after butylated hydroxytoluene (Kehrer and Klein-Szanto, 1985).

13. THE FUTURE

Because current antitumor agents are toxic to both malignant and non-malignant cells, a major chemotherapeutic goal is to make available selective therapy regimens having limited potential to injure normal cells. Rapidly proliferating cells are major targets, and selectivity continues to be a major problem. However, some cells lack such a high mitotic index and yet are highly susceptible to injury, e.g. endothelial cells found in endothelium (Lazo, 1986). CENU toxicity to endothelial cells and pulmonary fibrosis needs further investigation. Such studies could utilize very effectively the availability of CENUs with varying alkylating and carbamoylating capabilities to establish which reactive moiety is important in dose-limiting toxicity of these drugs.

The ability of the nitrosoureas to cross the blood–brain barrier, while many antitumor drugs fail to do so, has resulted in much interest in the lipophilic character of the nitrosoureas. Based on cancer quantitative structure–activity relationship (QSAR), some guidelines for the design of new nitrosoureas have been advanced. After an extensive study of a QSAR for 90 nitrosoureas against L1210 leukaemia in mice, it was concluded that the lipophilic character of the nitrosoureas is the most important parameter determining their antitumor activity (Hansch et al., 1980). P-values were measured for 43 nitrosoureas and efforts to make nitrosourea congeners somewhat more hydrophilic became a central point in the study. Justified concern was expressed about the limitation of functional groups such as COOH, which are almost completely ionized at physiological pH, pH 7–4, to confer greater hydrophilicity when unionized functional groups showed a better correlation. Making the R group more polar yet unionized with a disaccharide was suggested (Hansch el al., 1980). Interestingly, at about the same time, this approach was being tested with three nitrosoureas containing either a β-maltosyl, β-lactosyl, or β-cellobiosyl R group (Suami et al., 1979). Testing of these congeners against various types of tumors is continuing.

Increasing evidence supports the concept that carbamoylation capability remains an important factor in the design of new nitrosourea congeners. DNA alkylation events have a greater chance for cell killing when the rate of DNA repair is decreased. Day et al. (1980) have identified a group of eight (among 39) human tumor cell strains that are deficient in DNA repair ability. This deficiency is being studied in regard to susceptibility to DNA crosslinks caused by CNU, BCNU, and CCNU (Day et al., 1980; Erickson et al., 1980). Eisenbrand et al. (1976) have designed and synthesized a congener series of 1,1′-polymethylene bis-3-(2-chloroethyl)-3-nitrosoureas as transport forms of polymethylene diisocyanates. These compounds may cause some interesting crosslinking reactions primarily with proteins. Studies with these and other new nitrosoureas have led Eisenbrand and coworkers (1981) to conclude that the non-alkylating part of the CENU is important for the biological effects of these drugs. More recent work on hydroxylated CENUs by this group indicates that carcinogenicity and mutagenicity are closely related to induction of DNA single-strand breaks that result from hydroxyethylation (Zeller et al., 1989). Lea (1987) concluded from a review of the literature that the carbamoylation capability of some CENUs has importance in inhibition of DNA repair and possibly metabolite uptake by tumors.

Certain nitrosoureas have been shown to cause a prolonged in vivo depression of cytochrome

P450 content and cytochrome P450-dependent enzyme activities of liver microsomes when measured in vivo (Reed and May, 1978; Litterst, 1981). A single non-lethal dose of CCNU in vivo decreased liver cytochrome P450 content and drug metabolism of rat liver microsomes 40–70% for up to 6 weeks. This unique suppression is without parallel by any other drug and cannot be explained, except for possible persistent alkylation and/or carbamoylation effects by the degradation intermediates of the nitrosoureas.

14. CONCLUSIONS

Nitrosourea cytotoxicity remains a very complex effect with unique characteristics. Much more needs to be understood at the molecular level to provide even rudimentary explanation of the chemical modifications caused by the alkylations and carbamylating events of the nitrosoureas. If potent toxicity of the nitrosoureas could be ameliorated without sacrificing tumor cell cytotoxicity, the clinical impact of these drugs would be enormous.

Acknowledgements—The author wishes to acknowledge support by Grant CH 109 from the American Cancer Society and Grant ES00210.

REFERENCES

ALI-OSMAN, F., GIBLIN, J., BERGER, M., MURPHY, M. J., JR and ROSENBLUM, M. L. (1985) Chemical structure of carbamoylating groups and their relationship to bone marrow toxicity and antiglioma activity of bifunctionally alkylating and carbamoylating nitrosoureas. *Cancer Res.* **45:** 4185–4191.

ANDERSON, T., MCMENAMIN, M. G. and SCHEIN, P. S. (1975) Chlorozotocin, 2[3-(2-Chloroethyl)-3-nitrosoureido]-D-glucopyranose, an antitumor agent with modified bone marrow toxicity. *Cancer Res.* **35:** 761–765.

BABSON, J. R. and REED, D. J. (1978) Inactivation of glutathione reductase by 2-chloroethyl nitrosourea-derived isocyanates. *Biochem. biophys. Res. Commun.* **83:** 754–762.

BARTOSEK, I., CORADA, M., DALLARDA, S., LUCAS, C., DELOFFRE, P. and GUAITANI, A. (1991) Pharmacokinetic profile of fotemustine in rat plasma by electrochemical detection. *Xenobiotica* **21:** 235–242.

BEDFORD, P. and EISENBRAND, G. (1984) DNA damage and repair in the bone marrow of rats treated with four chloroethylnitrosoureas. *Cancer Res.* **44:** 514–518.

BODELL, W. J., AIDA, T. and RASMUSSEN, J. (1985a) Comparison of sister-chromatid exchange induction caused by nitrosoureas that alkylate or alkylate and crosslink DNA. *Mutat. Res.* **149:** 95–100.

BODELL, W. J., GEROSA, M., AIDA, T., BERGER, M. S. and ROSENBLUM, M. L. (1985b) Investigation of resistance to DNA crosslinking agents in 9L cell lines with different sensitivities to chloroethylnitrosoureas. *Cancer Res.* **45:** 3460–3464.

BODELL, W. J., MORGAN, W. F., RASMUSSEN, J., WILLIAMS, M. E. and DEEN, D. F. (1985c) Potentiation of 1,3-bis(2-chloroethyl)-1-nitrosourea (BCNU)-induced cytotoxicity in 9L cells by pretreatment with 6-thioguanine. *Biochem. Pharmac.* **34:** 515–520.

BODELL, W. J., TOSHIMITSU, A., BERGER, M. S. and ROSENBLUM, M. L. (1985d) Repair of O^6-(2-chloroethyl)guanine mediates the biological effects of chloroethylnitrosoureas. *Environ. Health Persp.* **62:** 119–126.

BODELL, W. J., TOKUDA, K. and LUDLUM, D. B. (1988) Differences in DNA alkylation products formed in sensitive and resistant human glioma cells treated with *N*-(2-chloroethyl)-*N*-nitrosourea. *Cancer Res.* **48:** 4489–4492.

BRENT, T. P. (1984) Suppression of crosslink formation in chloroethylnitrosourea-treated DNA by an activity in extracts of human leukemic lymphoblasts. *Cancer Res.* **44:** 1887–1892.

BRENT, T. P., HOUGHTON, P. J. and HOUGHTON, J. A. (1985) O^6-Alkylguanine-DNA alkyltransferase activity correlates with the therapeutic response of human rhabdomyosarcoma xenografts to 1-(2-chloroethyl)-3-(*trans*-4-methylcyclohexyl)-1-nitrosourea. *Proc. Nat. Acad. Sci. U.S.A.* **82:** 2985–2989.

BRISCOE, W. T., ANDERSON, S. P. and MAY, H. E. (1990) Base sequence specificity of three 2-chloroethylnitrosoureas. *Biochem. Pharmac.* **40:** 1201–1209.

BRODIE, A. E., BABSON, J. R. and REED, D. J. (1980) Inhibition of tubulin polymerization by nitrosourea-derived isocyanates. *Biochem. Pharmac.* **29:** 652–654.

BROWN, W. E. and WOLD, F. (1973a) Alkyl isocyanates as active-site-specific reagents for serine proteases. Identification of the active-site serine as the site of reaction. *Biochemistry* **12:** 835–840.

BROWN, W. E. and WOLD, F. (1973b) Alkyl isocyanates as active-site-specific reagents for serine proteases. Reaction properties. *Biochemistry* **12:** 828–834.

BRUBAKER, W. F., JR, ZHAO, H. P. and PRUSOFF, W. H. (1986) Measurement of carbamoylating activity of nitrosoureas and isocyanates by a novel high-pressure liquid chromatography assay. *Biochem. Pharmac.* **35:** 2359–2365.

BRUNDRETT, R. B. (1980) Chemistry of nitrosoureas. Intermediacy of 4,5-dihydro-1,2,3-oxadiazole in 1,3-bis(2-chloroethyl)-1-nitrosourea decomposition. *J. med. Chem.* **23:** 1245–1247.

BRUNDRETT, R. B., COWENS, J. W., COLVIN, M. and JARDINE, I. (1976) Chemistry of nitrosoureas. Decomposition of deuterated 1,3-bis(2-chloroethyl)-1-nitrosourea. *J. med. Chem.* **19:** 958–961.

BYRNE, P., TEW, K., JEMIONEK, J., MACVITTIE, T., ERICKSON, L. and SCHEIN, P. (1984) Cellular and molecular mechanisms of the bone marrow sparing effects of the glucose chloroethylnitrosourea chlorozotocin. *Blood* **63:** 759–767.

CADDY, B., IDOWU, O. R. and STUART, J. F. (1982) A high pressure liquid chromatographic procedure for monitoring 1-(2-chlorethyl)-3-(4-*trans*-methylcyclohexyl)-1-nitrosourea levels in body fluids. *Ther. Drug Mon.* **4:** 389–395.

CARTER, S. K., SCHABEL, F. M., JR., BRODER, L. S. and JOHNSON, T. P. (1972) 1,3-bis(2-chloroethyl)-1-nitrosourea (BCNU) and other nitrosoureas in cancer treatment: a review. *Adv. Cancer Res.* **16:** 273–332.

COLVIN, M., COWENS, J. W., BRUNDRETT, R. B., KRAMER, B. S. and LUDLUM, D. B. (1974) Decomposition of BCNU [1,3bis(2chloroethyl)1nitrosourea] in aqueous solution. *Biochem. biophys. Res. Commun.* **60:** 515–520.

DAY, R. S., III, ZIOLKOWSKI, C. H. J., SCUDIERO, D. A., MEYER, S. A., LUBINIECKI, A. S., GIRARDI, A. J., GALLOWAY, S. M. and BYNUM, G. D. (1980) Defective repair of alkylated DNA by human tumour and SV40-transformed human cell strains. *Nature* **288:** 724–727.

DEAN, S. W., TEW, K. D., CLARK, A. E. and SCHEIN, P. S. (1985) DNA repeal length in chromatin from murine bone marrow and L1210 leukaemia cells. *Br. J. Cancer* **52:** 377–382.

DIKSIC, M., SAKO, K., FEINDEL, W., KATO, A., YAMAMOTO, Y. L., FARROKHZAD, S. and THOMPSON, C. (1984) Pharmacokinetics of positron-labeled 1,3-bis(2-chloroethyl)nitrosourea in human brain tumors using positron emission tomography. *Cancer Res.* **44:** 3120–3124.

DIVE, C., WORKMAN, P. and WATSON, J. V. (1988) Inhibition of intracellular esterases by antitumour chloroethylnitrosoureas. Measurement by flow cytometry and correlation with molecular carbamoylation activity. *Biochem. Pharmac.* **37:** 3987–3993.

EISENBRAND, G. (1984) Anticancer nitrosoureas: investigations on antineoplastic, toxic and neoplastic activities. *IARC Sci. Publ.* **57:** 695–708.

EISENBRAND, G., FIEBIG, H. H. and ZELLER, W. J. (1976) Some new congeners of the anticancer agent 1,3-bis-(2-chloroethyl)-1-nitrosourea (BCNU). Synthesis of bifunctional analogs and water soluble derivatives and preliminary evaluation of their chemotherapeutic potential. *Z. Krebsforsch* **86:** 279–286.

EISENBRAND, G., HABS, M., ZELLER, W. J., FIEBIG, H., BERGER, M., ZELESMY, O. and SCHMAHL, D. (1981) New nitrosoureas—therapeutic and long-term toxic effects of selected compounds in comparison to established drugs. In: *Nitrosoureas in Cancer Treatment*, pp. 175–191, SERROU, B., SCHEIN, S. P. and IMBACH, J. L. (eds). Elsevier Publishers, New York.

ELLIS, M. E., WEISS, R. B. and KRUPERMINC, M. (1985) Nephrotoxicity of lomusine: a case report and literature review. *Cancer Chemother. Pharmac.* **15:** 174–175.

ERICKSON, L. C., LAURENT, G., A., S. N. and KOHN, K. W. (1980) DNA crosslinking and monoadduct repair in nitrosourea-treated human tumour cells. *Nature* **288:** 727–729.

FARHI, J. J., BENNOUN, M., TAPIERO, H., WANG, A. L. and TEW, K. D. (1984) Biochemical and cytotoxic properties of the isomeric forms of *N,N'*-bis[*N*-2-chloroethyl)-*N*-nitrosocarbamoyl] cystamine. *Biochem. Pharmac.* **33:** 2575–2580.

FARMER, P. B., FOSTER, A. B., JARMAN, M., ODDY, M. R. and REED, D. J. (1978) Synthesis, metabolism, and antitumor activity of deuterated analogs of 1-(2-chloroethyl)-3-cyclohexyl-1-nitrosoureas. *J. med. Chem.* **21:** 514–520.

FOSTER, A. B., JARMAN, M., COE, P. L., SLEIGH, P. and TATLOW, J. C. (1980) Fluorinated analogs of 1-(2-chloroethyl)-3-cyclohexyl-1-nitrosourea: an attempt to control metabolism. *J. med. Chem.* **23:** 1226–1229.

FOSTER, D. O. and PARDEE, A. B. (1969) Transport of amino acid by confluent and nonconfluent 3T3 and polyoma virus-transformed 3T3 cells growing on glass cover slips. *J. biol. Chem.* **244:** 2675–2681.

FREED, B. R., MCQUINN, R. L., TILBURY, R. S. and DIGENIS, G. A. (1982) Distribution of 13N in rat tissues following intravenous administration of nitroso-labeled BCNU. *Cancer Chemother. Pharmac.* **10:** 16–21.

FRISCHER, H. and AHMAD, T. (1977) Severe generalized glutathione reductase deficiency after antitumor chemotherapy with BCNU [1,3-bis(chloroethyl)-1-nitrosourea]. *J. Lab. clin. Med.* **89:** 1080–1089.

FUJIMOTO, S. and OGAWA, M. (1985) Toxicological study on a new nitrosourea derivative, 1-(2-chloroethyl)-3-isobutyl-3-(beta-maltosyl)-1-nitrosourea. *Jap. J. Cancer Res.* **76:** 651–656.

GARRETT, E. R., GOTO, S. and STUBBINS, J. F. (1965) Kinetics of solvolyses of various *N*-alkyl-*N*-nitrosoureas in neutral and alkaline solutions. *J. Pharm. Sci.* **54:** 119–123.

GIBSON, N. W., HARTLEY, J. A., STRONG, J. M. and KOHN, K. W. (1986) 2-Chloroethyl (methylsulfonyl)methanesulfonate (NSC-338947), a more selective DNA alkylating agent than the chloroethylnitrosoureas. *Cancer Res.* **46:** 553–557.

GODENECHE, D., MADELMONT, J. C., MOREAU, M. F., DUPRAT, J., CHABRAD, J. L., PLAGNE, R. and MEYNIEL, G. (1985) Metabolic disposition of 2-chloroethyl nitrosocarbamoylcystamine in rats. *Drug Metab. Disp.* **13:** 220–226.

GODENECHE, D., MADELMONT, J. C., MOREAU, M. F., DUPRAT, J., PLAGNE, R. and MEYNIEL, G. (1986)

Metabolism of 2-chloroethyl nitrosocarbamoylcystamine by rat liver subcellular fractions. *Drug Metab. Disp.* **14:** 112–117.

GORDON, B. H., RICHARDS, R. P., HILEY, M. P., GRAY, A. J., INGS, R. M. J. and CAMPBELL, D. B. (1989) A new method for the measurement of nitrosoureas in plasma: an HPLC procedure for the measurement of fotemustine kinetics. *Xenobiotica* **19:** 329–339.

GREEN, D., AHLGREEN, J. D. and SCHEIN, P. S. (1981) A molecular basis for differences in nitrosourea bone marrow toxicity. In: *Nitrosoureas in Cancer Treatment*, pp. 49–59, SERROU, B., SCHEIN, P. S. and IMBACH, J. L. (eds). Elsevier Publishers, New York.

GREENE, M. O. and GREENBERG, J. (1960) The activity of nitrosoguanidine against ascites tumors in mice. *Cancer Res.* **20:** 1166–1171.

GUENGERICH, F. P., CRAWFORD, W. M., JR, DOMORADZKI, J. Y., MACDONALD, T. L. and WATANABE, P. G. (1980) In vitro activation of 1,2-dichloroethane by microsomal and cytosolic enzymes. *Toxic. appl. Pharmac.* **55:** 303–317.

HABRAKEN, Y., CARTER, C. A., KIRK, M. C., RIORDAN, J. M. and LUDLUM, D. B. (1990) Formation of N,3-ethanoguanine in DNA after in vitro treatment with the therapeutic agent, *N*-(2-chloroethyl)-*N'*-cyclohexyl-*N*-nitrosourea. *Carcinogenesis* **11:** 223–228.

HABRAKEN, Y., CARTER, C. A., SEKIGUCHI, M. and LUDLUM, D. B. (1991) Release of N,3-ethanoguanine from haloethylnitrosoureatreated DNA by *Escherichia coli* 3-methyladenine DNA glycosylase II. *Carcinogenesis* **12:** 1971–1973.

HANSCH, C., LEO, A., SCHMIDT, C., JOW, P. Y. C. and MONTGOMERY, J. A. (1980) Antitumor structure–activity relationships. Nitrosoureas vs L1210 leukemia. *J. med. Chem.* **23:** 1095–1101.

HARTLEY, J. A., GIBSON, N. W., KOHN, K. W. and MATTES, W. B. (1986) DNA sequence selectivity of guanine-N7 alkylation by three antitumor chloroethylating agents. *Cancer Res.* **46:** 1943–1947.

HILL, D. L., KIRK, M. C. and STRUCK, M. F. (1975) Microsomal metabolism of nitrosoureas. *Cancer Res.* **35:** 296–301.

HILL, S. A. and SIEMANN, D. W. (1984) Chemopotentiation in vivo: no loss of sensitization with fractionation. *Br. J. Cancer* **50:** 509–517.

HILL, S. A., BAUER, K. D., KENG, P. C. and SIEMANN, D. W. (1984a) The effect in the KHT sarcoma of CCNU and MISO on cell cycle progression evaluated by flow cytometry. *Intl. J. Radiat. Oncol. Biol. Phys.* **10:** 1619–1622.

HILL, S. A., KENG, P. C. and SIEMANN, D. W. (1984b) Survival in subpopulations of cells derived from solid KHT sarcomas by centrifugal elutriation following treatment with CCNU and MISO. *Int. J. Radiat. Oncol. Biol. Phys.* **10:** 1615–1618.

HILTON, J. and WALKER, M. D. (1975) Hydroxylation of 1(2-chloroethyl)-3-cyclohexyl-1-nitrosourea. *Biochem. Pharmac.* **24:** 2153–2158.

IMBACH, J. L., MARTINEZ, J., OIRY, J., BOURUT, C., CHENU, E., MARAL, R. and MATHE, G. (1981) New nitrosoureas derivatives and related compounds. In: *Nitrosoureas in Cancer Treatment*, pp. 123–127, SERROU, B., SCHEIN, P. S. and IMBACH, J. L. (eds). Elsevier Publishers, New York.

INGS, R. M., GRAY, A. J., TAYLOR, A. R., GORDON, B. H., BREEN, M., HILEY, M., BROWNSILL, R., MARCHANT, N., RICHARDS, R., WALLACE, D., HUGHES, T., THOMAS, R., WILLIAMS, J., LUCAS, C. and CAMPBELL, D. B. (1990) Disposition, pharmacokinetics, and metabolism of ^{14}C-fotemustine in cancer patients. *Eur. J. Cancer* **26:** 838–842.

JENSEN, D. E. (1978) Reaction of DNA with alkylating agents. Differential alkylation of poly[dA-dT] by methylnitrosourea and ethylnitrosourea. *Biochemistry* **17:** 5108–5113.

JENSEN, D. E. and REED, D. J. (1978) Reaction of DNA with alkylating agents. Quantitation of alkylation by ethylnitrosourea of oxygen and nitrogen sites on poly [dA-dT] including phosphotriester formation. *Biochemistry* **17:** 5098–5107.

JOHNSTON, T. P., MCCALEB, G. S. and MONTGOMERY, J. A. (1963) The synthesis of anti-neoplastic agents. XXXII. *N*-Nitrosoureas. I. *J. med. Chem.* **6:** 669–681.

JOHNSTON, T. P., MCCALEB, G. S., OPLIGER, P. S. and MONTGOMERY, J. A. (1966) The synthesis of potential anticancer agents. XXXVI. *N*-nitrosoureas. II. Haloalkyl derivatives. *J. med. Chem.* **9:** 892–911.

JOHNSTON, T. P., MCCALEB, G. S. and MONTGOMERY, J. A. (1975) Synthesis of chlorozotocin, the 2-chloroethyl analog of the anticancer antibiotic streptozocin. *J. med. Chem.* **18:** 104–106.

JOHNSTON, T. P., KUSSNER, C. L., CARTER, R. L., FRYE, J. L., LOMAX, N. R., PLOWMAN, J. and NARAYANAN, V. L. (1984a) Studies on synthesis and anticancer activity of selected *N*-(2-fluoroethyl)-*N*-nitrosoureas. *J. med. Chem.* **27:** 1422–1426.

JOHNSTON, T. P., MCCALEB, G. S., ROSE, W. C. and MONTGOMERY, J. A. (1984b) *Cis*4[[[(2-chloroethyl)nitrosoamino]carbonyl]methylamino]cyclohexanecarboxylic acid, a nitrosourea with latent activity against an experimental solid tumor. *J. med. Chem.* **27:** 97–99.

KEHRER, J. P. and KLEIN-SZANTO, A. J. (1985) Enhanced acute lung damage in mice following administration of 1,3-bis(2-chloroethyl)-1-nitrosourea. *Cancer Res.* **45:** 5707–5713.

KOBAYASHI, S., HOSHINO, T., DOUGHERTY, D. V. and ROSENBLUM, M. L. (1984) Variable response to 1,3-bis(2-chloroethyl)-1-nitrosourea of human glioma cells sorted according to DNA content. *J. Neurooncol.* **2:** 5–11.

KOHLHEPP, S. J., MAY, H. E. and REED, D. J. (1981) Urinary metabolites of 1-(2-chloroethyl)-3-cyclohexyl-1-nitrosourea and 1-(2-chloroethyl)-3-*trans*-4-methylcyclohexyl)-1-nitrosourea. *Drug Metab. Disp.* **9:** 135–141.

KOHN, K. W. (1977) Interstrand crosslinking of DNA by 1,3-bis(2-chloroethyl)-1-nitrosourea and other 1-(2-haloethyl)-1-nitrosoureas. *Cancer Res.* **37:** 1450–1454.

KOHN, K. W., ERICKSON, L. C. and LAURENT, G. (1981) DNA alkylation, crosslinking and repair. In: *Nitrosoureas in Cancer Treatment*, pp. 33–48, SERROU, B., SCHEIN, P. S. and IMBACH, J. L. (eds). Elsevier Publishers, New York.

KRAMER, R. A. (1989) Cytochrome P450-dependent formation of alkylating metabolites of the 2-chloroethylnitrosoureas MeCCNU and CCNU. *Biochem. Pharmac.* **38:** 3185–3192.

KRAMER, R. A., BOYD, M. R. and DEES, J. H. (1986) Comparative nephrotoxicity of 1-(2-chloroethyl)-3-(*trans*-4-methylcyclohexyl)-1-nitrosourea (MeCCNU) and chlorozotocin: functional–structural correlations in the Fischer 344 rat. *Toxic. appl. Pharmac.* **82:** 540–550.

KROES, R. A., ABRAVAYA, K., SEIDENFELD, J. and MORIMOTO, R. I. (1991) Selective activation of human heat shock gene transcription by nitrosourea antitumor drugs mediated by isocyanateinduced damage and activation of heat shock transcription factor. *Proc. natn. Acad. Sci. U.S.A.* **88:** 4825–4829.

LABARRE, P., GODENECHE, D., MADELMONT, J. C., TRIANA, K., MATHE, G. and VEYRE, A. (1987) Qualitative and quantitative analysis of a new sulphur-containing nitrosourea in blood by high-performance liquid chromatography. *J. Chromatog.* **419:** 381–387.

LAZO, J. S. (1986) Endothelial injury caused by antineoplastic agents. *Biochem. Pharmac.* **35:** 1919–1923.

LEA, M. A. (1987) Effects of carbamoylating agents on tumor metabolism. *Crit. Rev. Oncol. Hematol.* **7:** 329–371.

LEMOINE, A., LUCAS, C. and INGS, R. M. J. (1991) Review. Metabolism of chloroethylnitrosoureas. *Xenobiotica* **21:** 775–791.

LEVIN, V. A. (1981) Clinical pharmacology of the nitrosoureas. In: *Nitrosoureas: Current Status and New Developments*, pp. 171–180, PRESTAYKO, C. A. W., CROOKE, S. T., BAKER, L. H., CARTER, S. K. and SCHEIN, P. S. (eds). Academic Press, New York.

LEVIN, V. A., KABRA, P. A. and FREEMAN-DOVE, M. A. (1978) Relationship of 1,3-bis(2-chloroethyl)-1-nitrosourea (BCNU) and 1-(2-chlorethyl)-3-cyclohexyl-1-nitrosourea (CCNU) pharmacokinetics of uptake, distribution, and tissue/plasma partitioning in rat organs and intracerebral tumors. *Can. Chem. Pharmac.* **1:** 233–242.

LEVIN, V. A., STEARNS, J., BYRD, A., FINN, A. and WEINKAM, R. J. (1979) The effect of phenobarbital pretreatment on the antitumor activity of 1,3-bis(2-chloroethyl)-1-nitrosourea (BCNU, 1-(2-chloroethyl)-3-cyclohexyl-1-nitrosourea (CCNU) and 1-(2-chloroethyl)-3-(2,6-dioxo-3-piperidyl)-1-nitrosourea (PCNU), and on the plasma pharmacokinetics and biotransformation of BCNU. *J. Pharmac. exp. Ther.* **208:** 1–6.

LEVIN, V. A., BYRD, D., CAMPBELL, J., GIANNINI, D. D., BORCICH, J. K. and DAVIS, R. L. (1985) Central nervous system toxicity and cerebrospinal fluid pharmacokinetics of intraventricular 3-(4-amino-2-methyl-5-pyrimidinyl)ethyl-1-(2-chloroethyl)-1-nitrosoureas and other nitrosoureas in beagles. *Cancer Res.* **45:** 3803–3809.

LIN, T. S., BRUBAKER, W. F., JR, WANG, Z. H., PARK, S. and PRUSOFF, W. H. (1986) Antineoplastic activity of 3′-(chloroethyl)nitrosourea analogs of 2′-deoxyuridine and 2′-deoxy-5-fluorouridine. *J. med. Chem.* **29:** 862–865.

LITTERST, C. L. (1981) Prolonged depression of hepatic microsomal drug metabolism and hemoprotein levels following a single dose of 1-(2-chloroethyl)-3-cyclohexyl-1-nitrosourea (CCNU). *Biochem. Pharmac.* **30:** 1014–1016.

LOHRER, H. and KRAUTH-SIEGEL, R. L. (1990) Purification and characterization of lipoamide dehydrogenase from *Trypanosoma cruzi. Eur. J. Biochem.* **194:** 863–869.

LOWN, J. W. and CHAUHAN, S. M. S. (1981) Synthesis of specifically ^{15}N- and ^{13}C-labeled antitumor (2-haloethyl)nitrosoureas. The study of their conformations in solution by nitrogen-15 and carbon-13 nuclear magentic resonance and evidence for stereoelectronic control in their aqueous decomposition. *J. med. Chem.* **24:** 5309–5321.

LOWN, J. W., MCLAUGHLIN, L. W. and CHANG, Y.M. (1978) Mechanism of action of 2-haloethylnitrosoureas on DNA and its relation to their antileukemic properties. *Bioorg. Chem.* **7:** 97–110.

LOWN, J. W., JOSHUA, A. V. and MCLAUGHLIN, L. W. (1980) Novel antitumor nitrosoureas and related compounds and their reactions with DNA. *J. med. Chem.* **23:** 798–805.

LOWN, J. W., KOGANTY, R. R., TEW, K. D., OIRY, J. and IMBACH, J. L. (1985) Mechanism of action of 2-haloethylnitrosoureas on deoxyribonucleic acid. Pathways of aqueous decomposition and pharmacological characteristics of new anticancer disulfide-linked nitrosoureas. *Biochem. Pharmac.* **34:** 1015–1024.

LUDLUM, D. B. (1977) Alkylating agents and the nitrosoureas. In: *Cancer, A Comprehensive Treatise*, Vol. 5, pp. 285–307, BECKER, F. F. (ed.). Plenum Press, New York.

LUDLUM, D. B. (1990) DNA alkylation by the haloethylnitrosoureas: nature of modifications produced and their enzymatic repair or removal. *Mutat. Res.* **223:** 117–126.

LUDLUM, D. B. and TONG, W. P. (1981) Modification of DNA and RNA bases by the nitrosoureas. In: *Nitrosoureas in Cancer Treatment*, pp. 21–81, SERROU, B., SCHEIN, P. S. and IMBACH, J. L. (eds). Elsevier/North-Holland Biomedical Publishers, Amsterdam.

LUDLUM, D. B., KRAMER, B. S., WANG, J. and FENSELAU, C. C. (1975) Reaction of 1,3-bis(2-chloroethyl)-1-nitrosourea with synthetic polynucleotides. *Biochemistry* **14:** 5480–5485.

MACFARLAND, J. G., KIRK, M. C. and LUDLUM, D. B. (1990) Mechanism of action of the nitrosoureas-IV. Synthesis of the 2-haloethylnitrosourea-induced DNA cross-link 1-(3-cytosinyl),2-(1-guanyl)ethane. *Biochem. Pharmac.* **39:** 33–36.

Machinami, T., Nishiyama, S., Kikushi, K. and Suami, T. (1975) Synthesis of (2-chloroethyl)-nitrosourea derivatives of carbohydrate. *Bull. Chem. Soc. Jap.* **48:** 3763–3764.

Madelmont, J. C., Godeneche, D., Parrv, D., Duprat, J., Chabard, J. L., Plagne, R., Mathe, G. and Meyniel, G. (1985) New cysteamine (2-chloroethyl)nitrosoureas. Synthesis and preliminary antitumor results. *J. med. Chem.* **28:** 1346–1350.

Mann, D. M. and Vanaman, T. C. (1988) Modification of calmodulin on Lys-75 by carbamoylating nitrosoureas. *J. biol. Chem.* **263:** 11284–11290.

May, H. E., Boose, R. and Reed, D. J. (1974) Hydroxylation of the carcinostatic 1-(2-chloroethyl)-3-cyclohexyl-1-nitrosourea (CCNU) by rat liver microsomes. *Biochem. biophys. Res. Comm.* **57:** 426–433.

May, H. E., Boose, R. and Reed, D. J. (1975) Microsomal monooxygenation of the carcinostatic 1-(2-chloroethyl)-3-cyclohexyl-1-nitrosourea. Synthesis and identification of *cis* and *trans* monohydroxylated products. *Biochemistry* **14:** 4723–4730.

May, H. E., Kohlhepp, S. J., Boose, R. B. and Reed, D. J. (1979) Synthesis and identification of products derived from the metabolism of the carcinostatic 1-(2-chloroethyl)-3-(*trans*-4-methylcyclohexyl)-1-nitrosourea by rat liver microsomes. *Cancer Res.* **39:** 762–772.

Meer, L., Schold, S. C. and Kleihues, P. (1989) Inhibition of the hepatic O^6-alkylguanine-DNA alkyltransferase in vivo by pretreatment with antineoplastic agents. *Biochem. Pharmac.* **38:** 929–934.

Montgomery, J. A. (1976) Chemistry and structure–activity studies of the nitrosoureas. *Cancer Treat. Rep.* **60:** 651–664.

Montgomery, J. A. and Mayo, J. G. (1974) Quantitative structure–activity relationships in anticancer agents. Activity of selected nitrosoureas against a solid tumor, the Lewis lung carcinoma. *J. med. Chem.* **17:** 477–480.

Montgomery, J. A., James, R., McCaleb, G. S. and Johnston, T. P. (1967) The modes of decomposition of 1,3-bis-(2-chloroethyl)-1-nitrosourea and related compounds. *J. med. Chem.* **10:** 668–674.

Montgomery, J. A., James, R., McCaleb, G. S., Kirk, M. C. and Johnston, T. P. (1975) Decomposition of *N*-(2-chloroethyl)-*N*-nitrosoureas in aqueous media. *J. med. Chem.* **18:** 568–571.

Moriconi, W. J., Taylor, S., Slavik, M., Belt, R. J., Haas, C. D. and Hoogstraten, B. (1985) Phase I evaluation of chlorozotocin (NSC-178248): weekly schedule. *Invest. New Drugs* **3:** 57–62.

Muggia, F. M., Louie, A. C. and Sikic, B. I. (1983) Pulmonary toxicity of antitumor agents. *Cancer Treat. Rev.* **10:** 221–243.

Nishigaki, T., Nakamura, K., Kinoshita, T., Kuwano, H. and Tanaka, M. (1985a) Identification of major urinary metabolites of ACNU, 3-[(4-amino-2-methyl-5-pyrimidinyl)methyl]1-(2-chloroethyl)-1-nitrosourea hydrochloride in rats. *J. Pharmacobiodyn.* **8:** 401–408.

Nishigaki, T., Nakamura, K. and Tanaka, M. (1985b) in vitro metabolism of ACNU, 3-[(4-amino-2-methyl-5-pyrimidinyl)-methyl]-1-(2-chlorethyl)-1-nitroso urea hydrochloride. 1. Water-soluble antitumor nitrosourea. *J. Pharmacobiodyn.* **8:** 409–416.

Polacek, J., Gunnarsson, P. O. and Brandin, S. (1988) Determination of tauromustine, a nitrosourea-based antitumor agent, in plasma by high-performance liquid chromatography. *J. Chromatog.* **425:** 424–428.

Potter, D. W. and Reed, D. J. (1980) Loss of methylcyclohexyl stereospecificity during cytochrome P450-dependent monooxygenation. In: *Microsomes, Drug Oxidations, and Chemical Carcinogenesis*, Vol. 2, pp. 371–374, Coon, M. J., Conney, M. H., Estabrook, R. W., Gelboin, H. V., Gillette, J. R. and O'Brien, P. J. (eds). Academic Press, New York.

Potter, D. W. and Reed, D. J. (1981) Denitrosation of carcinostatic nitrosoureas by NADPH dependent microsomal catalysis to yield nitric oxide under anaerobic conditions. *Pharmacologist* **23:** 168.

Reed, D. J. (1981) Metabolism of nitrosoureas. In: *Nitrosoureas. Current Status and New Developments*, pp. 57–67, Prestayko, A. W., Crooke, S. T., Baker, L. H., Carter, S. K. and Schein, P. S. (eds). Academic Press, New York.

Reed, D. J. (1984) Synthesis and characterization of nitrosoureas. In: *Anticancer and Interferon Agents: Synthesis and Properties*, pp.177–202, Ottenbrite, R. M. and Butler, G. B. (eds). Marcel Dekker, New York.

Reed, D. J. (1985) Nitrosoureas. In: *Oxidative Stress*, pp. 115–130, Sies, H. (ed.). Academic Press, London.

Reed, D. J. and May, H. E. (1975) Alkylation and carbamoylation intermediates from the carcinostatic 1-(2-chloroethyl)-3-cyclohexyl-1-nitrosourea (CCNU). *Life Sci.* **16:** 1263–1270.

Reed, D. J. and May, H. E. (1977) Formation of alkylation and carbamylation intermediates and cytochrome P450 catalyzed monooxygenation of the 2-chloroethylnitrosoureas CCNU and methyl CCNU. In: *Microsomes and Drug Oxidations*, pp. 680–687, Ullrich, V., Roots, I., Hildebrandt, A., Estabrook, R. W. and Conney, A. H. (eds). Pergamon Press, New York.

Reed, D. J. and May, H. E. (1978) Cytochrome P450 interactions with the 2-chloroethylnitrosoureas and procarbazine. *Biochimie* **60:** 989–995.

Reed, D. J., May, H. E., Boose, R. B., Gregory, K. M. and Beilstein, M. A. (1975) 2-Chloroethanol formation as evidence for a 2-chloroethyl alkylating intermediate during chemical degradation of 1-(2-chloroethyl)-3-cyclohexyl-1-nitrosourea and 1-(2-chloroethyl)-3-(*trans*-4-methylcyclohexyl)-1-nitrosourea. *Cancer Res.* **35:** 568–576.

Robins, P., Harris, A. L., Goldsmith, I. and Lindahl, T. (1983) Cross-linking of DNA induced by chloroethyl nitrosourea is prevented by O^6-methyl guanine-DNA methyl transferase. *Nucleic Acid Res.* **11:** 7743–7758.

Sariban, E., Erickson, L. C. and Kohn, K. W. (1984) Effects of carbamoylation on cell survival and DNA repair in normal human embryo cells (IMR-90) treated with various 1-(2-chloroethyl)-1-nitrosoureas. *Cancer Res.* **44:** 1352–1357.

SCHALLREUTER, K. U., GEASON, F. K. and WOOD, J. M. (1990) The mechanism of action of the nitrosourea antitumor drugs on thioredoxin reductase, glutathione reductase and ribonucleotide reductase. *Biochim. biophys. Acta* **1054:** 14–20.

SEIDEGARD, J., GRONQUIST, L. and GUNNARSSON, P. O. (1990) Metabolism of a novel nitrosourea, tauromustine, in the rat. *Biochem. Pharmac.* **39:** 1431–1436 .

SKIPPER, H. E., SCHABEL, F. M., JR, TRADER, M. W. and THOMSON, J. R. (1961) Experimental evaluation of potential anticancer agents. VI. Anatomical distribution of leukemic cells and failure of chemotherapy. *Cancer Res.* **21:** 1154–1164.

SMITH, A. C. and BOYD, M. R. (1984a) Effects of bis-chloronitrosourea (BCNU) on pulmonary and serum angiotensin converting enzyme activity in rats. *Biochem. Pharmac.* **32:** 3719–3722.

SMITH, A. C. and BOYD, M. R. (1984b) Preferential effects of 1,3-bis-(2-chloroethyl)-1-nitrosourea (BCNU) on pulmonary glutathione reductase and glutathione/glutathione disulfide ratios: possible implications for lung toxicity. *J. Pharmac. exp. Ther.* **229:** 658–663.

SMITH, R. G. and CHEUNG, L. K. (1982) Determination of two nitrosourea antitumor agents by chemical ionization gas chromatography-mass spectrometry. *J. Chromatog.* **229:** 464–469.

SMITH, R. G., BLACKSTOCK, S. C., CHEUNG, L. K. and LOO, T. L. (1981) Analysis for nitrosourea antitumor agents by gas chromatography-mass spectrometry. *Anal. Chem.* **53:** 1205–1208.

SMITH, R. G., CHEUNG, L. K., FEUN, L. G. and LOO, T. L. (1983) Determination of 1-(2-chloroethyl)-3-(2,6-dioxo-3-piperididyl)-1-nitrosourea in plasma by negative chemical ionization mass spectrometry. *Biomed. Mass Spectrom.* **10:** 404–407.

SOSNOVSKY, G. and LI, S. W. (1985) In the search for new anticancer drugs. XII. Synthesis and biological evaluation of spin labeled nitrosoureas. *Life Sci.* **36:** 1479–1483.

SRIVENUGOPAL, K. S. and ALI-OSMAN, F. (1990) Stimulation and inhibition of 1,3-bis-(2-chloroethyl)-1-nitrosourea-induced strand breaks and interstrand cross-linking in Col E1 plasmid deoxyribonucleic acid by polyamines and inorganic cations. *Biochem. Pharmac.* **40:** 473–479.

STAHL, W. and EISENBRAND, G. (1991) Comparative study on the influence of two 2-chloroethylnitrosoureas with different carbamoylating potential towards glutathione and glutathione-related enzymes in different organs of the rat. *Free Radic. Res. Commun.* **14:** 271–278.

STAHL, W., KRAUTH-SIEGEL, R. L., SCHIRMER, R. H. and EISENBRAND, G. (1987) A method to determine the carbamoylating potential of 1-(2-chloroethyl)-1-nitrosoureas. *IARC Sci. Publ.* **84:** 191–193.

SUAMI, T., MACHINAMI, T. and HISAMATSU, T. (1979) Synthesis and activities of antitumor agents. *J. med. Chem.* **22:** 247–250.

TEW, K. D. (1981) A molecular rationale for nitrosourea induced cytotoxicity. In: *Nitrosoureas in Cancer Treatment*, pp. 61–77, SERROU, B., SCHEIN, P. S. and IMBACH, J. L. (eds). Elsevier Publishers, New York.

TOFILON, P. J., WILLIAMS, M. E. and DEEN, D. F. (1984) The effects of X-rays on BCNU-induced DNA crosslinking. *Radiat. Res.* **99:** 165–174.

TONG, W. P. and LUDLUM, D. B. (1978) Mechanism of action of the nitrosoureas. 1. Role of fluoroethylcytidine in the reaction of bis-fluoroethylnitrosourea with nucleic acids. *Biochem. Pharmac.* **27:** 77–81.

TONG, W. P. and LUDLUM, D. B. (1981) Formation of the crosslinked base, diguanylethane, in DNA treated with *N,N'*-bis-(2-chloroethyl)-*N*-nitrosourea. *Cancer Res.* **41:** 380–382.

WEINKAM, R. J. and DOLAN, M. E. (1983) An analysis of 1-(2-chloroethyl)-1-nitrosourea activity at the cellular level. *J. med. Chem.* **26:** 1656–1659.

WEINKAM, R. J., WEN, J. H. C., FURST, D. E. and LEVIN, V. A. (1978) Analysis for 1,3-bis-(2-chloroethyl)-1-nitrosourea by chemical ionizalion mass spectrometry. *Clin. Chem.* **24:** 45–49.

WEINKAM, R. J., LIU, T.Y. J. and LIN, H.S. (1980) Protein mediated chemical reactions of chloroethylnitrosoureas. *Chem. Biol. Interact.* **31:** 167–177.

WEISS, R. B. and POSTER, D. S. (1982) The renal toxicity of cancer chemotherapeutic agents. *Cancer Treat. Rev.* **9:** 37–56.

WEISS, R. B., POSTER, D. S. and PENTA, J. S. (1981) The nitrosoureas and pulmonary toxicity. *Cancer Treat. Rev.* **8:** 111–125.

WEISS, R. B., POSADA, J. G., JR, KRARNER, R. A. and BOYD, M. R. (1983) Nephrotoxicity of semustine. *Cancer Treat. Rev.* **67:** 1105–1112.

WHEELER, G. P. and CHUMLEY, S. (1967) Alkylating activity of 1,3-bis-(2-chloroethyl)-1-nitrosourea and related compounds. *J. med. Chem.* **10:** 259–261.

WHEELER, G. P., BOWDEN, B. J., GRIMSLEY, J. A. and LLOYD, H. H. (1974) Interrelationships of some chemical, physicochemical, and biological activities of several 1-(2-haloethyl)-1-nitrosoureas. *Cancer Res.* **34:** 194–200.

YEAGER, R. L., OLDFIELD, E. H. and CHATTERJI, D. C. (1984) Quantitation of 1,3-bis-(2-chloroethyl)-1-nitrosourea in plasma using high-performance liquid chromatography. *J. Chromatog.* **305:** 496–501.

ZELLER, W. J., FRUHAUF, S., CHEN, G., EISENBRAND, G. and LIJINSKY, W. (1989) Biological activity of hydroxylated chloroethylnitrosoureas. *Cancer Res.* **49:** 3267–3270.

Garth Powis, editor.
(1994) *Anticancer Drugs: Reactive Metabolism and Drug Interactions*,
Pergamon Press Ltd, pp. 209–227
Printed in the United Kingdom

CHAPTER 6

METABOLISM OF THE HYDRAZINE ANTICANCER AGENT, PROCARBAZINE

JOHN M. ERIKSON,* DONALD J. TWEEDIE† AND RUSSELL A. PROUGH

Department of Biochemistry, University of Louisville School of Medicine, Louisville, KY 40292, U.S.A.

1. INTRODUCTION

Procarbazine [*N*-isopropyl-α-(2-methylhydrazino)-*p*-toluamide] has been shown to serve as a methylating agent (Kreis et al., 1966) and it is this property which has been assumed to lead to its cytotoxic activity. To date, a number of reviews have been published describing the history, pharmacology, and mode of action of procarbazine as an anticancer agent (Oliverio, 1973; Reed, 1975; Weinkam and Shiba, 1982). Reed (1975) surveyed much of the literature regarding the anticancer activity of the compound in rodents and discussed its presumed mode of action as it was understood at that time. In particular, that review contains an extensive survey of the experiments in which methylhydrazine derivatives were successfully used against a number of tumors in rodents. The present chapter will focus on recent developments related to the metabolism, toxicity, and carcinogenicity of the drug. Finally, the routes of metabolism of procarbazine and the nature of its metabolic activation to chemically reactive methylating species will be discussed.

2. HISTORY

Hydrazine derivatives were among a number of chemical compounds screened in the early 1960s as potentially useful inhibitors of monoamine oxidase (Zeller et al., 1963). Subsequent studies demonstrated that some of these compounds, in particular methyl-substituted hydrazines, exhibited antitumor activity (Bollag, 1963, 1964). Structure–activity studies of these agents revealed an absolute requirement for the presence of the *N*-methyl group in order to elicit antitumor activity. In addition, the presence of an electron-withdrawing group *para* to the methyl hydrazine moiety conveys a chemical stability which also reduces the toxic side effects of the compound. *N*-Isopropyl-α-(2-methylhydrazino)-*p*-toluamide hydrochloride (Procarbazine, Matulane, natulan, ibenzmethyzin, Ro46467, NSC-77213) was shown to be effective against a number of animal tumors (Bollag and Grunberg, 1963), but lacked the degree of overt hepatotoxicity displayed by its parent analog, 1-methyl-2-benzylhydrazine. Procarbazine was first used successfully in clinical trials against malignant lymphomas by Martz et al. (1963). It has subsequently been used with varying degrees of success in the treatment of other tumors. However, it has been most widely adopted as an adjunct in combination therapy for the treatment of Hodgkin's disease.

3. ANTITUMOR ACTIVITY

3.1. ANIMAL STUDIES

Procarbazine has been successfully tested as a therapeutic agent in a number of animal tumor systems (reviewed by Reed, 1975). It was shown to be effective against both solid tumors and ascites tumors of rats (e.g. Walker 256 carcinosarcoma and Ehrlich's carcinoma; Bollag and Grunberg,

*Current address—Department of Medicine, Division of Cardiology, The University of Texas Southwestern Medical School, 5323 Harry Hines Blvd., Dallas, TX 75235, U.S.A.
†Current address—Drug Metabolism Department, Pfizer Inc., Central Research, Groton, CT 06340, U.S.A.

1963), mammary tumors of mice (Gelzer and Loustalot, 1967; Kreis, 1970a,b), advanced mast cell P815 (Oliverio et al., 1964) and LPC-1 tumors (Abraham et al., 1967) in mice, and Dunning leukemia in rats (Oliverio et al., 1964). The Walker 256 carcinosarcoma tumors were shown to be extremely sensitive to treatment with procarbazine. A 100% inhibition of tumor growth was obtained at doses of procarbazine above 20 mg/kg (Bollag, 1963; Bollag and Grunberg, 1963). Procarbazine was also effective in the treatment of an intracranially implanted L1210 leukemia in mice (Oliverio et al., 1964). One advantageous property of the drug appears to be its distribution into cerebrospinal fluid (Dorr and Fritz, 1980; Oliverio et al., 1964). Based on these animal studies, the therapeutic efficacy of procarbazine against brain tumors in human patients has been considered (see Section 3.2). Bollag and Grunberg (1963) noted that Ehrlich ascites carcinoma cells could develop a resistance to procarbazine after 7–9 passages. Despite this complication of drug efficacy, the response of the animal tumor models to this drug made human studies desirable.

3.2. Human Studies

Procarbazine does not display a similar therapeutic effect against solid tumors in humans. While Martz and co-workers reported the first successful use of procarbazine as an antitumor agent against lymphomas (Martz et al., 1963), they also observed that procarbazine was ineffective against solid tumors in patients. With carcinomas of the lung, the drug has been demonstrated to have a noticeable, but limited effectiveness in combination therapy (Trovo et al., 1982; Bitran et al., 1978; Poplin et al., 1982). Pedersen et al. (1982) noted that when procarbazine was administered alone, it was ineffective against lung carcinoma. However, the agent was only used after alternative combination therapy had failed. Procarbazine has also been used less frequently, but with some success, for the treatment of non-Hodgkin's lymphoma, malignant melanoma and bronchogenic carcinoma in adults, and also for treatment of brain tumors in children and adults (Chamberlen and Levin, 1990; Coyle et al., 1990; Dorr and Fritz, 1980; Newton et al., 1990; Reed, 1975; Schuler et al., 1988).

The most consistently effective use of procarbazine has been in the treatment of Hodgkin's disease. Bonadonna et al. (1969) observed a 46% objective improvement of patients with generalized Hodgkin's disease following procarbazine therapy. They also reviewed a number of cases of patients with Hodgkin's disease in which procarbazine had been used as part of the treatment regimen (Bonadonna et al., 1969). These studies showed a 46–100% positive response. In addition, Miller (1970) reported a 57% response to procarbazine treatment in patients with Hodgkin's disease, 95% of whom had become refractory to other forms of therapy. The use of the MOPP combination therapy consisting of *mechlorethamine* (nitrogen mustard), *oncovin* (vincristine), *procarbazine*, and *prednisone* has become a standard treatment for Hodgkin's disease. The MOPP protocol has been the treatment of choice since 1964 for the management of advanced Hodgkin's lymphoma (Stages III and IV) and in combination with radiotherapy in earlier stages (Stages I and II) (DeVita et al., 1969, 1970; DeVita and Hellman, 1982). The drugs are given in accordance with the schedule shown in Table 1. The cycle is repeated every four weeks for a minimum of six cycles or until complete remission is documented. Two further cycles of chemotherapy are then given to consolidate the remission. DeVita et al. (1969, 1970) reported that 81% of the patients administered the combination therapy achieved complete remission, with a 29–42 month median duration of remission following completion of treatment. The MOPP regimen was also reported by Lowenbraun et al. (1970) to produce remission in patients with generalized lymphosarcoma and reticulum cell sarcoma. It should be noted that the dosages (based on mg/kg body weight) given to humans are much lower than those which were effective in animals. An alternative approach to therapy has been developed which consists of treating patients with

TABLE 1. *The Composition of the Standard MOPP Cancer Treatment Regimen**

Nitrogen mustard	6 mg/m^2	day 1 and 8
Vincristine	1.4 mg/m^2	day 1 and 8
Procarbazine	100 mg/m^2	day 1 through 14
Prednisone	40 mg/m^2	day 1 through 14, cycle 1 and 4 only

*Taken from DeVita and Hellman (1982).

alternating cycles of non-cross-resistant combinations such as MOPP and ABVD (*adriamycin, bleomycin, vinblastine,* and *dacarbazine*) (Calabresi and Parks, 1985).

4. TOXICITY

Several studies have addressed the toxicity and morbidity of procarbazine in animals. Miller (1970) reported that the oral LD_{50} value for the mouse was approximately 700 mg/kg and for the rat was 1400 mg/kg. Other studies at the Roche Laboratories determined LD_{50} doses of 1320 mg/kg body weight for mice, 785 mg/kg for rats and 145 mg/kg for rabbits (Roche Laboratories, 1969). These discrepancies may be due to strain differences in the mice and rats used.

In human patients, a number of toxic side effects have been observed, including nausea, vomiting, and as the treatment progresses, depression of bone marrow and decreases in sperm viability (DeVita et al., 1970). Hematological toxicity is carefully monitored during treatment as procarbazine can also cause leukopenia resulting in a loss of immune function and thrombocytopenia which can lead to anemia (Stolinsky et al., 1970). The immunosuppressive effects of procarbazine were also noted as early as 1963 by Bollag and have been confirmed in a number of graft vs host studies (Reed, 1975). These parameters, i.e. white cell and platelet count, are determining factors in the duration of treatment with the maximal dose of procarbazine. The recommended maximum dose of 300 mg/day is reduced if the white cell count falls below 4000/mm^3 or if the platelet count falls below 100,000/mm^3 (DeVita and Hellman, 1982; Roche Laboratories, 1969).

The neurotoxic effects of procarbazine are often manifested as depression, confusion, somnolence, depressed reflexes, and agitation (Weiss et al., 1974). The neurotoxicity may be related to the ease with which this drug enters the cerebrospinal fluid (Oliverio et al., 1964) and its ability to act as an inhibitor of monoamine oxidase (DeVita et al., 1965; Zeller et al., 1963). These processes probably alter the levels of biogenic amines in various portions of the brain. In addition, Chabner et al. (1969) have described a depression of the levels of pyridoxal phosphate in whole brain. Adverse effects due to the decreased levels of vitamin B_6 and its analogs have been suggested to occur in humans, including enhanced secondary carcinogenesis possibly due to the drug itself (Draudin-Krylenko et al., 1989).

The spermatotoxicity observed in human patients may result in irreversible azoospermia (Chapman, 1984). Animal studies have shown decreases in spermatogenesis and testicular atrophy ultimately result in permanent sterility (Reed, 1975). Procarbazine was shown to promote unscheduled DNA synthesis in the early spermatid stages in mice (Sotomayor et al., 1982) and to induce gene mutations in the spermatogonial and postspermatogonial stages. No mutations were detected in early spermatid or meiotic spermatocyte stages (Ehling and Neuhauser, 1979). Spermatozoa and cells in the late spermatid stage were shown to have little or no DNA repair capacity (Ehling and Neuhauser, 1979). Consequently, it has been suggested that the inability to repair mutations in the various stages of spermatogenesis may be an important factor in spermatotoxicity (Sotomayor et al., 1982). However, the chemical mechanism of procarbazine-induced spermatotoxicity has not been elucidated. Recent work reported by Horstman et al. (1987) suggests the importance of chemically reactive intermediate(s) formed during procarbazine metabolism in vivo. Recent studies have shown impaired gonadal function in humans for up to 10 years after treatment, but sexual maturation in boys was apparently attained without need for androgen replacement (Ortin et al., 1990). The pronounced azoospermia continued for up to 11 years and only 20% of the subjects studied regained fertility. Menstrual function in girls appeared to be normal and maintenance of gonadal function following combination treatment was more apparent in girls than boys. The progeny of the patients appear to be normal with no observed fetal growth retardation (Ortin et al., 1990). Other studies have recommended use of in vitro fertilization using frozen sperm of male Hodgkin patients to overcome the infertility of young adult males (Tournaye et al., 1991).

Occasional allergic dermatosis and infrequent pleuropulmonary reactions with fever were reported by Jones et al. (1972). A recent study by Lewis (1984) also demonstrated a procarbazine-associated irritation of the lung tissue of humans. A flushing syndrome observed in patients administered procarbazine who were consuming alcohol, suggests a possible inhibition of alcohol metabolism (Weiss et al., 1974). Studies evaluating possible food–drug interactions of procarbazine, particularily with food containing high levels of tryptophan, found no significant toxic effects of the drug (Maxwell, 1980). No drug–drug interactions for procarbazine with other alkylating agents have been described other than somnolence and CNS depression, which makes it a useful adjunct for combination therapy.

5. MUTAGENICITY AND CARCINOGENICITY

Procarbazine has been shown to be carcinogenic in laboratory animals. Pulmonary epithelial neoplasia, mammary adenocarcinomas, sarcomas of the kidney, and lymphocytic leukemias have been observed after exposure to the drug (Kelly et al., 1969; Sieber et al., 1978; Bacchi et al., 1982). Unlike other hydrazines, procarbazine rarely produces hepatic tumors, but causes significant hepatotoxicity. In addition, procarbazine causes teratogenesis (Chaube and Murphy, 1969; Schmid et al., 1982). It was suggested that metabolic activation of this drug as a teratogen required factors found in the intact cell (Schmid et al., 1982). Rutishauser and Bollag (1963) observed chromosomal breaks produced by procarbazine, and recently, Erikson et al. (1986, 1989) used alkaline elution techniques to demonstrate single-strand breaks and alkali-labile sites in the DNA of cultured L1210 tumor cells treated with the azoxy derivatives of procarbazine. These metabolites were also shown to be responsible for the cytotoxic effects of procarbazine (Erikson et al., 1989; Swaffar et al., 1989). The parent drug and its azo metabolite were not as effective in causing DNA damage in the tumor cells as were the azoxy isomers.

Binding of the methyl group of procarbazine to nucleic acids, DNA and RNA, has also been observed, both in studies in vitro (Brookes, 1965; Schold et al., 1989) and in vivo (Kreis et al., 1966; Wiestler et al., 1984; Fong et al., 1990; Souliotis et al., 1990). Methyl-labelled procarbazine was shown by Wiestler et al. (1984) to predominantly alkylate the N^7- and O^6-positions of guanine in DNA isolated from maternal and neonatal rat tissues. It has also been suggested that these adducts may result, in part, from incorporation of components of the C_1 pool into the base (Kreis et al., 1966). However, Souliotis et al. (1990) observed time- and dose-dependent accumulation of O^6-methylguanine adducts in lymphocyte DNA of humans and rodents administered procarbazine. An interesting inverse correlation between levels of O^6-methylquanine DNA adducts with levels of lymphocyte O^6-methylguanine-DNA methyltransferase was observed in all patients suggesting an active role of the O^6-methyltransferase in DNA repair. It has been suggested (Sagher et al., 1988; Strauss et al., 1990) that patients who have therapy-related neoplastic diseases such as acute nonlymphocytic leukemia after MOPP therapy have lower lymphocyte O^6-methyltransferase levels than other patients. The role of this DNA repair enzyme in the tissues of patients successfully treated by this therapy remains to be fully tested.

Although procarbazine has been demonstrated to be a potent carcinogen in vivo (BlijLeven and Vogel, 1977; Bayer, 1978; Ehling and Neuhauser, 1979; Lee and Dixon, 1978), the results from mutagenicity testing in vitro have been more equivocal. In the absence or presence of activating enzymes found in postmitochondrial supernatants (S9 fraction), procarbazine yielded false negatives in the standard Ames test (McCann et al., 1975). The absence of an *rfa* mutation in strains of *Salmonella typhimurium* was shown to be essential for procarbazine mutagenesis (Gatehouse and Paes, 1983; Pueyo, 1979). Procarbazine has also been demonstrated to be mutagenic to *Escherichia coli* D494 in a forward mutation fluctuation assay (Gatehouse and Paes, 1983). They concluded that S9 fractions contained only low levels of enzymes capable of activating procarbazine to mutagens. Malavielle et al. (1983) successfully used hepatocytes to activate procarbazine to a mutagen. Comparing the mutagenicity of procarbazine with 1,2-dimethylhydrazine in different bacterial strains of *S. typhimurium*, they suggested that the relative uptake of hydrophilic, reactive metabolites may be an important factor in the mutagenicity of both hydrazines. Mutagenicity studies in the yeast strain *Saccharomyces cerevisiae* D4 showed that procarbazine was more toxic and mutagenic at low doses in log phase cells than at high doses. In stationary phase cells, both high and low dosages were not toxic, but were mutagenic (Frezza and Bianchi, 1984). The lack of information about the routes of metabolism and the chemical nature of the reactive intermediates formed may have contributed to the equivocal results seen in such screening assays in the past.

6. CHEMISTRY OF PROCARBAZINE AND ITS METABOLITES

6.1. Hydrazine Derivatives

Procarbazine is a symmetrically- or 1,2-disubstituted hydrazine derivative (Fig. 1) whose physical form as the hydrochloride salt is a white crystalline powder. It is soluble in aqueous solutions and is rapidly oxidized in the presence of oxygen and redox active metals to yield the azo derivative and hydrogen peroxide (Reed, 1975). Metalloproteins, e.g. siderophilin, myoglobin, and hemoglobin, also catalyze the oxidation of procarbazine to its azo and hydrazone derivatives (Berneis et al., 1963; Aebi et al., 1965a,b). Figure 1 shows some of the biological and chemical products of procarbazine and their trivial names used in this chapter. The two adjacent heteroatom nitrogens provide a unique chemistry which is responsible for the biological reactivity of the molecule (Smith, 1966). For example, the *N*-isopropylamide function at the *para*-position of the benzyl group apparently causes the hydrazine moiety to be less easily oxidized to either the hydrazone or azo derivatives (D. L. Dunn and R. A. Prough, unpublished results). This property is important in the preparation and storage of the compound, as the parent analog, 1-methyl-2-benzylhydrazine, is far more easily oxidized than procarbazine. Electron-withdrawing groups at the *para*-position of the ring [—CN, —CO—NH—CH(CH_3)] decrease the ease of oxidation of the hydrazine, while electron-donating groups [—H, —NH_2] increase the ease of chemical oxidation. This decrease in reactivity with metal-catalyzed oxidation reactions may be an important factor for prolonging the shelf-life of the compound and in decreasing its toxicity relative to 1-methyl-2-benzylhydrazine.

A final note regarding structure can be drawn from early studies of the effect of various hydrazine derivatives on cell cytotoxicity. Bollag (1963, 1964) demonstrated that the biological activity was

CH_3-NH-NH-CH_2-R•HCl

PROCARBAZINE
N-ISOPROPYL-α-(2-METHYLHYDRAZINO)-*p*-TOLUAMIDE HYDROCHLORIDE

CH_3-N=N-CH_2-R

AZO PROCARBAZINE
N-ISOPROPYL-α-(2-METHYLAZO)-*p*-TOLUAMIDE

CH_3-NH-N=CH-R

HYDRAZONE
N-ISOPROPYL-*p*-FORMYLBENZAMIDE METHYLHYDRAZONE

O
|
CH_3-N=N-CH_2-R

BENZYLAZOXY
N-ISOPROPYL-α-(2-METHYL-NNO-AZOXY)-*p*-TOLUAMIDE

O
|
CH_3-N=N-CH_2-R

METHYLAZOXY
N-ISOPROPYL-α-(2-METHYL-ONN-AZOXY)-*p*-TOLUAMIDE

H-CO-R

ALDEHYDE
N-ISOPROPYL-*p*-FORMYLBENZAMIDE

HO-CO-R

TAC
N-ISOPROPYLTEREPHTHALAMIC ACID

H_3C-R

N-ISOPROPYL-*p*-TOLUAMIDE

$HOCH_2R$

N-ISOPROPYL-*p*-HYDROXYMETHYLBENZAMIDE

Fig. 1. The structure of procarbazine and its derivatives. R, —C_6H_4—CO—NH—CH$(CH_3)_2$.

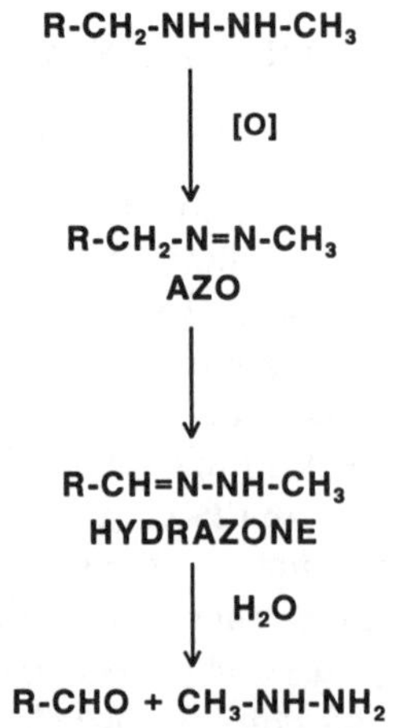

FIG. 2. The pathway for chemical degradation of procarbazine. R, —C_6H_4—CO—NH—$CH(CH_3)_2$.

absolutely dependent on the *N*-methyl group of the molecule. In the intervening years, no definitive data has emerged to satisfactorily link the metabolism of procarbazine to its biological activity.

6.2. AZO AND HYDRAZONE DERIVATIVES

Upon oxidation with chemical oxidants such as HgO, $K_3Fe(CN)_6$ or Fe^{3+}, procarbazine is converted to its azo and hydrazone products as shown in Fig. 2 (Dunn et al., 1979). Normally, the azo derivative [*N*-isopropyl-α-(2-methyl-azo)-*p*-toluamide] is formed in higher yields in the presence of chemical oxidants, but it is slowly converted to the hydrazone tautomer [*N*-isopropyl-*p*-formylbenzamide methylhydrazone]. This tautomerization reaction is potentiated at lower pH values. At pH 1, the hydrazone is hydrolyzed to form methylhydrazine and *N*-isopropyl-*p*-formylbenzamide (Dunn et al., 1979). However, in aprotic solvent, the azo derivative is relatively stable when compared to the monoazo compounds formed during the oxidation of alkyl- or arylhydrazines (Smith, 1966).

As commercially prepared, procarbazine hydrochloride is very pure. However, in aqueous preparations of procarbazine stored at room temperature for 2–6 hr, there are measurable amounts of oxidation products, i.e. the azo and hydrazone derivatives of procarbazine (R. A. Prough, unpublished results; Swaffer et al., 1991a,b). As procarbazine is an air-sensitive compound and the hydrazone derivative is most likely toxic, care must be taken in the formulation and storage of the compound. It is not known whether some of the toxic problems of procarbazine are due to the parent drug itself or its oxidation products.

6.3. AZOXY DERIVATIVES

The azoxy derivatives [*N*-isopropyl-α-(2-methyl-NNO-azoxy)-*p*-toluamide (benzylazoxy) and *N*-isopropyl-α-(2-methyl-ONN-azoxy)-*p*-toluamide (methylazoxy)] can be formed by oxidation of azo procarbazine with peracid oxidants such as *m*-chloroperbenzoic acid. These compounds are relatively stable in organic solvents. The methylazoxy derivative is, however, unstable in protic solvents. This isomer would be expected to undergo fascile oxidation of the benzylic carbon by metals (K. G. Taylor, personal communication). HPLC and GC-MS procedures have been described for separation, identification, and quantitation of the chemical and biological azoxy metabolites of procarbazine (Dunn et al., 1979; Gorsen et al., 1980; Shiba and Weinkam, 1982; Weinkam and Shiba, 1978; Wiebkin and Prough, 1980).

7. METABOLISM IN VIVO AND DISPOSITION

7.1. Animals

Excretion and distribution studies using ^{14}C-labelled procarbazine demonstrated that the radioactivity accumulated mainly in the liver, kidney, intestine and skin of rats and mice (Schwartz et al., 1967). A rapid distribution into cerebrospinal fluid also occurs (Oliverio et al., 1964). The half-life of the radioactive label in the systemic circulation was found to be 7 min in humans, 12 min in dogs and 24 min in rats (Raaflaub and Schwartz, 1965). Excretion and expiration of radioactivity occurred mainly over the first 24 hr (Baggiolini et al., 1965; Schwartz, 1966; Schwartz et al., 1967). In a comparative study in rats, Schwartz et al. (1967) demonstrated, using ^{14}C-*carbonyl* labelled procarbazine that approximately 70% of the radioactive label was excreted in the urine within 24 hr, whereas administration of ^{14}C-*methyl* labelled procarbazine resulted in the urinary excretion of only 32% of radioactive label. Expiration of $^{14}CO_2$ from ^{14}C-*methyl* labelled procarbazine could account for most of the difference, i.e. approximately 30% (Gescher and Raymont, 1981). By day four of the study, 4–12% of the administered [^{14}C-*carbonyl*]procarbazine radioactivity was excreted in the feces, while 8–12% was retained in the tissues of rats and dogs. Oliverio et al. (1964) also reported the presence of an unspecified glucuronide conjugate from mouse urine, although they could not find a similar conjugate in dog urine.

The primary circulating metabolite of procarbazine is the azo derivative (Raaflaub and Schwartz, 1965; Kuttab et al., 1982; Weinkam and Shiba, 1978), while the major urinary metabolite was shown to be *N*-isopropylterephthalamic acid (Oliverio et al., 1964). A comparison of metabolism in vivo and in an isolated, perfused liver preparation provided evidence that the liver was most likely the tissue primarily responsible for the oxidation of procarbazine (Baggiolini et al., 1965). Schwartz (1966) later demonstrated that the metabolism of procarbazine could be inhibited in vivo by SKF 525A, an inhibitor of cytochrome P450. The involvement of cytochrome P450 was further implicated by the observed prolongation of barbiturate-induced sleeping time by procarbazine (Eade et al., 1972; Lee and Lucier, 1976). Both methane (Dost and Reed, 1967; Schwartz et al., 1969) and formaldehyde (Schwartz, 1966) have been isolated as in vivo oxidation products of procarbazine.

7.2. Humans

The information available in the literature would support the contention that humans metabolize procarbazine, azo procarbazine, and the azoxy isomers in a manner similar to that seen in rats (Oliverio et al., 1964; Raaflaub and Schwartz, 1965; Schwartz et al., 1967; Shiba and Weinkam, 1983; Wolff et al., 1985). The early metabolic work of Schwartz and coworkers (Raaflaub and Schwartz, 1965; Schwartz et al., 1967) also demonstrated the presence of *N*-isopropylterephthalamic acid as a major urinary metabolite and $^{14}CO_2$ as a respired product in both rodents and humans. This result was confirmed in subsequent studies which have also demonstrated the formation of the azo and azoxy metabolites of procarbazine in man (Shiba and Weinkam, 1983). We have observed that human liver microsomes and mitochondria metabolize procarbazine to azo procarbazine in reactions catalyzed by cytochrome P450 and monoamine oxidase (M. I. Brown, M. L. Coomes, and R. A. Prough, unpublished results). In addition, Wolff et al. (1985) have reported that human liver microsomes metabolize azo procarbazine to azoxy procarbazine metabolites.

8. METABOLISM IN VITRO

8.1. Oxidative Transformation

Procarbazine is oxidized in aqueous solutions containing oxygen and metal ions, such as ferric ion, to yield azo procarbazine and its hydrazone tautomer as shown in Fig. 2 (Oliverio et al., 1964; Weinkam and Shiba, 1978). The other product formed is hydrogen peroxide. Early studies on the mode of action of the drug suggested that it was hydrogen peroxide which served as the DNA-damaging species (Berneis et al., 1963). However, Gale et al. (1967) demonstrated, using cultured Ehrlich ascites tumor cells, that the amount of hydrogen peroxide formed was not sufficient to account for the DNA damage seen in biological systems. The drug was shown to cause inhibition of DNA and RNA synthesis with cultured L5178Y ascites cells (Sartorelli and Tsunamura, 1966).

Although the rates of chemical degradation of procarbazine (Fig. 2) are slow, many of the breakdown products are also formed by biological systems both in vivo and in vitro during the metabolism of procarbazine (Prough, 1985; Reed and May, 1978). In general, the rate of formation of the azo, hydrazone, and aldehyde derivatives by chemical processes is less than 5–15% of that seen with enzyme-catalyzed reactions.

Methane is formed in vivo and in vitro as a minor metabolite of procarbazine and can be observed as a respired metabolite when administered to animals. Alkylhydrazines have been shown to yield alkane products both in vitro and in vivo (Moloney and Prough, 1983; Prough et al., 1969). Some confusion exists as to the route of formation of methane from procarbazine. It must be pointed out that this product is relatively unique for procarbazine, as 1,2-dimethylhydrazine does not yield methane either in vivo (Dost et al., 1966) or in vitro (Prough, 1973) in the amounts observed with procarbazine. The pathway leading to methane formation from procarbazine in vitro has been elucidated by Moloney and Prough (1983). Previous suggestions that methane was produced via methylhydrazine formation, after hydrolysis of the hydrazone tautomer of azo procarbazine, were not supported on the basis of kinetic and inhibitor studies. The V_{max} and apparent K_m values for methane formation from the hydrazone derivative and from methylhydrazine demonstrated that the hydrazone derivative had a lower apparent K_m and a higher V_{max} value than did methylhydrazine. This result clearly indicates that the hydrazone is a better substrate for methane production than is methylhydrazine. The inhibition studies employed methimazole and ethylhydrazine as specific inhibitors of azo and hydrazone metabolism in vitro, respectively. While methimazole could inhibit methane formation from procarbazine and azo procarbazine, it stimulated methane formation from methylhydrazine and the hydrazone. Ethylhydrazine strongly inhibited methane formation from methylhydrazine and the hydrazone, but had less effect on methane formation from procarbazine or azo procarbazine. Thus, formation of the hydrazone tautomer or methylhydrazine would not appear to contribute significantly to methane production from either procarbazine or its azo metabolite in vivo or in vitro.

Moloney and Prough (1983) also demonstrated a lag in the production of methane from procarbazine which would be consistent with the formation of methane from a metabolite of procarbazine, namely, azo procarbazine (Baggiolini et al., 1969; Dewald et al., 1969; Dost and Reed, 1967). Methane is not produced from either of the two azoxy isomers (Moloney and Prough, 1983), and although methane can be produced in the hydrazone pathway, the isomerization of azo to hydrazone is not fast enough to account for this reaction. In addition, little hydrazone is formed during the biological *N*-oxidation reaction (Moloney and Prough, 1983). Based on the chemical literature (Smith, 1966), one must assume that the methane formed from azo procarbazine is derived from some putative diazene or a *C*-hydroxyazo intermediate (Fig. 3).

Sinha (1984) has demonstrated that radicals are formed during the metabolism of procarbazine. The decomposition products of the diazene intermediate, i.e. a methyl free radical, apparently can either bind to cellular macromolecules or can abstract a proton, e.g. from reduced protein thiols or from the intracellular thiol, glutathione, to yield methane (Moloney and Prough, 1983; Moloney et al., 1985; Spearman et al., 1985). Albano and coworkers have utilized radical trapping reagents to demonstrate that the azo and hydrazone derivatives are better substrates for cytochrome P450 in forming methyl radicals than is procarbazine (Iannone et al., 1991; Goria-Gatti et al., 1992). However, the azoxy isomers were not metabolized by either microsomal or cytosolic enzymes to yield methyl radicals.

CO_2, an expired product of procarbazine metabolism (Gescher and Raymont, 1981), was suggested to be released during the metabolism of methylhydrazine, a chemical degradation product of the hydrazone derivative of procarbazine (Dewald et al., 1969; Raaflaub and Schwartz, 1965). However, further studies by Baggiolini and Dewald (Baggiolini et al., 1965; Dewald et al., 1969) comparing the metabolism of methylhydrazine to that of procarbazine, both in the rat in vivo and in the isolated rat liver, showed that there were significant differences in the rates of CO_2 production from these two compounds, suggesting that methylhydrazine was not an intermediate

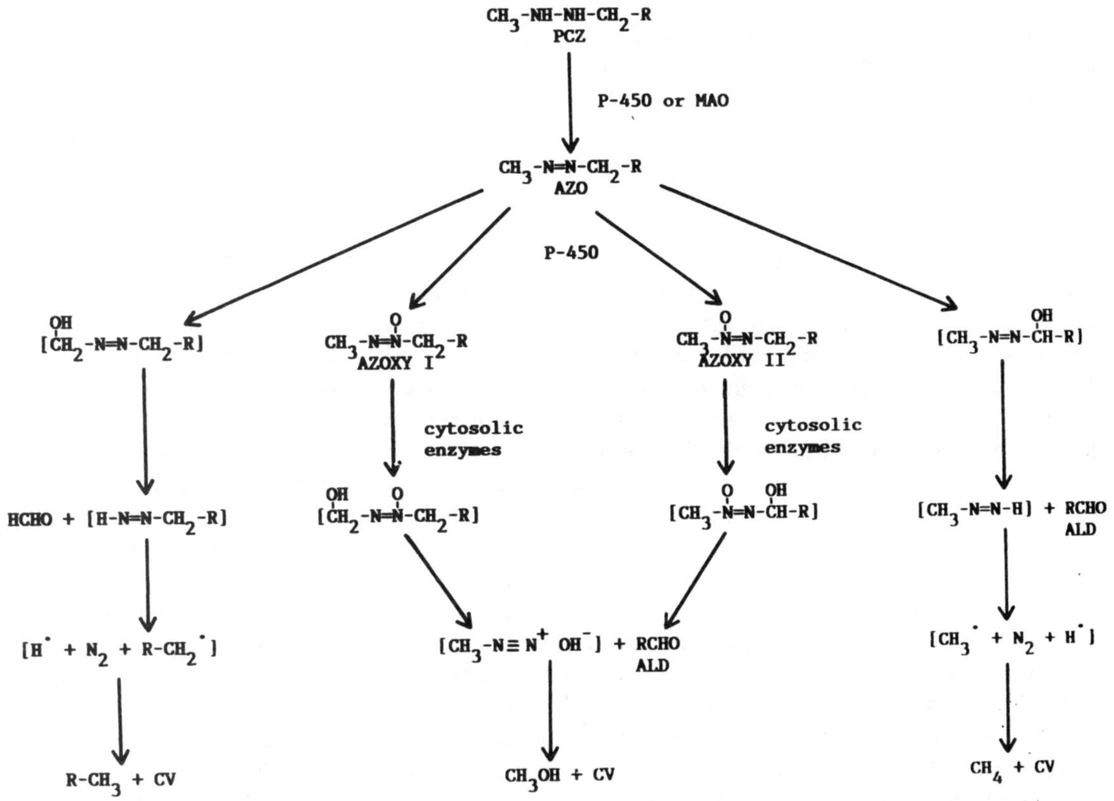

FIG. 3. The metabolic pathway of procarbazine activation. CV, covalent binding. R, —C_6H_4—CO—NH—$CH(CH_3)_2$.

in conversion of procarbazine to CO_2. These differences were substantiated by observations of differential effects with the monooxygenase inhibitor, SKF 525A, and inducing agents for cytochrome P450; namely, phenobarbital and 3-methylcholanthrene.

HPLC isolation and mass spectral analysis of both in vivo (Weinkam and Shiba, 1978) and in vitro (Dunn et al., 1979; Weinkam and Shiba, 1978; Wiebkin and Prough, 1980) products of procarbazine metabolism have provided evidence for additional pathways of metabolic activation of procarbazine. Two additional metabolites have been detected in the plasma of rats after i.p. administration of procarbazine and in incubation mixtures which contained either postmitochondrial supernatant fractions or microsomes. These products appear to be the result of the *N*-oxidation of the azo derivative to yield the two azoxy procarbazine isomers, benzylazoxy procarbazine [*N*-isopropyl-α-(2-methyl-NNO-azoxy)-*p*-toluamide] and methylazoxy procarbazine [*N*-isopropyl-α-(2-methyl-ONN-azoxy)-*p*-toluamide].

Further metabolism of the azoxy isomers by *C*-hydroxylation in vitro was suggested based on the metabolic activation pathway proposed for 1,2-dimethylhydrazine by Druckrey (1970) in which methylazoxymethanol was shown to be formed (Fiala, 1977). It was proposed that degradation of the putative *C*-hydroxy-azoxy metabolite would yield the aldehyde derivative and possibly diazomethane or formaldehyde (Weinkam and Shiba, 1978). The diazomethane formed may then decompose to form a methyl carbonium ion which can either alkylate cellular nucleophiles or undergo solvolysis to form methanol. Carbon dioxide may be formed from oxidation of methanol and formaldehyde in vivo. Also, the aldehyde derivative has been shown to be converted in vitro and in vivo to the terephthalamic acid derivative by cytosolic aldehyde dehydrogenase. In reaction mixtures containing washed microsomes (containing little or no aldehyde dehydrogenase), the aldehyde derivative is the ultimate metabolite (Weinkam and Shiba, 1978; Tweedie et al., 1991). With this overview, we will focus on the enzymology of the oxidative transformation of this drug and its metabolites.

8.2. ENZYMOLOGY

Wittkop et al. (1969) demonstrated that an *N*-demethylase activity for procarbazine existed in the microsomal fraction of the liver. Several lines of evidence indicated that the *N*-demethylase activity was dependent on cytochrome P450. For example, procarbazine *N*-demethylase activity could be induced by phenobarbital or methylcholanthrene treatment in vivo and inhibited in vitro by addition of carbon monoxide, steapsin or cholate. Addition of procarbazine to suspensions of liver microsomes yielded a Type II substrate interaction spectrum with microsomal cytochrome P450. Although other alkylhydrazines were converted to their parent alkanes by microsomal cytochrome P450, procarbazine was a poor substrate for alkane production (Moloney and Prough, 1983; Prough et al., 1969). This suggested that procarbazine was not a good substrate for the alkylhydrazine oxidase which yielded alkane products described by Prough et al. (1969).

The conversion of procarbazine to the azo derivative was shown to be mediated by liver microsomal cytochrome P450 based upon its dependence on NADPH, O_2, and NADPH-cytochrome P450 reductase. Additional evidence was provided by the action of various inhibitors and inducers of cytochrome P450 on this reaction (Dunn et al., 1979; Prough et al., 1977; Wittkop et al., 1969). Colorimetric and HPLC assays were devised to accurately measure the rates of metabolism of procarbazine to azo procarbazine (Dunn et al., 1979). The rate of conversion was approximately 10–18 nmol product/min/mg microsomal protein; a value similar to those obtained with the best drug substrates of cytochrome P450. The *N*-demethylase activity reported by Wittkop et al. (1969) was much lower than azo procarbazine formation. These results confirmed the contentions of others that the liver is the main site of metabolism of procarbazine and suggests that its disposition may be one of first pass kinetics.

The metabolism of procarbazine to azo procarbazine by an NADPH-independent mechanism was discovered using isolated rat hepatocytes (Coomes and Prough, 1983). Dilution of the cytosolic pool of NADPH by sonication of the hepatocytes did not greatly reduce the rate of procarbazine oxidation, whereas rates of biphenyl hydroxylation, a cytochrome P450 mediated reaction, were markedly decreased. This oxidase activity was localized in the mitochondrial fraction of the cells, was inhibited by the monoamine oxidase (MAO) inhibitor, *N,N*- dimethylpropargylamine, and was not linked to mitochondrial electron transport. The activity also co-purified with benzylamine oxidase activity. The product of procarbazine metabolism by MAO was the azo derivative, but azo procarbazine was shown not to be a substrate of MAO (Prough et al., 1983).

Based on the specific activity of both the NADPH-dependent (cytochrome P450) and NADPH-independent (MAO) reactions, it was estimated that in the non-induced rat hepatocyte, MAO is responsible for at least 40% of the total procarbazine oxidation to azo procarbazine, while in the phenobarbital (PB)-induced hepatocyte, the contribution of MAO was decreased to less than 25% (Coomes and Prough, 1983). The relative contributions of these two enzyme systems in the metabolism of procarbazine in rat liver and lung has been studied (Erikson and Prough, 1986). MAO oxidized the N–N bond of all classes of hydrazines, while cytochrome P450 preferentially oxidized the N–N bond of 1,2-disubstituted hydrazines, including procarbazine. Other hydrazines, such as monoalkylhydrazines appeared to be oxidized across the N–C bond by cytochrome P450. There did not appear to be any substrate specificity for either of the two isoforms of MAO (MAO-A or MAO-B). Unlike other hydrazine compounds (Patek and Hellerman, 1974), procarbazine does not inactivate MAO, but serves as a competitive substrate against benzylamine or kynurenine oxidase activity (Coomes and Prough, 1983). In contrast to other methyl-substituted hydrazines, procarbazine is not a good substrate for another flavoprotein, the microsomal FAD-containing (amine oxidase) monooxygenase (Prough et al., 1981; Prough and Ziegler, 1977).

Multiple forms of cytochrome P450 have been implicated in both the oxidation of procarbazine to azo procarbazine (Dunn et al., 1979) and in the subsequent *N*-oxygenation of azo procarbazine (Prough et al., 1984; Wiebkin and Prough, 1980). This is manifested by the stereoselective induction of microsomal *N*-oxygenation activity by PB and polycyclic aromatic hydrocarbons (PAH). For example, microsomes from PAH-treated rats preferentially *N*-oxidized the nitrogen atom closest to the methyl group of azo procarbazine (methylazoxy derivative: Dunn et al., 1979; Wiebkin and Prough, 1980); a 20:1 product ratio of methylazoxy/benzylazoxy as noted. In addition, microsomes from either untreated or PB-pretreated rats had identical product ratios for the two isomeric azoxy metabolites, but animal treatment with PB increased the total rate of azoxy synthesis 3- to 5-fold. The methylazoxy derivative was formed in a 5.5-1 ratio to benzylazoxy (azoxy with N–O bond closest to benzyl group). Based on these results, a subsequent set of experiments were performed with purified, reconstituted cytochromes P450 and with antibodies directed toward various purified forms of cytochrome P450. Of the 8 hepatic isozymes of the heme protein studied (Guengerich et al., 1982), most of the activity ($>80\%$) involved in the *N*-oxidation of azo procarbazine was mediated by either a minor form, P450IIC6 or a major form, P450IA1. A small portion of the activity was also noted with another major form, P450IIB1. The product ratios of the two azoxy isomers formed with the purified, reconstituted isozymes or with microsomes from the same pretreatment regimens were similar. Experiments using specific inhibitory antibodies supported these contentions of isozyme specificity.

Preliminary experiments on the metabolism of the azoxy metabolites suggested that cytochrome P450 might further metabolize these compounds. Weinkam and Shiba (1978) demonstrated that in ether extracts of incubation mixtures containing procarbazine and rat liver microsomes or post-mitochondrial supernatants, an unknown compound could be observed, based on a mass spectra with a parent ion at m/e 252. This structure corresponds to that of a putative *C*-hydroxy azoxy metabolite. The methylazoxy derivative possesses a readily oxidizable methylene C–H bond and decomposes chemically at appreciable rates in aqueous solutions (Moloney et al., 1985; K. G. Taylor, personal communication). The products of this chemical decomposition reaction are the aldehyde derivative, *N*-isopropyl-*p*-formylbenzamide and a protein-binding species, probably a methyl carbonium ion (Moloney et al., 1985).

The metabolism of these azoxy compounds can be accelerated in the presence of purified cytosolic protein(s) which produce the aldehyde derivative as the major metabolite and an uncharacterized alkylating species (Tweedie et al., 1991). We have observed two cytosolic proteins in rat liver which catalyze the conversion of the methylazoxy isomer of procarbazine to *N*-isopropyl-*p*-benzamide: NAD^+-specific aldehyde dehydrogenase (phenobarbital inducible) and xanthine oxidase. The aldehyde dehydrogenase does not require NAD^+ to catalyze this reaction, but the enzyme appears to utilize another site on its surface to catalyze this reaction. Both rat liver and milk xanthine oxidase oxidize methylazoxy procarbazine to the aldehyde derivative, albeit at a lower rate than the aldehyde dehydrogenase. In the presence of the cytosolic NADH-dependent aldehyde dehydrogenase and NAD^+, the aldehyde derivative formed is rapidly converted to the organic acid, *N*-isopropylterephthalamic acid (TAC). This NAD^+-dependent reaction, no doubt, accounts for the formation of TAC as the major urinary metabolite observed by others (Oliverio et al., 1964; Weinkam and Shiba, 1978). The covalent binding of the methyl group of azoxy II procarbazine may result from the metabolism of the metabolite to form a *C*-hydroxy metabolite described by Weinkam and Shiba (1978).

8.3. Pathways for Metabolic Activation

The proposed pathways of procarbazine metabolism, based on the literature, are summarized in Fig. 3. The reactive intermediates shown may contribute to the toxic and/or carcinogenic action of the drug. The formation of the first oxidative metabolite of procarbazine, the azo derivative, has been well documented. It appears to have little chemical reactivity (Prough, 1985). Tautomerization of the azo derivative to its hydrazone form is a very minor pathway and no evidence exists demonstrating the conversion of the hydrazone to azoxy metabolites. However, azo procarbazine, the hydrazone tautomer and methylhydrazine can all be metabolized by cytochrome P450 to yield methane as a product. Based on the studies by Moloney and Prough (1983), it would seem unlikely that the methane formed during the metabolism of procarbazine in vivo involves the intermediacy of the hydrazone derivative or methylhydrazine. Moloney et al. (1985) have demonstrated a correlation between methane formation and covalent binding of the methyl group of azo procarbazine to microsomal protein, without involvement of the azoxy metabolites. The presence of a free radical intermediate may provide a rationale for more than one potential mechanism of reactivity of procarbazine besides the azoxy pathway described below. Similar conclusions were made regarding the spermatogenic toxicity (Yost et al., 1985) and anticancer activity of procarbazine metabolites (Horstman et al., 1987).

Weinkam and Shiba (1978) have demonstrated the existence of two additional minor metabolites of procarbazine in the presence of postmitochondrial fractions; namely, *N*-isopropyl-*p*-toluamide and *N*-isopropyl-*p*-hydroxymethylbenzamide. It was postulated that these products may be the result of oxidation of azo procarbazine to give a benzyl radical. Sinha (1984) demonstrated that in the presence of NADPH, oxygen, and rat liver microsomes, measurable amounts of the benzyl radical metabolite could be detected by electron spin resonance. Little methyl radical was seen in the presence of liver microsomes. Sinha (1984) suggested that the methyl radical was far more reactive than the benzyl radical and could not be detected by spin resonance techniques. The work of Iannone et al. (1991) and Moloney and Prough (1983) have only accounted for the methyl radicals or methane produced during the metabolism of procarbazine and its metabolites. Wiebkin and Prough (1980) demonstrated that the methyl group of azo procarbazine is preferentially bound to microsomal protein during metabolism relative to the benzyl group. The benzyl radical could be terminated by various mechanisms to give the *N*-isopropyl-*p*-toluamide and *N*-isopropyl-*p*-hydroxymethylbenzamide (Weinkam and Shiba, 1978). Cummings et al. (1982) measured the formation of *N*-isopropyl-*p*-toluamide, *N*-isopropyl-*p*-formylbenzamide, and *N*- isopropyl-*p*-hydroxymethylbenzamide from azo procarbazine in the presence of rat liver microsomes. From these studies, it was determined that little *N*-isopropyl-*p*-toluamide was formed and nearly all of the *N*-isopropyl-*p*-hydroxymethylbenzamide present was derived from the reduction of *N*-isopropyl-*p*-formylbenzamide.

Further *N*-oxidation of azo procarbazine leads to formation of the two isomeric azoxy metabolites. The presence of a *C*-hydroxylated metabolite of the methylazoxy intermediate was proposed based on mass spectral data presented by Weinkam and Shiba (1978) and by analogy to the metabolism of 1,2-dimethylhydrazine (Fiala, 1977). As the methylazoxy isomer possesses a readily oxidizable C–H bond, it is presumed that this oxidation product is the *C*-hydroxylated derivative. The presence of this metabolite has not been further documented by other groups.

The amount of covalent binding of the terminal methyl group of methylazoxy procarbazine to microsomal protein (chemical decomposition) was judged by Moloney et al. (1985) not to be as large as that produced during metabolism of azo procarbazine in the presence of NADPH and oxygen (enzymatic decomposition). However, a portion of the covalent binding of either azo or azoxy procarbazine to liver microsomal protein, and presumably to other cellular nucleophiles, could be due to a chemical decomposition reaction of methylazoxy procarbazine. We have also demonstrated that azoxy isomers can be metabolized by a cytosolic protein to form the aldehyde derivative (Tweedie et al., 1991). This pathway could also lead to biologically-generated, chemically-reactive intermediates, since the background rate of methylazoxy procarbazine decomposition in aqueous solutions is estimated to be less than one-third of the protein-associated rate. This situation is similar to that shown by Feinberg and Zedeck (1980) for methylazoxymethanol conversion to reactive methylation agents in the presence of several alcohol dehydrogenases.

8.4. CHEMICAL INSTABILITY OF AZOXY ISOMERS

Recent studies by Yost and coworkers (Swaffar et al., 1992a,b) and by our group (Tweedie et al., 1991) on metabolism of the azoxy isomers of procarbazine in tumor cells and various proteins of rat liver have shown that the methylazoxy derivative of procarbazine displays significant chemical instability leading to the formation of *N*-isopropyl-*p*-formylbenzamide and other metabolites. In our studies with cytosolic enzymes (Tweedie et al., 1991), the rate of chemical decomposition of methylazoxy procarbazine was approximately 15–25% as large as that of the biological oxidation reaction. Swaffar et al. (1992a,b) have demonstrated that in aqueous solutions of culture media or suspensions of tumor cells containing redox active metals, procarbazine is oxidized to its azo product and hydrogen peroxide; addition of metal chelating agents to these reaction mixtures suppresses this oxidation reaction. The two products, azo procarbazine and hydrogen peroxide, were also shown to react further forming both azoxy isomers. During prolonged reaction times, the amount of the methylazoxy derivative in aqueous solution decreased relatively more rapidly than the benzylazoxy derivative. This supports the contention that the C–H bond of the benzylic carbon of methylazoxyprocarbazine is easily oxidized and may lead to formation of the putative, unstable *C*-hydroxy-azoxyprocarbazine intermediate. One other product was observed which could

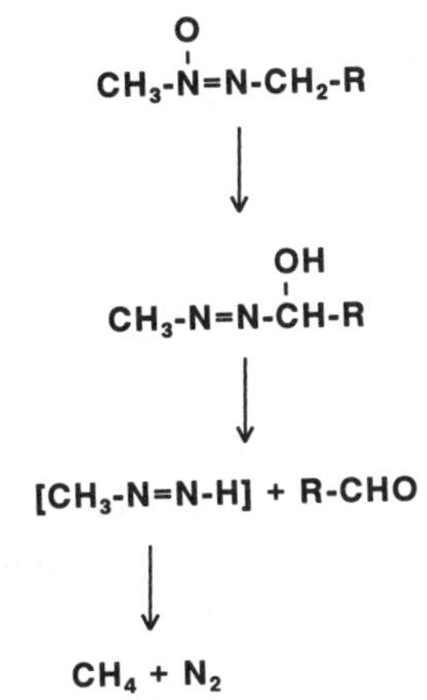

FIG. 4. Rearrangement of *N*-isopropyl-α-(2-methyl-ONN-azoxy)-*p*-toluamide R, —C_6H_4—CO—NH—$CH(CH_3)_2$.

be derived from migration of the oxygen atom from the N–O group to the benzylic carbon yielding a putative, unstable α-hydroxy-azoprocarbazine (Fig. 4; Swaffar et al., 1992b); this intermediate would yield methyl radical via methyldiazene as a reactive intermediate. Based on the work of both groups the methylazoxy derivative itself may be, in part, the ultimate reactive species, decomposing to chemically reactive intermediates at rates which approach those of the biological oxidation reactions catalyzed by cytosolic enzymes. Further study will be required to elucidate the role of chemical decomposition in the action of the azoxy derivatives of procarbazine.

In conclusion, three potential mechanisms lead to reactive chemical intermediates which may account for the mode of action of procarbazine. The following reactive intermediates can be visualized based on the scheme shown in Fig. 3: a methyl free radical (diazene) metabolite from azo procarbazine, a direct chemical reactivity of methylazoxy procarbazine during decomposition, and a reactive *C*-hydroxyazoxy metabolite formed from the azoxy derivatives. However, insufficient evidence is available at present to unambiguously state which mode of action of the drug contributes to its cytotoxic or carcinogenic activity. Indeed, future experimentation may demonstrate a separate mechanism for the cytotoxic and carcinogenic activities described in Sections 4 and 5.

9. FACTORS MODULATING ANTICANCER ACTIVITY

The biochemical studies of a number of groups (Dunn et al., 1979; Moloney et al., 1985; Moloney and Prough, 1983; Prough et al., 1984; Shiba and Weinkam, 1982, 1983; Reed 1975, 1976; Weinkam and Shiba, 1978, 1982; Wiebkin and Prough, 1980) have provided several pieces of information which may be useful for the modulation of the anticancer activity of procarbazine. For example, Prough et al. (1984) and Wiebkin and Prough (1980) have demonstrated in vitro that only certain forms of cytochrome P450 catalyze the *N*-oxidation of azo-procarbazine to form the isomeric azoxy derivatives. In addition, these various forms of the enzyme result in different ratios of the two isomeric azoxy metabolites. The work from Yost's group and our group suggest that methylazoxy procarbazine, the predominant metabolite, may have more chemical reactivity than does the benzyl azoxy I derivative (Erikson et al., 1989; Swaffer et al., 1989). Not only does pretreatment of mammals with inducing agents for the various forms of cytochrome P450 increase the metabolism to the azoxy metabolites, but certain agents (namely, PB and the PAH, β-naphthoflavone) cause the preferential formation of the methylazoxy isomer.

Wiestler et al. (1984) observed lower levels of DNA alkylation in newborn rat tissues compared to adult tissues, following a single dose of ^{14}C-*methyl*-labelled procarbazine. It was postulated that the difference seen was due to postnatal maturation of activating enzymes in the adult liver. A number of other workers have also proposed that the activation of procarbazine to mutagenic/toxic species requires enzymes other than those present in microsomes (Schmid et al., 1982; Malavielle et al., 1983). These observations suggest that the use of barbituates or other nontoxic inducing agents to increase the potency of the drug by enhancing the formation of proximal metabolites may be an effective method of altering the cytotoxicity of the drug.

Shiba and Weinkam (1983) examined the effect of inducing agents of cytochrome P450 on the antitumor activity of procarbazine against L1210 ascites leukemia cells in CDF_1 mice. Their results demonstrated that diphenylhydantoin and PB pretreatment of the mice prior to challenge with procarbazine resulted in a significant increase in lifespan of the mice implanted with the L1210 cells. Methylprednisolone, administered with procarbazine in treatment of human brain tumors (Levin et al., 1976), had no effect on lifespan. Interestingly, prior treatment with procarbazine itself caused a small, but significant increase in life span. Procarbazine does not directly affect cytochrome P450 function in vitro (Moloney et al., 1984), but may be an inducer of certain forms of cytochrome P450 in vivo or of some other enzyme(s) involved in the metabolic activation of procarbazine and/or its metabolites.

The possibility of modulating the metabolic activation of procarbazine or its metabolites to form the cytotoxic species holds some promise for future work in altering the effectiveness of this unique anticancer drug. Unlike other antitumor agents (e.g. nitrosoureas, folate antagonists), only one chemical form of the drug has been shown to be useful for treatment, the methyl-substituted derivative. In addition, the drug has selectivity in only a limited number of tumors in humans. Therefore, it is possible that little can be done to enhance the use of the drug beyond the experimental approaches provided in the past. However, this possibility justifies more focused studies on the metabolism and mechanism of action of procarbazine.

Acknowledgement—The work cited in this chapter from our laboratory was supported in part by American Cancer Society Grant BC-336.

REFERENCES

ABRAHAM, D., CARBONE, P. P. and VENDITTI, J. M. (1967) Evaluation of chemical agents against the plasma cell tumor LPC-1 in mice. *Biochem. Pharmac.* **16:** 665–673.

AEBI, H., DEWALD, B. and SUTER, H. (1965a) Autoxydation N^2-substituierter methylhydrazine beeinflesshung der cu und fe katalyse durch proteine. *Helv. Chim. Acta* **48:** 656–662.

AEBI, H., DEWALD, B. and SUTER, H. (1965b) Peroxidbildung bei der autoxydation N^2-substituierter methylhydrazine. *Helv. Chim. Acta* **48:** 1380–1394.

BACCHI, M., CAVALIERE, A. and FRATINI, D. (1982) Lung carcinogenesis by procarbazine chlorate in BALB/c mice. *Carcinogenesis* **3:** 71–73.

BAGGIOLINI, M., BICKEL, M. H. and MESSIHA, F. S. (1965) Demethylation in vivo of Natulan, a tumour-inhibiting methylhydrazine derivative. *Experientia (Basel)* **21:** 334–336.

BAGGIOLINI, M., DEWALD, B. and AEBI, H. (1969) Oxidation of *p*-(N^1-methyl hydrazino methyl)-*N*-isopropyl benzamide (procarbazine) to the methylazo derivative and oxidative cleavage of the N^2-C bond in the isolated perfused rat liver. *Biochem. Pharmac.* **18:** 2187–2196.

BAYER, U. (1978) The in vivo induction of sister chromatid exchanges in the bone marrow of the Chinese hamster. II. *N*-Nitrosodiethylamine (DEN) and *N-isopropyl*-α-(2-methylhydrazine)-*p*-toluimide (Natulan), two carcinogenic compounds with specific mutagenicity problems. *Mutat. Res.* **56:** 305–309.

BERNEIS, K., KOFLER, M., BOLLAG, W., KAISER, A. and LANGEMANN, A. (1963) The degradation of deoxyribonucleic acid by new tumor inhibiting compounds: the intermediate formation of hydrogen peroxide. *Experientia (Basel)* **19:** 132–133.

BITRAN, J. D., DRESSER, R. K., DE MEESTER, T. R., SHAPIRO, C. R., BILLINGS, C. R., RUBENSTEIN, L., EVANS, R., COLMAN, M., RAO, Y., GRIEM, M. and GOLOMB, H. M. (1978) Combined modality therapy for stage III M_0 non-oat cell bronchogenic carcinoma. *Cancer Treat. Rep.* **62:** 327–332.

BLIJLEVEN, W. G. H. and VOGEL, E. (1977) The mutational spectrum of procarbazine in *Drosophila melanogaster*. *Mutat. Res.* **45:** 47–59.

BOLLAG, W. (1963) The tumor-inhibitory effects of the methylhydrazine derivative Ro 4-6467/1 (NSC-77213). *Cancer Chemother. Rep.* **33:** 1–4.

BOLLAG, W. (1964) Investigations with methylhydrazine derivatives. In: *Chemotherapy of Cancer*, pp. 191–197, PLATTNER, P. A. (ed.) Elsevier, Amsterdam.

BOLLAG, W. and GRUNBERG, E. (1963) Tumour inhibitory effects of a new class of cytotoxic agents: methylhydrazine derivatives. *Experientia (Basel)* **19:** 130– 131.

BONADONNA, G., MONFARDINI, S. and OLDINI, C. (1969) Comparative effects of vinblastine and procarbazine in advanced Hodgkin's disease. *Eur. J. Cancer* **5:** 393–402.

BROOKES, P. (1965) Studies of the mode of action of ibenzmethyzin. In: *Natulan (Ibenzmethyzin)*, pp. 9–12, JELLIFFE, A. M. and MARKS, J. (eds) John Wright and Sons, Bristol.

CALABRESI, P. and PARKS, R. E., JR (1985) Antiproliferative agents and drugs used for immunosuppression. In: *Goodman and Gilman's The Pharmacological Basis of Theraputics*, 7th edn, pp. 1247–1306, GILMAN, A. G., GOODMAN, L. S., RALL, T. W. and MURAD, F. (eds) MacMillan Publishing Co., New York.

CHABNER, B. A., DEVITA, V., CONSIDINE, N. and OLIVERIO, V. T. (1969) Plasma pyridoxal phosphate depletion by the carcinostatic procarbazine. *Proc. Soc. exp. Biol. Med.* **132:** 1119–1122.

CHAMBERLAIN, M. C. and LEVIN, V. A. (1990) Adjuvant chemotherapy for primary lymphoma of the central nervous system. *Arch. Neur.* **47:** 1113–1116.

CHAPMAN, R. M. (1984) Effect of cytotoxic therapy on sexuality and gonadal function. In: *Toxicity of Chemotherapy*, pp. 343–363, PERRY, M. C. and YARBRO, J. W. (eds) Grune and Stratton, New York.

CHAUBE, S. and MURPHY, M. L. (1969) Fetal malformations produced in rats by *N*-isopropyl-α-(2-methylhydrazino)-*p*-toluamide hydrochloride (procarbazine). *Teratology* **2:** 23–31.

COOMES, M. W. and PROUGH, R. A. (1983) The mitochondrial metabolism of 1,2-di-substituted hydrazines, procarbazine and 1,2-dimethylhydrazine. *Drug Metab. Disp.* **11:** 550–555.

COYLE, T., BAPTISTA, J., WINFIELD, J., CLARK, K., POIESZ, B., KIRSHNER, J., SCALZO, A., NEWMAN-PALMER, N., KING, R. and GRAZIANO, S. (1990) Mechlorethamine, vincristine, and procarbazine chemotherapy for recurrent highgrade glioma in adults: a phase II study. *J. clin. Oncol.* **8:** 2014–2018.

CUMMINGS, S. W., GUENGERICH, F. P. and PROUGH, R. A. (1982) The characterization of *N*-isopropyl-*p*-hydroxymethylbenzamide formed during the oxidative metabolism of azo-procarbazine. *Drug Metab. Disp.* **10:** 459–464.

DEVITA, V. T. and HELLMAN, S. (1982) Hodgkin's disease and non-Hodgkin's lymphomas. In: *Cancer: Principles and Practice of Oncology*, pp. 1331–1401, DEVITA, V. T., HELLMAN, S. and ROSENBERG, S. A. (eds) J. P. Lippincott Co., Philadelphia, PA.

DEVITA, V. T., HAHN, M. A. and OLIVERIO, V. T. (1965) Monoamine oxide inhibition by a new carcinostatic agent *N*-isopropyl-*p*-hydroxymethylbenzamide. *Proc. Soc. exp. Biol. Med.* **120:** 561–565.

DEVITA, V. T., SERPICK, A. A. and CARBONE, P. P. (1969) Combination chemotherapy of advanced Hodgkin's disease (HD): the NCI program, a progress report. *Proc. Am. Ass. Cancer Res.* **10**, 19.

DEVITA, V. T., SERPICK, A. A. and CARBONE, P. P. (1970) Combination chemotherapy in the treatment of advanced Hodgkin's disease. *Ann. intern. Med.* **73:** 881–895.

DEWALD, B., BAGGIOLINI, M. and AEBI, H. (1969) N-Demethylation of *p*-(N^1-methylhydrazino methyl)-*N*-isopropyl benzamide (procarbazine), a cytostatically active methylhydrazine derivative, in the intact rat and in the isolated perfused rat liver. *Biochem. Pharmac.* **18:** 2179–2186.

DORR, R. T. and FRITZ, W. L. (1980) Procarbazine. In: *Cancer Chemotherapy Handbook*, pp. 593–601, Elsevier, New York.

DOST, F. N. and REED, D. J. (1967) Methane formation in vivo from, *N*-iso-propyl-α-(2-methylhydrazino)-*p*-toluamide hydrochloride, a tumor-inhibiting methylhydrazine derivative. *Biochem. Pharmac.* **16:** 1741–1746.

DOST, F. N., REED, D. J. and WANG, C. H. (1966) The metabolic fate of monomethylhydrazine and unsymmetrical dimethylhydrazine. *Biochem. Pharmac.* **15:** 1325–1332.

DRAUDIN-KRYLENKO, V. A., BUKIN, IU. V. and NIKONOVA, T. V. (1989) Anticarcinogenic action of vitamins PP and B_6 in the natulan initiation of malignant growth in mice. *Vopr. Onkol.* **35:** 34–38.

DRUCKREY, H. (1970) Production of colonic carcinomas by 1,2-dimethylhydrazines and azo alkanes. In: *Carcinoma of the Colon and Antecedent Epithelium*, pp. 267–279, BURDETTE, W. J. (ed.) C. C. Thomas, Springfield, IL.

DUNN, D. L., LUBET, R. A. and PROUGH, R. A. (1979) Oxidative metabolism of *N*-isopropyl-α-(2-methylhydrazino)-*p*-toluamide hydrochloride (procarbazine) by rat liver microsomes. *Cancer Res.* **39:** 4555–4563.

EADE, N. R., MACLEOD, S. M. and RENTON, K. W. (1972) Inhibition of hepatic microsomal drug metabolism by the hydrazines R0 4-4602, MK 486, and procarbazine hydrochloride. *Can. J. Physiol. Pharmac.* **50:** 721–724.

EHLING, U. H. and NEUHAUSER, A. (1979) Procarbazine-induced specific locus mutations in male mice. *Mutat. Res.* **59:** 245–256.

ERIKSON, J. M. and PROUGH, R. A. (1986) Oxidative metabolism of some hydrazine derivatives by rat liver and lung tissue fractions. *J. Biochem. Toxicol.* **1:** 41–52.

ERIKSON, J. M., DUCORE, J. M. and PROUGH, R. A. (1986) Potential of procarbazine (*N*-isopropyl-α-(2-methylhydrazino)-*p*-toluamide) and its metabolites to damage DNA in L1210 cells. *Pharmacologist* **28:** 174.

ERIKSON, J. M., TWEEDIE, D. J., DUCORE, J. M. and PROUGH, R. A. (1989) Cytotoxicity and DNA damage caused by the azoxy metabolites of procarbazine in L1210 tumor cells. *Cancer Res.* **49:** 127–133.

FEINBERG, A. and ZEDECK, M. S. (1980) Production of a highly reactive alkylating agent from the organospecific carcinogen methylazoxymethanol by alcohol dehydrogenase. *Cancer Res.* **40:** 4446–4450.

FIALA, E. S. (1977) Investigations into the metabolism and mode of action of the colon carcinogens 1,2-dimethylhydrazine and azoxymethane. *Cancer* **40:** 2436–2445.

FONG, L. Y., JENSEN, D. E. and MAGEE, P. N. (1990) DNA methyl-adduct dosimetry and O^6-alkylguanine-DNA alkyl transferase activity determinations in rat mammary carcinogenesis by procarbazine and *N*-methylnitrosourea. *Carcinogenesis* **11:** 411–417.

FREZZA, D. and BIANCHI, V. (1984) Genetic effects of procarbazine in the yeast *Saccharomyces cerevisiae*, strain D4. *Teratogen. Carcinogen. Mutagen.* **4:** 201–210.

GALE, G. R., SIMPSON, J. G. and SMITH, A. B. (1967) Studies of the mode of action of *N*-isopropyl-α-(2-methylhydrazino)-*p*-toluamide. *Cancer Res.* **27:** 1186–1191.

GATEHOUSE, D. G. and PAES, D. J. (1983) A demonstration of the in vitro bacterial mutagenicity of procarbazine, using the microtitre fluctuation test and large concentrations of S9 fraction. *Carcinogenesis* **4:** 347–352.

GELZER, J. and LOUSTALOT, P. (1967) Biological and chemotherapeutic studies on primary mammary tumors in C3H and C3HO mice. *Int. J. Cancer* **2:** 179–187.

GESCHER, A. and RAYMONT, C. (1981) Studies of the metabolism of *N*-methyl containing antitumour agents. $^{14}CO_2$ breath analysis after administration of ^{14}C-labelled *N*-methyl drugs, formaldehyde and formate in mice. *Biochem. Pharmac.* **30:** 1245–1252.

GORSEN, R. M., WEISS, A. J. and MANTHEI, R. W. (1980) Analysis of procarbazine and metabolites by gas chromatography-mass spectrometry. *J. Chromatog.* **221:** 309–318.

GORIA-GATTI, L., IANNONE, A., TOMASI, A., POLI, G. and E. ALBANO (1992) In vitro and in vivo evidence for the formation of methyl radical from procarbazine: a spin-trapping study. *Carcinogenesis* **13:** 799–805.

GUENGERICH, F. P., DANNAN, G. A., WRIGHT, S. T., MARTIN, M. V. and KAMINSKY, L. S. (1982) Purification and characterization of liver microsomal cytochromes P450: electrophoretic, spectral, catalytic, and immunochemical properties and inducibility of eight isozymes isolated from rats treated with phenobarbital and β-naphthoflavone. *Biochemistry* **21:** 6019–6030.

HORSTMAN, M. G., MEADOWS, G. G. and YOST, G. S. (1987) Separate mechanisms for procarbazine spermatotoxicity and anticancer activity. *Cancer Res.* **47:** 1547–1550.

IANNONE, A., ALBANO, E., GORIA-GATTI, L., TOMASI, A. and VANNINI, V. (1991) In vivo spin trapping of methyl free radical following the administration of procarbazine to the rat. *Proc. Am. Ass. Cancer Res.* **32:** 425.

JONES, S. E., MOORE, M., BLANK, N. and CASTELLINO, R. (1972) Hypersensitivity to procarbazine (Matulane) manifested by fever and pleuropulmonary reaction. *Cancer* **29:** 498–500.

KELLY, M. G., O'GARA, R. W., YANCEY, S. T., GADEKAR, K., BOTKIN, C. and OLIVERIO, V. T. (1969) Comparative carcinogenicity of *N*-isopropyl-α-(2-methylhydrazino)-*p*-toluamide HCl (procarbazine hydrochloride), its degradation products, other hydrazines, and isonicotinic acid hydrazide. *J. natn. Cancer Inst.* **42:** 337–344.

KREIS, W. (1970a) Metabolism of an antineoplastic methylhydrazine derivative in a P815 mouse neoplasm. *Cancer Res.* **30:** 82–89.

KREIS, W. (1970b) Mechanism of action of procarbazine. In: *Proceedings of the Chemotherapy Conference on Procarbazine* (*Matulane*: *NSC* 77213): *Development and Application*, pp. 35–44, CARTER, S. K. (ed.) Government Printing Office, Washington, D. C.

KREIS, W., PIEPHO, S. B. and BERNHARD, H. V. (1966) Studies on the metabolic fate of the ^{14}C-labeled methyl group of a methylhydrazine derivative in P815 mouse leukemia. *Experientia* **22:** 431–433.

KUTTAB, S. H., TANGLERTPAIBUL, S. and VOUROS, P. (1982) Studies on the metabolism of procarbazine by mass spectrometry. *Biomed. Mass Spectrom.* **9:** 78–84.

LEE, I. P. and DIXON, R. L. (1978) Mutagenicity, carcinogenicity, and teratogenicity of procarbazine. *Mutat. Res.* **55:** 1–14.

LEE, I. P. and LUCIER, G. W. (1976) The potentiation of barbiturate-induced narcosis by procarbazine. *J. Pharmac. exp. Ther.* **196:** 586–593.

LEVIN, V. A., CRAFTS, D. C., WILSON, C. B., SCHULTZ, M. J., BOLDREY, E. B., ENOT, K. J., PISCHER, T. L., SEAGER, M. and ELASHOFF, R. M. (1976) BCNU (NSC-409962) and procarbazine (NSC-77213) treatment for malignant brain tumors. *Cancer Treat. Rep.* **60:** 243–249.

LEWIS, L. D. (1984) Procarbazine associated alveolitis. *Thorax* **39:** 206–207.

LOWENBRAUN, S., DEVITA, V. T. and SERPICK, A. A. (1970) Combination chemotherapy with nitrogen mustard, vincristine, procarbazine, and prednisolone in lymphosarcoma and reticulum cell sarcoma. *Cancer* **25:** 1018–1025.

MALAVIELLE, C., BRUN, G. and BARTSCH, H. (1983) Studies on the efficiency of the *Salmonella*/rat hepatocyte assay for the detection of carcinogens as mutagens: activation of 1,2-dimethylhydrazine and procarbazine into bacterial mutagens. *Carcinogenesis* **4:** 449–455.

MARTZ, G., D'ALESSANDRI, A., KEEL, H. J. and BOLLAG, W. (1963) Preliminary clinical results with a new antitumor agent Ro 4-6467 (NSC-77213). *Cancer Chemother. Rep.* **33:** 5–14.

MAXWELL, M. B. (1980) Reexamining the dietary restrictions with procarbazine (an MAOI). *Cancer Nursing* **3:** 451–457.

MCCANN, J., CHOI, E., YAMASAKI, E. and AMES, B. N. (1975) Detection of carcinogens as mutagens in the Salmonella/microsome test: assay of 300 chemicals. *Proc. natn. Acad. Sci. U.S.A.* **72:** 5135–5139.

MILLER, E. (1970) Development of procarbazine. In: *Procarbazine* (*Matulane*: *NSC*-77213): *Development and Application*, pp. 3–8, CARTER, S. K. (ed.) Cancer Therapy Evaluation Branch, National Cancer Institute, Bethesda.

MOLONEY, S. J. and PROUGH, R. A. (1983) Studies on the pathway of methane formation from procarbazine, a 2-methylbenzylhydrazine derivative, by rat liver microsomes. *Arch. Biochem. Biophys.* **221:** 577–584.

MOLONEY, S. J., SNIDER, B. J. and PROUGH, R. A. (1984) The interactions of hydrazine derivatives with rat-hepatic cytochrome P450. *Xenobiotica* **14:** 803–814.

MOLONEY, S. J., WIEBKIN, P., CUMMINGS, S. W. and PROUGH, R. A. (1985) Metabolic activation of the terminal

N-methyl group of *N*-isopropylα-(2-methylhydrazino)-*p*-toluamide hydrochloride (procarbazine). *Carcinogenesis* **6:** 397–401.

NEWTON, H. B., JUNCK, L., BROMBERG, J., PAGE, M. A. and GREENBERG, H. S. (1990) Procarbazine chemotherapy in the treatment of recurrent malignant astrocytomas after radiation and nitrosourea failure. *Neurology* **40:** 1743–1746.

OLIVERIO, V. T. (1973) Derivatives of triazenes and hydrazines. In: *Cancer Medicine*, pp. 806–817, HOLLAND, J. F. and FREI, E. (eds) Lea and Febiger, Philadelphia.

OLIVERIO, V. T., DENHAM, C., DEVITA, V. T. and KELLY, M. G. (1964) Some pharmacologic properties of a new antitumor agent, *N*-isopropyl-α-(2-methylhydrazino)-*p*-toluamide, hydrochloride (NSC-77213). *Cancer Chemother. Rep.* **42:** 1–7.

ORTIN, T. T., SHOSTAK, C. A. and DONALDSON, S. S. (1990) Gonadal status and reproductive function following treatment for Hodgkin's disease in childhood: the Stanford experience. *Int. J. Radiat. Oncol. Biol. Phys.* **19:** 873–880.

PATEK, D. R. and HELLERMAN, L. (1974) Mitochondrial monoamine oxidase. Mechanism of inhibition by phenylhydrazine and by aralkylhydrazines. Roles of enzymatic oxidation. *J. biol. Chem.* **249:** 2373–2380.

PEDERSEN, A. G., SORENSON, S., AABO, K., DOMBERNOWSKY, P. and HANSEN, H. H. (1982) Phase II study of procarbazine in small cell carcinoma of the lung. *Cancer Treat. Rep.* **66:** 273–275.

POPLIN, E. A., AISNER, J., VAN ECHO, D. A., WHITACRE, M. and WIERNIK, P. H. (1982) CCNU, vincristine, methotrexate, and procarbazine treatment of relapsed small cell lung carcinoma. *Cancer Treat. Rep.* **66:** 1557–1559.

PROUGH, R. A. (1973) The *N*-oxidation of alkylhydrazines catalyzed by the microsomal mixed-function amine oxidase. *Arch. Biochem. Biophys.* **158:** 442–444.

PROUGH, R. A. (1985) The biological *N*-oxidation of hydrazines and azo-compounds. In: *Biological Oxidation of Nitrogen in Organic Molecules*, Ch. 29, pp. 267–277, GORROD, J. W. and DAMANI, L. A. (eds) Ellis Horwood, Chichester.

PROUGH, R. A. and ZIEGLER, D. M. (1977) The relative participation of liver microsomal amine oxidase and cytochrome P450 in *N*-demethylation reactions. *Arch. Biochem. Biophys.* **180:** 363–373.

PROUGH, R. A., WITTKOP, J. A. and REED, D. J. (1969) Evidence for the hepatic metabolism of some monoalkylhydrazines. *Arch. Biochem. Biophys.* **131:** 369–373.

PROUGH, R. A., COOMES, M. L. and DUNN, D. L. (1977) The microsomal metabolism of carcinogenic and/or therapeutic hydrazines. In: *Microsomes and Drug Oxidations*, pp. 500–507, ULLRICH, V., ROOTS, I., HILDEBRANDT, A., ESTABROOK, R. W. and CONNEY, A. H. (eds) Pergamon Press, Oxford.

PROUGH, R. A., FREEMAN, P. C. and HINES, R. N. (1981) The oxidation of hydrazine derivatives catalyzed by the purified liver microsomal FAD-containing monooxygenase. *J. biol. Chem.* **256:** 4178–4184.

PROUGH, R. A., BROWN, M. I., AMRHEIN, C. A. and MARNETT, L. J. (1983) Metabolism of azo and hydrazine derivatives to reactive intermediates. In: *Extrahepatic Drug Metabolism and Chemical Carcinogenesis*, pp.489–498, RYDSTROM, J., MONTELIUS, J. and BENGTSSON, M. (eds) Elsevier, Amsterdam.

PROUGH, R. A., BROWN, M. I., DANNAN, G. A. and GUENGERICH, F. P. (1984) Major isozymes of rat liver microsomal cytochrome P450 involved in the *N*-oxidation of *N*-isopropyl-α-(2-methylazo)-*p*-toluamide, the azo derivative of procarbazine. *Cancer Res.* **44:** 543–548.

PUEYO, C. (1979) Natulan induces forward mutations to L-arabinose-resistance in *Salmonella typhimurium*. *Mutat. Res.* **67:** 189–192.

RAAFLAUB, J. and SCHWARTZ, D. E. (1965) Uber den Metabolismus eines cytostatisch wirksamen Methylhydrazin-Derivats (Natulan). *Experientia (Basel)* **21:** 44–45.

REED, D. J. (1975) Procarbazine. In: *Handbook of Experimental Pharmacology, Antineoplastic and Immunosuppressive Agents*, Vol. 38/2, Ch. 70, pp. 747–765, SARTORELLI, A. C. and JOHNS, D. G. (eds) Springer Verlag, New York.

REED, D. J. (1976) Effects in vivo of lymphoma ascites tumors and procarbazine, alone and in combination, upon hepatic drug-metabolizing enzymes of mice. *Biochem. Pharmac.* **25:** 153–156.

REED, D. J. and MAY, H. E. (1978) Cytochrome P450 interactions with 2-chloroethylnitrosoureas and procarbazine. *Biochimie* **60:** 989–995.

ROCHE LABORATORIES (1969) Information supplied with Matulane capsules. Nutley, New Jersey, Hoffman-La Roche, Inc.

RUTISHAUSER, A., and BOLLAG, W. (1963) Cytological investigations with a new class of cytotoxic agents: methylhydrazine derivatives. *Experientia* **19:** 131–132.

SAGHER, D., KARRISON, T., SCHWARTZ, J. L., LARSON, R., MEIER, P. and STRAUSS, B. (1988) Low O^6-alkylguanine DNA alkyltransferase activity in the peripheral blood lymphocytes of patients with therapy-related acute nonlymphocytic leukemia. *Cancer Res.* **48:** 3084–3089.

SARTORELLI, A. C. and TSUNAMURA, S. (1966) Studies on the biochemical mode of action of a cytotoxic methylhydrazine derivative, *N*-isopropyl-α-(2-methylhydrazino)-*p*-toluamide. *Molec. Pharmac.* **2:** 275–283.

SCHMID, B. P., TRIPPMACHER, A. and BIANCHI, A. (1982) Teratogenicity induced in cultured rat embryos by the serum of procarbazine treated rats. *Toxicology* **25:** 53–60.

SCHOLD, S. C., JR, BRENT, T. P., VON-HOFE, E., FRIEDMAN, H. S., MITRA, S., BIGNER, D. D., SWENBERG, J. A. and KLEIHUES, P. (1989) O^6-alkylguanine-DNA alkyltransferase and sensitivity to procarbazine in human brain-tumor allografts. *J. Neurosurg.* **70:** 573–577.

SCHULER, D., SOMLO, P., BORSI, J., PARAICZ, E., REVESZ, T., KARDOS, G. and KOOS, R. (1988) New drug combination for the treatment of relapsed brain tumors in children. *Pediat. Hematol. Oncol.* **5:** 153–156.

SCHWARTZ, D. E. (1966) Comparative metabolic studies with natulan, methyl hydrazine and methylamine in rats. *Experientia (Basel)* **22:** 212–213.

SCHWARTZ, D. E., BOLLAG, W. and OBRECHT, P. (1967) Distribution and excretion studies of procarbazine in animals and man. *Arzneim.-Forsch.* **17:** 1389–1393.

SCHWARTZ, D. E., BRUBACHER, G. B. and VECCHI, M. (1969) Metabolic formation of methane from *N*-methyl-substituted hydrazine compounds and carcinostatic activity. *J. Label. Comp.* **111:** 487–488.

SHIBA, D. A. and WEINKAM, R. J. (1982) Quantitative analysis of procarbazine, procarbazine metabolites and chemical degradation products with application to pharmacokinetic studies. *J. Chromatog.* **229:** 397–407.

SHIBA, D. A. and WEINKAM, R. J. (1983) The in vivo cytotoxic activity of procarbazine and procarbazine metabolites against L1210 ascites leukemia cells in CDF_1 mice and the effects of pretreatment with procarbazine, phenobarbital, diphenylhydantoin, and methylprednisolone upon in vivo procarbazine activity. *Cancer Chemother. Pharmac.* **11:** 124–129.

SIEBER, S. M., CORREA, P., DALGARD, D. W. and ADAMSON, R. H. (1978) Carcinogenic and other adverse effects of procarbazine in nonhuman primates. *Cancer Res.* **38:** 2125–2134.

SINHA, B. K. (1984) Metabolic activation of procarbazine. Evidence for carbon-centered free radical intermediates. *Biochem. Pharmac.* **33:** 2777–2781.

SMITH, P. A. S. (1966) *The Chemistry of Open-chain Organic Nitrogen Compounds*, Vol. 2, pp. 119–209, W. A. Benjamin, Inc., New York.

SOTOMAYOR, R. E., CHAUHAN, P. S. and EHLING, U. H. (1982) Induction of unscheduled DNA synthesis in the germ cells of male mice after treatment with hydrazine or procarbazine. *Toxicology* **25:** 201–211.

SOULIOTIS, V. L., KAILA, S., BOUSSIOTIS, V. A., PANGALIS, G. A. and KYRTOPOULOS, S. A. (1990) Accumulation of O^6-methylguanine in human blood leukocyte DNA during exposure to procarbazine and its relationships with dose and repair. *Cancer Res.* **50:** 2759–2764.

SPEARMAN, M. E., FRANCK, T. G., MOLONEY, S. J. and PROUGH, R. A. (1985) Influence of cytosolic factors on hydrazine and hydrazide metabolism. In: *Biological Oxidation of Nitrogen in Organic Molecules*, Ch. 30, pp. 290–296, GORROD, J. W. and DAMANI, L. A. (eds) Ellis Horwood, Chichester.

STOLINSKY, D. C., SOLOMON, J., PUGH, R. P., STEVENS, A., JACOBS, E., IRWIN, L., WOOD, D., STEINFELD, J. and BATEMAN, J. (1970) Procarbazine HCl in Hodgkins disease, reticulum cell sarcoma, and lymphosarcoma. *Cancer* **26:** 984– 990.

STRAUSS, B., SAGHER, D., KARRISON, T., SCHWARTZ, J., LARSON, R. and WILLIAMS, S. (1990) Methyl transferase activity in secondary leukemia. *Basic Life Sci.* **53:** 277–289.

SWAFFAR, D. S., HORSTMAN, M. G., JAW, J. Y., THRALL, B. D., MEADOWS, G. G., HARKER, W. G. and YOST, G. S. (1989) Methylazoxyprocarbazine, the active metabolite responsible for the anticancer activity of procarbazine against L1210 leukemia. *Cancer Res.* **49:** 2442–2447.

SWAFFAR, D. S., POMERANTZ, S. C., HARKER, W. G. and YOST, G. S. (1992a) Nonenzymatic bioactivation of procarbazine to active cytotoxic species. *Oncol. Res.* **4:** 49–58.

SWAFFAR, D. S., HARKER, W. G., POMERANTZ, S. C., LIM, H.-K. and YOST, G. (1992b) Isolation, purification, and characterization of two new chemical decomposition products of methylazoxyprocarbazine. *Drug Metab. Disp.* **20:** 632–642.

TOURNAYE, H., CAMUS, M., BOLLEN, N., WISANTO, A., VAN STEIRTEGHEM, A. C. and DEVROEY, P. (1991) In vitro fertilization techniques with frozen–thawed sperm: a method for preserving the progenitive potential of Hodgkin patients. *Fertil. Steril.* **55:** 443–445.

TROVO, M. G., TIRELLI, U., DE PAOLI, A., FRANCHIN, G., RONCADIN, M., MAGRI, M. D., GALLIGIANO, E., VERONESI, A., TUMOLO, S., CARBONE, A. and GRIGOLETTO, E. (1982) Combined radiotherapy and chemotherapy with cyclophosphamide, adriamycin, methotrexate, procarbazine (CAMP) in 64 consecutive patients with epidermoid bronchogenic carcinoma, limited disease: a prospective study. *Int. J. Radiat. Oncol. Biol. Phys.* **8:** 1051–1054.

TWEEDIE, D. J., FERNANDEZ, D., SPEARMAN, M. E., FELDHOFF, R. C. and PROUGH, R. A. (1991) Metabolism of azoxy derivatives of procarbazine by aldehyde dehydrogenase and xanthine oxidase. *Drug Metab. Disp.* **19**, 783–803.

WEINKAM, R. J. and SHIBA, D. A. (1978) Metabolic activation of procarbazine. *Life Sci.* **22:** 937–946.

WEINKAM, R. J. and SHIBA, D. A. (1982) Nonclassical alkylating agents. Procarbazine. In: *Pharmacologic Principles of Cancer Treatment*, Ch. 15, pp. 340–362, CHABNER, B. (ed.) Saunders, Philadelphia.

WEISS, H. D., WALKER, M. D. and WIERNIK, P. H. (1974) Neurotoxicity of commonly used antineoplastic agents. *New Engl. J. Med.* **291:** 127–133.

WIEBKIN, P. and PROUGH, R. A. (1980) Oxidative metabolism of *N*-isopropyl-α-(2-methylazo)-*p*-toluamide (azoprocarbazine) by rodent liver microsomes. *Cancer Res.* **40:** 3524–3529.

WIESTLER, O. D., KLEIHUES, P., RICE, J. M. and IVANKOVIC, S. J. (1984) DNA methylation in maternal, fetal and neonatal rat tissues following perinatal administration of procarbazine. *Cancer Res. Clin. Oncol.* **108:** 56–59.

WITTKOP, J. A., PROUGH, R. A. and REED, D. J. (1969) Oxidative demethylation of *N*-methylhydrazines by rat liver microsomes. *Arch. Biochem. Biophys.* **134:** 308– 315.

WOLFF, T., DISTLERATH, L. M., WORTHINGTON, M. T., GROOPMAN, J. D., HAMMONS, G. J., KADLUBAR, F. F., PROUGH, R. A., MARTIN, M. V. and GUENGERICH, F. P. (1985) Substrate specificity of human liver cytochrome P450 debrisoquine hydroxylase probed using immunochemical inhibition and chemical modeling. *Cancer Res.* **45:** 2116–2122.

YOST, G. S., HORSTMAN, M. G., EL WALILY, A. F., GORDON, W. P. and NELSON, S. D. (1985) Procarbazine spermatogenesis toxicity: deuterium isotope effects point to regioselective metabolism in mice. *Toxic. appl. Pharmac.* **80:** 316– 322.

ZELLER, P., GUTMANN, H., HEGEDUS, B., KAISER, A., LANGEMANN, A. and MULLER, M. (1963) Methylhydrazine derivatives, a new class of cytotoxic agents. *Experientia* (*Basel*) **19:** 129.

Garth Powis, editor.
(1994) *Anticancer Drugs: Reactive Metabolism and Drug Interactions*,
Pergamon Press Ltd, pp. 229–271
Printed in the United Kingdom

CHAPTER 7

CHEMICAL REACTIONS OCCURRING BETWEEN METAL-CONTAINING ANTINEOPLASTIC DRUGS AND BIOLOGICAL MOLECULES

CHARLES L. LITTERST

Developmental Therapeutics Branch, Division of AIDS, National Institute of Allergy and Infectious Diseases, Bethesda, MD 20892, U.S.A.

1. GENERAL INTRODUCTION

The introduction into human chemotherapy of a platinum-containing drug for the treatment of human neoplasia in the early 1970s represented the first time that metallic complexes had been widely utilized in this capacity. The outstanding success of this agent—cisplatin—has prompted a far-reaching search for analogs of cisplatin with a greater therapeutic efficacy, or chemicals containing other metals with similar—or dissimilar but equally effective—physicochemical properties. Dozens of metallic or metalloid elements have been screened for antineoplastic activity in animal screening systems. Thus early transition metals (titanium, vanadium, molybdenum), group IB metals (copper, silver, gold), group IIIA metals (gallium, indium, aluminum), other group VIII metals (palladium) as well as miscellaneous other metals (ruthenium, rhodium, nickel) have all been tested either in vitro or in vivo for their antitumor activity. Relatively few of the thousands of chemical compounds that have been tested in animals have had sufficient properties to warrant consideration for clinical trials. Unfortunately little success was seen with most of the clinical trials when they were conducted and in spite of numerous examples of metal-containing drugs exhibiting antitumor activity, either in vitro or in animal test systems, none except for several analogs of cisplatin have been found to have composite characteristics suitable for clinical trials. There were two major exceptions to this lack of success. One was a drug containing gallium that had a long history of clinical use to study bone diseases, and the other was a novel organic chemical structure discovered in the early 1980s and containing germanium. Most recently the antiarthritic gold complexes have been screened for antitumor activity and some were found to be consistently positive, although no clinical trials have yet been proposed for these agents.

The extent of testing of metal-containing compounds was highlighted by Dr Barnett Rosenberg during his remarks following presentation to him of the Galileo Galilei medal of the University of Padua (Italy) at the 5th International Symposium of Metal-Containing Anticancer Drugs. Dr Rosenberg called attention to the fact that a total of 56 metal or metalloid elements have been tested for in vivo antitumor activity in animals (Sadler, 1982b). Some elements have had only a few compounds tested for in vivo antitumor activity in animals (Y = 10, Ho = Tm = Lu = 11) while others have had greater than a thousand compounds tested (Sn = 1400, As = 1200, Pt = Cu = 1100). By 1980, 988 metal-containing chemicals containing 35 different metals had sufficient in vitro anticancer activity to be considered positive in the National Cancer Institute (USA) antitumor drug screen (Sadler, 1982b), but as mentioned above, only a handful of these compounds have been tested for clinical activity or toxicity.

Once reproducible antitumor activity has been documented and clinical efficacy has been established, the mechanism of action of drugs is then pursued. This chapter will examine one aspect of that mechanism of action—the reactivity with biological molecules that takes place with several metals found in antineoplastic drugs. Because of its more widespread use and more extensive study, the majority of our information in this area is associated with platinum, but even with that element our understanding of the molecular action that produces either antitumor activity or other biological activity is still not firmly established. Other metals discussed in detail in addition to platinum are gold, metallocene halides, and gallium. Palladium and copper are discussed as far as our knowledge of their chemical interactions will allow.

2. PLATINUM

Cis-diamminedichloroplatinum-II (*cis*Pt) is a widely used cancer chemotherapeutic agent with clinical activity against numerous solid tumors. Its efficacy and potential are indicated by the fact that it now may be the most widely utilized drug in the chemotherapy of cancer. The chemical was first synthesized and described in the mid-19th century and its antibacterial activity discovered in the mid 1960s (Rosenberg et al., 1965, 1967). Shortly thereafter it was reported to have antitumor activity in murine solid and leukemia tumor systems (Rosenberg et al., 1969; Rosenberg and VanCamp, 1970) and clinical trials to investigate the antitumor effect in humans were initiated in the early 1970s. In spite of its clinical utility, its exact mechanism of action, both on tumor growth and on normal cells and tissues is not yet firmly established. This chapter will attempt to summarize the reactions that *cis*Pt undergoes with biologically relevant molecules and to call attention to similar interactions that occur with other platinum-containing experimental antineoplastic drugs.

2.1. Chemical Decomposition

2.1.1. *Enzyme-mediated*

Drug decomposition in biological systems frequently is mediated by endogenous enzymes, either hydrolytic, oxidative–reductive, or conjugative. Metal-containing compounds represent a general exception to this rule, although there is some biologically mediated metabolism of some metal compounds such as cadmium and mercury. In spite of 25 years of active research into the mechanism of *cis*Pt action, no evidence has been discovered to support the enzyme-mediated alteration in the *cis*Pt molecule. Numerous studies have investigated the effect of *cis*Pt on various endogenous enzymes (Aull et al., 1979; Aggarwal and Niroomand-Rad, 1983) including classic drug metabolizing enzymes (Litterst et al., 1982a, 1983) but no work has appeared in the literature which has addressed the question of enzyme-mediated metabolism of *cis*Pt. This may be due in part to the general lack of enzymatic metabolism of metal-containing compounds and in part to the extensive spontaneous decomposition of *cis*Pt addressed in the next section. Another reason for the lack of information on enzyme-mediated decomposition of *cis*Pt may be the analytical difficulty in detecting and identifying *cis*Pt metabolites. Numerous techniques are available for separation of the various *cis*Pt decomposition products (Daley-Yates and McBrien, 1983; Riley et al., 1983; Johnson et al., 1980; Rahn et al., 1983; Eastman, 1982; Rahn, 1984) but there is an embarrassing dearth of studies that unequivocally establish the identity of these separated chemicals. The use of nuclear magnetic or paramagnetic resonance techniques, circular dichroism studies or other specific analytical techniques which have been widely used to identify the products of *cis*Pt binding to DNA, have yet to be applied to identifying the nature of *cis*Pt decomposition products in physiological fluids or even in aqueous solutions. The lack of use of these identification techniques, in addition to the large number of spontaneous decomposition products formed in solutions may have discouraged investigators from searching for enzyme mediated metabolism of this drug. Clearly, this is an area for further investigation.

The only insight into metabolic decomposition that has appeared is a report demonstrating no difference in platinum–DNA adducts between castrated and normal rats of both sexes (Litterst et al., 1988). Frequently drugs that are metabolized by a cytochrome P450-dependent monooxygenase pathway demonstrate sex hormone dependent changes in biological activity. These negative results may be interpreted to support the lack of a mixed function oxidase-mediated metabolism of *cis*Pt.

In addition there are reports of *cis*Pt being mutagenic without prior metabolic activation (Zwelling et al., 1979; Johnson et al., 1980; Plooy et al., 1984). For this interpretation of these studies, however, one must assume that proper controls with and without metabolic activation systems were utilized, which was not true in all of these studies.

2.1.2. *Spontaneous Decomposition*

*Cis*Pt is a square planar coordination complex of divalent platinum in which the coordination number is 4 and the four coordination bonds are occupied by two ammine residues and two chlorine atoms arranged in a *cis* configuration in a plane around the central platinum atom (Fig. 1). The square planar configuration is characteristic of the platinum-II molecules, and numerous studies have demonstrated that the *cis* configuration of the leaving groups is an absolute requirement for biological activity (Cleare, 1974; Thomson et al., 1972). For both thermodynamic and kinetic reasons the platinum–nitrogen bond is stable but the chlorine–platinum bond is quite labile, making the chlorine atoms leaving groups and susceptible to replacement by a variety of potential nucleophiles. Potential incoming nucleophiles present in high concentration in biological milieu are water, sulfur, nitrogen, oxygen, and chlorine, with the order of stability of the ultimate complexes being CN > S > Cl > N > O. Numerous studies both theoretical based on thermodynamic and kinetic principles, and experimental done both in vitro and in vivo have established that the chlorine atoms are initially replaced with water molecules and this aquated *cis*Pt molecule then decomposes through loss of protons to form the mono- and dihydroxy species (Fig. 2). At 37°C the chlorines are lost sequentially with a rate constant of $1.1–1.5 \times 10^{-4}$ sec^{-1} for the loss of the first chlorine atom and a rate constant of $3.3–4.2 \times 10^{-5}$ sec^{-1} for loss of the second chlorine atom (Segal and LePecq, 1985; LeRoy, 1975; Reishus and Martin, 1961). This difference in rate constant means that in aqueous medium, a large majority (90%) of the *cis*Pt will be in the form of the monochloro–monoaquo complex (Johnson et al., 1980). These aquated/hydroxylated forms of *cis*Pt are reactive intermediates that may then be further exchanged with other incoming nucleophiles, commonly sulfur or nitrogen. It has been this particular order of replacement of the final ligand that led early platinum chemists to suggest that the interaction with sulfur on methionine and other low molecular weight substances, and the nitrogen or oxygen atoms of bases in nucleic acid would be likely reactions to occur in vivo. It also has been postulated that the dihydroxy form will spontaneously polymerize to form dimers and trimers (Martin, 1983; Rosenberg, 1978), both of which possess very high toxicity (Rosenberg, 1978; Cleare et al., 1978).

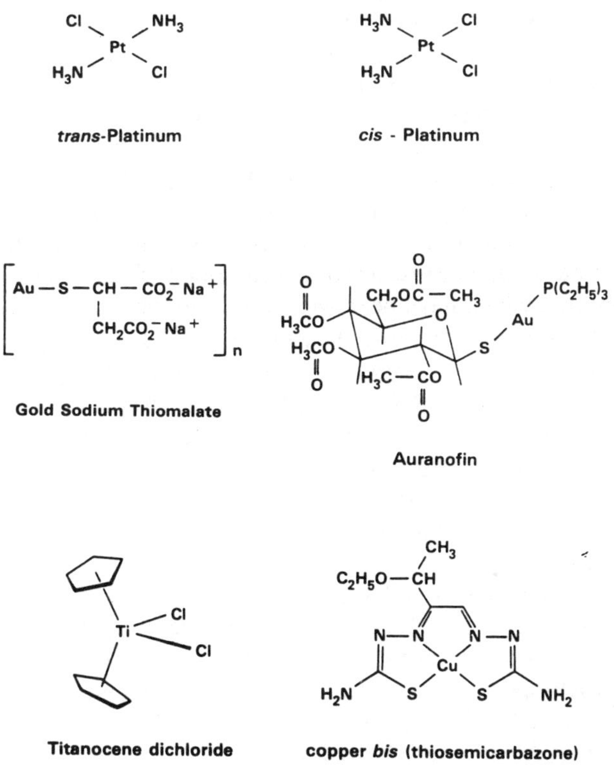

FIG. 1. Structures of chemicals discussed in the text.

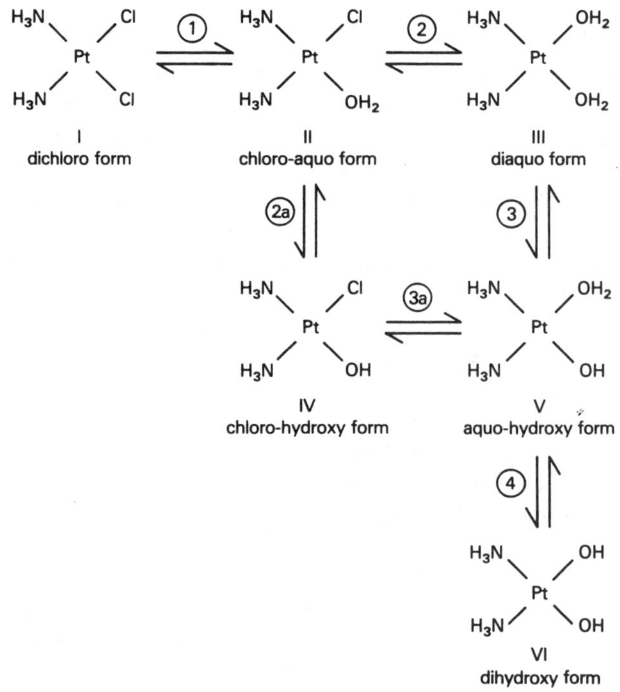

FIG. 2. Hydrolysis (aquation) scheme for *cis*-diamminedichloroplatinum-II.

Although the reaction scheme portrayed in Fig. 2 in all likelihood occurs in vivo, it should be reemphasized that the reaction products have not yet been identified from either in vitro reaction mixtures or from body tissues or fluids in vivo following administration of *cis*Pt to animals or patients. The reaction products isolated from reaction mixtures containing *cis*Pt and a variety of nucleotide fragments, however, are consistent with the scheme postulated above and could proceed via reactive intermediates such as the aqua and hydroxy derivatives. The exact mechanism by which the products are formed, however, is not known with certainty, although indirect evidence supports the formation of final bifunctional ligands formed via the aquated intermediates rather than by direct substitution (Thomson, 1974).

The exchange reaction of chloride ligands with nucleophiles can take place either as a characteristics SN_2 direct substitution reaction between chloride and the nucleophile, where reaction rate depends primarily on the reactivity of the replacing nucleophile, or as an SN_1 reaction, in which a relatively slow first order reaction produces a reactive intermediate (the monochloro–monoaquo derivative), which then reacts more quickly with the ultimate nucleophile. The SN_1 reaction proceeds with a first order rate constant of 2.5×10^{-5} sec^{-1} (25°C). The first order rate constant at 35°C is $7.6 - 10^{-5}$ sec^{-1}, which means that at physiologic temperature, the half time for the aquation reaction is about 2.5 hr (Knox et al., 1986) and the half time for the nucleophilic exchange is about 1.7 hr (Rosenberg, 1978). Clearly, these times are substantially too long for a reaction that apparently produces methionine adducts within minutes after *cis*Pt administration to animals or to patients (Daley-Yates and McBrien, 1984), or the extensive protein binding that takes place within the first hour after administration to animals or people. To account for the rapid formation of these adducts with strong nucleophiles in tissue, therefore, the SN_2-type of reaction must be invoked.

Leroy and Thompson (1989) have conducted elegant studies investigating the relative kinetics between aquation and binding of *cis*Pt. They measured free and bound charged and uncharged platinum species in human plasma and in solutions of bovine albumin. Their results show that two consecutive first order reactions take place: the initial rate limiting aquation step, and a subsequent binding reaction of the aquated *cis*Pt to protein. This is the reaction order that has been presumed throughout most of the previous decade of work in this area, but the first time a careful study has established relative quantities of reactive, reacted, and nonreactive species, and their relative rate constants. An interesting sidelight of this study was the discovery that when the *trans* isomer was used, prior aquation was not requisite for protein binding to occur; this occurred apparently by direct nucleophilic attack, without the need for prior metabolism.

The reaction sequence just discussed and portrayed in Fig. 2 proceeds optimally in a medium with no free chlorine atoms. Because water is a very weak nucleophile (weaker even than chlorine) the presence of even small concentrations of chloride ions in solution will be enough to suppress the replacement of two labile chloride ligands and the dichloro structure will be retained. Thus at chlorine concentrations present in blood (ca 104 mM) the hydrolysis reactions are presumed to be insignificant. Direct replacement of chlorines with a strong nucleophile such as sulfur is possible in plasma, however, and is one explanation for the strong binding that occurs between *cis*Pt and albumin. The parent *cis*Pt molecule (Fig. 1) is uncharged and as such apparently is readily absorbed across membranes into cells. Because of the much lower intracellular chloride concentration (ca 4 mM) the hydration or aquation reactions discussed above occur, with resulting interaction of the reactive intermediates with intracellular receptors on both macromolecules and lower molecular weight compounds. It has been estimated that the relative intracellular amount of the various platinum species present would be a 1:1 equilibrium of the monoaquo-monohydroxy, and the dihydroxy species in the absence of binding to stronger nucleophiles (LeRoy, 1975). As qualified by the author, however, this condition is unrealistic due to the very high concentration of numerous strong nucleophiles such as sulfur on amino acids and proteins, and the nitrogen and oxygen atoms present on nucleic acids and elsewhere within the cell. The importance of relatively modest concentrations of chloride ions is indicated by reports of less than 5% decomposition of *cis*Pt solution prepared in 75 mM NaCl. The reaction reaches equilibrium when ca. 45% of the total chlorides have exchanged (Perumareddi and Adamson, 1968). The chemical reactivity of *cis*Pt when dissolved in distilled water is very high, with extensive aquation to reactive products that can be presumed to be intermediates in the formation of nucleophilic products that have the potential to bind to reactive sites in macromolecules. These reactive aquation products have been shown to have greater biological activity than *cis*Pt (Kohl et al., 1978; Rosenberg, 1978). Kinetic studies in vitro suggest that under ideal (i.e. 'pure') conditions the predominant intracellular form of *cis*Pt will be the monoaquo–monochloro form because the rate constant for removal of the second chlorine atom is such that the appearance of the diaquo form would occur only a chloride concentrations well below 1 mM. It has been suggested that this concentration might occur in the nucleus (Segal and LePecq, 1985). However, under physiological conditions the monoaquo–monohydroxy species predominate (Reedijk et al., 1984).

Experimental data obtained from in vivo studies, however, tend to complicate our understanding of this apparently simple reaction scheme. Thus, the plasma half life of *cis*Pt declines very rapidly, due in part to a very extensive and rapid excretion of the parent *cis*Pt molecule (Litterst et al., 1976). Thus within 1 hr of administration, 50–70% of the administered dose of *cis*Pt can be recovered in rabbit urine (Bertolero and Litterst, 1982; Litterst, 1984b) and nearly 70% is excreted within the first 5 min in guinea pigs (Litterst and Schweitzer, 1988a). By 24 hr after dosing only trace amounts appear in urine, although platinum is still detectable up to 30 days following injection (Litterst et al., 1979). Additionally there is a rapid and extensive binding of the *cis*Pt molecule directly to plasma proteins. Although it has long been thought that platinum bound to protein with direct substitution of strongly nucleophilic sites on protein with no intermediate aquation reaction occurring, more recent results mentioned above (LeRoy and Thompson, 1989) demonstrate the necessity of aquation prior to binding. In addition, however, there have been reports of extensive and very early formation of a large number of discrete but unfortunately poorly-characterized platinum-containing 'metabolites' in plasma as early as 5 min after *cis*Pt administration (Daley-Yates and McBrien, 1984). This result suggests that our understanding of the chemical interactions that *cis*Pt undergoes in biological solutions is as yet incomplete and needs additional work.

The complexity of the reaction of *cis*Pt under intracellular conditions of substrate (reactants) and substrate concentration is indicated by the report demonstrating the formation of phosphate and carboxylate complexes of *cis*Pt formed from interaction with endogenous substrates such as citrate, glutamate and phosphate groups on nucleic acids and nucleotides (Segal and LePecq, 1985). These interactions would be predicted by the anionic nature of the replacing groups displacing the chloride ion on the *cis*Pt molecule. At relatively modest concentrations of acetate or phosphate (1–10 mM) the aquated form of *cis*Pt will react with those anions to yield acetate or phosphate complexes. The reactivity of these complexes is similar to that of the chloro–aquo form and therefore less than that of the diaquo form. Furthermore, *cis*Pt will bind to DNA no faster than it binds to the oligonucleotide Ap_4A, which may influence the rate of the reaction of *cis*Pt with DNA in the presence of any significant concentration of phosphate containing nucleotides (Segal and LePecq, 1985).

Although it is generally assumed that phosphate groups are not involved in the *cis*Pt-DNA binding, there is evidence to the contrary. Thus Pedersen et al. (1985) have shown a decrease in T_4 phage inactivation ability of *cis*Pt in phosphate buffer and have suggested this decrease in biological activity is due to the formation of a platinum–phosphate complex. Further, platinum is thermodynamically able to form phosphate complexes in vitro (Bose et al., 1984), even though this is not considered to be significant in vivo (Lippard, 1982). Sarrazin et al. (1986) have shown that platinum binds to adenosine nucleotides through bidentate complexation at N-7 of the adenosine, with the other bond involving the phosphate group. Phosphate, however, has been shown to be not involved with platinum binding to adenosine itself (Kong and Theophanides, 1975; Sarrazin et al., 1986). Finally, Drobnick and Horacek (1973) have postulated that *cis*Pt interacts initially with phosphate groups on DNA and then subsequently with the nucleobase. This hypothesis was based on the observation that *cis*Pt reacted more rapidly with nucleotides than with nucleosides. Most recently Segal and LePecq (1985) have suggested that the interaction between *cis*Pt and the Ap_4A polynucleotide is through a phosphate complex.

2.2. DNA INTERACTIONS

The demonstration by Rosenberg et al. (1965) that platinum compounds could alter the replication of bacteria without altering their survival was the first suggestion that the antitumor mechanism of this drug involved DNA. The involvement of DNA with *cis*Pt mechanism of action has been inferred not only from the studies indicating noncytotoxic inhibition of bacterial cell replication but also from several additional lines of evidence. *Cis*Pt is mutagenic (Perera et al., 1990; Plooy et al., 1984; Zwelling et al., 1979), an effect which is intimately related to DNA integrity. Cells deficient in DNA repair mechanisms are more sensitive to *cis*Pt that those with normal repair mechanisms (Plooy et al., 1985b), suggesting that a repairable DNA lesion may be involved. Finally, the inhibition of DNA synthesis by *cis*Pt has been shown to occur earlier and at lower doses than the *cis*Pt-induced inhibition of RNA and protein synthesis (Pascoe and Roberts, 1974; Harder and Rosenberg, 1970; Howle and Gale, 1970). Subsequent studies have devoted much time and effort to establishing with certainty how *cis*Pt interacts with DNA and what the subsequent biochemical and cellular consequences of the interaction are.

After early suggestions that the mechanism of action of *cis*Pt as an antitumor agent might involve DNA synthesis, several investigators documented that, in fact, DNA synthesis in animals was inhibited at doses of drug which had little effect on protein or RNA synthesis (Harder and Rosenberg, 1970; Howle and Gale, 1970). The mechanism by which *cis*Pt altered DNA synthesis was then pursued and it was shown that platinum bound to nucleobases and not to phosphate groups in the DNA rich in guanosine and cytosine residues (Stone et al., 1974; Scovell and Kroos, 1982; Macquet et al., 1980).

Oswald and Hall (1989) have established that the inhibition of DNA synthesis by *cis*Pt does not result from a primary effect on de novo purine, pyrmidine or deoxynucleotide synthesis. However, *cis*Pt does cause a decrease in DNA polymerase activity in the nucleus, an effect also observed with several *cis*Pt analogs. Inhibition of DNA synthesis, therefore, is apparently due to *cis*Pt binding to DNA bases, with a binding ratio of about 1 platinum atom per 1500–3000 bases. As discovered previously, chloro leaving ligands cause considerably more strand breakage and subsequently slower adduct formation than is observed with nonchloro ligands. Additional work to investigate the role of polymerase inhibition in blocking DNA synthesis was also conducted by these authors (Oswald et al., 1990). In these studies, DNA polymerase alpha was found to be sensitive to *cis*Pt, but not to analogs which do not significantly affect DNA synthesis. Binding of *cis*Pt to the polymerase appears to be through the apoprotein moiety because dGTP could reverse the binding and partially restore activity. Although the role of inhibition of DNA polymerase alpha appears to be substantial, the authors conclude that inhibition of this enzyme is likely to be not the only mechanism of action of *cis*Pt in inhibiting DNA synthesis.

The location of the platinum binding on the DNA strand was initially determined to be at sites that were rich in guanine (G) and cytosine (C) residues because of results from density gradient centrifugation studies with platinated and nonplatinated DNA. It was found that platinated DNA had a greater density than nonplatinated DNA and this increase in density was discovered to be directly proportional to the C–G content of the DNA and also to the ratio of drug to nucleotide. For example, when the synthetic polymer polyG–polyC was utilized, a 5-fold increase in density was observed after *cis*Pt exposure.

Although there are numerous reports that the cytotoxic effects of *cis*Pt are not cell cycle dependent, Roberts and Fraval (1978) showed that with both Chinese hamster and HeLa cells the binding of platinum to DNA was greater in G_1 than in either mid-S phase or in asynchronous cultures, and that mid-S phase cells were least susceptible to *cis*Pt cytotoxicity. It is known that DNA that is synthesized in early S phase has a C–G content that is greater than the C–G content of DNA synthesized in late S phase. The increased sensitivity of cells in G_1 might therefore be related to the higher platinum binding due to higher C–G content DNA at that stage relative to the DNA that was synthesized later in S phase, thus supporting the involvement of the C–G content in platinum–DNA binding and cytotoxicity.

The manner in which platinum binds to intact purified or cellular DNA has been uniquely determined by the use of endonucleases, enzymes which cleave DNA in a known and regular manner (Inagaki et al., 1984). In the presence of platinum binding, the activity of the enzyme is blocked and by determining the base pair sequence of the resulting oligonucleotide fractions and the nucleotides present at the cut ends of the sequences it is possible to deduce the nucleotides to which the drug is bound. When these studies were conducted it was found that platinum bound to fragments terminating at oligo G–oligo C sequences. These studies therefore further support a preferential binding of *cis*Pt to GC regions of the DNA chain.

It is now well-established that *cis*Pt, due to the bifunctional nature conferred on it by the two leaving chloride ligands, reacts initially by loss of a chlorine atom and the formation of a platinum–nitrogen bond to the N-7 nitrogen of a guanine base. This monofunctional adduct has been studied in vitro and in vivo and is found to be relatively transient in both situations, even though it represents a relatively high percentage of platinum bound to DNA (Plooy et al., 1985b). The site of this monofunctional binding can be typically any of the reactive sites on nucleobases which would be thermodynamically favored for metal interaction. Thus the N-7 atom of guanine, because of its high electron density, is a likely theoretical candidate whose involvement has, in fact, been demonstrated both in vitro and in vivo (Polissiou et al., 1985; Scovell and O'Connor, 1977; Fichtinger-Schepman et al., 1982; Mansy et al., 1973). Because of the lability of the second chlorine atom and the subsequent reactivity this confers on the *cis*Pt molecule, a second reaction then takes place with the replacement of the second chlorine with a second tissue ligand. It is presumed that this second reaction is with the N-7 of guanine but other sites are theoretically possible.

Thus the N-1 site of guanine, which is thermodynamically stable due to protonation at physiologic pH, becomes much more labile once an N-7 site is occupied by *cis*Pt. This reaction deprotonates the N-1 site and makes binding of the second reactive site on *cis*Pt theoretically possible (Martin, 1983; Kistenmacher et al., 1983). This would create a chelate structure, with the platinum atom bound to two nitrogen atoms from the same guanine.

Another possible reactive site is the O-6 of guanine, which has received little recent attention but which is theoretically possible, particularly under certain physiological conditions. An elegant hypothesis for the mechanism of interaction of *cis*Pt with nucleobases that was well supported with in vitro cytotoxicity data has been proposed, based on formation of N-7 and O-6 bidendate bonds with *cis*Pt (Rosenberg, 1978; Macquet et al., 1978). However, subsequent studies failed to find significant evidence for involvement of the O-6 bond in the binding of *cis*Pt to guanine (Hitchcock et al., 1983).

The importance of the bifunctional reaction in establishing the *cis*Pt mechanisms of action is illustrated by the fact that the ethylenediamine analog has little antitumor activity and does not for stearic reasons form bifunctional adducts (Macquet et al., 1983).

There are three potential results of this bifunctional binding. After the first bond forms with the DNA molecule, the establishment of a second bond to the platinum atom can form between ligands on protein, forming a DNA–protein crosslink. Alternatively, the second bond can form on a nucleobase on the second strand of DNA in the same helix as the first reacted strand, forming an interstrand crosslink. Finally the second reaction can occur with a second ligand on the same strand of DNA as the first reaction, forming an intrastrand crosslink. The relative proportion of these three reactants is reasonably well established, but their relative importance as the critical lesion caused by *cis*Pt is still a matter of conjecture.

Most workers in the field have evolved to the opinion that the principle lesion producing the antitumor effect and other biological activities of *cis*Pt is the intrastrand crosslink. This conclusion originally was based on largely circumstantial evidence, but eventually X-ray crystal structures of platinum bonded intramolecularly to purine bases on DNA were published (Admiraal et al., 1987; Sherman et al., 1985). However, the relationship between intrastrand links and antitumor activity has yet to unequivocally demonstrated, although realistic theoretical mechanisms have been proposed.

The DNA–protein crosslink has been demonstrated with both *cis*Pt and *trans*Pt, but the *cis*Pt link is repaired more rapidly and therefore is less persistent than the protein link formed from *trans*Pt (Ciccarelli et al., 1985). Because the *trans* configuration results in an inactive antitumor agent, the significance of the DNA–protein crosslink for antitumor activity is questionable. However, recent work has demonstrated extensive formation of interstrand crosslinks with DNA in a series of bis platinum complexes (Roberts et al., 1989). These complexes have two *cis* diammine platinum groups linked by an alkylamine and thus are potentially tetrafunctional. Interstrand crosslinks with DNA are more than 200-fold more prevalent with these compounds than with other *cis*Pt analogs. In vivo antitumor activity has yet to be demonstrated.

The interstrand crosslink has been very widely studied, in part because the analytical techniques available for their isolation and quantitation have been more readily available. Because of their widely studied nature, many correlations have been drawn between biological activity and formation rate and stability of these adducts. However, numerous studies have shown this adduct to be 1% of the total DNA–Pt adducts formed from *cis*Pt (Pascoe and Roberts, 1974; Eastman, 1982; Plooy et al., 1985a,b). Although it is certainly possible that such a specific and rare adduct may be responsible for the cytotoxicity and antitumor activity of *cis*Pt, conclusions should be carefully drawn until experiments are conducted which quantitate both inter- and intrastrand crosslinks in the same study and results are correlated with appropriate biological response parameters.

Studies with interstrand crosslinks demonstrated that the formation of these bonds occurred with a time lag of 6–12 hr (Zwelling et al., 1978), suggesting that time was required to form the second bond. These results were interpreted to indicate that the second bond formed in a time-dependent fashion. Similar studies have demonstrated the same time lag in the formation of intrastrand crosslinks (Filipski et al., 1980).

Several studies were directed at establishing the importance of the interstrand crosslink in biological activity of *cis*Pt and showed a correlation between rate and extent of interstrand crosslink formation and cell kill (Pascoe and Roberts, 1974; Zwelling et al., 1979; Plooy et al., 1985b). However, other results in *cis*Pt resistant tumor cell lines have not been consistent with the importance of interstrand links and other evidence argues against the importance of this adduct. One such line of evidence is the lack of correlation between interstrand crosslinks and levels of resistance in platinum resistant cell lines (Rawlings and Roberts, 1986). Furthermore, early work showed a lack of correlation between interstrand links and phage inactivation (Shooter et al., 1972), results which were confirmed later (Filipski et al., 1980). These authors showed that when interstrand crosslinked DNA was separated from noninterstrand crosslinked DNA after exposure of phage to *cis*Pt, the noninterstrand crosslinked DNA was inactive. When *trans*Pt was studied, the noninterstrand crosslinked DNA was still active in transfection. These results support the claim that *trans*Pt is inactive biologically because it cannot form the intrastrand crosslinks formed by *cis*Pt.

The interaction between the second chlorine atom and a guanine residue on the same strand of DNA has been proposed as the mechanism for the formation of the intrastrand crosslinks that comprise the overwhelming majority of the platinum–DNA adducts formed (Metzler, 1986). It appears as if the reaction can be between two adjacent guanines in a base sequence that contains a –G–C– sequence, or between two guanines separated by any other base such as a sequence that contains –G–X–C–, where X is adenine or another cytosine. There is also evidence that both G–A and G–C adducts also form.

Most of our knowledge of the reaction of *cis*Pt with DNA derives from in vitro studies. Initially investigators pursued the thermodynamic reactions that occur when *cis*Pt is added to a relatively simple (i.e. pure water) solution containing a single other solute, in most cases a potential reactive component of nucleic acids such as nucleosides or nucleotides. The results of these studies established that thermodynamically *cis*Pt could complex with cystosine (C), guanine (G) and adenosine (A), but not with thymidine (T). Later, more complex studies utilized purified di- and polynucleotides and other nucleotide sequences and demonstrated that platinum bound to GG or GC sequences and rarely to sequences containing A, but not to sequences containing T (Fesen and Harder, 1986). It was appreciated very early, however, that contamination of the thermodynamic reaction studies by using common buffers such as acetate or phosphate gave conflicting results and the ability of the acetate or phosphate groups to compete with the nucleotide of interest for the reactive binding site of the *cis*Pt molecule was demonstrated. Studies of increasing complexity then utilized whole purified DNA isolated from viruses, bacteria or other procaryotes and showed binding of Pt to normal or neoplastic cells that were exposed in vitro to *cis*Pt. Finally, binding was demonstrated to DNA of tissues from animals and patients treated with *cis*Pt (Fichtinger-Schepman et al., 1987; Reed et al., 1987).

When *cis*Pt was incubated with a tetranucleoside with CCGG sequence, the binding product was shown to contain one platinum atom per 4-base sequence, suggesting the binding of platinum to either two adjacent cytosine residues, two adjacent guanine residues, or to both cytosine and guanine. Further work with a trinucleoside showed one platinum atom for each GCG residue. The authors concluded that because of pH dependencies of the base proton shift and temperature dependency of the reaction, the binding was to the two guanine residues rather than to the guanine and cytosine, which would have been theoretically possible. This result supports the claim that platinum can bind to two guanines when they are separated by a third base. Thus platinum can bind to intrastrand guanines in one or two ways in vitro and the relevance of this binding in vivo is important. When *cis*Pt was exposed to DNA and then enzymes were used to degrade the DNA to small nucleotide fragments, both types of binding were found to occur at about equal frequency (Fichtinger-Schepman et al., 1987). The formation of this bifunctional adduct on the same DNA strand causes severe distortion in the spatial conformation of the strand, leading to an inability to replicate properly.

One of the early mysteries in platinum–DNA chemistry was the fact that *trans*Pt, the structural analog of *cis*Pt with the two chlorine atoms on opposite corners of the planar configuration from each other, was inactive as an antitumor agent but bound more DNA per unit dose than did the active *cis* configuration. One explanation for this inactivity of the *trans* configuration is that it cannot form the bifunctional complex with two guanines on the same DNA strand due to conformational hindrance of the molecule because the two reactive leaving groups are on opposite sides of the molecule. Further support for this mechanism is the similarity between the distance between the chlorines on the *cis*Pt molecule (3.3 Å) and the distance between the reactive nitrogen atoms on the DNA base sequence (3.4 Å).

Although the stereochemistry of *trans*Pt suggests its inability to form a bifunctional adduct, recent studies have isolated a platinum–DNA adduct formed between N-7 on 2 guanine molecules, a lesion exactly similar to that formed with *cis*Pt and DNA under similar reaction conditions, and theoretically unlikely to form due to the *trans* configuration of the molecule. This occurred at a very high Pt:nucleotide ratio of 0.1, however, which may be thermodynamically possible in an isolated system but unlikely in the cell in vivo.

One other reason for the inactivity of the *trans* isomer is related not to reaction of the molecules themselves, but to the apparent inability of the cell to repair the *cis*-derived bifunctional intrastrand adduct, and to extensively repair the adduct formed by the *trans*Pt. In several elegant papers Roberts and colleagues have discussed the role of DNA repair in the mechanism of action of *cis*Pt. Two cell lines which have the same capacity for excision repair (HeLa and Chinese Hamster) were shown to have different cytotoxic response to, and DNA binding of *cis*Pt, and that sensitivity was further increased in the most sensitive strain (HeLa) in the presence of the repair-inhibiting compound caffeine (Roberts and Fraval, 1978). Further, xeroderma pigmentosa cells, which are genetically deficient in DNA repair mechanisms, showed enhanced sensitivity to the effects of *cis*Pt, suggesting the presence of an intracellular mechanism to remove by excision the platinum–DNA lesion and that the most sensitive cells in vitro (and presumably in vivo also) are those with deficient excision repair processes (Plooy et al., 1985a). Interestingly, however, in bacterial systems differing in excision repair pathways, there does not appear to be differential sensitivities to *cis*Pt (Drobnik and Horacek, 1973).

Although most experimental effort has been devoted to studying the interaction of *cis*Pt with DNA as the most consequential molecular interaction, there are, however, several lines of evidence that are inconsistent with primary effect on DNA as being responsible for the biological activity. Under several experimental conditions, *cis*Pt is found to be essentially equal to *trans*Pt in its inhibition of DNA replication (Cleare, 1974; Thomson et al., 1972). In addition, *cis*Pt can induce giant cells with polyploid nuclei in *Physarum* sp. at drug concentrations which permit growth but have no effect on DNA synthesis (Wright et al., 1984). Finally, several groups have shown in vivo that at equitoxic doses, greater than 10 times more *trans*Pt than *cis*Pt binds to nuclear DNA and, at equivalent antitumor doses, greater than 100 times more *trans*Pt than *cis*Pt DNA adducts are observed. Although these results do not negate the myriad results implicating DNA binding as the critical lesion, they point out dramatically that the mere demonstration of drug–DNA binding may not always be sufficient to establish a true cause–effect relation and the conclusions that we draw from platinum–DNA adduct studies should be drawn with caution. Hence one possible mechanism that is consistent with the findings mentioned above is that platinum in some way preferentially disrupts the normal cell division process, rather than the DNA synthetic pathway, perhaps by interacting with tubulin to prevent its involvement in the division cycle. Tubulin has been investigated for its in vitro interaction with *cis*Pt, but effects were observed only at concentrations that were several orders of magnitude above those achievable physiologically (Peyrot et al., 1983).

In addition, recent evidence demonstrates that in one cell culture system, mammalian cells in culture had equal rates of repair of DNA adducts following both *cis*Pt and *trans*Pt even though the *cis*Pt adduct was associated with a greater inhibition of DNA synthesis. On the other hand, Olinski et al. (1983) have recently demonstrated that although Pt–protein crosslinking was more efficient with *trans*Pt, the *cis*Pt-induced protein link was more persistent.

The ultimate demonstration of the mechanism of *cis*Pt reaction with DNA must derive from studies where a Pt–DNA complex is isolated from cells of animals that have received *cis*Pt. The analytical difficulty in this endeavor is indicated by the realization that platinum appears to be active in inhibiting RNA polymerase function at a platinum:DNA base ratio of ca. 1:2500 (Srivastava et al., 1978), suggesting a very small amount of platinum bound to DNA may be sufficient to produce cytotoxic effects in vivo. This Pt:DNA base ratio is consistent with that reported by Oswald et al. (1990). Our current level of analytical sensitivity of atomic absorption spectroscopic determination of platinum is about 1 μg platinum per injection. This translates to a limit of sensitivity of about $1–5 \times 10^{-6}$ platinum atoms per DNA for both radiochemical or atomic absorption spectrophotometric methods (Macquet et al., 1983). The sensitivity of immunochemical methods, however, approaches 10^{-12} mol platinum per μg DNA (Plooy et al., 1985a; Poirier et al., 1982).

Frequently, in vitro studies of Pt binding are conducted at very high platinum:nucleotide ratios (e.g. 0.1). In order to achieve the kind of resolution of platinum:DNA adducts necessary at the extremely low concentration of platinum present in animal DNA it was necessary to await the development of an antibody to the DNA–Pt complex. Studies with such a DNA–Pt specific antibody have now been conducted by several laboratories using both polyclonal (Poirer et al., 1985; Plooy et al., 1985b) and monoclonal antibodies. This work has contributed immensely to furthering our understanding of the mechanism and ultimate reactants involved in the binding of *cis*Pt to DNA.

Work with antibodies to the *cis*Pt–DNA adduct has shown that in cell cultures the major Pt–DNA adducts are platinum bound monofunctionally to guanine (38%), and an intrastrand crosslink between two adjacent guanines (35%) (Plooy et al., 1985b). An intrastrand crosslink between guanine and adenine accounts for a large majority of the remaining adducts (Fichtinger-Schepman et al., 1987). During the 24 hr after exposure, approximately 75% of the monofunctional adduct disappears and the bifunctional GG adduct predominates (ca. 50%). This result is different from that observed when *cis*Pt is incubated with purified salmon sperm DNA in vitro, where the monofunctional adduct represents only about 10% of the adducts and the bifunctional GG adduct represented greater than 60%. It therefore appears as if the second step in the reaction between *cis*Pt and DNA occurs much more slowly in vivo than in vitro and that the thermodynamics of binding in vitro cannot be assumed to be relevant in vivo. Even these elegant studies to identify the in vivo Pt–DNA adducts fail to identify the biological significance of each adduct, except to demonstrate that the monofunctional adduct is relatively rapidly removed and therefore not very stable and that this adduct is extremely common in DNA exposed to the biologically inactive *trans* isomer.

The antibody originally was thought to be specific for a bifunctional adduct of *cis*Pt bound to two adjacent deoxyguanosine residues on the same DNA strand representing approximately 70% of the total DNA-bound platinum. More recent work, however, suggests that the antibody also recognizes adducts between G and C and now represents in excess of 80% of the Pt–DNA adducts. It is interesting to note that the author concludes that the adduct recognized by the antibody is probably not that which is responsible for DNA shortening (Lippard et al., 1983). The involvement of other indicators of biological activity of the adduct recognized by the antibody is now under intensive investigation but circumstantial evidence points to some relevance. Thus Reed et al. (1987) showed a correlation between Pt–DNA adducts recovered from blood of patients and response to *cis*Pt chemotherapy, and Fichtinger-Schepman et al. (1987) demonstrated that adduct presence in patients was dose-related, but subject to large interindividual variation.

The ultimate effect of DNA–platinum complex formation is to produce a block in cell division, presumably by blocking the replication of DNA. The exact mechanism producing this block, however, is unknown. It is known that binding of platinum to double stranded circular supercoiled DNA produces conformational changes that unwind the DNA (Scovell et al., 1983). Both *cis*Pt and *trans*Pt produce this effect, however, although the bis platinum complexes which form a majority of interstrand crosslinks, do not unwind supercoiled DNA (Roberts et al., 1989). It is also known that the changes in conformation produce changes in electrophoretic mobility that can be interpreted to result from the shortening of the DNA chain due to crosslinking, and to alter the migration of single stranded DNA by an amount that is parallel to the amount of platinum bound.

DNA binding has been the primary focus of investigations into *cis*Pt interactions with nucleic acids. Theoretically, however, the binding sites on deoxyribonucleosides found in DNA should be similar to those found in their ribonucleotide analogs found in RNA. Relatively little work has been conducted on the binding of *cis*Pt to RNA, however. Roberts and Pera (1983) showed that the quantity of platinum bound to RNA was greater than that bound to DNA, in part because the binding coefficient of platinum to RNA is greater than to DNA. However, the much larger molecular weight of DNA means that substantially more platinum atoms can be bound per molecule of DNA than is true with RNA. In addition, the mode of binding of *cis*Pt to RNA was found to be monodentate and to the N-7 atom of guanine (Rubin et al., 1983). No intrastrand crosslinks between guanines of RNA were reported. This finding undoubtedly has direct relevance to the mechanism of action of platinum on DNA structural integrity and probably contributes to the lack of pursuit by investigators of specific binding sites and mechanism and kinetics of platinum–RNA binding.

Baudin et al. (1989) investigated the binding of *trans*Pt to ribosomal RNA from *Xenopus* and identified preferential binding to 3 RNA regions centered around the hinge region at the junction of the 3 helical domains of the ribonucleoprotein particle. Previous work has suggested that the only difference in binding between the *cis* and *trans* forms of *cis*Pt was stability of the bond. If so, it therefore is likely that *cis*Pt might bind at similar sites on human ribonucleoprotein.

Danenberg et al. (1991) reacted *Tetrahymena* self-splicing rRNA (ribozyme) with *cis*Pt and found a loss of self-splicing ability and formation of several platinated RNAs. One species containing interstrand crosslinks was resistant to RNase digestion, and correlated closely with the loss of self-replication. This is interesting in light of the recognized importance of the DNA intrastrand crosslinks in *cis*Pt mechanism of action. The interaction was characteristic of affinity labeling, rather than a bimolecular interaction, and after treatment with urea, the RNA did not react with *cis*Pt, indicating that the native structure of the nucleic acid is required for interaction. Therefore, the secondary and/or tertiary structure of the RNA is necessary for *cis*Pt interaction, suggesting the importance of crosslinking in the mechanism of action.

Recent interest in mechanisms of resistance has also included investigations of *cis*Pt. Fichtinger-Schepman et al. (1989) have investigated the DNA adducts formed in resistant and susceptible tumors. Resistant tumors showed levels of total platinum, and platinum adducts that were similar to those observed in the susceptible tumor. However, the resistant tumor demonstrated a more rapid decrease in platinum levels and in levels of adducts than was seen in the sensitive tumors, suggesting that tissue turnover of platinum might be important in conferring resistance to therapy. It would have been interesting to have measured protein synthesis rates, or to have reported differential growth rates in the two tumors.

Chan et al. (1988) isolated satellite DNA from the heterochromatin of chromosomes from two sensitive human cell lines and from sublines made *cis*Pt resistant by exposure to increasing concentrations of *cis*Pt. Sequence analysis was conducted on cloned DNAs in order to investigate the hypothesis that resistance might be due to a shift in base composition favoring the less favorable binding nucleotides A and T. Their results, however, showed that resistance was *not* the result of a general alteration in DNA base sequences from C and G, to A and T. This is consistent with the results of Perera et al. (1990) who showed that when human DNA was isolated from *cis*Pt patients, the pattern of nine different oncogene protein products remained the same as those for non-*cis*Pt treated patients. This suggests that although *cis*Pt is a known mutagen, the base sequences are not significantly altered by exposure to *cis*Pt, and the slight oncogenic potential appears to derive not from changes in oncogene expression.

2.3. Protein Interactions

2.3.1. *Plasma*

Most of the research effort directed toward an understanding of the intracellular binding of *cis*Pt has focused on the interaction of *cis*Pt with DNA, as discussed above. From the perspective of toxic side effects—particularly to the kidney—the binding of platinum to proteins is perhaps of equal or greater importance. The binding of *cis*Pt to plasma proteins—notably albumin—has been extensively studied both in vitro and in vivo. In virtually all animal species, platinum binds to high molecular weight plasma components (commonly assumed to be albumin) when the drug is incubated in vitro at 37°C with freshly isolated plasma. The reaction takes place in a time-dependent fashion (Fig. 3) and the in vitro half-life of platinum not bound to high molecular weight components is on the order of 100 min depending on the species (Litterst, 1984a). Within a relatively narrow range of physiologically relevant concentrations the binding also has been demonstrated to be concentration dependent (LeRoy et al., 1979). The binding is also temperature dependent (Fig. 3). In vivo, the binding of *cis*Pt to high molecular weight components of plasma also occurs in a time-dependent fashion. The half-life, however, is substantially shorter, being in the order of 10 min (α) to 90 min (β) (Litterst et al., 1977). This is undoubtedly due to the fact that large quantities of unbound *cis*Pt are also being excreted during this time and thus the quantity of platinum neither excreted nor bound decreases very rapidly.

It is generally assumed that *cis*Pt binds mainly to albumin. However, definitive studies to identify other binding protein(s) have not been conducted. Manaka and Wolf (1978) showed, however, that 5 min after injection of radioactive *cis*Pt to rats, 40% of the radioactivity was associated with gamma globulins when protein electrophoresis was done, and that 35 min later 40% of the radioactivity was in the albumin fraction. The kinetics of this association have not been investigated but binding to globulins as well as albumin apparently occurs.

An analogous situation may exist with binding of gold compounds to plasma proteins, where

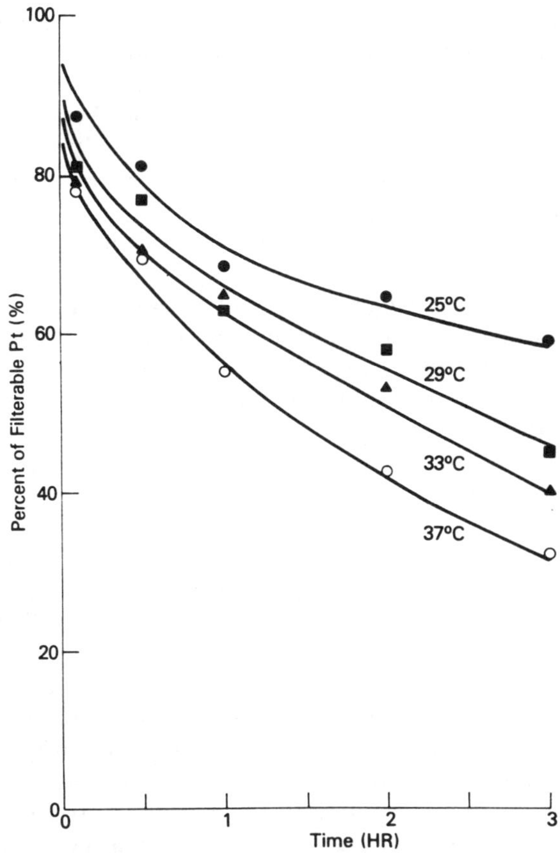

FIG. 3. Temperature dependent binding of platinum to fresh rat plasma in vitro.

binding to both albumin and globulin is reported (see below). The globulin-bound fraction represents a relatively greater quantity at later time (2 hr) than at earlier times (1 hr) because the binding is apparently more stable (Danpure et al., 1979). Thus albumin-bound gold is apparently exchangeable and decreases with time while globulin-bound gold is stable and is more constant with time, thus accounting for a larger percentage of total plasma gold at later time. Whether such kinetics are present with *cis*Pt is unknown, but would be consistent with the data that are available.

A specific globulin has been implicated in *cis*Pt binding. It has been shown that the activity of α_2 macroglobulin, a high molecular weight (ca. 750,000) plasma protein protease inhibitor, was inhibited by *cis*Pt by a mechanism that was initially suggested to be due to crosslinking of globulin subunits (Gonias and Pizzo, 1983). Subsequent studies (Pizzo et al., 1986), however, showed a specific interaction with a methionine residue on the α_2 macroglobulin surface which resulted in lack of recognition by the cellular α_2 macroglobulin receptor rather than a direct crosslinking of subunits as originally proposed.

*Cis*Pt interaction with the methionyl residue of alpha 2 macroglobulin produces extensive crosslinking and results in blockage of receptor recognition sites, and loss of proteinase activity (Pizzo et al., 1988). Reaction of *cis*Pt with alpha 1 proteinase inhibitor results in binding of platinum to methionine 358 at the reactive site of the enzyme. Methionyl binding of platinum on alpha 2 macroglobulin has been shown to occur at sites other than the active site. These authors further showed that *cis*Pt binds specifically to cysteine 34 of albumin in approximately a 1:1 molar ratio. *Trans*Pt, while binding to a greater extent to both albumin and to alpha 1 proteinase, did not possess the high degree of amino acid binding specificity seen with the *cis* isomer.

The actual binding sites for *cis*Pt on high molecular weight components of plasma are largely unknown. It has been suggested that *cis*Pt binds nonspecifically to all plasma proteins (Cole and Wolf, 1980), a mechanism that is consistent with the observation of binding to gamma globulin as well as albumin. However, one study reported the specific binding of *cis*Pt to the free cysteine residue on albumin (Gonias and Pizzo, 1983). This result is consistent with the theoretical reaction of *cis*Pt discussed above wherein the relatively high chloride concentration plasma would retard the aquation reaction and the replacement of chloride ligand would occur only with ligands of much higher nucleophilicity than water. The free sulfur of cysteine meets such a requirement. More recent work cited above clearly identifies the binding to the cys-34 site on albumin (Pizzo et al., 1988). Other proteins containing free sulfhydryl groups have been shown to similarly react with *cis*Pt in vitro (Aull et al., 1977; Howe-Grant and Lippard, 1983) although no noticeable consequences of this binding have ever been demonstrated in vivo.

Another large molecular weight plasma protein that has been implicated in *cis*Pt binding is cobalamine. Cobalamine is an essential cofactor for several enzymes involved in endogenous synthetic reactions, notably those involving myelin and vitamin B_{12}. In vitro the diaquo analog of *cis*Pt was shown to complex with several alkylcobalamines through the N-3 of the dimethylbenzimidazole moiety (Hogenkamp et al., 1980; Trugman et al., 1985). However, in conditions of *cis*Pt induced neurotoxicity, where inactivation of cobalamine-requiring enzymes might be expected, no change in serum B_{12} levels or in B_{12} binding capacity was observed and there was no change in urinary excretion of cobalamine metabolites suggesting that in vivo there was no change in cobalamine activity or synthesis in the presence of *cis*Pt (Trugman et al., 1985), although binding to the enzyme of *cis*Pt with no change in activity cannot be ruled out by the studies that were conducted.

*Cis*Pt was also found to bind to transferrin, the high molecular weight (80,000) metal-transporting glycoprotein most active in iron transport in vivo. When incubated at 4°C in bicarbonate buffer solution with iron-free transferrin for up to 2 weeks, only 5% of the incubated platinum bound to transferrin, but the platinum had the ability to displace gallium from transferrin binding sites (Stjernholm et al., 1978; Sykes et al., 1985; Tonini et al., 1986). In contrast nearly 20% of incubated K_2PtCl_4, and greater than 80% of incubated gallium, bound to transferrin. Approximately 1–2 atoms of platinum were bound per transferrin molecule, which is consistent with the binding of two iron atoms per molecule. Thus it appears thermodynamically possible for platinum from *cis*Pt to bind to transferrin, but whether this occurs to any appreciable extent in vivo has not been determined. It would be unlikely, however, that such a small quantity of metal bound to transferrin over the extremely long time course studied in vitro would significantly alter platinum kinetics or pharmacology in vivo.

Most of the work investigating the binding of *cis*Pt to plasma proteins—most specifically albumin—has utilized ultrafiltration techniques to separate protein-bound from nonprotein-bound platinum. The wording in reports of results of many of these studies reporting the amount of platinum binding to high molecular weight plasma components frequently suggests an unequivocal distinction between 'bound' and 'free' *cis*Pt with all of the attendant consequences for reactivity. It should be emphasized, however, that these studies usually separate free from bound *cis*Pt by means of a membrane with a molecular weight cutoff between 25,000 and 50,000. This means that although high molecular binding is relatively distinct from non-high molecular weight binding the latter fraction may—and in all likelihood does—contain platinum bound to substances with molecular weights below the membrane cutoff, and perhaps considerably below that level, and therefore does not represent free and unreacted (i.e. parent) *cis*Pt, but rather *cis*Pt which may be either in the dichloro form, or in any uncharacterized form in which it is bound to very low molecular weight substances. Thus Daley-Yates and McBrien (1984) showed the formation of a number of low molecular weight platinum-bound species when *cis*Pt was incubated in vitro at extremely high and unphysiological concentration of *cis*Pt. Although none of these complexes were positively identified, one of them had the same retention time in the authors' high pressure liquid chromatography assay as a complex formed when *cis*Pt was incubated in vitro with methionine. Similarly, other authors have shown the binding of *cis*Pt to reduced glutathione (Litterst et al., 1982a) and to metallothionein in vitro (Endresen et al., 1984) and in tissue homogenates and cytosolic fractions from animals treated with *cis*Pt (Litterst, 1984a; Litterst et al., 1986; Kraker et al., 1985; Parti and Wolf, 1990). It is assumed that these adducts must also form in plasma as well. It should therefore be cautioned that *cis*Pt appears to be bound to very low molecular weight plasma components as well as very high weight components and this binding occurs very soon after the administration of *cis*Pt to animals or rapidly in *in vitro* incubations.

Several authors have investigated the potential interaction between *cis*Pt and other drugs that are known to be protein bound and found that the kinetics and binding of *cis*Pt was unaffected by concomitant treatment with trimetrexate (Hudes et al., 1991), etoposide (O'Dwyer et al., 1991), IL-2 (Gandara et al., 1989), and methotrexate (el-Yazigi et al., 1989), and there is no difference with difference routes of administration (Shani et al., 1989). As might be expected, complexing of *cis*Pt with carboxymethyl-dextrans of different molecular weights led to differing plasma half-lives, plasma levels of free drug, and rates of protein binding, depending on the molecular size of the dextran complex (Schechter et al, 1989). Efficacy was measured in vitro however, so true efficacy or bioavailability of such complexes are still unknown.

2.3.2. *Tissue Protein Binding*

Although the binding of *cis*Pt to plasma proteins has been relatively widely studied, the binding to nonspecific tissue proteins has been as widely neglected. Numerous studies have shown reaction with proteins—mostly enzymes—in vitro (Aull et al., 1977; Howe-Grant and Lippard, 1983; Uozumi and Litterst, 1985), but similar reactions in vivo have not been demonstrated (Litterst et al., 1982a; Uozumi and Litterst, 1986). In fact, the in vivo relevance of such in vitro interactions is questionable because the concentrations and incubations conditions are highly artificial relative to physiological concentrations, temperature and times of incubation. When comparable studies monitored ATPase in vivo, no effects were detectable (Uozumi and Litterst, 1985).

Involvement of protein kinase C (PKC) has been implicated in *cis*Pt's mechanism of action. In a paper by Isonishi et al. (1990), it was discovered that pretreatment of tumor bearing animals with tetradecanoylphorbal acetate, which activates PKC, increased the susceptibility of the tumor to *cis*Pt, while producing no change in cellular accumulation of platinum. Treatment with phorbol, which has no effect on PKC, did not alter the sensitivity of the tumor to *cis*Pt. When animals were pretreated with staurosporine, an inhibitor of PKC, the increased sensitivity of the tumor to *cis*Pt was lost. This effect was observed in both a *cis*Pt sensitive and *cis*Pt resistant tumor line, and suggests the involvement of PKC in *cis*Pt sensitivity of tumors.

*Cis*Pt binding to tissue components—in all probability proteins—has been recognized since the first studies of distribution of platinum following *cis*Pt administration to animals demonstrated high concentrations of platinum existing for very long times in most tissues (Litterst et al., 1976). Farris et al. (1985) calculated that the half-time of the tissue bound platinum was similar enough to the biological half-time of the tissue proteins to suggest that the only way tissue platinum could be removed was by the normal catabolism of the protein to which it was bound. This prediction has recently been supported by studies in both animals and patients which showed platinum persistence for weeks and months. In these studies (Poirier et al., 1992) persistence was demonstrated of both platinum, and platinum–DNA adducts for up to 14 days (the longest time studied) in animals, and for 7–15 months after the most recent *cis*Pt dose in patients.

The issue of *cis*Pt binding by a specific tissue transport protein has been raised by the suggestion of countercurrent platinum secretion in the proximal tubule of the nephron. Although *cis*Pt is clearly secreted in the nephron, a receptor has never been identified. An interesting finding by Binks and Dobrota (1990) was that *cis*Pt is absorbed across the rat everted small intestine. The oral absorption of *cis*Pt was established nearly two decades ago, but never investigated further until this study. According to the authors absorption was quantitatively similar to, if not actually greater than, that of the orally active carboplatin. These authors demonstrated that there was no active transport mechanism for either drug and that both were passively absorbed by a process that followed the expected first order kinetics. A similar mechanism might be operative in the renal tubule. Although not specifically mentioned, *cis*Pt might be less active orally than is carboplatin because the highly acidic conditions in the stomach cause such rapid aquation that an uncharged species exists for too short a time to be effectively absorbed. This theory is supported by their data which showed that at low pH, carboplatin absorption was substantially increased.

Recently, covalent binding of platinum to proteins in cellular organelles from kidney and other organs has been demonstrated (Litterst and Schweitzer, 1988a,b), with half-times of covalently bound platinum ranging from 33 to 186 hr depending on the organelle (Litterst and Schweitzer, 1988a). This finding should come as no surprise due to the extensive plasma protein binding of *cis*Pt and the very long tissue half-life of platinum discussed above. The authors had hoped to relate covalent binding to the sensitivity of the kidney to *cis*Pt, but differences between kidney and other organs were of questionable magnitude to be responsible for the sensitivity of this organ. However, in studies with *cis*Pt-sensitive and *cis*Pt-resistant guinea pigs, they reported a 2-fold greater amount of platinum covalently bound in renal subcellular fractions of platinum-sensitive relative to platinum-resistant guinea-pigs (Litterst and Schweitzer, 1988b). However, the involvement of covalently bound platinum in the mechanism of renal failure is still unknown, as is the specific proteins to which the platinum is covalently bound.

Ewen et al. (1988) tried to correlate platinum tissue concentration with renal toxicity and discovered that although total renal concentrations of platinum were similar for *cis*Pt and several nonrenal toxic analogs, the concentration in the pars recta of the cortex was greater for *cis*Pt than for the analogs, and that concentration and/or localization within the segment of the nephron may explain the lower renal toxicity of second generation platinum analogs.

The association of platinum with cytoplasmic proteins was shown for $Pt(NH_3)_2Cl_4$ as early as 1967 (Renshaw and Thomson, 1967). More recently, it was shown by gel chromatography that liver and kidney cytosol from animals treated with *cis*Pt contains platinum associated with several high molecular weight peaks as well as very low molecular weight peaks (Litterst, 1984a). Thus complexes with high molecular weight proteins as well as low molecular weight substances such as amino acids or free nucleobases also can occur. The binding site or mode of association of this platinum in tissue has not been investigated until recently, however. Recent results from our laboratory showed that nearly all hepatic and renal platinum present during the first 24 hr after treatment was covalently bound to protein, in the classic sense of being stable when a trichloroacetic acid-insoluble pellet was exhaustively extracted with hot methanol (Litterst and Schweitzer, 1988b). The binding is apparently complete by 1 hr after dosing but decays very slowly, with a half-life of 196 hr in kidney cytoplasm.

One unique aspect of this finding is the temporal difference between *cis*Pt binding to protein and *cis*Pt binding to DNA. It has been shown that the binding of *cis*Pt to DNA requires 6–12 hr to completely form the bifunctional adduct (Zwelling et al., 1978; Filipski et al., 1980) presumably due to the time required for the monofunctional adduct to be converted to a bifunctional adduct. However, the results with covalent binding of *cis*Pt to tissue proteins show this binding to be essentially complete by 1 hr (Litterst and Schweitzer, 1988a,b) and suggests a potentially different mode of binding of *cis*Pt to protein nucleophiles than to DNA and supports the SN_2 type of direct and relatively immediate binding of Pt directly to a strong nucleophile, similar to what was discussed above in the context of Pt-protein binding in plasma. It may well be that the monofunctional platinum–nucleophile adduct in proteins is stable enough to be resistant to solvent extraction and the covalent binding to tissue proteins reflects the presence of a monofunctional adduct rather than the bifunctional adduct which is present in DNA.

Although *cis*Pt has been shown to bind covalently to transferrin (Sykes et al., 1985), some data argue against covalent binding. For example diethyl-dithiocarbamate (DDC), a strong nucleophile, has the ability to remove platinum from tissue binding sites in the renal tubules (Bodenner et al., 1986). This suggests that the nature of the Pt–protein bond is a coordination complex, where nucleophilic interaction under physiological conditions would be unlikely. This question of different modes of binding also addresses the question of the difference in DNA binding between *cis*Pt and *trans*Pt, which has frequently been attributed to different 'modes' of binding on the same receptor to explain the different spectra of biological activities.

In addition to plasma proteins, *cis*Pt also has been shown to bind to histone and nonhistone proteins in the nucleus (Banjar et al., 1984; Nazimiec et al., 1982). Early work showed protein–protein crosslinks formed when *trans*Pt was incubated with nucleosomal core particles but *cis*Pt produced mainly DNA binding (Lippard and Hoeschele, 1979). At high Pt:nucleosome ratios and after relatively long times (2 days), *cis*Pt also formed protein–protein crosslinks. Subsequent work also failed to find histone crosslinks with *cis*Pt and reported mainly protein–DNA adducts (Houssier et al., 1983). Although several specific and distinct proteins were shown to bind *trans*Pt the exact identity of these proteins were not determined except to designate by relative elution fraction (Nazimiec et al., 1982).

Parti and Wolf (1990) showed that a significant amount of platinum was incorporated into chromosomal protein following administration of *cis*Pt to rats. This may be related to the increased number of mutational events (Sister Chromatid Exchanges) reported from blood cells of patients treated with *cis*Pt (Perera et al., 1990). Hayes and Scovell (1991b) investigated the influence of *cis*Pt when bound to chromatin or the nucleosome core particle. Binding of *cis*Pt to chromatin disrupts its structure sufficiently to retard the rate of nuclease digestion and alter the digestion profile. Binding to the core particle had no such effect. It therefore appears as if *cis*Pt binding does not disrupt DNA structure within the core particle, but has a major effect on internucleosomal DNA. The reason for this preferential binding was not elucidated, but one possibility mentioned by the authors is that the intrastrand crosslinks may show preference for adjacent guanines in the linker region, but this then raises the unanswered question of why the specificity for the linker region. The covalent protein–protein crosslinks in chromatin apparently involve nucleosomal low mobility proteins. Further work by these authors (Hayes and Scovell, 1991a) showed that nuclease digestion profiles were different from those of DNase I digestion profiles, indicating that the covalent crosslink between DNA and the high mobility proteins is inaccessible to DNase. Results of these and other studies have established that the predominant modification produced by platinum binding on core particle DNA is such that the helical structure of the nucleic acid backbone is not modified by complexing with *cis*Pt. Perez et al. (1991) also have reported results that establish the stability of the DNA helix after binding by *cis*Pt.

*Cis*Pt has been shown to depress protein synthesis both in vitro and in vivo (Harder and Rosenberg, 1970), but the mechanism of this inhibition has been assumed to be through the *cis*Pt effect on DNA replication rather than on a direct binding or interaction with the protein synthetic mechanism (e.g. ribosomes) itself.

All too frequently the biological relevance of in vitro studies utilizing metals is questionable due to the artificial conditions employed to generate metal–ligand complexes. Frequently concentrations of metals in such reaction mixtures are orders of magnitude above those predicted or found physiologically, the temperature under which the reactions are conducted are considerably above physiological temperatures, or the length of time the reactions are allowed to run in order to generate reaction products are many hours, or even days, long. In addition reaction mixtures from in vitro studies are tightly controlled and frequently contain only the substrate (metal) and the proposed receptor molecule. The presence of small molecules such as electrolytes, bicarbonate ions, phosphate groups etc., all of which are present in relatively large concentrations in vivo, is largely ignored in such studies. This combination of artificial conditions frequently makes the in vivo relevance of such studies questionable. In addition, because hydrogen ions compete competitively with the cationic metal complexes or metal ions, pH may have a major significant effect on the interactions of platinum or other metals. Frequently in vitro studies are conducted at pH which favors a particular reaction rather than one which accurately reflects the biological milieu in which the reaction will proceed in vivo. Many of the above objections pertain to early, and some subsequent, studies on the reaction of *cis*Pt with nucleic acids and proteins, notably enzymes. Results of these kinds of studies are valuable for providing information on the thermodynamics of drug–receptor interactions but are frequently found to have little relevance to situations and conditions that prevail in vivo. In the case of nucleic acids, however, the in vitro results have largely been confirmed by recent in vivo studies where antibodies to DNA–Pt adducts have been utilized to demonstrate the same platinum–guanine adducts that were shown to be formed in vitro are formed in vivo as well.

The reaction of *cis*Pt with sulfhydryl groups on proteins may be a relatively nonspecific reaction and thereby not likely to be directly involved in tissue mechanism of action. Gonias and Pizzo (1983) showed that *cis*Pt reacted with the cysteine of albumin but concluded that sulfhydryl groups represented only a small percentage of potentially reactive nucleophilic sites. This is similar to the nonspecific protein binding that occurs with a wide variety of therapeutic agents and to the mechanism of other metals when they interact with tissue sulfhydryl protein, where Clarkson (1986) reported that less than 0.1% of the potentially available protein binding sites in fact interacted with mercury to produce mercury-induced renal failure. This is almost exactly the same binding as has been shown for platinum binding to protein (Roberts and Pera, 1983). Tissue protein concentrations of platinum in the range of μg/mg (Litterst et al., 1976; Farris et al., 1985) may be several orders of magnitude too great for tissue protein binding to be realistically considered as directly relevant to *cis*Pt mechanisms of action. This is also suggested by the fact that enzyme inhibition studies when conducted in vitro have required extremely high concentrations of *cis*Pt or elevated temperatures or exposure times before enzyme inhibition can be demonstrated. The only time that in vivo enzyme studies were conducted in parallel to in vitro studies was when inhibition of ATPases was investigated. In that case (Uozumi and Litterst, 1985) no detectable change in ATPase activity was observed in vivo. It therefore seems unlikely that a direct effect of *cis* Pt tissue binding—particularly with respect to enzymes—is significant enough to be responsible for target organ toxicity of *cis* Pt.

Binding to low and intermediate weight tissue components is also recognized, however. Thus metallothionein and glutathione have been shown by several investigators to be the site of *cis* Pt interaction in both kidney and liver. The interaction of platinum with endogenous low molecular weight compounds such as glutathione has attracted attention due to the observation that *cis* Pt toxicity appeared to correlate with endogenous concentrations of glutathione. This low molecular weight (ca. 300) protein is a strong nucleophile due to its free sulfhydryl group and should therefore represent a likely site of *cis* Pt interaction. In addition, subcellular distribution of platinum following *cis* Pt administration to animals shows strong localization of platinum in cell compartments such as cytosol which are known to contain high concentrations of glutathione. Recent studies in animals have shown that *cis* Pt toxicity is directly related to concentrations of glutathione (Litterst et al., 1986). However, decreases in lethality and renal toxicity of a dramatic nature do not correlate with the magnitude or localization of changes in intracellular platinum distribution that might be expected if glutathione was the molecular target of *cis* Pt action (Litterst et al., 1986). Thus, a more likely explanation is that this tripeptide represents a nonspecific binding site for *cis* Pt by virtue of its highly nucleophilic sulfhydryl group. A similar lack of effect on intracellular concentrations of platinum following apparent binding is also observed with sodium thiosulfate (STS), where doses of STS that provide dramatic protection against renal toxicity and lethality result in nonbiologically significant changes in subcellular distribution or localization of platinum (Uozumi and Litterst, 1986), suggesting that the localization of platinum in subcellular organelles may not be a critical determinant in *cis* Pt induced renal toxicity or lethality.

An interesting study in this regard was that of Levi et al. (1980) who studied the effect of *cis* Pt administration on sulfhydryl concentration in rat kidney. These authors showed that nephrotoxic doses of *cis* Pt produced only very small (14%) decreases in sulfhydryl concentration and they concluded that *cis* Pt does not react directly with sulfhydryl groups. This conclusion was based in part on the lack of reaction with cysteine in vitro. Similarly, work by Litterst et al. (1982a) showed that there was no decrease in renal, and relatively small decreases in hepatic, glutathione levels following administration of *cis* Pt to rats. Both of these studies were conducted at times beginning 24 hr after drug administration, so no information was available about effects at earlier times. Leyland-Jones et al. (1983), however, looked at renal glutathione levels as early as 5 min after treatment of rats with *cis* Pt and found no change in total glutathione during the first 4 hr after drug treatment. Thus it appears from these studies that the reaction of *cis* Pt with renal sulfhydryls, including glutathione, may not be a primary effect, but may merely be a nonspecific interaction that occurs following interaction of *cis* Pt with the primary receptor.

Another strong nucleophile that has all the potential of interacting with *cis* Pt is metallothionein (MT). This small protein (ca. 6000 MW) is composed of an amino acid sequence that contains 30% cysteine. After the initial demonstration that platinum could bind to a MT-like protein (Litterst, 1984a) several other laboratories subsequently confirmed the work and more firmly established the nature of the binding protein (Mason et al., 1984; Zelazowski et al., 1984). However, no one has yet definitely established by amino acid sequence that MT is the binding protein. Theoretical support for the involvement of MT in the *cis* Pt mechanisms of action derives from in vitro studies which showed that the MT content was greater in platinum-resistant cells in culture than in platinum-sensitive cells (Bakka et al., 1981). In vivo work, however, showed that when cadmium pretreatment was used as an inducing regimen to increase MT content of liver and kidney in vivo, the amount of platinum bound to MT was also increased (Litterst, 1984a) even though *cis* Pt itself did not produce an increase in MT levels. However, induction of MT did not always lead to decrease in toxicity or altered effectiveness of *cis* Pt (Naganuma et al., 1985). Thus it appears as if MT may also represent only a site of nonspecific binding for *cis* Pt rather than a critical molecule involved in the mechanism of action of *cis* Pt.

In contrast to several other works reported above, Suzuki and Cherian (1990) found no increase in either renal or hepatic MT following either a single high dose, or multiple daily injections of lower doses for a week. These authors found only 20% of platinum associated with low molecular weight compounds in renal cytosol. When MT was induced with injections of zinc, MT increased in both kidney and liver but there was no localization of platinum in a column chromatographic fraction containing MT. These authors similarly found that pretreatment with buthionine sulfoximine, an inhibitor of glutathione synthesis, produced no change in *p*-aminohippuric acid uptake by kidney, suggesting no involvement with glutathione in *cis*Pt-mediated renal dysfunction. In direct contrast to these results, Bongers et al. (1988) have calculated the molar ratio of platinum bound to purified equine MT and found that at neutral pH, a monomer is formed that contains 7 mol of platinum per mol MT. At extreme acid pH, however, a polymer apparently is formed that contains 17 mol platinum per mol of MT. These studies utilized highly purified MT, and platinum from a 20-fold molar excess of K_2PtCl_4, rather than using physiologically relevant ratios of MT and *cis*Pt.

The effect on toxicity of binding to low molecular weight components is not yet resolved, although Daley-Yates and McBrien (1984) have shown high toxicity from one of their low molecular weight complexes. However, these same authors also showed that the methionine adduct that formed in their system was in fact not toxic, although injection of a mixture of their low molecular weight adducts was more toxic than the parent *cis*Pt. This may reflect the presence of the aquo and/or hydroxy species in relatively high concentrations, however, and these products are known to be highly reactive and therefore toxic (Rosenberg, 1978). The lack of toxicity of the protein bound *cis*Pt can be assumed from classic pharmacology if the protein to which the platinum binds is not the ultimate site of action. In fact Cole and Wolf (1980) showed that when a *cis*Pt–protein adduct was allowed to form in vitro, isolated and then injected into rats, it produced neither elevations of BUN nor histological evidence of renal damage.

Whereas binding to proteins has occupied most of the attention of investigators, binding to other receptors also is possible. Thus Sarna et al. (1988) have shown that exposure to *cis*Pt liberates sialic acid residues from the surface of fibrosarcoma cells. These cells were less tumorigenic when injected into mice than were similar cells not exposed to *cis*Pt. This result suggest that *cis*Pt has the ability to unmask antigenic sites on cell surfaces, thus increasing the immunogenicity of the cells, and potentially making them less virulent. Other authors also have found antigenic receptors modified following exposure to *cis*Pt. Roche et al. (1988b) found that exposure to *cis*Pt resulted in nearly an order of magnitude less binding of a monoclonal antibody to alpha 2 macroglobulin than was seen before *cis*Pt exposure, suggesting a modification of the antigenic recognition site on the macroglobulin by *cis*Pt. The reaction with platinum does not occur at the methionyl residue of the antigen receptor site because in other work using a form of alpha 2 macroglobulin in which this site was conformationally not exposed, these same authors (Roche et al., 1988a) showed that platinum was still bound to the macroglobulin molecule even though the receptor was unavailable for binding. This interaction prevented a conformational change that is deemed necessary for interaction with a neoantigen.

2.4. Protective Mechanisms

One of the serious impediments to the broader efficacy of *cis*Pt is the dose-limiting renal toxicity that is seen. In early clinical studies the incidence of severe nephrotoxicity was in excess of 75% in patients receiving two courses of therapy and was 33% when only one course was given (Higby et al., 1973). The simple use of high volume hydration with or without diuretics dramatically reduced the incidence of renal failure to manageable levels (Cvitkovic et al., 1977), as long as total doses did not exceed approximately 100 mg/M^2. Above that dose, both incidence and severity of renal toxicity increased to unacceptable levels. The chemical reactivity of the *cis*Pt molecule has been exploited by enterprising clinicians in an attempt to find chemical means of avoiding or reversing the systemic toxicity of *cis*Pt, while hopefully not affecting the antitumor activity. Thus a large number of chemicals and drugs have been tested as potential antidotes for *cis*Pt-induced toxicity. Three methods have found clinical acceptance to a greater or lesser degree and the chemical basis for these three will be discussed in this section.

The most widely utilized technique for blocking the renal toxicity of *cis*Pt is the administration of the drug in a high concentration of NaCl (Ozols et al., 1984). The rationale for this technique was based on the fact that the high chloride concentration would force the aquation reaction (Fig. 2) strongly to the left and prevent the formation of the toxic aquo and hydroxy derivatives.

The technique was initially demonstrated in vivo using a rodent model (Litterst, 1981) and resulted in a dramatic decrease in lethality and renal toxicity that correlated with the amount of chloride ion present in the vehicle of administration. Antitumor efficacy was maintained in a murine tumor model, although subsequent work has questioned this aspect of the study (Aamdal et al., 1984). Clinically the procedure has permitted doses nearly twice as high as traditionally allowable, with no increase in renal toxicity. Hearing loss and peripheral neuropathy, however, are apparently not protected (Ozols et al., 1984). An apparent increased response concomitant with the increased dose has not been reported in early clinical studies (Ozols et al., 1984). Although the theoretical rationale for the high chlorine concentrations is reasonable, the in vivo mechanism is not as clearly obvious. The excessive chloride concentration should be quickly diluted in the circulation and the rationale for differential protection of only the kidney, while not sparing the ear, peripheral nerves or tumor is difficult to understand. Subsequent authors have postulated a chlorouresis as being involved in the renal protection (Earhart et al., 1983). While the increased clinical efficacy is indisputable and probably related to the increased dose, the actual mechanism for the renal sparing effect may not be that which was originally proposed.

Fulco et al. (1990) have pursued the question of how salt reduces the toxicity of *cis*Pt by investigating the protein binding of *cis*Pt in mice after pretreatment with 0.9% NaCl (NS) or distilled water and found that NS decreased the amount of platinum bound to plasma proteins. They postulated that the decrease in toxicity of *cis*Pt in the presence of salt results in a reduced binding of aquated *cis*Pt products to tissue and plasma proteins. Dumas et al. (1990) came to similar conclusions when a similar study was conducted in patients. Whether this effect is in addition to, or in place of, the previously proposed change in quantity and rate of aquation resulting from salt presence, was not addressed.

A second protective mechanism of clinical relevance is the use of STS. The theoretical mechanism of this protective effect is the preferred interaction of the strongly nucleophilic sulfhydryl groups on STS with the highly labile chlorides on the *cis*Pt molecule to form an inactive complex (Howell and Taetle, 1980; Ishizawa et al., 1981; Elferink et al., 1986). The clinical use of this procedure is mainly in therapeutic regimens which utilize *cis*Pt intraperitoneally for cancers restricted to the abdominal cavity, and STS intravenously to prevent systemic toxicity of *cis*Pt that is absorbed from the peritoneal reservoir into the systemic circulation (Howell, et al., 1982). Success has been shown by response in several solid tumors, with no renal or bone marrow toxicity at doses of *cis*Pt three times greater than traditionally utilized. The success of this method is based on the predictable first order absorption of *cis*Pt from the peritoneal cavity into the systemic circulation (Howell et al., 1982; Litterst et al., 1982c), which means the absorbed *cis*Pt can be easily inactivated by relatively modest circulating levels of STS.

Hasuda et al. (1989) have combined sodium thiosulfate with angiotensin-II (AT) in rats, and concluded that this combination was superior to STS alone as an antidote for *cis*Pt renal toxicity. Their postulated mechanism for this effect is that the AT-induced hypertension reduces delivery of platinum to the kidney, thus reducing exposure and binding. This conclusion derived from observations that renal concentrations were reduced by approximately one third, while tumor concentrations were increased by nearly 50% under the influence of AT.

Perhaps the most exciting use of *cis*Pt chemical reactivity to potentially antidote *cis*Pt toxicity is the use of DDC. It has been observed that the use of DDC after *cis*Pt administration had the ability to reverse the renal and gastrointestinal toxicities of *cis*Pt (Borch and Pleasants, 1979; Khandekar, 1983). The unique aspect of this finding was the ability to reverse the *cis*Pt toxicity when DDC was given up to 2 hr after *cis*Pt, in contrast to the other mechanisms discussed, where STS or NaCl had to be given before or simultaneously with *cis*Pt. The exciting finding of these studies was the ability of DDC to apparently reverse the binding of *cis*Pt to renal tubule cells (Bodenner et al., 1986), although early studies did not monitor renal platinum levels. DDC does not alter antitumor efficacy in animal models. Subsequent work has established that DDC has the ability to reverse the monofunctional binding of platinum to guanine and the bifunctional binding to adenosine, but to be unable to alter the bifunctional interaction between platinum and guanine (Bodenner et al., 1986). This accounts for the ability to reverse the effect of bound platinum and is consistent with the time course of platinum binding to nucleobases discussed earlier. All of the work detailing mechanism of action was done on interstrand binding at exaggerated conditions

(50°C for 48 hr) but may be applicable to the more prevalent intrastrand crosslinks and physiological conditions. It is disappointing that clinical results with this procedure have yet to be published.

Intensive work continues in an attempt to develop/discover an antidote that can ameliorate the adverse effects of *cis*Pt on the kidney, peripheral nervous system and ear, without blocking the efficacy of the drug. A major focus of these studies has been sulfhydryl interactions. Leeuwenkamp et al. (1990), using a highly theoretical method for calculating inactivation of *cis*Pt, calculated that under conditions of their simulation thiosulfate inactivated *cis*Pt better than did mesna or diethyldithiocarbamate, which both were about equivalent in their protective ability. Goel et al. (1990) estimated the metabolism of *cis*Pt and the potential for protection by DDC in patients. Their results indicate the following a bolus, or short term infusion of *cis*Pt, the majority of platinum in plasma for a period up to 4 hr still can react with DDC, but as these reactive species are eliminated (or are bound), they are replaced with longer lived, but nonreactive species. A further highlight of this work is the finding that the potential for neutralization of *cis*Pt by DDC is apparently not sufficient to account for the extensive protection afforded by this antidote. This latter finding was supported by other clinical studies in which the authors measured changes in creatinine clearance (Goel et al., 1989).

An extremely promising clinical finding is the potential ability of glutathione to reduce the toxicity of *cis*Pt (Oriana et al., 1988). It is known that animals pretreated with glutathione (GSH), are highly resistant to the toxicity of a subsequent dose of *cis*Pt, as measured by both mortality and BUN elevation (Litterst et al., 1986). Clinical investigators in Italy have pretreated a small number of patients ($n = 15$) with GSH followed 15 min later by a 30 min infusion of *cis*Pt (90 mg/M^2) with total treatment doses of near 800 mg/M^3. There were no observable increases in creatinine (Oriana et al., 1988) or signs of ototoxicity or neuropathy (M. Tedeschi, personal communication). Complete remissions were obtained in five out of six advanced ovarian carcinoma patients. If these results are confirmed by other, more extensive clinical trials, the potential for expanding the use and efficacy of *cis*Pt may be extensive.

Boogaard et al. (1991) have investigated the ability of methylthiobenzoic acid (MTBA) to block renal toxicity of *cis*Pt and have found that the aquated form of *cis*Pt reacts with the methylthio sulfur atom by nucleophilic attack. The effect was demonstrated in the ability of a relatively low dose of MTBA to completely block the renal toxicity of a toxic dose of *cis*Pt. However, these studies, and those done in vitro to show transport of MTBA into proximal renal tubular cells, were done with pretreatment. It would be interesting to see similar studies conducted after treatment with *cis*Pt, similar to the work previously discussed with diethyldithiocarbamate, which apparently has the ability to reverse platinum–protein bonds.

3. GOLD

In the early 1980s several publications appeared reporting the ability of Auranofin, an antiarthritic drug containing the noble metal gold, to inhibit the growth of tumor cells in tissue culture with a greater efficacy than was found with the anticancer drug cisplatin (Simon et al., 1979). Later, Aranofin was shown to inhibit the growth of P388 murine leukemia cells in animals, with increases in life span ranging from 30 to 120%, depending on the treatment regimen (Simon et al., 1981). These discoveries have produced an increased interest in the clinical potential of gold complexes in the treatment of human malignancies. Unfortunately, Auranofin, an Au-I phosphine complex, has been found to have antitumor activity in only one out of 15 animal tumor systems screened in vivo for response (Mirabelli et al., 1985), thus suggesting that the P388 system is somehow unique in its sensitivity to this compound. A diphenylphosphine–gold chloride complex, however, is active against several solid tumor systems in vivo (Berners-Price et al., 1986), although this activity may be due to the phosphine moiety rather than to the gold atom. It is also enlightening to note that when diphenylphosphine gold chloride was tested against P388 tumor grown intraperitoneally in mice, it was active only when injected i.p. and was inactive when injected i.v., s.c., or p.o. (Berners-Price et al., 1986), thus suggesting that its antitumor effect may be merely a cytotoxic effect manifested when cells in suspension come into direct contact with the highly reactive gold complex. Although not yet approved for clinical trials, gold containing drugs have the potential of being useful in human chemotherapy. The long history of use of the water soluble gold thiolates in arthritis treatment has recently been supplemented by the introduction of orally active gold phosphine complexes, most notably Auranofin. The historical experience with these agents in human medicine will certainly provide an incentive for promoting clinical trials in cancer therapy as well as providing an incentive for promoting our understanding of the biochemical and pharmacological effects of these agents. An overview of gold-containing drugs is therefore included here because of the awakening interest in their anticancer potential, mainly from in vitro activity. This brief review will concentrate on gold-I, because of its proven clinical usefulness in arthritis therapy, and gold-III because of the numerous similarities in chemistry and biological activity with the highly successful platinum-containing anticancer drugs discussed above.

3.1. CHEMISTRY

Gold (Au) can exist in any one of three common oxidation states—Au-0, Au-I, and Au-III. The three oxidation states are apparently readily interchangeable with each other in solution, with the final chemical state dependent on the solvent, upon the various ligands attached to the gold atom, and upon the general reaction conditions, most critical being pH. The rate of ligand exchange, particularly on the Au-III molecule, will be dependent on not only pH, but also on chloride ion composition, and the concentration of both the gold complex, and the concentration of any replacing ligands. Even though less biologically reactive than the Au-I complexes, the Au-III complexes nonetheless can oxidize thiols to disulfides and can even oxidize Au-0 to Au-I in the presence of thiols. One possible explanation for this reactivity is due to the solution chemistry of Au-III compounds. The reason that these complexes have never found clinical application is because of their high toxicity (Shaw, 1979). In acid solution in the presence of chloride ions Au-III complexes tend to dissociate to form $HAuCl_4$, a strong oxidizing agent which is able to oxidize the sulfur of methionine to the sulfoxide and the sulfur of cysteine completely to sulfonic acid. This latter oxidation step includes the oxidation of disulfide bonds to sulfonic acid. This destruction of disulfide bonds would have serious consequences on the structure of proteins, including enzymes. Shaw (1979) has postulated that this local denaturation of protein structure is responsible for the greater inhibition of enzyme activity exhibited by the Au-III, relative to that of the Au-I, complexes. Once in solution the various species formed are highly labile and the solution composition therefore varies with time. A complex dissociation of Au-III compounds into aquated and hydroxylated species has been illustrated by several authors using schemes that are similar to those postulated for *cis*Pt and discussed in the preceding section. The $HAuCl_4$ exists as a mixture of the $AuCl_2(OH)_2$ anion (hydroxy form) and the $AuCl_2(H_2O)_2$ cation (aquo form), with the relative quantities of these two intermediates determined by the pH and by chloride ion concentration (Mandal and Nandi, 1978).

The chemical structures of the various gold complexes are such that the classical gold thiolates apparently do not exist in solution as monomers, but tend to polymerize and form long chains with a gold–sulfur backbone and ligands attached as shown in Fig. 1 (Sadler, 1982a). Auranofin on the other hand apparently exists in solution as a discrete monomer.

Au-I, which is the oxidation state of the gold thiolates and phosphines currently utilized clinically in arthritis therapy, is a highly reactive oxidation state that appears to be more common, or at least more widely studied (Allaudeen et al., 1985; Mirabelli et al., 1986a), than Au-III compounds. The Au-III compounds, however, are chemically more closely related to the chemistry of the platinum-II drugs (e.g. *cis*Pt) which were discussed earlier. Thus the Au-III molecule forms a square planar structure with four coordination bonds, exactly similar to the structure of *cis*Pt, and loses its ligands sequentially in interaction that result ultimately in bonds to sulfhydryl groups, both free in the cell and protein bound. Because of the relative reaction rates of the two major oxidation states, the ligand exchange rate is slower with Au-III than with Au-I, even though this relatively slow rate of reaction is generally more rapid than for platinum-II.

The composition of the ligands attached to the gold atom is of critical importance in determining biological activity and chemical stability of the gold complex. Unfortunately no widely applicable general rule can be applied to predict which ligands will provide the ideal combination of optimum stability and maximum biological activity. Thus, Moustatih and Garnier-Suillerot (1989) have produced a complex of gold (III) with the antineoplastic drug streptonigrin, which is extremely stable as long as the gold remains in the trivalent state. However, in vivo Au (III) is slowly converted to Au (I), which is displaced from the complex. The loss of the trivalent gold atom coincides with a decrease in antitumor efficacy and increase in toxicity of the complex. Thus, it appears from these studies that the Au (III) complex may have greater biological activity as an antitumor agent than the Au (I) complex, although it is difficult to determine whether activity results from the intact complex or from the gold ions that are generated in solution. One report even suggests that the gold atom is responsible for stabilizing the phosphine ligand, which may itself be the actual moiety active in antineoplastic activity of the gold phosphine complexes (Razi et al., 1983).

The thermodynamic stability of gold-ligand bonds is similar to that of platinum-II. Thus CN and the sulfur of cysteine form substantially more stable bonds with gold than do the sulfur of methionine and the nitrogen of histidine, which in turn form more stable bonds with gold than does chloride (Sadler, 1982a). The stability of Au-I is substantially less in the presence of thiol groups, because the gold atom will exchange one of its ligands for the competing thiol. Gold-III complexes exchange two of their four ligands and the two that are exchanged are those *trans* to teach other on opposite sides of the gold atom, a result of the labilizing *trans* influence of the ligands (Shaw, 1979).

3.2. Protein Binding

Au-III binds strongly to plasma proteins. The major protein implicated in the binding is albumin, even though binding to other proteins also has been reported. Although the specific binding site on protein has not yet been conclusively demonstrated the occurrence of a gold–sulfur bond in the presence of gold complex and proteins has been reported (Brown and Smith, 1983), thus strengthening claims for gold–sulfur binding of Au-III complexes. It is interesting to note that Au-I does not bind to sulfur groups and does not undergo thiol substitution reactions in aqueous systems. In plasma, Au-III binds to albumin at the cysteine-34 sulfhydryl (Crooke, 1982), as has been shown to be true for platinum-II. The linkage is a linear one, with the protein separated from the gold center through the sulfur atom, rather than formation of a chelate structure, wherein the gold would be joined to both sulfur and protein in a ring. This linear binding is consistent with the *trans* influence chemistry of the Au-III atom mentioned above.

Several authors have studied the binding of gold to protein and are agreed that the binding curves are representative of a single high affinity, but relatively low capacity, site and one or more low affinity sites with higher binding capacity (Mason, 1977; Biggs et al., 1979). The suggestion of more than one binding site on protein suggests binding to other reactants than sulfur-34 of cysteine. It has been suggested that for aurothiomalate this alternate binding may be through electrostatic bonds of the anionic carboxyl groups of the drug and various cationic groups on the protein (Mason, 1977). Penicillamine, which has traditionally been used as an antidote for gold overdose due to its strong chelating ability, was found to have little effect on protein-bound gold (Biggs et al., 1979), even at molar ratios two orders of magnitude greater than that of the bound gold. This is intriguing in the light of reports that extracellular thiols such as glutathione can actually increase the efflux of gold from red bloods cells and cellular binding has been shown to be decreased in the presence of mercaptoethanol and dithiothreitol (Mirabelli et al., 1985).

Some early authors claimed that gold was bound exclusively to albumin, although consistently gold has been shown to bind to other high molecular weight plasma components as well. Some of the discrepancy between reported binding to albumin relative to other plasma components may be related to the manner in which the authors reported their results. Thus, McQueen and Dykes (1969) reported gold binding to be "virtually confined to" albumin, although their data show an average of 16% of the recovered gold bound to various globulins but with greater than 80% bound to albumin. These authors apparently considered 5–10% on each of several alternate sites to be biologically insignificant, even though their generalization may have been misleading. Similar wording in other papers may have further confounded the early literature.

In addition to albumin, gold has been shown to bind to globulins, with molecular ratios of gold binding to be less than an order of magnitude different among the four globulins IgM, IgA, IgG and IgE (Lorber et al., 1972). When total gold binding capacity is considered, however, binding to IgG is substantially greater than any of the other three fractions. Also of interest is the strength of binding of the gold atom to protein vs gold binding of globulins. It has been shown that the albumin/globulin ratio of bound gold changes with time after dosing (Danpure et al., 1979) and several studies have led to the conclusion that there is in fact a more rapid loss of gold from the albumin molecule than from the globulin. The molecular basis for this difference in binding is unknown. Furthermore, when serum from patients treated with gold-containing drugs was incubated with red blood cells from nontreated normal volunteers the gold from patients treated with Auranofin (Au-I–phosphine) more rapidly and more completely transferred to the red cells than the gold from plasma of patients treated with myocrisine, a standard gold thiolate used in arthritis therapy (Brown and Smith, 1983). This also illustrates the significance of the ligands in determining biological activity and chemical reactivity. These results support the assertion that binding and other interactions of gold are highly dependent on the ligands associated with the coordination sphere of the gold atom and the valence state of the atom itself.

Novotna et al. (1991) used the known ability of gold to bind collagen as the basis for investigating the interaction between gold in gold sodium thiosulfate and a collagen-containing component (Clq) of complement. After determining the kinetics of the gold–Clq binding, they conducted efficacy studies in an animal model of arthritis. They conclude that a possible explanation for gold action may be the blocking of the activation of the complement system based on binding to complement components.

It was traditionally assumed that all gold present in blood was associated with the cellular fraction (Shaw, 1979; Razi et al., 1983). Recently, however, several papers have shown binding to the red cell fraction, with amounts varying from 15 to 55% depending on the specific gold compound utilized and the time after administration that the gold content was determined (Walz et al., 1979; Gottlieb, 1982; Intoccia et al., 1982). Detectable but small quantities of gold also occur in white blood cells and platelets (Walz et al., 1979). The localization of gold in blood cells may be more prevalent after parenteral administration of gold compounds. One study reported that one third of patients receiving Auranofin had gold present in erythrocytes in amounts ranging from 25–55% of the total blood gold. Of the gold present in the red cells, an overwhelming proportion is present in the cytosol rather than in the cellular ghosts (Gottlieb, 1982). This is analogous to the situation with *cis*Pt, where an overwhelming percentage (92–96%) is found in plasma, but of that small percentage associated with cells, most (94–98%) is present in the cytosol (Litterst, 1984a). An abstract has reported the presence of a gold–glutathione complex in red blood cells, which may represent the intracellular form of gold (cited in Brown and Smith, 1983).

Binding of gold to tissue proteins also occurs, with numerous authors reporting the near-universal binding of gold to all tissue fractions (Brown and Smith, 1983) and to all cytosolic proteins (Schmitz et al., 1980; Thompson et al., 1978). In this general context, gold has been found to inactivate various enzymes in vitro, presumably by direct binding to the enzyme at sulfhydryl groups. The concentration of gold, however, which produces inhibition is quite high and has been proposed as too high (mM) to be of therapeutic importance (Crooke et al., 1986). The mechanism of enzyme inactivation is alleged to be the formation of coordination bonds between sulfhydryl groups on the proteins, with subsequent formation of inter- or intraprotein crosslinks. The interprotein links are thought to occur only at very high protein concentrations and probably very high gold concentrations as well. Sufficiently high numbers of these links might cause local denaturation of the protein and if this occurred on membranes, a site where relatively high concentration of protein occur and which therefore favor denaturation, alteration in membrane stability and function might be expected to occur. These possible membrane changes would be consistent with the fact that gold complexes—particularly Au-I—are known to cause cytolysis at concentrations of gold which produce no dramatic inhibition in nucleic acid or protein synthesis or apparent effects on DNA structure (Berners-Price et al., 1986). Auranofin has been shown to exert little effect on enzyme activity, possibly because of its lower sulfhydryl reactivity.

Simon et al. (1979), however, have shown that the membrane transport mechanism for deoxyglucose is intact following a 4 hr exposure to 1 μg/mL Auranofin in cells, suggesting that membrane integrity had not been disrupted by this relatively high concentration of gold. The membrane bound transport enzyme Na/K ATPase is also inhibited by Auranofin in vitro, but only by high concentration (2×10^{-4} M) (Hardcastle et al., 1986). These high inhibitory concentrations suggest that there may be minimal effects in vivo, thus further reaffirming that membrane integrity may be undistributed by gold in vivo.

Lee et al. (1989) investigated the inhibition of several purified enzymes by gold (I) and gold (III) compounds in an attempt to understand the relative roles of charge vs stearic factors on the formation of covalent bond formation. Equilibrium constants were several orders of magnitude less for the gold (I) compounds, suggesting a stronger interaction from the more highly charged gold ion and the active site on the enzyme. However, covalent bond formation was found to be as much an influence of the stearic configuration of the active site, as the gold ion charge.

Other specific enzymes also have been studied and shown to be affected by gold treatment. Thus Allaudeen et al. (1985) showed that gold had the ability to inhibit purified nucleic acid polymerases in vitro by a mechanism that appeared to be related to gold binding to enzyme sulfhydryl groups. The inhibition occurred at very high drug concentrations (i.e. cytotoxic concentrations) and could be blocked by the presence of thiol groups, thus indicating how strongly these complexes bind to thiols. There was no ability to inhibit intracellular polymerases, however, when the effect was studied in vivo (Allaudeen et al., 1985). An interesting distinction was observed between Au-I and Au-III complexes in their mechanism of inhibition of polymerases in vitro. In the presence of DNA, the inhibition of polymerases by Au-I complexes was noncompetitive, while in the presence of a similar concentration of DNA, Au-III complexes inhibited DNA polymerases competitively (Allaudeen et al., 1985). Gold complexes have also been shown to inhibit the activity of cathepsin and other lysosomal enzymes, but again the effect was observable only in vitro and was not observed when studied in tissues or cells in vivo (Lewis et al., 1980).

Inhibition of collagenase isolated from human neutrophils has been studied by Mallya and Van Wart (1989), and found to be noncompetitive and reversible by zinc. Collagenase exists in both a latent form and a form activated by *p*-chloromercuribenzoate (PCMB). The noncompetitive inhibition occurs by binding of gold to a zinc-associate binding site. However, these authors also found that PCMB potentiates the inhibition of the latent collagenase by gold (I) compounds, apparently by complexing with thiol moieties to promote the release of the gold (I) ion which binds to collagenase. This binding is to a different binding site than that associated with zinc on the activated enzyme.

Froscio et al. (1989) have shown that Auranofin directly inhibits the activity of PKC. Their results preclude an effect on the regulatory domain of the enzyme, and suggest a direct interaction with thiol groups at the enzyme active site. The importance of the interaction of gold in the PKC pathway has been established by Lison et al. (1989), who showed that Auranofin inhibits the induction of plasminogen activator activity in murine macrophages, but has no effect on that activity in Lewis lung cells, which are PKC deficient. Thus Auranofin may work in reducing inflammation by inhibiting this enzyme which has a central role in degradation of the extracellular matrix.

For a complete list of the enzymes studied and found to interact with gold in vitro the reader is referred to the review of Shaw (1979).

The strong affinity of gold complexes for thiol groups is indicated by the change in the protein binding and biological activity observed when fetal calf serum was added to incubation mixtures (Berners-Price et al., 1986; Snyder et al., 1986). Thus the protein binding of Auranofin increased to 100% when 10% fetal calf serum was included in the incubation medium and presumably the biological activity against RAW 264.7 cells was correspondingly decreased. The involvement of tissue sulfhydryls in vivo was originally shown by Thompson et al. (1978), who homogenized kidneys from gold-treated animals and showed that gold eluted from a liquid chromatography column in fractions that were nearly identical to the elution fraction sulfhydryl content. These authors further showed that some gold eluted at a very low molecular weight and by adding cysteine to their preparations in vitro they increased the size of the sulfhydryl peak and diluted the concentration of gold, suggesting strongly that gold bound to free cysteine that was presumably intracellular.

In addition to binding to high molecular weight plasma and tissue proteins, gold complexes also have been shown to bind to low molecular weight compounds, particularly thiols as has been suggested by comments above concerning the ability of thiols to alter the stability and biological activity of gold complexes. Lewis et al. (1980) showed that when an Au-III complex interacted with either glutathione or cysteine at neutral pH, an insoluble complex was quickly formed. The difference in reactivity between Au-III and Au-I compounds and the significance of the ligands is indicated by the fact that aurothiomalate, a soluble Au-I complex, interacted more slowly with glutathione to form a soluble complex, but interacted with cysteine to form an insoluble complex (Lewis et al., 1980). The gold phosphine derivatives, however, are totally unreactive, presumably because of their low water solubility. The aurothiomalate complex has been shown to enter red blood cells and to participate in a very slow exchange with intracellular glutathione to form a Au-*S*-glutathione complex, even though Berners-Price et al. (1986) showed that the diphenylphosphine gold complex did not bind to glutathione and was unable to displace the ligand from gold to form a complex similar to the aurothiomalate.

Snyder et al. (1986) showed that membrane thiols competed with the tetraacetylthioglucose (TATG) moiety on Auranofin to form a coordination bond between the thiol and the gold atom, and that extracellular thiols had the ability to compete in this reaction. The gold–thiol bond thus formed in the membrane was labile in the presence of extracellular thiols. The competition between TATG and extracellular thiols for the gold coordination sphere means that the gold–thiol complex first forms extracellularly and then must exchange again to form the gold–membrane complex. When *N*-ethyl maleimide, a sulfhydryl group alkylating agent, was added to in vitro incubates, a decrease was observed in the association of gold with cell membranes, thus supporting the role of thiol binding in gold mechanism of action at the level of cell membranes (Snyder et al., 1986). Razi et al. (1983), however, showed that there was little exchange of TATG when Auranofin was dissolved in a solution of glutathione and concluded that TATG was a poor leaving group on the Auranofin and that little replacement should occur with TATG. Within the cell Auranofin apparently leaves its TATG moiety behind bound to either extracellular or membrane protein. This may be the reason that Snyder et al. (1986) proposed the exchange of TATG with extracellular thiols prior to potential exchange with intracellular glutathione.

These same authors (Snyder et al., 1986) have extrapolated this scheme for Auranofin-based thiol exchange and binding to gold compounds in general and have suggested that any gold complexes capable of interacting with sulfhydryls may be bound to cell membranes in a similar way. Furthermore these authors suggest that a similar sulfhydryl exchange process may result in intracellular distribution of Auranofin by an exchange of the membrane-bound gold to cytosolic sulfhydryl groups. This mechanism is proposed to occur via direct exchange of cytosolic sulfhydryls at the site originally occupied by the TATG moiety. An alternative mechanism involves the removal of the triethylphosphine moiety from the membrane bound gold and then binding to cytosolic sulfhydryls prior to actual dissociation from the membrane. Removal of gold from cells is postulated to occur by a simple reversal of the above mechanism, suggesting that the entire scheme may be in equilibrium.

In addition, it has been shown that efflux of gold from cells can be promoted by addition of extracellular glutathione (Crooke et al., 1986), although whether or not the intracellular gold was protein bound or not was not established. In addition, Mirabelli et al. (1985) reported that the addition of mercaptoethanol and dithiothreitol will dissociate cell-associated gold, but details of their work were not provided.

All of these results presume a direct interaction between gold and thiols, although in most cases other interpretations of the data presented are possible. In only one case, however, has the direct formation of a gold–sulfur complex been conclusively demonstrated (Brown and Smith, 1983).

In addition to glutathione binding, gold has been shown to interact nonspecifically with MT. MT is a relatively low MW (ca. 6000 Da), heat-stable protein with a unique 30% of its amino acid sequence composed of cysteine. The protein has been shown to bind a variety of metals, including cadmium and copper, and is implicated in endogenous zinc homeostasis. The likelihood of interaction between gold and MT was suggested by the broad spectrum of metals that are known to bind to MT-like proteins (e.g. Cd, Be, Pt, Cu, Zn). When purified MT was reacted in vitro with sodium thiomalate it was found that gold at a gold to cadmium ratio of 2:1 was able to preferentially displace 78% of zinc but no cadmium from MT binding sites (Schmitz et al., 1980). At a higher gold ratio of 5:1, 50% of the cadmium was displaced and all of the zinc displaced. Even at a ratio of 25:1, all of the cadmium was not displaced by gold, indicating a stronger affinity of MT for cadmium than for gold. In vivo, when gold was injected into rats and the gold content of MT determined, it was found that only 5% of the protein-bound gold was associated with MT, however. The authors (Schmitz et al., 1980) suggest that the bond is linear, with MT joined to the Au-MT complex via a SH group. Although no work was done with Au-III complexes, binding to Au-III also was suggested as likely, and that Au-III, because of its increased toxicity, might be able to produce a stress-associated induction of MT with a resulting increase in binding.

Hu et al. (1988) have shown that gold in the form of aurothioglucose interacts strongly with both metallothionein-like proteins, and with selenium in both liver and kidney of rats. Whether the interaction is a direct binding of the two metals, or whether both metals bind to the same protein was not resolved, but the possible direct interaction of these two metals was not precluded. In addition, their results further implicate the ability of gold to induce the synthesis of metallothionein-like proteins in vivo.

3.3. DNA Binding

Even though the antineoplastic effect of gold complexes is limited to phosphine stabilized complexes, there has been a surprisingly large amount of work done on the DNA interaction of various gold complexes. However, as recently as 1982 it was admitted that nothing was known about the effects of Auranofin or other gold complexes on nucleic acids, either in vitro or in vivo (Crooke, 1982). This is because many early studies on nucleic acid interactions with gold complexes utilize $HAuCl_4$ as the source of Au-III, presumably on the assumption that this was the active species formed in aqueous solution. In addition, early work did not anticipate the interest in Au-I phosphine compounds which are only now being carefully studied.

Early work showed that gold bound preferentially to RNA, rather than to DNA, and that given the choice between native and denatured DNA, gold would bind preferentially to the latter (Pillai and Nandi, 1978). It was proposed by several different authors that Au-III interacts with the nucleic acids in biphasic manner. It has even been suggested that reactions of the amine chloroaurate complexes are of the classic SN_2 alkylation type (Gibson et al., 1971). The first step in the reaction is the production in solution of a gold cation by a mechanism best hypothesized by Snyder et al. (1986). This cation permits the approach of the gold atom to the anionic phosphate groups in the DNA molecule. Because of the fact that these phosphates are hard bases, a firm complex would not be expected, although at relatively low gold:nucleotide ratios some interaction does occur. After this initial reaction brings the gold center into proximity with the nucleic acid chain, a second reaction then takes place that results in the strong association between gold and a nucleophilic site on the purine bases on the nucleic acid. This reaction occurs most probably with adenine or thymine because studies with synthetic DNAs of various base composition have shown a preferential binding to DNA rich in these two bases (Pillai and Nandi, 1978). Other studies have established that the preferred bases for binding are adenine > guanine > cytosine > thymine and that the bonds occur at the N-1 and N-7 and/or C-(6)-O of guanine, because these are the sites generally found most favorable for protonation by metal ions. This binding is reversible with triethylphosphine gold complexes and does not result in denaturation with that compound. Classic Au-III complexes, however, form crosslinks—probably interstrand—that result in changes in base orientation in the chain as indicated by hyperchromatic changes in UV spectral studies. These changes most probably result in disturbances in DNA replication and subsequent inhibition of DNA replication and cell death.

Simon et al. (1979) showed a dose-dependent and irreversible inhibition of protein and nucleic acid synthesis in HeLa cells at clinically achievable gold concentrations following exposure to Auranofin, and suggested that DNA was the most sensitive synthetic pathway of the three that were studied. Other workers also showed Auranofin-induced inhibition of DNA synthesis (Simon et al., 1979). Other work showed DNA and protein synthesis to be inhibited about equally by Auranofin (Walz et al., 1979) and still other work showed a greater effect on RNA and protein synthesis than on DNA synthesis by Auranofin (Berners-Price et al., 1986). What was consistently observed, however, was that although Au-I complexes appeared to inhibit DNA synthesis, the only gold complexes that were shown to interact directly with DNA were the Au-III compounds. These studies were conducted with several compounds of each gold valence state. The most recent investigations, however, have shown that both Au-I and Au-III complexes demonstrate direct binding to DNA when studied in vitro at basic pH. It is interesting to note that at an in vitro pH which approximates physiologic pH (ca. 7.1) most complexes of Au-I gave negative results (Mirabelli et al., 1986b). Even when positive results were obtained, however, they occurred at drug:nucleotide ratios in excess of 5, which is unrealistically high. In similar studies with *cis*Pt, drug:receptor ratio of 0.1 are considered high and values of 0.0004 are more realistic. This extensive study, however, again reinforces the importance of ligands when studying biological activity of any of the gold complexes.

Crooke (1982) reported that Au-III complexes bind to purine bases and to both nucleosides and nucleotides. It was further shown that the binding of Au-III complexes to purine bases was to the nitrogen atom and that the ability of Au-III to inhibit DNA replication was not caused by an inhibition of DNA polymerase activity, which is similar to what has been established for *cis*Pt action (Harder et al., 1976).

Berners-Price et al. (1986) showed that Auranofin did not cause DNA or chromatin damage at doses that were rapidly cytotoxic and that this cytotoxicity was apparently not due to inhibition of either nucleic acid or protein synthesis. It was shown that Auranofin and other Au-I phosphines do not bind to DNA, but other phosphine complexes have been shown to bind to it. The reason for this apparent discrepancy is related to the strength of the gold–ligand bond. If the two leaving groups are strong binding ligands (soft bases like RS or ethylphosphine) then no interaction with DNA would be expected. If, however, one ligand is relatively weak (i.e. a hard base such as chloride or phosphate) displacement can be expected to occur and the resulting cation would bind to DNA. For those phosphine complexes that have been shown to interact with DNA, the binding moiety is apparently the triethylphosphine group (Blank and Dabrowiak, 1984).

Although much less work has been done to identify the atomic interactions between the purine bases on DNA and the gold atom than has been done with *cis*Pt, the probable binding sites of Au-III have been tentatively identified as the N-1 and N-7 atoms of adenine, the N-7 and C-(6)-O atoms of guanine, and the N-3 atom of both cytosine and thymine. This is similar to what was reported for *cis*Pt binding (see above) and reflects the general affinity of these sites for metals. In contrast, Au-I apparently binds only at the N-7 site (Hadjiliadis et al., 1981). Both Au-III and Au-I have been shown to form interstrand crosslinks (Mirabelli et al., 1986c). Because of the similarity between the pattern of changes in the electrophoretic mobility of DNA between platinum and gold treated nucleic acids it has been postulated that the Au-III complexes can also form intrastrand crosslinks due to the analogy with the structure of the platinum–DNA adducts. This appears to be a reasonable postulate whose proof awaits further analytical work. These intrastrand crosslinks, however, have not yet been demonstrated and absolute proof will probably have to await the preparation of an antibody to the gold–DNA adduct much the way that a platinum–DNA antibody has recently clarified our understanding of platinum–DNA interactions (Lippard et al., 1983). Auranofin, the oral Au-I complex highly successful in arthritis therapy, has been shown to have no interaction at all with DNA (Mirabelli and Crooke, 1983). This lack of interaction has been postulated as being due to the stronger affinity of gold for the phosphine moiety than for the nitrogen on the purine bases of the DNA chain (Crooke, 1982).

The gold phosphine complexes were shown to produce dose-related increases in single strand DNA breaks that continued to form even after drug was removed (Mirabelli et al., 1986c). This suggests a monofunctional-to-bifunctional adduct formation sequence similar to that proposed for the mechanism of platinum–DNA adduct formation. A similar continual increase in crosslinks after drug removal was shown to be true with platinum. The formation of DNA-protein crosslinks was not similarly dose related, and occurred at a relatively steady state level that did not further increase when drug was removed.

The Au-III compound $AuCl_4$ reacts with the nucleotides cytosine and inosine. Although $AuCl_4$ formed insoluble complexes with adenosine and adenine, the reaction formed soluble complex with the mono-, di- and triphosphates of adenosine and the monophosphate of guanine.

4. METALLOCENES

Perhaps the most exciting new group of metal-containing compounds that have been investigated for antitumor activity and found positive are the metallocene dihalides. In these complexes, a central metal atom is bound to two cyclopentadienyl rings and to two halide atoms in a twisted tetrahedron configuration (Fig. 1). The metal atom is usually an early transition metal and titanium and vanadium have been the most effective, although many others have been tested but found less active (molybdenum, hafnium, zirconium, tungsten). The chemical similarity between these complexes and *cis*Pt is most obvious if one envisions the two rings as being analogous to the two ammine residues in *cis*Pt (i.e. tightly bound, nonleaving ligands) and the halides, which in the most active cases are chlorines, as analogous to the chlorine leaving ligands on the *cis*Pt molecule. In the metallocene dihalides the central metal appears to be the structural component most important in determining biological activity, although the ability of the halide ligand to be readily dissociable is also important. Thus, complexes with strongly bonded halide ligands have little or no antitumor activity (Kopf and Kopf-Maier, 1983). The cyclopentadienyl rings apparently act as stabilizing and transport components. In aqueous solution, the complexes readily dissociate, much as is the case with *cis*Pt, to form oxo-bridged dimers. In addition, pH functions to affect the formation of diaquo and aquo-hydroxy species and the dimer formed from these monomers. Interestingly, these hydrolysis products appear to be less biologically active than do their parent compounds (Kopf and Kopf-Maier, 1983). Thus hydrolysis or aquation appears to be not a necessary requisite for biological activity with the metallocene halides as it apparently is with *cis*Pt.

The mechanism of action of these complexes appears to be inhibition of DNA synthesis. Metal from the complexes accumulates in heterochromatin, the nuclear protein which is richest in DNA. Subcellular distribution studies of titanocene dichloride in Ehrlich Ascites Tumor (EAT) cells demonstrated low concentrations also in euchromatin and in the nucleolus, but no metal atoms are found elsewhere within the cell (Kopf-Maier and Krahl, 1981). However, as is known for *cis*Pt, chromatin binding can be to protein as well as to DNA, so direct metallocene involvement with DNA is still presumptive. Further presumptive evidence for this involvement is from the fact that giant cells are formed in EAT cells in vivo after metal exposure with both vanadium and titanium (Kopf-Maier, 1982).

Metallocene halides also alter the synthesis of RNA, but at concentrations of metal complex that are much greater than those required to decrease DNA synthesis. In addition, the vanadium complex has been shown to alter the UV absorption spectra of both DNA and RNA, indicating a change in the secondary structure of these two macromolecules. Protein synthesis is also reduced in the presence of metallocenes, but at two orders of magnitude greater concentration of drug than are required to significantly alter DNA synthesis.

As discussed above in the context of platinum–DNA interaction, the bond distance between the *cis* chlorines in the *cis*Pt molecule (3.35 Å) is nearly equal to the distance between two DNA nucleobase atoms that would have to be bridged in order to form a crosslink on the DNA strand. For all effective antitumor metallocene dihalide molecules, a similar chlorine–chlorine atomic distance is also observed (3.24–3.47 Å). The implication is that the metallocene–DNA binding is by a mechanism that must be structurally similar to that observed with Pt–DNA, although evidence to support this hypothesis has not yet been published.

5. GALLIUM

Perhaps the metal with the longest history of use in human chemotherapy is the group IIIA element gallium (Ga). In the late 1940s Ga salts were found to preferentially localize in bone and this element was then promoted as an agent useful in diagnosing neoplastic and other diseases of bone. In the late 1960s it was discovered that gallium nitrate [$Ga(NO_3)_3\ H_3$] would distribute preferentially into solid tumors. Thus radioactive gallium nitrate has been used as a diagnostic agent in cancer detection. Early studies then demonstrated the antitumor activity of gallium nitrate against the Walker 256 carcinosarcoma in rats (Hart et al., 1971), and Hart and Adamson (1971) showed impressive antitumor activity in three subcutaneously implanted animal solid tumors in rats. This latter finding was significant because the drug expressed its activity when administered by a route different from that of tumor inoculation. In part because of this impressive animal antitumor activity and in part because the drug expressed its activity when administered by a route different from that of tumor inoculation, gallium nitrate was entered into clinical trials in the 1970s. Ga has subsequently been found useful in a relatively limited number of human tumors and unfortunately has generated little interest in establishing its interactions with biologically relevant molecules.

Observations that Ga had no apparent effect on populations of rapidly dividing cells except at supralethal doses in animals (Hart et al., 1971) suggested that this metal acted by some mechanism other than an effect on nucleic acid synthesis or cell replication. The early finding that Ga administration resulted in the release from hydroxyapatite crystals of a number of calcium atoms equivalent to the number of Ga atoms subsequently fixed within the crystal (Anghileri, 1971) suggested a mechanism of action related to competition by Ga for metal binding sites in tissue proteins. Similar results were obtained for gallium/calcium exchange in ketoglutarate, and in tissue proteins from tumor homogenate (Anghileri, 1971). It was later found that Ga would exchange with calcium in both RNAase and DNAase (Anghileri and Heidbreder, 1977). In addition to calcium, magnesium has also been found to exchange readily with Ga (Anghileri, 1973). It therefore appears as if one of the major chemical interactions that Ga undergoes is a simple competitive replacement of alkaline earth cations in biological macromolecules. The high concentrations of calcium and magnesium in tumors would therefore account for the concentration of Ga in tumor tissue by this mechanism. The interaction with tumor tissue to produce an antitumor effect can be inferred from this finding, but demonstration of the true mechanism of action awaits further investigation.

Extensive studies have been conducted on the binding of Ga to nucleic acids and proteins using conductivity titration to indicate binding (Bandurski et al., 1977). Although sufficient for qualitative estimations of binding, this method makes quantitative studies difficult. It was found that Ga bound most strongly to DNA, apparently through the phosphate groups of the deoxynucleotides in a metal:phosphate ratio of about 3:1. An interesting biphasic shift in the conductivity curve was noted that was not observed with either indium or aluminum in the same study. The second change in slope was attributed to a change in DNA conformation, but in retrospect one might wonder whether this also suggests a bidentate complexation similar to what is observed with cisplatinum. Ga was found to bind RNA at about the same metal:nucleic acid ratio as was found with DNA (i.e. 3:1). This fact has been used to support the claim of binding through the phosphate groups, this time with ribonucleotides. Ga also bound to proteins, but about forty times less avidly on a weight basis than its binding with nucleic acids. Thus Ga bound to transferrin at a molar ratio of about 1:21 and to hemoglobin at a molar ratio of 1:7.7 (Bandurski et al., 1977). Binding to serum albumin was not strongly indicated by the conductivity titration but the authors suggest that this possibility should not be ruled out. One caution in this entire study is the relatively high pH at which the binding curves were determined. Gallium nitrate hydrolyzes very rapidly in all but extremely acid solutions (i.e. pH 3) so that exact species that was bound is probably not known. However, this situation is exactly similar to what is seen with *cis*Pt, where ill-defined aquated/hydroxylated species are responsible for actual binding but the exact species can only be inferred from empirical data. The problem of the instability of gallium nitrate has been solved clinically by using a citrated form of gallium nitrate.

It is known that Ga is cytotoxic through a blockade of the synthesis of DNA. Chitambar and Narasimhan (1991) have shown that this block is due to the blockage of cellular iron uptake and utilization at the level of ribonucleotide reductase. They showed a marked inhibition of the electron spin resonance signal from the M2 subunit of the enzyme, and the intracellular concentrations of iron-59 were reduced in the presence of gallium nitrate. Cells made resistant to Ga were also resistant to growth inhibition by an antitransferrin monoclonal antibody, further supporting the theory that Ga acts by blocking the transferrin-mediated intracellular uptake of iron.

However, Ohkubo et al. (1990) showed that Ga transport into inflammatory cells was not mediated by transferrin. Thus when intracellular transport of Ga was studied into inflamed livers of CCl4 treated mice, uptake of Ga was nearly an order of magnitude greater than the increase in transferrin levels and activity. Thus it appears as if transferrin is active in the transport of Ga into normal, but not inflamed cells.

In addition to nucleic acid binding, gallium nitrate has been shown to effectively inhibit DNA polymerase activity in a specific manner. DNA polymerases B and D from Walker 256 tumor were inhibited by 40% and 30% respectively, but there was no effect on the A and C forms from the same source (Adamson et al., 1975). In addition, the reverse transcriptase (DNA polymerase) from Rauscher murine leukemia virus has also been shown to be sensitive to gallium nitrate and its activity was shown to be inhibited by 59%. The mechanistic significance of the Ga-induced inhibition of polymerases, and the binding of Ga to DNA, has not been addressed, but the inability of the polymerase to function properly may be because the template—DNA—is ineffective because of the Ga bound to it, rather than a direct interaction of Ga with the enzyme. This situation would be analogous to that which is observed with the *cis*Pt-induced inactivation of DNA polymerases (Harder et al., 1976).

In the blood, Ga is highly bound to high molecular weight substances in plasma, with little or no association with cellular elements. The binding location has been extensively investigated and found to be mainly transferrin (Clausen et al., 1974; Gunasekera et al., 1972), although significant binding to haptoglobin has also been reported. Small amounts of Ga are also bound to globulin and lipoprotein. Only about 30% of the plasma protein binding is reported to be albumin (Gunasekera et al., 1972). Both haptoglobin and transferrin have been identified using specific antisera (Clausen et al., 1974). Nearly 70% of the protein-bound Ga is associated with the protein through noncovalent bonds, as indicated by the fact that the metal can be removed by dialysis. The remaining 30% can be removed by dialysis in PO_4^{3-}(Gunasekera et al., 1972). It has been calculated that the transferrin molecule contains 14 Ga binding sites (Clausen et al., 1974).

In tissue homogenates, Ga is preferentially bound to protein, with only about 20% of homogenate Ga associated with lipid (Clausen et al., 1974). Most of the protein with which the Ga is bound appears to be membrane-associated, although a small amount is associated with ferritin. In addition, a large amount appears to be free in the cytoplasm (Glickson et al., 1973). For example, when a tumor homogenate from a patient was assayed by acrylamide gel electrophoresis for the site of Ga accumulation, 30% of the Ga was associated with a mobility similar to that of transferrin. It has been alleged that the Ga is bound to transferrin by Van der Waals forces and hydrophobic bonds (Clausen et al., 1974), although the evidence for this conclusion was circumstantial.

Lactoferrin, a transferrin-like molecule in human breast milk, has been found to bind Ga even more strongly than does transferrin at physiological pH (Hofer et al., 1977). A similar binding was absent from milk of dogs and rabbits.

Ga is known to mimic lead in its ability to interfere with heme synthesis. In this regard, the mechanism of Ga inhibition of delta aminolevulinic acid dehydratase has been investigated by Goering and Rehm (1990). Lineweaver–Burke analysis of binding data for both renal and hepatic enzymes established that inhibition is noncompetitive, with a K_i that is similar to that for lead. Further studies then showed that zinc could block the inhibitory effects of gallium, and the authors postulate that Ga inhibition of enzyme activity may result from displacement or blockage of zinc from the sulfhydryl group of the active site on the enzyme.

6. COPPER

Complexes of copper, a member of group IB of the Periodic Table, have seen extensive testing in animal tumor systems. Thus more than 1100 copper complexes have been tested for activity in vitro and in vivo (Sadler, 1982b). In one study, however, only one copper complex out of many tested produced greater than a 50% increase in the life span of tumored animals (Sadler et al., 1984). Copper I complexes are extremely reactive and can be utilized only in those situations where the Cu-I has been stabilized by appropriate binding ligands. Activity in both valence states has been found only with ligands that exchange slowly. Cu-II complexes may be expected to form square planar structures with four short bond distances and two longer axial bonds like those found with gold-III and platinum-II. Two of the most active compounds in several in vivo tumor systems are Cu-I and Cu-II complexes containing either 6-mercaptopurine or thioguanine as ligands (Sadler et al., 1984). Interestingly, both of these ligands are active antitumor agents in themselves. This raises the possibility that these copper compounds are actually prodrugs that act by releasing moieties with antitumor activity. One of the most active copper complexes tested in vivo at the National Cancer Institute is a complex where the copper atom is chelated between four nitrogen atoms in a porphyrin-like structure (Sadler et al., 1984). Cu-II is readily reduced to Cu-I, which is the more stable, but does not possess the planar configuration of the Cu-II form. Thus, the antitumor activity of copper-containing agents may be related to the energy released by shifting valence states within the individual molecules.

Only recently has evidence been generated to support the interaction between copper-containing drugs and nucleic acids. Prutz et al. (1990) have studied the binding of copper (I) to DNA and to the model compounds poly (dG-dC), poly (dA-dT) and poly (I). Calculated rate constants of association and dissociation show a stronger binding to poly (dG-dC) and poly (I), but with a very slow dissociation of copper bound to native but not heat denatured DNA. Rate constants for interactions of copper ions with Cu–Zn superoxide dismutase also have been determined and the role of pH in affecting the activity of superoxide dismutase in dismutation of superoxide anion are discussed by the authors in the context of moderating intracellular redox reactions.

Percival and Harris (1990) studied the transport of the strongly bound copper from ceruloplasmin into human erythroleukemia cells. At 4°C ceruloplasmin-associated copper bound nonspecifically to cells in a stoichiometric fashion with protein, and was easily removed by washing. At 37°, however, copper, but not protein, from ceruloplasmin was incorporated into cells. Thus it appears as if normal cells have the ability to extract bound copper from ceruloplasmin and incorporate it independent of the protein moiety.

The possible involvement of copper with steroid hormone receptors has been demonstrated by Hutchens and Li (1988) using bovine uterine estrogen receptor proteins. Although the role of this interaction is still speculative, the authors suggest that these receptors may in fact be metalloproteins, and the metal may play a previously unrecognized essential role in the structure or function of these proteins.

Copper complexes of (bis)thiosemicarbazone (bTS) were found to be active antitumor agents whose activity depended entirely on the presence of the copper atom. Thus when bTS was administered to animals on a copper free diet, the complex was an inactive antitumor agent (Petering et al., 1967). However, when copper was present in the diet, the bTS became highly active, suggesting that bTS can chelate copper from its surrounding environment and form the active antitumor agent Cu-bTS. The crystal structure of the Cu-bTS is such that a planar configuration is formed, which is consistent with the activity of planar complexes of both platinum and gold.

Copper complexes typically react chemically by forming adducts with Lewis bases, by undergoing ligand substitution reactions, and by participating in oxidation–reduction reactions (Petering, 1980). The activity of the Cu–bTS complex apparently involves a single electron reduction to an intermediate that then reacts to oxidize intracellular thiols. The rates at which various copper complexes oxidize cellular thiols correlate well with in vitro cytotoxicity (Petering, 1980). In animals, copper is apparently transported into the cell as the thiosemicarbazone. The metal atom is then released or exchanged with other metal atoms in the cell but the bTS moiety diffuses out of the cell and equilibrates in the extracellular fluid (Booth and Sartorelli, 1967). The intracellular copper concentration correlates with the observed decrease in intracellular thiol concentrations (Minkel and Petering, 1978). The distribution of copper within the cell appears to be uniform with no apparent localization in any one cellular compartment. Within 5 min of exposure to a copper bTS complex, inhibition of DNA synthesis is observed (Chan-Stier et al., 1976). The cytotoxic reactant has not been identified but several realistic alternatives to a copper–nucleic acid complex have been proposed (Booth and Sartorelli, 1967). In addition high concentrations of reactive oxygen radicals have been observed and may be involved with the mechanism of action (Petering, 1980), as might be the depletion or oxidation of cellular thiols.

In contrast to the thiosemicarbazone complexes, there are also copper complexes of heterocyclic carboxyaldehyde thiosemicarbazones (CATS) that have been identified as cytotoxic and possessing strong DNA inhibiting capabilities (Saryan et al., 1979). The DNA inhibiting activity has been related to the binding of the heterocyclic CATS moiety to the active site on a molecule of ribonucleotides reductase, a central enzyme in the DNA synthetic pathway. This binding involves an iron atom in the reductase molecule, but whether the copper atom interacts directly with the iron atom is unknown. An alternative mechanism of inhibition of DNA synthesis is the strong but indirect inhibition of thymidine kinase produced by the CATS complexes (Booth and Sartorelli, 1967).

Redox reactions also occur with CATS complexes but adduct formation plays a more important role in their reactivity, in contrast to that of the bTS complex. Glutathione has been shown to form a coordination complex with the CATS molecule and this is assumed to be indicative of CATS complex formation with cellular thiol-containing compounds. Oxygen radicals are also formed from the strong redox reactions that occur. The CATS penetrates cells readily and intracellularly retain their structure, again in contrast to the bTS complex. Reaction is primarily with the cellular thiols but in formation of a coordination complex formation as distinct from the thiol oxidation that occurs with bTS. Both complexes cause DNA inhibition at quite low concentrations, however.

However, copper is known to be bound to the low molecular weight protein chelatin, and to interact with MT. Serafini et al. (1989) investigated the interaction of copper (II) with glutathione reductase and found that inhibition was competitive when the substrate is oxidized glutathione, but noncompetitive when the substrate was NADPH, at levels up to 8 μM. Copper did not effectively inhibit glucose 6-phosphate dehydrogenase.

Furst and Hamer (1989) have further defined the interaction of copper (I) with the ACE1 transcription factor of the MT gene. It has been known that copper ions activate MT gene transcription by altering the conformation and hence the DNA binding activity of this transcription factor. These authors now show that this change occurs in an all-or-none cooperative fashion, and analysis of the subunit composition indicates that the cooperativity results from binding of multiple copper ions to the cysteine-rich DNA binding domain, and that the effect on DNA binding is primarily kinetic, rather than thermodynamic. The effect is that a relatively small change in extracellular metal concentration can result in a relatively larger change in expression of this gene.

In another study, a series of Cu(II) complexes was prepared where the reacting ligands were salicylates. In this instance the cytotoxic effect was attributed to a complex stimulation of the immune system with subsequent immune-mediated regression of the tumor (reported in Sadler et al., 1984). The rationale for this argument was that the copper complex was an active antitumor agent at doses that were an order of magnitude less than the median lethal dose of the complex. Although not considered by the authors, the known ability of salicylates to affect the immune system might also have been involved.

It is known that copper (II) binds to bovine lactalbumin (LAB) at both a histidyl residue and at a deprotonated amide group. Tieghem et al. (1991) showed that only poor binding occurs in human LAB, which is deficient in the HIS 68 histidyl suggesting that the predominant binding site is through the histidyl residue. Goat LAB has a conformationally restricted histidyl site, and copper binding to goat LAB is intermediate between the other two species, further supporting this conclusion.

Eaton et al. (1990) investigated the binding of accessory ions to copper (II) complexed with lactoferrin and transferrin, and found that carbon from carbonate, and the nitrogen from the imidazole group of histidine bound copper in the complex with similar binding constants, and the binding was about 5-fold greater than binding of these atoms to iron (III). This is similar to results generated by Taniguchi et al. (1990) using Cu (II) binding to ovotransferrin, where they showed binding to both carbon and nitrogen were approximately the same. These authors conclude that the preference of copper for the nitrogen binding site was therefore due to a more rapid dissociation of the copper–carbon bond.

Zgirski and Frieden (1990) have studied the binding and association of Cu (II) ions in ceruloplasmin from various sources. They found that in addition to the prosthetic copper atoms normally recognized as being bound to ceruloplasmin, there apparently are also exogenous copper atoms that are less covalently associated with the molecule and can be removed by Chelex-100 filtration or dialysis. The role of these exogenous copper atoms is not known.

7. PALLADIUM

Palladium-containing compounds have also been widely screened for their potential antitumor activity in vitro and in vivo because palladium is a group VIII B metal like platinum. Palladium complexes are similar to platinum complexes in oxidation state, coordination number, structural geometry and ligand affinities, although the palladium compounds are generally less stable and thus have less extensive chemical interactions. Generally, however, results of in vivo screening tests have been negative. The explanation for this lack of antitumor activity is that the palladium salts are much more reactive than platinum salts and thus form more stable aquated products more quickly than is the case with platinum complexes. Gill (1984) synthesized a series of hydroxy-bridged oligomeric palladium complexes that demonstrated impressive antitumor activity against ascites sarcoma 10 in mice. In one entire series, it was found that the *trans* isomer had greater antitumor activity than did the *cis* isomers. The activity of these oligomeric, charged species of palladium was attributed to an intracellular equilibrium which included highly reactive monomeric aquated forms, which have the ability to interact with nucleic acids.

It has also been found that a palladium–piperidine complex was highly active in inhibiting DNA synthesis in L1210 cells in culture at concentrations that were minimally 20 times less than those required for similar activity using the analogous platinum–piperidine complex (Kirschner et al., 1975). The same complex was 80% as active as *cis*Pt in inducing filamentous growth in *E. coli*. These results suggest that at least this one palladium complex has the ability to inhibit DNA synthesis in vitro and thus may be able to produce a similar effect in vivo. Other palladium complexes were inactive in the same test systems. There is also evidence that palladium, like platinum, binds to thiamine through the N-1 atom (Hadjiliadis et al., 1975). If this is true in vitro then binding of palladium complexes to nucleobases through nitrogen atoms may be likely in vivo.

REFERENCES

AAMDAL, S., FOSTAD, O., KAALHUS, O. and PIHL, A. (1984) Reduced antineoplastic activity in mice of *cis*-diamminedichloroplatinum administered with high salt concentration in the vehicle. *J. natn. Cancer Inst.* **73:** 743–752.

ADAMSON, R. H., CANELLOS, G. P. and SIEBER, S. M. (1975) Studies on the antitumor activity of gallium nitrate (NSC-15200) and other group IIIa metal salts. *Cancer Chemother. Rep.* **59** (Part 1): 599–610.

ADMIRAAL, G., VAN DER VEER, J. L., DE GRAAFF, R. A. G., DEN HARTOG, J. H. J. and REEDJIK, J. (1987) Intrastrand bis(guanine) chelation of d (CpGpG) to *cis*-platinum: an X-ray single-crystal structure analysis. *J. Am. Chem. Soc.* **109:** 592–594.

AGGARWAL, S. K. and NIROOMAND-RAD, I. (1983) Effect of cisplatin on the plasma membrane phosphatase activities in ascites sarcoma-180 cells: a cytochemical study. *J. Histochem. Cytochem.* **31:** 307–317.

ALLAUDEEN, H. S., SNYDER, R. M., WHITMAN, M. H. and CROOKE, S. T. (1985) Effects of coordinated gold compounds on in vitro and in situ DNA replication. *Biochem. Pharmac.* **34:** 3243–3250.

ANGHILERI, L. J. (1971) Studies on the accumulation mechanisms of radioisotopes used in tumor diagnostic. *Strahlentherapie* **142:** 456–461.

ANGHILERI, L. J. (1973) ^{67}Ga-citrate accumulation by tumours: importance of magnesium and calcium metabolism. *Strahlentherapie* **146:** 359–366.

ANGHILERI, L. J. and HEIDBREDER, M. (1977) On the mechanism of accumulation of ^{67}Ga by tumors. *Oncology* **34:** 74–77.

AULL, J. L., RICE, A. C. and TEBBETTS, L. A. (1977) Interactions of platinum complexes with the essential and nonessential sulfhydryl groups of thymidylate synthetase. *Biochemistry* **16:** 672–677.

BAKKA, A., ENDRESEN, L. JOHNSEN, A. B. S., EDMINSEN, P. D. and RUGSTAD, H. E. (1981) Resistance against *cis*-dichlorodiammineplatinum in cultured cells with a high content of metallothionein. *Toxic. appl. Pharmac.* **61:** 215–219.

BANDURSKI, M., POLLOCK, R. J., ROSENBERG, B. and SHAPIRO, G. (1977) Interaction of anticancer salts of Group IIIA elements with biomacromolecules. *J. clin. Hematol. Oncol.* **7:** 411–426.

BANJAR, Z. M., HNILICA, L. S., BRIGGS, R. C., STEIN, J. and STEIN, G. (1984) *Cis*- and *trans*-diamminedichloroplatinum (II)-mediated cross-linking of chromosomal nonhistone proteins to DNA in HeLa cells. *Biochemistry* **23:** 1921–1926.

BAUDIN, F., ROMBY, P., ROMANIUK, P. J., EHRESMANN, B. and EHRESMANN, C.(1989) Crosslinking of transcription factor TFIIIA to ribosomal 5S RNA for *X. laevis* by *trans*-diamminedichloroplatinum (II). *Nucleic Acids Res.* **17:** 10035–10046.

BERNERS-PRICE, S. J., MIRABELLI, C. K., JOHNSON, R. K., MATTERN, M. R., MCCABE, F. L., FAUCETTE, L. F., SUNG, C-M., MONG, S.-M., SADLER, P. J. and CROOKE, S. T. (1986) In vivo antitumor activity and in vitro cytotoxic properties of bis[1,2-bis(diphenylphosphino)-ethane]gold(I) chloride. *Cancer Res.* **46:** 5486–5493.

BERTOLERO, F. and LITTERST, C. L. (1982) Changes in renal handling of platinum in cisplatinum-treated rats following induction of metabolic acidosis or alkalosis. *Res. Commun. Chem. Path. Pharmac.* **36:** 273–285.

BIGGS, D. F., BOLAND, D. M., DAVIS, P. and WAKARUK, J. (1979) In vitro binding and pharmacokinetics of gold salts in plasma proteins and chelating agents. *J. Rheumat.* **6** (Suppl. 5): 68–73.

BINKS, S. P. and DOBROTA, M. (1990) Kinetics and mechanism of uptake of platinum-based pharmaceuticals by the rat small intestine. *Biochem. Pharmac.* **40:** 1329–1336.

BLANK, C. E. and DABROWIAK, J. C. (1984) Absorption and circular dichroism studies of a gold (I)–DNA complex. *J. Inorg. Biochem.* **21:** 21–29.

BODENNER, D. L. DEDON, P. C., KENG, P. C. and BORCH, R. F. (1986) Effect of diethyldithiocarbamate on *cis*-diamminedichloroplatinum(II)-induced cytotoxicity, DNA cross-linking and γ-glutamyl transpeptidase inhibition. *Cancer Res.* **46:** 2745–2750.

BONGERS, J., BELL, J. U. and RICHARDSON, D. E. (1988) Platinum (II) binding to metallothioneins. *J. Inorg. Biochem.* **34:** 55–62

BOOGAARD, P. J., LEMPERS, E. L., MULDERS, G. J. and MEERMAN, J. H. (1991) 4-Methylthiobenzoic acid reduces cisplatin nephrotoxicity in rats without compromising anti-tumor activity. *Biochem. Pharmac.* **41:** 1997–2003.

BOOTH, B. A. and SARTORELLI, A. C. (1967) Metabolic effects of copper in intact cells: comparative activity of cupric chloride and the cupric chelate of kethoxal bis thiosemicarbazone. *Molec. Pharmac.* **3:** 290–302.

BORCH, R. F. and PLEASANTS, M. E. (1979) Inhibition of *cis*-platinum nephrotoxicity by diethyldithiocarbamate rescue in a rat model. *Proc. natn. Acad Sci. U.S.A.* **76:** 6611–6614.

BOSE, R. N., VIOLA, R. E. and CORNELIUS, R. D. (1984) Phosphorus-31 NMR and kinetic studies of the formation of ortho-, pyro, and triphosphato complexes of *cis*-dichlorodiammineplatinum(II). *J. Am. Chem. Soc.* **106:** 3336–3343.

BROWN, D. H. and SMITH, W. E. (1983) Gold thiolate complexes in vitro and in vivo. In: *Platinum, Gold, and Other Metal Chemotherapeutic Agents*, pp. 401–418, LIPPARD, S. J. (ed.) American Chemical Society, Washington, D. C.

CHAN, V., ELLIOTT, K. E., HERMAN, T. S. and TEICHER, B. A. (1988) Alphoid DNA nucleotide sequences from two human cell lines and the corresponding *cis*-diamminedichloroplatinum (II)-resistant sublines. *Cancer Lett.* **43:** 219–225.

CHAN-STIER, C. H., MINKEL, D. and PETERING, D. H. (1976) Reactions of bis(thiosemicarbazonato) copper(II) complexes with tumor cells and mitochondria. *Bioinorg. Chem.* **6:** 203–217.

CHITAMBAR, C. R. and NARASIMHAN, J. (1991) Targeting iron-dependent DNA synthesis with gallium and transferrin-gallium. *Pathobiology* **59:** 3–10.

CICCARELLI, R. B., SOLOMON, M. J., VARSHAVSKY, A. and LIPPARD, S. J. (1985) In vivo effects of *cis*- and *trans*-diamminedichloroplatinum(II) on SV40 chromosomes: differential repair, DNA–protein crosslinking, and inhibition of replication. *Biochemistry* **24:** 7533–7540.

CLARKSON, T. W. (1986) General principles of toxic action. In: *Handbook of Toxicology of Metals*, Vol. 1, Ch. 6, pp. 128–148, FRIBERG, L., NORDVEG, G. and VOUK, V. (eds) Elsevier, NY.

CLAUSEN, J., EDELING, C.-J. and FOGH, J. (1974) ^{67}Ga binding to human serum proteins and tumor components. *Cancer Res.* **34:** 1931–1937.

CLEARE, M. J. (1974) Transition metal complexes in cancer chemotherapy. *Coordin. Chem. Rev.* **12:** 349–405.

CLEARE, M. J., HYDES, P. C., MALERBY, B. and WATKINS, D. M. (1978) Anti-tumor platinum complexes: relationships between chemical properties and activity. *Biochimie* **60:** 835–850.

COLE, W. C. and WOLF, W. (1980) Preparation and metabolism of cisplatin/serum protein complex. *Chem.-Biol. Interact.* **30:** 223–235.

CROOKE, S. T. (1982) A comparison of the molecular pharmacology of gold and platinum complexes. *J. Rheumat.* **9** (Suppl. 8): 61–70.

CROOKE, S. T., SNYDER, R. M., BUTT, T. R., ECKER, D. J., ALLAUDEEN, H. S., MONIA, B. and MIRABELLI, C. K. (1986) Cellular and molecular pharmacology of auranofin and related gold complexes. *Biochem. Pharmac.* **35:** 3423–3431.

CVITKOVIC, E., SPAULDING, J., BETHUNE, V., MARTIN, J. and WHITMORE, W. F. (1977) Improvement of *cis*-dichlorodiammineplatinum (NSC 119875): therapeutic index of an animal model. *Cancer* **39:** 1357–1361.

DALEY-YATES, P. T. and MCBRIEN, D. C. H. (1983) Cisplatin metabolites: a method for their separation and for measurement of their renal clearance in vivo. *Biochem. Pharmac.* **32:** 181–184.

DALEY-YATES, P. T. and MCBRIEN, D. C. H. (1984) Cisplatin metabolites in plasma, a study of their pharmacokinetics and importance in the nephrotoxic and antitumor activity of cisplatin. *Biochem. Pharmac.* **33:** 3063–3070.

DANENBERG, P. V., SHEA, L. C., DANENBERG, K. D., and HORIKOSHI, T. (1991) Inactivation of *Tetrahymena* rRNA self-splicing by *cis*-platin proceeds through dissociable complexes. *Nucleic Acids Res.* **19:** 3123–3128.

DANPURE, C. J., FYFE, D. A. and GUMPEL, J. M. (1979) Distribution of gold among plasma fractions in rheumatoid arthritis patients undergoing chrysotherapy compared with its distribution in plasma incubated with aurothiomalate in vitro. *Ann. Rheumat. Dis.* **38:** 364–370.

DROBNIK, J. and HORACEK, P. (1973) Specific biological activity of platinum complexes contribution to the theory of molecular mechanism. *Chem.-Biol. Interact.* **7:** 223–229.

DUMAS, M., DE GISLAIN, C., D'ATHIS, P., CHADOINT-NOUDEAU, V., ESCOUSSE, A., GUERRIN, J. and AUTISSIER, N. (1990) Influence of hydration on ultrafilterable platinum kinetics and kidney function in patients treated with *cis*-diamminedichloroplatinum (II). *Cancer Chemother. Pharmac.* **26:** 278–282.

EARHART, R. H., MARTIN, P. A., TUTSCH, K. D., ETURK, E., WHEELER, R. J. and BULL, F. E. (1983) Improvement in the therapeutic index of cisplatin by pharmacologically induced chloruresis in the rat. *Cancer Res.* **43:** 1187–1194.

EASTMAN, A. (1982) Separation and characterization of products resulting from the reaction of *cis*-diamminedichloroplatinum(II) with deoxyribonucleosides. *Biochemistry* **21:** 6732–6736.

EATON, S. S., DUBACH, J., EATON, G. R., THURMAN, G. and AMBRUSO, D. R. (1990) Electron spin echo envelope modulation evidence for carbonate binding to iron (III) and copper (II) transferrin and lactoferrin. *J. biol. Chem.* **265:** 7138–7141.

ELFERINK, F., VAN DE VUGH, W. J. F., KLEIN, I. and PINEDO, H. M. (1986) Interaction of cisplatin and carboplatin with sodium thiosulfate: reaction rates binding. *Clin. Chem.* **32:** 641–645.

EL-YAZIGI, A., AMER, M. and MARTIN, C. R. (1989) Pharmacokinetics of platinum in cancer patients treated with carboplatin in combination with high-dose methotrexate. *Pharm. Res.* **6:** 492–496.

ENDRESEN, L., SCHJEVEN, L. and RUGSTAD, H. E. (1984) Tumours from a cell strain with a high content of metallothionein show enhanced resistance against *cis*-dichlorodiammineplatinum. *Acta Pharmac. Toxic.* **55:** 183–187.

EWEN, C., PERERA, A., HENDRY, J. H., MCAULIFFE, C. A., SHARMA, H. and FOX, B. W. (1988) An autoradiographic study of the intrarenal localization and retention of cisplatin, iproplatin, and paraplatin. *Cancer Chemother. Pharmac.* **22:** 241–245.

FARRIS, F. F., KING, F. G., DEDRICK, R. L. and LITTERST, C. L. (1985) Physiological model for the pharmacokinetics of *cis*-dichlorodiammine-platinum(II) (DDP) in the tumored rat. *J. Pharmacokin. Biopharmaceut.* **13:** 13–39.

FESEN, M. and HARDER, H. C. (1986) The effects of *cis*-dichlorodiammine platinum on alkaline density gradient centrifugation of poly(dA) poly(dT). *Chem.-Biol. Interact.* **57:** 123–128.

FICHTINGER-SCHEPMAN, A. M. J., LOHMAN, P. H. M. and REEDJIK, J. (1982) Detection and quantification of adducts formed upon interaction of diamminedichloroplatinum (II) with DNA, by anion exchange chromatography after enzymatic digestion. *Nucleic Acid Res.* **10:** 5345–5356.

FICHTINGER-SCHEPMAN, A. M. J., VAN OOSTEROM, A. T., LOHMAN, P. H. M. and BERENDS, F. (1987) *Cis*-diamminedichloroplatinum(II)-induced DNA adducts in peripheral leukocytes from seven cancer patients: quantitative immuno-chemical detection of the adduct induction and removal after a single dose of *cis*-diamminedichloroplatinum(II). *Cancer Res.* **47:** 3000–3004.

FICHTINGER-SCHEPMAN, A. M., VENDRIK, C. P., VAN DIJK-KNIJNENBURG, W. C., DE JONG, W. H., VAN DER MINNEN, A. C., CLAESSEN, A. M., VAN DER VELDE-VISSAR, S. D., DE GROOT, G., WUBS, K. L. and STEERENBERG, P. A. (1989) Platinum concentrations and DNA adduct levels in tumors and organs of cisplatin-treated LOU/M rats inoculated with cisplatin-sensitive or -resistant immunoglobulin M immunocytoma. *Cancer Res.* **49:** 2862–2867.

FILIPSKI, J., KOHN, K. W. and BONNER, W. M. (1980) Nature of inactivating lesions produced by platinum(II) complexes in phage lambda DNA. *Chem-Biol. Interact.* **32:** 321–330.

FROSCIO, M., MURRAY, A. W. and HURST, N. P. (1989) Inhibition of protein kinase C activity by the antirheumatic drug auranofin. *Biochem. Pharmac.* **38:** 2087–2089.

FULCO, R. A., VANNOZZI, M., COLLECCHI, P., MERLO, F., PARODI, B., CIVALLERI, D. and ESPOSITO, M. (1990) Effect of normal saline on cisplatin pharmacokinetics and antitumor activity in mice bearing P388 leukemia. *Anticancer Res.* **10:** 1603–1610.

FURST, P. and HAMER, D. (1989) Cooperative activation of a eukaryotic transcription factor: interaction between Cu (I) and yeast ACE1 protein. *Proc. natn. Acad. Sci. U.S.A.* **86:** 5267–5271.

GANDARA, D. R., PEREZ, E. A., DENHAM, A., WIEBE, V. J. and DEGREGORIO, M. W. (1989) Pharmacokinetics of cisplatinum in patients receiving interleukin-2-containing treatment regimens. *Cancer Chemother. Pharmac.* **24:** 135–136.

GIBSON, D. W., BEER, M. and BARNETT, R. J. (1971) Gold(III) complexes of adenine nucleotides. *Biochemistry* **10:** 3669–3678.

GILL, D. S. (1984) Structure–activity relationship of antitumor palladium complexes. In: *Platinum Coordination Complexes in Cancer Chemotherapy*, pp. 267–278, HACKER, M. O., DOUPLE, E. B. and KRAKOFF, I. H. (eds) M. Nijhoff, Boston.

GLICKSON, J. D., RYEL, R. B., BORDENCA, M. M., KIM, K. H. and GAMS, R. A. (1973) In vitro binding of ^{67}Ga to L1210 cells. *Cancer Res.* **33:** 2706–2713.

GOEL, R., CLEARY, S. M., HORTON, C., KIRMANI, S., ABRAMSON, I., KELLY, C. and HOWELL, S. B. (1989) Effect of sodium thiosulfate on the pharmacokinetics and toxicity of cisplatin. *J. natn. Cancer Inst.* **81:** 1552–1560.

GOEL, R., ANDREWS, P. A., PFEIFLE, C. E, ABRAMSON, I. S., KIRMANI, S. and HOWELL, S. B. (1990) Comparison of the pharmacokinetics of ultrafilterable cisplatin species detectable by derivitization with diethyldithiocarbamate or atomic absorption spectroscopy. *Eur. J. Cancer* **26:** 21–27.

GOERING, P. L. and REHM, S. (1990) Inhibition of liver, kidney, and erythrocyte delta-aminolevulinic acid dehydratase (porphobilinogen synthase) by gallium in the rat. *Environ. Res.* **53:** 135–151.

GONIAS, S. L. and PIZZO, S. V. (1983) Complexes of serum albumin and *cis*-dichlorodiammineplatinum(II). The role of cysteine 34 as a nucleophile entering group and evidence for reaction between platinum and a second macromolecule. *J. biol. Chem.* **258:** 5764–5769.

GOTTLIEB, N. L. (1982) Comparative pharmacokinetics of parenteral and oral gold compounds. *J. Rheumat.* **9** (Suppl. 8): 99–109.

GUNASEKERA, S. W., KING, L. J. and LAVENDER, P. J. (1972) The behavior of tracer gallium-67 towards serum proteins. *Clinica chim. Acta* **39:** 401–406.

HADJILLIADIS, N., MARKAPOULOS, J., PNEUMATIKAKIS, G. and KATANIS, D. (1975) Interaction of thiamine and its phosphate esters with Pt (II) and Pd (II). *J. clin. Hematol. Oncol.* **7:** 289–292.

HADJILLIADIS, N., PNEUMATIKAKIS, G. and BASOSI, R. (1981) Gold complexes of purine and pyrimidine nucleosides. *J. Inorg. Biochem.* **14:** 115–126.

HARDCASTLE, J., HARDCASTLE, P. T., KELLEHER, D. K., HENDERSON, L. S. and FONDACARO, J. D. (1986) Effect of auranofin on absorptive processes in the rat small bowel. *J. Rheumat.* **13:** 541–546.

HARDER, H. C. and ROSENBERG, B. (1970) Inhibitory effects of anti-tumor platinum compounds on DNA, RNA, and protein synthesis in mammalian cells in vitro. *Int. J. Cancer* **6:** 207–216.

HARDER, H. C., SMITH, R. G. and LEROY, A. F. (1976) Template primer inactivation by *cis*- and *trans*-dichlorodiammine platinum for human DNA polymerase, and Rauscher murine leukemia virus reverse transcriptase, as a mechanism of cytotoxicity. *Cancer Res.* **36:** 3821–3829.

HART, M. M. and ADAMSON, R. H. (1971) Antitumor activity and toxicity of salts of inorganic group IIIa metals: aluminum, gallium, indium, and thallium. *Proc. natn. Acad. Sci. U.S.A.* **68:** 1623–1626.

HART, M. M., SMITH, C. F., YANCEY, S. T. and ADAMSON, R. H. (1971) Toxicity and antiumor activity of gallium nitrate and periodically related metal salts. *J. natn. Cancer Inst.* **47:** 1121–1127.

HASUDA, K., KOBAYASHI, H., AOKI, K., TANIGUCHI, S., and BABA, T. (1989) Efficacy of two-route chemotherapy using *cis*-diamminedichloroplatinum (II) and its antidote, sodium thiosulfate, in combination with angiotensin-II for rat liver tumor. *Int. J. Cancer* **44:** 373–377.

HAYES, J. and SCOVELL, W. M. (1991a) Cis-diamminedichloroplatinum (II) modified chromatin and nucleosomal core particle probed with DNase I. *Biochim. biophys. Acta* **1088:** 413–418.

HAYES, J. and SCOVELL, W. M. (1991b) Cis-diamminedichloroplatinum (II) modified chromatin and nucleosomal core particle. *Biochim. biophys. Acta* **1089:** 377–385.

HIGBY, D. J., WALLACE, H. J. and HOLLAND, J. F. (1973) *Cis*-diamminedichloroplatinum (NSC-119875): a Phase I study. *Cancer Chemother. Rep.* **57:** 459–463.

HITCHCOCK, A. P., LOCK, C. J. L., PRATT, W. M. C. and LIPPERT, B. (1983) Platinum complexes with DNA bases, nucleotides, and DNA. In: *Platinum, Gold, and Other Metal Chemotherapeutic Agents*, pp. 209–227. LIPPARD, S. J. (ed.) American Chemical Society, Washington, D. C.

HOFER, P. B., HUBER, J. and KYAHAM-BASHI, H. (1977) The association of Ga-67 and lactoferrin. *J. nucl. Med.* **18:** 713–717.

HOGENKAMP, H. P. C., KOHLMILLER, N. A., HOWSINGER, R., WALKER, T. E. and MITWIYOFF, N. A. (1980) Interaction of *cis*-diamminediaquoplatinum(II) with adenosylcobalamin and alkylcobalamin. *J. chem. Soc.* **9:** 1668–1673.

HOUSSIER, C., DEPAUW-GILLET, M. C., HACHA, R. and FREDERICQ, E. (1983) Alteration in the nucleosome and chromatin structures upon interaction with platinum coordination complexes. *Biochim. biophys. Acta* **739:** 317–325.

HOWE-GRANT, M. E. and LIPPARD, S. J. (1983) Aqueous platinum (II) chemistry: binding to biological molecules. In: *Metal Ions in Biological Systems*, pp. 63–125. SIGEL, H. (ed.) Marcel Dekker, NY.

HOWELL, S. B. and TAETLE, R. (1980) Effect of sodium thiosulfate on *cis*-dichlorodiammineplatinum(II) toxicity and antitumor activity in L1210 leukemia. *Cancer Treat. Rep.* **64:** 611–616.

HOWELL, S. B., PFEIFLE, C. L., WUNG, W. E., OLSHEN, R. A., LUCASE, W. E., YON, J. A. and GREEN, M. (1982) Intraperitoneal cisplatin with systemic thiosulfate protection. *Ann. intern. Med.* **97:** 845–851

HOWLE, J. A. and GALE, G. R. (1970) *Cis*-dichlorodiammineplatinum(II): persistent and selective inhibition of DNA synthesis in vivo. *Biochem. Pharmac.* **19:** 757–762.

HU, M.-L., VILJOEN, A. J. and TAPPEL, A. L. (1988) Interactions of gold with cytosolic selenium-containing proteins in rat kidney and liver. *J. Inorg. Biochem.* **32:** 281–290.

HUDES, G. R., LACRETA, F., WALCZAK, J., TINSLEY, P., LITWIN, S., COMIS, R. L. and O'DWYER, P. J. (1991) Pharmacokinetic study of trimetrexate in combination with cisplatin. *Cancer Res.* **51:** 3080–3087.

HUTCHENS, T. W. and LI, C. M. (1988) Estrogen receptor interaction with mobilized metals. Differential molecular recognition of Zn^{2+}, Cu^{2+} and Ni^{2+} and separation of receptor isoforms. *J. molec. Recog.* **1:** 80–92.

INAGAKI, K., KASAYA, K. and KIDANI, Y. (1984) Determination of platinum binding bases in oligonucleotides. Application of exonuclease digestion method. *Inorg. Chim. Acta* **91:** L13–L15.

INTOCCIA, A. P., FLANAGAN, T. L., WALZ, D. T., GUTZANT, L. SWAGZDIS, J. E., FLAGIELLO, J. HWANG, B. Y.-H., DEWEY, R. H. and NOGUCHI, H. (1982) Pharmacokinetics of auranofin in animals. *J. Rheumat.* **9** (Suppl. 8): 90–98.

ISHIZAWA, M., TANIGUCHI, S. and BABA, T. (1981) Protection by sodium thiosulfate and thiourea against lethal toxicity of *cis*-diamminedichloroplatinum(II) in bacteria and mice. *Jap. J. Pharmac.* **31:** 883–889.

ISONISHI, S., ANDREWS, P. A. and HOWELL, S. B. (1990) Increased sensitivity to *cis*-diamminedichloroplatinum (II) in human ovarian carcinoma cells in response to treatment with 12-O-tetradecanoylphorbol 13-acetate. *J. biol. Chem* **265:** 3623–3627.

JOHNSON, N. P. HOESCHELE, J. D. and RAHN, R. O. (1980) Kinetic analysis of the in vitro binding of radioactive *cis*- and *trans*-dichlorodiammeplatinum(II) to DNA. *Chem.-Biol. Interact.* **30:** 151–169.

KHANDEKAR, J. D. (1983) Improved therapeutic index of *cis*-diamminedichloroplatinum by diethyldithiocarbamate in rodents. *Res. Commun. Chem. Path. Pharmac.* **40:** 55–66.

KIRSCHNER, S., MAURER, A. and DRAGULESCU, C. (1975) Potential antitumor activity of platinum and palladium complexes with sulfur and nitrogen ligands. *J. clin. Hematol.* **7:** 190–196.

KISTENMACHER, T. J., ORBELL, J. D. and MARXILLI, L. G. (1983) Conformation properties of purine and pyrimidine complexes of *cis*-platinum. Implications for platinum-II DNA crosslinking modes. In: *Platinum, Gold and Other Metal Chemotherapeutic Agents*, pp. 191–207, LIPPARD, S. J. (ed.) American Chemical Society, Washington, D. C.

KNOX, R. J., FRIEDLOS, F., LYDALL, D. A. and ROBERTS, J. J. (1986) Mechanism of cytotoxicity of anticancer platinum drugs: evidence that *cis*-diamminedichloroplatinum(II) and *cis*-diammine-(1,1-cyclobutanedicarboxylato)platinum(II) differ only in kinetics of their interaction with DNA. *Cancer Res.* **46:** 1972–1979.

KOHL, H. H., FRIEDMAN, M. E., MELIUS, P., MORA, E. C. and MCAULIFFE, C. A. (1978) Enhanced inhibition of both cellular protein synthesis and malate dehydrogenase by aged aquoplatinum(II) complexes. *Chem.-Biol. Interact.* **24:** 209–215.

KONG, P.-C. and THEOPHANIDES, T. (1975) Platinum complexes of nucleotides. *Bioinorg. Chem.* **5:** 51–58.

KOPF, H. and KOPF-MAIER, P. (1983) Tumor inhibition by metallocene dihalides of early transition metals. Chemical and biological aspects. *Am. chem. Soc. Symp. Ser.* **209:** 315–333.

KOPF-MAIER, P. (1982) Development of necroses, virus activation and giant cell formation after treatment of Ehrlich ascites tumor with metallocene dichlorides. *J. Cancer Res. clin. Oncol.* **103:** 145–164.

KOPF-MAIER, P. and KRAHL, D. (1981) Intracellular distribution of titanium after treatment with the antitumor agent titanocene dichloride: an electron energy loss spectroscopic study. *Naturwissenschaften* **68:** 273– 274.

KRAKER, A., SCHMIDT, J., KREZOSKI, S. and PETERING, D. H. (1985) Binding of *cis*-dichlorodiammine platinum (II) to metallothionein in Ehrlich cells. *Biochem. biophys. Res. Commun.* **130:** 786–792.

LEE, M. T., AHMED, T., HADDAD, R. and FRIEDMAN, M. E. (1989) Inhibition of several enzymes by gold compounds. II. Beta-glucuronidase, acid phosphatase, and L-malate dehydrogenase by sodium thiomalatoaurate (I), sodium thiosulfatoaurate (I) and thioglucosoaurate (I). *J. Enzym. Inhib.* **3:** 35–47.

LEEUWENKAMP, O. R., VAN DER VIJGH, W. J., NEIJT, J. P. and PINEDO, H. M. (1990) Reaction kinetics of cisplatin and its monoaquated species with the (potential) renal protecting agents (di)mesna and thiosulfate. Estimation of the effect of protecting agents on the plasma and peritoneal AUCs of CDDP. *Cancer Chemother. Pharmac.* **27:** 111–114.

LEROY, A. F. (1975) Interactions of platinum metals and their complexes in biological systems. *Environ. Health Perspect.* **10:** 73–83.

LEROY, A. F. and THOMPSON, W. C. (1989) Binding kinetics of tetrachloro-1,2-diaminocyclohexaneplatinum (IV) (tetraplatin) and *cis*-diamminedichloroplatinum (II) at 37°C with human plasma proteins and with bovine serum albumin. Does aquation precede protein binding? *J. natn. Cancer Inst.* **81:** 427–436.

LEROY, A. F., LUTZ, R. J., DEDRICK, R. L., LITTERST, C. L. and GUARINO, A. M. (1979) Pharmacokinetic study of *cis*-dichlorodiammineplatinum(II) (DDP) in the beagle dog: thermodynamic and kinetic behavior of DDP in a biologic mileu. *Cancer Treat. Rep.* **63:** 59–71.

LEVI, J., JACOBS, C., KALMAN, S. M., MCTIGUE, M. and WEINER, M. W. (1980) Mechanism of *cis*-platinum nephrotoxicity: I. Effects of sulfhydryl groups in rat kidneys. *J. Pharmac. exp. Ther.* **213:** 545–550.

LEWIS, A. J. COTTNEY, J. WHITE, D. D., FOX, P. K., MCNEILLIE, A., DUNLAP, J., SMITH, W. E. and BROWN, D. H. (1980) Action of gold salts in some inflammatory and immunological models. *Agents Actions* **10:** 63–67.

LEYLAND-JONES, B., MORROW, C., TATE, S., URMACHER, C., GORDON, C. and YOUNG, C. W. (1983) *Cis*-diamminedichloroplatinum(II) nephrotoxicity and its relationship to renal γ-glutamyl transpeptidase and glutathione. *Cancer Res.* **43:** 6072–6076.

LIPPARD, S. J. (1982) New chemistry of an old molecule: *cis*-$Pt(NH_3)_2Cl_2$. *Science* **218:** 1075–1082.

LIPPARD, S. J. and HOESCHELE, J. D. (1979) Binding of *cis*- and *trans*-dichlorodiammineplatinum(II) to the nucleosome core. *Proc. natn. Acad. Sci. U.S.A.* **76:** 6091–6095.

LIPPARD, S. J., USHAY, H. M., MERKEL, C. M. and POIRIER, M. C. (1983) Use of antibodies to probe the sterochemistry of antitumor platinum drug binding to deoxyribonucleic acid. *Biochemistry* **22:** 5165–5168.

LISON, D., KNOOPS, B., COLLETTE, C. and LAUWERYS, R. (1989) Comparison of the effects of auranofin and retinoic acid on plasminogen activator activity of peritoneal macrophages and Lewis lung carcinoma cells. *Biochem. Pharmac.* **38:** 2107–2112.

LITTERST, C. L. (1981) Alterations in the toxicity of *cis*-dichlorodiammineplatinum-II and in tissue localization of platinum as a function of NaCl concentration in the vehicle of administration. *Toxic. appl. Pharmac.* **61:** 99–108.

LITTERST, C. L. (1984a) Cisplatinum: a review, with special reference to cellular and molecular interactions. *Agents Action* **15:** 520–524.

LITTERST, C. L. (1984b) Plasma pharmacokinetics, urinary excretion, and tissue distribution of platinum following i.v. administration of cyclobutanedicarboxylatoplatinum-II and *cis*-platinum to rabbits. In: *Platinum Coordination Complexes in Cancer Chemotherapy*, pp. 71–81, HACKER, M. P., DOUPLE, E. B. and KRAKOFF, I. H. (eds) Nijhoff, Boston.

LITTERST, C. L. and SCHWEITZER, V. G. (1988a) Covalent binding of platinum to kidney subcellular fractions

from guinea pig strains sensitive and resistant to cisplatin toxicity. In: *Platinum and Other Metal Coordination Complexes in Cancer Chemotherapy*, pp. 207–215, NICOLINI, M. (ed.) M. Nijhoff, Boston.
LITTERST, C. L. and SCHWEITZER, V. G. (1988b) Covalent binding of platinum to renal protein from sensitive and resistant guinea pits treated with cisplatin: Possible role in nephrotoxicity. *Res. Commun. Chem. Path. Pharmac.* **61:** 35–48.
LITTERST, C. L., GRAM, T. E., DEDRICK, R. L., LEROY, A. F. and GUARINO, A. M. (1976) Distribution and disposition of platinum following intravenous administration of *cis*-diamminedichloroplatinum(II) (NSC 119875) to dogs. *Cancer Res.* **36:** 2340–2344.
LITTERST, C. L., TORRES, I. J. and GUARINO, A. M. (1977) Plasma levels and organ distribution of platinum in the rat, dog, and dogfish shark following single intravenous administration of *cis*-dichlorodiammineplatinum(II). *J. clin. Hematol. Oncol.* **7:** 169–179.
LITTERST, C. L., LEROY, A. F. and GUARINO, A. M. (1979) Disposition and distribution of platinum following parenteral administration of *cis*-dichloro-diammineplatinum(II) to animals. *Cancer Treat. Rep.* **63:** 1485–1492.
LITTERST, C. L., TONG, S., HIROKATA, Y. and SIDDIK, Z. H. (1982a) Alterations in hepatic and renal levels of glutathione and activities of glutathione *S*-transferases from rats treated with *cis*-dichlorodiammineplatinum-II. *Cancer Chemother. Pharmac.* **8:** 67–71.
LITTERST, C. L., TORRES, I. J., ARNOLD, S., MCGUNAGLE, D., FURNER, R., SIKIC, B. I. and GUARINO, A. M. (1982b) Absorption of antineoplastic drugs following large-volume i.p. administration to rats. *Cancer Treat. Rep.* **66:** 147–155.
LITTERST, C. L., TONG, S., HIROKATA, Y. and SIDDIK, Z. (1983) Stimulation of microsomal drug oxidation in liver and kidney of rats treated with the oncolytic agent *cis*-dichlorodiammineplatinum (II). *Pharmacology* **26:** 46–53.
LITTERST, C. L., BERTOLERO, F. and UOZUMI, J. (1986) The role of glutathione and metallothionein in the toxicity and subcellular binding of cisplatin. In: *Biochemical Mechanisms of Platinum Antitumor Drugs*, pp. 227–254, MCBRIEN, D. C. H. and SLATER, T. F. (eds) IRL Press, Oxford.
LITTERST, C. L., POIRER, M. C. and REED, E. (1988) Factors influencing the formation and persistence of platinum–DNA adducts in tissues of rats treated with cisplatin. In: *Organ Directed Toxicities of Anticancer Drugs*, pp. 172–189, HACKER, M., LAZO, J. and TRITTON, T. (eds) M. Nijhoff, Boston.
LORBER, A., BOVY, R. A. and CHANG, C. C. (1972) Relationship between serum gold content and distribution to serum immunoglobulins and complement. *Nature New Biol.* **236:** 250–252.
MACQUET, J. P., BUTOUR, J. L. and JOHNSON, N. P. (1978) Modifications of the DNA secondary structure upon platinum binding: a proposed model. *Biochemie* **60:** 901–914.
MACQUET, J. P., JANKOWSKI, K. and BUTOUR, J. L. (1980) Mass spectrometry study of DNA–cisplatin complexes: perturbation of guanine-cytosine base pairs. *Biochem. biophys. Res. Commun.* **82:** 68–74.
MACQUET, J. P., BUTOUR, J. L. and JOHNSON, N. P. (1983) Physicochemical and structural studies of the in vitro interactions between platinum(II) compounds and DNA. In: *Platinum, Gold, and Other Metal Chemotherapeutic Agents*, pp. 75–100, LIPPARD, S. J. (ed.) American Chemical Society, Washington, D. C.
MALLYA, S. K. and VAN WART, H. E. (1989) Mechanism of inhibition of human neutrophil collagenase by gold (I) chrysotherapeutic compounds. Interaction at a heavy metal binding site. *J. biol. Chem.* **264:** 1594– 1601.
MANAKA, R. C. and WOLF, W. (1978) Distribution of *cis*-platin in blood. *Chem.-Biol. Interact.* **49:** 165–176.
MANDAL, C. and NANDI, U. S. (1978) Kinetic studies on the interaction of gold (III) with nucleic acids. IV. RNA-Au(III) system. *Chem.-Biol. Interact.* **21:** 125–134.
MANSY, S., ROSENBERG, B. and THOMSON, A. J. (1973) Biding of *cis*- and *trans*-dichlorodiammineplatinum(II) to nucleosides. I. Location of binding sites. *J. Am. chem. Soc.* **95:** 1633–1640.
MARTIN, R. B. (1983) Hydrolytic equilibria and N7 versus N1 binding in purine nucleosides of *cis*-diamminedichloroplatinum(II). Palladium(II) as a guide to platinum(II) reactions at equilibrium. In: *Platinum, Gold, and Other Metal Chemotherapeutics Agents*, pp. 231–244, LIPPARD, S. J. (ed.) American Chemical Society, Washington, D. C.
MASON, R. W. (1977) The binding of aurothiomalate to plasma proteins in vitro. *Pharmacology* **15:** 536–544.
MASON, R., EDWARDS, I. R. and MCLAREN, S. J. (1984) Interaction of platinum with metallothionein-like ligands in the rat kidney after administration of *cis*-dichlorodiammineplatinum-II. *Chem.-Biol. Interact.* **49:** 165–176.
MCQUEEN, E. G. and DYKES, P. W. (1969) Transport of gold in the body. *Ann. Rheum. Dis.* **28:** 437–442.
METZLER, M. (1986) DNA adducts of medicinal drugs: some selected examples. *J. Cancer Res. clin. Oncol.* **112:** 210–215.
MINKEL, D. T. and PETERING, D. H. (1978) Initial reaction of 3-ethoxy-2-oxobutyraldehyde bis (thiosemicarbazonato)copper (II) with Ehrlich ascites tumor cells. *Cancer Res.* **38:** 117–123.
MIRABELLI, C. K. and CROOKE, S. T. (1983) Pharmacology of auranofin—a review and future perspective. In: *Auroanofin*, pp. 71–31, CAPELL, H. A., COLE, D. S., MANGHANI, K. K. and MORRIS, R. W. (eds) Excerpta Medica, Amsterdam.
MIRABELLI, C. K., JOHNSON, R. K., SUNG, C. M., FAUCETTE, L. F., MUIRHEAD, K. and CROOKE, S. T. (1985) Evaluation of the in vivo antitumor activity and in vitro cytotoxic properties of auranofin, a coordinated gold compound, in murine tumor models. *Cancer Res.* **45:** 32–39.
MIRABELLI, C. K., JOHNSON, R. K., HILL, D. T., FAUCETTE, L. F., GIRARD, G. R., KUO, G. Y., SUNG, C. M. and

CROOKE, S. T. (1986a) Correlation of the in vitro cytotoxic and in vivo antitumor activities of the gold(I) coordination complexes. *J. med. Chem.* **29:** 218–223.

MIRABELLI, C. K., SUNG, C. M., ZIMMERMAN, J. P., HILL, D. T., MONG, S. and CROOKE, S. T. (1986b) Interactions of gold coordination complexes with DNA. *Biochem. Pharmac.* **35:** 1427–1433.

MIRABELLI, C. K., ZIMMERMAN, J. P., BARTUS, H. R., SUNG, C. M. and CROOKE, S. T. (1986c) Inter-strand crosslinks and single-strand breaks produced by gold(I) and gold(III) coordination complexes. *Biochem. Pharmac.* **35:** 1425–1443.

MOUSTATIH, A. and GARNIER-SUILLEROT, A. (1989) Bifunctional antitumor compounds: synthesis and characterization of a Au (III)-streptonigrin complex with thiol-modulating properties. *J. med. Chem.* **32:** 1426–1431.

NAGANUMA, A., SATOH, M., KOYAMA, Y. and IMURA, N. (1985) Protective effect of metallothionein inducing metals on lethal toxicity of *cis*-diamminedichloroplatinum in mice. *Toxic. Lett.* **24:** 203–207.

NAZIMIEC, M., CROOKE, S. T. and PRESTAYKO, A. W. (1982) Effects of *cis*-diamminedichloroplatinum (CDDP) on HeLa cell nonhistone nuclear proteins. *Cancer Chemother. Pharmac.* **9:** 36–40.

NOVOTNA, J., MITEROVA, L., KRABCOVA, M., DEYL, Z. and ADAM, M. (1991) Contribution to the mode of action of univalent gold. *Z. Rheumat.* **50:** 99–102.

O'DWYER, P. J., LACRETA, F., HOGAN, M., ROSENBLUM, N., O'DWYER, J. L. and COMIS, R. L. (1991) Pharmacologic study of etoposide and cisplatin by the intraperitoneal route. *J. clin. Pharmac.* **31:** 253–258.

OHKUBO, Y., SASAYAMA, A., TAKEGAHARA, I., KATOH, S., ABE, K., KOHNO, H. and KUBODERA, A. (1990) 67-Ga in transferrin-unbound form is taken up by inflamed liver of mouse treated with CCl4. *Ann. Nucl. Med.* **4:** 89–93.

OLINSKI, R., WIADERKIEWICZ, R. and WALTER, Z. (1983) Estimation of *cis*-diamminedichloroplatinum(II) binding to purine bases of calf thymus DNA using [^{14}C]methylbromphevinphos. *J. Biochem. biophys. Meth.* **7:** 171–173.

ORIANA, S., SPATTI, G. B., BOHM, S., OGNELLA, S., TEDESCHI, M., ZUNINO, F. and DI RE, G. (1988) A preliminary clinical study of reduced glutathione as a protective agent against cisplatin-induced toxicity. In: *Organ Directed Toxicities of Anticancer Drugs*, p. 240, HACKER, M., LAZO, J. and TRITTON, T. (eds) M. Nijhoff, Boston.

OSWALD, C. B. and HALL, I. H. (1989) The inhibition of P388 lymphocytic leukemia DNA polymerase alpha activity by *cis*-diamminedichloroplatinum (II) and related derivatives. *Anticancer Res.* **9:** 915–922.

OSWALD, C. B., CHANEY, S. G. and HALL, I. H. (1990) Inhibition of nucleic acid synthesis in P388 lymphocytic leukemia cells in culture by *cis*-platinum derivatives. *Biomed. Biochim. Acta* **49:** 579–587.

OZOLS, R. F., CORDEN, B. J., JACOB, J., WESLEY, M. N., OSTCHEGA, Y. and YOUNG, R. C. (1984) High-dose cisplatin in hypertonic saline. *Ann. intern. Med.* **100:** 19–24.

PARTI, R., and WOLF, W. (1990) Quantitative subcellular distribution of platinum in rat tissues following i.v. bolus and i.v. infusion of cisplatin. *Cancer Chemother. Pharmac.* **26:** 188–192.

PASCOE, J. M. and ROBERTS, J. J. (1974) Interactions between mammalian cell DNA and inorganic platinum compounds-I. DNA interstrand cross-linking and cytotoxic properties of platinum(II) compounds. *Biochem. Pharmac.* **23:** 1345–1357.

PEDERSEN, H. B., JOSEPHSEN, J. and KERZMAN, G. (1985) Phosphate buffer and salt medium concentrations affect the inactivation of T4 phage by platinum(II) complexes. *Chem.-Biol. Interact.* **54:** 1–8.

PERCIVAL, S. S. and HARRIS, E. D. (1990) Copper transport from ceruloplasmin: characterization of the cellular uptake mechanism. *Am. J. Physiol.* **258:** C140–146.

PERERA, F., FISCHMAN, H. K., HEMMINKI, K., BRANDT-RAUF, P., NIMAN, H. L., SMITH, S., TOPOROFF, E., O'DOWD, K., TANG, M. X. and TSAI, W. Y. (1990) Protein binding, sister chromatid exchange and expression of oncogene proteins in patients treated with cisplatinum-based therapy. *Arch. Toxic.* **64:** 401–406.

PEREZ, J. M., NAVARRO-RANNINGER, M. C., REQUENA, J. M., JIMENEZ-RULZ, A., PARRONDO, E., CRACIUNESCU, D., LOPEZ, M. C. and ALONSO, C. (1991) DNA binding properties and antileukemic (L1210) activity of a Pt-pentamidine complex. *Chem.-Biol. Interact.* **77:** 341–355.

PERUMAREDDI, J. R. and ADAMSON, A. W. (1968) Photochemistry of complex ions. V. The photochemistry of some square-planar platinum(II) complexes. *J. phys. Chem.* **72:** 414–420.

PETERING, D. H. (1980) Carcinostatic copper complexes. In: *Metal Ions in Biological Systems*, pp. 197–229, SIGEL, H. (ed.) Marcel Dekker, N.Y.

PETERING, H. G., BUSKIRK, H. H. and CRIM, J. A. (1967) Effect of dietary mineral supplements of the rat on the antitumor activity of 3-ethoxy-2- oxobutyraldehyde bis (thiosemicarbazone). *Cancer Res.* **27:** 1115–1121.

PEYROT, V., BRIAND, C., CREVAT, A., BRAGUER, D., CHAUVET-MONGES, A. M. and SARI, J. C. (1983) Action of hydrolyzed cisplatin and some analogs on microtubule assembly inhibition by *cis*-dichlorodiammine-platinum(II). *Biochem. Pharmac.* **35:** 371–375.

PILLAI, C. K. S. and NANDI, U. S. (1978) Interaction of metal ions with nucleic acids and related compounds. II. Studies on Au (III)-nucleic acid system. *Biopolymers* **17:** 709–729.

PIZZO, S. V., ROCHE, P. A., FELDMAN, S. R. and GONAS, S. L. (1986) Further characterization of the platinum-reactive component of the α_2-macroglobulin-receptor recognition site. *Biochem. J.* **238:** 217–225.

PIZZO, S. V., SWAIM, M. W., ROCHE, P. A. and GONIAS, S. L. (1988) Selectivity and stereospecificity of the reactions of dichlorodiammineplatinum (II) with three purified plasma proteins. *J. Inorg. Biochem.* **33:** 67–76.

PLOOY, A. C. M., VAN DIJK, M. and LOHMAN, P. H. M. (1984) Induction and repair of DNA cross-links in chinese hamster ovary cells treated with various platinum coordination compounds in relation to platinum binding to DNA, cytotoxicity, mutagenicity and antitumor activity. *Cancer Res.* **44:** 2043–2051.

PLOOY, A. C. M., FICHTINGER-SCHEPMAN, A. M. J., SCHUTTE, H. H., VAN DIJK, M. and LOHMAN, P. H. M. (1985a) Quantitative detection of various Pt-DNA adducts in Chinese hamster ovary cells treated with cisplatin: application of immunochemical techniques. *Carcinogenesis* **6:** 561–566.

PLOOY, A. C. M., VAN DIJK, M., BERENDS, F. and LOHMAN, P. H. M. (1985b) Formation and repair of DNA interstrand cross-links in relation to cytotoxicity and unscheduled DNA synthesis induced in control and mutant human cells treated with *cis*-diamminedichloroplatinum(II). *Cancer Res.* **45:** 417–4184.

POIRIER, M. C., LIPPARD, S. J., ZWELLING, L. A., USHAY, H. M., KERRIGAN, D., THILL, C. C., SANTELLA, R. M., GRUNBERGER, D. and YUSPA, S. H. (1982) Antibodies elicited against *cis*-diamminedichloroplatinum(II)-modified DNA are specific for *cis*-diamminedichloroplatinum(II)-DNA adducts formed in vivo and in vitro. *Proc. natn. Acad. Sci. U.S.A.* **79:** 6443–6447.

POIRIER, M. C., REED, E., ZWELLING, L. A., OZOLS, R. F., LITTERST, C. L. and YUSPA, S. H. (1985) Polyclonal antibodies to quantitate *cis*-diamminedichloroplatinum(II)–DNA adducts in cancer patients and animal models. *Environ. Health Perspec.* **62:** 89–94.

POIRIER, M. C., REED, E., LITTERST, C. L., KATZ, D. and GUPTA-BURT, S. (1992) Persistence of platinum-ammine–DNA adducts in gonads and kidneys of rats and multiple tissues from cancer patients. *Cancer Res.* **52:** 149–153.

POLISSOIU, M., VIET, M. T. P., ST. JACQUES, M. and THEOPHANIDES, T. (1985) Binding study of the drug *cis*-dichlorodiammineplatinum(II) to $G^{5'}_{p}$ and $dG^{5'}_{p}$ by high resolution proton and carbon-13 NMR spectroscopy. *Inorg. Chim. Acta* **107:** 203–210.

PRUTZ, W. A., BUTLER, J. and LAND, E. J. (1990) Interaction of copper (I) with nucleic acids. *Int. J. Radiat. Biol.* **58:** 215–234.

RAHN, R. O. (1984) Chromatographic analysis of the adducts formed in DNA complexed with *cis*-diamminedichloroplatinum(II). *J. Inorgan. Biochem.* **21:** 311–321.

RAHN, R. O., CHANG, S. S. and HOESCHELE, J. D. (1983) Adducts formed between deoxyguanosine and *cis*-diamminedichloroplatinum(II): separation by means of cation-exchange chromotography. *J. Inorgan. Biochem.* **18:** 279–290.

RAWLINGS, C. J. and ROBERTS, J. J. (1986) Walker rat carcinoma cells are exceptionally sensitive to *cis*-diamminedichloroplatinum (II) (cisplatin) and other difunctional agents but not defective in the removal of platinum–DNA adducts. *Mutat. Res.* **166:** 157–168.

RAZI, M. T., OTIKO, G. and SADLER, P. J. (1983) Ligand exchange reactions of gold drugs in model systems and in red cells. In: *Platinum, Gold and Other Metal Chemotherapeutic Agents*, pp. 371–384, LIPPARD, S. J. (ed.) American Society, Washington, D.C.

REED, E., LITTERST, C. L., THILL, C. C., YUSPA, S. H. and POIRIER, M. C. (1987) *Cis*-diamminedichloroplatin-um(II)–DNA adduct formation in renal, gonadal, and tumor tissues of male and female rats. *Cancer Res.* **47:** 718–722.

REEDIJK, J., DEN HARTOG, J. H. J., FICHTINGER-SCHEPMAN, A. M. J. and MARCELIS, A. T. M. (1984) Specific binding of *cis*-platinum compounds to DNA and DNA fragments. In: *Platinum Coordination Complexes in Cancer Chemotherapy*, pp. 39–50, HACKER, M. P., DOUPLE, E. B. and KRAKOFF, I. H. (eds) M. Nijhoff, Boston.

REISHUS, J. W. and MARTIN, D. S. JR. (1961) *Cis*-dichlorodiammineplatinum(II). Acid hydrolysis and isotopic exchange of the chloride ligands. *J. Am. chem. Soc.* **83:** 2457–2462.

RENSHAW, E. and THOMSON, A. J. (1967) Tracer studies to locate the site of platinum ions within filamentous and inhibited cells of *Escherichia coli. J. Bact.* **94:** 1915–1918.

RILEY, C. M., STERNSON, L. A., REPTA, A. J. and SLYTER, S. A. (1983) Monitoring the reactions of cisplatin with nucleotides and methionine by reversed-phase high-performance liquid chromatography using cationic and anionic pairing ions. *Analyt. Biochem.* **130:** 203–214.

ROBERTS, J. D., VAN HOUTEN, B., QU, Y. and FARRELL, N. P. (1989) Interaction of novel bis(platinum) complexes with DNA. *Nucleic Acids Res.* **17:** 9719– 9733.

ROBERTS, J. J. and FRAVAL, H. N. A. (1978) The interaction of antitumor platinum compounds with cellular DNA in cultured cells and animal tissues: relationship to DNA cellular repair processes. *Biochimie* **60:** 869–877.

ROBERTS, J. J. and PERA, M. P., JR (1983) Action of platinum antitumor drugs. In: *Molecular Aspects of Anti-cancer Drug Action*, pp. 183–231, NEIDLE, S. and WARING, M. J. (eds) Verlag Chemi, Basel.

ROCHE, P. A., JENSEN, P. E. H. and PIZZO, S. V. (1988a) Intersubunit cross-linking by *cis*-dichlorodiammine-platinum (II) stabilizes an alpha-2 macroglobulin "nascent" state: evidence that thiol ester bond cleavage correlates with receptor recognition site exposure. *Biochemistry* **27:** 759–764.

ROCHE, P. A., STRICKLAND, D. K., ENGHILD, J. J. and PIZZO, S. V. (1988b) Evidence that the platinum-reactive methionyl residue of the alpha-2 macroglobulin receptor recognition site is not in the carboxyl terminal receptor binding domain. *J. biol. Chem.* **263:** 6715–6721.

ROSENBERG, B. (1978) Platinum complex-DNA interaction and anticancer activity. *Biochimie* **60:** 859–867.

ROSENBERG, B. and VANCAMP, L. (1970) The successful regression of large solid sarcoma 180 tumors by platinum compounds. *Cancer Res.* **30:** 1799–1802.

ROSENBERG, B., VANCAMP, L. and KRIGAS, T. (1965) Inhibition of cell division in *E. coli* by electrolysis products from a platinum electrode. *Nature* **205:** 698–699.

ROSENBERG, B., RENSHAW, E., VANCAMP, L., HARGWICK, J. and DROBNIK, J. (1967) Platinum-induced filamentous growth in *E. coli*. *J. Bact.* **93:** 716–721.

ROSENBERG, B., VANCAMP, L., TROSKO, J. and MANSEUR, V. H. (1969) Platinum compounds: a new class of potent antitumor agents. *Nature (Lond.)* **222:** 385–386.

RUBIN, J. R., SABAT, M. and SUNDARALINGAM, M. (1983) Similar binding of the carcinostatic drugs *cis* $[Pt(NH_3)_2Cl_2]$ and $[Ru(NH_3)_5Cl]$ Cl_2 to $tRNA^{phe}$ and a comparison with the binding of the inactive *trans*-$[Pt(NH_3)_2Cl_2]$ complex—reluctance in binding to Watson–Crick base pairs within double helix. *Nucleic Acids Res.* **11:** 6571–6586.

SADLER, P. J. (1982a) The comparative evaluation of the physical and chemical properties of gold compounds. *J. Rheumat.* **9:** 71–78.

SADLER, P. J. (1982b) Inorganic pharmacology. *Chem. Br.* **18:** 12–14.

SADLER, P. J., NASR, M. and NARAYAN, V. L. (1984) Design of metal complexes as anti-cancer drugs. In: *Platinum Coordination Complexes in Cancer Chemotherapy*, pp. 290–306, HACKER, M. P., DOUPLE, E. B. and KRAKOFF, I. H. (eds) M. Nijhoff, Boston.

SARNA, S., BHOLA, R. K., and SODHI, A. (1988) Release of protein bound sialic acid from fibrosarcoma cells after *cis*-dichlorodiammineplatinum (II) treatment: the possible role in tumor regression. *Pol. J. Pharmac. Pharm.* **40:** 295–302.

SARRAZIN, M., PEYROT, V. and BRIAND, C. (1986) NMR studies of the interaction of *cis*-diamminedichloroplatinum(II) and corresponding hydrolysis products with adenosine phosphates. *Inorgan. Chim. Acta* **124:** 87–96.

SARYAN, L. A., ANKEL, E., KRISHNAUMURTI, C. and PETERING, D. H. (1979) Comparative cytotoxic and biochemical effects of ligands and metal complexes of alpha-*N*-heterocyclic carboxaldehyde thiosemicarbazones. *J. med. Chem.* **22:** 1218–1221.

SCHECHTER, B., ROSING, M. A., WILCHECK, M. and ARNON, R. (1989) Blood levels and serum protein binding of *cis*-platinum (II) complexed to carboxymethyl-dextran. *Cancer Chemother. Pharmac.* **24:** 161–166.

SCHMITZ, G., MINKEL, D. T., GINGRICH, D. and SHAW, C. F., III (1980) The binding of gold(I) to metallothionein. *J. Inorg. Biochem.* **12:** 293–306.

SCOVELL, W. M. and KROOS, L. R. (1982) *Cis*-diamminedichloroplatinum(II) modification of SV40 DNA occurs preferentially in (G + C) rich regions. Implications into the mechanism of action. *Biochem. biophys. Res. Commun.* **108:** 16–23.

SCOVELL, W. M. and O'CONNOR, T. (1977) Interaction of aquated *cis*-$[(NH_3)_2Pt^{II}]$ with nucleic acid constituents. I. Ribonucleosides. *J. Am. chem. Soc.* **99:** 120–126.

SCOVELL, W. M., KROOS, L. R. and CAPPONI, V. J. (1983) Model for the interaction of *cis*-diamminedichloroplatinum(II) with simian virus 40DNA. In: *Platinum, Gold and Other Metal Chemotherapeutic Agents*, pp. 102–121, LIPPARD, S. J. (ed.) American Chemical Society, Washington, D. C.

SEGAL, E. and LEPECQ, J. B. (1985) Role of ligand exchange processes in the reaction kinetics of the antitumor drug *cis*-diamminedichloroplatinum(II) with its targets. *Cancer Res.* **45:** 492–498.

SERAFINI, M. T., ROMEU, A. and AROLA, L. (1989) Zn (II), Cd (II), and Cu (II) interactions on glutathione reductase and glucose-6-phosphate dehydrogenase. *Biochem. Int.* **18:** 793–802.

SHANI, J., BERTRAM, J., RUSSELL, C., DAHALAN, R., CHEN, D. C., PARTI, R., AHMADI, J., KEMPF, R. A., KAWADA, T. K. and MUGGIA, F. M. (1989) Noninvasive monitoring of drug biodistribution and metabolism: studies with intraarterial Pt-195m-cisplatin in humans. *Cancer Res* **49:** 1877–1881.

SHAW, C. F., III (1979) The mammalian biochemistry of gold: an inorganic perspective of chrysotherapy. *Inorg. Persp. Biol. Med.* **2:** 287–355.

SHERMAN, S. E., GIBSEN, D., WANG, A. H. J. and LIPPARD, S. J. (1985) X-ray structure of the major adduct of the anticancer drug cisplatin with DNA: *cis*-$Pt(NH_3)_2$ d(pGpG). *Science* **230:** 412–417.

SHOOTER, K. V., HOUSE, R., MERRIFIELD, R. K. and ROBINS, A. B. (1972) Interaction of platinum-II compounds with bacteriophage T7 and R17. *Chem.-Biol. Interact.* **5:** 289–307.

SIMON, T. M., KUNISHIMA, D. H., VIBERT, G. J. and LORBER, A. (1979) Inhibitory effects of a new oral gold compound on HeLa cells. *Cancer* **44:** 1965–1975.

SIMON, T. M., KUNISHIMA, D. H., VIBERT, G. J. and LORBER, A. (1981) Screening trial with the coordinated gold compound auranofin using mouse lymphocytic leukemia P388. *Cancer Res.* **41:** 94–97.

SNYDER, R. M., MIRABELLI, C. K. and CROOKE, S. T. (1986) Cellular association, intracellular distribution, and efflux of auranofin via sequential ligand exchange reactions. *Biochem. Pharmac.* **35:** 923–932.

SRIVASTAVA, R. C., FROEHLICH, J. and EICHHORN, G. L. (1978) The effect of platinum binding on the structure of DNA and its function in RNA synthesis. *Biochimie* **60:** 879–891.

STJERNHOLM, R., WARNER, F. W., ROBINSON, J. W., EZEKIEL, E. and KATAYAMA, N. (1978) Binding of platinum to human transferrin. *Bioinorg. Chem.* **9:** 277–280.

STONE, P. J., KELMAN, A. D. and SINEX, F. M. (1974) Specific binding of antitumor drug *cis*-Pt $(NH_3)_2Cl_2$ to DNA rich in guanine and cytosine. *Nature* **251:** 736–737.

SUZUKI, C. A. and CHERIAN, M. G. (1990) The interactions of *cis*-diamminedichloroplatinum with metallothionein and glutathione in rat liver and kidney. *Toxicology* **64:** 113–127.

SYKES, T. R., STEPHENS-NEWSHAM, L. G. and NOUJAIM, A. A. (1985) In vitro binding of platinum compounds to human transferrin. *Res. Commun. Chem. Path. Pharmac.* **50:** 387–394.

TANIGUCHI, T., ICHIMURA, K., KAWASHIMA, S., YAMAMURA, T., TACHIIRI, Y., SATAKE, K. and KIHARA, H. (1990)

Binding of Cu (II), Tb (III), and Fe (III) to chicken ovotransferrin. A kinetic study. *Eur. Biophys. J.* **18:** 1–8.

THOMPSON, H. O., BLASZAK, J. KNUDTSON, C. J. and SHAW, C. F., III (1978) Characterization of gold in the cytosol of rat-kidney cortex cells. *Bioinorg. Chem.* **9:** 375–388.

THOMSON, A. J. (1974) The interactions of platinum compounds with biological molecules. *Rec. Res. Cancer Res.* **48:** 38–62.

THOMSON, A. J., WILLIAMS, R. J. P. and RESLOVA, S. (1972) Chemistry of complexes related to *cis*$Pt(NH_3)_2Cl_2$, an antitumor drug. *Struct. Bond.* **11:** 1–46.

TIEGHEM, E., VAN DAEL, H. and VAN CAUWELAERT, F. (1991) Comparison of the Cu2+ binding to bovine, goat and human alpha-lactalbumin. *Biochem. Int.* **23:** 119–126.

TONINI, G. P., PARODI, M. T., BOLOGNA, R., PERSICI, P. and CORNAGLIA-FERRARIS, P. (1986) Cisplatin induces modulation of transferrin receptor during cellular differentiation in vitro. *Cancer Chemother. Pharmac.* **18:** 92.

TRUGMAN, J., HOGENKAMP, H. P. C., ROELOPS, R. and HRUSHESKY, H. J. M. (1985) Cisplatin neurotoxicity: failure to demonstrate vitamin B_{12} inactivation. *Cancer Treat. Rep.* **69:** 453–455.

UOZUMI, J. and LITTERST, C. L. (1985) The effect of cisplatin on renal ATPase activity in vivo and in vitro. *Cancer Chemother. Pharmac.* **15:** 93–96.

UOZUMI, J. and LITTERST, C. L. (1986) Effect of sodium thiosulfate on subcellular localization of platinum in rat kidney after treatment with cisplatin. *Cancer Lett.* **32:** 279–283.

WALZ, D. T., GRISWOLD, D. E., DIMARTINO, M. J. and BUMBIER, E. (1979) Distribution of gold in blood following administration in auranofin (SK and FD 39162). *J. Rheumat.* **6** (Suppl. 5): 56–60.

WRIGHT, M., LACORRE-ARESCALDINO, I., MACQUET, J. P. and DAFFE, M. (1984) Induction of polyploid nuclei in the plasmodium of *Physarum polycephalum* by platinum antitumor compounds. *Cancer Res.* **44:** 777–783.

ZELAZOWSKI, A. J., GARVEY, J. S. and HOESCHELE, J. D. (1984) In vivo and in vitro binding of platinum to metallothionein. *Arch. Biochem. Biophys.* **229:** 246–252.

ZGIRSKI, A. and FRIEDEN, E. (1990) Binding of Cu (II) to nonprosthetic sites in ceruloplasmin and bovine serum albumin. *J. Inorg. Biochem.* **39:** 137–48.

ZWELLING, L. A., KOHN, K. W., ROSS, W. E., EWIG, R. A. G. and ANDERSON, T. (1978) Kinetics of formation and disappearance of DNA cross-linking effect in mouse leukemia L1210 cells treated with *cis*- and *trans*-diamminedichloroplatinum(II). *Cancer Res.* **38:** 1762–1768.

ZWELLING, L. A., BRADLEY, M. O., SHARKEY, N. A., ANDERSON, T. and KOHN, K. W. (1979) Mutagenicity, cytotoxicity and DNA cross-linking in V79 Chinese hamster cells treated with *cis*- and *trans*-platinum (II) diamminedichloride. *Mutat. Res.* **67:** 271–280.

Garth Powis, editor.
(1994) *Anticancer Drugs: Reactive Metabolism and Drug Interactions*,
Pergamon Press Ltd, pp. 273–386
Printed in the United Kingdom

CHAPTER 8

METABOLISM AND REACTIONS OF QUINOID ANTICANCER AGENTS

GARTH POWIS

Arizona Cancer Center, University of Arizona, 1515 North Campbell Avenue, Tucson, AZ 85724, U.S.A.

1. INTRODUCTION

Quinoid compounds (compounds containing the chromatophoric quinoid group) are widely distributed in nature. They are found in bacteria, fungi, higher plants and, in the animal kingdom, in arthropods, echinoderms and as components of the respiratory system (Moore, H.W. et al., 1986; Morton, 1965; Nohl et al., 1986; Thompson, 1971). A number of quinoid types are possible containing combinations of oxygen (=O), sulfur (=S), carbon (=CH_2), and nitrogen (=NH) in the terminal positions. Quinoid compounds containing oxygen (quinones), nitrogen (quinonediimines), or both oxygen and nitrogen (quinoneimines) are more stable than quinoid compounds containing carbon (quinonemethides) or sulfur (quinonethiides) (Coopinger and Bauer, 1963). Quinones represent, by far, the largest class of quinoid compounds. There are three main groups of naturally occurring quinones (in order of increasing size); benzoquinones, naphthoquinones and anthraquinones. In addition to naturally occurring quinones large numbers of simple and more complex quinones have been synthesized (Bruce, 1974). The quinone structure is well represented among agents currently used to treat cancer which have been selected from an enormous number of compounds randomly screened for antitumor activity in a variety of animal test systems. In the U.S.A. the National Cancer Institute's Drug Research and Development Program has tested more than 600,000 natural and synthetic products since 1955 (Staquet et al., 1983), including over 1500 quinones (Driscoll et al., 1974). As a general rule simple quinones without reactive or complex side chains lack appreciable antitumor activity (Driscoll et al., 1974). The clinically useful anticancer quinones are *p*-benzoquinones with reactive or heterocyclic groups, or extensively substituted anthraquinones.

The other group of quinoid compounds which will be considered in this review are quinoneimines and quinonediimines which have many of the same chemical properties as quinones (Bruce, 1974). Quinoneimines and quinonediimines do not occur widely in nature but some naturally occurring quinoneimines and a number of synthetic quinoneimines and quinonediimines have been shown to possess antitumor activity in animals and man (Auclair and Paoletti, 1981; Brockmann, 1969; Hodnett et al., 1978; Hodnett and Prakash, 1984; Tong et al., 1979).

This chapter will cover the reactions and metabolism of antitumor quinoid compounds in animals and man, focusing on compounds that are, or have been, used to treat human cancer. Emphasis will be placed on the relationship between metabolism and the biological effects of quinoid compounds, which includes their antitumor activity and toxic side effects. Because of the complex structure of most antitumor quinoid compounds it is often difficult to separate the contributions of chemical reactivity and the different pathways of metabolism to overall biological activity. By studying simple quinoid compounds it is possible to obtain important clues to the way complex quinoid compounds act. The first part of this chapter will, therefore, deal briefly with the chemistry and metabolism of simple quinoid compounds.

2. SIMPLE QUINOIDS

2.1. Chemical reactions

Quinones readily undergo addition and substitution reactions and can react directly with cellular nucleophiles such as thiols. The addition and substitution reactions of simple benzo- and naphthoquinones have been comprehensively reviewed by Finley (1974) and Brunmark and Cadenas (1989). The majority of the reactions are reductive additions of the Michael type which result in the formation of a hydroquinone adduct (Fig. 1, reaction 1). Depending on the nature of the substituent the hydroquinone adduct can be oxidized to a quinone adduct by oxygen, with the formation of hydrogen peroxide (Fig. 1, reaction 2), by an added oxidant or, with a hydroquinone adduct with an electron donating substituent, by the parent quinone (Fig. 1, reaction 3). Higher polycyclic quinones do not usually show such addition reactions.

Quinones also undergo facile reduction and oxidation. One-electron reduction of a quinone gives a semiquinone radical (Fig. 1, reaction 4), while two-electron reduction gives a hydroquinone (Fig. 1, reaction 5). Protonation of the quinone or the semiquinone radical facilitates reduction since the charge on the molecule does not repel the reducing electron. Whether a quinone or its reduced species is protonated at physiologic pH depends upon its pK value. A semiquinone radical can also be formed by a comproportionation reaction between a hydroquinone and a quinone (Fig. 1, reaction 6) (Michaelis, 1946). In the reverse reaction two molecules of a semiquinone radical disproportionate to give one molecule each of a quinone and a hydroquinone. Under physiological

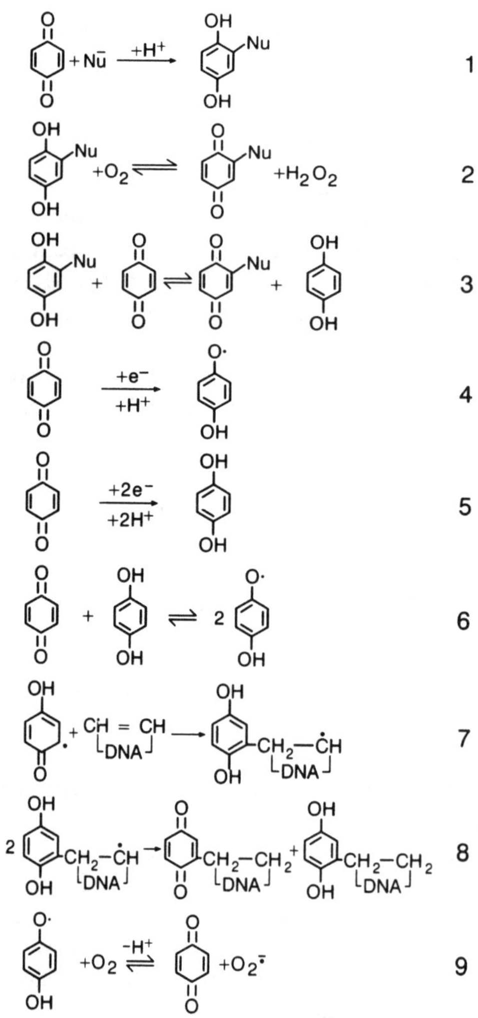

Fig. 1. Addition and reduction reactions of simple quinones. Nu represents a nucleophile.

conditions electrons for the reduction of a quinone can come from the reduced form of a less electron affinic quinone (Fendler and Fendler, 1974), from a non-quinone radical such as superoxide anion radical ($O_2^{\cdot-}$) (Winterbourn et al., 1978; Youngman and Elstner, 1984), from reduced pyridine nucleotide usually by an enzyme catalyzed reaction (see Section 2.2), or from a cellular nucleophile such as a thiol (Gant et al., 1986; Gause et al., 1967).

Once formed a semiquinone radical can be oxidized back to the quinone by transferring its electron to a suitable acceptor. Biologically important electron acceptors include oxygen, which is reduced to superoxide anion radical (Halliwell and Gutteridge, 1984), cytochrome c (Yamazaki, 1977), methemoglobin (Winterbourn et al., 1978) and cytochrome b_5 (Iyanagi and Yamazaki, 1969). Semiquinone radicals can also bind covalently to DNA and other cellular macromolecules (Mason, 1979, Morrison et al., 1984; Sinha, 1980). A possible mechanism is shown in Fig. 1, reaction 7, where a semiquinone radical forms a carbon-centered radical which adds to a double bond in, for example, a pyrimidine of DNA. Disproportionation of the radical product leads to a mixture of the hydroquinone and quinone adducts (Fig. 1, reaction 8). A hydroquinone may undergo spontaneous oxidation by transferring either one or two electrons to oxygen. For example, menadiol, the hydroquinone of menadione (2-methyl-1,4-naphthoquinone), undergoes air auto-oxidation to form predominantly hydrogen peroxide and menadione (Nickerson et al., 1963; Ross et al., 1985). Ubiquinol, the hydroquinone of ubiquinone (2-deca(3-methylbut-2-enylene)-5,6-dimethoxy-3-methyl-*p*-benzoquinone), forms almost exclusively superoxide anion radical and the ubiquinone semiquinone radical (Cadenas et al., 1977).

As will become clear from later discussions the potential for rapid electron transfer between the fully and partly reduced forms of a quinoid, as well as for electron transfer with biological oxidants and reductants can make it difficult to determine which metabolic pathway and which form of the quinoid is responsible for biological activity.

2.2. Metabolism

Pathways for the metabolism and reactions of simple quinoid compounds in the cell are shown in Fig. 2. Most simple quinones undergo flavoenzyme catalyzed reduction in the presence of a suitable electron donor. Some flavoenzymes catalyze only single-electron reduction of quinones resulting in the formation of a semiquinone radical. They include NADPH-cytochrome P-450 reductase (E.C.1.6.2.3), NADH-cytochrome b_5 reductase (E.C.1.6.2.2) (Iyanagi and Yamazaki, 1969), NADPH:ubiquinone oxidoreductase (E.C.1.6.5.3) and ferredoxin-NADP$^+$ reductase (E.C.1.6.7.1) (Iyanagi and Yamazaki, 1970). Other flavoenzymes, such as quinone reductase (NAD(P)H:(quinone-acceptor)oxidoreductase, E.C.1.6.99.2), formerly known as DT-diaphorase, catalyze only two-electron reduction of quinones resulting in the formation of a hydroquinone

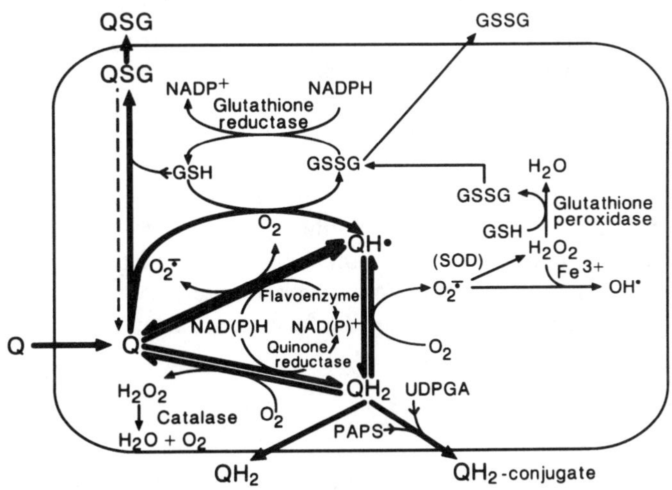

FIG. 2. Cellular quinone metabolism and some of its consequences. Q, quinone; QH, semiquinone; QH_2, hydroquinone. For an explanation see the text.

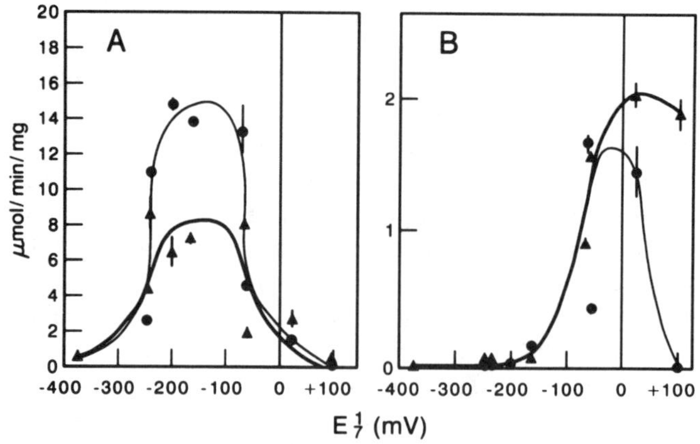

FIG. 3. Metabolism of various simple quinones by A, NADPH-cytochrome P-450 reductase and B, NADH-cytochrome b_5 reductase. (▲) NAD(P)H oxidation; (●) superoxide anion radical formation. Bars are S.E. $E^1/7$ is the one-electron reduction potential at pH 7.0 of the quinone/semiquinone couple. Adapted from Powis and Appel (1980).

(Iyanagi and Yamazaki, 1970). Enzymes that simultaneously catalyze both one- and two-electron reduction of quinones include xanthine oxidase (xanthine:oxidase oxygen oxidoreductase, E.C.1.2.3.2) (Nakamura and Yamazaki, 1973), NADH:lipoamide oxidoreductase (E.C.1.6.4.3) (Nakamura and Yamazaki, 1972) and xanthine dehydrogenase (Yamazaki, 1977).

Flavoenzymes accept a wide variety of artificial electron acceptors as substrates including quinones (Bilmoria and Kamin, 1973; Iyanagi and Yamazaki, 1969; Nishibayashi et al., 1967). A factor in determining the rate of flavoenzyme catalyzed single-electron reduction of quinones is the single-electron reduction potential (at pH 7.0, E^1_7) of the quinone/semiquinone radical couple (Powis and Appel, 1980). Although reduction potentials are only truly meaningful in determining equilibria they can have significance for rates of metabolism. The rate of reduction of simple quinones has been found to decrease markedly at E^1_7 values below -250 mV for NADPH-cytochrome P-450 reductase and below -100 mV for NADH-cytochrome b_5 reductase (Miller et al., 1986; Powis and Appel, 1980) (Fig. 3). The decreased rate of quinone reduction at negative E^1_7 values is probably related to a slower rate of electron transfer to the quinone from the reduced-flavin prosthetic group of the flavoenzyme, $FMNH_2$ in NADPH-cytochrome P-450 reductase and $FADH_2$ in NADH cytochrome b_5 reductase (Powis and Appel, 1980). An unexpected finding was a decreased rate of quinone reduction at positive E^1_7 values. A possible explanation for this finding is product inhibition of the flavoenzyme by the semiquinone radical. Electrochemical studies of hydroxylated 1,4-naphthoquinones and 9,10-anthraquinones have shown that a hydroxyl group to the quinone group raises the reduction potential and stabilizes the semiquinone radical, probably by increased delocalization due to exchange of the hydroxyl hydrogen between the two neighboring oxygen atoms (Ashnager et al., 1984).

Quinone reductase catalyzes two-electron reduction of quinones to the hydroquinone. There does not appear to be a simple relationship between the half-wave reduction potential or E^1_7 of quinones and published rates (Ernster, 1967) metabolism by quinone reductase. Hydroquinones are generally less reactive than semiquinone radicals and are conjugated with glucuronic acid or sulfate, and eliminated from the cell. It has been suggested that quinone reductase is a cellular protection mechanism against the toxic consequences of single-electron reduction of quinones (see Section 2.4). In hepatic microsomes quinone reductase competes with NADPH-cytochrome P-450 reductase for reduction of quinones and decreases the formation of semiquinone radicals (Lind et al., 1982).

2.3. Oxygen Radical Formation

A semiquinone radical is capable of transferring an electron to molecular oxygen to form the superoxide anion radical and, in the process, regenerating the parent quinone (Fig. 1, reaction 9). The repetitive reduction and reoxidation of a quinone under aerobic conditions with generation of superoxide anion radical (the sum of reactions 4 and 9) is known as redox cycling. The reaction of a semiquinone radical with oxygen is generally very rapid, for example, the rate of reaction of 2,5-dimethylbenzosemiquinone radical with oxygen is $k = 4.8 \times 10^6\ \text{M}^{-1}\ \text{sec}^{-1}$ (Ilan et al., 1976). Most semiquinone radicals have a short lifetime and diffuse only short distances under physiological conditions. The half-life of 2,5-dimethylbenzosemiquinone radical at a concentration of 1 μM in air-saturated medium has been calculated to be 0.6 msec which gives it a mean diffusion distance of only 0.7 μm (Powis et al., 1981). The E_7^1 for the oxygen/superoxide anion radical couple is − 155 mV (Wardman, 1977). However, even quinones more electropositive than − 155 mV can transfer an electron to oxygen to form the superoxide anion radical, probably because of rapid removal of superoxide anion radical from the system by its spontaneous dismutation to hydrogen peroxide which serves to pull reaction 9 to the right. The limiting factor in the rate of superoxide anion radical formation during redox cycling of simple quinones by flavoenzymes appears to be the rate of quinone reduction and not the transfer of electrons to molecular oxygen (Powis et al., 1981) (Fig. 3). The same is true for quinone metabolism by intact cells (Powis et al., 1981). The superoxide anion radical has a short lifetime in aqueous solution; k for reaction 10 where protonated superoxide radical reacts with superoxide anion radical (the predominating reaction at neutral pH) is $1.0 \times 10^8\ \text{M}^{-1}\ \text{sec}^{-1}$ (Bielski, 1978).

$$HO_2^{\cdot} + O_2^{\bar{\cdot}} \longrightarrow HO_2^- + O_2 \xrightleftharpoons{H_2O} O_2 + H_2O_2 + OH^- \qquad (10)$$

$$O_2^{\bar{\cdot}} + H_2O_2 \xrightarrow{\text{Fe Salt}} O_2 + HO^- + HO\cdot \qquad (11)$$

$$H_2O_2 + (Fe(II)) \xrightarrow{\text{catalysis}} HO^- + HO\cdot + Fe(III) \qquad (12)$$

$$QH\cdot + Fe(III) \xrightarrow{-H^+} Fe(II) + Q \qquad (13)$$

The superoxide anion radical formed by redox cycling of a quinone is not a particularly reactive species but can give rise to hydroxyl radical (HO·), a powerful oxidizing species that can cause oxidation of polyunsaturated fatty acids, degradation of DNA and protein damage, among other things (Halliwell and Gutteridge, 1984). Hydroxyl radical is formed from superoxide anion radical only in the presence of catalytic amounts of a transition metalion, in biological systems usually provided by iron salts. The first step is spontaneous dismutation of two molecules of superoxide anion radical (or its protonated form) to give hydrogen peroxide (reaction 10). Hydrogen peroxide then reacts with superoxide anion radical in the presence of trace amounts of iron salts to form hydroxyl radical (reaction 11). This reaction is sometimes referred to as an iron catalyzed Haber–Weiss reaction (Halliwell and Gutteridge, 1984). Inhibition of hydroxyl radical formation by the enzyme superoxide dismutase, which catalyzes reaction 10 at a faster rate than the spontaneous dismutation, is due to a lowered steady state concentration of superoxide anion radical. This pulls reaction 9 (Fig. 1) to the right so that the steady state concentration of the semiquinone radical is also lowered by superoxide dismutase (Winterbourn et al., 1978). Superoxide dismutase does not always inhibit quinone-induced hydroxyl radical formation (Gutteridge and Quinlan, 1985). In this case the superoxide anion radical may be serving as a precursor for hydrogen peroxide which reacts with Fe(II) ion to generate hydroxyl radical by a Fenton Reaction (reaction 12). Fe(III) ion is reduced to Fe(II) ion, probably by the semiquinone radical (QH: in reaction 13). Singlet oxygen (ΔgO_2), another potentially toxic species, is also generated during redox cycling of quinones (Wefers and Sies, 1986).

2.4. Metabolism and Cytotoxicity

Important insights into the way metabolism of simple quinones might lead to damage and death of cells has been provided by the studies of Orrenius and his colleagues with menadione (2-methyl-1,4-naphthoquinone) and isolated hepatocytes. Menadione-induced hepatocyte toxicity is preceded by depletion of intracellular glutathione and protein thiol groups (DiMonte et al.,

1984a,b; Thor et al., 1982) and can occur without an alteration in the redox state of cellular pyridine nucleotides (Thor et al., 1982). Menadione-induced oxidation of mitochondrial pyridine nucleotides is, however, more usually accompanied by their hydrolysis and depletion (Frei et al., 1986; Moore, et al., 1986). In mitochondria menadione is reduced by several enzymes including NAD(P)H:(quinone-acceptor) oxidoreductase (quinone reductase), and NADH:(quinone-acceptor)-oxidoreductase (Frei et al., 1986). Mitochondrial NADH dehydrogenase does not appear to participate in menadione reduction. Depletion of the cellular thiols by menadione is a consequence of two processes, oxidative stress and adduct formation. In oxidative stress reactive oxygen species formed by redox cycling of menadione lead to oxidation of glutathione and protein thiol groups (Armstrong and Buchanan, 1978; Lin and Armstrong, 1977). Hydrogen peroxide is removed from the cell by glutathione peroxidase with concomitant conversion of glutathione to its oxidized form (Wendel, 1981) (Fig. 2). Oxidized glutathione can be reduced back to glutathione by glutathione reductase and NADPH (Fig. 2), but the loss of oxidized glutathione by excretion from the cell and, at high menadione concentrations, depletion of reduced pyridine nucleotides, means that this reaction is limited (Eklow et al., 1981). Menadione also forms adducts with cellular nucleophiles such as glutathione and protein thiol groups. When menadione and glutathione are mixed, a 3-*S*-glutathionyl-menadione adduct, thiodone, is formed (DiMonte et al., 1984b; Ross et al., 1985). Brunmark and Cadenas (1989) have pointed out that while the formation of glutathionyl-substituted hydroquinones upon reaction of glutathione with quinones has little affect upon the reduction potential of the quinoid, it causes a loss of the electrophilic character of the quinone and greatly increases its hydrophilicity, thus, affecting its subsequent reactivity and disposition within the cell. Thus, thiodone has an E_7^1 similar to that of menadione (Wilson et al., 1986) and undergoes flavoenzyme-mediated redox cycling with formation of oxygen radicals in a similar manner to menadione (Wefers and Sies, 1983). However, thiodone is rapidly transported out of the cell (DiMonte et al., 1984b) and glutathione adduct formation may be a protective mechanism against quinone toxicity. Glutathione can directly reduce naphthoquinones to the semiquinone free radical (Gant et al., 1986) and with menadione there is redox cycling with stimulation of oxygen utilization, and formation of superoxide anion radical and hydrogen peroxide (DiMonte et al., 1984a,b; Ross et al., 1985).

1,4-Benzoquinone is reduced by hepatocytes to the ESR detectable 1,4-benzosemiquinone and 2-3-glutathionyl-1,4-benzosemiquinone free radicals (Rao et al., 1988). 1,4-Benzoquinone is an inherently reactive compound and undergoes direct reduction the semiquinone by reduced glutathione, as well as conjugation and reduction to the glutathionyl free radical. The 2,5-glutathionyl-1,4-benzosemiquinone free radical reacts relatively slowly with oxygen allowing its detection by ESR spectroscopy.

Other simple naphthoquinones are metabolized in a similar manner to menadione. 1,4-Naphthoquinone undergoes redox cycling by rat liver microsomes and NADPH (Miller et al., 1986). It reacts readily with, and depletes, cellular glutathione and is toxic to hepatocytes. 3-Dichloro-1,4-naphthoquinone undergoes redox cycling by rat liver mitochondria with formation of superoxide anion radical and hydrogen peroxide, and depletion of mitochondrial thiol groups (Pritsos et al., 1982; Pritsos and Pardini, 1984). 2,3-Dimethyl- and 2,3-diethyl-1,4-naphthoquinone undergo redox cycling by rat liver microsomes and NADPH, although at a slower rate than menadione, but do not form adducts with nucleophiles such as glutathione (Miller et al., 1986; Ross et al., 1986). Both compounds are toxic to hepatocytes, although at considerably higher concentrations than menadione. These findings have led to the suggestion that metabolism and oxidative stress may be a more important determinant of the toxicity of simple naphthoquinones than adduct formation (DiMonte et al., 1984b; Ross et al., 1986).

Because quinones undergo redox cycling under aerobic conditions it has not been possible to separate the effects of quinone reduction from those of oxygen radical formation on quinone toxicity. The contribution of adduct formation to quinone toxicity is also unclear because quinones that are less active at forming adducts and are less toxic to hepatocytes also undergo less redox cycling (Miller et al., 1986; Ross et al., 1986). In order to study the relative contributions of metabolism, oxygen radical formation and adduct formation to quinoid toxicity we have used quinoneimines and quinonediimines (Powis et al., 1987a). These compounds undergo one-electron reduction by hepatic microsomal flavoenzymes and NADPH or NADH, and form semiquinoneimine or semiquinone diimine radicals (Mason, 1982; Powis et al., 1987a). Some, but not all, semiquinoneimines and semiquinonediimines redox cycle to form oxygen radicals (Powis et al., 1987a). Compounds that undergo rapid one-electron reduction by hepatic microsomal flavoenzymes but that do not stimulate oxygen utilization and do not form superoxide anion radical or hydrogen peroxide are *N*-acetyl-*p*-benzoquinoneimine, the putative hepatotoxic metabolite formed from acetaminophen (Powis et al., 1984), 2,6-dichloroindophenol (Lyakhovich et al., 1977), 2,3′,6-trichloroindophenol, *N,N*-dimethylindo-aniline and *N,N′*-dichloro-2-chloro-1,4-benzoquinone-diimine (Powis et al., 1987a). The toxicity of a series of quinoneimines and quinonediimines to hepatocytes was found to be greater with compounds that were rapidly metabolized, but toxicity was not related to the formation of reactive oxygen species or to the rate of adduct formation with glutathione (Powis et al., 1987a). The results suggest that, for quinoneimines and quinonediimines at least, metabolism per se may be more important for cytotoxicity than oxygen radical formation or chemical reactivity. Subsequent events in quinoneimine and quinonediimine toxicity may be similar to those involved in quinone toxicity. Quinoneimines and quinonediimines at toxic concentrations decrease intracellular glutathione to the same extent as does menadione (K.S. Santone and G. Powis, unpublished observations).

A protective role has been proposed for quinone reductase against quinone toxicity. This was first suggested by Lind et al. (1982) and subsequently by other workers (Ames, 1983; Benson et al., 1980; Chesis et al., 1984; Lind et al., 1978; Morrison et al., 1984; Smart and Zannoni, 1984; Thor et al., 1982). Evidence that supports a role for quinone reductase in protecting cells against quinone toxicity is the potentiation of quinone toxicity by dicumarol, a potent inhibitor of quinone reductase (Ernster, 1967). Dicumarol increases the toxicity of menadione to hepatocytes from control and phenobarbital pretreated rats (Powis et al., 1987b; Thor et al., 1982), to cultured human fibroblasts (Morrison et al., 1985), to A204 human rhabdomyosarcoma tumor cells and to Chinese hamster ovary cells (Powis, et al., 1987b). Ackman et al. (1985) found that dicumarol potentiated the cytotoxicity of menadione to murine L1210 leukemia cells but proposed a mechanism that did not involve inhibition of quinone reductase by dicumarol. Dicumarol has been reported to decrease the toxicity of halogenated dimethylnaphthoquinones to *Salmonella typhimurium TA97* (Talcott et al., 1983) and to human tumor and murine bone marrow cells (Berger et al., 1986), suggesting a role for quinone reductase in the activation of these compounds. Glutathionyl-quinoid conjugates are known to substrates for reduction by quinone reductase and it has been reported that the resulting glutathionyl-hydroquinone conjugate autooxidizes at rates far above the parent hydroquinone (Brunmark and Cadenas, 1988; Buffinton et al., 1989). It is, thus, possible that quinone reductase could be a protective enzyme against the cytotoxicity of some quinones but might lead to the activation of other quinones, in particular those that form glutathionyl conjugates in the cell. Quinoneimines are also substrates for quinone reductase and dicumarol increases the toxicity of a number of quinoneimines to hepatocytes from phenobarbital pretreated rats, although not to hepatocytes from control rats (Powis et al., 1987b). Dicumarol has been reported not to protect hepatocytes against the toxicity of the quinoneimines, *N*-acetyl-*p*-benzoquinoneimine (Albano et al., 1985). *N*-acetyl-3,5-dimethyl-*p*-benzoquinoneimine or *N*-acetyl-2,6-dimethyl-*p*-benzoquinoneimine (Rundgren et al., 1988). Dicumarol does not significantly modify the response of A204 human rhabdomyosarcoma or Chinese hamster ovary cells to growth inhibition caused by quinoneimines (Powis et al., 1987b).

The link between menadione-induced oxidative stress and subsequent cell death has been suggested to be an increase in intracellular free Ca^{2+}. An increase in intracellular free Ca^{2+} has been associated with the toxic effects of many compounds (Trump et al., 1984). Cell injury following a rise in intracellular free Ca^{2+} may be due to an activation of Ca^{2+}-dependent autolytic systems such as phospholipases and proteases (Orrenius, 1985). Depletion of cellular thiols by menadione precedes a sustained increase in intracellular free Ca^{2+} (DiMonte et al., 1984a) due to a release of Ca^{2+} from mitochondria (Bellomo et al., 1982), an impaired ability of mitochondria and microsomes to sequester Ca^{2+} (Bellomo et al., 1982; Jones et al., 1983; Thor et al., 1982) and a decreased extrusion of Ca^{2+} from the cell (DiMonte et al., 1984a). The primary mechanism for maintaining intracellular free Ca^{2+} at submicromolar levels is the high affinity plasma membrane Ca^{2+}-ATPase pump which has been shown to be inhibited by exposure of hepatocytes to menadione (Nicotera et al., 1985). The inhibition can be reversed by subsequent treatment of the hepatocytes with dithiothreitol or treatment of the plasma membrane fraction with reduced glutathione. This suggests that the inhibition of Ca^{2+}-ATPase by menadione is due to oxidation of protein sulfhydryl groups subsequent to depletion of cellular thiols. 2,5-Di(*tert*-butyl)-1,4-benzohydroquinone has been claimed to be a relatively selective inhibiter of ATP-dependent Ca^{2+} sequestration by rat liver microsomes without affecting liver mitochondrial Ca^{2+} fluxes (Moore et al., 1987). The increase in hepatocyte intracellular free Ca^{2+} produced by menadione is associated with alterations in the cytoskeleton and characteristic small blebs appear on the surface of menadione-treated hepatocytes (Thor et al., 1982).

2.5. Metabolism and Antitumor Activity

Menadione inhibits the growth of a number of tumor cells in vitro (Akman et al., 1985; Chlebowski et al., 1983, 1985; Harrison, 1970; Powis et al., 1987b; Prasad et al., 1981) and in vivo (Gold, 1986). Menadione, sodium bisulfite (Synkavit), has been used in combination with radiation to treat human malignancies producing a small but significant beneficial effect (Deeley, 1962; Krishanamurthi et al., 1971; Mitchell et al., 1965), and in combination with warfarin and 5-fluorouracil to treat colon cancer (Chlebowski et al., 1983). The mechanism of menadione's antitumor activity is not known. In a preliminary report, Chlebowski et al. (1981) have indicated that compounds related to menadione may affect salvage pathway synthesis of pyrimidine nucleotides necessary for DNA synthesis. Menadione is mutagenic (Chesis et al., 1984) which suggests that it, or a metabolite, reacts with DNA. Such a reaction could lead to inhibition of cell division. Incubation of [^{3}H]-menadione with hepatic microsomes and NADH or NADPH results in covalent binding of radioactivity to added DNA (Morrison et al., 1984). The nature of the reactive menadione metabolite(s) was not established but binding to DNA was blocked by glutathione and it was suggested that the reactive species might be the menadione semiquinone radical. Quinone reductase did not catalyze binding of [^{3}H]-menadione to DNA. Akman et al. (1985) have presented evidence that depletion of cellular NADPH and glutathione may be responsible for the inhibition of L1210 leukemia cell growth by menadione. The growth inhibition could be prevented by adding cysteine or glutathione to the medium, in the latter case without repletion of the cellular glutathione pool. This suggests that the cytotoxic effect of menadione could be mediated at, or near to, the cell surface. It is interesting that reactive oxygen species generated by thiol-dependent redox cycling of simple quinones, including 1,2-naphthoquinone and menadione, but not daunorubicin, lead to tyrosine-specific phosphorylation of rat liver plasma membrane proteins (Chan et al., 1986). Simple quinones such as 1,4-benzoquinone, 1,4-naphthoquinone and menadione, although not complex quinones such as anthracyclines and lapachol, inhibit the binding of epidermal growth factor to its cell surface receptors by a process that appears to require metabolism of the quinone (Shoyab and Todaro, 1980). It is known that the activated intracellular component of the epidermal growth factor receptor is closely homologous to the protein product of the *erb*-B (erythro-blastosis) oncogene (Downward et al., 1984). This raises the intriguing possibility that the metabolism of quinones at, or near to the cell surface might be toxic to a transformed cell through a mechanism involving protein phosphorylation and the functioning of an oncogene product.

2.6. Bioreductive Alkylation

Attempts have been made to exploit the enzymatic reduction of quinones in the design of so-called bioreductive alkylating agents. The concept of bioreductive alkylation was developed by Sartorelli and his colleagues (Lin et al., 1972) based on the observation that human solid tumors contain cells that are remote from the vascular supply and most likely deficient in oxygen. Hypoxic cells are an obstacle to the effective treatment of cancer because they are relatively resistant to treatments aimed at killing rapidly dividing cells. It was hypothesized that hypoxic cells might have a greater capacity for reductive metabolism than euoxic cells and that it might be possible to exploit this feature of hypoxic cells by synthesizing prodrugs which become cytotoxic after reduction. It had been shown in the early 1970s that the antitumor quinone antibiotic mitomycin C required reduction in order to alkylate DNA and it was hypothesized that an *o*-quinonemethide might be

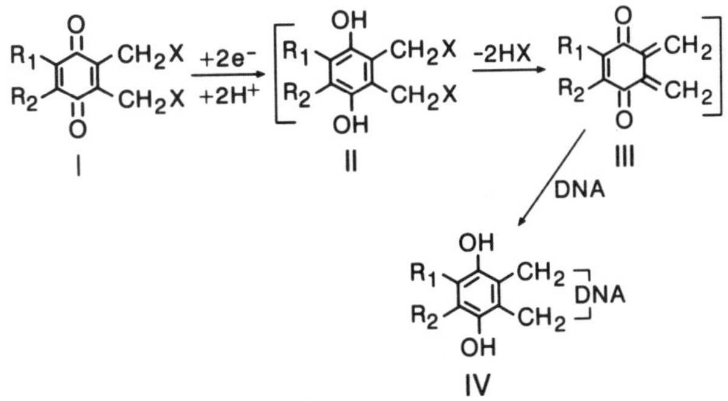

FIG. 4. Proposed mechanism for reductive activation of substituted benzoquinones. I is the parent benzoquinone with two potential leaving groups (X) which is reduced to the hydroquinone II. This decomposes to form a reactive quinone methide III which alkylates cellular DNA to form the adduct IV (Lin et al., 1973).

an intermediate in this process (Lin et al., 1972). Quinonemethides exhibit high reactivity to electrophiles as well as nucleophiles and generally occur only as intermediates (Wagner and Gompper, 1974). The enzymatic process for mitomycin C reduction was known to be relatively non-substrate specific (Iyer and Szybalski, 1964) and it seemed likely that other quinone compounds would be reduced by the same system. To test their hypothesis Sartorelli and his colleagues synthesized and tested a series of benzonaphthoquinones and anthraquinones with one or two side chains that were visualized as being reduced by hypoxic cells to highly reactive quinonemethide intermediates which would alkylate critical sites within the cell (Lin et al., 1972, 1973, 1974, 1982). The agents synthesized were found to be potent inhibitors of nucleic acid synthesis in tumor cells and to have antitumor activity in rodent models, but also to be fairly toxic to the host. The proposed pathway for reductive activation of the substituted quinones is shown in Fig. 4.

Chemical evidence supports the formation of a quinonemethide during the reduction of substituted 1,4-benzoquinone derivatives (Lin and Sartorelli, 1973). However, direct evidence for quinonemethide formation in the biological activity of these compounds has not been presented. Indirect evidence is a correlation between the quinone half-wave reduction potential and antitumor activity of the substituted quinones, with agents having the lowest reduction potential having the greatest activity (Hodnett et al., 1983; Lin et al., 1974). Pulse radiolysis studies suggest that the loss of the leaving group from a bioreductive quinone occurs upon two-electron reduction to the hydroquinone and not at the level of the semiquinone radical (Wilson et al., 1986). To date, the best example of bioreductive alkylation involving a quinonemethide intermediate is mitomycin C which is discussed in Section 5.4.4. The concept of bioreduction alkylation has received theoretical treatment by Moore and his colleagues (Moore, 1977; Moore and Czerniak, 1981; Moore, H. W. et al., 1986) who pointed out that among quinones simple quinonemethides and vinylogous quinonemethides would be expected to be good alkylating agents.

Studies on the metabolism of a representative bioreductive alkylating agent 2,3-(chloromethyl)-1,4-naphthoquinone have shown that it is reduced by mitochondria of S-180 tumor cells, binds to mitochondrial proteins, releases mitochondrial respiratory control and depresses cellular ATP (Biagini et al., 1979, 1981; Cosby et al., 1976).

Although the adduct resulting from alkylation by a substituted quinone shown in Fig. 4 is a hydroquinone it is likely that it would rapidly auto-oxidize in air to the level of quinone. This raises the possibility that quinone group covalently bound to DNA could undergo redox cycling with formation of reactive oxygen species in close vicinity to the DNA leading, possibly, to selective damage to the DNA. Support for such a mechanism comes from the finding that compounds possessing a quinone group and an active alkylating group cause more DNA strand breaks and show greater in vitro cytotoxicity than can attribute to either group alone (Begleiter, 1983, 1985).

3. ANTHRACYCLINES

3.1. Historical Perspective

The anthracycline glycosides represent the largest class of clinically useful antitumor quinoids. They were first studied in the late 1950s as pigmented antibiotics produced by different strains of *Streptomyces* (Brockmann, 1963). The era of antitumor anthracyclines began with the almost simultaneous reports in 1963 of the isolation of daunomycin from *S. peucetius* by workers at Farmitalia in Italy (DiMarco et al., 1963) and rubidomycin from *S. coeroleorubidus* by workers at Rhône-Poulenc in France (DuBost et al., 1963). When both antibiotics were found to be the same the name daunorubicin was adopted to indicate its dual origin. The rubomycin complex of antibiotics isolated in Russia at about the same time (Gause, 1964) was later found to contain daunorubicin. The potent antileukemic activity of daunorubicin led to the search for other anthracyclines with antitumor activity and in 1969 doxorubicin was isolated from a chemically mutated strain *S. peucetius* var. *caesius* (Arcamone et al., 1969). This new antibiotic had an enlarged spectrum of activity and greater efficacy against solid tumors than daunorubicin. Since its introduction for clinical use in the early 1970s more than 2 million patients have received doxorubicin (Arcamone, 1985). In excess of 1000 analogs of daunorubicin and doxorubicin have been obtained by partial or total synthesis and tested in experimental tumor models in an attempt to improve on the biological activity of the parent compounds (Arcamone, 1977, 1984; Henry, 1979; Naff et al., 1982; Weiss et al., 1986). In 1975 Japanese investigators isolated a substantially different type of anthracycline named aclacinomycin A from *S. galilaeus* (Oki et al., 1975). Instead of a single sugar attached to the aglycone portion of the molecule, as with daunorubicin and doxorubicin, aclacinomycin A has three sugars linked in a carbohydrate chain. Since the discovery of aclacinomycin A other anthracyclines with carbohydrate chains containing two or three saccharides, such as musettamycin and marcellomycin, have been isolated (Nettleton et al., 1977; Oki, 1977). So far, 17 anthracyclines have been tested clinically but doxorubicin and daunorubicin are by far the most widely used (Casazza, 1986).

3.2. Structure–Activity Relationships

Active anthracyclines are composed of a tetracyclic aglycone chromophore, usually red, orange or yellow in color, linked to a mono-, di- or tri-saccharide carbohydrate chain. The structures of some anthracyclines of clinical and experimental importance are shown in Fig. 5. Changes in the structure of the aglycone moiety of anthracyclines, with the exception of alterations in the C-9 acyl group, frequently result in inactive compounds (Brown, 1978; Arcamone, 1977). The C-4 methoxy group of daunorubicin and doxorubicin is not, however, essential for antitumor activity and many active semisynthetic compounds have a C-4 hydroxyl group. The saccharide most frequently found attached to the anthracycline aglycone moiety is daunosamine, as in daunorubicin and doxorubicin, while a carbohydrate chain may contain as constituents L-rhodosamine, L-rhodinose, 2-deoxy-L-fucose, L-cinerulose A, L-cinerulose B, D-cinerulose A, L-amicetose and L-aculose (Oki et al., 1977). Structural changes in the carbohydrate moiety of anthracyclines are compatible with retention of antitumor activity. 4′-Epidoxorubicin is an epimer of doxorubicin with a different configuration of the C-4′ hydroxyl group of daunosamine. *N*-Trifluoro-acetyl doxorubicin 14-valerate (AD32) has a trifluoroacetyl group attached to the amino nitrogen of daunosamine. Incorporation of the amino nitrogen of daunosamine into a morpholino ring yields compounds that are more potent anti-tumor agents than the parent anthracycline. One such compound, 3′-deamino-3′-(3″-cyano-4″-morpholinyl)-doxorubicin (MRA-CN), has a potency up to 1000 times greater than doxorubicin in vitro and in vivo (Acton et al., 1984; Johnston et al., 1983). Superior potency is also exhibited by MRA-CN against in vivo tumors and tumor cell lines that are resistant to doxorubicin. Complete removal of the carbohydrate moiety from anthracyclines usually gives compounds that are devoid of antitumor activity (Henry, 1979). Menogaril is an active semisynthetic derivative of the naturally occurring anthracycline nogalomycin and is unusual in having no C-7 carbohydrate moiety (McGovern et al., 1984). Instead menogaril has a dimethylamine saccharide (glucopyranose) attached to the anthracycline D ring through both carbon–oxygen and carbon–carbon bonds.

A functional classification of anthracyclines based on their relative abilities to inhibit DNA and

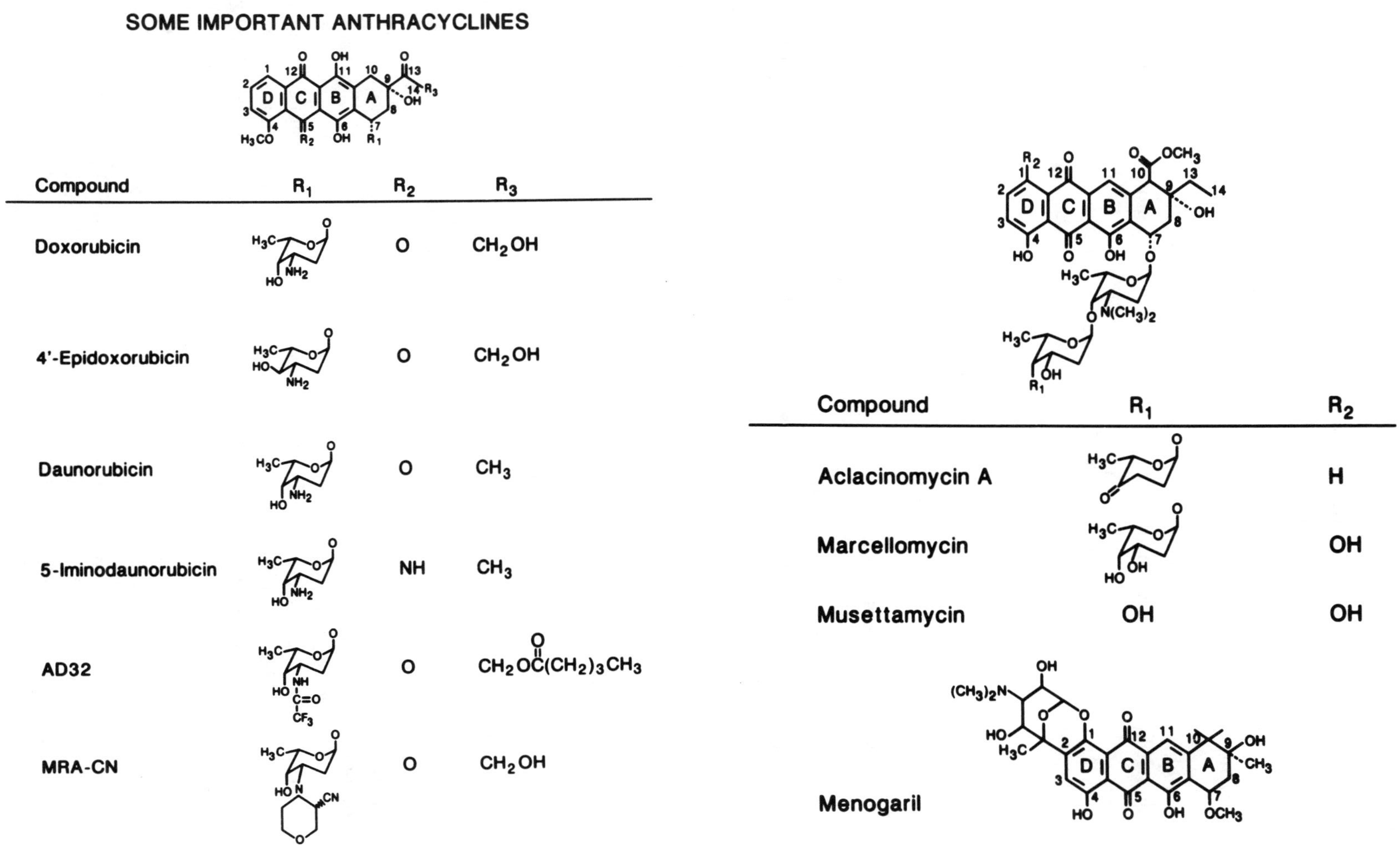

FIG. 5. Structure of some important anthracyclines.

nuclear RNA synthesis has been proposed by Crooke et al. (1978). Class I anthracyclines, which includes daunorubicin, doxorubicin and carminomycin, inhibit DNA and RNA synthesis at similar concentrations, while Class II anthracyclines preferentially inhibit ribosomal RNA synthesis at concentrations several hundred-fold lower than required to inhibit DNA synthesis and interfere equally with the transcription of the proximal and distal DNA regions of the gene for rRNA (Schwartz and Maher, 1986). Class II anthracyclines have a C-10 carbomethoxy group and a di- or tri-saccharide carbohydrate chain (DuVernay et al., 1979; DuVernay and Crooke, 1980). Removal of the C-10 carbomethoxy group decreases the inhibition of nucleolar RNA synthesis as well as the in vitro and in vivo toxicity of Class II anthracyclines (Oki et al., 1977). Because this classification of anthracyclines was originally devised based on a functional property of a limited number of anthracyclines it is not surprising that compounds have been discovered whose structures do not fit within the above guidelines. The extremely potent morpholinyl anthracyclines do not have a C-10 carbomethoxy group or a di- or tri-saccharide chain but preferentially inhibit RNA compared to DNA synthesis (Johnston and Glazer, 1983). Because some of the morpholinyl anthracyclines bind irreversibly to DNA it has been suggested that they should be considered a new class of anthracyclines (Casazza, 1986).

3.3. Clinical Activity

Since the first clinical trials of daunorubicin and doxorubicin more than two decades ago they have gained rapid acceptance as major therapeutic agents in the treatment of cancer. Both drugs are widely used as part of combination chemotherapy regimens for the effective treatment of acute non-lymphocytic leukemia, Hodgkin's and non-Hodgkin's lymphomas, breast cancer and sarcomas (Young et al., 1981). Doxorubicin has shown a wide range of activity in human solid tumors including those of the breast, lung, ovary, head and neck, bladder, endometrium and prostate and it is the most effective single agent against soft-tissue sarcomas in adults, although it is rarely curative in the advanced disease. The use of doxorubicin for adjuvant chemotherapy of soft-tissue sarcomas is being actively studied.

Toxic effects of anthracyclines include myelosuppression, cardiomyopathy, nausea and vomiting, hair loss and, if the drug accidentally extravasates during administration, tissue necrosis (Young et al., 1981). Myelosuppression, mainly in the form of neutropenia, is the acute dose-limiting toxicity of daunorubicin and doxorubicin while cardiomyopathy is the cumulative dose-limiting toxicity. There are unique pathological changes in the heart with swelling of the sarcoplasmic reticulum and myofibrillar dropout. Initially focal, these changes become diffuse as the damage progresses (Von Hoff et al., 1979). The most marked biochemical change is an increase in total myocardial calcium content with sequestration of calcium by heart mitochondria (Billingham et al., 1978) and an increase in the slowly exchanging calcium pool size (Revis and Marusic, 1979). The incidence of congestive heart failure is proportional to the dose of anthracycline. With doses of doxorubicin of 400 mg/m^2 or less the incidence of cardiomyopathy is under 2%, for cumulative doses in excess of 700 mg/m^2 the incidence is increased to greater than 20% (Olson et al., 1974). Even asymptomatic patients who received a total dose of doxorubicin of 480–550 mg/m^2 were found upon radionucleide angiography to have a 63% incidence of abnormal scans (Gottdiener et al., 1981). The cardiac damage produced by doxorubicin does not undergo significant repair and once clinically overt cardiomyopathy is present the prognosis is grave, with mortality rates as high as 48% (Pratt et al., 1978). Total dose limits for doxorubicin of 500–550 mg/m^2 have been suggested for patients with no underlying cardiac disease and, because of the risk of interactions with thoracic radiation or cyclophosphamide, total doses of 450 mg/m^2 have been recommended in patients receiving combined methods of therapy. Weekly, as opposed to every three weeks, administration of doxorubicin may produce less cardiotoxicity (Weiss and Manthel, 1977), as may continuous infusion of doxorubicin (Legha et al., 1982). The cardiotoxicity of daunorubicin and doxorubicin has provided the main rationale for the extensive isolation and synthetic programs for anthracycline anthracyclines that have been reported to have less cardiotoxicity and other toxicities in experimental animals than daunorubicin or doxorubicin include 4′-epidoxorubicin, 4′-deoxydoxorubicin, 4-demethoxydaunorubicin, 4-demethyldaunorubicin, aclacinomycin A, menogaril, 5-iminodaunorubicin, AD-32 and MRA-CN. It remains to be seen whether these agents will be better tolerated clinically and whether they will be as effective antitumor agents as daunorubicin and doxorubicin.

3.4. Metabolism

There are three types of anthracycline metabolic reactions, keto reduction, cleavage reactions and conjugation. In addition, during anthracycline cleavage to aglycone an anthracycline radical is formed which, in the presence of molecular oxygen, undergoes redox cycling to form reactive oxygen species. The metabolism of anthracyclines by each pathway will be reviewed from the viewpoint of both in vitro and in vivo studies. Radical formation and alkylation will be dealt with separately.

3.4.1. *In Vitro Metabolism*

3.4.1.1. *Keto reduction.* All rat tissues studied, except plasma, contain a soluble enzyme that, in the presence of NADPH, is capable of reducing anthracyclines and anthracycline aglycones with a C-13 keto group to the corresponding C-13 alcohol (Bachur and Cradock, 1970; Bachur and Gee, 1971). A C-13 anthracycline alcohol is designated by the suffix ol, for example, the C-13 alcohol of daunorubicin is daunorubicinol and the C-13 alcohol of doxorubicin is doxorubicinol. Liver, lung and kidney show the highest daunorubicin C-13 keto reductase activity. The enzyme has a molecular weight of 39,000 Da (Felsted et al., 1974) and belongs to a group of widely distributed enzymes classified as $NADP^+$ oxidoreductases (E.C.1.1.1.2) (Felsted et al., 1977; Turner and Hick, 1976). Activity of the enzyme is noncompetitively inhibited by barbiturates, warfarin and diphenylhydantoin. The enzyme exhibits extensive activity with a variety of natural and foreign aldehydes but has only limited activity with ketones as substrates. In fact, daunorubicin and doxorubicin are the only ketones so far found to undergo reduction at a significant rate. Except for daunorubicin and doxorubicin, which have a pH optimum of 8.5, other substrates have a pH optimum of 6.0 (Felsted et al., 1977). Daunorubicin is a much better substrate for C-13 keto reduction than doxorubicin. The K_m of daunorubicin for the purified enzyme is 0.06 mM and the k_{cat} 1.5 sec^{-1}, while the K_m of doxorubicin is 0.19 mM and the k_{cat} 0.07 sec^{-1} (Felsted et al., 1974). 4-Demethoxy-daunorubicin is a better substrate than doxorubicin for C-13 keto reduction by rat liver homogenate (Riggs and Schrader, 1985). 4′-Epidoxorubicin and 4′-deoxydoxorubicin have been reported to be better (Weenen et al., 1984b) and poorer (Riggs and Schrader, 1985; Sweatman et al., 1986) substrates than doxorubicin for C-13 keto reduction by rat and human liver preparations.

Human and rabbit liver cytosol contain in addition to the pH 8.5 aldehyde daunorubicin reductase found in rodent liver, a pH 6.0 ketone daunorubicin reductase (Ahmed et al., 1978a,b, 1981). The enzyme has different properties to the pH 8.5 aldehyde daunorubicin reductase on isoelectric focusing, ion exchange and gel filtration chromatography and is not inhibited by barbiturates, although it is inhibited by the alkaloid quercitrin. Human normal lymphocytes, myelocytes and erythocytes contain both the pH 8.5 aldehyde daunorubicin reductase and the pH 6.0 ketone daunorubicin reductase, while myeloblasts from patients with acute myelogenous leukemia and human myeloid leukemia cell lines may lack one or other enzyme (Ahmed, 1985). Work by Schwartz and Parker (1981) and by Dodion et al. (1986a) suggests there may also be an anthracycline C-13 keto reductase in the rat hepatic microsomal fraction that is not removed by extensive washing. The properties of this enzyme have not been characterized.

The C-4‴ keto group of the terminal L-cinerulose of aclacinomycin A undergoes stereoselective reduction by cytosolic and microsomal reductases in rat liver (Komiyama et al., 1978, 1979c). Cytosolic cinerulose reductase requires NADPH and converts L-cinerulose to L-amicetose and L-rhodinose. Microsomal cinerulose reductase requires NADH and converts L-cinerulose to L-rhodinose only. Neither enzyme is capable of reducing the C-13 keto group of daunorubicin (Oki et al., 1981).

The C-13 keto reduced metabolites of daunorubicin and doxorubicin, and the C-14‴ keto reduced metabolites of aclacinomycin A retain antitumor activity comparable to that of the parent compounds (Henry, 1979; Oki et al., 1981).

3.4.1.2. *Cleavage reactions. C-7 Cleavage (Aglycone Formation).* DiMarco et al. (1967) first reported that daunorubicin incubated with homogenates of rat liver and kidney formed a much less polar metabolite and suggested that it might be a modified aglycone of daunorubicin. Bachur and Cradock (1970) found that the formation of the less polar metabolite from daunorubicin by rat tissues slices was preceded by the formation of a more polar metabolite which was a precursor for the less polar metabolite. In 1971 Bachur identified the less polar metabolite as 7-hydroxydaunorubicinol aglycone and suggested it was formed by hydrolytic cleavage of daunorubicinol (Bachur, 1971; Bachur and Cradock, 1970). Bachur and Gee (1971) reported that the enzyme responsible for the hydrolytic cleavage of daunorubicin was found in the liver microsomal fraction, required NADPH but not NADH and, significantly, was equally active under aerobic or anaerobic conditions. However, Asbell et al. (1972) found that under anaerobic conditions different aglycone metabolites were formed from daunorubicin by NADPH fortified rat liver and kidney homogenates. The aglycones were the products of reductive cleavage of daunorubicin and daunorubicinol, 7-deoxydaunorubicin aglycone and 7-deoxydaunorubicinol aglycone, respectively. Doxorubicin formed corresponding 7-deoxyaglycone metabolites. The enzyme responsible for reductive cleavage was located in the liver microsomal fraction, required NADPH but not NADH, was induced by phenobarbital, was not inhibited by the classical inhibitors of cytochrome P-450, SKF-525A (β-diethyl-aminoethyldiphenyl-propyl acetate) and carbon monoxide, and was reversibly inhibited by oxygen above about 35 torr (Bachur and Gee, 1972, 1976). The latter observation explained why previous studies conducted under aerobic conditions had not seen 7-deoxyaglycone formation. Formation of 7-hydroxyaglycones is now recognized as a minor pathway of anthracycline metabolism and may result from hydroxyl radical produced during redox cycling of anthracyclines reacting with radical precursors of the 7-deoxyaglycone (Schwartz and Paul, 1984). It is now also realized that anthracyclines are unstable in biological fluids and hydrolyze to aglycones if samples are left too long before assay (Maniez-Devos et al., 1986a).

Bachur and Gee (1976) concluded that the microsomal enzyme catalyzing anthracycline 7-deoxyaglycone formation was not a typical microsomal drug metabolizing enzyme and termed it a reductive glycosidase. However, a clue to the true identity of the enzyme came in the same year when Handa and Sato (1976) found that catalytic amounts of daunorubicin and doxorubicin stimulated the oxidation of NADPH by a partly purified preparation of microsomal NADPH cytochrome P-450 reductase. Confirmation that the microsomal enzyme responsible for reductive cleavage of anthracyclines was indeed NADPH-cytochrome P-450 reductase was provided by Oki et al. (1977) who showed that the purified enzyme catalyzed the conversion of a number of anthracyclines to the 7-deoxyaglycones (Table 1). The enzyme had a broad substrate specificity and also reduced 7-hydroxyaglycones to 7-deoxyaglycones, although Bachur and Gee (1976) had earlier reported that 7-hydroxyaglycones were not substrates for reduction by rat liver microsomes. 4′-Epidoxorubicin, 4′-deoxydoxorubicin, 4-demethoxydaunorubicin (Riggs and Schrader, 1985), *N*-benzyldaunorubicin, *N,N*-dibenzyldauno-rubicin and *N*-benzyldaunorubicinol (Gordon and Kashiwase, 1981) are reductively cleaved by rat liver microsomes more slowly than doxorubicin. *N,N*-dimethyl-daunorubicin and *N,N*-dimethyldaunorubicinol are cleaved at about the same rate as doxorubicin (Gordon and Kashiwase, 1981), while 11-deoxyanthracycline analogs are more

TABLE 1. *Reductive Cleavage of Anthracycline Antibiotics by NADPH-Cytochrome P-450 Reductase*

Substrate	Products	Rate (relative to daunorubicin)
Daunorubicin	7-Deoxydaunorubicin aglycone	1.00
Doxorubicin	7-Deoxydoxorubicin aglycone	0.46
Aclacinomycin A	7-Deoxyaklavinone aglycone	0.04
	7-Deoxyaklavinone aglycone	0.04
Daunorubicinol	7-Deoxydaunorubicin aglycone	0.30
Aklavinone	7-Deoxyaklavinone aglycone	0.12
	7-Deoxyaklavinone aglycone dimer	0.17
7-Hydroxydaunorubicin aglycone	7-Deoxydaunorubicin aglycone	0.40
7-Hydroxydaunorubicin aglycone	7-Deoxydoxorubicin aglycone	0.71

Date from Oki et al. (1977).

rapidly cleaved than daunorubicin (Barchielli et al., 1986). 5-Iminodaunorubicin shows negligible reduction by NADPH cytochrome P-450 reductase (Scheulen, 1985), probably because hydrogen bonding between the imine nitrogen and adjacent hydroxyl group makes the compound difficult to reduce (Lown et al., 1979). 6-Deoxy-4-demethoxydaunorubicin is not reductively cleaved by rat liver preparations (Arcamone, 1985; Barchielli et al., 1986) although its quinone group is reduced (Barchielli et al., 1986). This confirms expectations from electrochemical reduction studies where compounds such as 10-β-methoxydauno-rubicin and 11-deoxydaunorubicin, with the same conformation of the A ring as daunorubicin, are readily reduced in a two step process to the corresponding 7-deoxyaglycones, while 10-methoxy-daunorubicin and 6-deoxydaunorubicin, with a β conformation of the A ring, do not undergo reductive deglycosidation and in polar solvents form only the hydroquinone glycosides (Malatesta et al., 1984). The reason for the different behavior of β-anthracyclines is thought to be the lack of conjugative electron delocalization due to the large dihedral angle with respect to the π-type orbital(s) of the anthraquinone system compared to α-anthracyclines. Only anthracyclines with a C-7 glycoside group undergo reductive cleavage upon electrochemical reduction (Berg et al., 1982). Anthracyclines with a C-10 glycoside group undergo reversible reduction to the hydroquinone without glycoside cleavage.

As has been discussed previously, an important factor determining the rate of enzymatic reduction of quinones is the quinone one-electron reduction potential (E^1_7) (Powis and Appel, 1980). E^1_7s for several anthracyclines have been measured and are all around -300 mV (Land et al., 1983; Powis and Svingen, 1981; Svingen and Powis, 1981). Thus, E^1_7 is probably not a major factor determining the relative rates of reduction of different anthracyclines by NADPH-cytochrome P-450 reductase.

Other flavoenzymes that catalyze single electron reduction will support reductive cleavage of anthracyclines under anaerobic conditions. The enzymes include xanthine oxidase, mitochondrial NADH-dehydrogenase (E.C.1.6.99.3) and nitrate reductase from *Neurospora* (E.C.1.6.6.3) (Komiyama et al., 1979a, 1986; Pan and Bachur, 1980; Pan et al., 1981b; Schwartz, 1983). Flavoenzymes catalyzing two electron reduction have been reported not to support reductive cleavage of anthracyclines (Pan et al., 1981b), although Komiyama et al. (1979a) reported that quinone reductase cleaved doxorubicin to 7-deoxydoxorubicin aglycone.

C-7 reductive cleavage of anthracyclines is associated with formation of a semiquinone radical intermediate. Radical formation from anthracyclines is discussed further in Section 3.4.1.4. Although the formation of a semiquinone radical appears to be an obligatory step the exact mechanism of enzymatic anthracycline C-7 reductive cleavage is not known. Mason (1979) and Sinha (1980) have suggested a mechanism involving a C-7 carbon centered anthracycline radical. Other workers have suggested that enzymatic anthracycline C-7 reductive cleavage involves the anthracycline hydroquinone (Anne and Moiroux, 1985; Berg et al., 1982; Fisher et al., 1985; Houée-Levin et al., 1984). Evidence for such a mechanism comes from the observation that chemical reduction of a number of anthracyclines gives unstable hydroquinones which lose the glycoside group by heterolytic bond cleavage (Fisher et al., 1983; Kleyer et al., 1984; Kleyer and Koch, 1984). Anne and Moiroux (1985) have reported that during electrochemical reduction of daunorubicin in aprotic media glycoside elimination occurs only after addition of the second electron and not at the level of the semiquinone radical. It may be, as suggested by Houée-Levin et al. (1984), that the enzymatically formed anthracycline semiquinone radical has first to disproportionate to the hydroquinone before losing its glycoside group.

C-4 cleavage. Schwartz and his colleagues (Schwartz and Parker, 1981; Schwartz and Paul, 1984) have shown C-4 cleavage as an additional pathway of anthracycline metabolism by rat liver microsomes and NADPH under anaerobic conditions. Daunorubicin aglycone undergoes C-4 reductive cleavage to 4-deoxydaunorubicin aglycone, as well as C-4-*O*-demethylation to 4-hydroxydauno-rubicin aglycone. Both reactions require NADPH and because they are inhibited by SKF-525A it has been suggested that anthracycline C-4 reductive cleavage and C-4-O demethylation are catalyzed by microsomal cytochrome P-450 (Schwartz and Parker, 1981; Schwartz and Paul, 1984). SKF-525A is not, however, a specific inhibitor of cytochrome P-450 catalyzed reactions (Netter, 1980) and it is possible that other microsomal enzyme(s) are involved in C-4 cleavage.

A complete reaction sequence for formation of aglycone metabolites from daunorubicin by rat liver microsomes as proposed by Schwartz and Paul (1984) is shown in Fig. 6. The first step, based

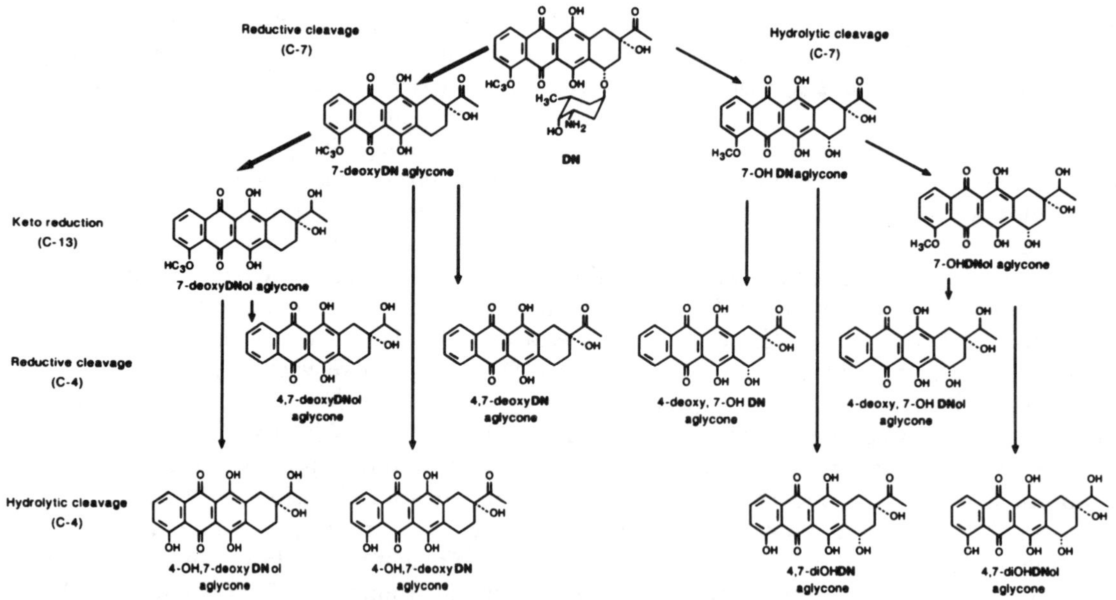

FIG. 6. Formation of aglycone metabolites of daunorubicin by rat liver microsomes and NADPH under anaerobic conditions. Dark arrows indicate major pathways. Adapted from Schwartz and Paul (1984).

on kinetic evidence, is C-7 reductive cleavage of daunorubicin to 7-deoxydaunorubicin aglycone with smaller amounts of C-7 hydrolytic cleavage to 7-hydroxydaunorubicin aglycone. This is followed by C-13 keto reduction and C-4 cleavage.

3.4.1.3. *Miscellaneous reactions.* A 7,7′-dimer of 7-deoxyalkylavin aglycone has been identified as one of the products of the reductive cleavage of aclacinomycin A by purified NADPH cytochrome P-450 reductase and NADPH (Oki et al., 1977), and by xanthine oxidase and xanthine (Komiyama et al., 1979b). The reaction is thought to proceed through an aclacinomycin A semiquinone radical intermediate. Electrochemical studies have shown that only anthracyclines lacking a C-11 hydroxyl group form 7,7′-dimers (Berg et al., 1982). Aclacinomycin A also undergoes C-4‴ keto reduction of the terminal L-cinnerulose of the carbohydrate chain (see Section 3.4.1.1) as well as C-7 reductive and hydrolytic cleavage. A suggested reaction sequence for in vitro metabolism of aclacinomycin A by NADPH fortified rat tissue homogenates is shown in Fig. 7. Marcellomycin undergoes similar metabolism to aclacinomycin A forming 7-deoxypyrromycin aglycone, bisanhydropyrromycin aglycone, and probably the 7,7′-dimer of 7-deoxypyrromycin aglycone (Dodion et al., 1986b).

Xanthine oxidase with xanthine as an electron donor converts 7-deoxydaunorubicin aglycone to a nonfluorescent metabolite (Dodion et al., 1987). Analogy to the metabolism of dihydroxyanthraquinone which is converted by the same system to tetrahydroxy-anthracene suggests that the nonfluorescent metabolite of 7-deoxydaunorubicin aglycone might be a dihydroquinone derivative. Marcellomycin is converted to a nonfluorescent metabolite upon prolonged incubation under anaerobic conditions with NADPH fortified rat liver microsomes, mitochondria, nuclei or cytosol (Chang et al., 1983; Dodion et al., 1986b). A yellow nonfluorescent metabolite is formed from the marcellomycin metabolite 7-deoxypyrromycin aglycone under anaerobic conditions by xanthine oxidase and xanthine, by rat liver microsome and NADPH, by rat liver cytosol and NADPH or NADH, but not by purified NADPH cytochrome P-450 reductase and NADPH. The metabolite was tentatively identified as 7-deoxypyrromycin dihydroquinone aglycone (Dodion et al., 1987).

A glutathione-anthracycline adduct has been claimed to be formed when glutathione is included in anaerobic incubations of daunorubicin or doxorubicin with NADPH and rat liver microsomes (Sinha and Gregory, 1981). Adduct formation was suggested to proceed through a free radical intermediate.

Menogaril is a nogalomycin analog with a dimethylamine glycoside attached to the anthracycline D ring (Fig. 5). Rat liver homogenate and NADPH under aerobic conditions catalyzes *N*-demethy-

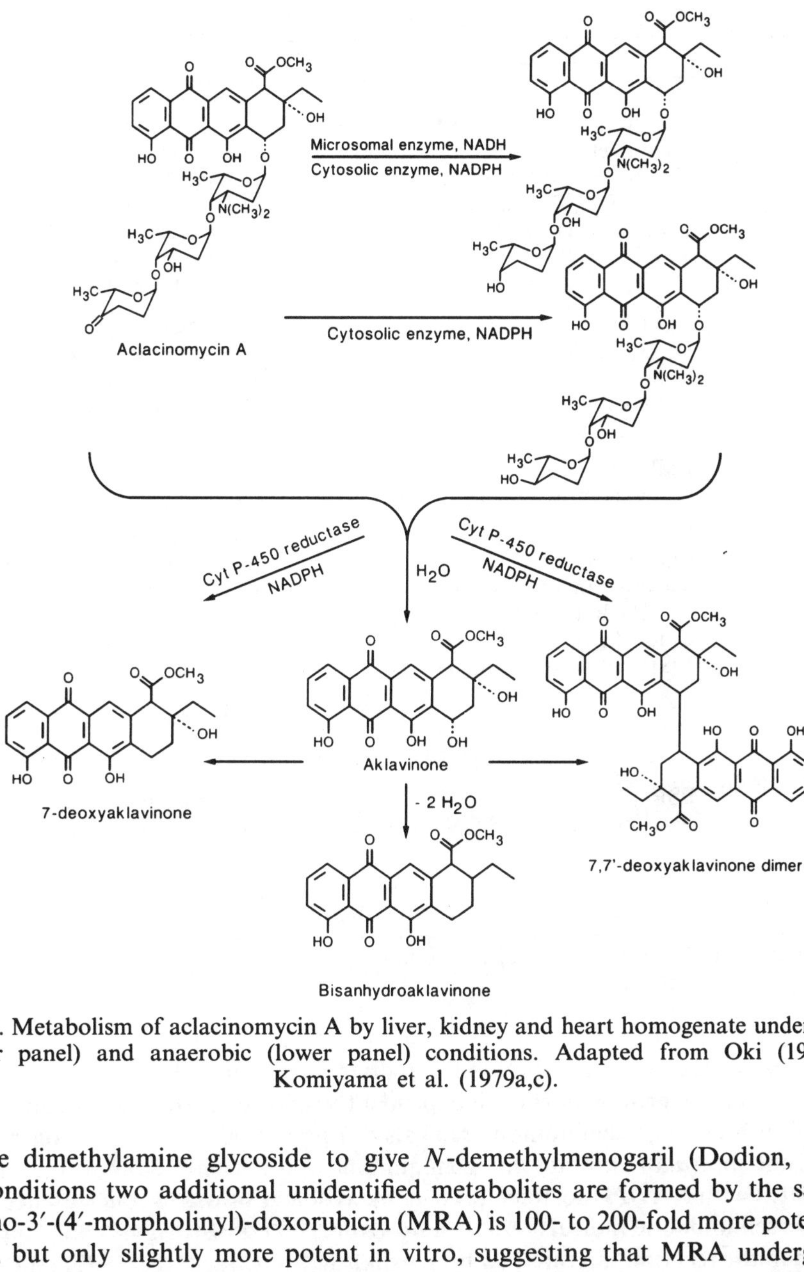

FIG. 7. Metabolism of aclacinomycin A by liver, kidney and heart homogenate under aerobic (upper panel) and anaerobic (lower panel) conditions. Adapted from Oki (1977) and Komiyama et al. (1979a,c).

lation of the dimethylamine glycoside to give *N*-demethylmenogaril (Dodion, 1986c). Under anaerobic conditions two additional unidentified metabolites are formed by the same system.

3′-Deamino-3′-(4′-morpholinyl)-doxorubicin (MRA) is 100- to 200-fold more potent in vivo than doxorubicin, but only slightly more potent in vitro, suggesting that MRA undergoes metabolic activation in vivo. The cytotoxicity of MRA to the human ovarian carcinoma cell line ES-2 as well as DNA cross links are potentiated by coincubation with human liver microsomes and NADPH (Lau et al., 1989). The most likely mechanism for metabolic activation of MRA suggested by the authors of this work was hydroxylation of one or both of the α-carbons attached to the nitrogen of the morpholino ring. Cyanomorpholinodoxorubicin (MRA-CN) was not activated under the same conditions. Cyanomorpholinodaunorubicin undergoes spontaneous elimination of cyanide giving a postively charged reactive species, possibly an iminium cation, that reacts with DNA (Westendorf et al., 1988; Peters et al., 1988).

Kolodziejczyk et al. (1989) have demonstrated the oxidation of 5-iminodaunorubicin, but not daunorubicin, by horseradish peroxidase to form an ESR detectable nitrogen centered free radical.

3.4.1.4. *Radical formation.* Anthracyclines, as might be expected, undergo flavoenzyme catalyzed one-electron reduction and form radicals. Handa and Sato (1975) first reported that daunorubicin and doxorubicin incubated with rat liver microsomes and NADPH under aerobic conditions formed a radical that was capable of initiating sulfite oxidation. Inhibition of the reaction by

TABLE 2. *Free Radical Formation by Anthracyclines*

Compound	Drug Radical	Oxygen Radical
Doxorubicin	ESR (Basra et al., 1985, 1984; Bachur et al., 1978b; Berlin and Haseltine, 1981; Pietronigro et al., 1979, 1983; Pollakis et al., 1984; Sato et al., 1977; Sinha and Chignell, 1979)	ERS/spin trap (Davies et al., 1983; Gutierrez et al., 1983; Goormaghtigh and Ruysschaert, 1983; Kalyanaraman et al., 1980, 1984; Komiyama et al., 1982; Nohl and Jordan, 1983; Sinha et al., 1994; Thornalley et al., 1986)
		chemical (Adachi et al., 1983; Doroshows 1983a,b; Komiyama et al., 1982; Powis et al., 1981; Tobia et al., 1985)
N-acetyldoxorubicin	ESR (Pollakis et al., 1984)	
Daunorubicin	ESR (Bachur et al., 1977; Kalyanaraman et al., 1984; Pan and Bachur, 1980; Sinha and Chignell, 1979, Lown and Chen, 1981; Schreiber et al., 1987)	ESR/spin trap (Kalyanaraman et al., 1980, 1984)
		chemical (Doroshow, 1983a,b)
Aclacinomycin A	ESR (Bachur et al., 1978b; Kodama et al., 1983)	ESR/spin trap (Komiyama et al., 1982)
Rubidazone		chemical (Doroshow, 1983a,b)

Techniques used to demonstrate free radical formation are electron spin resonance (ESR), with or without spin trapping, and chemical assay.

superoxide dismutase suggested that the radical species being formed was the superoxide anion radical. Two years later two groups working independently reported ESR spectroscopic evidence for the formation of anthracycline semiquinone radicals during anthracycline metabolism. Sato et al. (1977) reported ESR spectra of anthracycline semiquinone radicals when daunorubicin and doxorubicin were incubated with NADPH fortified rat liver microsomes or with Ehrlich ascites tumor cells. The anthracycline semiquinone radicals rapidly auto-oxidized and ESR signals only appeared when dissolved oxygen in the reaction mixture had been exhausted. Bachur et al. (1977) reported an ESR signal when daunorubicin was incubated with NADPH fortified rat liver microsomes under conditions where dissolved oxygen in the incubation medium was probably depleted. Subsequently, a number of anthracyclines have been shown to undergo enzymatic one-electron reduction to form ESR detectable semiquinone radicals (Table 2). The ESR spectra obtained by reduction of anthracyclines can be observed for up to several hours. The long duration of the signal is probably due to disproportionation–comproportionation equilibrium between the anthracycline and the hydroquinone, which continually destroys and reforms the semiquinone radical.

Aqueous solutions of doxorubicin spontaneously form the doxorubicin semiquinone radical at physiologic pH, although the rate is much slower than the enzyme catalyzed rate (Pietronigro et al., 1979). Spontaneous semiquinone radical formation is probably due to intramolecular electron transfer between the anthracycline hydroquinone B ring and the quinone C ring analogous to the intermolecular comproportionation of quinone and hydroquinone.

Intercalation of doxorubicin and other anthracyclines into double-stranded DNA prevents its enzymatic reduction (Berlin and Haseltine, 1981; Kalyanaraman et al., 1980; Peters et al., 1986; Rowley and Haliwell, 1983; Sato et al., 1977). This is not due to a loss of the redox properties of

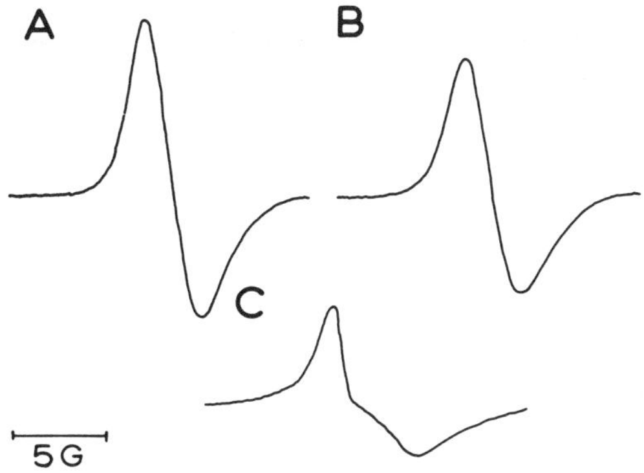

FIG. 8. Electron spin resonance signals obtained when 5 mM daunorubicin was incubated with rat liver microsomes, 1 mg/mL, and a 1 mM NADPH generating system in 0.1 M potassium phosphate buffer, pH 7.4 at 23°, showing progressive immobilization of the signal. (A) 10 min, (B) 30 min, (C) 120 min.

the anthracycline but rather to steric hindrance since doxorubicin bound to DNA can still be reduced by a small reductant such as sodium borohydride (Lown et al., 1977), COO^- free radicals (Houée-Levin et al., 1990; Rouscilles et al., 1989), or superoxide anion radical (Youngman and Elstner, 1984).

An unusual feature of the ESR spectra of doxorubicin and daunorubicin is that they change with time (Kalyanaraman et al., 1980; Pan et al., 1980, 1981a; Pollakis et al., 1984; Sinha et al., 1984). This is shown for doxorubicin in Fig. 8. The first signal that appears is symmetrical with a spectroscopic splitting constant (g) of 2.0036 (Kalyanaraman et al., 1980; Pan et al., 1980, 1981a). With time the spectrum evolves into one with asymmetry and g anisotropy, $g_1 = 2.0046$–2.0052, $g_1 1 = 2.0023$ (Gutierrez et al., 1983; Kalyanaraman et al., 1980; Pan et al., 1981b), characteristic of a highly immobilized radical. Kalyanaraman et al. (1980) suggested that the immobilized radical might be the 7-deoxyaglycone semiquinone radical or the radical of an anthracycline polymerization product. Evidence that the anisotropic signal is that of the 7-deoxyaglycone semiquinone radical is the appearance of anthracycline 7-deoxyaglycone in the incubation mixture preceding the appearance of the anisotropic signal (Gutierrez et al., 1983). In addition, the fully developed anisotropic signal has the same parameters as the signal obtained with the 7-deoxyaglycone as substrate (Pan et al., 1980). Other anthracyclines, such as *N*-acetyldoxorubicin, also give an ESR signal that shows anisotropy with time (Pollakis et al., 1984). Daunosamine, the sugar cleaved from the anthracycline, does not give rise to an ESR signal (Pan et al., 1980).

The properties of anthracycline semiquinone radicals have been studied by pulse radiolysis. In this technique an aqueous solution of anthracycline is irradiated with a short burst of high energy electrons in the presence of a trapping agent to remove oxidizing species formed by the radiolysis of water. The anthracycline is reduced by aqueous electrons to a semiquinone radical whose decay can be followed spectrophotometrically (Svingen and Powis, 1981). E^1_7 for the anthracycline can be calculated from the rates of electron transfer between the anthracycline and a redox indicator of known E^1_7. Measurements made by an approach to equilibrium method have given E^1_7 for daunorubicin as −305 mV and doxorubicin as −292 mV (Svingen and Powis, 1981). Measurements made at equilibrium have given E^1_7 for doxorubicin as −328 mV (Land et al., 1983). Mukherjee et al. (1989) have reported an E^1_7 for both doxorubicin and daunorubicin of −341 mV and a second one-electron reduction potential (E^2_7) of −260 mV calculated from equilibrium measurements using several redox indictors. An E^1_7 of −430 mV has been calculated from the rate of disproportionation of doxorubicin semiquinone (Houée-Levin et al., 1985). Values in this range indicate that anthracyclines such as doxorubicin and daunorubicin have a low E^1_7 compared to simple quinones which may explain the relatively slow rate of reduction of anthracyclines by NADPH-cytochrome P-450 reductase and other flavoenzymes, compared to simple quinones (Svingen and Powis, 1981). Pulse radiolysis studies have also shown that the doxorubicin semiquinone free radical reacts rapidly with oxygen with a bimolecular rate constant of 3×10^8 M^{-1} sec^{-1} (Butler et al., 1985; Land et al., 1985).

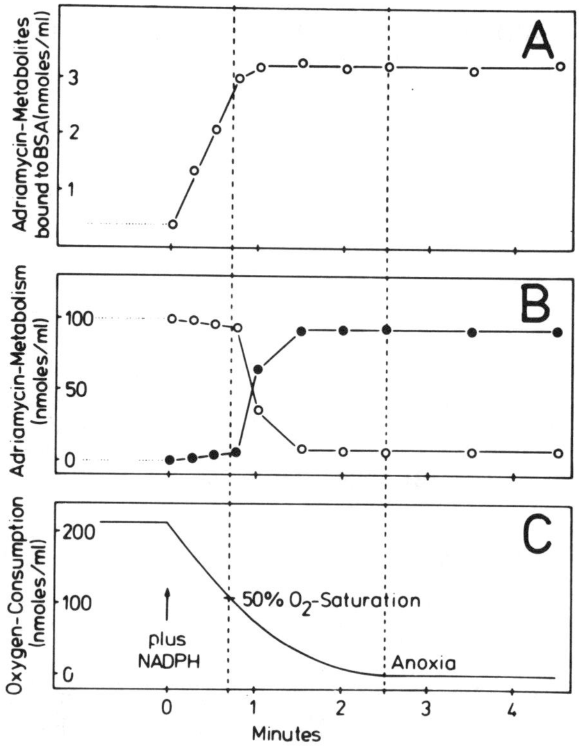

FIG. 9. Simultaneous determination of (A) covalent binding of [^{3}H]-doxorubicin metabolites to bovine serum albumin (B) formation of 7-deoxydoxorubicin aglycone (●) from doxorubicin (○) and (C) oxygen consumption when [^{3}H]-doxorubicin 0.1 mM was incubated with rat liver microsomes 2 mg/mL, bovine serum albumin 0.2 mM and a NADPH generating system. Reprinted from Scheulen et al. (1982) with permission of the authors and the copyright holder, Springer, Berlin.

Catalytic amounts of anthracycline stimulate NADPH oxidation and oxygen utilization by microsomes from liver (Goodman and Hochstein, 1977; Bachur et al., 1977; Peters et al., 1986) and a variety of other tissues including murine L1210 and P388 tumor cells (Bachur et al., 1978b; Peters et al., 1987), heart (Doroshow, 1983a; Mimnaugh et al., 1982), kidney (Bachur et al., 1982b; Mimnaugh et al., 1983), lung (Mimnaugh et al., 1983), spleen (Bachur et al., 1978b), red blood cells (Bannister and Thornalley, 1983; Pedersen et al., 1990), as well as by purified NADPH-cytochrome P-450 reductase (Handa and Sato, 1975; Bachur et al., 1979). The levels of anthracycline remain constant until all the dissolved oxygen has been depleted when there is rapid conversion of anthracycline to the 7-deoxyaglycone (Fig. 9). These, and other observations discussed previously, are consistent with the concept of redox cycling of the anthracycline to the semiquinone radical and back, with molecular oxygen as the final electron acceptor. Anne and Moiroux (1984) have studied the electrochemical reduction of substituted hydroxyanthraquinones in aprotic media and found that oxidation of the hydroxyanthrasemiquinone radical does not give the parent hydroxyanthraquinone directly but probably precedes through a conjugated hydroxyanthraquinone base, formed by proton transfer between the hydroxyanthrasemiquinone and superoxide anion radical, which is then converted to the parent hydroxyanthraquinone. A similar mechanism may occur with the anthracycline glycosides.

The initial oxygen species formed by reduction of molecular oxygen by the anthracycline semiquinone radical is the superoxide anion radical. Formation of superoxide anion radical has been shown by chemical assays and by ESR studies using dimethyl-1-pyrroline-1-oxide (DMPO) to spin trap the superoxide anion radical as a stable adduct (Table 2). Small amounts of a DMPO-hydroxyl radical adduct are also occasionally seen (Kalyanaraman et al., 1980). Using another spin trapping agent, α-phenyl-*N*-tert-butylnitrone (PBN), only a hydroxyl radical adduct is seen (Komiyama et al., 1982; Sugioka et al., 1984). Studies using anthraquinonyl glucosaminosides as model compounds have shown that superoxide anion radical formation by rat heart sarcosomes and NADPH increases with the addition of successive hydroxyl groups to the anthraquinone nucleus (Abramson et al., 1986).

Aqueous air-saturated solutions of daunorubicin and doxorubicin at physiologic pH spontaneously form oxygen radicals at a slow rate. A solution of doxorubicin incubated with PBN gives an ESR signal that has been attributed to either the superoxide anion radical or hydroxyl radical adduct (Dickinson et al., 1984). Photoirradiation of an aqueous solution of daunorubicin or doxorubicin at 438 nm stimulates the formation of superoxide anion radical, detected as the spin trapped adduct with 4-(*N*-methylpyridinium)-tert-butylnitrone, and of hydroxyl radical, detected as the spin trapped adduct with DMPO (Carmichael et al., 1983). In these studies the DMPO-hydroxyl radical adduct was not formed by direct reaction of hydroxyl radical with DMPO and was probably formed by decomposition of a DMPO superoxide anion radical adduct.

The superoxide anion radical is a common respiratory intermediate of aerobic cells (Fridovich, 1976), and it has been pointed out that the superoxide anion radical might react with anthracycline to give rise to biologically important reactive intermediates (Nakazawa et al., 1985; Sawyer et al., 1983). Studies of the interaction of superoxide anion radical with daunorubicin and its aglycones in aprotic media have shown that superoxide anion radical can extract a proton from one of the weakly acidic anthracycline C-6 or C-11 phenolic groups to generate a phenolate anion (Nakazawa et al., 1985). The phenolate anion is then oxidized by molecular oxygen to give a B ring semiquinone radical, or breaks down to unidentified products. This interpretation of the interaction between superoxide anion radical and anthracycline is in contrast to earlier studies where the interaction was attributed to direct electron transfer from superoxide anion radical to the anthracycline to give a C ring semiquinone radical (Afanas'ev et al., 1980). It is possible that superoxide anion radical, formed spontaneously or drug induced, could react with anthracycline bound to DNA or in a hydrophobic region of the cell, for example, a lipid bilayer, to give rise to species important for the biological activity of the anthracycline.

The superoxide anion radical formed by redox cycling of anthracycline can give rise, by an iron salt catalyzed reaction, to a hydroxyl radical that leads to oxidation of polyunsaturated fatty acids (Goodman and Hochstein, 1977; Mimnaugh et al., 1983), degradation of deoxyribose (Bates and Winterbourn, 1982; Gutteridge and Quinlan, 1985) and DNA strand breaks (Rowley and Halliwell, 1983; Sinha et al., 1984; Sugioka et al., 1984). Hemoproteins may be able to replace iron salts in catalyzing anthracycline-induced hydroxyl radical formation from superoxide anion radical (Komiyama et al., 1985). Hydroxyl radical can also be formed by the direct reaction of anthracycline semiquinone radical with hydrogen peroxide without the need for iron catalysis. Several organic radicals react with hydrogen peroxide in this way to give a hydroxyl radical-like species (Elstner et al., 1980; Youngman and Elstner, 1981; Youngman et al., 1982a). Simple *o*-semiquinone radicals do not, however, react with hydrogen peroxide (Kalyanaram et al., 1984). Winterbourn and her colleagues (Bates, 1982; Bates and Winterbourn, 1982; Winterbourn, 1981) first demonstrated the reaction of doxorubicin semiquinone radical with hydrogen peroxide under aerobic conditions to give a species with reactivity similar to that of hydroxyl radical. Formation of this species was not inhibited by chelating agents, thus ruling out a Haber–Weiss or Fenton type reaction, but was inhibited by oxygen. This is apparently because the rate of reaction of doxorubicin semiquinone radical with hydrogen peroxide, 10^4–10^5 $M^{-1}sec^{-1}$ (Kalyanaraman et al., 1984), cannot effectively compete with the reaction of oxygen with doxorubicin semiquinone radical to form superoxide anion radical, 3×10^8 M^{-1} sec^{-1} (Land et al., 1985). Evidence that the species formed by reaction of doxorubicin semiquinone radical with hydrogen peroxide might be hydroxyl radical comes from the observation that doxorubicin semiquinone radical and hydrogen peroxide at low oxygen concentrations degrade methional to ethylene, a reaction known to require hydroxyl radical (Paur et al., 1984). Other evidence suggesting the formation of hydroxyl radical is ESR spin trapping of a hydroxyl radical adduct with DMPO (Bannister and Thornalley, 1983; Kalyanaraman et al., 1984). However, unlike the breakdown of deoxyribose produced by other hydroxyl radical generating systems, breakdown of deoxyribose by doxorubicin semiquinone radical and hydrogen peroxide is not inhibited by hydroxyl radical scavenging agents (Winterbourn and Sutton, 1984). This suggests that an intermediate species with a more limited reactivity than hydroxyl radical may be formed. The formation of a species which mimics the hydroxyl radical but is more discriminating in its reactivity has been described for the reaction of paraquat anion radical

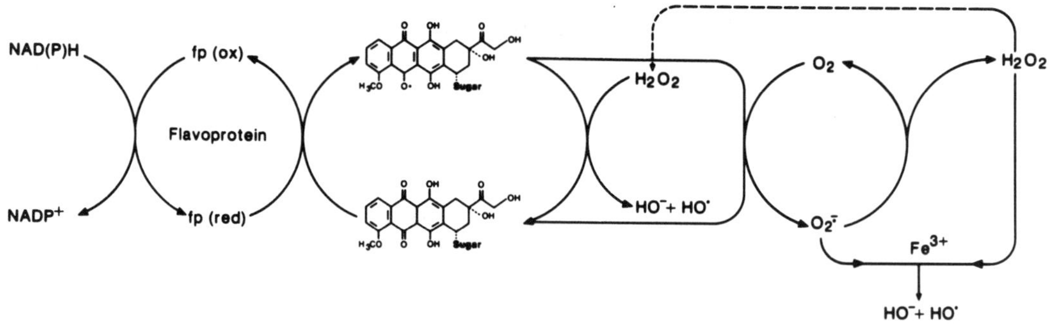

FIG. 10. Pathways for formation of oxygen radicals during redox cycling of doxorubicin. For an explanation see the text. Reprinted from Powis (1987) with permission of the copyright holder, Taylor and Francis, London.

(Youngman and Elstner, 1981) and nitrofurantoin radical (Youngman et al., 1982b) with hydrogen peroxide under limiting oxygen concentrations. The species has been termed a crypto-hydroxyl radical. A similar species may be formed by reaction of doxorubicin semiquinone free radical with hydrogen peroxide. A summary of the pathways for the formation of oxygen radicals during metabolism of anthracyclines is shown in Fig. 10.

3.4.1.5. *Anthracycline metal complexes.* Several studies have indicated that anthracycline-mediated lipid peroxidation only occurs in the presence of trace amounts of iron (Doroshow, 1983a,b; Mimnaugh et al., 1983; Sterrenberg et al., 1984; Sugioka et al., 1981; Sugioka and Nakano, 1982; Minotti, 1989). The iron in such systems might be catalyzing a Haber–Weiss type or Fenton reaction to form hydroxyl radical as already discussed. Alternatively, a mechanism involving direct reaction of iron with the anthracycline could be involved as suggested by the fact that a mixture of doxorubicin and ferric chloride stimulates lipid peroxidation without the need for redox cycling of doxorubicin (Gutteridge, 1983, 1984a; Sterrenberg et al., 1984; Sugioka et al., 1981). Anthracyclines, such as doxorubicin, daunorubicin, carminomycin and 5-iminodaunorubicin, form very strong complexes with Fe(III) in which three molecules of anthracycline are bound to one Fe(III), each anthracycline molecule probably being chelated through one carbonyl and one phenolate oxygen to form a six membered ring (Beraldo et al., 1985; Fantine and Garnier-Suillerot, 1986; Fiallo and Garnier-Suillerot, 1985). The stability constant of such a complex is around 10^{28}–10^{34} (Beraldo et al., 1985; Fantine and Garnier-Suillerot, 1985; Fiallo and Garnier-Suillerot, 1985), which is among the highest reported for any Fe(III) complex. Doxorubicin can even extract iron from ferritin, the major storage form of iron in cells (Demant, 1984) and from transferrin (Lvstad, 1988). The release of the Fe(III) from ferritin has been reported to be facilitated by its reduction to Fe(II) by anthracycline semiquinone radical or superoxide anion radical (Thomas and Aust, 1986). It has been claimed that anthracycline iron complexes dissociate in vivo in the presence of serum or at the cell surface (Gelvan and Samuni, 1988; Kessel, 1988). To play a role in the cytotoxicity of the anthracyclines, the iron complex would have to be formed intracellularly. Doxorubicin and daunorubicin also form complexes with other metal ions including Pd(II) which has a stability constant around 10^{22} (Fiallo and Garnier-Suillerot, 1986). Unlike free anthracyclines, anthracycline–Fe(III) and Pd(II) complexes are poor stimulants of superoxide anion radical formation by redox cycling with mitochondrial NADH dehydrogenase (Beraldo et al., 1985; Fiallo and Garnier-Suillerot, 1986).

A consequence of Fe(III) chelation is a dramatic increase in anthracycline electrophilicity. Sugioka et al. (1981) first proposed that a doxorubicin–Fe(III) complex might undergo self-reduction to a Fe(II) complex by a process involving intramolecular electron transfer. ESR evidence for such a mechanism has been provided by Zweier (1983, 1985). Doxorubicin slowly reduces bound Fe(III) to Fe(II) giving a complex with a one-electron oxidized doxorubicin semiquinone radical (Gianni et al., 1983b; Zweier, 1983, 1985). In the presence of oxygen bound Fe(II) is rapidly oxidized back to Fe(III) (Hasinoff, 1989). Oxygen is presumed to bind to Fe(II) and an electron transferred from Fe(II) to oxygen (Zweier, 1983). The rate-limiting step in the redox cycle is reduction of Fe(III) to Fe(II) by doxorubicin which may explain why preparations of Fe(II) or Fe(III) added to doxorubicin in air give only the Fe(III)–doxorubicin complex. Doxorubicin undergoes accelerated degradation in the presence of iron resulting in a complex with increased affinity for iron but decreased toxicity (Gelvan et al., 1990). When added to vesicles of dimyristoyl phosphatidylcholine the doxorubicin–Fe(III) complex has been reported to be slowly converted to a new form which lacks a daunosamine sugar group but differs from normal doxorubicin aglycones (Samuni et al., 1986).

In the presence of thiols such as cysteine or glutathione (Gianni et al., 1983b; Myers et al., 1982), or membrane protein thiol groups (Muindi et al., 1985a) the doxorubicin–Fe(III) complex is rapidly reduced and catalyzes oxygen consumption and the formation of superoxide anion radical and hydrogen peroxide. Catalysis is inhibited by the specific Fe(II) chelator 4,7-diphenyl-1,10-phenanthroline sulfonate indicating that Fe(II) is formed during the catalytic cycle (Gianni et al., 1983b). When a doxorubicin–Fe(III) complex is reduced by thiol no oxidized doxorubicin semiquinone radical ESR signal is seen, suggesting that glutathione reduces Fe(III) directly by-passing the doxorubicin mediated reduction step (Zweier, 1985). Unlike the enzymatic reduction of doxorubicin to 7-deoxydoxorubicin aglycone, reduction of doxorubicin–Fe(III) complex by glutathione is not associated with a loss of doxorubicin or with aglycone formation (Myers et al., 1982). Reactive oxygen species generated by doxorubicin–Fe(III) complex in the presence of thiols lead to cell membrane lipid peroxidation (Myers et al., 1982). Superoxide dismutase and catalase are weak inhibitors of this membrane lipid peroxidation while the hydroxyl radical scavengers dimethylsulfoxide and mannitol are more effective inhibitors suggesting the involvement of a hydroxyl radical-like species (Myers et al., 1982; Muindi et al., 1985a).

The doxorubicin–Fe(III) complex preferentially alkylates DNA on guanine sequences leading to the termination of transcription (Phillips et al., 1989). The doxorubicin–Fe(III) complex also cleaves DNA (Muindi et al., 1985b) by a process that is stimulated by thiol (Eliot et al., 1983). DNA cleavage is inhibited by catalase suggesting the involvement of hydrogen peroxide (Eliot et al., 1983; Muindi et al., 1985b) probably generated by reduction of iron by doxorubicin (Zweier, 1983). ESR spectroscopy and spin trapping with DMPO have demonstrated the formation of small amounts of free hydroxyl radical when hydrogen peroxide is mixed with doxorubicin–Fe(III) complex (Muindi et al., 1984). The hydroxyl radical scavengers ethanol and dimethylsulfoxide inhibit this DMPO-hydroxyl radical adduct formation. The complex formed between 5-iminodaunorubicin and Fe(III) is much less reactive than that of doxorubicin–Fe(III), which may explain the lower cardiotoxicity of 5-iminodaunorubicin (Myers et al., 1987). 5-Iminodaunorubicin–Fe(III) complex and hydrogen peroxide also give a DMPO-hydroxyl radical adduct, but ethanol and dimethylsulfoxide do not inhibit adduct formation (Lown et al., 1982). The yield of hydroxyl radical is far less than obtained with the doxorubicin–Fe(III) complex and declines at high 5-iminodaunorubicin-iron ratios (Myers et al., 1987). A close parallel has been claimed between DNA cleavage and hydroxyl radical formation by 5-iminodaunorubicin–Fe(III) complex (Myers et al., 1987). Lown et al. (1982), however, found no cleavage of DNA by 5-iminodaunorubicin–Fe(III) complex. Addition of DNA stimulates hydroxyl radical formation by doxorubicin–Fe(III) complex and hydrogen peroxide over 250% (Muindi et al., 1984, 1985b; Lown et al., 1982). Stimulation of hydroxyl radical formation by DNA is also seen with iron complexes of 4-demethoxydaunorubicin and 4-demethyldaunorubicin, but not with daunorubicin (Muindi et al., 1985b) or 5-iminodaunorubicin (Lown et al., 1982). Since all of these anthracyclines form a ternary complex with DNA and iron (Muindi et al., 1985b) this ability alone cannot explain why DNA enhances hydroxyl radical formation. Doxorubicin may be released from its strong coordination with Fe(III) on binding with DNA and intercalate between the base pairs of DNA (Beraldo et al., 1985). The importance of a complex of drug, Fe(III) and DNA for cleavage of DNA remains to be established.

Unlike doxorubicin–Fe(III) complex-dependent cleavage of DNA, doxorubicin–Fe(III) complex-dependent degradation of deoxyribose is not inhibited by catalase or superoxide dismutase (Gutteridge, 1984a). Furthermore, the process is inhibited by some hydroxyl radical scavengers, such as mannitol and thiourea, but not by others, such as benzoate and formate. The reactive oxygen species responsible for cleavage of deoxyribose by doxorubicin–Fe(III) complex might be a crypto-hydroxyl radical rather than free hydroxyl radical.

$$\mathrm{Dox\,H_2 + Fe(III) \longrightarrow Dox^{\bar{\cdot}}\text{-}Fe(III) + 2H^+}$$

$$\mathrm{Dox^{\bar{\cdot}}\text{-}Fe(III) \longleftrightarrow Dox^{\cdot}\text{-}Fe(II) \longleftrightarrow Fe(II) + Dox^{\cdot}}$$

$$\mathrm{Fe(II)\ (or\ Dox^{\cdot}\text{-}Fe(II)) + O_2 \longrightarrow Fe(III)\text{-}O_2^{\bar{\cdot}}}$$

$$\mathrm{Fe(III)\text{-}O_2^{\bar{\cdot}} \longrightarrow Fe(III) + O_2^{\bar{\cdot}}}$$

$$\mathrm{2O_2^{\bar{\cdot}} + 2H^+ \longrightarrow H_2O_2 + O_2}$$

$$\mathrm{Fe(II)\ (or\ Dox^{\cdot}\text{-}Fe(II)) + H_2O_2 \longrightarrow Fe(III) + HO^- + [HO\cdot]}$$

$$\mathrm{Dox^{\cdot} + H_2O_2 \xrightarrow[catalysis]{Fe} Dox^+ + HO^- + [HO\cdot]}$$

Fig. 11. Reactions contributing to the reactivity of the doxorubicin–iron complex (Gutteridge, 1984a). $DoxH_2$ is doxorubicin; Dox· the semiquinone radical formed by oxidation of doxorubicin; [HO·] is hydroxyl radical or a species with similar reactivity to hydroxyl radical. The first two reactions are the self-reduction of doxorubicin-Fe(III) complex described by Sugioka and Nakano (1982).

A summary of possible pathways for formation of reactive oxygen species by anthracycline iron complexes is given in Fig. 11. The exact nature of the oxygen radical species, whether a free hydroxyl or a hydroxyl radical-like species, remains to be established. The relationship of the reactions shown in Fig. 11 to anthracycline antitumor activity is not known, although Gianni et al. (1983a) have hypothesized that doxorubicin–Fe(III) complex might be the active form of the drug.

The metal ions Zn(II), Mg(II), Ca(II), Yb(III) and Cu(II) can substitute for Fe(III) and Fe(II) in the thiol-dependent degradation of DNA by doxorubicin (Mariam and Glover, 1986). Cu(II) is considerably more potent than Fe(III) or Fe(II) in stimulating thiol-dependent DNA degradation in a reaction inhibited by catalase but not by superoxide dismutase. Doxorubicin forms a 1:1 complex with Cu(II) with a stability constant of 10^{12}–10^{16} (Beraldo et al., 1983). Doxorubicin–Cu(II) complex is capable of reducing molecular oxygen to superoxide anion radical and of causing oxygen radical-dependent lipid peroxidation (Wallace, 1986a) as well as DNA degradation (Someya and Tanaka, 1979). In contrast to the doxorubicin–Fe(III) complex which is activated by glutathione, the doxorubicin–Cu(II) complex is inactivated by glutathione due to the formation of free doxorubicin (Hasinoff and Davey, 1988). Although Cu(II) forms a weaker complex with anthracyclines than Fe(III) it has been suggested that the anthracycine–Cu(II) complex may be the physiologically important form of the drug in blood because of the relative abundance of free copper and the limited availability of free iron (Phillips and Carlyle, 1981; Wallace, 1986a).

It is interesting that a combination of doxorubicin and iron has received clinical trial, under the name quelamycin, because of claims of reduced cardiotoxicity and other toxicities (Brugarolas et al., 1978). Unfortunately, quelamycin was found to produce severe noncardiac as well as cardiac toxicity (Brugarolas et al., 1978; Cortes-Funes et al., 1979). Quelamycin is a colloidal mixture of doxorubicin–Fe(III) complex and polymeric ferric hydroxide (Bachur et al., 1984; Beraldo et al., 1985) rather than a distinct triferric–doxorubicin complex as originally claimed (Gosalvez et al., 1978). Quelamycin probably acts as an intravascular slow release form of doxorubicin (Bachur et al., 1984) which might explain indications of less extensive metabolism of quelamycin than doxorubicin, with less C-13 keto reduction and less aglycone formation (Reich and Gordon, 1977).

3.4.1.6. *Alkylation by anthracyclines.* In addition to forming radicals when reduced anthracyclines also alkylate proteins, lipids and DNA. Figure 12 shows the proposed pathways for formation of alkylating species by either one- or two-electron reduction of anthracyclines. Single-electron reduction of daunorubicin and doxorubicin with a limiting amount of sodium borohydrate under anaerobic conditions (Sinha and Chignell, 1979), or reduction by NADPH fortified rat liver or heart microsomes under aerobic or anaerobic conditions (Scheulen et al., 1982; Sinha, 1980; Sinha and Gregory, 1981) results in covalent binding of anthracycline residues to microsomal proteins and to added DNA. Incubation of doxorubicin with rat hepatic nuclei and NADPH under aerobic or anaerobic conditions also results in covalent binding of anthracycline residues to nuclear DNA (Sinha et al., 1984; Wallace and Johnson, 1987). The addition of microsomal protein to intact nuclei under aerobic conditions increases the binding of doxorubicin to DNA, but almost completely abolishes DNA binding under anaerobic conditions (Wallace and Johnson, 1987). A possible explanation for this affect is that under anaerobic conditions more highly reactive doxorubicin intermediates are formed that bind to the microsomal surface in the immediate vicinity of their generation without being able to diffuse to the nucleus. Two-electron reduction of doxorubicin with an excess of sodium borohydride also results in covalent binding of anthracycline residues to DNA, although less than with single- electron reduction (Sinha and Chignell, 1979). Covalent binding of doxorubicin residues to cardiolipin has been demonstrated in a reconstituted system of doxorubicin, cardiolipin, mitochondrial NADH-cytochrome c reductase and NADH (Goormaghtigh et al., 1983; Pollakis et al., 1983). 5-Iminodaunorubicin which is not reduced by NADH-cytochrome c reductase shows minimal binding to cardiolipin under the same conditions. Glutathione, which has no effect on the formation of anthracycline semiquinone radicals (Sinha and Gregory, 1981), considerably decreases drug binding to protein (Scheulen et al., 1982) and DNA (Sinha and Gregory, 1981). This has been reported to be accompanied by the formation of a glutathione anthracycline adduct suggesting that glutathione reacts with a species derived from the anthracycline semiquinone radical thereby reducing the concentration available for alkylation (Sinha and Gregory, 1981). Scheulen et al. (1982) have reported that covalent binding of [^{3}H]-doxorubicin to bovine serum albumin by NADPH fortified rat liver microsomes occurs most readily under aerobic conditions before there is formation of 7-deoxydoxorubicin aglycone, showing that covalent binding can compete effectively with oxygen for the common intermediate (see Fig. 9). The nature of the anthracycline residue in anthracycline–DNA adducts has not been elucidated (Sinha, 1980). Activated doxorubicin has a greater affinity for DNA than activated daunorubicin and gives adducts with one drug molecule bound per 12–15 nucleotides, compared to one drug molecule per 135 nucleotides with daunorubicin (Sinha, 1980). Studies with synthetic polynucleotides suggest that activated anthracyclines have a high preference for guanine and cytosine regions of DNA. A carbon centered C-7 anthracycline radical has been proposed to be a common intermediate in

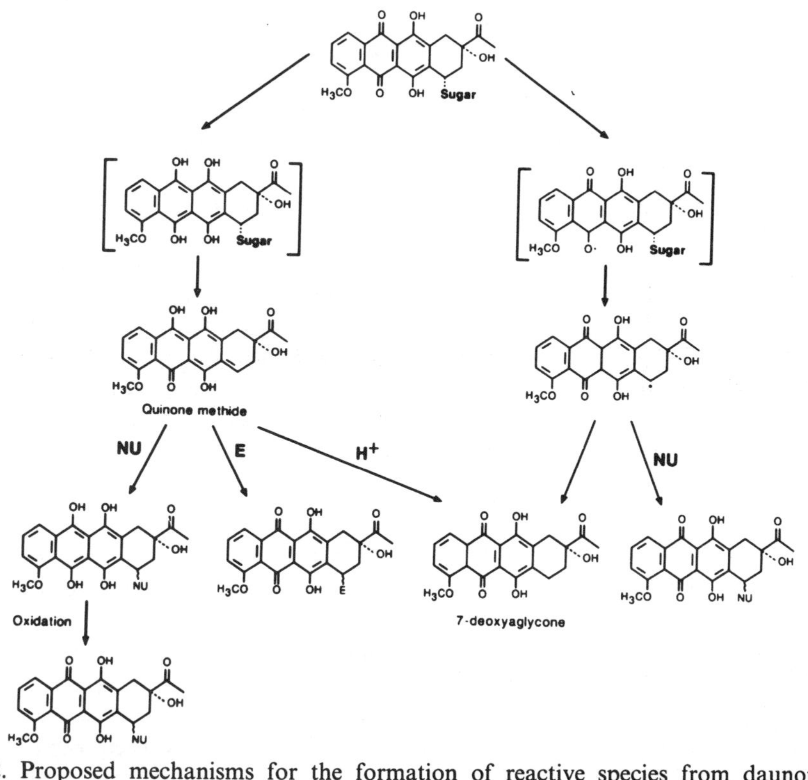

FIG. 12. Proposed mechanisms for the formation of reactive species from daunorubicin through either (on the left) two-electron reduction to the quinonemethide or (on the right) through one-electron reduction to the semiquinone radical. Nu is a nucleophile, E is an electrophile. The nature of the drug adducts has not been elucidated. See text for further explanation.

covalent binding and in reductive cleavage of anthracyclines to deoxyaglycones (Mason, 1979; Sinha, 1980). However, the postulated reactivity of the C-7 anthracycline semiquinone radical enabling it to bind covalently to cellular macromolecules has been questioned on chemical grounds (Abdella and Fisher, 1985).

Moore (1977) originally proposed a mechanism for activation of anthracyclines involving two-electron reduction to the anthracycline hydroquinone. In the process the C-7 sugar group is converted from a stable functional group in the quinone to a stable leaving group in the hydroquinone. Intramolecular loss of the C-7 group gives a quinonemethide intermediate. Koch and colleagues (Kleyer et al., 1984; Kleyer, and Koch, 1983, 1984) have demonstrated that a quinonemethide is formed upon reduction of anthracyclines in organic solvent. Claims have been made that the blue intermediates (V_{max} 540–600 nm) seen on anaerobic reduction of anthracyclines by spinach NADPH:ferredoxin oxidoreductase (E.C.1.6.7.1) in aqueous solution are quinone methides (Fisher et al., 1985). The half-life of the blue intermediate formed from daunorubicin (at pH 8.0 and 30°) is 15 sec and from doxorubicin 23 sec. The intermediate formed from aclacinomycin A has a more rapid decay while no blue intermediates are formed with nogalomycin and menogaril. The putative anthracycline quinonemethide is seen as behaving as a nucleophile or an electrophile to yield a C-7 functionalized hydroquinone. Abdella and Fisher (1985) have pointed out that stable adduct formation via the latter route requires conversion of the hydroquinone adduct to the oxidation level of quinone. This could be accomplished by comproportionation of the bound anthracycline hydroquinone with quinone. All anthracyclines so far studied exhibit nucleophilic character but only 11-deoxydaunorubicin (Ramakrishnan and Fisher, 1983) and aclacinomycin A (Kleyer et al., 1984) have clearly been shown to exhibit both nucleophilic and electrophilic character. It has proved remarkably difficult to demonstrate electrophilic character for daunorubicin and doxorubicin. Ramakrishnan and Fisher (1986) have recently reported electrophilic addition of daunorubicin activated by spinach NADPH:ferredoxin oxidoreductase and NADPH to thiol nucleophiles such as *N*-acetylcysteine, with utilization of substoichiometric amounts of NADPH, thus providing evidence for autocatalytic hydroquinone adduct formation. The quinonemethide may react with a solvent proton acting as an electrophile to form a 7-deoxyaglycone and, in some cases, it may react with itself to form a 7,7′-dimer. The variable and unexpectedly low reactivity of the putative quinonemethide intermediates has led Abdella and Fisher (1985) to suggest that if quinonemethide formation is involved in the biological activity of the anthracyclines the anthracycline must bind to its cellular target prior to reduction which would enforce a common reactivity on all quinonemethides.

Evidence for the enzymatic generation of a C-7 quinonemethide has been sought in the ability of rat liver cytosol and NADPH to covalently link daunorubicin and doxorubicin to DNA under anaerobic conditions, on the presumption that cytosol contains only reductases that catalyze two-electron reduction of quinones (Sinha and Gregory, 1981). Binding with cytosol was found to be almost as great as with a microsomal system and the two-electron activation of anthracycline was ascribed to quinone reductase (Sinha and Gregory, 1981). However, cytosol may contain other enzymes that reduce anthracyclines and most important, dicumarol, an inhibitor of quinone reductase, produced only slight inhibition of covalent binding. Covalent binding of anthracycline due to metabolism by cytosol might involve a free radical mechanism. The slow formation of an ESR detectable anthracycline semiquinone free radical signal has been reported when daunorubicin is incubated with rat liver cytosol and NADPH under anaerobic conditions (Sinha and Gregory, 1981). This could be due to comproportionation of the anthracycline with its hydroquinone formed by two-electron reduction by an enzyme such as quinone reductase, to give an anthracycline semiquinone radical.

3.4.2. *In Vivo Metabolism*

The in vivo pharmacokinetics of anthracyclines is characterized by their rapid and extensive uptake from plasma into tissues followed by slow re-release back into the plasma. Metabolism is an important route for the elimination of most anthracyclines with the exception of doxorubicin and in humans, at least, menogaril. Excretion of anthracyclines and anthracycline metabolites occurs predominantly in the bile with smaller amounts being excreted in urine. The metabolism

TABLE 3. *Pharmacokinetic Parameters of Some Anthracyclines in Human*

Compound	Half-lives $t_{1/2\alpha}$ min	$t_{1/2\beta}$ hr	$t_{1/2\gamma}$ hr	Vd_{dses} L/m²	Cl L/mg/m²	Dose mg/m²	Reference
Doxorubicin	10	—	30.2	1088*	0.51	75	Greene et al., 1983
	—	—	20.0	310*	0.33*	75–85	Robert et al., 1985
	4.6	2.5	70.0	533	—	75	Oosterbaan et al., 1982
	4.4	1.6	40.7	—	0.49*	40	Natale et al., 1983
Daunorubicin	5.4	3.5	14.4	1297	1.8	60	Rahman et al., 1984
	3.4	0.5	16.6	—	0.4	—	Natale et al., 1983
4′-Epidoxorubicin	—	—	18.3	516	0.56	75–100	Robert et al., 1985
	4.8	2.6	38.0	794	—	75–90	Weenan et al., 1983
	3.1	1.2	30.1	—	0.41	—	Natale et al., 1983
	18.0	0.5	15.3	575*	0.71	40–56	Mross et al., 1988
4′Demethoxy-daunorubicin	12.0	—	27.0	2485*	1.19	10	Lu et al., 1986
	9.4	3.8	24.8	—	—	—	Daghestani et al., 1985
	10.0	3.2	34.7	200	0.82	15	Smith et al., 1987
4′-Deoxydoxorubicin	1.3	1.7	90.6	2994	0.44*	10–30	Stanton et al., 1985
	—	—	20.4	—	0.45†	20–40	Dodion et al., 1984c
4-Demethyl-daunorubicin	60.0	8	—	—	—	20	Comis et al., 1982
	—	—	—	—	1.70	7.5–18	Weenen et al., 1984b
	6.6	1.03	20.4	139	—	15	Reich et al., 1981
4′-*O*-tetrahydro-pyronyldoxorubicin	3.1	0.72	16.0	1468	1.55	20	Robert et al., 1988
	1.4	0.30	13.0	2124	1.90	30–70	Miller and Schmidt, 1987
Menogaril	11.4	13.2	—	370	0.47	3–56	Egorin et al., 1986
	3.0	10.5	—	231	0.34	8–140	Grochow et al., 1985
	—	11.9	—	197	0.20	42–126	Long et al., 1985
Aclacinomycin A	2.5	0.33	2.7	998	4.01	60	Malspeis et al., 1981
	6.6	—	13.3	2072	2.51	65	Karanes et al., 1983
Marcellomycin	—	—	19.1	—	1.50	40–50	Dodion et al., 1985d

*Calculated, based on a 1.8 m², 70 kg individual.
†Reported as 45.4 but probably a mistake.

of a number of anthracyclines has been studied in both animals and human. These anthracyclines will be discussed first. Other anthracyclines have not yet received clinical use and their metabolism has been studied only in animals. It is not the intent of this review to deal in depth with the pharmacokinetics of anthracyclines, for which the reader is referred to other excellent reviews (see Riggs and Bachur, 1983; Young et al., 1981). However, a summary of the pharmacokinetic parameters of some of the more clinically important anthracyclines is given in Table 3. The noticeable features of the pharmacokinetic parameters of the anthracyclines is their long terminal half-life and their large volume of distribution, indicating extensive tissue uptake.

3.4.2.1. *Daunorubicin (daunomycin).* Daunorubicin is rapidly cleared from plasma by uptake into tissues in all species so far examined, including mouse, rat, hamster, rabbit, dog and man (Alberts et al., 1971; Huffman et al., 1972; Maniez-Devos et al., 1986a,b; Yesair et al., 1972; Zini et al., 1986). The drug is then slowly excreted, mostly as metabolites, in bile and in smaller amounts in urine. In rats 10–16% of a dose of daunorubicin fluorescence is excreted in the bile within 8 hr of administration and 6–10% in the urine (Cradock et al., 1973; Yesair et al., 1972). Studies with [14-^{14}C]-daunorubicin in rat have shown that 70% of the administered radioactivity is excreted in the feces over 72 hr, 14% in urine while 0.3% is expired as $^{14}CO_2$ (Zini et al., 1986). In rabbit 17% of daunomycin fluorescence is excreted in the bile in 8 hr and 2% in the urine (Bachur et al., 1974). In human 7–17% of daunomycin fluorescence is excreted in the urine in 24 hr (Alberts et al., 1971; Huffman et al., 1972).

The primary metabolite of daunorubicin in all species is daunorubicinol. In rat daunorubicinol accounts for 53% of daunorubicin-derived fluorescent compounds excreted in the bile, unchanged drug for 32% and polar metabolites for a further 13% (Cradock et al., 1973). In rat urine daunorubicinol accounts for 57% of fluorescent compounds, unchanged drug for 40%, aglycones for 1%, with no measurable polar metabolites. Using [^{14}C]-daunorubicin the corresponding values for excretion in bile over 8 hr are 38% as unchanged drug, 34% as daunorubicinol, 23% as polar metabolites, 5% as free aglycones; and in urine over 72 hr 32% as unchanged drug, 64% as daunorubicinol and 4% as aglycone (Zini et al., 1986). Treatment of the polar metabolites from rat bile with β-glucuronidase has been reported to give increased levels of daunorubicin, daunorubicinol and the 7-hydroxy and 7-deoxyaglycones of daunorubicin, suggesting that all are excreted as glucuronide conjugates (Cradock et al., 1973). However, studies with isolated hepatocytes from rat and rabbit have failed to show the formation of glucuronide conjugates of daunorubicin (Gewirtz and Yanovich, 1986a). Glucuronide conjugates, if formed, would be degraded in the gastrointestinal tract and only aglycones of daunorubicin are found in the feces. Indirect evidence for the formation of a glucuronide conjugate of daunorubicinol by murine leukemia P-388 daunorubicin-resistant cells has been reported by Gessner et al. (1990). Dog and rabbit excrete an even greater fraction of metabolites as daunorubicinol than does rat (Bachur et al., 1974; Maniez-Devos et al., 1986b; Yesair et al., 1972). In rabbit Bachur et al. (1973) using TLC found daunorubicinol to account for 84% of daunorubicin-derived fluorescent compounds in bile, unchanged daunorubicin for 1.3%, polar metabolites for 12.4% and aglycones for 0.2%. Maniez-Devos et al. (1986b) using HPLC found daunorubicinol to account for 94% of daunorubicin-derived fluorescent compounds in rabbit bile, daunorubicin for 5%, with only trace amounts of aglycone. There is no significant reabsorption of daunorubicin or its metabolites from the gastro-intestinal tract. Urinary excretion of daunorubicin-derived radioactivity is 13% over 100 hr, 92% as daunorubicinol, 4% as parent drug and the remainder as aglycones. No glucuronide or sulfate conjugates have been found in rabbit bile or urine.

Tissues of animals administered daunorubicin contain substantial quantities of daunorubicinol but aglycone metabolites are found only in liver, kidney and small intestine (Asbell et al., 1972; Bachur et al., 1973, 1974; Zini et al., 1986). The tissues showing greatest retention of radioactivity 72 hr after a dose of [^{14}C]-daunorubicin to rat are bone marrow, thymus, lymph nodes, hypophysis and spleen (Zini et al., 1986).

The major daunorubicin metabolite found in the plasma of patients receiving the drug is daunorubicinol, generally at concentrations higher than those of parent drug (Bolanowska et al., 1983; Huffman et al., 1972). Also found in plasma in smaller amounts are 7-deoxydaunorubicinol and 7-deoxydaunorubicin aglycone. Gessner et al. (1987) have reported higher levels of daunorubicin aglycone metabolites in plasma of patients with acute nonlymphocytic leukemia who did not enter remission than in patients who entered remission, suggesting that resistance to the chemotherapeutic effects of daunorubicin might be related to enhanced metabolism to aglycones. Takanashi and Bachur (1975) have reported a number of fluorescent metabolites of daunorubicin in the 5 day urine of patients receiving daunorubicin. Separation by TLC and comparison to reference compounds showed the presence of daunorubicinol, 7-hydroxydaunorubicinol aglycone, 7-deoxydaunorubicin aglycone, 7-deoxydaunorubicinol aglycone and C-4-*O*-demethyl-7-deoxydaunorubicinol aglycone, while the results of enzymatic hydrolysis with β-glucuronidase and aryl sulfatase were taken to indicate the presence of the conjugates 7-deoxydauno-rubicinol aglycone-13-*O*-β-glucuronide, C-4-*O*-demethyl-7-deoxydaunorubicinol aglycone-4-*O*-β-glucuronide and C-4-*O*-demethyl-7-deoxydaunorubicinol aglycone-4-*O*-sulfate. Other metabolites were purified but not identified. The pathways proposed by Takanashi and Bachur (1975) to explain formation at these metabolites are shown in Fig. 13. While the pathways for the formation of most daunorubicin metabolites are well worked out the formation of daunorubicin glucuronide and sulfate conjugates in vivo have been reported by only one group. Furthermore, the evidence for formation of these daunorubicin conjugates is indirect based on an increase in free anthracyclines after enzymatic

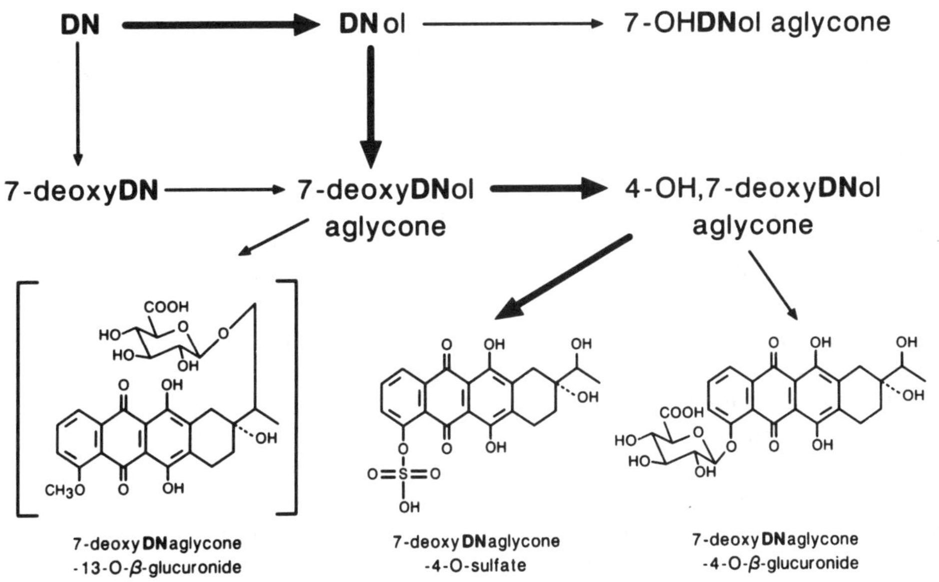

FIG. 13. Proposed pathways for daunorubicin metabolism in man. DN is daunorubicin, DNol is daunorubicinol. Dark arrows indicate major pathways. Adapted from Takanashi and Bachur (1975).

hydrolysis. It would be desirable to have confirmation of these findings using newer analytical techniques to allow unequivocal identification of daunorubicin glucuronide and sulfate conjugates, if they are formed.

3.4.2.2. *Doxorubicin (adriamycin).* Clearance of doxorubicin from plasma and tissues is slower than for daunorubicin, and doxorubicin undergoes less metabolism than daunorubicin (Bachur et al., 1973, 1974; DiFronzo et al., 1971; Hartman et al., 1982; Maniez-Devos et al., 1986b; Mhatre et al., 1972; Oosterbaan et al., 1984; Rosso et al., 1972; Yesair et al., 1972). Approximately 10% of a dose of doxorubicin is excreted as fluorescent compounds in rat bile over 24 hr and 6% in urine (Yesair et al., 1972). In some early studies no evidence could be found for doxorubicin metabolism in rat or mouse (Bachur et al., 1973; DiFronzo et al., 1971; Yesair et al., 1972). However, subsequent studies using improved analytical techniques with fluorescence detection of metabolites have shown low but detectable levels of doxorubicin metabolism. In the rat small amounts of doxorubicinol are formed from doxorubicin by isolated rat hepatocytes (Ballet et al., 1986; Hartman et al., 1982; Gewirtz and Yanovich, 1986a), are excreted in bile and urine, and are found in plasma (Broggini et al., 1980; Hartman et al., 1982; Israel et al., 1978; Shinozawa and Oda, 1981). Hartman et al. (1982) found that 2.5 hr after administration of doxorubicin to rat 8.4% of the dose was excreted as unchanged drug in bile, 0.9% as doxorubicinol, 0.6% as 7-deoxydoxorubicin aglycone and 0.5% as 7-deoxydoxorubicinol aglycone. Conjugated metabolites were not measured in this study. Work with [14-^{14}C]-doxorubicin has also shown unchanged drug to be the major compound excreted in rat bile and urine, with very low levels of doxorubicinol (Arcamone et al., 1984). Unchanged doxorubicin was 10% of the radioactivity excreted in urine over 48 hr, doxorubicinol 1%, polar metabolites 1% and aglycones 0.1%. Interestingly, expired air contained about 5% of the total radioactivity as $^{14}CO_2$ indicating degradation of the C-14 side chain. One-third of the radioactivity administered was excreted in bile in 22 hr, mostly as unchanged drug, with some doxorubicinol but no aglycones. Hydrolysis of bile with β-glucuronidase suggested that there might be low levels of conjugated aglycone metabolites. Studies of the metabolism of doxorubicin by the isolated perfused rat liver has shown it to be a low extraction ratio drug (<0.24). The only metabolites detected were in the perfusate, with doxorubicinol accounting for less than 4% of the total AUC after 3 hr, and doxorubicin aglycones which remained within the liver representing up to 30% of the total fluorescence after 3 hr (Ballet et al., 1987). Despite the fact that up to one-third of the doxorubicin was excreted in the bile, only 1% was excreted as doxorubicinol. In rat isolated hepatocytes the primary intracellular metabolite of doxorubicin is deoxydoxorubicin aglycone with lesser amounts of deoxydoxorubicinol aglycone but very little doxorubicinol (Gewirtz and Yanovich, 1987). Vrignaud et al. (1986) reported very little deoxyaglycones formed by freshly isolated or cultured rat heptocytes.

Other animal species metabolize doxorubicin more extensively than rat but again to a lesser extent than daunorubicin. 7-Deoxydoxorubicinol aglycone is found in serum of tumor-bearing mice within a few minutes of administration of doxorubicin at concentrations greater than those of parent drug, together with smaller amounts of doxorubicinol (Cummings et al., 1986a). 7-Deoxydoxorubicin aglycone and 7-deoxydoxorubicinol aglycone are found in mouse heart and liver, doxorubicinol in liver and tumor. Isolated hepatocytes from rabbit form appreciable amounts of doxorubicinol and 7-deoxydoxorubicinol aglycone but little 7-deoxydoxorubicin aglycone (Gewirtz and Yanovich, 1986a). Rabbits excrete 17% of a dose of doxorubicin fluorescence in bile over 8 hr, 21% over 100 hr; and 2% in urine over 8 hr, 12% over 100 hr (Bachur et al., 1973; Maniez-Devos, 1986b). Studies by Bachur et al. (1973) using TLC and fluorescence to identify metabolites found that 60% of doxorubicin-derived fluorescence in rabbit bile was doxorubicinol, 30% unchanged drug, 7% polar metabolites and the remainder aglycones. Maniez-Devos et al. (1986b) using HPLC found that 71% of the doxorubicin-derived fluorescence was unchanged drug with the rest being doxorubicinol and only traces of aglycone. Bachur et al. (1973) reported that 60% of the fluorescence in rabbit urine was unchanged drug, 35% doxorubicinol and 2% polar metabolites. Maniez-Devos et al. (1986b) reported that 67% of the urinary fluorescence was unchanged drug, 32% doxorubicinol and 1% aglycones. No glucuronide or sulfate conjugates of doxorubicin were found in rabbit bile or urine (Maniez-Devos et al., 1986b). Doxorubicinol is the major metabolite of doxorubicin found in rabbit plasma and occurs at concentrations not exceeding more than one-third those of parent drug (Johansen et al., 1984; Maniez-Devos et al., 1986b).

Doxorubicinol is the major metabolite of doxorubicin found in human plasma and is present at concentrations well below those of parent drug (Andrews et al., 1980; Pierce and Jatlow, 1979; Bolanowska et al., 1983; Gill et al., 1983). There are low levels of other doxorubicin metabolites in human plasma including 7-hydroxydoxorubicin aglycone, 7-deoxydoxorubicin aglycone and 7-deoxydoxorubicinol aglycone (Brenner et al., 1985; Cummings, 1985; Cummings and McArdle, 1986; Cummings et al., 1986b), as well as other unidentified nonpolar metabolites (Brenner et al., 1985), with marked inter-patient variability (Cummings et al., 1986a). 7-Deoxydoxorubicin aglycone and 7-deoxydoxorubicinol aglycone have been found in resected normal liver of patients administered a sub-therapeutic dose of doxorubicin 30 min previously (Cummings and McArdle, 1986). No doxorubicin metabolites could be detected in tumor tissue or normal intestinal mucosa. Biliary excretion of doxorubicin in human is 50% of the dose over 5 days and urinary excretion 10% of the dose (Benjamin et al., 1973, 1974). Takanishi and Bachur (1976) have reported a qualitatively similar pattern of doxorubicin metabolites in human urine as for daunorubicin. This was except for the absence of a 7-deoxydoxorubicinol aglycone 13-*O*-β-glucuronide and the presence of 7-hydroxydoxorubicin aglycones. The formation of 7-hydroxyaglycones was considered to be an artifact due to the chemical breakdown of the parent glycosides. While with daunorubicin the amount of the 4-*O*-sulfated conjugate of C-4-*O*-demethyl-7-deoxydaunorubicinol aglycone exceeded 4-*O*-glucuronide conjugate nearly 2-fold, with C-4-*O*-demethyl-7-deoxydoxorubicinol aglycone almost equal amounts of 4-*O*-glucuronide and 4-*O*-sulfate conjugates were found (Takanashi and Bachur, 1976). In contrast to the report of Takanashi and Bachur (1976), where β-glucuronidase hydrolysis was used to identify glucuronide conjugates, a study by Cassinelli et al. (1984) using improved extraction procedures for glucuronides has found no evidence for glucuronide conjugates of doxorubicin or doxorubicinol in urine of patients receiving the drug. Furthermore, no evidence could be found for formation of doxorubicin glucuronides by isolated human hepatocytes (Ballet et al., 1986). The formation of glucuronide conjugates of doxorubicin, if it occurs at all, appears to be a very minor pathway of metabolism in human.

3.4.2.3. *4′-Epidoxorubicin (epirubicin).* 4′-Epidoxorubicin is a second generation anthracycline which has activity against anthracycline responsive and resistant tumors in animals equivalent to that of doxorubicin, but is less cardiotoxic than doxorubicin (Arcamone et al., 1984). Clinical studies have shown that 4′-epidoxorubicin is active against a number of tumor types, perhaps having a greater spectrum of activity than doxorubicin, and have confirmed that 4′-epidoxorubicin is less cardiotoxic than doxorubicin (Cersosimo and Hong, 1986).

Studies using [^{14}C]-4′-epidoxorubicin in rat have shown a similar pattern of metabolism to doxorubicin, except that bile contains less unchanged 4′-epidoxorubicin and large amounts of 4′-epidoxorubicin glucuronide (Arcamone et al., 1984). Very little, if any, 4′-epidoxorubicin glucuronide was detected in the plasma of a number of animal species given epidoxorubicin, but large species variation in the formation of epidoxorubicinol and 7-deoxydoxorubicinol aglycone was observed (Maessen et al., 1987). 4′-Epidoxorubicin administered as an i.v. bolus or 24 hr infusion to rats is primarily excreted in the bile with 40–50% of the dose being eliminated in 55 hr, and less than 5% of the dose excreted in the urine in 60 hr (Sweatman and Israel, 1987). Studies in patients receiving 4′-epidoxorubicin have shown the formation of 4-*O*-demethyl-4′-epidoxorubicinol, 7-deoxydoxorubicin aglycone, 7-hydroxydoxorubicin aglycone, 7-deoxydoxorubicinol aglycone, as well as 4′-epidoxorubicin glucuronide conjugates (Camaggi et al., 1986, 1988; Cassinelli et al., 1984; Deesen and Leyland-Jones, 1984; Robert et al., 1985; Speth et al., 1986a; Speyer et al., 1982; Vrignaud et al., 1985; Weenen et al., 1983, 1984a; Mross et al., 1988). Human hepatocytes incubated with 4′-epidoxorubicin form 4′-epidoxorubicin glucuronide as the major metabolite with smaller amounts of 4′-epidoxorubicinol and 4′-epidoxorubicinol glucuronide (Ballet et al., 1986). Rat hepatocytes did not form glucuronide conjugates of 4-epidoxorubicin (LeBot et al., 1988). 4′-Epidoxorubicin glucuronide is the major metabolite of 4′-epidoxorubicin in plasma of patients receiving the drug with an area under the plasma concentration–time curve (AUC) almost equal to that of 4′-epidoxorubicin (Robert et al., 1985; Vrignaud et al., 1985). Attachment of the glucuronide group in 4′-epidoxorubicin glucuronide has been shown by Cassinelli et al. (1984) to be at the C-4′-hydroxyl of daunosamine, which in 4′-epidoxorubicin is in an equatorial orientation. Steric hindrance of the axial C-4′-hydroxyl of doxorubicin by the adjacent *cis* equatorial 3′-amino group may explain the lack of glucuronide formation by doxorubicin compared to 4′-epidoxorobucin (Cassinelli et al., 1984). In human urine collected up to 48 hr after administration of 4′-epidoxorubicin unchanged drug accounts for approximately 6% of the dose (Casinelli et al., 1984; Vrignaud et al., 1985; Weenen et al., 1983, 1984b). Of the total 4′-epidoxorubicin-derived fluorescence in urine 57% is 4′-epidoxorubicin, 32% 4′-*O*-(β-D-glucuronyl)-4′-epidoxorubicin, 7% 4′-epidoxorubicinol and 3% 4′-*O*-(β-D-glucuronyl)-4′-epidoxorobucinol (Cassinelli et al., 1984). Biliary excretion of 4′-epidoxorubicin in patients with percutaneous biliary drainage is 22% of the dose over 96 hr, 4′-epidoxorubicinol 6%, 4′-*O*-(β-D-glucuronyl)-4′-epidoxorubicin 5% and 4′-O-(β-D-glucuronyl)-4′-epidoxorubicinol 2% (Camaggi et al., 1986). Sulfate conjugates of 4′-epidoxorubicin have not been detected (Deesen and Leyland-Jones, 1984). It has been suggested that glucuronidation may enhance the rate of elimination of 4′-epidoxorubicin compared to doxorubicin (Weenen et al., 1984b) and may be related to a lower incidence of toxic side effects seen with 4′-epidoxorubicin (Arcamone, 1985). Considerable interpatient variability in the formation of 4-epidoxorubicin glucuronide was reported by Robert et al. (1988). Low glucuronidation was associated with hepatic dysfunction and a better response to the treatment.

3.4.2.4. *4-Demethoxydaunorubicin (idarubicin).* 4-Demethoxydaunorubicin is a completely synthetic analog of daunorubicin possessing antitumor activity in animals superior to that of daunorubicin, and reduced cardiotoxicity (Ganzina et al., 1986). 4-Demethoxydaunorubicin is a more potent antitumor agent than doxorubicin or daunorubicin and, an advantage over both these agents, is active when administered orally. Clinical studies have shown that 4-demethoxydaunorubicin is a potent antileukemic agent and has low cardiotoxicity (Villani et al., 1989). It has activity against breast cancer (Ganzina et al., 1986). 4-Demethoxydaunorubicin is more slowly eliminated from plasma and tissues of tumored mice than daunorubicin and has a plasma half-life of 23 hr (Broggini et al., 1984; Formelli et al., 1979). 4-Demethoxydaunorubicin is metabolized in mice and rabbit to 4-demethoxydaunorubicinol which appears in the plasma and in tumors at concentrations approximately 20% those of parent drug (Broggini et al., 1984, 1986). The disposition and metabolism of [^{14}C]-4-demethoxydaunorubicin has been studied in rat by Zini et al. (1986). More than 80% of the radioactivity was found in the feces over 72 hr after intravenous administration indicating extensive biliary excretion. Only 16% of the radioactivity was found in urine over the same period. Seven percent of the radioactivity excreted in the bile over 8 hr was unchanged drug, 11% 4-demethoxy-daunorubicinol, 77% polar metabolites, at least one of which appeared to be a glucuronide or sulfate conjugate of 7-deoxy-4-demethoxydaunorubicinol, and 5% free aglycones. More than 60% of the total radioactivity excreted in urine over 72 hr was 4-demethoxydaunorubicin, 20% 4-demethoxydaunorubicin, 18% polar metabolites, a small fraction of which was aglycone glucuronide or sulfate conjugates, and approximately 2% free aglycones. After oral administration of 4-demethoxydaunorubicin there was a large increase in the relative proportion of polar metabolites in the urine. Tissues contained predominantly 4-demethoxydaunorubicinol 72 hr after intravenous drug administration with small amounts of aglycones in the liver and kidney. The highest total radioactivity was found in the bone marrow lymph nodes, thymus, spleen, kidney and liver.

Studies in patients receiving 4-demethoxydaunorubicin by either the intravenous or oral routes have shown extensive formation of 4-demethoxydauno-rubicinol with a prolonged retention in plasma at concentrations greater than those of parent drug (Arcamone, 1985; Berman et al., 1983; Daghestani et al., 1985; Kaplan et al., 1984; Lu et al., 1986; Tan et al., 1987; Moro et al., 1983; Pannuti et al., 1986). The terminal half-life of 4-demethoxydaunorubicin in plasma is 15–24 hr and 4-demethoxydaunorubicinol 40–72 hr (Daghestani et al., 1985; Kaplan et al., 1984; Lu et al., 1986; Pannuti et al., 1986; Robert et al., 1986; Speth et al., 1986b). Lu et al. (1986) reported that 5% of an intravenous of 4-demethoxydaunorubicin is excreted as unchanged drug in urine over 24 hr and 8% as 4-demethoxydaunorubicinol. Biliary excretion of 4-demethoxydaunorubicin studied in patients with percutaneous biliary drainage has shown that only 4% of the administered dose is excreted as 4-demethoxydoxorubicin and 4-demethoxydoxo-rubicinol over 7 days (Kaplan et al., 1984). Urinary excretion of 4-demethoxydaunorubicin in these patients was 0.5% of an oral dose over 72 hr with 4% as 4-demethoxydaunorubicinol. 4-Demethoxydaunorubicin is converted at a rate of 3% per hr to its aglycone when subjected to acid conditions likely to be found in the stomach after oral administration (Cummings and Milroy, 1986).

3.4.2.5. *4′-Deoxydoxorubicin (esorubicin).* 4′-Deoxydoxorubicin is a semisynthetic daunorubicin analog with a high and apparently broad spectrum of activity against animal tumors combined with a low cardiotoxicity (Arcamone, 1984). 4′-Deoxydoxorubicin is undergoing clinical evaluation. Mouse studies have shown that 4′-deoxydoxorubicin is eliminated more rapidly from tissues than doxorubicin (Formelli et al., 1981). The mouse metabolizes 4′-deoxydoxorubicin to 7-hydroxydoxorubicinol aglycone and 7-deoxydoxorubicinol aglycone which is found in plasma and the tissues (Fumagalli et al., 1985). Mouse urine contains 15% of an administered dose of 4′-deoxydoxorubicin as unchanged drug over 2 days, 1.7% as 4′-deoxydoxorubicinol and no detectable aglycones. In patients receiving 4′-deoxydoxorubicin the drug is metabolized to 4′-deoxydoxorubicinol which is present in plasma at levels well below those of parent drug (Cummings, 1985; Dodion et al., 1984d, 1985a; Stanton et al., 1985), together with small amounts of 7-deoxydoxorubicin aglycone (Cummings, 1985) and 7-deoxydoxorubicinol aglycone (Stanton et al., 1985). Biliary excretion of 4′-deoxydoxorubicin and the metabolites has been studied in a single patient where excretion of unchanged 4′-deoxydoxorubicin over 5 days was 8% of the administered dose and 4′-deoxydoxorubicinol 14% (Stanton et al., 1985). Urinary excretion of 4′-deoxydoxorubicin and 4′-deoxydoxorubicinol in human is low (Dodion et al., 1985a; Stanton et al., 1985). Approximately 5.9% of a dose is excreted as unchanged drug in urine over 2 days and 1.4% as 4′-deoxydoxorubicinol (Dodion et al., 1985a).

3.4.2.6. *4-Demethyldaunorubicin (carminomycin).* 4-Demethyldaunorubicin is a naturally occurring anthracycline antibiotic initially isolated from *Actinomadura carminata* in the U.S.S.R. (Gause et al., 1975). It has antitumor activity against a number of animal tumors following both i.v. and oral administration, and is less cardiotoxic than doxorubicin (Crooke, 1977). Clinical trials of 4-demethyldaunorubicin have been conducted in the U.S.S.R., Europe and the U.S.A. Antitumor activity similar to that doxorubicin has been reported against a variety of tumors (Comis, et al., 1982; Crooke, 1977). The dose-limiting toxicity of 4-demethyldaunorubicin is leukopenia and nonspecific cardiac abnormalities have been seen in some patients.

4-Demethyldaunorubicin slowly eliminated from plasma with a half-life in dog of 86 hr (Reich et al., 1981) and in patients of 6–20 hr (Comis et al., 1982; Reich et al., 1981; Weenen et al., 1984b). 4-Demethyldaunorubicin is rapidly metabolized to 4-demethyldaunorubicinol which can be detected in plasma within 5 min of administration and is slowly eliminated with a half-life of over 50 hr (Comis et al., 1982; Reich et al., 1981; Weenen et al., 1984b). Less than 2% of a dose of 4-demethyldaunorubicin is excreted in urine over 48 hr as unchanged drug and 6% as 4-demethyldaunorubicinol (Comis et al., 1982).

3.4.2.7. *Menogaril.* Menogaril is a semisynthetic analog of the anthracycline antibiotic nogalomycin. Menogaril is unusual in not having a C-7 carbohydrate group but instead has a glucopyranose group attached to the anthracycline D ring (Fig. 5). Animal studies suggest that menogaril is less cardiotoxic than doxorubicin (McGovern et al., 1979). Early clinical trials have shown the dose-limiting toxicity of menogaril administered as an intermittent intravenous bolus to be myelosuppression (Brown et al., 1985) and venous irritation when administered by continuous infusion (Long et al., 1985).

Animal studies have shown that menogaril is extensively metabolized or taken up by tissues. First pass elimination of orally administered menogaril by the liver and/or intestine of mouse reduces its bioavailability to 30% of an i.v. administered dose (Pratt et al., 1982). Two fluorescent metabolites of menogaril have been seen in mouse plasma (Dodion et al., 1984c; Pratt et al., 1982) and three fluorescent metabolites in dog plasma (Pratt and Adams, 1983) following i.v. administration of the drug. In both species one of the metabolites has been found to have an HPLC retention time identical to that of *N*-demethylmenogaril and to be present at concentration approximately one-tenth those of parent drug. Tissue distribution studies in the mouse have shown that there is extensive uptake of menogaril by lung and all other tissues except brain (Dodion et al., 1984c). An unidentified metabolite was present in all tissue except brain. In the liver this metabolite accounted for more than 80% of all fluorescent compounds between 4 and 16 hr after administration of the drug. The rabbit metabolizes menogaril more slowly than mouse and fluorescent metabolites have not been detected in rabbit plasma following intravenous administration of menogaril (Dodion et al., 1985d). Urinary excretion of menogaril and its metabolites in rabbit is less than 2% of the dose over 8 hr and biliary excretion less than 4%. Four fluorescent metabolites have been found in rabbit urine and six in bile. One of these metabolites is *N*-demethylmenogaril while in bile two other metabolites have been tentatively identified as 7-deoxynogarol and *N*-demethyl-7-deoxynogarol formed by the reductive cleavage of the C-7 methoxy group. In rabbit liver, small intestine and kidney the predominant metabolite is 7-deoxynogarol with smaller amounts of *N*-demethylmenogaril in liver and kidney (Dodion et al., 1985c).

Menogaril is only slowly metabolized in human. Only one metabolite, *N*-demethylmenogaril has been identified in plasma and urine (Dodion et al., 1986c; Egorin et al., 1986; Grochow et al., 1985; Zanette et al., 1986). Urinary excretion of menogaril administered by continuous infusion over 72 hr is 17.3% as parent drug and 0.5% as *N*-demethylmenogaril (Egorin et al., 1986; Long et al., 1985). Small amounts of a more polar metabolite have been seen in urine of some patients (Long et al., 1985) but glucuronide or sulfate conjugates of menogaril have not been found (Zanette et al., 1986). Studies of biliary excretion of menogaril in patients with bile tract drains have shown 2–4% of the daily dose of menogaril to be excreted in bile, initially as unchanged menogaril but by 24 hr approximately 40% of bile drug fluorescence is *N*-demethylmenogaril (Egorin et al., 1986). Menogaril elimination appears to be unaltered in patients with hepatic dysfunction (Van Echo et al., 1986). *N*-Demethylmenogaril has a decreased antitumor activity and greater potency than menogaril (Pratt et al., 1982), however, the low rate of menogaril metabolism in humans makes it unlikely that *N*-demethylation makes a significant contribution toward the antitumor activity of menogaril.

3.4.2.8. *Aclacinomycin A.* C-4‴ keto-reduced metabolites of aclacinomycin A with a terminal L-amicetase or a L-rhodinase residue have been found as the major metabolites in plasma of rabbit and dog administered aclacinomycin, with smaller amounts of the aglycone metabolites 7-deoxyaklavinone, bisanhydroaklavinone and the 7,7′-dimer of 7-deoxyaklavinone (Kitamura et al.,

1978; Ogasawara et al., 1981). Bisanhydroaklavinone, 7-deoxyaklavinone and the 7,7′-dimer of 7-deoxyaklavinone, are found in liver and kidney of mice administered the drug (Dodion et al., 1985c). Plasma of patients receiving aclacinomycin A has been shown to contain, in addition to parent drug, the more slowly eliminated L-amicetose glycoside metabolite (Ando et al., 1986; Oki et al., 1981; Smith et al., 1983), bisanhydroaklavinone (Egorin et al., 1982; Smith et al., 1983) and an unidentified metabolite (Egorin et al., 1982). Urinary excretion of unchanged aclacinomycin A in human is 0.6% of the dose over 24 hr and 4% as glycoside metabolites (Oki et al., 1981). Egorin et al. (1983) analyzed the urine of patients given aclacinomycin A and found 11 metabolites, including the metabolites identified in vitro by Oki et al. (1977) and Komiyama et al. (1979a,b) (Fig. 7). An additional metabolite was identified as bisanhydroaklavinic acid, probably resulting from hydrolysis of the methyl ester of bisanhydroaklavinone, while another metabolite was converted to bisanhydroaklavinic acid by incubation β-glucuronidase, suggesting it to be a glucuronide conjugate. The previously unidentified plasma metabolite was shown to be identical with the urinary metabolite identified as bisanhydroaklavinic acid.

3.4.2.9. *Marcellomycin.* Marcellomycin is metabolized by mouse to 4 fluorescent metabolites in plasma. Dodion et al. (1984a) assigned structures to these metabolites as musettamycin, pyrromycin, 7-hydroxypyrromycin aglycone and 7-deoxypyrromycin aglycone. A contaminant present with the parent drug, possibly with a rhodinose sugar replacing the terminal deoxyfucose of marcellomycin, was also present in plasma. In liver an aglycone tentatively identified as 7-deoxypyrromycin aglycone was observed, initially at concentrations equal to those of parent drug but falling rapidly to be undetectable by 8 hr. In other organs 7-deoxypyrromycin aglycone was observed in smaller quantities. In human marcellomycin undergoes metabolism to an aglycone, probably bisanhydropyrromycinone, and a conjugate, both of which are found in plasma. The conjugate resists hydrolysis by arylsulfatase and β-glucuronidase but is converted by acid hydrolysis to marcellomycin. Seven to 8% of a dose of marcellomycin is excreted in the urine over 72 hr in human with parent drug being the predominant component at a high dose, and bisanhydropyrromycinone the predominant component at a lower dose (Dodion et al., 1985d).

3.4.2.10. *4′-O-Tetrahydropyranyldoxorubicin (pirarubicin).* 4′-*O*-Tetrahydropyranyldoxorubicin is an epimeric doxorubicin analog with a tetrahydropyranyl moiety attached to the 4′ position of the daunosamine sugar. It has activity superior to doxorubicin against murine leukemia L1210 and is less cardiotoxic than doxorubicin in animals (Umezawa et al., 1979). Clinical studies have shown 4′-O-tetrahydropyranyldoxorubicin to have activity against hematologic and solid tumors, with leukopenia to be the dose-limiting toxicity (Majima, 1986; Ogawa et al., 1986). Some cardiac abnormalities have been seen in patients given 4′-*O*-tetrahydropyranyldoxorubicin. Metabolites found in plasma, tissues and bile of mice following administration of 4′-*O*-tetrahydro-pyranyldoxorubicin are doxorubicin, doxorubicinol, 7-deoxydoxorubicinol aglycone and 7-deoxydoxorubicin aglycone (Iguchi et al., 1985; Fujita et al., 1986). Urinary excretion of 4′-*O*-tetrahydropyranyldoxorubicin and metabolites in mouse is less than 1.2% of the administered dose. Biliary excretion of 4′-*O*-tetrahydropyranyldoxorubicin in patients is 20% of a dose over 48 hr, mostly as metabolites, and urinary excretion 6% (Majima, 1986; Robert et al., 1988). The main metabolites in plasma are doxorubicin which can exceed the concentrations of parent drug, and low concentrations of 4-*O*-tetrahydropyranyl-doxorubicinol and doxorubicinol (Robert et al., 1988; Miller and Schmidt, 1987).

3.4.2.11. *N,N-Disubstituted anthracyclines.* The amino group of daunosamine is important for binding of anthracyclines to DNA and a number of *N,N*-alkyl and aryl disubstituted anthracycline analogs have been synthesized in an attempt to alter this binding. *N,N*-Dimethyl and *N,N*-dibenzyl substituted anthracycline analogs have been found to have greater antitumor efficacy and less cardiotoxicity in animal models than the parent compounds (Acton, 1980).

The metabolism and disposition of *N,N*-dimethyldaunorubicin and *N,N*-dimethyldoxorubicin have been studied in mouse and rabbit by Egorin et al. (1980). Both compounds show increased persistence of tissue fluorescence *N*-benzyldaunorubicin and *N*-benzyldaunorubicinol. Daunorubicin can be detected in the liver and lung. Liver is the only tissue to contain appreciable levels of aglycone metabolites, principally 7-hydroxydaunorubicin aglycone, 7-deoxydaunorubicin aglycone and 7-deoxydaunorubicinol aglycone. *N,N*-Dibenzyldaunorubicin is nearly inactive as a cytotoxic agent in in vitro test systems but has high antitumor efficacy and low potency in vivo (Peters et al., 1983). This can be explained by *N,N*-dibenzyldaunorubicin acting as a prodrug with conversion in vivo to active glycosidic metabolites.

3.4.2.12. *4-Demethoxy-4′-O-methyldoxorubicin.* 4-Demethoxy-4′-*O*-methyldoxorubicin was synthesized to exploit the known high potency and low cardiotoxicity of 4-demethoxy analogs of daunorubicin and doxorubicin. The compound has marked activity against disseminated murine leukemia L1210 compared to doxorubicin and is active after oral administration (Arcamone, 1984). 4-Demethoxy-4′-*O*-methyldoxorubicin is eliminated from plasma of tumor bearing mice at a rate slightly faster than doxorubicin. It is converted to a polar metabolite, presumed to be 4-demethoxydoxorubicin, by demethylation at position 4′ of the amino sugar (Formelli et al., 1986a). The amount of tissue fluorescence due to the metabolite ranges from 25% in the tumor to 50% in the liver.

3.4.2.13. *5-Iminodaunorubicin.* Introduction of an imino group in place of the C-5 carbonyl of daunorubicin yields 5-iminodaunorubicin, a quinoneimine that undergoes reduction with considerable difficulty compared to other anthracyclines (Davies et al., 1983; Doroshow and Davies, 1983; Lown et al., 1979; Scheulen, 1985). The compound is remarkably active against murine leukemia P-388, although an order of magnitude less potent than daunorubicin, and is less cardiotoxic than daunorubicin (Arcamone, 1984) compared to the parent anthracyclines. Following administration of *N,N*-dimethyldaunorubicin to rabbit or mouse kidney, lung, spleen and liver show the highest maintained levels of fluorescence due, in large part, to a metabolite presumed to be *N*-methyldaunorubicinol. Small amounts of aglycone metabolites including 7-deoxydaunorubicinol aglycone are found in the liver and kidney. Biliary excretion of *N,N*-dimethyldaunorubicin-derived fluorescence in rabbit is 4% of the dose over 8 hr consisting exclusively of metabolites. Initially, the major metabolite is *N*-methyldaunorubicinol with the later appearance of three unidentified polar metabolites. Significantly, no daunorubicin or daunorubicinol have been found suggesting that complete *N*-demethylation of the daunosamine sugar does not occur. *N,N*-Dimethyldoxorubicin persists even longer in tissues than *N,N*-dimethyldaunorubicin and shows only minor metabolism. Biliary excretion of *N,N*-dimethyldaunorubicin-derived fluorescence over 8 hr in rabbit is 5% of the dose, mostly as *N,N*-dimethyldoxorubicinol. There is very little urinary excretion of *N,N*-dimethyldoxorubicin-derived fluorescence. Unlike *N,N*-dimethyldaunorubicin, *N,N*-dimethyldoxorubicin does not undergo *N*-demethylation.

Metabolism of 5-iminodaunorubicin has been studied in rat (Peters et al., 1984). The major metabolite in plasma is 5-iminodaunorubicinol which achieves concentrations similar to those of the parent drug. Significant amounts of an unidentified fluorescent metabolite were found in plasma after intravenous but not after intraperitoneal or oral administration of 5-iminodaunorubicin. Small amounts of 5-imino-7-hydroxydaunorubicin aglycone and 5-imino-7-hydroxydaunorubicin aglycone are found in plasma, stomach and liver. The major fluorescent compound in tissues is 5-iminodaunorubicinol. The failure to detect significant levels of 7-deoxyaglycone metabolites is consistent with in vitro findings that 5-iminodaunorubicin is a poor substrate for NADPH-cytochrome P-450 reductase and does not undergo C-7 reductive cleavage (Scheulen, 1985). The failure to detect daunorubicin shows also that 5-iminodaunorubicin is not a prodrug of daunorubicin.

3.4.2.14. *AD-32.* AD-32 is *N*-trifluoroacetyl-doxorubicin-14-valerate. It is relatively insoluble in water and does not intercalate with DNA. AD-32 is less cardiotoxic in animals than doxorubicin (Henderson et al., 1978). Metabolism of AD-32 has been studied in animals only. The drug is extensively excreted in the bile in the rat with 80% of the administered dose appearing in the bile over 24 hr and 2% in urine (Israel et al., 1978). AD-32 undergoes rapid deesterification of the C-14 side chain to *N*-trifluoroacetyldoxorubicin by nonspecific esterases in rat serum (Israel et al., 1976). Approximately 18–22% of a dose is excreted in bile as *N*-trifluorouroacetyldoxorubicin and 18–23% as *N*-trifluoroacetyldoxorubicinol (Israel et al., 1976, 1981). Glucuronide conjugates form the major fraction of biliary metabolites with about 20% as unidentified polar metabolites. Only small amounts of aglycone metabolites have been detected (Israel et al., 1976, 1981) although studies in rat with AD-32 labelled with ^{14}C at the carbonyl carbon on the *N*-trifluoroacetyl group have shown relatively large amounts of nonfluorescent radioactive metabolites in plasma and tissues, thought to be *N*-trifluoroacetyldaunosamine. This would suggest extensive C-7 reductive cleavage of AD-32. In rats given AD-32 only a small amount of doxorubicin, less than 0.2% of the total dose, has been detected in urine (Israel et al., 1978) and tissue extracts (Zini et al., 1984). AD-32 is not considered a prodrug of doxorubicin.

3.4.2.15. *AD-143.* AD-143 is *N*-trifluoroacetyldoxorubicin-14-*O*-hemiadipate. It was synthesized as a more water soluble analog of AD-32. Metabolism of AD-143 has been studied in the rat by Israel and Sweatman (1983). Bile contains 17% of an administered dose of AD-143 as unchanged drug over 60 hr, 20% as *N*-trifluoroacetyldoxorubicin, 2% as doxorubicin, together with small amounts of *N*-trifluoroacetyldoxorubicinol and an unidentified fluorescent metabolite. No aglycone metabolites of AD-143 have been detected in bile. Urinary excretion of AD-143 and metabolites is very low, with only 0.3% of the administered dose being excreted over 36 hr, mostly as *N*-trifluoroacetyldoxorubicin and *N*-trifluoroacetyldoxorubicinol.

3.4.2.16. *Doxorubicin octanoylhydrazone.* Doxorubicin octanoylhydrazone is reported to be less cardiotoxic in animals than doxorubicin. Metabolism of doxorubicin octanoylhydrazone has been studied in mice and rabbits by Egorin et al. (1981). Following administration of doxorubicin octanoylhydrazone to mice the liver and and kidney were found to contain relatively large amounts of doxorubicin, equal to or greater than the amount of parent drug, together with small amounts of 7-hydroxydoxorubicin aglycone and 7-deoxydoxorubicin aglycone. The major pathway for metabolism of doxorubicin and octanoylhydrazone is hydrolysis to doxorubicin which, in rabbit contributes 10–15% of the total fluorescence in plasma, with 1–5% as doxorubicinol and less than 1% as aglycone. There is no detectable urinary excretion of doxorubicin octanoylhydrazone-derived fluorescence. Biliary excretion of doxorubicin octanoylhydrazone-derived fluorescence in rabbit is 25% of the dose over 8 hr the majority as unchanged drug, with small amounts of doxorubicin, doxorubicinol and about 1% as aglycones.

3.4.2.17. *4′-Deoxy-4′-iododoxorubicin.* 4′-Deoxy-4-iododoxorubicin is a lipophilic doxorubicin analogue with activity against a variety of experimental tumors following both oral and intravenous administration, and is less cardiotoxic than doxorubicin in mice (Barbieri et al., 1987). Studies in mice have shown that 4′-deoxy-4-iododoxorubicin is eliminated from plasma more rapidly than doxorubicin with a terminal half-life of 5 hr (Formelli et al., 1986b, 1987). Ten metabolites of 4′-deoxy-4-iododoxorubicin have been detected in liver, the major metabolite being 4′-deoxy-4-iododoxorubicinol (Giuliani et al., 1986).

3.4.2.18. *AD-198.* (*N*-benzyldoxorubicin-14-valerate) is a prodrug form of *N*-benzyldoxorubicin. Administration of AD-198 to rat results in plasma *N*-benzyldoxorubicin concentrations in excess of parent drug at all times from 2.5 min to 24 hr (Israel et al., 1986). Other metabolites in plasma and liver have been tentatively identified as 4-*O*-demethyl-*N*-benzyldoxorubicin, 4-*O*-demethyl-*N*-benzyldoxorubicinol, and in liver *N*-benzyldoxorubicinol and its aglycones. Little or no doxorubicin is seen in liver or plasma. The metabolism of *N,N*-dibenzyldaunorubicin has been studied in rat by Peters et al. (1983). Sequential debenzylation of *N,N*-dibenzyldaunorubicin to *N*-benzyldaunorubicinol and daunorubicin is accompanied by the usual pattern of anthracycline C-13 keto reduction and C-7 hydrolytic and reductive cleavage. Plasma and tissues contain appreciable quantities of parent drug together with *N,N*-dibenzyldaunorubicinol.

3.4.3. *Metabolism by Tumor Cells*

Anthracyclines are cytotoxic to cultured tumor cells in vitro at therapeutically achievable concentrations. It is, therefore, of interest to investigate anthracycline metabolism by tumor and other cells to see if cytotoxicity might be modified by metabolism. Some studies have found very low or undetectable levels of anthracycline metabolism by normal and tumor cells (DeGregorio et al., 1984; Skovsgaard, 1977; Yesair et al., 1980; Zenebergh et al., 1984) while other studies have reported variable but measurable levels of anthracycline metabolism. There is between 5 and 30% conversion of daunorubicin to daunorubicinol after 4–24 hr incubation with Ehrlich ascites cells (Londos-Gagliardi et al., 1982), murine leukemia L1210 cells (Baurain et al., 1980; Yesair et al., 1980), human HeLa cervix carcinoma, LoVo and HT-29 colon carcinoma cells (Geroni et al., 1986), human promyelocytic HL-60 cells and leukemic cells from patients with acute nonlymphocytic leukemia (DeGregorio et al., 1982). Aglycones, when formed, account for 1% or less of intracellular anthracyclines (Baurain et al., 1980). However, nodules of A549 human lung adenocarcinoma cells metabolize doxorubicin efficiently to both doxorubicinol and aglycone derivative (Chevillard et al., 1990). After 24 hr incubation doxorubicinol accounts for 18% and the aglycone for 27% of the intracellular anthracycline. Aglycone formation may be enhanced because of relatively hypoxic conditions within the nodule compared to cells in monolayer culture. It has been claimed that the cytotoxicity of daunorubicin to human myeloid leukemic cells is lower in cell lines that do not metabolize daunorubicin to daunorubicinol (Ahmed, 1985). This led to the suggestion that intracellular production of the less lipophilic and, it was assumed, better retained daunorubicinol favors cell killing. No difference in daunorubicinol formation has been found between daunorubicin resistant and sensitive cell lines (Baurain et al., 1980). Doxorubicin is poorly metabolized by tumor cell lines and doxorubicin analogs are less well metabolized than corresponding daunorubicin analogs (Geroni et al., 1986). No consistent pattern has emerged of the levels of daunorubicin reductases in a number of murine and human tumor cell lines (Vasanthakumar and Ahmed, 1985). Claims have been made for a positive correlation between daunorubicin reductase in leukemic myeloblasts and the response of the patients of chemotherapy (Gola, 1979; Huffman and Bachur, 1972), and it has been suggested that levels of daunorubicin and its metabolites in leukemic cells may be of more relevance in evaluating clinical outcome than monitoring plasma levels of drug (DeGregorio et al., 1982). Such suggestions are intriguing but need further evaluation before their worth can be judged. The weight of available evidence suggests that cellular metabolism of anthracyclines to C-13 alcohols is not a major factor in determining cytotoxicity.

3.4.4. *Influence of Other Drugs on Anthracycline Metabolism*

The numerous pathways of anthracycline metabolism offer considerable potential for interaction with other drugs that could affect the metabolism and, possibly, biological activity of the anthracyclines. The interaction that has received most attention is between doxorubicin and cyclophosphamide. These drugs are used in combination in several clinically useful regimens (Davis and Davis, 1979). Cyclophosphamide is known to decrease the activity of several hepatic drug metabolizing enzymes including microsomal NADPH-cytochrome P-450 reductase (Marinello et al., 1981) which, as has been discussed, is responsible for C-7 reductive cleavage of anthracyclines. Hartman et al. (1982) studied the effects of cyclophosphamide pretreatment upon the hepatic metabolism and biliary excretion of doxorobucin metabolites in rat. Despite a 40% decrease in hepatic microsomal NADPH cytochrome P-450 reductase by cyclophosphamide pretreatment there was no change in the formation of anthracylcine aglycone metabolites by isolated hepatocytes, or in the biliary excretion of aglycone metabolites in the intact animal. Dodion et al. (1984e) found no change in the formation of 7-deoxydoxorubicin aglycone from doxorubicin by rat liver microsomes from cyclophosphamide pretreated rats incubated with NADPH under anaerobic conditions. There was, however, a decrease in the formation of 7-deoxydoxorubicinol aglycone due to inhibition of microsomal anthracycline C-13 keto reductase by the cyclophosphamide pretreatment. At the same time there was no inhibition of the more abundant cytosolic anthracycline C-13 keto reductase by cyclophosphamide pretreatment. In the rat, at least, NADPH-cytochrome P-450 reductase does not appear to be rate-limiting in the formation of anthracycline aglycone metabolites.

The H_2-receptor blocker and cytochrome P-450 inhibitor cimetidine given to rabbits at therapeutic doses significantly decreases the clearance of doxorubicin but did not affect the conversion to doxorubicinol or 7-deoxyrubicinol aglycone (Brenner et al., 1986a). Similar effects were seen using ranatidine (Harris et al., 1988). Phenytoin increases the elimination of doxorubicinol in rabbit, without affecting the conversion of doxorubicin to doxorubicinol (Cusack et al., 1988). Hepatic necrosis in the rabbit induced by allyl alcohol has little effect on the conversion of doxorubicin to doxorubicinol but decreases the elimination of doxorubicinol (Brenner et al.,

1986b). Hepatic necrosis in the rat caused by carbon tetrachloride significantly decreases the excretion of doxorubicin in the bile, while phenobarbital pretreatment increases the biliary excretion of doxorubicin (Wosilait and Ryan, 1987). Bromosulphthalein and rifampicin administered acutely decrease the biliary excretion of doxorubicin. The Ca^{2+} channel antagonist verapamil, which can overcome acquired resistance to doxorubicin in vitro, dramatically decreases the plasma clearance of daunorubicin 9-fold in rat (Nooter et al., 1987). In patients receiving oral verapamil, there is a small decrease in the clearance of doxorubicin, from 53.6 to 36.1 L/hr, and an increase in the steady state volume of distribution, but no change in the levels of doxorubicinol in plasma (Kerr et al., 1986).

Relatively few drug interactions involving anthracycline metabolism have been reported but it is likely that more will be found. It remains to be seen whether such interactions have an effect on the biological activity of the anthracyclines, particularly under clinical conditions. Since tissue uptake is the major determinant of plasma anthracycline concentration alterations in anthracycline metabolism are unlikely to have a marked effect on plasma anthracycline concentrations and may thus have little effect on the biological activity of the anthracyclines, unless excretion is also affected. A change in anthracycline biological activity resulting from a drug interaction appears more likely to occur as a result of a direct effect on the target tissue metabolism of the anthracycline. The relationship between metabolism and biological activity of the anthracyclines is discussed in the next section.

3.5. Metabolism and Biological Activity

3.5.1. *Antitumor Activity*

Three mechanisms have been proposed to account for the cytotoxicity of anthracyclines and full expression of an anthracycline's antitumor activity may represent a combination of one or more of these mechanisms. The first and most studied mechanism is the high affinity binding of anthracyclines to DNA through intercalation of the aglycone moiety between adjacent base pairs in the DNA double helix (Pigram et al., 1972) leading to blockage of DNA, RNA and protein synthesis, DNA protein-associated strand breaks and inhibition of DNA repair (Painter, 1978). A general relationship exists between the ability of anthracyclines to bind to DNA and in vitro cytotoxicity and in vivo toxicity (Arcamone et al., 1982). However, DNA intercalation does not appear to be a primary mechanism of anthracycline toxicity (Myers, 1982). No correlation has been found between inhibition of DNA or RNA synthesis by doxorubicin and extent of cell survival, except at very high drug concentrations (Aubel-Sadron and Landas-Gagliandi, 1984; Siegfried et al., 1983). A second mechanism for anthracycline cytotoxicity has focused on cell membrane effects of the anthracyclines leading to altered membrane fluidity (Hickman et al., 1985; Tritton et al., 1978; Tritton and Hickman, 1985) and altered ion permeability (Santone et al., 1986; Solie and Yuncker, 1978). The third possible mechanism for anthracycline cytotoxicity involves generation of reactive radicals.

Bachur et al. (1978b, 1979) first proposed that activation of anthracyclines to semiquinone radicals by NADPH cytochrome P-450 reductase or other flavoenzymes might lead to site-specific damage to nuclear DNA. Intercalation of the semiquinone radical with DNA was seen as leading to an increased likelihood of damage to DNA by direct reaction of the semiquinone radical in close proximity to the double stranded DNA, or by generation of reactive oxygen species within the DNA helix. A problem with this mechanism is that since most flavoenzymes are located outside the nucleus the anthracycline semiquinone radical would have to be stable enough to diffuse from its site of formation outside the nucleus to its presumed site of action within the nucleus (Bachur et al., 1982b; Svingen and Powis, 1981). Most semiquinone free radicals and oxygen free radicals have very short lifetimes under physiological conditions (Hutchinson, 1957). Pulse radiolysis studies suggest that the doxorubicin semiquinone free radical decays rapidly under anaerobic conditions with a lifetime as short as < 0.1 msec (Svingen and Powis, 1981). Transient equilibrium of the anthracycline quinone and the hydroquinone could stabilize the semiquinone radical for up to 20 msec (Land et al., 1985; Houée-Levin et al., 1985) and in this case a semiquinone radical might conceivably have time to diffuse from its site of formation to a critical site within a cell. However, the doxorubicin semiquinone radical reacts rapidly with oxygen to form superoxide anion radical

(Butler et al., 1985; Land et al., 1985) which further reduces the distance a doxorubicin semiquinone radical is likely to travel in the cell. Kalyanaram et al. (1980) have calculated that the half-life of an anthracycline semiquinone radical, even at an oxygen concentration as low as 1 μM which might be found in some poorly perfused tumors, is of the order of 6 msec. The authors concluded that with the exception of electron transfer reactions, most chemical reactions of semiquinones will be too slow to be of significance at in vivo oxygen concentrations. Oxygen radicals formed by redox cycling of anthracyclines are unlikely to diffuse any further than the drug radicals themselves. The mean effective radius for the action of oxygen radicals produced by ionizing radiation, principally hydroxyl radical and superoxide anion radical, in cells is 30 Å (Hutchinson, 1957). It appears, therefore, that if anthracycline radicals or anthracycline-derived oxygen radicals are to produce an effect on DNA in the nucleus they will have to be formed in close proximity to the nucleus. It has been shown that this can occur. Isolated nuclei in the presence of NADPH can activate doxorubicin and daunorubicin to ESR detectable semiquinone radicals (Sinha et al., 1984; Bachur et al., 1982b; Mimnaugh et al., 1985) and, in the presence of oxygen, form superoxide anion radical and hydroxyl radical (Sinha et al., 1984; Mimnaugh et al., 1985). The rate of anthracycline metabolism by isolated nuclei is slower and less complete than metabolism by the microsomes, apparently because of binding of the anthracycline to nuclear DNA in a form unavailable for metabolism (Wallace, 1986b). Despite this, nuclear anthracycline metabolism leads to nuclear membrane lipid peroxidation (Mimnaugh et al., 1985), covalent binding of anthracycline to DNA (Sinha et al., 1984) and DNA strand breakage (Berlin and Haseltine, 1981).

As an alternative to damage to nuclear DNA, Nudd and Wilkie (1983) have proposed that mitochondrial DNA is a target for anthracycline cytotoxicity. An attraction of this suggestion is that mitochondria rapidly metabolize anthracyclines to anthracycline semiquinone radical and oxygen radicals (Doroshow, 1983a,b). It should also be noted that mitochondrial DNA can migrate to the nucleus (Fox, 1983) which might transfer some damage originating in the mitochondria to the nucleus.

There is some evidence that hydroxyl radicals are involved in the cytotoxic effects of anthracyclines. Scavengers of hydroxyl radicals, such as dimethylsulfoxide, diethylurea, thiourea and sodium benzoate; iron chelators such as deferoxamine and 2,2-bipyridine; and catalase and superoxide dismutase have all been reported to reduce the cytotoxicity of doxorubicin and other anthracyclines to cells in vitro (Doroshow, 1985; Doroshow and deVries, 1984; Henriksson and Grankvist, 1988). The effects of these agents has been suggested to relate to effects on iron-dependent generation of hydroxyl radical by doxorubicin (Doroshow and deVries, 1984; Doroshow, 1985, 1986a,b). In the same system radical scavengers did not affect the cytotoxicity of 5-iminodaunorubicin which does not form hydroxyl radical. A dose–response relationship between doxorubicin induced hydroxyl radical formation and doxorubicin cytotoxicity in a human breast cancer cell line has been reported (Sinha et al., 1985). Hydroxyl radical formation, measured by ESR spectroscopy and DMPO-hydroxyl radical adduct formation, has been reported to be much greater in the doxorubicin sensitive MCF-7 breast cancer cell line than in the resistant cell line. The difference was ascribed to increased levels of glutathione peroxidases in the resistant cell line leading to lower levels of hydrogen peroxide (Sinha et al., 1986b, 1987a, 1989a,b; Akman et al., 1990). An interesting feature of these studies was that more than half the DMPO-hydroxyl radical adduct formation appeared to be extracellular since it was stimulated by added NADH and NADPH. This was later confirmed by the use of an extracellular spin-broadening agent, poly(ethylene)glycol (Sinha et al., 1987b). Mimnaugh et al. (1989) reported that doxorubicin-resistent MCF-7 human breast cancer cells also tolerated superoxide dismutase and hydrogen peroxide better than doxorubicin sensitive MCF-7 cells. They showed an increase in superoxide dismutase and in glutathione peroxidase in the resistant cells. Scheulen et al. (1987) correlated increased levels of glutathione reductase with doxorubicin resistance in Ehrlich ascites tumor cells. Recent spin-trapping studies by Alegria et al. (1989) using doxorubicin resistant human MCF-7 breast cancer cells and Chinese hamster ovary cells reported comparable levels of doxorubicin semiquinone formation under anaerobic conditions, and DMPO-hydroxyl radical formation under aerobic conditions, by resistant and sensitive cells, thus, differing from the results of Sinha et al. (1986, 1989a). In the study by Alegria et al. (1989), the DMPO-hydroxyl radical signal was completely abolished by tris(oxaloto)chromate, an extracellular line broadening agent, apparently ruling out any contribution to the signal by intracellular spin adduct formation. The results led Alegria et al. (1989) to conclude that ESR detectable oxygen-derived radicals were unlikely to play a role in doxorubicin antitumor activity. Meijer et al. (1987) could find no increased capacity for the detoxification of free radicals between doxorubicin resistant and sensitive human small cell lung cancer cells. Doroshow (1986b) has presented evidence that intracellular generation of hydrogen peroxide may be important for the cytotoxicity of a number of anticancer quinones including doxorubicin. Catalase and PZ 51 (2-phenyl-1,2-benziso-selenazol-3(2H)-one), a selenium compound that possesses glutathione peroxidase-like activity for intact cells and can detoxify hydrogen peroxide in the presence of glutathione (Müller et al., 1984), protected Ehrlich tumor cells against doxorubicin, mitomycin C and diaziquone cytotoxicity. Doxorubicin resistant MCF-7 human breast cancer cells have been reported to have lower glucose-6-phosphate dehydrogenase activity and to show a decreased stimulation of the pentose phosphate shunt by doxorubicin than the wild type cells (Yeh et al., 1986, 1988; Jamis-Dow et al., 1988). A decreased capacity to generate NADPH in the doxorubicin resistant cells could lead to decreased activation of doxorubicin and decreased glutathione peroxidase stimulation of the pentose phosphate shunt in these cells. It should be noted that doxorubicin resistant MCF-7 cells also show increased expression of *p*-glycoprotein which is an effective cell membrane efflux pump for the anthracyclines (Kramer and Zahker, 1988). *p*-Glycoprotein expression appears to act together with altered redox metabolism to decrease the sensitivity of MCF-7 cells to doxorubicin (Kramer and Zahker, 1988). In contrast, Gessner et al. (1990) reported elevated activity of glucose-6-phosphate dehydrogenase and of the pentose phosphate shunt in daunorubicin resistant murine leukemia P-388 cells. These cells also had elevated glucuronyltransferase activity and showed formation of daunorubicinol glucuronide, which could contribute to the daunorubicin resistence. Dusre et al. (1989) reported that buthionone sulfoximine, a specific inhibitor of α-glutamylcysteine synthetase, which lowers reduced glutathione levels in cells increased doxorubicin cytotoxicity and increased the formation of hydroxyl radicals in doxorubicin-resistant MCF-7 cells. Based on their results the authors concluded that reduced glutathione plays a role in protecting the cells against the cytotoxic effects of doxorubicin via the scavenging of hydrogen peroxide by glutathione peroxidase. Mimnaugh et al. (1985) have emphasized a role for oxygen radical-induced nuclear membrane lipid peroxidation in the cytotoxicity of anthracyclines and have suggested that it may contribute to biochemical and morphological alterations in the nucleus following anthracycline treatment. The authors pointed out that such a mechanism could explain why anthracyclines such as AD-32 that do not bind to DNA and apparently do not enter the nucleus (Egorin et al., 1980) can cause protein associated DNA strand breaks and DNA–protein cross-links in tumor cells (Levin et al., 1981). Evidence against a role for oxygen radicals as a general mechanism for cytotoxicity of anthracyclines is the low oxygen radical formation by both 5-imino substituted anthracyclines and by morpholinyl anthracyclines which can be considerably more potent cytotoxic agents than the parent anthracyclines (Peters et al., 1986).

An intriguing observation is that anthracyclines immobilized on the surface of polymeric beads retain some cytotoxicity to cultured cells (for a review see Tritton, 1991). This has been interpreted to indicate a cell surface action for the immobilized anthracyclines. Panneerselyam et al. (1987) found that a combination of dimethylsulfoxide, catalase and superoxide dismutase decreased to cytotoxicity of immobilized doxorubicin to murine L1210 leukemia and human SK-MEL melanoma cell lines, suggesting that oxygen radicals are responsible for the cytotoxicity of immobilized anthracycline. 5-Iminodaunorubicin, which does not form oxygen free radicals, exhibited very little cytotoxicity when bound to the surface of beads. If reactive oxygen species are involved in the cytotoxicity of the anthracyclines it might be expected that exposing cells to anthracyclines under hypoxic conditions would decrease anthracycline cytotoxicity. Conversely, if the anthracycline semiquinone radical is important for cytotoxicity the absence of oxygen should increase the drug effect because there is no longer competition for the anthracycline semiquinone radical by oxygen. Unfortunately, the reported effects of hypoxia on anthracycline cytotoxicity are equivocal. Doxorubicin has been reported to be both less toxic (Martin and McNally, 1979; Powis et al., 1987a; Sciandra et al., 1985; Smith et al., 1980; Tannock and Guttman, 1981; Tannock, 1982), to be equally toxic, and to be more toxic (Gupta and Kishnan, 1982; Kennedy et al., 1983; Teicher et al., 1981; Gupta and Constanzi, 1987) to cells under hypoxic conditions. Reviewing the different reports it is clear that the effect of hypoxia on the response of cells to cytotoxic agents depends in part upon the cell line employed (Keyes et al., 1984b; Ludwig et al., 1984; Rauth et al., 1983), although different workers have reported different effects with the same cell lines (Harris and Shrieve, 1979; Ludwig et al., 1984; Rauth et al., 1983; Teicher et al., 1981). Part of the variability may also relate to the extent and duration of hypoxia achieved under the experimental conditions in different laboratories and to metabolic adaptation by the cells. Sartorelli and his co-workers (Kennedy et al., 1983; Teicher et al., 1981) found that the increased sensitivity of sarcoma 180 cells to doxorubicin caused by hypoxic conditions was not reversed until at least 18 hr of reoxygenation, suggesting metabolic adaptation by the hypoxic cells. Sciandra et al. (1985) reported doxorubicin resistance in cells exposed to hypoxia for 12 hr and suggested that this was due to the synthesis of a special class of proteins called oxygen regulated proteins. In the light of such findings interpretation of the effects of hypoxia on the response of cells to cytotoxic agents goes beyond simple considerations of hypoxia's effects on drug redox cycling and provides little direct information as to how redox active drugs such as anthracyclines might be producing their cytotoxic effects.

DNA strand breakage after exposure to anthracycline has been observed in DNA isolated from tumors in mice (Schwartz, 1975) and in DNA of cultured cells (Kanter and Schwartz, 1979). DNA is known to undergo degradation by superoxide anion radical generating systems almost entirely due to the formation of hydroxyl radical from superoxide anion radical in the presence of trace amounts of iron salts (Brawn and Fridovich, 1981; Rowley and Halliwell, 1983). It has been suggested that oxygen radicals formed by redox cycling of anthracycline bound to DNA may produce selective damage to the DNA (Lown et al., 1982). Intercalation of doxorubicin and other anthracyclines into double stranded DNA prevents their enzymatic reduction and greatly decreases the yield of superoxide anion and hydroxyl radicals (Sato et al., 1977; Kalyanaraman et al., 1980; Rowley and Halliwell, 1983; Berlin and Haseltine, 1981; Peters et al., 1986). Because of this, it has been argued that oxygen radicals are unlikely to be responsible for doxorubicin-induced DNA damage in vivo (Rowley and Halliwell, 1983). However, DNA-intercalated doxorubicin can still be reduced by diffusible reductant species Houée-Levin et al., 1990; Rouscilles et al., 1989) including superoxide anion radical (Youngman and Elstner, 1984), presumably because the small species such as superoxide anion radical can gain access where a large enzyme cannot. It is possible, therefore, that activation of DNA-bound anthracycline by a diffusible cellular reductant could lead to the formation of oxygen radical species in close proximity to the DNA. Another possibility is that the covalently bound anthracycline becomes attached at a different site on the DNA to intercalated drug and is still available for enzymatic reduction leading to formation of anthracycline semiquinone and oxygen radicals in close proximity to DNA.

A number of anthracyclines including doxorubicin (Capranico et al., 1986a; Potmesil et al., 1984), 11-deoxydaunorubicin, 4-demethoxydauno-rubicin, 4-demethoxy-11-deoxy-4′-epidaunorubicin, 4-demethyl-6-*O*-methyldoxorubicin (Capranico et al., 1986a), 5-iminodaunorubicin (Pommier et al., 1985) and AD-32 (Levin et al., 1981) produce protein-associated DNA breaks at therapeutic concentrations of anthracycline. Several other antitumor agents produce protein associated DNA breaks by a mechanism that does not involve free radical formation or even binding of the drug to DNA (Younes et al., 1985). Protein-associated DNA breaks are thought to arise from interference by the drug with the action of the enzyme DNA topoisomerase II (E.C.5.99.1.3.) (Nelson et al., 1984). Protein-associated DNA breaks induced by anthracyclines probably occurs by a similar mechanism. 5-Imino-substituted anthracyclines undergo very little redox cycling and do not form oxygen radicals (Peters et al., 1986; Pollakis et al., 1984) but 5-iminodaunorubicin will bind to DNA and causes protein-associated DNA breaks (Pommerier et al., 1985). There are also anthracyclines such as AD-32 and its metabolites that do not bind to DNA but still produce protein associated DNA breaks (Levin et al., 1981). Anthracyclines probably stabilize the topoisomerase II–DNA complex in an open (cleaved) conformation of DNA (Pommier et al., 1985; Tewey et al., 1984).

Potmesil et al. (1984) have reported that although doxorubicin produces nonprotein associated DNA single strand breaks in L1210 leukemia cells, thought to be due to oxygen radicals, this only occurs at concentrations of doxorubicin of 2.8 μM and greater, which are above concentrations achievable therapeutically. At lower concentrations of doxorubicin only protein-associated DNA breaks are seen (Potmesil et al., 1983, 1984). In contrast, Goldenberg et al. (1986) found nonprotein associated DNA single strand breaks in leukemia P-388 cells exposed to doxorubicin concentrations of 0.1–2 μM. DNA double strand breaks were also seen and appeared to be a better index of cytotoxicity than DNA single strand breaks. There is a preliminary report by Potmesil et al. (1986) that DNA protein associated single strand breaks and DNA–protein crosslinks persist in cultured cells for 24 hr after 1 hr exposure to the *N*-alkyl doxorubicin analogs, *N*-benzyldoxorubicin-14-valerate and *N,N*-dimethyldoxorubicin-14-valerate, but disappear after only 1 hr on exposure to the *N*-acyl doxorubicin analogs, *N*-trifluoroacetyl-doxorubicin-14-valerate (AD-32) and *N*-trifluoroacetyl-doxo-rubicin-14-*O*-hemi-adipate (AD-143). The loss of DNA lesions is associated with rapid disappearance from cells of the *N*-acyl analogs and their metabolite *N*-trifluoroacetyldoxorubicin, whereas metabolites of the *N*-alkyl analogs persist for a long time in the cells, presumably associated with DNA, maintaining their ability to cleave DNA. Despite intensive study, it has not been possible to show a simple correlation between cytotoxicity and induction of DNA strand breaks by different anthracycline analogs (Capranico et al., 1986a,b; Zwelling et al., 1982), and a relationship between anthracycline-induced DNA breaks and anthracycline cytotoxicity has yet to be established.

In summary, although intriguing, the hypothesis that anthracycline metabolism leading to formation of anthracycline radicals or oxygen radicals is important for the cytotoxicity of anthracyclines is unproven. The evidence for a relationship is incomplete and often contradictory. Studies showing a relationship between anthracycline radical or anthracycline-induced oxygen radical formation by intact cells and the growth inhibitory effects anthracyclines would be useful evidence to support such a hypothesis. It is also clear the other actions of the anthracyclines at the level of DNA, such as DNA binding or inhibition of DNA-dependent enzymes, do not wholly explain the cytotoxic activity of the anthracyclines. Multiple actions of anthracyclines at the level of DNA or actions at other critical sites in the cell, perhaps the plasma membrane, are probably also important for anthracycline cytotoxicity.

3.5.2. *Cardiotoxicity*

The cumulative-dose limiting toxicity of the anthracyclines is congestive cardiomyopathy (Green et al., 1984). The risk of doxorubicin cardiomyopathy increases as the total dose of drug increases (Von Hoff et al., 1979). With doses of doxorubicin less than 550 mg/m^2, the incidence of cardiomyopathy is less than 1% (Bonadonna et al., 1975; Praga et al., 1979) but this increases to about 30% at doses above this amount. However, even asymptomatic patients receiving total doses of doxorubicin of 480–550 mg/m^2 have abnormal radionucleide angiography scans (Gottdiener et al., 1981). The pathological findings of doxorubicin cardiomyopathy give little clue as to its cause and include loss of myofibrils, cytoplasmic vacuolization, swollen mitochondira, enlarged nuclei, increased numbers of lysosomes and lipid accumulation (Powis, 1991; Billingham, 1979; Goormaghtigh et al., 1980). Monitoring left ventricular function with radionuclide angiography before and during anthracycline therapy appears to be the most successful noninvasive method for predicting drug-induced cardiomyopathy (Fantine and Garnier-Suillerot, 1986; Schwartz et al., 1987). A number of mechanisms have been suggested to account for the cardiotoxicity of anthracyclines, including the ability of anthracyclines to delocalize iron from cardiac ferritin stores (Thomas and Aust, 1986), disturbances of cardiac mitochondrial function such as ATP synthesis (Bachmann et al., 1975; Mailer and Petering, 1976; Gosalvez et al., 1974; Iwamoto et al., 1974), alterations in cardiac mitochondrial calcium translocation (Moore et al., 1977; Revis and Marusic, 1979) and damage to the cardiac microtubule structure (Rabkin and Sunga, 1987; Colombo and Milzani, 1987. However, the cardiotoxicity of anthracyclines is most frequently linked to their ability to undergo redox cycling to form reactive oxygen species (Adachi et al., 1983; D'Alessandro et al., 1980; Doroshow, 1983a; Doroshow and Davies, 1986; Goodman and Hochstein, 1977; Thayer, 1977). There are several pieces of evidence favoring such an association.

Doxorubicin, daunorubicin and other cardiotoxic anthracyclines stimulate the formation of superoxide anion radical, hydrogen peroxide and hydroxyl radical by heart subcellular fractions (Adachi et al., 1983; Doroshow, 1983a,b; Doroshow and Davies, 1986; Gutierrez et al., 1983; Thayer, 1977). Complex I of the mitochondrial electron transport chain, probably the NADH dehydrogenase, is the major site of anthracycline-induced oxygen radical formation in the heart (Adachi et al, 1983; Davies et al., 1983; Davies and Doroshow, 1986; Doroshow, 1983a; Thornalley et al., 1986). Unlike the liver, where superoxide anion radical is the primary oxygen species formed, ESR spin trap studies suggest that in the heart hydroxyl radical may be a major oxygen radical species produced by redox cycling of anthracyclines. Pollakis et al. (1984), using an ESR flow technique with respiring heart mitochondria or heart submitochondrial particles incubated with anthracycline, observed short lived DMPO spin trapped adducts of hydroxyl radical and superoxide anion radical. Superoxide anion was the predominated species formed by intact mitochondria and hydroxyl radical the predominant species formed by sonicated mitochondria. Thornalley and Dodd (1985) could not detect superoxide anion radical formation by rat heart sarcosomas incubated with NADPH and doxorubicin using ESR and spin trapping with DMPO, although they could detect formation of hydroxyl radical. Hydroxyl radical formation was strongly inhibited by catalase, although not by superoxide dismutase, suggesting a direct reduction of hydrogen peroxide to hydroxyl radical. The authors assumed, however, that hydrogen peroxide was being formed via superoxide, and that their failure to detect superoxide was due to the much greater efficiency of trapping of hydroxyl radicals compared to superoxide anion radicals by DMPO . Nohl and Jordan (1983) were also unable to find ESR evidence for formation of superoxide anion radical by respiring rat heart mitochondria and doxorubicin using DMPO as a spin trap. A doxorubicin-derived semiquinone radical signal was seen which was stable even in the presence of oxygen. The signal disappeared on addition of hydrogen peroxide and concomitantly there appeared a DMPO-hydroxyl radical adduct signal. The authors interpreted their results to indicate that a doxorubicin semiquinone radical was produced during mitochondrial respiration, probably at the lipophilic phase of the mitochondrial inner membrane, in a way which precluded electron transfer to oxygen. This then allowed reaction of the anthracycline semiquinone radical with hydrogen peroxide, probably present at relatively high concentrations in heart because of low levels of catalase (Herzog and Fahimi, 1974), to form hydroxyl radical. Studies by the same group have suggested that the oxygen-insensitive semiquinone radical is that of doxorubicin aglycone semiquinone incorporated into the phospholipid of the mitochondrial inner membrane (Nohl et al., 1986). Controlled disruption of the phospholipid membrane exposes the semiquinone radical allowing it to react with oxygen and generate superoxide anion radical. More recently a heart specific NADH-oxidoreductase located on the cytosolic face of the inner mitochondrial membrane has been identified as a probable site of anthracycline semiquinone radical formation in rat heart cells (Nohl, 1988).

A second piece of evidence linking anthracycline-cardiotoxicity to oxygen radical formation is the finding that newer less cardiotoxic anthracycline analogs undergo less redox cycling. Studies by Lown et al. (1982) have shown a positive correlation between the cardiotoxicity of a series of anthracyclines in rat and generation reactive oxygen species by electrochemically reduced anthracyclines. The ease of generation of reactive oxygen species appeared to be related to the ease with which the reduced anthracycline was reoxidized. 5-Iminodaunorubicin, which is less cardiotoxic in animals than either daunorubicin or doxorubicin (Tong et al., 1979; Zbinden et al., 1978), does not form an anthracycline semiquinone radical (Doroshow and Davies, 1986; Pollakis et al., 1984) and does not produce superoxide anion radical or hydroxyl radical (Doroshow, 1983b; Doroshow and Davies, 1986; Peters et al., 1986; Pollakis et al., 1984). The decreased tendency of 5-iminodaunorubicin to undergo redox cycling is because of hydrogen bonding between the imine nitrogen and adjacent hydroxyl groups which makes the compound more difficult to reduce and much more difficult to reoxidize (Lown et al., 1979). 5-Iminodaunorubicin, but not daunorubicin, undergoes oxidation by hydrogen peroxidase and horse radish peroxidase to give a nitrogen-centered free radical species (Kolodzieczyke et al., 1989). 4′-Deoxydoxorubicin and 4-demethoxydaunorubicin, which in animals have a lesser tendency for producing cardiotoxicity than the parent anthracyclines, do not generate oxygen free radicals spontaneously in aerated aqueous solution unlike the parent anthracyclines (Dickinson et al., 1984, 1985). Both compounds are, however, equally active as doxorubicin in stimulating oxygen utilization when incubated with liver microsomes and NADPH (Peters et al., 1986).

The heart appears to have a decreased capacity to detoxify oxygen radicals compared to other tissues which may make it susceptible to anthracycline induced oxygen radical damage. Compared to other tissues the heart has low levels of superoxide dismutase (Adachi et al., 1983; Doroshow et al., 1980), catalase (Thayer, 1977; Doroshow et al., 1980) and nonselenium dependent glutathione peroxidase (Doroshow et al., 1980; Revis and Marusic, 1978). Administration of doxorubicin also produces a selective decrease in cardiac glutathione peroxidase (Doroshow et al., 1980), a depletion of cardiac glutathione (Julicher et al., 1986; Olson et al., 1980), and an increase in cardiac superoxide dismutase and catalase, although with no change in the superoxide dismutase and catalase of liver and kidney (Adachi et al., 1983; D'Alessandro et al., 1980), perhaps as a response to oxidative stress.

It has been suggested by Pollakis et al. (1983) that generation of anthracycline semiquinone radicals in the heart might damage mitochondrial membranes by a covalent interaction of the anthracycline semiquinone radical with the mitochondrial membrane (Pollakis et al., 1983). Alternatively, reactive oxygen species could lead to damage to heart mitochondria or other organelles. Activation of doxorubicin by heart NADH dehydrogenase with formation of hydroxyl radical has been shown to lead to inhibition of Ca^{2+} uptake by heart sarcoplasmic reticulum (Harris and Doroshow, 1985). Evidence was presented that the effect might be related to radical oxidation of critical thiol groups since *N*-acetylcysteine and glutathione protected against the damage. Lipid peroxidation is another mechanism by which oxygen radicals damage critical macromolecules. Studies with rat heart microsomes and NADPH have shown that anthracyclines stimulate lipid peroxidation, but only if the microsomes are prepared from rats fed a diet deficient in α-tocopherol (Mimnaugh et al., 1981, 1982). Mouse heart microsomes, on the other hand, have low endogenous levels of α-tocopherol and exhibit a marked increase in lipid peroxidation in the presence of anthracyclines (D'Alessandro et al., 1980; Mimnaugh et al., 1983). Some workers have found that it is necessary to add Fe(II) ions to obtain appreciable levels of doxorubicin-stimulated lipid peroxidation in mouse heart microsomes (Daugherty et al., 1982). Low concentrations of 5-iminodaunorubicin inhibit cardiac lipid peroxidation without affecting the rate of NADPH oxidation and inhibit doxorubicin-stimulated NADPH-dependent cardiac microsomal lipid peroxidation (Mimnaugh et al., 1982). The high affinity of 5-iminodaunorubicin for iron might explain its inhibition of lipid peroxidation (Myers et al., 1987). The doxorubicin–Fe(III) complex is a more potent inhibitor of mitochondrial function than doxorubicin alone (Demant, 1983). This has been attributed to a combined effect by doxorubicin–Fe(III) complex of inhibition of mitochondrial electron transfer and increased lipid peroxidation. Doxorubicin–Fe(III) complex is, however, less toxic to cardiac myocytes in vitro than doxorubicin (Lampidis et al., 1987). An increase in phospholipase activity secondary to increased lipid peroxidation has been suggested to be the cause of doxorubicin cardiomyopathy (Ogawa et al., 1987). Even though anthracyclines stimulate lipid peroxidation by subcellular fractions lipid peroxidation may not be a primary effect of anthracyclines in the intact heart. Julicher et al. (1986) found no increase in lipid peroxidation in α-tocopherol deficient rat hearts treated with doxorubicin despite being able to see doxorubicin-dependent lipid peroxidation in heart mitochondrial and microsomal fractions from the same animals. Singal and Pierce (1986) found that increased lipid peroxidation in rat isolated ventricular wall only occurred at concentrations of doxorubicin of 10 μM, which is considerably in excess of therapeutic concentrations, and became maximal at 1 mM doxorubicin. Reports of increased in vivo lipid peroxidation following anthracycline administration using malondialdehyde as an indicator of lipid peroxidation (D'Alessandro et al., 1980; Lenzhofer et al., 1983; Llesuy et al., 1985; Myers et al., 1977; Stuart et al., 1978; Yamanaka et al., 1979; Griffin-Green et al., 1988) have to be treated with caution because malondialdehyde formation is not a good indicator of in vivo lipid peroxidation (Bus and Gibson, 1979). It has been reported that 4′-epidoxorubicin, which is less cardiotoxic than doxorubicin in mice, does not increase malondialdehyde formation by mouse heart in vivo (Llesuy et al., 1985). Praet et al. (1986) have shown that both doxorubicin and 4′-epidoxorubicin increase malondialdehyde formation by mouse heart mitochondria in vitro but that when administered to intact mice 4′-epidoxorubicin produces a much smaller increase in heart mitochondrial malondialdehyde than doxorubicin. The lower levels of lipid peroxidation seen with 4′-epidoxorubicin in vivo may be due to a pharmacokinetic difference between 4′-epidoxorubicin and doxorubicin, perhaps due to 4′-epidoxorubicin glucuronide formation and more rapid elimination of 4′-epidoxorubicin (see Section 3.4.2.3). Studies by Muliawan et al. (1980) using ethane expiration, which is generally regarded as a more reliable indicator of lipid peroxidation in vivo, have failed to show an increase in lipid peroxidation in rats given lethal doses of doxorubicin. However, several compounds that are believed to exert their toxic effects through generation of active oxygen species and lipid peroxidation, for example nitrofurantoin, paraquat, diquat and menadione, also do not increase ethane production in vivo in this system (Younes et al., 1985). Only when animals were pretreated with a low doses of Fe(II) salts was there an increase in ethane production by these compounds. Thus, the failure to demonstrate increased ethane production by doxorubicin in vivo cannot be taken as conclusive evidence for a lack of lipid peroxidation in vivo, particularly at a specific organ site such as the heart.

While selective uptake of anthracycline probably explains their acute toxicity for heart muscle compared to other muscle (Doroshow et al., 1985; Chen et al., 1987; Sazuka et al., 1987) some studies have suggested a link between the cardiotoxicity of anthracyclines and the formation and accumulation in the heart of C-13 anthracycline alcohols (del Tacca et al., 1985). Doxorubicinol has been reported to be more cardiotoxic than doxorubicin in vivo (Olsen et al., 1988) and more inhibitory of the sarcoplasmic reticulum Ca^{2+} pump in vitro (Boucek et al., 1987; Olson et al., 1988). Other studies have found doxorubicinol to be less cardiotoxic than doxorubicin in vivo (Danesi et al., 1986, 1988) and, at present, the role of C-13 anthracycline metabolites in anthracycline cardiotoxicity is unresolved (Powis, 1991).

Numerous agents have been tested for their ability to protect animals against acute and chronic anthracycline cardiotoxicity (reviewed in Powis, 1991). Free radical scavenging agents such as α-tocopherol (Myers et al., 1976; Mimnaugh et al., 1979), butylated hydroxy toluene (Daugherty et al., 1982), glutathione (Yoda et al., 1986), ascorbate (Fujita et al., 1982) and ubiquinone (Bertazzoli et al., 1975; Folkers et al., 1978; Tábora et al., 1986), and the redox agent methylene blue (Hrushesky et al., 1985) protect animals against the acute cardiotoxicity of doxorubicin. The level of cellular glutathione, which is an endogenous free radical scavenger, also appears to be important in anthracycline cardiotoxicity. Pretreatment of mice with diethylmaleate, which lowers cellular glutathione, increases the lethality of doxorubicin (Olson et al., 1980), while concurrent administration of cysteamine (Freeman et al., 1980; Olson et al., 1980) and *N*-acetylcysteine pretreatment (Doroshow et al., 1982) protect mice against doxorubicin lethality. Redox cycling of anthracyclines in the heart leading to depletion of cardiac NADPH might be the cause of cardiotoxicity, rather than reactive oxygen species. It has been reported that both niacin, a precursor of $NADP^+$, and isocitrate, the major substrate for NADPH-regeneration in the heart, decrease acute doxorubicin cardiotoxicity in the mouse, without affecting antitumor activity (Schmitt-Graff and Scheulen, 1986).

It is important to distinguish two kinds of doxorubicin cardiotoxicity. First, there is acute cardiotoxicity which occurs within minutes of drug administration and is characterized by the occurrence of cardiac arrhymias and nonspecific electrocardiographic changes (Cortes et al., 1973). Second, there is irreversible congestive heart failure which occurs after the cumulative dose of anthracyclines has been reached (Cortes et al., 1973; Jaenke, 1976). Chronic anthracycline cardiotoxicity may be related to the extent of anthracycline accumulation in cardiac tissue (Jaenke et al., 1980). While the free radical scavenger α-tocopherol can protect animals against acute doxorubicin cardiotoxicity it does not protect against delayed (Mimnaugh et al., 1979) and chronic doxorubicin cardiotoxicity (Breed et al., 1980; Van Vleet et al., 1980). In clinical trials α-tocopherol did not protect patients against a progressive decline of cardiac function caused by doxorubicin (Weitzman et al., 1980; Legha et al., 1982; Whitaker and Al-Ismail, 1984). Similarly, *N*-acetylcysteine did not protect dogs against chronic doxorubicin cardiotoxicity (Unverferth et al., 1985). Protection against chronic doxorubicin cardiotoxicity has been reported in animals by ubiquinone (Domae et al., 1981) and ascorbate (Fujita et al., 1982). Clinical studies have shown that ubiquinone decreases the degree of anthracycline cardiotoxicity in patients with normal cardiac function and allows increased doses of anthracycline to be given before cardiotoxicity is seen. The most promising protective agent against doxorubicin cardiotoxicity in clinical trials has been ICRF-187 [(+)-1,2-bis(3,5-dioxopiperazinyl-1-ye)propane]. This is a lipid soluble analog of EDTA that forms a mixed ligand complex with doxorubicin–Fe(III) or Cu(II) followed by the ring-opening hydrolysis of ICRF-187 and the displacement of the metal ion from its complex with doxorubicin (Hasinoff, 1990). Both ICRF-187 and, before that, its less water soluble racemate ICRF-159, were shown to protect animals against chronic anthracycline cardiotoxicity (Herman and Ferrans, 1983,1986;

Herman et al., 1985). Clinical trials have shown that ICRF-159 may indeed offer protection against anthracycline cardiotoxicity (Green et al., 1984; Speyer et al., 1987, 1988). Other agents that have been tested clinically, with only limited success for their ability to protect against doxorubicin cardiotoxicity, are digoxin (Whitaker and Al-Ismail, 1984), the Ca^{2+} channel blockers verapamil (Ozols et al., 1987; Garbrecht and Müllerleile, 1986) and nifedipine (Lenzhofer et al., 1983), prenylamine, an antianginal drug (Milei et al., 1988) and L-carnitine (DeLeonardis et al., 1985, 1987).

In summary, the evidence suggests that anthracycline-induced oxygen radicals and lipid peroxidation are important factors in the acute cardiotoxicity of anthracyclines, although other factors may also play a role. It is less likely that oxygen radicals and lipid peroxidation are the cause of chronic, and clinically more relevant, cardiotoxicity of anthracyclines. It is possible that the anthracycline semiquinone radical itself is important for this chronic cardiotoxicity.

3.5.3. *Skin Toxicity*

Accidental infiltration of doxorubicin into the area around an i.v. infusion site in patients can cause severe ulceration. The necrosis increases in severity over several weeks and results in slowly healing ulcers that can be a source of severe pain and even functional impairment for patients. Between 0.5 and 6% of patients receiving doxorubicin are affected (Svingen et al., 1981). A free radical mechanism for the ulcerogenic activity of doxorubicin is suggested by the ability of topically applied free radical scavenging agents, such as dimethylsulfoxide (Desai and Teres, 1982; Svingen et al., 1981), α-tocopherol (Nobbs and Barr, 1983; Svingen et al., 1981) and butylated hydroxytoluene (Daugherty and Khurana, 1985), or pretreating with butylated hydroxytoluene (Upton et al., 1986) to prevent the ulceration in some, although not all (Dorr and Alberts, 1983), animal species. Dimethylsulfoxide (Lawrence and Goodnight, 1983; Lawrence et al., 1989; Olver and Schwarz, 1983) and a mixture of dimethylsulfoxide and α-tocopherol (Ludwig et al., 1987) have been reported to protect patients against skin ulceration following anthracycline extravasation.

4. BIS(SUBSTITUTED AMINOALKYLAMINO)ANTHRAQUINONES

4.1. Historical Perspective

The problem of the dose-limiting cardiotoxicity associated with the use of anthracyclines has led to the search for new classes of antitumor agents with the ability to bind to DNA but without cardiotoxic side effects. In 1974 Adamson proposed, on the basis of then available information on the structure–activity relationships of anthracyclines, that antitumor activity required both the anthracycline ring and the basic amino group of the daunosamine sugar, whereas cardiotoxicity was due to the daunosamine sugar which permitted the anthracycline to be taken up by cardiac muscle. The logical extension of this suggestion was that replacement of the daunosamine sugar with a basic amino or alkylamino side chain might lead to compounds that still bound to DNA and had antitumor activity, but lacked cardiotoxicity. About this time the Allied Chemical Corporation in the U.S.A. provided the National Cancer Institute with a number of colored compounds for screening for antitumor activity in the new drug program. One of these compounds, 1,4-bis(2-[(2-hydroxyethyl)amino]-ethyl-amino)-9,10-anthracenedione (HAQ; Fig. 14), originally developed to be used as blue ink for ballpoint pens, had the structural characteristics suggested by Adamson (1974) and showed significant activity against murine leukemia P-388 (Traganos, 1983). Zee-Cheng and Cheng (1978), who were contractors for the National Cancer Institute at the Midwest Research Institute, synthesized and tested 14 analogs based on HAQ and found 1,4-dihydroxy-5,8-bis-(2-[(2-hydroxyethyl)amino]-ethylamino)-9,10-anthracenedione (DHAQ, Fig. 14) to be the most active compound (Cheng et al., 1979; Johnson et al., 1979; Zee-Cheng and Cheng, 1978). Meanwhile, Murdock and his colleagues working independently at Lederle Laboratories in New York synthesized 56 bis(substituted aminoalkylamino)anthra-quinone derivatives based on the moderate antitumor activity of their lead compound 1,4-bis[(2-(dimethylamino)-ethyl)amino]-9,10-anthracenedione, and found the dihydrochloride salt of DHAQ (DHAD or mitoxantrone) to be most active in animal models (Murdock et al., 1979; Wallace et al., 1979). Over

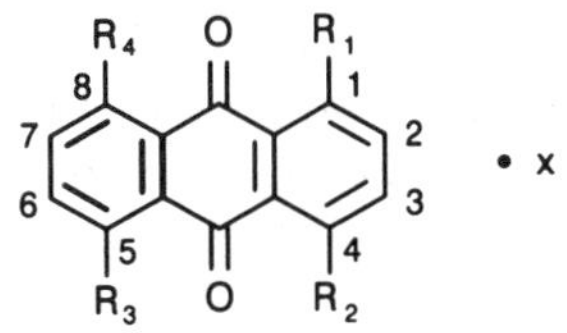

Compound	R_1, R_2	R_3, R_4	x
DHAD (Mitoxantrone)	$NH(CH_2)_2NH(CH_2)_2OH$	OH	2HCl
DHAQ	$NH(CH_2)_2NH(CH_2)_2OH$	OH	
HAQ (Ametantrone)	$NH(CH_2)_2NH(CH_2)_2OH$	H	$2CH_3COOH$

FIG. 14. Structure of some bis(substituted aminoalkylamino) anthraquinones.

300 bis(substituted aminoalkylamino) anthraquinones have since been synthesized and tested in animals for antitumor activity (Krapcho et al., 1986; Uyeki et al., 1981; White and Durr, 1985; Zee-Cheng and Cheng, 1982).

4.2. Structure–Activity Relationships

The structure–antitumor activity relationships of the bis(substituted aminoalkylamino)anthraquinones have been studied by several groups of workers (Johnson et al., 1979; Murdock et al., 1979; Zee-Cheng and Cheng, 1978, 1982). Good antitumor activity requires the ethylenediamine substitutents at positions C-1 and C-4 of the anthracenedione nucleus. Substitutions at positions C-1 and C-5 gives inactive compounds. The presence of two basic side chains is not an absolute requirement for antitumor activity and compounds where one-side chain is replaced by a hydroxyl group retain significant activity. Both basic N atoms of the side chain are essential for activity but increasing the distance between the N atoms, adding additional basic N centers, or adding bulky substituent groups to the terminal N atom decreases activity. The exception is that adding a hydroxyethyl substituent to the terminal N atom increases activity, presumably by imparting hydrophilic character to the molecule which overcomes the decreased activity caused by an ethyl group alone. Hydroxyl groups at positions C-5 and C-8 of the anthracenedione nucleus increase antitumor activity but other nuclear substituents do not. Despite the fact that the bis(substituted aminoalkyl-amino)anthraquinones were synthesized to be DNA binding agents a poor correlation has been found between the compounds' DNA binding capacity, inhibition of DNA and RNA synthesis, and in vivo antitumor activity (Johnson et al., 1979).

4.3. Clinical Activity

DHAQ is administered clinically as the dihydrochloride salt and in this form is known as DHAD or mitoxantrone. Mitoxantrone has shown activity against breast cancer, acute leukemias and non-Hodgkin's lymphoma (Poirier, 1986; Smith, 1983; Young and Raymond, 1986). Marginal activity has been reported against non-small cell lung cancer, Hodgkin's lymphoma, myeloma and cancer of the liver, prostate, bladder, head and neck. The dose-limiting toxicity of mitoxantrone is myelosuppression, usually leukopenia but sometimes thrombocytopenia. In leukemic patients who receive more frequent doses of mitoxantrone stomatitis is the dose-limiting toxicity. Mitoxantrone was developed to be less cardiotoxic than the anthracyclines and in preclinical testing in dogs was found to be devoid of cardiotoxic effects (Sparano et al., 1982). Mitoxantrone does, however, cause cardiotoxicity in humans with an incidence of between 3% in adults and 6% in children (Poirier, 1986). Large scale comparative trials of previously anthracycline non-treated patients has shown the incidence of congestive heart failure with mitoxantrone to be 0.9%, compared to 3.0% with doxorubicin (Dukart et al., 1986). The risk of cardiotoxicity with mitoxantrone appears to increase above a cumulative dose of 160 mg/m^2, which is equivalent to 800 mg/m^2 doxorubicin (Posner et al., 1985). This translates into an improved therapeutic index for DHAD compared to doxorubicin (Saleton, 1987). HAQ is administered clinically as the diacetate salt known as ametantrone and has received limited clinical trials (Gams et al., 1985;

Piccart et al., 1981). The dose-limiting toxicity of ametantrone is myelosuppression, principally leukopenia. Ametantrone, like mitoxantrone, is a dark blue compound. A reversible blue skin discoloration has been observed in some patients receiving ametantrone although this is not seen with mitoxantrone. Insufficient data is available to evaluate the clinical antitumor activity of ametantrone.

4.4. Metabolism

The bis(substituted aminoalkylamino)anthraquinones have the potential for three types of metabolism; reduction-oxidation of the quinone group, modification of aminoalkylamino side chains and modification of the anthraquinone ring.

4.4.1. *Free Radical Formation*

The bis(substituted aminoalkylamino)anthraquinones, as might be expected, undergo redox cycling, but compared to anthracyclines and other antitumor quinones they are poor substrates for flavoprotein-mediated reduction. HAQ is metabolized by NADPH-cytochrome P-450 reductase and NADPH at only 6% the rate of doxorubicin and mitomycin C, and at 2% the rate of diaziquone (Svingen and Powis, 1981). This may be due to the low E^1_7 for HAQ of -348 mV compared to -292 mV for doxorubicin and -168 mV for diaziquone. A low rate of HAQ metabolism by NADPH cytochrome P-450 reductase and NADPH, and by phenobarbital-induced rabbit liver microsomes and NADPH has also been reported by Kharasch and Novak (1981, 1983c, 1985). DHAD is metabolized by NADPH-cytochrome P-450 reductase and NADPH at 15% the rate of doxorubicin (Kharasch and Novak, 1981, 1983c, 1985). Superoxide anion radical formation is only marginally stimulated when DHAD is incubated with rat liver microsomes and NADPH, with NADPH cytochrome P-450 reductase and NADPH, or with NADH dehydrogenase and NADH, while HAQ has no effect or even inhibits the basal levels of superoxide anion radical formation (Basra et al., 1984, 1985; Kharasch and Novak, 1983c, 1985; Sinha et al., 1983). HAQ is such a poor substrate for redox cycling that it inhibits doxorobucin-stimulated superoxide anion radical production by NADPH-cytochrome P-450 reductase and NADPH, and by NADH dehydrogenase and NADH (Kharasch and Novak, 1983c). DHAD inhibits oxygen consumption by cardiac sarcoplasmic reticulum and NADPH, and by mitochondrial NADH dehydrogenase and NADH, with no increase in superoxide anion radical formation (Doroshow, 1983a,b; Doroshow and Davies, 1983).

HAQ is a weak non-competitive inhibitor of hepatic microsomal oxidative drug metabolism with a K_i around 3.0 mM (Kharasch and Novak, 1982b). DHAD also inhibits microsomal oxidative drug metabolism (Kharasch and Novak, 1983b). Unlike quinones such as menadione which act as an electron sink for NADPH-cytochrome P-450 reductase and inhibit oxidative drug metabolism by diverting electron flow from cytochrome P-450, HAQ is a direct inhibitor of NADPH-cytochrome P-450 reductase (Kharasch and Novak, 1982b). Bis(substituted aminoalkylamino)anthraquinones show high affinity binding for FAD and FMN, and form bimolecular complexes. This may explain HAQ's inhibition of NADPH cytochrome P-450 reductase which contains both FAD and FMN in the prosthetic group (Kharasch and Novak, 1984).

Despite being poor substrates for metabolism by NADPH cytochrome P-450 reductase both DHAD and HAQ have been reported to give an ESR detectable semiquinone radical signal, $g = 2.0036–2.0042$, when incubated under anaerobic conditions with NADPH and liver microsomes from rat (Sinha et al., 1983), mouse (Basra et al., 1984) and human (Basra et al., 1985). A semiquinone radical signal is also formed by DHAD and HAQ incubated under anaerobic conditions with mouse liver nuclei and NADPH (Basra et al., 1984). A feature of the ESR signal obtained by enzymatic reduction of DHAD and HAQ is that, unlike anthracyclines where the signal appears within 1–2 min of starting the incubation, it takes 15–20 min for the DHAD or HAQ semiquinone radical signal to appear (Basra et al., 1984; Sinha et al., 1983). The delay has been attributed to formation of the semiquinone radical from the hydroquinone following two electron reduction of the bis(substituted aminoalkylamino)anthraquinone (Sinha et al., 1983). However, NADPH-cytochrome P-450 reductase is an obligate one-electron transferring enzymes (Mason,

1979) and the delay may simply represent the time it takes for the semiquinone radical to reach to detectable concentrations.

Nguyen and Gutierrez (1990) have suggested that the free radical signal obtained upon incubation of DHAD with microsomes and NADPH may in fact be due to oxidation of DHAD. These authors found no free radical formation upon incubation of DHAD with purified NADP-cytochrome P-450 reductase and NADPH but there was free radical formation when incubated with horseradish peroxidase and hydrogen peroxide. Reszka et al. (1989) identified the product of horseradish peroxidase catalyzed oxidation of DHAD as a substituted hexahydronaphtho[2,3-f]-quinoxaline-7,12-dione in which one side chain has cyclized to the chromophore. The initial oxidation of DHAD is irreversible but the cyclic metabolite can undergo reversible oxidation to the unstable fully oxidized diimino compound (Kolodziejczyk et al., 1988). Admixture of the fully oxidized diimino compound with the reduced cyclic metabolites generates an ESR detectable radical cation by disproportionation-comproportionation.

4.4.2. *Side Chain Metabolism*

DHAD breaks down in plasma or buffer with a half-life of about 24 hr by an oxidative process that is prevented by low pH and ascorbic acid (Reynolds et al., 1981). The breakdown products of DHAD have not been identified but appear to be different to the metabolites formed in vivo. Reynolds et al. (1981) suggested that spontaneous DHAD breakdown is due to oxidation of the phenylenediamine function of the substituted anthraquinone ring to a quinoneimine. Ehninger et al. (1984) studied DHAD metabolism by perfused rat liver and found that 26% of the DHAD was excreted in the bile, 80% as a major metabolite with two minor metabolites. In a preliminary account of a study using ^{14}C-labeled DHAD (the position of the label was not specified) Avramis (1982) reported an unidentified metabolite of DHAD in the plasma, urine and bile of rat. Ten to 21% of the radioactivity was excreted in the bile over 3 hr and 8% in urine over 72 hr. Chiccarelli et al. (1984) used (side chain-^{14}C)-DHAD in rat and found that biliary excretion of radioactivity was 32% of the dose over 51 hr and urinary excretion 7% over 48 hr. Half the radioactivity, in both cases, was unchanged drug. Lu et al. (1984) reported that in beagle dog given [2-hydroxyethyl-^{14}C]-DHAD only 65% of the radioactivity in plasma was unchanged drug. In this study urinary excretion of total radioactivity was 4.9% of the dose over 48 hr, with almost half the activity as unchanged DHAD. Biliary excretion of total radioactivity was 4% of the dose over 5 hr, with 75% as unchanged DHAD. Wolf et al. (1986) have reported that when DHAD is incubated with UDPGA and hepatic microsomes from rats pretreated with Araclor 1254 or with 3-methylcholanthrene to increase the levels of glucuronyl transferase, a glucuronide conjugate of DHAD is formed. Glucuronide conjugation was presumed to have occurred on one of the N atoms of the DHAD side chains. Glucuronide metabolites of DHAD have not been found in vivo (Smyth et al., 1984, 1986).

Bile appears to be the major route for elimination of DHAD and metabolites in human. Alberts et al. (1985a,b) reported that 18% of the radioactivity in a patient given [side chain ^{14}C]-DHAD was excreted in the feces over 5 days. Savaraj et al. (1982a,b) found that only 5.0% of a dose of [2-hydroxyethyl-^{14}C]-DHAD was excreted in the bile over 96 hr but this patient had abnormal liver function. Urinary excretion of DHAD is low and ranges from 3–6% of the dose (Alberts et al., 1985a,b; Ehninger et al., 1985b; Macpherson et al., 1984; Savaraj et al., 1982a,b; Smyth et al., 1984). Polar metabolites has been reported in the bile (Savaraj et al., 1982a,b) and in the urine (Alberts et al., 1983, 1985a; Chiccarelli et al., 1986; Ehninger et al., 1985a,b; MacPherson et al., 1984; Smyth et al., 1984) of patients receiving DHAD. Smyth and his colleagues (Macpherson et al., 1984; Smyth et al., 1984, 1986) found that β-glucuronidase or sulfatase treatment of urine of patients receiving DHAD did not change the amount of two polar metabolites they detected indicating that these metabolites, at least, were not glucuronide or sulfate conjugates. Ehninger et al. (1985b) used HPLC and comparison with reference compounds to identify two of four colored urinary metabolites of DHAD as the mono- and dicarboxylic acid derivatives resulting from oxidation of the terminal hydroxyl groups of the side chains of DHAD. The urine of patients given DHAD collected over 48 hr contained 4.4% of the dose as unchanged DHAD, 0.5% as the dicarboxylic acid metabolite and 0.3% as the monocarboxylic acid metabolite (Ehninger et al., 1985a). Chiccarelli et al. (1986) used HPLC and mass spectrometry together with comparison to reference compounds, to identify the mono- and dicarboxylic acid metabolites of DHAD in patient urine. Both the mono- and dicarboxylic acid derivatives of DHAD were inactive when tested for antitumor activity against murine leukemia L1210.

4.4.3. *Anthraquinone Ring Metabolism*

Although no anthraquinone ring modified metabolites of bis(substituted aminoalkylamino)anthracenediones have been reported there is a precedent for the formation of such metabolites. Martin et al. (1983) studied the metabolism of a closely related compound 1-methylaminoanthraquinone (MAAQ), an intermediate material in vat dye synthesis, in sheep. Analysis of the urine using TLC, mass spectrometry and NMR techniques showed products resulting from three pathways of metabolism: *N*-demethylation, C-2 and C-4 ring hydroxylation and glucuronide formation. The predominant urinary metabolite of MAAQ was the glucuronide conjugate of 2-hydroxy-1-amino-anthraquinone which formed 19% of an oral dose over 96 hr, with a further 5.4% as the glucuronide conjugate of unchanged MAAQ and 1.2% as the glucuronide conjugate of 1-aminoanthraquinone. Parent MAAQ, 1-aminoanthraquinone and 2- and 4-hydroxy-1-aminoanthraquinone each formed less than 1% of the administered dose. It remains to be seen whether ring hydroxylation of bis(substituted aminoalkylamino)anthracenediones can occur. Clearly, 4-hydroxylation of 1,4-bis(substituted aminoalkylamino)anthracenediones is not possible and steric hindrance may prevent hydroxylation at position C-2.

A perplexing study has been reported by Wolf et al. (1986) who found that DHAD incubated with rat liver microsomes, NADPH and glutathione formed two unidentified metabolites. Without the added glutathione no metabolites were formed. Metabolism was inhibited by metyrapone and carbon monoxide which led the authors to suggest that the initial step in metabolism of DHAD involved cytochrome P-450. Metabolism of DHAD was not, however, induced by pretreating the animals with phenobarbital, 3-methylcholanthrene or Aroclor 1254, suggesting that if an isozyme of cytochrome P-450 was involved in metabolism it was a form not induced by these compounds. Inhibition of metabolite formation by 1-chloro-2,4-dinitrobenzene, a substrate for microsomal and cytosolic glutathione transferase, suggested that the second step of metabolism might be by conjugation with glutathione. Adding cytosol as a source of glutathione transferase did not, however, affect the rate of metabolite formation.

4.4.4. *Pharmacokinetics*

DHAD is rapidly taken up from the plasma into tissues from where it is slowly released for elimination, mostly as metabolites, in the bile and to a lesser extent in the urine. The plasma elimination half-life for unchanged DHAD in rat is 87 hr (Avramis, 1982) and in beagle dog 28 hr (Lu et al., 1984). The large apparent volume of distribution of DHAD, 12.1 L/kg in rat and 27 L/kg in dog indicate extensive tissue uptake or binding of the drug. Tissue distribution studies conducted in dog 5 hr after giving [2-hydroxy-ethyl-^{14}C]-DHAD showed highest radioactivity in the liver, with 50% as unchanged drug, followed by the small intestine, kidneys, and lung, spleen and stomach (Lu et al., 1984).

The plasma elimination half-life of DHAD in patients has been reported to be from 17–46 hr (Alberts et al., 1983, 1985a,b; Macpherson et al., 1984; Savaraj et al., 1982a,b; Stewart et al., 1982; Smyth et al., 1984, 1986; Van Belle et al., 1986). Ehninger et al. (1985a,b), using an improved HPLC assay with increased sensitivity reported a terminal half-life for DHAD of 215 hr. The apparent volume of distribution of DHAD in human is 2000 L/m^2 (approximately 51 L/kg) (Alberts et al., 1983, 1985a,b; Ehninger et al., 1985b; Van Belle et al., 1986), again suggesting extensive distribution of DHAD into a deep tissue compartment. There is a report of detectable levels of DHAD in the heart, liver, spleen and kidney of a patient who died nine days after the last dose of DHAD (Roboz et al., 1984). Alberts et al. (1985a,b) found that 15% of a dose of radioactivity was present in the tissues of a patient who died 35 days after receiving [side chain ^{14}C]-DHAD, with the highest activity in liver, pancreas, thyroid, spleen and heart.

HAQ appears to be less well taken up by tissues and much more rapidly eliminated than DHAD. Studies in dog have shown a terminal plasma half-life for HAQ of 115 min and an apparent volume of distribution of 0.69 L/kg (equivalent to the volume of total body water) with 24% of the administered dose being excreted unchanged in urine over 5 hr and 39% in bile (Lu and Loo, 1980). Tissue levels of HAQ 5 hr after administering the drug were found to be highest in the liver followed by the kidney, pancreas, small intestine, stomach and spleen. Studies in patients have shown a rapid plasma elimination of HAQ with a half-life of 110 min and a volume of distribution of 26 L/m^2 (approximately 0.67 L/kg) (Gams et al., 1985). In this study urinary excretion of HAQ over 48 hr accounted for 10–33% of the dose (Piccart et al., 1981). No metabolites of HAQ have been reported.

4.5. Metabolism and Antitumor Activity

There are a number of mechanisms that might account for the cytotoxicity of bis(substituted aminoalkylamino)anthraquinones. Most bis(substituted aminoalkylamino)anthraquinones bind to DNA and inhibit DNA and RNA synthesis as would be expected of intercalating agents (Johnson et al., 1979; Lown et al., 1985). However, Bowden et al. (1985) using nucleoid sedimentation techniques have shown that DHAD does not induce changes in DNA supercoiling characteristic of classical intercalating agents but probably binds to the anionic exterior of the DNA. Whatever the mechanism, a poor correlation has been found between the DNA binding of bis(substituted aminoalkylamino)-anthraquinones and cytotoxicity (Johnson et al., 1979) suggesting that some other mechanism is important for cytotoxicity.

The low rate of metabolism of bis(substituted aminoalkylamino)anthraquinones might be thought to eliminate redox cycling as a mechanism of cytotoxicity. However, both DHAD and HAQ can be enzymatically reduced to a semiquinone radical (Basra et al., 1984, 1985; Sinha et al., 1983) and it may be that it is the site of radical formation in the cell rather than the absolute rate which is important for cytotoxicity. Kimler and Cheng (1984) have reported that modulation of intracellular thiol levels in Chinese hamster V79 cells with *N*-ethylmaleimide and cysteamine does not affect the cytotoxicity of DHAD. The authors suggested that free radicals were not involved in the cytotoxicity of DHAD based on their presumption that intracellular thiols protect cells against free radical damage. Duthie and Grant (1989) reached a similar conclusion using human Hep G2 hepatoma cells in which they inhibited glutathione reductase and catalase. There was no effect of inhibiting these enzymes on DHAD cytotoxicity, unlike menadione cytotoxicity which was potentiated. Inhibition of epoxide hydrolase activity potentiated DHAD cytotoxicity to the Hep G2 cells and the authors suggested that DHAD cytotoxicity might involve activation to an epoxide intermediate.

DHAD and HAQ when incubated with cells produce DNA single strand breaks, DNA double strand breaks and protein associated DNA double strand breaks (Bowden et al., 1985; Cohen et al., 1986; Fry et al., 1985; Locher and Meyn, 1983). Incubation of DHAD with isolated tumor cell nuclei in the absence of added NADPH does not give rise to DNA single strand breaks (Bowden et al., 1985). Similar studies were not conducted in the presence of NADPH and it is possible that DHAD-dependent DNA single strand breaks are caused by oxygen radicals formed during metabolism of DHAD. Crespi et al. (1986) have reported that DHAD is an inhibitor of topoisomerase II (Crespi et al., 1986; Smith et al., 1990) which could account for the occurrence of DNA double strand breaks. As with the anthracyclines there is a poor correlation between the frequency of protein associated DNA strand breaks and the level of bis(substituted aminoalkylamino)-anthraquinone cytotoxicity (Bowden et al., 1985). The importance of DNA strand breaks to the cytotoxicity of the bis(substituted aminoalkylamino)-anthraquinones remains to be established.

4.6. Metabolism and Cardiotoxicity

Although preclinical studies in animals showed an almost complete absence of DHAD cardiotoxicity clinical experience has shown that DHAD is cardiotoxic to humans, although probably to a lesser degree than doxorubicin (Dukart et al., 1986; Poirier, 1986). Considerable emphasis has been placed on the decreased formation of oxygen radicals by DHAD incubated with heart subcellular fractions compared to doxorubicin as an explanation for the lower cardiotoxicity of DHAD (Doroshow, 1983a; Doroshow and Davies, 1983, 1986; Kharasch and Novak, 1982a, 1983d; Novak and Kharasch, 1985). HAQ administered to rats does not increase lipid peroxidation, measured by malondialdehyde production, in liver and heart (Patterson et al., 1983). In particular, the dose dependent inhibition by DHAD and HAQ of basal and drug induced lipid peroxidation by heart sarcosomes and NADPH, and by heart mitochondria and NADH has been suggested to be related to the low cardiotoxicity of the bis(substituted aminoalkylamino)anthraquinones (Kharasch and Novak, 1982a, 1983a,b; Mimnaugh et al., 1983). Kharasch and Novak (1983d, 1985) reported that inhibition of lipid peroxidation by DHAD and HAQ was not because of decreased oxygen radical dependent initiation of lipid peroxidation but probably occurred by an inhibition of hydroperoxide-dependent initiation and propagation of lipid peroxidation. Despite the lack of effects of DHAD on cardiac tissue oxygen radical formation and lipid peroxidation Neri et al. (1984) showed that DHAD causes a significant impairment of respiratory control by rat heart slices and a decrease in ATP levels greater than caused by doxorubicin. The emerging picture of DHAD cardiotoxicity in humans without significant experimental oxygen radical formation or lipid peroxidation will necessitate the reevaluation of these processes as mechanisms for cardiotoxicity of all anthraquinone-type compounds.

5. MITOMYCINS

5.1. Historical Perspective

The mitomycin antibiotics were first isolated in 1956 from the culture fluid of *Streptomyces caespitosis* by Hata and his collaborators at the Kitasato Institute, Japan (Hata et al., 1956). Two compounds were isolated designated mitomycins A and B. They proved to be potent antibacterial and antitumor agents but were also very toxic in mice. Two years later Wakaki and his collaborators at the Kyowa Fermentation Institute, Japan, isolated a third mitomycin called mitomycin C from *S. caespitosis*, which had superior antitumor activity and less toxicity than the other mitomycins (Wakaki et al., 1958). Clinical trials established the antitumor activity of mitomycin C and it soon found widespread clinical use in Japan (Frank and Osterberg, 1960). The initial clinical trials of mitomycin C in the U.S.A. proved less promising (Jones, 1959) and the drug was not approved for standard clinical use in the U.S.A. until 1974. In 1960 an *N*-methyl derivative of mitomycin C, designated porfiromycin, was isolated by a group at the Upjohn Company in the U.S.A. from cultures of *S. ardus* (DeBoer et al., 1960). Clinical trials of porfiromycin showed it to be less active than mitomycin C (Izbicki et al., 1972) and it was not marketed. The total synthesis of mitomycins A and C, and porfiromycin was first achieved in 1977 (Fukuyama et al., 1977; Nakatsubo et al., 1977). A large number of semisynthetic analogs of mitomycin C have been prepared (Hodges et al., 1981; Iyengar et al., 1983; Kinoshita et al., 1971). Bradner et al. (1989) report that over 600 analogs of mitomycin C have been synthesized. Promising analogs are those with substituted ethylamines at position C-7, including 7-*N*-(dimethylaminomethylene)-mitomycin C (BMY-25282) (Bradner et al., 1984a), 7-cysteamino-mitomycin C (Bradner et al., 1984b) and various 7-aminoethyldisulfide analogs of mitomycin C (Bradner et al., 1986). 7-*N*-(*p*-hydroxyphenyl)-mitomycin C (KW 2083), which in animal studies was less myelotoxic than the parent compound (Kobayashi et al., 1981), has undergone clinical trial in Japan. Novel mitomycin C delivery forms are under development. For example, Steven et al. (1990) have reported mitomycin C linked to agmatine which binds with high affinity to a cell surface protease (quinidobenzoatase) on the surface of tumor cells. Sahin et al. (1990) reported that specific activation of the prodrug mitomycin A phosphate by a bispecific anti-CD30/anti-alkaline phosphatase monoclonal antibody bound with alkaline phosphatase produced selective toxicity to CD30 positive Hodgkin's lymphoma cell lines. Mitomycin C-conjugated prodrug forms with improved pharmacokinetic properties have been developed. Mitomycin C-dextran conjugates microparticles rapidly accumulate in the liver through binding to the surface hepatocytes (Nakane et al., 1988).

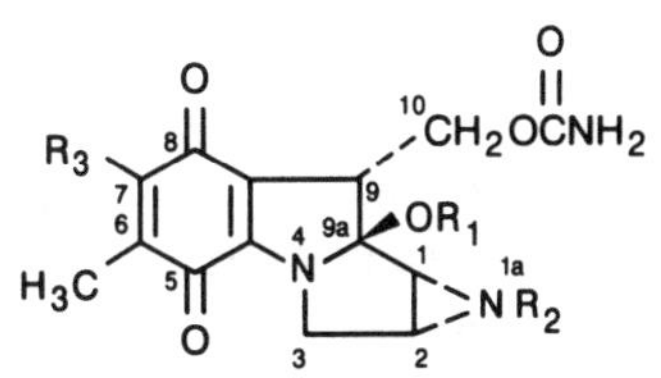

Compound	R_1	R_2	R_3
Mitomycin A	CH_3	H	OCH_3
Mitomycin B	H	CH_3	OCH_3
Mitomycin C	CH_3	H	NH_2
Porfiromycin	CH_3	CH_3	NH_2
KW 2083	CH_3	H	HN-⌬-OH
BMY-25282	CH_3	H	$N=CH-N(CH_3)_2$
BMY-25067	CH_3	H	$NH-CH_2-S-S$-⌬-NO_2
RR-150	CH_3	H	$NH-CH_2-CH_2-SH$

FIG. 15. Structure of some mitomycins.

5.2. Structure–Activity Relationships

The complete chemical structure of all the mitomycins was established in 1962 by Webb and his colleagues from Lederle Laboratories, U.S.A. (Webb et al., 1962) (Fig. 15). These structures were confirmed by X-ray crystallographic studies (Tulinsky, 1962) and by later independent analysis (Stevens et al., 1964). Structure–antitumor activity relationships have shown that the intact mitosane structure is necessary for activity. Myelosuppression, antitumor activity and potency do not parallel each other from one analog to the next. *N*-1a alkyl substitution (porfiromycin type compounds) offers little advantage and usually a loss of potency. A low quinone reduction potential which promotes facile enzymatic reduction, good water solubility and low lipophilicity enhance antitumor activity (Bradner et al., 1984b; Kinoshita et al., 1971; Remers, 1979a,c; Remers and Schempman, 1974).

5.3. Clinical Activity

As a single agent mitomycin C has shown activity against breast, stomach, pancreatic, head and neck cancers, and possible activity against lung, ovary, biliary tree and cervix cancers (Crooke and Bradner, 1976). Responses to mitomycin C are usually of short duration. Mitomycin C now is almost always used in combination with other agents, for example in the FAM regimen (5-fluorouracil, doxorubicin, mitomycin C). The contribution of mitomycin C to the various drug combination regimens has, in general, not been adequately defined (Doll et al., 1985). Mitomycin C as a single agent has found recent use for treating superficial bladder cancer by intravesicular instillation (Aeikens et al., 1982). The principal dose-limiting toxicity of mitomycin C is delayed cumulative myelosuppression. This toxicity discouraged early clinical use of the drug but the use of high dose intermittent regimens and other refinements in dose scheduling have resulted in a decrease in mylesuppression accompanying the use of mitomycin C. In many regimens an automatic dose reduction of mitomycin C is employed after two full doses. Other toxicities of mitomycin C include alopecia, rashes, gastrointestinal toxicities and if the drug accidently extravasates from the site of injection, tissue necrosis. Less frequent but potentially lethal toxicities are pulmonary fibrosis and microangiopathic hemolytic anemia with renal failure (Doll et al., 1985). In many respects mitomycin C must still be regarded as an investigational agent and is not recommended for use in the adjuvant setting. The early indications from clinical studies of 7-*N*-(*p*-hydroxylphenyl)mitomycin are that the dose-limiting toxicity is unpredictable myelosuppression with other toxicities similar to those of mitomycin C (Meguro et al., 1984).

5.4. Metabolism

5.4.1. *In Vitro Metabolism*

Early studies by Schwartz (1962) showed that rat liver homogenate and NADPH under anaerobic conditions catalyzed the disappearance of mitomycin C. Under aerobic conditions there was no loss of mitomycin C and NADH supported the anaerobic reaction poorly. The major part (87%) of the NADPH-dependent activity resided in the microsomal fraction. Kidney, spleen, brain and muscle homogenates were less active than liver homogenate at metabolizing mitomycin C (Schwartz and Philips, 1961). In 1964 Iyer and Szybalski, using bacterial lysates, showed that an NADPH-dependent microsomal enzyme activated mitomycin C to an alkylating species that cross-linked DNA. The activity was not inhibited by dicumarol, an inhibitor of quinone reductases. This remained the only work on the metabolism of mitomycin C for several years. Beginning in 1979 Sartorelli and his colleagues (Kennedy and Sartorelli, 1979; Kennedy et al., 1982) extended these original observations and found that NADPH-fortified mouse liver microsomes and nuclei catalyzed the disappearance of mitomycin C with the formation of an alkylating species that could be measured by reaction with 4-(*p*-nitrobenzyl)-pyridine. As before mitomycin C disappearance occurred only under anaerobic conditions. Phenobarbital pretreatment, but not pretreatment of the rats with 3-methylcholanthrene or ethanol, increased the rate of mitomycin C disappearance. The reaction was inhibited by carbon monoxide and the inhibition was reversed by light at a wavelength of 450 nm, suggesting the involvement of cytochrome P-450. Studies with a reconstituted system consisting of NADPH, NADPH-cytochrome P-450 reductase, cytochrome P-450 and phospholipid also showed conversion of mitomycin C to alkylating metabolites under anaerobic conditions (Kennedy et al., 1982). It was reported that neither NADPH-cytochrome P-450 reductase alone nor in combination with phospholipid, or substitution of cytochrome P-450 with cytochrome C resulted in activation of mitomycin C. The metabolism of mitomycin C by sonicates of two tumor cell lines, Sarcoma 180 and EMT6 mammary carcinoma, was also studied (Kennedy et al., 1980a). Both preparations activated mitomycin C to alkylating species in the presence of NADPH under anaerobic but not under aerobic conditions, in a reaction that was inhibited by carbon monoxide. The findings were considered to be of particular significance since in EMT6 carcinoma cells mitomycin C was considerably more toxic to chronically hypoxic cells than to cells maintained under oxygenated conditions (Kennedy et al., 1980a; Rockwell et al., 1982). Although Kennedy et al. (1982) reported there was no metabolism of mitomycin C to alkylating metabolites by purified NADPH-cytochrome P-450 reductase, Komiyama et al. (1979b) had earlier reported that mitomycin C disappeared from anaerobic incubations of purified NADPH-cytochrome P-450 reductase and NADPH, or xanthine oxidase and xanthine. Pan et al. (1984) confirmed that there was metabolism of mitomycin C by purified NADPH-cytochrome P-450 reductase and NADPH, and by xanthine oxidase and NADH. Further studies by Sartorelli and his colleagues (Keyes et al., 1984a) showed that purified NADPH cytochrome P-450 reductase could indeed metabolize mitomycin C under anaerobic conditions, although the reaction was increased up to 100% by the presence of cytochrome P-450 in a 1:1 ratio with the reductase. In contrast to the earlier studies carbon monoxide did not inhibit mitomycin C metabolism by cell sonicates. Vromans et al. (1990) also found that while purified NADPH-cytochrome P-450 reductase could reduce mitomycin C in a fully reconstituted system containing cytochrome P-450b or P-450c the reductase was much more effective. It appears, therefore, that cytochrome P-450 is not directly involved in the bioactivation of mitomycin C, but when present under certain in vitro conditions cytochrome P-450 may act to facilitate the metabolism of mitomycin C by NADPH-cytochrome P-450 reductase.

The other flavoenzyme whose role in the metabolism of mitomycin C has received considerable attention is quinone reductase. Keyes et al. (1984a) reported that inhibition of quinone reductase with dicumarol increased the formation of alkylating metabolites by sonicates of EMT6 carcinoma and V79 lung tumor cells and NADPH. These workers suggested that metabolism of mitomycin C by quinone reductase might protect cells from the cytotoxicity of mitomycin C by reducing the intracellular concentrations of the drug, as has been reported for other quinones (see Section 2.4). Evidence supporting this suggestion is the finding that dicumarol increases the toxicity of mitomycin C to hypoxic EMT6 carcinoma cells, although it decreases mitomycin C's toxicity to the euoxic cells (Keyes et al., 1985). Experiments with transplanted EMT6 tumor cells in mice have shown that dicumarol combined with radiation increases the toxicity of mitomycin C to hypoxic tumor cells without increasing the hematologic toxicity (Rockwell et al., 1989). Studies using purified rat and human quinone reductase have failed to show metabolism of mitomycin C by the enzyme (Schlager and Powis, 1988; Workman et al., 1989). Siegel et al. (1990) have reported that the metabolism of mitomycin C by purified rat quinone reductase increases at low pH and is over 10-fold greater at pH 5.8 than at pH 7.4. It remains to be determined whether metabolism of mitomycin C by quinone reductase can occur at intracellular pH. It is possible that dicumarol has other effects on cell metabolism that account for the increased toxicity of mitomycin C. Hodnick and Sartorelli (1991) have reported that NADH-cytochrome b_5 reductase can catalyze the reduction of mitomycin C and that this reduction is inhibited by dicumarol.

It is not known whether all mitomycins undergo equally facile enzymatic reduction. Work by Patrick et al. (1964) has shown that porfiromycin is much less readily chemically reduced than mitomycin B. Since both compounds have a similar redox potential it is not clear why differences should exist in their susceptibility to reduction.

Identification of the metabolites formed during metabolism of mitomycin C by the rat liver microsomes and NADPH under anaerobic conditions was reported by Tomasz and Lipman in 1981. The study was aided by previous work by the same authors on the spontaneous activation of mitomycin C to alkylating species at low pH in phosphate containing media which had provided a series of well characterized phosphate alkylation products (Tomasz and Lipman, 1979). Incubation of mitomycin C with NADPH and rat liver microsomes in phosphate buffer under anaerobic conditions, with exposure to air after the reaction was complete, gave five major metabolites identified as 1,2-*cis*- and 1,2-*trans*-2,7-diamino-mitosene-1-phosphates, 1,2-*cis*- and 1,2-*trans*-diaminono-1-hydroxymitosenes, and 2,7-diaminomitosene (Fig. 16). When inorganic phosphate was replaced by 5′-uridylic acid as the added nucleophile, 5′-uridylate alkylation products were obtained. Approximately equal amounts of 1,2-*cis*- and 1,2-*trans*-isomers were formed. These studies provided the first direct evidence that mitomycin C could function as a

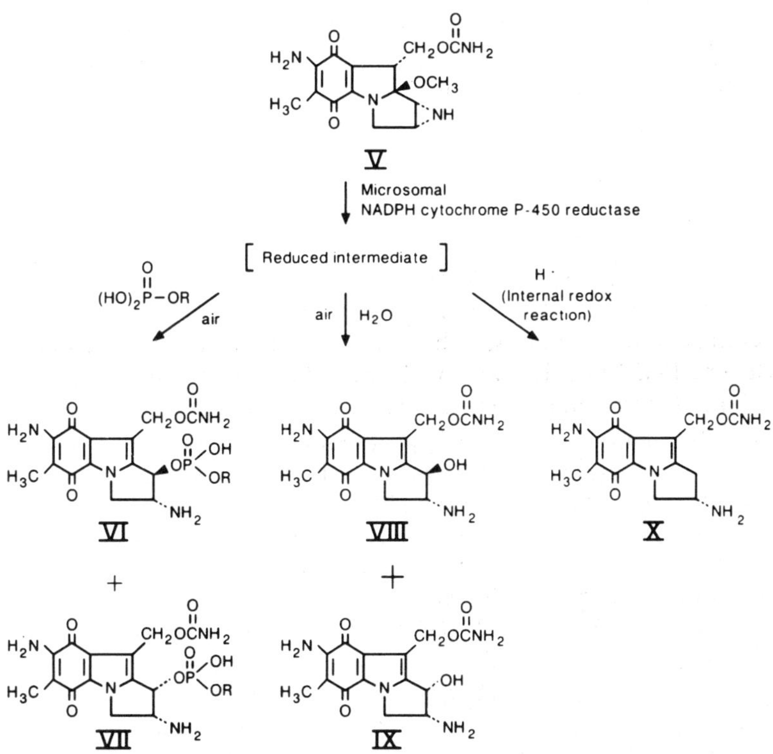

FIG. 16. Products formed by enzymatic reduction of mitomycin C (V) by rat liver microsomes and NADPH under anaerobic conditions. VI, 1,2-*trans*- and VII, 1,2-*cis*-2,7-diaminomitosene-1-phosphates, VIII, 1,2-*trans* and IX, 1,2-*cis*-2,7-diamino-1-hydroxymitosenes, and X, 2,7-diamino-mitosene (Tomasz and Lipman, 1981).

reductively activated alkylating agent. Pan et al. (1984) used HPLC followed by mass spectrometry to identify three major products of anaerobic mitomycin C metabolism by purified NADPH cytochrome P-450 reductase and NADPH, and by xanthine oxidase and NADH. They were 1,2-*cis* and 1,2-*trans*-2,7-diamino-1-hydroxymitosenes, at a ratio of 1:2 to 1:3, and 2,7-diaminomitosene. A further three metabolites were formed only in phosphate buffer and alkaline phosphate digestion showed two of them to be 1,2-*cis* and 1,2-*trans*-2,7-diaminomitosene-1-phosphates. A number of additional unidentified mitomycin C metabolites were seen. These may have been secondary metabolites of the five primary metabolites which were shown to be substrates for metabolism by the purified enzymes. Peterson and Fisher (1986) used yeast NADPH:(acceptor)-oxidoreductase (Old Yellow Enzyme, E.C.1.6.99.1) and NADPH to anaerobically reduce mitomycin C. HPLC and comparison to reference compounds was used to quantify and identify the products of metabolism as 45% *cis*- and 30% *trans*-2-hydroxy-2,7-diaminomitosene, 8% 2,7-diaminomitosene, and 5% as another product thought to be an NADPH-mitosene adduct whose formation had been suggested by Tomasz and Lipman (1981). There were also some minor unidentified products.

It will be noted that in Fig. 16 the exact form of the reduced mitomycin C intermediate is not specified. Some workers have suggested that the biologically active form of mitomycin C is the two electron-reduced hydroquinone. Iyer and Szybalski first proposed in 1964 that mitomycin C was reduced to the hydroquinone followed by the spontaneous loss of the C-9a methoxy group as methanol to give an indole hydroquinone intermediate. The indole hydroquinone intermediate was then seen as acting as a bifunctional alkylating agent with nucleophilic attack resulting in displacement of the C-1 aziridine and C-10 carbamate leaving groups. Moore (Moore, 1977; Moore and Czerniak, 1981) further developed this idea and suggested that after the initial two-electron reduction and formation of the indole hydroquinone intermediate the C-1 aziridine ring opens and by an elimination process gives a quinonemethide, followed by nucleophilic attack at C-1 and C-10 to give mitosene hydroquinone adducts (Fig. 17A). There is considerable evidence to support the reactivity of mitomycin C at the C-1 position (Tomasz and Lipman, 1979, 1981; Pan et al., 1984) but much less evidence for reactivity at the C-10 position. Hornemann et al. (1979) reported formation of a 1,10-bis-substituted adduct upon reductive activation of mitomycin C by sodium dithionite or Pd/C plus H_2 in the presence of the nucleophile ethylxanthate. No C-10 monosubstituted adduct was seen in this study which is consistent with the pathway proposed by Moore (1977) of a reactive center at C-1 preceding decarbamylation at C-10. Zein and Kohn (1986) presented evidence for both electrophilic and nucleophilic nature of the C-10 position in mitomycin C. Instead of direct substitution of the C-10 carbamate group by a nucleophile they showed initial loss of the C-10 carbamate group to form an iminium ion with a C-10 exocyclic methylene group across which the DNA adds. Recent evidence suggest that bifunctional reductive alkylation of DNA by mitomycin C may occur as a concerted reaction without involving the monofunctional adduct as an intermediate (Pan et al., 1986). Peterson and Fisher (1986) have presented evidence that autocatalytic oxidation of the C-1 mitosene hydroquinone adduct to the level of mitosene quinone stabilizes C-1 adduct formation while effectively preventing C-10 adduct formation which requires the hydroquinone oxidation state. In the reaction studied by Peterson and Fisher (1986) the majority of mitomycin C consumption was by an autocatalytic process following initial enzymatic reduction by yeast NADPH:(acceptor)oxido-reductase and NADPH. Support for the formation of a mitosene quinone from mitomycin C as proposed by Peterson and Fisher (1986) is found in the electrochemical studies of Rao et al. (1977a,b). Here, it was shown that mitomycin C hydroquinone has a very short half-life, around 0.07 sec, and rapidly and irreversibly breaks down to a second reducible species with a redox potential virtually identical to that of mitomycin C. The proposed mechanism involves loss of the C-9a methoxy group of mitomycin C to give an indole hydroquinone intermediate (compound XI, Fig. 17), followed by rapid aziridine ring opening and oxidation to the mitosene quinone form. Studies of the acid-catalyzed conversion of mitomycins to mitosenes using deutrium incorporation methods has provided evidence for spontaneous elimination of the C-9a methoxy group to form an aziridinomitosene (Iyengar and Remers, 1985). The first step in the acid-catalyzed reaction is protonation of the C-9a methoxy group which leaves as methanol to form an immonium ion (Fig. 18). Loss of the hydrogen at C-9 then gives an aziridinomitosene as suggested by Underberg and Lingeman (1983). Pulse radiolysis studies by Hoey et al. (1988) have provided evidence for reductive activation of mitomycin C occurring through the hydroquinone.

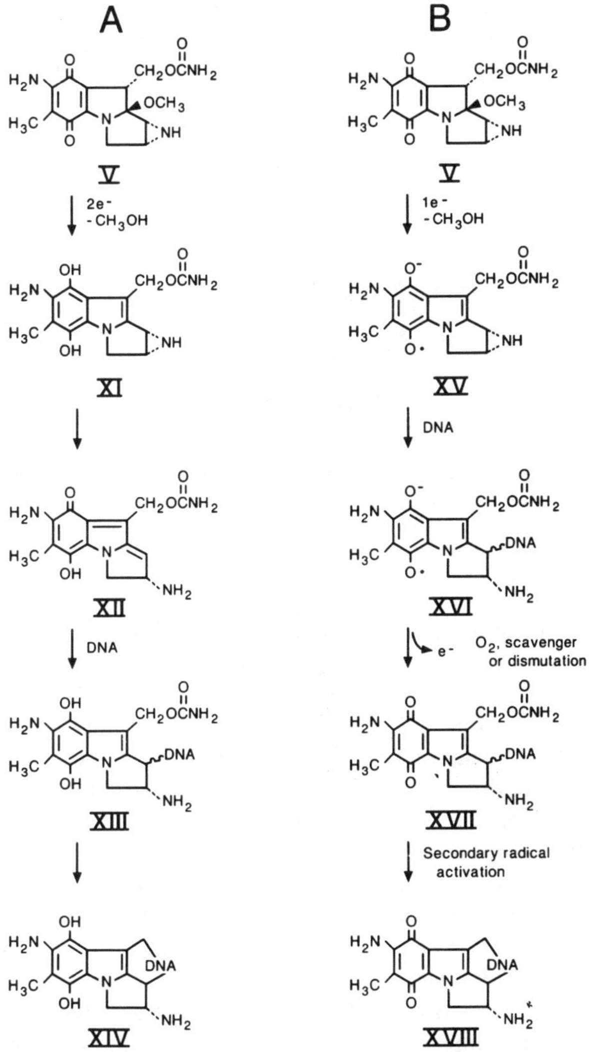

FIG. 17. Proposed pathways for biological activation of mitomycin C (V) involving (A), two-electron reduction to the hydroquinone with spontaneous loss of methanol to give an indole hydroquinone intermediate (XI) and, after aziridine ring opening, a quinonemethide (XII). Nucleophilic addition gives first a monofunctional (XIII) and then by intramolecular SN_2 displacement of carbamate, a bifunctional adduct (XIV) (Moore and Czerniak, 1981). (B), Single-electron reduction to the semiquinone with spontaneous loss of methanol to give an indole semiquinone (XV). Nucleophilic addition gives a monofunctional semiquinone adduct (XVI) which, after conversion to the quinone (XVII) undergoes secondary radical activation to a bifunctional adduct (XVIII).

As an alternative to the activation of mitomycin C through two-electron reduction to the hydroquinone, some workers have proposed that single-electron reduction serves to activate mitomycin C (Nagata and Matsuyama, 1970; Pan et al., 1984; Sartorelli, 1986) (Fig. 17). This suggestion is based on the observation that enzymes that active mitomycin C, namely, NADPH-cytochrome P-450 reductase and xanthine oxidase under the conditions employed, preferentially catalyze one-electron reduction of quinones (see Section 2.2). Under aerobic conditions enzymatic reduction of mitomycin C the semiquinone radical leads to redox cycling and formation of radicals (see Section 5.4.2) but under anaerobic conditions there is the formation of an alkylating species (Keyes et al., 1984a). It has been suggested (Pan et al., 1984; Sartorelli, 1986) that the semiquinone radical spontaneously looses a C-9a methoxy group to form an indole semiquinone radical that can undergo nucleophilic attack at the C-1 position to form a monofunctional mitomycin C adduct (Fig. 17B). Recent chemical evidence supports the notion that loss of the C-9a methoxy group

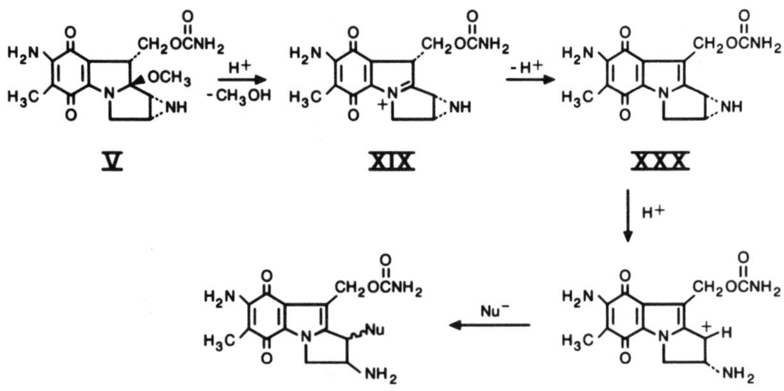

V XIX XXX XXXI XXXII

FIG. 18. Acid catalyzed conversion of mitomycin C (V) to mitosenes. It begins with protonation of the 9-methoxy group, which leaves as methanol and forms an immonium ion (XIX). Loss of the C-9 hydrogen then gives an aziridinomitosene (XXX). Protonation of the aziridine nitrogen results in ring opening to give a C-1 carbonium ion (XXXI) and the nucleophile (Nu) adds at C-1 to give a mitosene (XXXII) (Underberg and Lingeman, 1983).

occurs at the level of the semiquinone rather than the hydroquinone. Failure to recover the parent mitomycin by reoxidation after chemical reduction had been taken as evidence that mitomycin hydroquinones have a short lifetime and spontaneously loose the C-9a methoxy group (Remers, 1979b). However, Danishefsky and his colleagues (Danishefsky and Giufolini, 1984; Danishefsky and Egbertson, 1986) showed that it was possible to recover the parent mitomycin following chemical reduction of *N*-methylmitomycin A, mitomycin B and mitomycin C. Furthermore, when mitomycin quinone and hydroquinone were present together a mitomycin semiquinone radical was formed by comproportionation and it was the radical which lost the C-9a methoxy group (Danishefsky and Egbertson, 1986). Furthermore, evidence supporting a one-electron activation pathway of mitomycin C is provided by electrochemical studies where one-electron reduction of mitomycin C gives products very similar to those reported for enzymatic reduction whereas two-electron electrochemical reduction of mitomycin C gives products of the 10-decarbamoyl-mitosene type that are not seen with biochemical preparations (Andrews et al., 1983, 1986). Crosslinking of DNA by mitomycin C may involve secondary enzymatic reduction of the monofunctional *cis* or *trans* adduct of DNA to a second semiquinone radical and nucleophilic attack by the DNA, presumably at the C-10 position with loss of the carbamate side chain (Pan et al., 1984). Finally, it has to be considered that the single electron reduced semiquinone radical could undergo disproportionation to the hydroquinone so that alkylation might still proceed by the two-electron pathway shown in Fig. 17A.

5.4.2. *Free Radical Formation*

Like other quinones mitomycin C can undergo chemical and enzymatic single electron reduction to form a semiquinone radical. The semiquinone radical can then react with oxygen to form oxygen radicals and regenerate mitomycin C. Nagata and Matsuyama showed in 1970 that chemical reduction of an aqueous solution of mitomycin C by sodium borohydride under anaerobic conditions resulted in the formation of an intermediate species with a lifetime of 10 sec and a red shift in the maximum absorption to 518 nm. Flow ESR spectroscopy was used to demonstrate that the intermediate species was the mitomycin C semiquinone radical with an ESR signal of $g = 2.0034$. Studies by Lown et al. (1978) of the mitomycin C semiquinone radical formed by chemical reduction of an aqueous solution of mitomycin C with sodium borohydride in air gave a 36 line ESR spectrum, $g = 2.0046$ (Fig. 19). Similar studies using mitomycin B gave a 17 ESR line spectrum (Fig. 19). Early studies showed that mitomycin C stimulated NADPH oxidation and oxygen utilization by the hepatic microsomal fraction (Bachur et al., 1978b, 1982b; Handa and Sato, 1975, 1976) and that the enzyme responsible was NADPH-cytochrome P-450 reductase

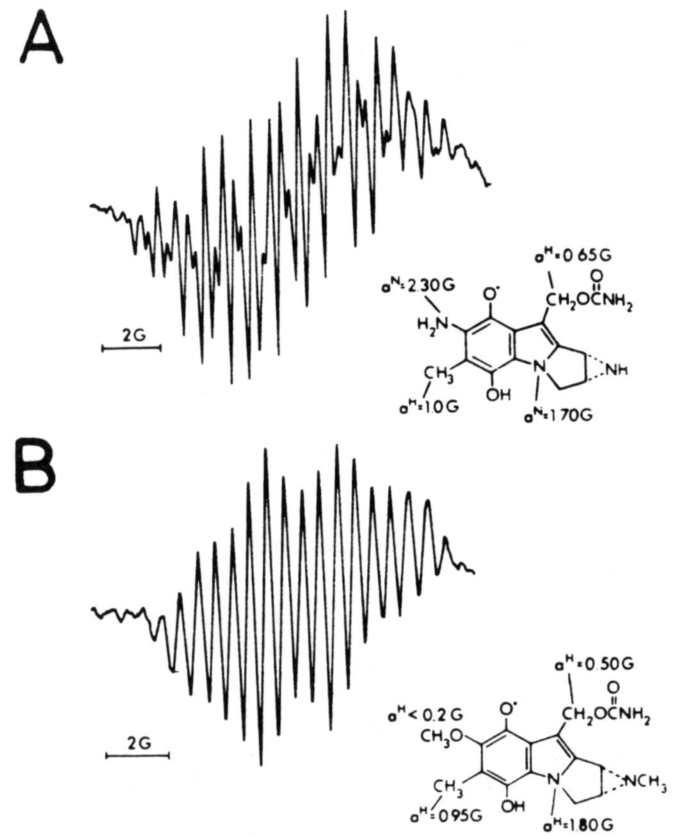

FIG. 19. Electron spin resonance signals of (A) mitomycin C, 2 mM and (B) mitomycin B, 1.5 mM in 10% dimethylsulfoxide and 60 mM potassium phosphate buffer, pH 7.0, reduced with a four-fold excess of sodium borohydride under aerobic conditions. Inserts are the computer calculated splitting constants for the mitomycins. Reprinted from Lown et al. (1978), with permission of the authors and the copyright holder, National Research Council of Canada, Ottawa.

(Handa and Sato, 1976). However, for a long time it was not possible to demonstrate an ESR signal of mitomycin C semiquinone radical during the enzymatic reduction of mitomycin C (Bachur et al., 1978b; Handa and Sato, 1976; Sato et al., 1977). An early report of a short lived mitomycin C signal by Bachur et al. (1979) was, in all probability, the ESR spectrum of NADPH-cytochrome P-450 reductase (Kalyanaraman et al., 1980). In 1980 Kalyanaraman et al. reported a transient ESR signal, $g = 2.0035$, formed by hepatic microsomal reduction of mitomycin C by NADPH under anaerobic conditions. The signal disappeared within 4 min which presumably explains why other workers had not been able to detect an ESR signal. Pan et al. (1984) later confirmed the formation of an ESR signal during enzymatic reduction of mitomycin C under anaerobic conditions.

Oxygen radical formation during microsomal NADPH-dependent redox cycling of mitomycin C was first shown by Handa and Sato (1975) who used initiation of sulfite oxidation to measure superoxide anion radical formation. Chemical assays have subsequently been used to show formation of the hydroxyl radical during redox cycling of mitomycin C (Doroshow, 1981; Komiyama et al., 1982, 1985; Pritsos et al., 1985; Tobia et al., 1985). An ESR detectable DMPO-superoxide radical adduct signal is obtained when mitomycin is incubated with hepatic microsomes, NADPH and DMPO under aerobic conditions (Kalyanaraman et al., 1980). A PBN-hydroxyl radical adduct signal is obtained, when mitomycin C is reduced under anaerobic conditions in the presence of PBN, either chemically (Lown et al., 1978), or enzymatically by NADPH and hepatic microsomes (Kalyanaraman et al., 1980) or NADPH and purified NADPH-cytochrome P-450 reductase (Hamana et al., 1985; Komiyama et al., 1982). Superoxide dismutase (Kalyanaraman et al., 1980) and catalase (Komiyama et al., 1982) block formation of the

PBN-hydroxyl radical adduct suggesting that hydroxyl radical is formed from superoxide anion radical generated by redox cycling of mitomcyin C. Unlike the anthracyclines, mitomycin C bound to DNA can still be enzymatically (Sinha and Chignell, 1979) as well as chemically reduced (Lown et al., 1978) to give oxygen radicals. This is important when considering the possible role of oxygen radicals in the biological activity of mitomycin C (see Section 5.4.4). Mitomycin C stimulates lipid peroxidation when incubated with pulmonary microsomes and NADPH through generation of reaction oxygen species (Trush et al., 1982).

5.4.3. *In Vivo Metabolism*

Early studies by Schwartz and Philips (1961) using a biological assay for mitomycin C showed that the drug disappeared rapidly from the plasma of dog and rat, with an approximate half-life of 7 min and that one-third or less of the drug was recovered unchanged in the urine. Five minutes after administration of mitomycin C to guinea pig, the kidney, eye, tongue, heart, lung and muscle contained appreciable amounts of drug, but none was detected in brain, spleen or liver (Fujita, 1971). Studies by Fujiwara et al. (1982) employing an enzyme immunoassay to quantify mitomycin C showed that about 80% of the drug was removed from serum of rat within the first 10 min after administration, followed by slower removal of the remaining drug. Approximately 25% of the drug was excreted unchanged in the urine in 1 hr. A number of specific HPLC techniques are now available for the analysis of mitomycin C (Beijnen et al., 1986) and have been used to study the pharmacokineics of mitomycin C in animals and human. Studies by van Hazel and Kovach (1982) in rabbit showed rapid plasma elimination of mitomycin C with a distributive half-life of 2 min and an elimination half-life of 9 min. Urinary excretion of mitomycin C was 14% in 4 hr. Beagle dog shows three phases of mitomycin C plasma elimination with half-lives of 2, 8 and 53 min. There have been a number of studies of mitomycin C pharmacokinetics in human using HPLC assays for unchanged mitomycin C (Table 4). These studies have not so far detected mitomycin C metabolites in plasma or urine. This could be due to limitations in the extraction and assay techniques used. Comparison of plasma cytotoxicity measured using a sensitive mitomycin C bioassay with plasma mitomycin C concentrations measured by HPLC have failed to detect activity other than that attributable to mitomycin C itself (Marshall et al., 1985). Thus, if metabolites of mitomycin C are present in plasma they are non-cytotoxic. No relation between clinical data and mitomycin C pharmacokinetics, nor between mitomycin AUC and bone marrow toxicity have been detected (Verweij et al., 1987).

TABLE 4. *Pharmacokinetics of Mitomycin C in Human*

Dose IV mg/m^2	Peak concentration μg/ml	Half-lives $t_{1/2\alpha}$ min	$t_{1/2\beta}$ min	V_{dss} L/m$_2$	Cl L/min/m^2	Urinary excretion %	References
11	1	25*	—	—	—	5	Tjaden et al., 1982
10–20	2	5	50	22*	0.30*	2–15	Den Hartigh et al., 1982
8–15	1	10	47	21	0.22	8	van Hazel and Kovach, 1982
20	0.9	10	86	—	—	3–19	Sarna et al., 1982
10	—	12	46	25*	0.39	—	Buice et al., 1983
0.4–4.0†	—	—	—	—	0.33–0.61*	—	Hu and Howell, 1983
7–14‡	0.3	—	66	—	—	12	Eksborg et al., 1983
7–14	1	13	50	—	—	—	Marshall et al., 1985
15–60§	0.4–2	—	45	39	0.56	3	Schilcher et al., 1984
6–20	—	8	52	36	0.33	8	van Hazel et al., 1983

*Estimated from data.
†Intraarterial infusion mg/m^2/hr.
‡Intrahepatic administration.
§60 min infusion.

5.4.4. *Metabolism and Antitumor Activity*

There are a number of different mechanisms by which mitomycin C might cause cell death. All of these mechanisms involve metabolic activation of mitomycin C and an action on DNA as the most likely target in the cell. Mitomycin C acts as an alkylating agent with cells in vivo (Berlin and Haseltine, 1981; Fracasso and Sartorelli, 1986; Iyer and Szybalski, 1963; Taniguchi et al., 1981). However, alkylation by mitomycin C in vitro requires its chemical or enzymatic reduction (Iyer and Szybalski, 1964; Schwartz et al., 1963). Reductively activated mitomycin C can act as either as a monofunctional alkylating agent and bind to DNA, RNA and protein (Weissbach and Lisio, 1965) or it can act as a bifunctional alkylating agent and crosslink complementary strands of DNA (Dorr et al., 1985; Fornace et al., 1979; Iyer and Szybalkski, 1963, 1964; Pan et al., 1986; Schwartz et al., 1963) or cross-link DNA with protein (Fornace et al., 1979; Meyn et al., 1982). Mitomycin C crosslinks DNA by alkylation through both the C-1 and C-10 positions of the drug (Tomasz et al., 1986). Chemical reduction of mitomycin C leads to binding to DNA at a ratio of one drug molecule to 5–12 nucleotide bases (Sinha and Chignell, 1979; Tomasz et al., 1974). Guanine residues appear to be important for both the monofunctional and bifunctional binding of mitomycin C to DNA (Lipsett and Weissbach, 1965; Tomasz et al., 1974). Hashimoto et al. (1982, 1983) using chemically activated mitomycin C reported that monofunctional DNA adducts were formed at the C-1 position of mitomycin C, and at the O-6 and *N*-2 positions of guanine and the *N*-6 position of adenine, in equal proportions. Pan et al. (1986) found that the preferred site for monofunctional alkylation of DNA by enzymatically activated mitomycin C was the O-6 position of guanine. A major adduct found after nuclease digestion of DNA was 2,7-diamminomitosene linked at the C-1 position to O-6 of deoxyguanosine. Tomasz et al. (1987a) found that while reductively activated mitomycin C alkylates the *N*-2 position of deoxyguanosine, acid-activated mitomycin C alkylates the *N*-7 position. The difference was ascribed to different electronic structures of acid and reductively activated mitomycin C. Phillips et al. (1989) found that mitomycin C reduced enzymatically by xanthine oxidase and NADPH bound almost exclusively to guanine residues measured by transcriptional blockage. Tomasz et al. (1986) identified the major mitomycin C-DNA adduct formed when mitomycin C was reduced be NADPH-cytochrome P-450 reductase and NADPH, xanthine oxidase and NADH or H_2 and P + O_2 as N^2-(2″β,7″-diaminomitosene-1″-α-yl)-2′-deoxyguanosine. N^2-(2″β,7″-diaminomitosene-1″-α-yl)-2′-deoxyguanosine hydrolyses spontaneously by two pathways; scission of the glycosidic bond to form N^2-(2″β,7″-diaminomitosene-1″-α-yl) guanine and its 1″β-isomer, and imidazolinium ring opening to generate three products 2,6-diamino-4-hydroxy-5-(*N*-formy)-2″β,7-diaminomitosene-1″,β-furanose, 1′α-furnanase and 1′β-pyranose (Tomasz et al., 1987b). Reductive activation of mitomycin C with sodium dithionite produces exclusively bisadduct formation with DNA (Tomasz et al., 1987b). Formation of bisadduct was also demonstrated after injection of rats with mitomycin C. Tomasz et al. (1988) have proposed that activation of mitomycin C proceeds sequentially with, first, reduction at the C-1 position, followed by reduction at the C-10 position. The second (bisadduct forming) reduction is susceptible to inhibition by kinetic factors or oxygen (Tomasz et al., 1988). Mitomycin C DNA crosslinking appears to be specific for the CG-CG duplex sequence due to the specific orientation of the monofunctionally attached mitomycin C in the minor groove (Borowy-Borowski et al., 1990). It is not known which type of alkylation by mitomycin C, monofunctional or bifunctional, might be more important for cytotoxicity and, indeed, there is no direct evidence as yet that either type of alkylation is responsible for the antitumor activity of the mitomycins.

The exact mechanism of bioreductive activation of mitomycin C is open to question. Mechanisms involving two-electron reduction to the mitomycin C hydroquinone and one-electron reduction to the mitomycin C semiquinone have been discussed previously (see Section 5.4.1). As noted, enzymes catalyzing bioreductive alkylation by mitomycin C are predominantly one-electron transferring flavoenzymes and direct two-electron enzymatic reduction of mitomycin C has so far not been demonstrated. While the mitomycin C semiquinone radical appears the most likely reduced form of mitomycin C to be generated in vivo it could disproportionate to the mitomycin C hydroquinone and either pathway of activation shown in Fig. 17 could be operative.

Whatever the mechanism of activation, because of the presumed short-lived nature of the reactive mitomycin C intermediate its site of its formation within the cell is important. Nuclei from normal and tumor cells have been shown to contain enzymes that in the presence of NADPH catalyze reductive activation of mitomycin C (Bachur et al., 1982b; Kennedy et al., 1982). There may, however, be differences in the reductive activation of mitomycin C by nuclei from normal and tumor cells. Kennedy et al. (1985b) presented evidence that activation of mitomycin C proceeds by a one-electron reduction pathway in EMT6 carcinoma cell nuclei and by a one- and two-electron reduction pathway in rat liver nuclei. Alkylating intermediates were trapped with either glutathione, which it was proposed reacts with both one- and two-electron reduced species, and with ethylxanthine, which it was proposed reacts only with the two-electron reduced species. While glutathione inhibited the formation of mitomycin C-derived alkylating species by both NADPH-fortified rat liver and EMT6 carcinoma cell nuclei, ethylxanthate inhibited formation of alkylating species by rat liver nuclei and NADPH, but not by EMT6 carcinoma cell nuclei and NADPH. It was also observed that dicumarol, an inhibitor of quinone reductase, did not affect formation of alkylating species from mitomycin C by rat liver nuclei but increased their formation by EMT6 carcinoma cell nuclei.

Mitomycin C can crosslink DNA at acid pH (pH 3.5) without the need for reduction (Lown, 1979; Lown et al., 1976; Tomasz and Lipman, 1979). This has led to the suggestion that acid catalyzed activation may play a role in the cytotoxicity of mitomycin C to tumor cells. Solid tumors contain many hypoxic cells and hypoxia is known to increase the activity of the enzymes of the glycolytic pathway (Robin et al., 1984). Anaerobic glycolysis leads to hydrolysis of ATP with accumulation of lactic acid (Busa and Nuccitelli, 1984). The average pH of a number of tumors has been found to be about 0.5 units lower than that of the surrounding normal tissue and may be associated with a lower intracellular tumor pH (for a review see Kennedy et al., 1985a). Kennedy et al. (1985a) have shown that there is increased DNA crosslinking by mitomycin C and increased cytotoxicity in EMT6 carcinoma cells incubated with mitomycin C under relatively moderate (pH 5.7–6.4) acid conditions.

Mitomycin C is generally more cytotoxic to hypoxic cells than to euoxic cells (Berlin and Haseltine, 1981; Fracasso and Sartorelli, 1986; Kennedy et al., 1980a,b, 1983; Keyes et al., 1984a; Rauth et al., 1983; Teicher et al., 1981) and any mechanism to explain the cytotoxicity of mitomycin C need to explain this observation. Proponents of the two-electron hydroquinone reduction pathway of mitomycin C activation have suggested that mitomycin C hydroquinone is spontaneously reoxidized under aerobic conditions, thus reducing the cytotoxicity of mitomycin C (Tomasz and Lipman, 1981). The semiquinone radical of mitomycin C also undergoes spontaneous reoxidation in the presence of oxygen which would reduce the steady state concentration of mitomycin C semiquinone and could result in a decreased cytotoxicity of mitomycin C under aerobic conditions. DNA crosslinking by mitomycin C in cells showing oxygen inhibition of mitomycin C cytotoxicity is decreased under euoxic compared to hypoxic conditions (Fracasso and Sartorelli, 1986). The rate at which mitomycin induced DNA crosslinks are formed is also slower and their removal more rapid under euoxic compared to hypoxic conditions. Porfiromycin, which is less cytotoxic than mitomycin C to euoxic cells, produces similar crosslinking to mitomycin C in hypoxic cells but relatively less crosslinking in euoxic cells.

As well as alkylating DNA mitomycin C can produce degradation of DNA both in vivo and in vitro (Hamana et al., 1985; Reich et al., 1961; Wakaki, 1961), although this has not been a universal finding (Dorr et al., 1984). Originally DNA degradation was proposed to be due to stimulation of exonuclease activity by mitomycin C (Nakata et al., 1961). Goodman et al. (1974) showed, however, that mitomycin C inhibits nuclease activity. More recently, generation of active oxygen species (Bachur et al., 1978b; Lown et al., 1976; Tomasz, 1976), in particular the hydroxyl radical (Bachur et al., 1978b; Hamana et al., 1985; Lown et al., 1976), has been suggested to be responsible for the degradation of DNA by mitomycin C. Hydroxyl radical scavengers and iron chelating agents have been reported to protect Ehrlich tumor cells against mitomycin C cytotoxicity in vitro (Doroshow, 1986b). Hamana et al. (1985) found that an ESR-detectable PBN-hydroxyl radical adduct was formed during redox cycling of mitomycin C by NADPH-cytochrome P-450 reductase and NADPH, but only in the presence of an iron chelate such as Fe(III)-ADP. Without the iron chelate a PBN-superoxide anion radical adduct was formed. Degradation of added DNA by enzymatically reduced mitomycin C was also only seen in the presence of an iron chelate, suggesting that superoxide anion radical or hydrogen peroxide alone could not cleave the DNA but that hydroxyl radical was the responsible species. Cu(II) ions promote the strand scission of bacteriophage øX174 DNA by mitomycin C and sodium dithionite (Ueda et al., 1980). However, a role for the Cu(II) ions in mitomycin cytotoxicity has been difficult to prove and no correlation has been found between the experimental antitumor activity and Cu(II) complexing ability of mitomycin C analogs (Iyengar et al., 1986). Gutteridge et al. (1984) have reported that mitomycin C dependent degradation of deoxyribose increases at low oxygen concentrations in a reaction that is inhibited by catalase, hydroxyl radical scavengers, iron chelators and superoxide dismutase. The authors suggested that, as with the anthracycline semiquinone radical (see Section 3.4.1.4), mitomycin C semiquinone radical reacts directly with hydrogen peroxide to form hydroxyl radical. The reaction is inhibited at oxygen concentration in air when superoxide anion radical is preferentially formed by electron transfer from the mitomycin C semiquinone radical to molecular oxygen. Such a mechanism, perhaps with generation of hydroxyl radical by mitomycin C bound to DNA, might explain the selective toxicity of mitomycin C to hypoxic cells.

The ability of a series of mitomycin analogs to generate oxygen radicals has been studied by Pritsos and Sartorelli (1986) using analogs such as BMY-25282 that are up to 10 times more cytotoxic than mitomycin C to euoxic tumor cells, but are only 4 times more cytotoxic to hypoxic cells (Keyes et al., 1984b). The analogs were found to be more rapidly reduced than mitomycin C and to generate more superoxide anion radical and hydroxyl radical when reduced by either tumor cell sonicates, NADPH-cytochrome P-450 reductase or mitochondria. Porfiromycin, which has greater toxicity than mitomycin C for hypoxic EMT6 carcinoma cells but less toxicity for euoxic cells, did not generate hydroxyl radical. The results suggest that the ability of the mitomycin analogs to generate oxygen radicals may be related to their cytotoxicity to euoxic tumor cells. Pan and Gonzalez (1990) studied a series of seven mitomycin C analogs and found that the less negative the one-electron reduction potential the more easily the analog was reduced by xanthine oxidase and NADPH-cytochrome P-450 reductase, and the more it augmented oxygen consumption. A relationship between the reduction potential of the analogs and cytotoxicity to HCT 116 human colon carcinoma cells was established. An interesting but unexplained observation by Marshall and Rauth (1986) is that ascorbic acid increases the toxicity of mitomycin C to Chinese hamster ovary cells and increases the generation of alkylating species from the drug by cell sonicates under aerobic but not under anaerobic conditions. The authors suggest that there might be two enzyme mechanisms responsible for activation of mitomycin C in cells, one of which is inhibited by oxygen and stimulated by ascorbic acid.

Cell lines made resistant to mitomycin C have provided insights to the mechanisms of mitomycin C cytotoxocity. Dulhanty et al. (1989) reported a series of Chinese hamster ovary cell lines in which mitomycin C resistance was due to deficient bioreduction (measured by dicumarol inhibited cytotoxicity) or to deficient DNA excision repair, alone or in combination. BMY 25282 has been reported to overcome the resistance of mitomycin C resistant human colonic carcinoma cells possessing deficient mitomycin C bioactivation (Chakrabaty et al., 1986; Chakrabarty and Brattain, 1987). Marshall and Rauth (1989) reported a human fibroblast cell line from the member of a cancer-prone family (3437t) that was six times more resistant to mitomycin C under aerobic conditions than an equivalent cell line from a normal donor (GM38). The 3437T cell line had substantially decreased levels of quinone reductase compared to GM 38 cells and dicumarol decreased the aerobic sensitivity of GM 38 but not 3437T cells to mitomycin C. Other studies have implicated decreased levels of NADPH-cytochrome P-450 reductase as a cause of resistance to mitomycin C. A Chinese hamster ovary cell line with induced resistance to mitomycin C under oxic conditions (but not hypoxic conditions) exhibited no change in quinone reductase activity but a decrease in NADPH-cytochrome P-450 reductase (Hoban et al., 1990). Similar results were obtained by Bligh et al. (1990) who also found that expression of NADPH-cytochrome P-450 reductase activity in *S. typhimurium* LR5000 sensitized the bacterium to mitomycin C cytotoxicity. These results tend to confirm that NADPH-cytochrome P-450 reductase activity contributes to mitomycin C cytotoxicity under aerobic conditions. Mitomycin C resistant cells with the multidrug resistance phenotype showing cross resistance to antracyclines, vinca alkaloids and methotrexate, and possessing P-glycoprotein have also been identified (Dorr et al., 1987; Dalton et al., 1986).

6. AZIRIDINYLBENZOQUINONES

6.1. Historical Perspective

The prototype antitumor aziridinylbenzoquinone is 2,5-bis(aziridinyl)-1,4-benzoquinone first studied in 1954 by Domagk et al. Based on the experimental antitumor activity of this compound Gauss and his colleagues at Farbenfabriken Bayer in Germany synthesized and tested a series of aziridinylbenzoquinones (Gauss, 1957, 1958). 2,3,5-Tris(aziridinyl)-1,4-benzoquinone (triaziquone, Trenimon, Fig. 20) was found to possess marked cytostatic and cytotoxic properties both in vivo and in vitro (Gerhartz, 1964). An attractive property of triaziquone for clinical chemotherapists at this time was its increased potency compared to most nitrogen mustards then available. Triaziquone underwent widespread clinical testing in Europe in the 1960s and while it showed some activity, particularly in hematological malignancies and ovarian cancer, it was also very toxic and proved difficult to administer (Gerhartz, 1964; Hartleib, 1974). 2,5-Bis(1-aziridinyl)-3-(2-carbamoyloxy-1-methoxyethyl)-6-methyl-1,4-benzoquinone (carbazilquone, carboquone, Fig. 20) was the most active compound in animal tumor models of a series of aziridinylbenzoquinones synthesized by Arakawa and Nakao at the Sankyo Company in Japan (Arakawa et al., 1970a,b; Nakao et al., 1972, 1975). Carbazilquinone has undergone clinical trial in Japan (Himori et al., 1983; Uzuka et al., 1982). In the U.S.A. between 1955 and 1971 the National Cancer Institute tested over 1500 quinones for antitumor activity in animal tumor models as part of its random screening program. Of several hundred purely synthetic quinones tested the aziridinylbenzoquinones were found to have the greatest activity in a number of murine tumor models (Driscoll et al., 1974). Several of the aziridinylbenzoquinones were subsequently found to be active against intracerebrally implanted murine leukemia L1210 which raised the possibility that they might also be active against brain tumors in man (Driscoll et al., 1974). The central nervous system active aziridinylbenzoquinones were all found to have a high lipid solubility and a low degree of ionization, properties which facilitate a compound's penetration across the blood–brain barrier (Rall and Zubrod, 1962). However, the same properties give a low water solubility and the aziridinylben zoquinones were difficult to formulate. A synthetic program was undertaken to prepare more water soluble aziridinylbenzoquinones that retained activity against intracerebrally implanted tumors. The culmination of this effort was the synthesis in 1976 by Driscoll and his collaborators at the National Cancer Institute of 2,5-bis(1-aziridinyl)-3,6-bis-(carboethoxy-amino)-1,4-benzoquinone (diaziquone, AZQ, Fig. 20) (Chou et al., 1976; Khan and Driscoll, 1976). Diaziquone has been tested clinically and has shown promising activity against primary brain tumors (Bender et al., 1983). Another aziridinylbenzoquinone synthesized by Driscoll and his collaborators was 2,5-bis(1-aziridinyl)-3,6-bis-(2-hydroxethylamino)-1,4-benzoquinone (BZQ, Fig. 20) (Chou et al., 1976). BZQ is more water soluble than diaziquone making it easier to formulate. BZQ has undergone clinical trial in the U.K. (Bosanquet and McLoughlin, 1985). There are other aziridinylbenzoquinones in the early stages of preclinical development (Driebergen et al., 1986).

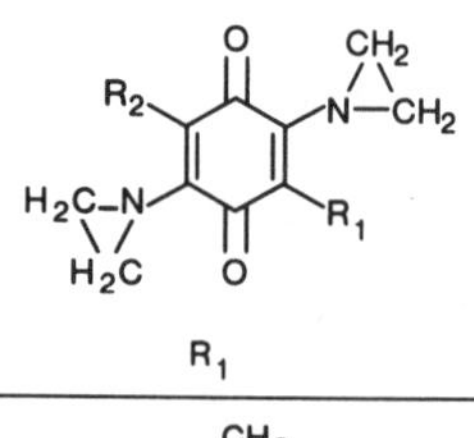

Compound	R_1	R_2
Triaziquone	$N<(CH_2)_2$	H
Carbazilquinone	CH_3	$CHCH_2OCONH_2$ / OCH_3
Diaziquone	NH $COOCH_2CH_3$	NH $COOCH_2CH_3$
BZQ	$NHCH_2CH_2OH$	$NHCH_2CH_2OH$

Fig. 20. Structure of some aziridinylbenzoquinones.

6.2. Structure–Activity Relationships

The structure–antitumor activity relationships of the aziridinylbenzoquinones have been extensively studied (Chou et al., 1976; Driscoll et al., 1974; Khan and Driscoll, 1976; Yoshimoto et al., 1979). The aziridine ring structure is essential, although by itself not sufficient, for antitumor activity. Substitution in the aziridinyl rings with 1 or 2 methyl groups results in a loss of antitumor activity. Di-, tri- and tetra-aziridinylbenzoquinones are all active but 2,5-diaziridinylbenzoquinones with various donor or electronically neutral functional groups in positions C-3 and C-6 are most active. Strong electron-attracting groups such as halogen atoms at positions C-3 and C-6 decrease antitumor potency. Compounds with a high lipophilicity have the greatest antitumor activity while more hydrophilic compounds have a greater chemotherapeutic index.

6.3. Clinical Activity

Triaziquone was the first aziridinylbenzoquinone to receive clinical trial, mostly in Europe. It was found to be useful for the local treatment of tumors and, administered either orally or intravenously, to have activity against myelocytic leukemia, Kaposi's sarcoma, Hodgkin's lymphoma, breast cancer, ovarian cancer, and polycythemia vera (Blacow, 1972; Gerhartz, 1964; Kyalwazi, 1968). These are conditions for which alkylating agents have generally proved to be most useful. The low therapeutic index of triaziquone made it a very difficult drug to use. Its use was associated with severe leucopenia, thrombocytopenia and a decrease in the number of red blood cells, often leading to a need for repeated transfusions. Carbazilquinone has received clinical trial in Japan. It has produced remissions in patients with malignant lymphoma, chronic myelogenous leukemia, chronic granulocytic leukemia and polycythemia vera (Uzuka et al., 1982), but has shown disappointing activity against solid tumors except for lung cancer (Himori et al., 1983; Nakoa et al., 1975). The dose-limiting toxicity of carbazilquinone is myelosuppression, predominantly leukopenia. Clinical trials of diaziquone have shown that it has activity against primary brain-tumors but little activity in other tumors (Bender et al., 1983; Maral et al., 1985). The dose-limiting toxicity of diaziquone is myelosuppression, primarily thrombocytopenia. A way to avoid the myelosuppressive effects of diaziquone in patients with meninigeal malignancies is to give the drug to patients intrathecally (Zimm et al., 1987).

6.4. Chemical Reactivity

The aziridinylbenzoquinones possess alkylating activity by virtue of the aziridine groups. Alkylation of a nucleophile can occur by activation of the aziridine group under neutral conditions or following protonation under acid conditions to give an aziridinium ion which may then form a carbonium ion intermediate (Fig. 21) (Khan and Ross, 1969; Linford, 1973). Mossoba et al. (1985) have provided NMR and electrochemical evidence that protonation of the aziridine ring of diaziquone under acid conditions facilitates ring opening by release of the strain energy of the aziridine ring.

Chemical breakdown of the aziridinylbenzoquinones in aqueous solution is determined by the reactivity of the aziridine groups. Mechanisms for the acid and base catalyzed degradation of aziridinylbenzoquinones are shown in Fig. 22. Studies with 2,5-bis(aziridinyl)-1,4-benzoquinone and 2,5-bis(aziridinyl)-3,6-diisopropoxy-1,4-benzoquinone under acid conditions have shown

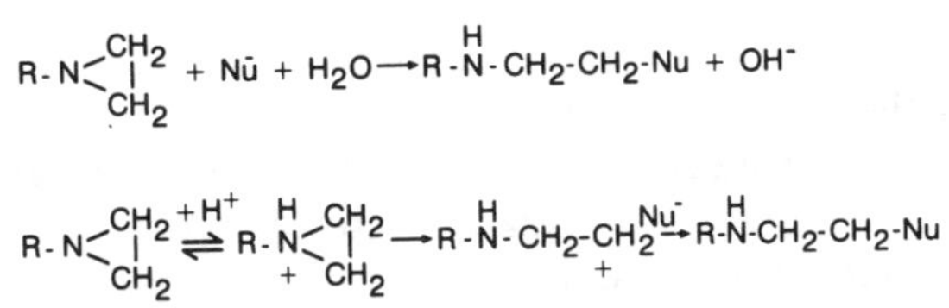

FIG. 21. Possible mechanisms of alkylation by aziridinylbenzoquinones. Upper panel, under neutral conditions; and lower panel, under acid conditions. Nu is a nucleophile.

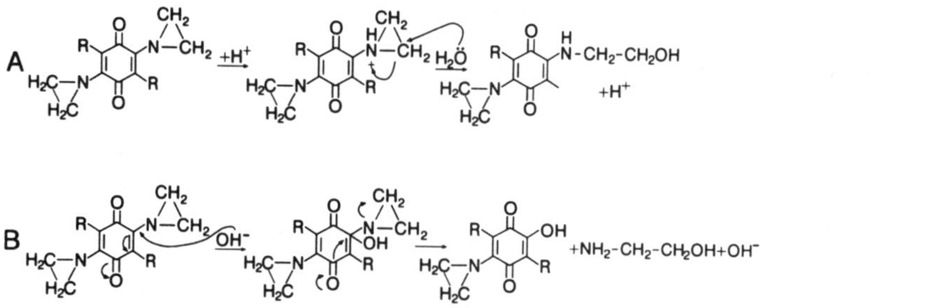

FIG. 22. Mechanisms for chemical degradation of aziridinylbenzoquinones. (A), The acid catalyzed breakdown of a bis(aziridinyl)benzoquinone to a 2′-hydroxyethylaminobenzoquinone derivative. This is followed by ring opening of the second aziridinyl group to give a bis(2′-hydroxy-ethyl-amino)benzoquinone derivative. (B), the base catalyzed substitution of an aziridinyl group by hydroxyl ion to give a hydroxybenzoquinone derivative. This is followed by subsitution of the second aziridinyl group to give the bis-hydroxybenzoquinone derivative. At neutral pH a combination of both reactions occurs.

nucleophilic attack by water leading to sequential hydrolytic cleavage of the aziridinyl rings to give, first, the 2-aziridinyl-5-(2′-hydroxyethylamino) derivative and then the 2,5-*bis*-(2′-hydroxyethylamino) derivative (Kusai et al., 1981). Under alkaline conditions 2,5-bis(aziridinyl)-1,4-benzoquinone undergoes sequential hydroxyl replacement of the aziridinyl rings to give first, 2-aziridinyl-5-hydroxy-1,4-benzoquinone and then, 2,5-dihydroxy-1,4-benzoquinone (Kusai et al., 1981). At neutral pH both ring opening and substitution reactions occur and 2,5-bis-(aziridinyl)-1,4-benzoquinone gives, in addition to the previous products, the mixed product 2-ethanolamino-5-hydroxy-1,4-benzoquinone. Carbazilquinone undergoes a similar pattern of chemical breakdown to 2,5-bis(aziridinyl)-1,4-benzoquinone with sequential hydrolytic cleavage of the aziridinyl rings at acid pH, sequential hydroxyl replacement of the aziridinyl rings at alkaline pH and a combination of the two mechanisms at neutral pH (Kusai and Ueda, 1984). Many more degradation products are formed from carbazilquinone than from 2,5-bis(aziridinyl)-1,4-benzoquinone because of the asymmetrical structure of carbazilquinone and not all the degradation products have been identified (Kusai et al., 1981; Kusai and Ueda, 1984). Diaziquone undergoes a similar pattern of chemical breakdown to 2,5-bis(aziridinyl)-1,4-benzoquinone. This has been shown by Poochikian and Kelley (1981) using HPLC and mass spectral techniques to characterize the products. Under acid to neutral conditions nucleophilic attack by water yields first 2-aziridinyl-5-(2′-hydroxyethylamino)-3,6-bis(carboethoxyamino)-1,4-benzoquinone then 2,5-bis(2′-hydroxyethylamino)-3,6-bis(carboethoxyamino)-1,4-benzoquinone. Nucleophilic attack by chloride ion gives the corresponding mono- and bis-(2′-chloroethylamino) derivatives. These derivatives, it will be noted, are mono- and bifunctional mustards. Under alkaline conditions diaziquone undergoes sequential hydroxyl ion replacement of the aziridine groups to give 2-aziridinyl-5-hydroxy-3,6-bis(carboethoxyamino)-1,4-benzoquinone and 2,5-dihydroxy-3,6-bis(carboethoxyamino)-1,4-benzoquinone.

The quinone group of aziridinylbenzoquinones is a second potential site for chemical reaction. Triaziquone can undergo reversible reduction by sodium borohydride and dithiothreitol (Linford, 1973). It has been suggested that the product of this reduction is the hydroquinone which in air is slowly reoxidized to the parent quinone (Linford, 1973). In contrast reduction of triaziquone with cysteine or glutathione results in the formation of non-auto-oxidizable derivatives, suggested to be the C-6-cysteine and C-6-glutathione hydroquinone adducts (Linford, 1973). It is interesting that the cysteine adduct of triaziquone was found to be a more active alkylating agent than the parent compound. However, the cysteine adduct of triaziquone does not readily cross the cell membrane and the role the adduct in the antitumor activity of triaziquone is not known. Electrochemical reduction of diaziquone has been studied by Mossoba et al. (1985). In aprotic media diaziquone undergoes single-electron reduction to give the diaziquinone semiquinone radical while in aqueous media there is two-electron reduction to diaziquone hydroquinone. The hydro quinone spontaneously oxidizes in air to form the semiquinone free radical and superoxide anion radical (Mossoba et al., 1985; Gutierrez, 1989).

6.5. Metabolism

6.5.1. *In Vitro Metabolism*

Aziridinylbenzoquinones stimulate both NADPH and NADH oxidation when incubated with hepatic microsomes (Handa and Sato, 1975). Stimulation of NADPH oxidation by carbazilquinone is due to reduction by microsomal NADPH cytochrome P-450 reductase (Komiyama et al., 1979b, 1982). Stimulation of NADH oxidation by aziridinylbenzoquinones does not involve direct reduction by microsomal NADH-cytochrome b_5 reductase, rather the aziridinylbenzoquinones act as electron carriers between cytochrome b_5 and molecular oxygen. Carbazilquinone stimulation of NADH oxidation and oxygen utilization by NADH-cytochrome b_5 reductase does not occur without cytochrome b_5 (Tamura and Sato, 1977). Under the same conditions doxorubicin, daunorubicin and mitomycin C do not stimulate NADH oxidation (Tamura and Sato, 1977). Diaziquone, and possibly other aziridinylben zoquinones, has a relatively high E^1_7 compared to other antitumor quinones (Svingen and Powis, 1981) which may enable aziridinylbenzoquinones to act as an electron receptor from cytochrome b_5. The anaerobic reduction of a series of 2,5-bis(aziridinyl)-1,4-benzoquinone derivatives with various 3,6 substituents, by xanthine oxidase was shown by Lusthof et al. (1990) to be related to quinone reduction potential as well as steric factors. Diaziquone undergoes metabolism by quinone reductase. The cytosol of HT-29 human colon carcinoma cells, which contains high levels of quinone reductase activity, catalyzes the removal of diaziquone in the presence of NADPH or NADH. Dicoumarol, an inhibitor of quinone reductase, inhibits removal of diaziquone (Ross et al., 1990). Fisher and Gutierrez (1991) reported dicumarol-inhibitable reduction of diaziquone by the post-mitochondrial superantant fraction of MCF-7 human breast cancer cells. Schlager and Powis (1990) showed that a cell density dependent increase in quinone reductase was associated with an increased sensitivity of mouse fibroblasts to diaziquone.

6.5.2. *Free Radical Formation*

Metabolism of carbazilquinone by hepatic microsomes and NADPH or NADH (Kikuchi and Sugiura, 1981; Sato et al., 1977), or by purified NADPH-cytochrome P-450 reductase and NADPH (Kikuchi and Sugiura, 1981) gives a 5 line ESR signal, $g = 2.004$–2.005, indicating formation of the carbazilquinone semiquinone radical. The signal is only detected when oxygen is excluded from the medium or when all the dissolved oxygen has been utilized by redox cycling of carbazilquinone (Kikuchi and Sugiura, 1981; Sato et al., 1977). The signal is not decreased by adding DNA (Sato et al., 1977). Formation of superoxide anion radical when carbazilquinone and triaziquone are incubated with rat hepatic microsomes and NADPH under aerobic conditions has been demonstrated by Handa and Sato (1975) using superoxide dismutase-inhibitable sulfite oxidation. Komiyama et al. (1982) used ESR and PBN spin trapping to demonstrate hydroxyl radical formation by carbazilquinone incubated with NADPH-cytochrome P-450 reductase and NADPH. Formation of the hydroxyl radical adduct was completely blocked by catalase and decreased by superoxide dismutase.

An excellent review on free radical formation by diaziquone has been prepared by Gutierrez (1989). Diaziquone stimulates NADPH or NADH oxidation, and oxygen utilization by rat hepatic microsomes, nuclei and purified NADPH-cytochrome P-450 reductase (Gutierrez et al., 1982; Svingen and Powis, 1981). ESR studies have shown the formation of a 5 line radical signal, $g = 2.005$, with relative line intensities of 1:2:3:2:1 (Gutierrez et al., 1982; Gutierrez and Bachur, 1983; Svingen et al., 1980) (Fig. 23). A similar ESR signal has been obtained by electrochemical reduction of diaziquone in aqueous media (Gutierrez et al., 1984, 1985b). Confirmation that the ESR signal is that of the diaziquone semiquinone radical has been provided by Gutierrez and Bachur (1983) who compared the signal with that obtained by enzymatic reduction of chlorine substituted diaziquone analogs (Gutierrez and Bachur, 1983). The hyperfine coupling seen in the ESR spectrum of the diaziquone semiquinone radical is due to coupling of the unpaired electrons with the nitrogens of the aziridine rings, and to a smaller extent with the nitrogen and imide hydrogen of the carboethoxyamino groups (Gutierrez and Bachur, 1983). Unresolved coupling and hindered rotation due to the bulky carboethoxyamino groups leads to line broadening in aqueous

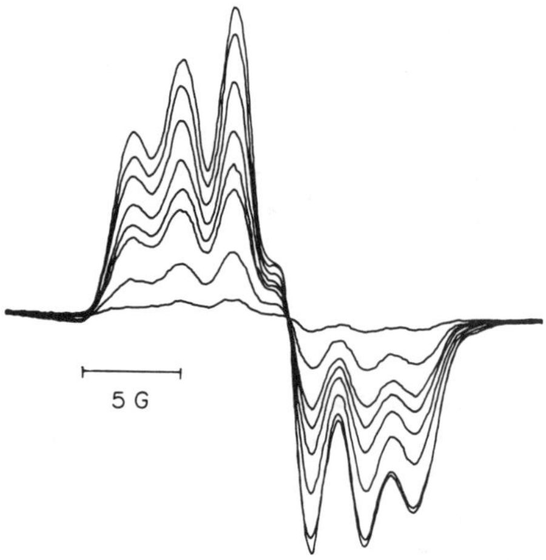

FIG. 23. Electron spin resonance signals obtained when 5 mM diaziquone was incubated with a rat liver microsomal fraction, 0.36 mg protein/mL in 0.15 M potassium phosphate buffer, pH 7.4, and a 1 mM NADPH generating system. Scans were recorded every 10 min and get progressively larger.

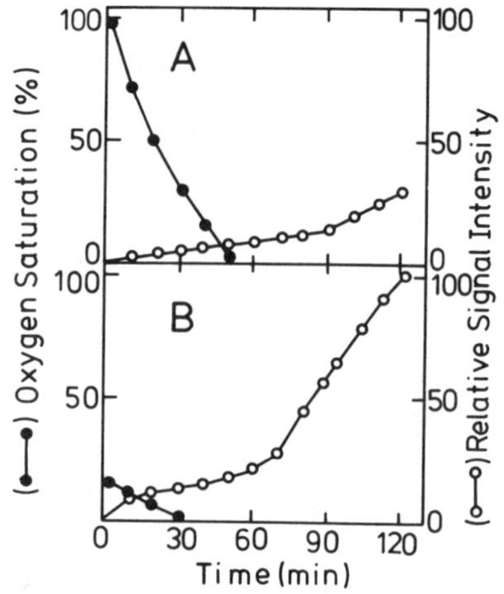

FIG. 24. Diaziquone semiquinone radical formation by rat hepatocytes. Hepatocytes were at 107 cells/mL and diaziquone 5 mM, in a closed cell, (A), initially under aerobic conditions; (B), under anaerobic conditions. The ESR spectrometer was operated in the kinetic mode and the relative signal growth (○) measured. Dissolved oxygen concentration (●) was measured under identical conditions.

solution. Diaziquone can be directly reduced to the semiquinone radical by NADPH in the millimolar concentration range (Gutierrez et al., 1985a). This is the NADPH concentration usually used in enzymatic systems to generate the diaziquione semiquinone radical and direct reduction of diaziquinone by NADPH may make a small contribution to the overall signal seen. Irradiation of anaerobic aqueous solutions of diaziquone by 500 nm visible light leads to the formation of an ESR detectable diaziquone semiquinone radical, while under aerobic conditions in the presence of DMPO a DMPO-hydroxyl radical adduct is formed (Mossoba and Gutierrez, 1985). Visible light at 500 nm potentiates the cytotoxicity of diaziquone to MCF-7 breast cancer cells (Al-Nabulsi and Gutierrez, 1991). Pulse radiolysis studies have shown the lifetime of the diaziquone semiquinone radical under anaerobic conditions to be 1 msec and that it reacts with oxygen (Svingen and Powis, 1981). These studies also showed the E^1_7 of diaziquone to be -168 mV. The relatively of high E^1_7 may explain why diaziquone is more rapidly metabolized by NADPH-cytochrome P-450 reductase than other antitumor quinones such as mitomycin C and anthracyclines, which have more negative E^1_7 values (Svingen and Powis, 1981). Butler et al. (1987) have reported an E^1_7 of -70 mV for diaziquone and -376 mV for BZQ. The study also found diaziquone semiquinone radicals could be produced by the reduction of diaziquone by superoxide anion radicals. BZQ semiquinone radicals reacted rapidly with oxygen.

Cysteine under anaerobic but not aerobic conditions directly reduces diaziquone to the semiquinone radical (Gutierrez et al., 1985a). In contrast glutathione does not reduce diaziquone to the semiquinone radical, either under anaerobic or aerobic conditions. Whether glutathione does not react with diaziquone or reacts, but does not form a semiquinone radical intermediate is not known. As previously noted, cysteine and glutathione react with triaziquone to give stable hydroquinone adducts (Linford, 1973). ESR studies have shown that diaziquone can be reduced to the semiquinone radical by several cells including isolated rat hepatocytes, human solid tumor cell lines (Svingen et al., 1980), Hep-2 cells (Gutierrez et al., 1986) and murine and human leukemic cell lines (Egorin et al., 1985; Gutierrez et al., 1985a). Formation of the diaziquone semiquinone radical by rat hepatocytes increases as dissolved oxygen in the incubation media is utilized (Fig. 24) although complete anaerobicity may not be required for diaziquone semiquinone radical formation by subcellular fractions or by whole cells (Gutierrez et al., 1985a). Red blood cells reduce diaziquone to an ESR detectable semiquinone radical which is then rapidly replaced by an ascorbyl radical signal due to reaction of diaziquone semiquinone with ascorbic acid in leukocytes of the buffy coat (Gutierrez, 1988). Diaziquone stimulates cellular oxygen consumption (Gutierrez et al., 1985a) and superoxide anion radical is released into the media surrounding the cells (Svingen et al., 1980). Opening of the aziridine ring of diaziquone by acid treatment gives compound(s) that do not stimulate oxygen utilization by murine leukemia L1210 cells and do not give an ESR semiquinone radical signal (Egorin et al., 1985). This may be because of the ring opened compound(s) are not taken up by the cells. BZQ does not produce a detectable ESR signal when incubated with L1210 and K502 leukemia cells, although toxic to both cell lines (Lea et al., 1988).

6.5.3. *Metabolites*

To date no metabolites of the aziridinylbenzoquinones have been identified although there is indirect evidence for metabolism of diaziquone from both in vitro and in vivo studies. Gutierrez and Bachur (1983) reported that there was no loss of diaziquone incubated with purified microsomal NADPH-cytochrome P-450 reductase and NADPH under aerobic conditions for 16 hr, compared to incubations containing no enzyme or without NADPH. However, the amount of NADPH used in these studies was probably limiting. Spiegel et al. (1982) reported loss of diaziquone incubated with mouse liver homogenates without added NADPH. The enzymatic nature of the loss was demonstrated by the fact that it did not occur at 4°, nor if boiled mouse liver homogenate was used. The nature of the product(s) formed was not investigated. Cytotoxic activation of diaziquone has been reported to occur with rat liver post-mitochondrial fraction and NADPH using rat 9L brain tumor cells as the target for cytotoxicity (Alhonen-Hongisto et al., 1984).

6.5.4. *In Vivo Metabolism*

In vivo studies suggest that metabolites and/or breakdown products of diaziquone are formed. Spiegel et al. (1982) reported that when [ring-^{14}C]-diaziquone was administered to mice, diaziquone, the only material extracted into chloroform, disappeared rapidly from plasma with a half-life of 1 hr. There remained a large amount of chloroform non-extractable radioactivity in plasma for at least 24 hr, presumably due to metabolites and/or breakdown products of diaziquone. Brain, heart, liver and muscle also contained large amounts of non-chloroform extractable radioactivity. Chloroform non-extractable radioactivity has been reported in the plasma and CSF of non-human primates receiving [ring-^{14}C]-diaziquone (Gormley et al., 1981), as well as in the plasma and tumor tissue of patients (Savaraj et al., 1983). Feun et al. (1983) found that following administration [ring-^{14}C]-diaziquone to beagle dogs 41% of the radioactivity was excreted in urine in 96 hr but that only 4% was unchanged [ring-^{14}C]-diaziquone. Lu et al. (1981, 1983) administered [ring-^{14}C]-diaziquone to patients and found that unchanged [ring-^{14}C]-diaziquone accounted for 9% of the administered radioactivity excreted in urine over 96 hr, while metabolites and/or breakdown products accounted for a further 10%. Up to three unidentified radioactive peaks were separated from urine by HPLC. Savaraj et al. (1983) found that only 18-45% of the radioactivity in brain tumor tissue and 30–56% of the radioactivity in plasma of patients receiving [ring-^{14}C]-diaziquone was parent drug.

Pharmacokinetic studies of unlabeled diaziquone in humans are consistent with the concept rapid metabolism and/or breakdown of the drug. There is rapid elimination of diaziquone from plasma with a terminal plasma half-life of 25–37 min, a total body clearance of 500 mL/min/m^2 and a 24 hr urinary recovery of unchanged drug of less than 1% (Bachur et al., 1982a; Bjornsson et al., 1985; Curt et al., 1983; Frytak et al., 1984; Griffin et al., 1982; Schilcher et al., 1983; Schilsky et al., 1982). Diaziquone appears to be retained in the tissues for a long time. Tissue samples from a patient who died 10 days after receiving [ring-^{14}C]-diaziquone studied for chloroform extractable radioactivity showed the highest levels in liver followed by kidney, spleen, adrenal gland, heart and ovary (Savaraj et al., 1983).

6.6. Metabolism and Antitumor Activity

The presence of both the quinone and aziridinyl functions offer a number of possible mechanisms for the cytotoxicity of aziridinylbenzoquinones. The aziridine group confer alkylating activity to the aziridinylbenzoquinones but this is a latent alkylating activity that, in most cases, needs special conditions for its expression. The quinone group allows semiquinone radical formation which could itself be a toxic species, while redox cycling leads to the formation of cytotoxic oxygen radicals. One, or a combination of these mechanisms could be responsible for the cytotoxicity of aziridinylbenzoquinones. In each case metabolism is required for the expression of cytotoxicity.

The aziridine group in aziridinylbenzoquinones represents a latent alkylating site. Appreciable alkylation of DNA, the presumed primary site of action of alkylating agents, only occurs with aziridinylbenzoquinones under acid conditions or following reduction. Akhtar et al. (1975) studied covalent crosslinking of phage DNA by a series of aziridinylbenzoquinones which included triaziquone. Crosslinking was slow under neutral conditions but became progressively more rapid under acid conditions to a pH of 4.5. A correlation was found between the number of DNA crosslinks per DNA molecule and the guanine and cytosine content of the DNA. A correlation was also found between the extent of DNA crosslinking and antitumor activity of the aziridinylbenzoquinones against murine leukemia L1210 and several solid tumors. Gupta et al. (1991) used a modification of the standard ^{32}P-postlabeling assay to detect relatively polar adducts of diaziquone reacted with DNA under acid conditions. Peak binding occurred at 2 hr but declined by 24 hr, indicating the instability of the adducts. The major DNA adduct as well as several minor ones were guanine derived. The aziridine rings of diaziquone were the main reactive sites, and the monaminoalcohol derivative showed as much DNA reactivity as diaziquone. However, the diaminoalcohol derivative showed no DNA reactivity. Covalent binding of carbazilquinone to DNA has been found to be negligible at neutral pH but to be increased at acid pH (Nakamura et al., 1974). In this study reducing agents such as sodium borohydride, 2-mercaptoethanol and dithiothreitol increased the covalent binding of carbazilquinone to DNA. DNA interstrand crosslinking by diaziquone requires acid or alkaline conditions and a reducing agent. Under acid conditions, sodium borohydride, NADH and NADPH support DNA interstrand crosslinking while under alkaline conditions sodium borohydride supports DNA crosslinking by diaziquone (King and Loo, 1983; King et al., 1984c). DNA crosslinking by diaziquone is not seen under neutral conditions even with a reducing agent, while anaerobic conditions decrease the amount of crosslinking. 2,5-bis(aziridinyl)-3,6-bis(chloro)-1,4-benzoquinone is an active alkylating agent in the oxidized state and is little affected by reduction with sodium borohydride, while diaziquone is inactive as an alkylating agent unless reduced with sodium borohydride. 2,5-bis(chloro)-3,6-bis(carboethoxy-amino)-1,4-benzoquinone, which has no aziridine rings is inactive as an alkylating agent whether oxidized or reduced. Szmigiero and Kohn (1984) reported that DNA interstrand crosslinks are formed by diaziquone incubated with nuclei isolated from tumor cells only in the presence of a reducing agent such as sodium borohydride or NADPH. In the same study the alkylating activity of diaziquone, measured by reaction with 4-(*p*-nitrobenzyl)pyridine, was stimulated by reducing agents and acid pH (Szmigiero and Kohn, 1984). Gutierrez et al. (1985b) found that although there is a close relation between quinone reduction and aziridine ring activation, in vitro cytotoxicity of diaziquone analogs does not correlate with the quinone reduction potential. Electrochemical studies of a series of aziridinylbenzoquinones by Driebergen et al. (1986) revealed that cytotoxicity correlates well with the ease of protonation of the aziridine ring(s) after quinone reduction. No correlation is found between cytotoxicity and the ease of protonation of the aziridines prior to quinone reduction or with the quinone reduction step itself.

DNA crosslinking is seen when aziridinylbenzoquinones are incubated with whole cells. Incubation of diaziquone with Chinese hamster ovary cells (King et al., 1984a), with human embryonic cells or with a variety of human and murine tumor cell results in DNA–protein crosslinks and DNA interstrand crosslinks (King et al., 1984a; Szmigiero et al., 1984). However, marked differences are found in the extent of DNA interstrand crosslinks in different cell types. For example, the normal human embryo fibroblast cell line, IMR-90 shows no detectable DNA crosslinking while HT-29, a human colon carcinoma cell line, has considerable DNA crosslinking (Szmigiero et al., 1984). The cytotoxicity of diaziquone to different cell lines has been found to correlate well with the degree of DNA crosslinking (Szmigiero et al., 1984). The requirement of oxygen for DNA crosslinking reported by King et al. (1984a) has been suggested by Mossoba et al. (1985) to reflect the necessity of oxidation of the hydroquinone form of aziridinylbenzoquinones to the semiquinone prior to aziridine ring opening (King et al., 1984b; Mossoba et al., 1985).

Aziridinylbenzoquinones incubated with a reducing agent such as sodium borohydride or thiols produces single strand breaks of DNA along with some double strand breaks (Gutierrez et al., 1986; King and Loo, 1983; Nakamura et al., 1974). Bacteriophage PM2 DNA strand scission by sodium borohydride-reduced diaziquinone is greatest at acid pH and is inhibited by catalase and glutathione, but not by superoxide dismutase (King and Loo, 1983). Cu(II) and Fe(II) enhance DNA cleavage by diaziquone but other divalent metal ions do not. Gutierrez et al. (1986) reported that superoxide dismutase offers partial protection against PM2 DNA strand breaks by sodium borohydride-reduced diaziquone under aerobic conditions. The finding of Gutierrez et al. (1986) that anaerobic conditions do not decrease DNA degradation by sodium borohydride-reduced diaziquone may be partly explained by the ability of sodium borohydride itself to cleave DNA under anaerobic conditions. The results suggest that hydrogen peroxide or hydroxyl radical formed from superoxide anion radical are involved in DNA cleavage by diaziquone. The diaziquone semiquinone free radical, generated by mixing electrochemically generated diaziquone hydroquinone and diaziquone in a 9:1 ratio, was directly cytotoxic to murine P-388 leukemia cells under aerobic conditions (Nguyenet al., 1988). Hydroxyl radical scavenging agents, as well as iron chelating agents, protect Ehrlich tumor cells against diaziquone cytotoxicity (Doroshow, 1986b). Szmigiero and Kohn (1984) found that when diaziquone was incubated with isolated nuclei and NADPH DNA single strand breaks were formed which could be completely prevented by superoxide dismutase. DNA single strand breaks have been reported in human and murine cell lines incubated with diaziquone (Szmigiero et al., 1984). As with DNA crosslinks considerable variability in DNA strand breakage between cell lines is seen. IMR-90 cells show large amounts of strand breakage while HT-29 cells show little or no strand breakage. Catalase, glycerol and dimethylsulfoxide decrease DNA strand breakage with intact cells while superoxide dismutase has little effect. This may be because of limited uptake of superoxide dismutase by the intact cells. In this study the cytotoxicity of diaziquone to the different cell lines did not correlate with the degree of DNA strand breaks.

Silva and O'Brien (1989) found that in rat hepatocytes diaziquone caused the stochiometric oxidation of reduced glutathione to glutathione disulfide and that cytotoxicity occurred when diaziquone concentrations were sufficient to completely deplete reduced glutathione. When catalase was inhibited by azide or cyanamide, diaziquone cytotoxicity was increased up to 100-fold if ascorbate was also present. The authors concluded that aerobic oxidation–reduction cycling of diaziquone with formation of hydrogen peroxide was responsible for cytotoxicity, and suggested a mechanism involving mitochondrial Ca^{2+} release. If oxygen radicals are important for cytotoxicity of aziridinylbenzoquinones exposing cells to the compounds in the absence of oxygen should lead to a decrease in cytotoxicity. On the other hand, if reduction of aziridinylbenzoquinone to the semiquinone radical is necessary for alkylation, as has been shown for chemically reduced diaziquone in vitro, the absence of oxygen should increase aziridinylbenzoquinone cytotoxicity by allowing a higher steady state concentration of semiquinone radical when there is no redox cycling. Studies with A204 human rhabdomyosarcoma cells and Chinese hamster ovary cells exposed to diaziquone in the presence or absence of air have shown no difference in the cytotoxicity of diaziquone (Powis et al., 1987b). Tannock (1983) has reported no selective toxicity of diaziquone for hypoxic mouse mammary tumor cells in vivo. These results suggest that if diaziquone semiquinone radical is important for cytotoxicity its concentration is not affected by oxygen at physiological conditions.

The work of Mossoba et al. (1985) discussed previously, shows that protonation of the aziridine rings at acid pH greatly facilitates reduction leading to aziridine ring opening. Acid conditions should, therefore, favor both spontaneous and biologic activation of aziridinylbenzoquinones. Attempts have been made to increase the antitumor activity of carbazilquinone by selectively lowering tumor cell intracellular pH. The approach was based on the hypothesis that glucose should selectively increases lactic acid production by tumor cells which tend to have a higher glycolytic activity than normal cells (Warburg, 1924). Glucose did indeed increase the in vitro (Handa and Sato, 1975; Kimura et al., 1974) and in vivo antitumor activity in mice of carbazilquinone (Handa and Sato, 1975; Kimura et al., 1974; Baba et al., 1979). However, neither intracellular nor extracellular pH was measured in these studies and the mechanism of the increased cytotoxicity of carbazilquinone in the presence of glucose remains to be established.

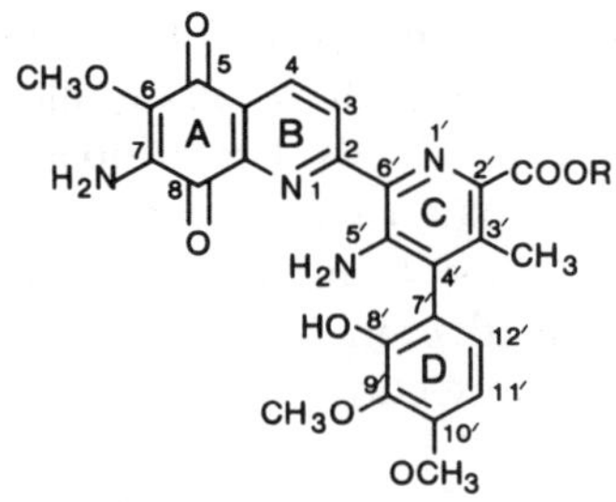

Compound	R
Streptonigrin	H
Methylstreptonigrin	CH_3

FIG. 25. Structure of some streptonigrins.

Butler et al. (1989) studied the alkylation of DNA in vitro by BZQ and concluded that BZQ functions as a bifunctional alkylating agent by an acid-assisted aziridine ring-opening and that other factors such as oxidation or reduction are much less important for cytotoxicity.

A mitochondrial site of action for diaziquone has been suggested by Obere-Greenwood et al. (1983) based on morphological evidence of early damage to mitochondria in glioma cells exposed to diaziquone. Mechanisms such as alkylation of mitochondrial DNA, interference with electron transport and disruption of the lipid layer of the mitochondrial inner membrane were suggested.

7. STREPTONIGRINS

7.1. Historical Perspective

Streptonigrin is an aminoquinone antibiotic first isolated in 1960 from *S. flocculus* by investigators at the Pfizer Company, U.S.A. (Rao and Cullen, 1960). Bruneomycin, isolated in the U.S.S.R. a number of years later, proved to be identical to streptonigrin (Brazhnikova et al., 1968). The structure of streptonigrin was determined by Rao et al. (1963) and later confirmed by Chiu and Lipscomb (1975) (Fig. 25). Streptonigrin was found to have broad-spectrum in vitro antibiotic and antiviral activity and significant antitumor activity in experimental animals (Oleson et al., 1961; Rao and Cullen, 1960). Clinical trials of streptonigrin showed that although it had some activity against human malignancies it also produced severe toxicity (Humphrey and Blank, 1961). Methylstreptonigrin was synthesized in an attempt to overcome the toxic side effects of streptonigrin but it offered no advantage over streptonigrin in clinical trials (Rivers et al., 1966).

7.2. Structure–Activity Relationships

A number of streptonigrin derivatives have been synthesized and tested for experimental antitumor activity (Driscoll et al., 1974; Inouye et al., 1985; Mizuno, 1967). Masking the quinone group, as in the monoxime, results in compounds with little or no antitumor activity (Rao, 1974). Replacement of the C-7 amino group also results in a loss of antitumor activity showing the importance of the aminoquinone structure, which is also found in mitomycins and actinomycin D (Rao et al., 1963). At least part of the linked amino substituted picolinic acid moiety is necessary for activity (Rao, 1974).

7.3. Clinical Activity

Streptonigrin given either intravenously and orally has been evaluated against a wide range of human tumors and shown to produce objective responses in patients with lymphoid malignancies (Kremer and Laszlo, 1975). The spectrum of activity of streptonigrin is similar to that of chlorambucil (Kuang et al., 1969), but the high degree of toxicity, in the form of severe nausea and vomiting, and delayed bone marrow suppression (Humphrey and Blank, 1961) led to the abandonment of streptonigrin for clinical use. Methylstreptonigrin was also subjected to clinical trials in the hope that it would have fewer toxic side effects than streptonigrin (Rivers et al., 1966). Responses to methylstreptonigrin were seen in patients with lymphoid malignancies but at higher doses than streptonigrin, and severe nausea and vomiting and bone marrow suppression led to the abandonment of methylstreptonigrin for clinical use.

7.4. Metabolism

The metabolism of streptonigrin in vivo has not been reported. Studies in vitro have shown that streptonigrins undergo redox cycling as do other quinones. Streptonigrin and methylstreptonigrin are reduced under aerobic conditions with an increase in oxygen utilization and formation of hydrogen peroxide by rat liver mitochondria and NADPH or NADH (Hochstein et al., 1965; Inouye et al., 1986; Kremer and Laszlo, 1967), by rat liver microsomes and NADPH (Bachur et al., 1978b) and by NADPH-cytochrome P-450 reductase and NADPH (Bachur et al., 1979). The hydrogen peroxide probably results from dismutation of superoxide anion radical which has been shown to be formed when streptonigrin is reduced by ferredoxin-NADPH reductase and NADPH under aerobic conditions (White et al., 1971). When streptonigrin is reduced under anaerobic conditions by intact bacteria (Ishizu et al., 1968; White and Dearman, 1965) and by rat liver microsomes and NADPH (Bachur et al., 1978b) an ESR radical signal is formed. Comparison of this ESR signal with the signal produced when streptonigrin is reduced by sodium borohydride has permitted its assignment as the streptonigrin semiquinone radical (Lown et al., 1978). A PBN-hydroxyl radical adduct is seen when streptonigrin semiquinone radical is mixed with PBN under aerobic conditions (Lown et al., 1978).

7.5. Metabolism and Biological Activity

The mechanisms of streptonigrin's cytotoxicity are poorly understood. Streptonigrin does not intercalate with DNA (Cone et al., 1976; Mizuno and Gilboe, 1970) although it does bind strongly to the cytosine moiety of DNA (Mizuno and Giboe, 1970). This binding has been suggested to be responsible for the inhibition of DNA synthesis and replication seen with streptonigrin (Mizuno and Gilboe, 1970). Streptonigrin also binds covalently to DNA when reduced chemically or enzymatically by hepatic microsomes and NADPH (Sinha, 1981). Binding to DNA is more extensive following enzymatic reduction than following chemical reduction. Zn(II) ions increase the chemical but not the enzymatic binding of streptonigrin to DNA. The nature of the alkylating species responsible for streptonigrin binding to DNA has not been determined.

Like mitomycin C the antibacterial action of streptonigrin requires its intracellular reduction (White and White, 1964), but unlike mitomcyin C streptonigrin does not crosslink DNA (Szybalski and Iyer, 1964). In vitro reduced streptonigrin produces DNA degradation and single strand breaks (White and White, 1966). The lethal effect of streptonigrin has been reported to correlate directly with the extent of DNA degradation. Studies of a series of aza and diaza bicyclicquinones related to the AB ring system of streptonigrin have shown that DNA degradation increases with increasing quinone reduction potential (Shaikh et al., 1986). In vivo streptonigrin degrades bacterial DNA to acid soluble components and produces DNA single strand breaks (Levine and Brothwick, 1963; Szybalski, 1964). When incubated with human leukocytes streptonigrin produces extensive chromosomal breaks and rearrangements (Cohen et al., 1963) as well as indications of DNA degradation (Miller et al., 1967). Lown and his colleagues (Cone et al., 1976; Lown and Sim, 1976) have found that a mixture of streptonigrin and NADH or NADPH cleaves closed circular DNA in a reaction that is inhibited by catalase, superoxide dismutase and potassium iodide, a hydroxyl radical scavenger. The authors ascribed DNA degradation to the slow reduction of streptonigrin by reduced pyridine nucleotide followed by auto-oxidation and formation of superoxide anion radical and hydroxyl radical. Studies with substituted 5,8-quinolinediones resembling streptonigrin have shown that hydroquinone auto-oxidation occurs most readily as a metalion complex (Lown and Sim, 1976). This finding led Cone et al. (1976) to suggest that auto-oxidation of reduced streptonigrin might be facilitated by metal complexation. Metal complexation has been reported to alter the redox of streptonigrin (Hadju and Armstrong, 1981) and coordination of the quinone oxygen with Cu(II) makes streptonigrin more readily chemically reducible (Lown, 1983). Cu(II) and Co(II) ions have been found to stimulate reduced streptonigrin-induced cleavage of DNA (Cone et al., 1976). Streptonigrin incubated with xanthine oxidase and hypoxanthine at low oxygen concentrations, although not in air, degrades deoxyribose (Gutteridge, 1984b). The degradation is inhibited by hydroxyl radical scavengers, catalase, and iron chelating agents, suggesting a role for a hydroxyl radical like species in the process.

Oxygen is required for the maximum antibacterial effect of streptonigrin and reactive oxygen species have been suggested to be responsible for the antibacterial activity of streptonigrin (White and White, 1964). *E. coli* grown in an atmosphere of oxygen has higher levels of superoxide dismutase than cells grown anaerobically, and the oxygen grown cells are more resistant to the lethal effects of a streptonigrin in the presence of oxygen than the anaerobically grown cells (Gregory and Fridovich, 1973). This difference disappears under anaerobic conditions. The results have been taken to indicate that the enhanced lethality of streptonigrin under aerobic conditions is due to generation of superoxide anion radical by redox cycling of streptonigrin. This interpretation appears to be supported by the observation that streptonigrin monoxime, which is not reduced and does not form superoxide anion radical, is not toxic to either superoxide dismutase induced or uninduced cells. However, Harley et al. (1982) have reported that *E. coli* grown in hyperbaric oxygen have even higher levels superoxide dismutase than *E. coli* grown in air, but that both cell types exhibit the same sensitivity to streptonigrin. On the basis of these results, Harley et al. (1982) concluded that superoxide dismutase was not involved in bacterial resistance to streptonigrin. Evidence suggesting a role of reactive oxygen species in the antitumor activity of streptonigrin is the greater cytotoxicity of streptonigrin to euoxic than to hypoxic EMT6 carcinoma or sarcoma 180 tumor cells (Kennedy et al., 1983; Teicher et al., 1981). Sinha (1981) has suggested that in addition to redox cycling as free drug, streptonigrin covalently bound to DNA might redox cycle with production of active oxygen species in close proximity to DNA.

Miller et al. (1967) has proposed that the cellular toxicity of streptonigrin is due uncoupling of mitochondrial oxidative phosphorylation and formation of hydrogen peroxide leading to depletion of cellular reduced pyridine nucleotides and ATP. The finding that methylstreptonigrin, which is more slowly metabolized by mitochondria than streptonigrin shows less toxicity in vitro and in vivo than streptonigrin has been taken as support for a mitochondrial action of streptonigrin (Kremer and Laszlo, 1967).

8. LAPACHOLS

8.1. Historical Perspective

Lapachol [2-(3-methyl-2-methyl-2-butenyl)-3-hydroxy-1,4-naphthoquinone] is a compound originally isolated from the roots of *Stereospermum suaveolens*. Lapachol has been known since 1858 and its structure (Fig. 26) was elucidated before the beginning of this century (Hooker, 1986). Synthesis of lapachol was reported by Fieser in 1927. The experimental antitumor activity of

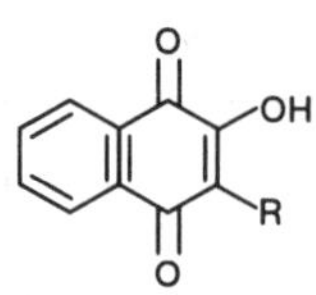

Compound	R
Lapachol	$CH_2-CH=C(CH_3)_2$
Dichloroallyl lawsone	$CH_2-CH=CCl_2$

Fig. 26. Structure of some lapachols.

lapachol was not recognized until 1968 (Rao et al., 1968). Clinical studies of lapachol in treatment of human cancer proved disappointing (Block et al., 1970, 1974) and a more lipid soluble compound, dichloroallyl lawsone (2-(3,3-dichloro-allyl)-3-hydroxy-1,4-naphthoquinone) (Fig. 26), was selected from a series of lapachol analogs for clinical development, but it also proved too toxic for human use.

8.2. Structure–Activity Relationships

A number of lapachol analogs have been tested for experimental antitumor activity (Driscoll et al., 1974; Rao, 1974). The structure of lapachol shows an almost unique specificity for biological activity. Blocking the quinone group with an oxime or a semicarbazone, removal of the hydroxyl group, or modification of the isoprenoid side chain all result in a loss of biological activity. Only if the terminal methyl groups of the isoprenoid side chain are replaced by halogen atoms, as in dichloroallyl lawsone, is there no loss of antitumor activity.

8.3. Clinical Activity

Lapachol has been subjected to limited clinical trials (Block et al., 1970, 1974). No tumor responses were seen and the toxic effects were nausea and vomiting, and an increased blood clotting time. Failure to achieve a favorable clinical response was ascribed to the low plasma levels of lapachol that were attained at the doses used in humans. The lack of signs of antitumor activity and the uncertain effects on antitumor activity of having to administer vitamin K to correct the prolonged blood clotting time led to discontinuation of the clinical use of lapachol (Block et al., 1974). Dichloroallyl lawsone was selected as a more lipid soluble lapachol derivative for clinical development. However, preclinical toxicity studies showed that dichloroallyl lawsone could cause cardiac arrest in the rhesus monkey (Oleson et al., 1967). Since this effect appeared to be related to the concentration of dichloroallyl lawsone in plasma preliminary pharmacokinetic studies with tracer doses of [^{14}C]-dichloroallyl lawsone were conducted in patients in an attempt to define the safe dose limits for clinical trials (McKelvey et al., 1979). The potential for cardiac toxicity, however, effectively prevented further clinical development of dichloroallyl lawsone.

8.4. Metabolism and Biological Activity

Lapachol is a relatively poor substrate for metabolism by rat liver microsomes compared to other antitumor quinones but it does increase NADPH oxidation and oxygen utilization (Bachur et al., 1978b, 1979; Preusch, 1986). Lapachol uncouples mitochondrial oxidative phosphorylation (Hadler and Moreau, 1969; Howland, 1963). Lapachol and dichloroallyl lawsone at toxic concentrations produce a small lowering of NADPH in murine leukemia L1210 cells but do not lower intracellular glutathione (Akmen et al., 1985). Lapachol is a potent reversible inhibitor of the coumarin anticoagulant-sensitive enzyme vitamin K epoxide reductase (Preusch and Suttie, 1984), and quinone reductase (Preusch, 1986).

In mice and monkey 30% of a dose of dichloroallyl lawsone is excreted in the urine, in rat and dog 10–15%, with 10% as unchanged drug (Loo et al., 1978). There is a report by Rao (1974), without supporting data, for three metabolites of lapachol in urine of dog. The metabolites were listed as 4′-hydroxylapachol, 4′-hydroxylapachol glucuronide and a side chain terminal monocarboxylic acid lapachol derivative (Rao, 1974). In human subjects receiving lapachol plasma concentrations of lapachol-derived fluorescence exceed those of parent drug by 2- or 3-fold, suggesting the formation of metabolites which have been proposed to include 4′-hydroxylapachol and the monocarboxylic derivative (Sieber et al., 1976). Urinary elimination of lapachol-derived fluorescence in human is 10% of the dose over 48 hr (Block et al., 1970). Administration of a tracer dose of [^{14}C]- or [^{14}C-4]-dichloroallyl lawsone to cancer patients has shown an initial plasma half-life for parent drug of 49 min and a terminal half-life of 20.3 hr (Loo et al., 1978; McKelvey et al., 1979). Initially 40% of the radioactivity in plasma is unchanged drug and this percent increases with time. The 24 hr urinary excretion of radioactivity is 33% of the dose with just over one-third as unchanged drug. Metabolites of dichloroallyl lawsone were not identified.

9. ACTINOMYCIN D

9.1. HISTORICAL PERSPECTIVE

In 1940 a red crystalline antibiotic complex, designated actinomycin A, was isolated from cultures of *S. antibioticus* by Waksman and Woodruff at Rutgers University, U.S.A. It had antibacterial activity but was too toxic for human use. A series of actinomycin complexes were isolated over the next decade and their polypeptide nature established (Dalgliesh and Todd, 1949). One of the complexes, actinomycin C, was found to have antitumor activity in animals (Hackmann, 1952) and activity against Hodgkin's lymphoma in human (Schulte, 1952). It was developed for clinical use by Farbenfabriken Bayer in Germany. In the U.S.A. another actinomycin complex, actinomycin D, or dactinomycin, was also shown to have activity against human tumors (Farber, 1958) and was developed for clinical use by Merck, Sharp and Dohme.

9.2. STRUCTURE–ACTIVITY RELATIONSHIPS

Many actinomycins are mixtures, for example, actinomycin C is a mixture of actinomycins C_2, C_3 and D (Waksman and Lechavalier, 1962). Actinomycin D, however, is a single component with just traces of other actinomycins. The structure of the actinomycins was determined by Brockmann and his colleagues (Brockmann and Grone, 1953; Brockmann and Muxfeldt, 1956). Actinomycins consist of two penta-peptide lactone rings attached to a quinoneimine containing chromophore known as actinocin (Fig. 27). Different actinomycins vary in the structure of the peptide chains which will not be considered here. Total synthesis of actinomycin D has been achieved (Brockmann and Lackner, 1961). More than 100 natural, semisynthetic and totally synthetic actinomycins are known but antitumor activity is available for less than half of these (Remers, 1979a). Modification of the chromophore has shown that methyl groups at C-4 and C-6 are essential for activity. This high degree of specificity appears to be because the C-4 and C-6 substituents must pass through the gap between the base pairs in DNA during binding of actinomycin D. Replacement of the 2-amino group by a chlorine, hydroxyl or alkyl group results in a loss of antitumor activity.

9.3. CLINICAL ACTIVITY

Actinomycin D has activity against rapidly growing tumors such as Wilm's tumor, Ewing's sarcoma and choriocarcinoma and is usually given in combination with other agents, and with radiation (Glaubiger and Ramu, 1982). Toxic side effects of actinomycin D include myelosuppression, skin rashes and oral and gastrointestinal mucositis.

9.4. METABOLISM

Actinomycin D produces an increase in oxygen consumption when incubated with rat liver microsomes and NADPH, or NADPH-cytochrome P-450 reductase and NADPH (Bachur et al., 1978a). Superoxide anion radical production is increased when actinomycin D is incubated with rat heart mitochondria, heart sarcomas and NADPH, or NADH-dehydrogenase and NADH

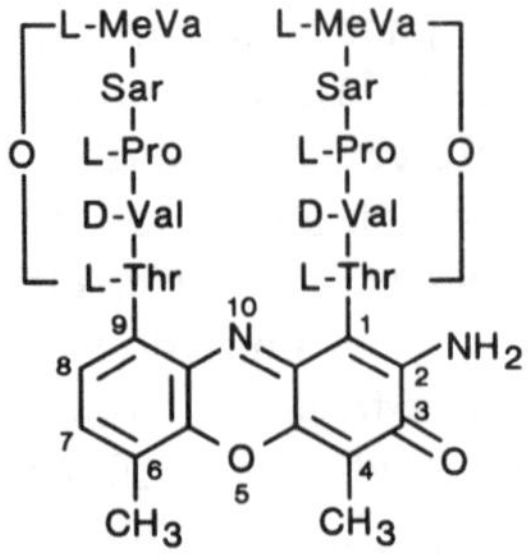

FIG. 27. Structure of actinomycin D. L-Thr, L-threonine; D-Val, D-valine; L-Pro, L-proline; Sar, sarcosine; L-MeVa, methylvaline.

(Doroshow, 1983a,b). Bachur et al. (1978a) reported an ESR radical signal, tentatively identified as that of actinomycin D semiquinoneimine radical, when actinomycin D was incubated with rat liver microsomes and NADPH under anaerobic conditions. Confirmation that the radical signal was that of the semiquinoneimine was provided by Nakazawa et al. (1981) who used chemical reduction of actinomycin D in aprotic solvent. The radical site on the actinomycin D semiquinoneimine radical has been assigned to the *N*-10 nitrogen rather than the C-3 oxygen.

Following its in vivo administration actinomycin D is rapidly removed from plasma by uptake into tissues, followed by its slow release and elimination. Studies with [^{3}H]-actinomycin D in dog, rat and monkey have shown a rapid initial phase of elimination of plasma radioactivity followed by a slower terminal phase (Galbraith and Mellett, 1975, 1976). The initial and elimination plasma half-lives of unchanged [^{3}H]-actinomycin D in rat are 2 and 180 min (Juliane and Stamp, 1978). Studies in dog employing a radioimmunoassay for measuring actinomycin D have shown an initial plasma half-life of 1 min and an elimination half-life of 208 min (Brothman et al., 1982). Following administration of [^{3}H]-actinomycin D to animals the highest tissue levels of radioactivity are found in spleen and submaxillary gland falling with a half-life of 30–50 hr (Galbraith and Mellett, 1975, 1976). No indication of actinomycin D metabolites have been found in the tissues of mice administered [^{3}H]-actinomycin D (Schwartz et al., 1968; Weissbach et al., 1966). The 24 hr urinary excretion of radioactivity following administration of [^{3}H]-actinomycin D to rat, monkey and dog is 31, 22 and 12%, and the 6 hr biliary excretion 12, 9 and 5%, respectively (Galbraith and Mellett, 1975). In these studies, analysis of the urine and bile failed to show the presence of metabolites of [^{3}H]-actinomycin D. Studies in patients receiving actinomycin D, where a radioimmunoassay was used to measure parent drug, have shown an initial plasma half-life of 2 min and an elimination half-life of 34 min (Brothman et al., 1982). Excretion of radioactivity in urine of patients receiving [^{3}H]-actinomycin D was found to be 5-13% of the dose over 24 hr (Tattersall et al., 1975). In a patient studied for 9 days 20% of the radioactivity was recovered in the urine and 14% in the feces. Paper electrophoresis of the urine revealed that 3–6% of the radioactivity was present as monolactones of actinomycin D with the remainder as unchanged drug. Since the sample of actinomycin D administered contained 2–5% monolactones, metabolism to monolactones was calculated to account for 1–4% of the dose. No actinomycinic acid was detected in the urine. In the same study it was reported that rat liver cells slowly cleaved actinomycin D to monolactones, but no data were given. It is possible the small amounts of metabolites of actinomycin D seen in human are formed by bacteria in the gastrointestinal tract since bacteria have been shown to possess an esterase that can hydrolyze the lactone ring of actinomycins to actinomycinic acid and actinomycin lactone (Perlman et al., 1967).

9.5. Metabolism and Antitumor Activity

The cytotoxic effect of actinomycin D is usually ascribed to its ability to intercalate into the helix of DNA thus interfering with transcription of RNA polymerase and preventing RNA synthesis (Glaubiger and Ramu, 1982). High concentrations of Cu(II) have been reported to prevent inhibition of proliferation of chick embryo blastoderm by actinomycin D (Iyengar and Lal, 1982). Bachur and his colleagues have suggested that the semiquinoneimine radical of actinomycin D may be the pharmacologically active and toxic form for DNA interaction and cardiac damage (Nakazawa et al., 1980, 1981). This is an interesting suggestion but a mechanism for the toxic effect of the semiquinoneimine radical remains to be established.

10. CONCLUSION AND FUTURE DIRECTIONS

The quinoid group is well represented among agents with antitumor activity and next to the chloroethyl group is the most common structural feature among clinically approved antitumor drugs in the U.S.A. In addition, there are several quinoid drugs in various stages of clinical development. A pertinent question to ask is why the quinoid group is such a common feature among anticancer drugs? Most of these drugs are natural products and as quinones are widely distributed in nature it would be expected that the quinone group would appear by chance in some compounds selected by a random screening process. Also, once an agent with promising antitumor activity has been identified great efforts are made to obtain analogs with improved therapeutic activity. This is certainly a reason for the large number of anthracycline and mitomycin compounds that have been developed, as well as new classes of antitumor agents such as the bis(substituted aminoalkylamino)anthraquinones. It seems unlikely, however, that chance and analog development are the only factors contributing to the large number of quinoid agents with antitumor activity.

Tumor cells are known to be deficient in several mechanisms that protect cell against radical damage. For example, tumor cells have low levels of cytosolic superoxide dismutase (Oberley and Buettner, 1979; Peskin et al., 1976) and, in some cases, have an almost complete absence of mitochondrial superoxide dismutase (Dionissi et al., 1975; Sahu et al., 1977). Cytosolic and mitochondrial glutathione peroxidase can also be decreased in tumor cells (Bozzi et al., 1976; Peskin et al., 1976; Pinto and Bartley, 1973). It might be relevant, in this regard, that the genes for superoxide dismutase and glutathione peroxidase are found on chromosomes that are frequently aberrant in neoplastic cells (Mitelman and Levan, 1978; Peskin et al., 1981; Shows and McAlpine, 1979). It is tempting to speculate that because of these enzyme deficiencies tumor cells are more susceptible to quinoid-dependent radical damage than are normal cells.

Quinoid compounds undergo two types of metabolism. There is metabolism important for elimination of the quinoid from the body, which can be termed pharmacokinetic metabolism, and there is metabolism which may be important for the biological effects of the quinoid, which can be termed pharmacodynamic metabolism. Pharmacokinetic metabolism depends, for the most part, upon the nature of the functional groups surrounding the quinoid nucleus. This is well exemplified by the anthracycline 4′-epidoxorubicin where a small change in the stereochemistry of the daunosamine sugar of doxorubicin results in large amounts of glucuronide conjugates being formed, while hardly any glucuronide conjugate is formed with doxorubicin. A feature common to nearly all the quinoid antitumor agents is rapid uptake from the plasma by the tissues followed by slow re-release into the plasma. Under such conditions pharmacokinetic metabolism will have relatively little effect upon the rate of quinoid elimination even though the compound may be extensively metabolized. Pharmacodynamic metabolism involves the quinone or quinoneimine group and is unique in that, despite extensive metabolism, there is little change in the total concentration of the compound under aerobic conditions because of redox cycling of the quinoid. A feature of pharmacodynamic metabolism of quinoid compounds is that all tissues, including the tumor, have enzymes for the reductive metabolism of quinoids and there is no need to postulate transport forms of quinoid cytotoxic metabolites. Only a small fraction of the total pharmacodynamic drug metabolism probably contributes to the cytotoxic effects of the drug. This can make it difficult to determine the true contribution of metabolism in quinoid cytotoxicity.

Considerable attention has been devoted to chemical pathways of alkylation by antitumor quinoids. A dichotomy is apparent between the chemical literature, where conditions favoring two-electron reduction are studied and mechanisms of quinoid alkylation involving two-electron reduction have been proposed, and the biological literature, where most enzymes responsible for quinoid reduction transfer only a single electron and mechanisms involving single-electron reduction leading to alkylation by quinoids have been proposed. The difference between the two approaches may be more apparent than real since an equilibrium exists between the reduced forms of a quinoid. This means that because a quinoid undergoes initial single-electron reduction, a two-electron alkylation mechanism is not ruled out and vice versa.

There appear to be two important factors for antitumor activity of quinoid compounds. First, metabolism of the quinoid group is necessary for cytotoxicity and second, antitumor activity is associated with binding of the compound to DNA or other sites in the cell. A general mechanism for the cytotoxicity and antitumor activity of quinoid compounds incorporating these features is

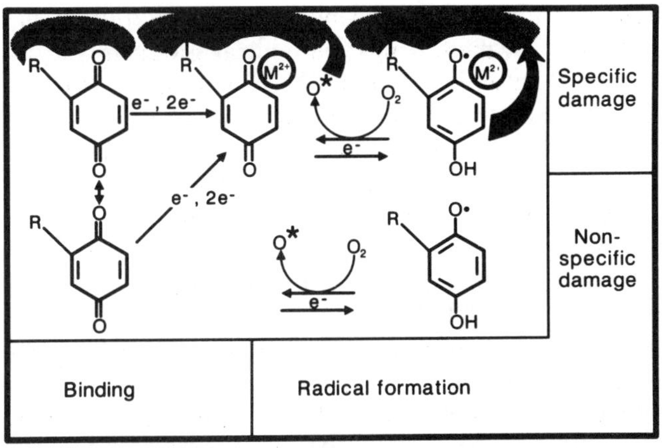

FIG. 28. Proposed mechanisms of non-specific and specific quinoid cytotoxicity. Quinoid compounds are reductively activated to alkylating species that bind covalently to critical macromolecular sites. Alkylation may occur after non-covalent binding of the compound leading to site-specific covalent binding. Binding is shown here through a substituent group but may be directly to the quinoid group. The covalently bound quinoid is reduced either enzymatically or by a diffusible reductant, to a semiquinoid radical which auto-oxidizes to give reactive oxygen species. M^{2+} indicates the stimulatory effect of divalent metal ions on the process. The large arrows show site specific damage to the cell caused by the semiquinoid radical or reactive oxygen species. Without binding of the quinoid formation of the semiquinoid radical and redox cycling with formation of reactive oxygen species leads to non-selective damage to the cell.

shown in Fig. 28. It represents a synthesis of a large number of observations and should only be regarded as a working hypothesis. It is unlikely to explain all the biologic effects of quinoid compounds. The anthracyclines, bis(substituted aminoalkylamin)anthraquinones, streptonigrin and actinomycin D bind reversibly to DNA while all the quinoids except bis(substituted aminoalkylamino)anthraquinones, lapachol and actinomycin D have been shown to bind covalently to DNA after chemical or enzymatic reduction. It is possible that in many cases non-covalent binding of quinoids precedes covalent binding leading to site-specific alkylation of DNA. However, alkylation of DNA by itself cannot explain the wide spectrum of antitumor activity of the quinoid compounds. In the proposed model covalently bound quinoid is seen as being reduced, either enzymatically or by a diffusible cellular reductant, leading to the formation of semiquinoid radical bound to the DNA. The semiquinoid radical then undergoes electron transfer reactions with suitable groups in the immediate vicinity, or auto-oxidizes to form reactive oxygen species. The consequence, in both cases, is site-specific damage to the DNA, its location determined by the specificity of the original binding reaction. According to this model the decreased cytotoxicity of quinoids such as mitomycin C under euoxic conditions could be due to decreased covalent binding of mitomycin C to the sensitive site because of auto-oxidation of the reductively activated binding species. A role for divalent metal ions such as Cu(II) or Fe(II) has been shown for DNA degradation by anthracyclines, mitomycins, aziridinylbenzoquinones and streptonigrin and is included in the proposed mechanism. In the case of the anthracyclines a ternary complex is formed between the quinoid, the divalent metal ion and DNA. Whether a complex is formed between DNA, divalent metal ions and other quinoids is not known.

The mechanism shown in Fig. 28 does not presuppose nuclear DNA as the site of action of antitumor quinoid compounds. It has been generally assumed that nuclear DNA is the site of action of antitumor quinoids because antitumor quinoids bind to DNA and produce measurable DNA damage. This may be part of a more general covalent binding of quinoid compounds with damage at other critical sites in the cell. These other sites could be solely responsible, or could contribute to the cytotoxic effects of the quinoid compounds. It is probable and indeed likely that more than one mechanism will be found to contribute to the antitumor activity of the quinoid compounds. Damage to mitochondrial DNA as a mechanism of cytotoxicity has received relatively little attention until now and is interesting because the mitochondrion contains several enzymes that metabolize quinoids. The cell surface membrane is another potential site for anticancer drug action (Hickman et al., 1985; Tritton and Hickman, 1985). Several quinoid-reducing flavoenzymes are located at the cell surface membrane (Green et al., 1980; Goldenberg, 1982) and there could be localized quinoid-dependent damage to the cell surface membrane. Inhibition of the cell surface receptor for epidermal growth factor during quinoid metabolism has been reported (Shoyab and Todaro, 1980).

Without binding to DNA or other cellular macromolecules quinoid compounds are seen as producing nonspecific cytotoxicity due to unfocused cellular metabolism with a disruption of the redox status of the cell. A similar mechanism may account for the cardiotoxicity of quinoid compounds where a high rate of oxidative metabolism in the heart makes it a prime target for quinoid-induced oxygen radical damage. Generation of oxygen radicals leading to peroxidation of lipid membranes is the currently favored mechanism for quinoid-induced cardiotoxicity. While this may be the mechanism of acute cardiotoxicity produced by quinoid compounds, it has yet to be demonstrated that lipid peroxidation plays a role in the clinically more relevant chronic cardiotoxicity of quinoid compounds. The observation that the poorly metabolized bis(substituted aminoalkylamino)-anthraquinones are cardiotoxic in humans despite the absence of cardiotoxicity in animals, suggests that quinoid-induced cardiotoxicity in humans may have a different basis to that seen in animal models.

The quinoid compounds are one of the most useful and, arguably, the most intriguing class of antitumor agents. We still do not know with certainty how they produce their effects although there is good evidence that metabolism is important for cytotoxic action. The quinoid compounds offer great potential for devising new agents and strategies to treat human cancer, independent of modifying the bodies own response to the disease. However, until we have a clearer understanding of how the antitumor quinoids act, we will not be able to embark upon a rational search for new quinoid compounds to treat human cancer. The future offers exciting challenges to chemists, pharmacologists, biochemists, molecular biologists, and others who would answer the question of how the quinoid class of antitumor agents produce their biological effects.

REFERENCES

Abdella, B. R. J. and Fisher, J. (1985) A chemical perspective on the anthracycline antitumor antibiotics. *Environ. Hlth. Perspect.* **64:** 3–18.

Abramson, H. N., Banning, J. W., Nachtman, J. P., Roginski, E. T., Sardessai, M., Wormser, H. C., Wu, J., Nagai, Z., Schroeder, R. R. and Bernardo, M. M. (1986) Synthesis of anthraquinonyl glucosaminosides and studies on the influence of aglycone hydroxyl substitution on superoxide generation. DNA binding, and antimicrobial properties. *J. Med. Chem.* **29:** 1709–1714.

Ackman, S., Dietrich, M., Chlebowski, R., Doroshow J. and Block, J. (1985) Menadione (K3) and dicumarol (D) synergy vs. leukemia 1210. *Proc. Am. Assoc. Cancer Res.* **26:** 325.

Acton, M. (1980) N-alkylation of anthracylines. In: *Anthracyclines, Current Status and New Developments*, pp. 15–25, Crooke, S. T. and Reich, S. D. (eds) Academic Press, New York.

Acton, M., Tong, G. L., Mosher, C. W. and Wolgemuth, R. L. (1984) Intensely potent morpholinyl anthracyclines. *J. Med. Chem.* **27:** 638–645.

Adachi, T., Nagae, T., Ho, Y., Hirano, K. and Sugiura, M. (1983) Relation between cardiotoxic effect of adriamycin and superoxide anion radical. *J. Pharmacobiodyn.* **6:** 114–123.

Adamson, R. H. (1974) Daunomycin (NSC-82151) and adriamycin (NSC-123127): a hypothesis concerning antitumor activity and cardiotoxicity. *Cancer Chemother. Rep.* **58:** 293–294.

Aiekens, B., Niermann, R. and Schindler, E. (1982) Investigation about the penetration depth in the normal bladder wall and tumor by local instillation of mitomycin into the urinary bladder. *Urol. Int.* **37:** 389–393.

Afanas'ev, I. B., Polozova, N. I. and Samokhvalov, G. I. (1980) Investigation of the interaction of superoxide ion with adriamycin and the possible origin of cardiotoxicity of the anthracycline anticancer antibiotics. *Bioorg. Chem.* **9:** 434–439.

Ahmed, N. K. (1985) Daunorubicin reductase activity in human normal lymphocytes, myeloblasts and leukemic cell lines. *Eur. J. Clin. Oncol.* **21:** 1209–1213.

Ahmed, N. K., Felsted, R. L. and Bachur, N. L. (1978a) Heterogeneity of anthracycline antibiotic carbonyl reductases in mammalian livers. *Biochem. Pharmac.* **27:** 2713–2719.

Ahmed, N. K., Felsted, R. L. and Bachur, N. R. (1978b) Comparison and characterization of mammalian xenobiotic ketone reductases. *J. Pharmac. Exp. Ther.* **209:** 12–19.

Ahmed, N. K., Felsted, R. L. and Bachur, N. R. (1981) Daunorubicin reduction mediated by aldehyde and ketone reductases. *Xenobiotica* **11:** 131–136.

AKHTAR, M. H., BEGLEITER, A., JOHNSON, D., LOWN, L. W., MACHAUGHLIN, L. and SIM, S. K. (1975) Studies relating to antitumor antibiotics. Part VI. Correlation of covalent crosslinking of DNA by bifunctional aziridinoquinones with their antineoplastic activity. *Can. J. Chem.* **53:** 2891–2905.

AKMAN, S. A., DIETRICH, M., CHLEBOWSKI, R., LIMBERG, P. and BLOCK, J. B. (1985) Modulation of cytotoxicity of menadione sodium busulfite versus leukemia L1210 by the acid soluble thiol pool. *Cancer Res.* **45:** 5257–5262.

AKMAN, S. A., FORREST, G., CHU, F. F., ESWORTHY, R. S. and DOROSHOW, J. H. (1990) Antioxidant and xenobiotic-metabolizing enzyme gene expression in doxorubicin-resistant MCF-7 breast cancer cells. *Cancer Res.* **50:** 1297–1402.

ALBANO, E., RUNDGREN, P. J., HARVISON, P. J., NELSON, S. D. and MOLDEUS, P. (1985) Mechanisms of *N*-acetyl-*p*-benzoquinoneimine cytotoxicity. *Molec. Pharmac.* **28:** 306–311.

ALBERTS, D. S., BACHUR, N. R. and HOLTZMAN, J. L. (1971) The pharmacokinetics of daunomycin in man. *Clin. Pharmac. Ther.* **12:** 96–104.

ALBERTS, D. S., PENG, Y. M., LEIGH, S., DAVIS, T. P. and WOODWARD, D. L. (1983) Disposition of mitoxantrone in patients. *Cancer Treat. Rev.* **20:** 23–27.

ALBERTS, D. S., PENG, Y. M., BOWDEN, G. T., DALTON, W. S. and MACKEL, C. (1985a) Pharmacology of mitoxantrone: mode of action and pharmacokinetics. *Invest. New Drugs* **3:** 101–107.

ALBERTS, D. S., PENG, Y. M., LEIGH, S., DAVIS, T. P. and WOODWARD, D. L. (1985b) Disposition of mitoxantrone in cancer patients. *Cancer Res.* **45:** 1879–1884.

ALHONEN-HONGISTO, L., DEEN, D. F. and MARTON, L. J. (1984) Decreased cytotoxicity of aziridinylbenzoquinone caused by polyamine depletion in 9L rat brain tumor cells *in vitro*. *Cancer Res.* **44:** 39–42.

AL-NABULSI, I. and GUTIERREZ, P. L. (1991) Photosensitization by diaziquone: correlation between diaziquone cytotoxicity and photoinduced free radicals in MCF-7 cells. *Proc. Am. Ass. Cancer Res.* **32:** 39.

ALEGRIA, A. E., SAMUNI, A., MITCHELL, J. B., RIESZ, P. and RUSSO, A. (1989) Free radicals induced by adriamycin-sensitive and adriamycin-resistant cells: a spin-trapping study. *Biochemistry* **28:** 8653–8658.

AMES, B. N. (1983) Dietary carcinogens and anticarcinogens. Oxygen radials and degenerative diseases. *Science* **221:** 1256–1264.

ANDO, S., NAKAMURA, T., KAGAWA, D., UEDA, T., NISHIMURA, T., KUBO, A., TSUTANI, H., SASADA, M. and UCHINO, H. (1986) Pharmacokinetics of aclarubicin and its metabolites in humans and their disposition in blood cells. *Cancer Treat. Rep.* **70:** 835–841.

ANDREWS, P. A., BRENNER, D. E., CHOU, F. T. E., KUBO, H. and BACHUR, N. R. (1980) Facile and definitive determination of human adriamycin and daunoribicin metabolites by high-pressure liquid chromatography. *Drug Metab. Disp.* **8:** 152–156.

ANDREWS, P. A., PAN, S., GLOVER, C. J. and BACHUR, N. R. (1983) Electrochemical reduction of mitomycin C to alkylating intermediates. *Proc. Am. Assoc. Cancer Res.* **24:** 246.

ANDREWS, P. A., PAN, S. and BACHUR, N. R. (1986) Electrochemical reductive activation of mitomycin C. *J. Am. Chem. Soc.* **108:** 4158–4166.

ANNE, A. and MOIROUX, J. (1984) One-electron reduction of variously substituted anthraquinones. Reactivity of the radical anions with oxygen in aprotic media. *Nouv. J. Chim.* **8:** 259–266.

ANNE, A. and MOIROUX, J. (1985) One-electron and two-electron reductions of daunomycin, *Nouv. J. Chim.* **9:** 83–89.

ARAKAWA, M., AOKI, T. and NAKAO, H. (1970a) The effect of carbaziliquinone on lymphoid leukemia. L1210. *Gann* **61:** 485–493.

ARAKAWA, M., NAKAO, H. and AOKI, T. (1970b) Effect of carbaziliquinone on transplantable and primary tumors in mice. *Gann* **61:** 535–539.

ARCAMONE, F. (1977) New antitumor anthracyclines. *Lloydia* **40:** 45–66.

ARCAMONE, F. (1984) Antitumor anthracyclines: recent developments. *Med. Res. Rev.* **4:** 153–158.

ARCAMONE, F. (1985) Properties of antitumor anthracyclines and new developments in their application: Cain Memorial Award Lecture. *Cancer Res.* **45:** 5995–5999.

ARCAMONE, F., FRANCESHCHI, G., PENCO, S. and SELVA, A. (1969) Adriamycin (14-hydroxydaunomycin), a novel antitumor antibiotic. *Tetrahedron Lett.* **13,** 1007–1016.

ARCAMONE, F., CASAZZA, A. M. and CASSEINELLI, G. (1982) Doxorubicin and related compounds. II. Structure-activity considerations. In: *Anthracycline Antibiotics in Cancer Therapy*, pp. 179–189, MUGGIA, F. M., YOUNG, C. A. and CARTER, S. K. (eds) Martinus Nijhoff, The Hague.

ARCAMONE, F., LAZZATI, M., VICARIO, G. P. and ZINI, G. (1984) Disposition of ^{14}C-labelled 4′-epidoxorubicin and doxorubicin in the rat. A comparative study. *Cancer Chemother. Rep.* **12:** 157–166.

ARMSTRONG, D. A. and BUCHANAN, J. D. (1978) Reactions of O_2^-, H_2O_2 and other oxidants with sulfhydryl enzymes. *Photochem. Photobiol.* **28:** 743–749.

ASBELL, M. A., SCHWARTZBACH, E., BULLOCK, F. J. and YESAIR, D. W. (1972) Daunomycin and adriamycin metabolism via glycoside cleavage. *J. Pharmac. Exp. Ther.* **182:** 63–69.

ASHNAGER, A., BRUCE, J. M., DUTTON, P. L. and PRINCE, R. C. (1984) One- and two-electron reduction of hydroxy-1,4-naphthoquinones and hydroxy-9,10-anthraquinones. *Biochem. biophys. Acta* **801:** 351–359.

AUBEL-SADRON, G. and LONDOS-GAGLIARDI, D. (1984) Daunorubicin and doxorubicin, anthracycline antibiotics, a physicochemical and biological review. *Biochimie* **66:** 333–352.

AUCLAIR, C. and PAOLETTI, C. (1981) Bioactivation of the antitumor drugs 9-hydroxyellipticine and derivatives by a peroxidase-hydrogen peroxide system. *J. Med. Chem.* **24:** 289–295.

Avramis, V. (1982) Pharmacokinetics of dihydroxyanthracenedione (DHAD) and its metabolite in rats. *Pharmacologist* **24:** 241.

Baba, T., Aoki, K., Kimura, N. T., Nishikawa, K. and Taniguchi, S. (1979) Potentiation of anticancer effect of carboquone *in vivo* by glucose pretreatment. *Gann* 70: 255–258.

Bachmann, Kamura, T., E., Weber, E. and Zbinden, G. (1975) Effects of seven anthracycline antibiotics on electrocardiogram and mitochondrial function of rat hearts. *Agents Actions* **5:** 383–390.

Bachur, N. R. (1971) Daunorubicinol, a major metabolite of daunorubicin; isolation from human urine and enzymatic reactions. *J. Pharmac. exp. Ther.* **177:** 573–578.

Bachur, N. R. and Cradock, J. C. (1970) Daunomycin metabolism in rat tissue slices. *J. Pharmac. exp. Ther.* **175:** 331–337.

Bachur, N. R. and Gee, M. (1971) Daunorubicin metabolism by rat tissue preparations. *J. Pharmac. exp. Ther.* **177:** 567–572.

Bachur, N. R. and Gee, M. (1972) Oxygen sensitive reductive cleavage of daunorubicin and adriamycin. *Fed. Proc.* **31:** 835.

Bachur, N. R. and Gee, M. (1976) Microsomal reductive glycosidase. *J. Pharmac. exp. Ther.* **197:** 681–686.

Bachur, N. R., Egorin, M. J. and Hildebrand, R. (1973) Daunorubicin and adriamycin metabolism in the golden Syrian hamster. *Biochem. Med.* **8:** 352–361.

Bachur, N. R., Hildebrand, R. C. and Jaenke, R. S. (1974) Adriamycin and daunorubicin disposition in the rabbit. *J. Pharmac. exp. Ther.* **191:** 331–340.

Bachur, N. R., Gordon, S. L. and Gee, M. L. (1977) Anthracycline antibiotic augmentation of microsomal electron transport and free radical formation. *Molec. Pharmac.* **13:** 901–910.

Bachur, N. R., Gee, M. V. and Gordon, S. L. (1978a) Enzymatic activation of actinomycin D (ACTD) to free radical state. *Proc. Am. Assoc. Cancer Res.* **19:** 75.

Bachur, N. R., Gordon, S. L. and Gee, M. V. (1978b) A general mechanism for microsomal activation of quinone anticancer agents to free radicals. *Cancer Res.* **38:** 1745–1750.

Bachur, N. R., Gordon, S. L., Gee, M. V. and Kon, H. (1979) NADPH cytochrome P-450 reductase activation of quinone anticancer agents to free radicals. *Proc. natn. Acad. Sci. U.S.A.* **76:** 954–957.

Bachur, N. R., Collins, J. M., Kelley, J. A., Van Echo, D. A., Kaplan, R. S. and Whitacre, M. (1982a) Diaziquone, 2,-5-diaziridinyl-3,6-*bis*carboethoxyamino-1,4-benzoquinone, plasma and cerebrospinal fluid kinetics. *Clin. Pharmac. Ther.* **31:** 650–655.

Bachur, N. R., Gee, M. V. and Friedman, R. D. (1982b) Nuclear catalyzed antibiotic free radical formation. *Cancer Res.* **42:** 1078–1081.

Bachur, N. R., Friedman, R. D. and Hollenbeck, R. G. (1984) Physicochemical characteristics of ferric adriamycin complexes. *Cancer Chemother. Pharmac.* **12:** 5–9.

Ballet, F., Robert, J., Bouma, M. E., Vrignaud, P. and Infante, R. (1986) Metabolism of doxorubicin and epirubicin in adult human hepatocytes in culture. *Pharmac. Res. Commun.* **18:** 343–347.

Ballet, F., Vrignaud, P., Robert, J., Rey, C. and Poupon, R. (1987) Hepatic extraction, metabolism and biliary excretion of doxorubicin in the isolated perfused rat liver. *Cancer Chemother. Pharmac.* **19:** 240–245.

Bannister, J. V. and Thornalley, P. J. (1983) The production of hydroxyl radicals by adriamycin in red blood cells. *FEBS Lett.* **157:** 170–172.

Barbieri, B., Giuliani, F. C., Bordoni, T., Casazza, A. M., Geroni, C., Bellini, O., Suarato, A., Gioia, B., Penco, S. and Arcamone, F. (1987) Chemical and biological characterization of 4′-iodo-4′-deoxydoxorubicin. *Cancer Res.* **47:** 4001–4006.

Barchielli, G., Malatesta, V., Penco, S., Sacchi, N. and Arcamone, F. (1986) Influence of the chromophore on the anthracycline reductive deglycosidation catalyzed by rat liver microsomes. *Proc. Am. Assoc. Cancer Res.* **27:** 24.

Basra, J., Brown, J. R. and Patterson, L. H. (1984) Free radical formation *in vitro* by cytotoxic anthraquinone derivatives; comparison with doxorubicin. *Invest. New Drugs* **2:** 117.

Basra, J., Wolf, C. R., Brown, J. R. and Patterson, L. H. (1985) Evidence for human liver mediated free-radical formation by doxorubicin and mitoxantrone. *Anticancer Drug Design* **1:** 45–52.

Bates, D. A. (1982) Evidence for the production of hydroxyl radicals from the adriamycin semiquinone and H_2O_2. *FEBS Lett.* **136:** 89–94.

Bates, D. A. and Winterbourn, C. C. (1982) Deoxyribose breakdown by the adriamycin semiquinone and H_2O_2: evidence for hydroxyl radical participation. *FEBS Lett.* **145:** 137–142.

Baurain, R., Masquelier, M., Deprez-DeCampaneere, D. and Trouet, A. (1980) Amino acid and dipeptide derivatives of daunorubicin. 2. Cellular pharmacology and antitumor activity on L1210 leukemia cells *in vitro* and *in vivo*. *J. Med. Chem.* **23:** 1171–1174.

Begleiter, A. (1983) Cytocidal action of the quinone group and its relationship to antitumor activity. *Cancer Res.* **43:** 481–484.

Begleiter, A. (1985) Studies on the mechanism of action of quinone antitumor agents. *Biochem. Pharmac.* **34:** 2629–2636.

Beijnen, J. H., Lingeman, H., Van Munster, H. A. and Underberg, W. J. M. (1986) Mitomycin antitumor agents: a review of their physico-chemical and analytical properties and stability. *J. Pharmac. Biomed. Anal.* **4:** 275–295.

Bellomo, G., Jewell, S. A. and Orrenius, S. (1982) The metabolism of menadione impairs the ability of rat liver mitochondria to take up and retain calcium. *J. biol. Chem.* **257:** 11,558–11,562.

BENDER, J. F., GRILLO-LOPEZ, A. J. and POSADA, J. G. (1983) Diaziquone (AZQ). *Invest. New Drugs* **1:** 71–84.

BENJAMIN, R. S., RIGGS, C. E. and BACHUR, N. R. (1973) Pharmacokinetics and metabolism of adriamycin in man. *Clin. Pharmac. Ther.* **14:** 592–600.

BENJAMIN, R. S., RIGGS, C. E., SERPICK, A. A. and BACHUR, N. R. (1974) Biliary excretion of adriamycin (A) in man. *Clin. Res.* **22:** 483A.

BENSON, A. M., HUNKELER, M. J. and TALALAY, P. (1980) Increase of NAD(P)H: quinone reductase by dietary antioxidants: possible role in protection against carcinogenesis and toxicity. *Proc. natn. Acad. Sci. U.S.A.* **77:** 5216–5220.

BERALDO, H., GARNIER-SUILLEROT, A. and TOSI, L. (1983) Copper(II)-adriamycin complexes. A circular dichroism and resonance raman study. *Inorg. Chem.* **22:** 4117–4124.

BERALDO, H., GARNIER-SUILLEROT, A., TOSI, L. and LAVELLE, F. (1985) Iron(III)-adriamycin and iron(III)-daunorubicin complexes: physicochemical characteristics, interaction with DNA, and antitumor activity. *Biochemistry* **24:** 284–289.

BERG, H., HORN, G. and IHN, W. (1982) Electrochemical reduction pathways of anthracycline antibiotics. *J. Antibiot.* **35:** 800–805.

BERGER, M. S., TALCOTT, R. E., ROSENBLUM, M. L., SILVA, M., ALI OSMAN, F. and SMITH, M. T. (1986) Use of quinones as brain-tumor therapy: preliminary results of preclincial laboratory investigations. *J.Toxicol. Env. Hlth* **16:** 713–719.

BERLIN, V. and HASELTINE, W. A. (1981) Reduction of adriamycin to a semiquinone-free radical by NADPH cytochrome P-450 reductase produces DNA cleavage in a reaction mediated by molecular oxygen. *J. biol. Chem.* **256:** 4747–4756.

BERMAN, E., WITTES, R. E., LEYLAND-JONES, B., CASPER, E. S., GRALLA, R. J., HOWARD, J., WILLIAMS, L., BONATZ, R. and YOUNG, C. W. (1983) Phase I and clinical pharmacology studies of intravenous and oral administration of 4-demethoxydaunorubicin in patients with advanced cancer. *Cancer Res.* **43:** 6096–6101.

BERTAZZOLI, C., SALA, L., SOLCIA, E. and GHIONE, M. (1975) Antagonistic action of ubiquinone on the experimental cardiotoxicity of adriamycin in isolated rabbit heart. *Int. Res. Commun. Sup. Med. Sci.* **3:** 467–472.

BIAGINI, R. E., PARDINI, R. S., LIN, A. J. and SARTORELLI, A. C. (1979) Effect of the bioreductive alkylating agent 2,3-bis(chloromethyl)-1,4-naphthoquinone on coupled mitochondria isolated from Sarcoma 180 ascites cells. *Cancer Biochem. Biophys.* **3:** 129–134.

BIAGINI, R. E., TILKA, M. A. and PARDINI, R. S. (1981) The inhibition by a series of potentially bioreductive naphthoquinones of rat liver mitochondria and Sarcoma 180 tumor cell respiration. *Res. Commun. Chem. Path. Pharmac.* **33:** 293–304.

BIELSKI, B. H. J. (1978) Reevaluation of the spectral and kinetic properties of HO_2 and H_2^- free radicals. *Photochem. Photobiol.* **28:** 645–649.

BILLINGHAM, M. E. (1979) Some recent advances in cardiac pathology. *Human Path.* **10:** 367–386.

BILLINGHAM, M. E., MASON, J. W., BRISTOW, M. R. and DANIELS, J. R. (1978) Anthracycline cardiomyopathy monitored by morphologic changes. *Cancer Treat. Rep.* **62:** 865–877.

BILMORIA, M. H. and KAMIN, H. (1973) The effect of high salt concentrations upon cytochrome c, cytochrome b_5, and iron-EDTA reductase activities of liver microsomal NADPH-cytochrome c reductase. *Ann. NY Acad. Sci.* **212:** 428–448.

BJORNSSON, T. D., SCHOLD, S. C., FRIEDMAN, H. S., SCHNIEDER, D. and FALLETTA, E. (1985) Pharmacokinetics of diaziquone after three different dosage regimens. *Cancer Treat Rep.* **69:** 1383–1385.

BLACOW, N. W. (1972) In: *Martindale, The Extra Pharmacopoeia*, 26th Edition, p. 1227, REYNOLDS, J. E. and PRASAD, A. B. (eds). The Pharmaceutical Press, London.

BLIGH, H. F. J., BARTOSZEK, A., ROBSON, C. N., HICKSON, I. D., KASPAR, C. B., BEGGS, J. D. and WOLF, C. R. (1990) Activation of mitomycin C by NadPH: cytochrome P-450 reductase. *Cancer Res.* **50:** 7789–7792.

BLOCK, J. B., SERPICK, A. A., WIERNIK, P., NAYAK, P. K. and MOLINS, D. (1970) Early clinical studies with lapachol. *Fed. Proc.* **29:** 682.

BLOCK, J. B., SERPICK, A. A., MILLER, W. and WIERNICK, P. H. (1974) Early clinical studies with lapachol. *Cancer Chemother. Rep.* **4**(Part 4): 27–28.

BOLANOWSKA, W., GESSNER, T. and PREISLER, H. (1983) A simplified method for determination of daunorubicin, adriamycin, and their chief fluorescent metabolites in human plasma by high-pressure liquid chromatography. *Cancer Chemother. Pharmac.* **10:** 187–191.

BONADONNA, G., BERETTA, G., TANCINI, G., BRAMBILLA, C., BAJETTA, E., DE PALO, G. M., DE LENA, M., FOSSATI, BELLCENI, F., GASPARINI, M., VALAGUSSA, P. and VERONESI, U. (1975) Adriamycin NSC 123127 studies at the Instituto Nasionale Tumori Milan. *Cancer Chemother. Rep.* **6:** 231–245.

BOROWY-BOROWSKI, H., LIPMAN, R. and TOMASZ, M. (1990) Recognition between mitomycin C and specific DNA sequences for cross-link formation. *Biochemistry* **29:** 2999–3006.

BOSANQUET, A. G. and MCLOUGHLIN, S. B. (1985) Stability of 2,5-diaziridinyl-3,6-*bis*(2-hydroxyethylamino)-1,4-benzoquinone (BZQ, NSC 224070) in aqueous solutions by high performance liquid chromatography. *Invest. New Drugs* **3:** 43–50.

BOUCEK, R. J., JR OLSON, R. D., BRENNER, D. E., OGUNBUNMI, E. M., INUI, M. and FLEISCHER, S. (1987) The major metabolite of doxorubicin in a potent inhibitor of membrane-associated ion pumps. A correlative study of cardiac muscle with isolated membrane fractions. *J. biol. Chem.* **262:** 15,851–15,856.

BOWDEN, G. T., ROBERTS, R., ALBERTS, D. S., PENG, Y. M and GARCIA, D. (1985) Comparative molecular pharmacology in leukemic L1210 cells of the anthracene anticancer drugs mitoxantrone and bisantrene. *Cancer Res.* **45:** 4915–4920.

Bozzi, A., Mavelli, I., Finazzi, A., Strom, R., Wolf, A. M., Mondovi, B. and Rotilio, G. (1976) Enzyme defense against reactive oxygen derivatives. II. Erythrocytes and tumor cells. *Molec. Cell Biochem.* **10:** 11–16.

Bradner, W. T., Rose, W. C., Schurig, J. E., Huftalen, J. B., Florczyk, A. P. and Vyas, D. (1984a) Experimental antitumor activity of the mitomycin analog BMY-25282. *Proc. Am. Assoc. Cancer Res.* **25:** 288.

Bradner, W. T., Rose, W. C., Schurig, J. E., Schlein, A. and Huftalen, J. B. (1984b) Antitumor activity and toxicity in animals of RR-150 (7-cysteaminomitosane), a new mitomycin derivative. *Cancer Res.* **44:** 5619–5623.

Bradner, W. T., Rose, W. C., Schurig, J. E., Huftalen, J. B., Florczyk, A. P., Rozencweig, M. and Vyas, D. (1986) Structure activity relationships among 7-aminothyldisulphide derivatives of mitomycin C. *Proc. Am. Assoc. Cancer Res.* **27:** 232.

Bradner, W. T., Remers, W. A. and Vyas, D. M. (1989) Structure-activity comparison of mitomycin C and mitomycin A analogues (review). *Anticancer Res.* **9:** 1095–1100.

Brawn, K. and Fridovich, I. (1981) DNA strand scission by enzymatically generated oxygen radicals. *Arch. Biochem. Biophys.* **206:** 414–419.

Brazhnikova, M. G., Ponomarenko, V. I. and Kavsharova, I. N. (1968) Issledovanie bruneominitsina, obrazuemogo *Act. albys* var. *bruneomycin*; ego identifikatsiia so streptonigrinom. *Antibiotiki* **13:** 99–102.

Breed, J. G., Zimmerman, A. N. E., Dormans, J. A. M. and Pinedo, H. M. (1980) Failure of the antioxidant vitamin E to protect against adriamycin-induced cardiotoxicity in the rabbit. *Cancer Res.* **40:** 2033–2038.

Brenner, D. E., Galloway, S., Cooper, J., Noone, R. and Hande, K. R. (1985) Improved high-performance liquid chromatography assay of doxorubicin: detection of circulating aglycones in human plasma and comparison with thin-layer chromatography. *Cancer Chemother. Pharmac.* **14:** 139–145.

Brenner, D. E., Collins, J. C. and Hande, K. R. (1986a) The effects of cimetidine upon the plasma pharmacokinetics of doxorubicin in rabbits. *Cancer Chemother. Pharmac.* **18:** 219–222.

Brenner, D. E., Harris, N. L., Anthony, L. B., Hatter, S., Collins, J. C. and Hande, K. R. (1986b) Effect of hepatic dysfunction upon doxorubicin pharmacology in rabbit. *Proc. Am. Assoc. Cancer Res.* **27:** 243.

Brockmann, H. (1963) Anthracyclinones and anthracyclines (Rhodomycinone and Pyrromycinone and their glycosides). *Fortschr. Chem. Org. Naturst.* **21:** 121–182.

Brockmann, H. (1969) Structural differences of the actinomycins and their derivatives. *Ann. NY Acad. Sci.* **89:** 323–335.

Brockmann, H. and Gröne, H. (1953) Abbau von actinomycin C zu actinocinin und desamino-actinocinylthreonin. *Chem. Ber.* **91:** 773–781.

Brockmann, H. and Lackner, H. (1961) Zur totalsynthese des actinomycins C_3. *Naturwissenschaften* **48:** 555.

Brockmann, H. and Muxfeldt, H. (1956) Constitution and synthesis of the actinomycin chromophore. *Angew. Chem.* **68:** 69–70.

Broggini, M., Colombo, T., Martini, A. and Danelli, M. G. (1980) Studies on the comparative distribution and biliary excretion of doxorubicin and 4′-epi-doxorubicin in mice and rats. *Cancer Treat. Rep.* **64:** 897–904.

Broggini, M., Italia, C., Colombo, T., Marmonti, L. and Donelli, M. G. (1984) Activity and distribution of iv and oral 4-demethoxydaunorubicin in murine experimental tumors. *Cancer Treat. Rep.* **68:** 739–747.

Broggini, M., Sommacampagna, B., Paolini, A., Dolfini E. and Donelli, M. G. (1986) Comparative metabolism of daunorubicin and 4-demethoxydaunorubicin in mice and rabbits. *Cancer Treat. Rep.* **70:** 697–702.

Brothman, A. R., Davis, T. P., Duffy, J. J. and Lindell, T. J. (1982) Development of an antibody to actinomycin D and its application for the detection of serum levels by radioimmunoassay. *Cancer Res.* **42:** 1184–1187.

Brown, J. R. (1978) Adriamycin and related anthracycline antibiotics. *Prog. Med. Chem.* **15:** 125–164.

Brown, T. D., Donehower, R. C., Grochow, L. B., Ettinger, D. S., Rice, A. P. and Waalkes, T. P. (1985) A Phase I study of menogaril (Men) in patients with advanced cancer. *Proc. Am. Soc. Clin. Oncol.* **4:** 32.

Bruce, J. M. (1974) Benzoquinones and related compound. In: *Rodd's Chemistry of Carbon Compounds*, 2nd Edition, Volume III, Part 4, pp. 1–306, Coffey, S. (ed.) Elsevier, Amsterdam.

Brugarolas, A., Pachon, N., Gosalvez, M., Llanderal, A. P., Lacave, A. I., Buesa, J. M. and Marco, M. G. (1978) Phase I clinical study of quelamycin. *Cancer Treat. Rep.* **62:** 1527–1534.

Brunmark, A. and Cadenas, E. (1988) Reductive addition of glutathione to p-benzoquinone, 2-hydroxy- and glutathionyl substituents on -penzohydroquinone autoxidation. *Chem.-Biol. Interact.* **12:** 273–398.

Brunmark, A. and Cadenas, E. (1989) Redox and addition chemistry of quinoid compounds and its biological implications. *Free Rad. Biol. Med.* **7:** 435–477.

Buffinton, G., Öllinger, K., Brunmark, A. and Cadenas, E. (1989) DT-diaphorase-catalyzed reduction of 1,4-naphthoquinone derivatives and glutathionyl-quinone conjugates. *Biochem. J.* **257:** 561–571.

Buice, R. G., Niell, H. B., Sidhu, P. and Gurley, B. J. (1983) Pharmacokinetics of intravenously-administered mitomycin C in non-oat cell carcinoma of the lung. *Cancer Chemother. Pharmac.* **13:** 1–4.

Bus, J. S. and Gibson, J. E. (1979) Lipid peroxication and its role in toxicology. In: *Reviews in Biochemistry and Toxicology*, pp. 5–149, Hodgson, E., Bend, J. R. and Philpot, R. M. (eds) Elsevier/North Holland, New York.

Busa, W. B. and Nuccitelli, R. (1984) Metabolic regulation via intracellular pH. *Am. J. Physiol.* **246:** R409–R438.

Butler, J., Hoey, B. M. and Swallow, A. J. (1985) Reactions of the semiquinone free radicals of anti-tumour agents with oxygen and iron complexes. *FEBS Lett.* **182:** 95–98.

Butler, J., Hoey, B. M. and Lea, J. S. (1987) The reduction of anti-tumour diaziridinyl benzoquinones. *Biochim. Biophys. Acta* **925:** 144–149.

Butler, J., Hoey, B. M. and Ward, T. H. (1989) The alkylation of DNA in vitro by 2,5-bis(2-hydroxyethylamino)-3,6-diaziridinyl-1,4-benzoquinone (BZQ)—I. *Biochem. Pharmac.* **38:** 923–927.

Cadenas, E., Boveris, A., Ragan, C. I. and Stoppani, A. O. M. (1977) Production of superoxide radicals and hydrogen peroxide by NADH-ubiquinone reductase and ubiquinol-cytochrome c reductase from beef heart mitochondria. *Arch. Biochem. Biophys.* **180:** 248–257.

Camaggi, C. M., Strocchi, E., Comparsi, R., Testoni, F., Angelelli, B. and Pannuti, F. (1986) Biliary excretion and pharmacokinetics of 4′-epidoxorubicin (epirubicin) in advanced cancer patients. *Cancer Chemother. Pharmac.* **18:** 47–50.

Cammagi, C. M., Comparsi, R., Strocchi, E., Testoni, F., Angelelli, B. and Pannuti, F. (1988) Epirubicin and doxorubicin comparative metabolism and pharmacokinetics—a cross-over study. *Cancer Chemother. Pharmac.* **21:** 221–228.

Capranico, G., Dasdia, T. and Zunino, F. (1986a) Comparison of doxorubicin-induced DNA damage in doxorubicin-sensitive and resistant P388 murine leukemia cells. *Int. J. Cancer.* **37:** 227–231.

Capranico, G., Soranzo, C. and Zunino, F. (1986b) Single-strand DNA breaks induced by chromophore-modified anthracyclines in P388 leukemia cells. *Cancer Res.* **46:** 5499–5503.

Carmichael, A. J., Mossoba, M. M. and Riesz, P. (1983) Photogeneration of superoxide by adriamycin and daunomycin. An electron spin resonance and spin trapping study. *FEBS Lett.* **164:** 401–405.

Casazza, A. M. (1986) Preclinical selection of new anthracyclines. *Cancer Treat. Rep.* **70:** 43–49.

Cassinelli, G., Configliacchi, E., Penco, S., Rivola, G., Arcamone, F., Pacciarini, A. and Ferrari, L. (1984) Separation, characterization, and analysis of epirubicin (4′-epidoxorubicin) and its metabolites from human urine. *Drug Metab. Disp.* **12:** 506–510.

Cersosimo, R. J. and Hong, W. K. (1986) Epirubicin: a review of the pharmacology, clinical activity, and adverse effects of an andriamycin analogue. *J. Clin. Oncol.* **4:** 425–439.

Chakrabarty, S. and Brattain, M. G. (1987) Molecular comparisons of acquired and native mitomycin C resistance in human colon carcinoma cells. *Cancer Lett.* **37:** 267–276.

Chakrabarty, S., Danels, Y. J., Long, B. H., Willson, J. K. V. and Brattain, M. G. (1986) Circumvention of deficient activation in mitomycin C-resistant human colonic carcinoma cells by the mitomycin C analogue BMY25282. *Cancer Res.* **46:** 3456–3458.

Chan, T. M., Chen, E., Tatoyan, A., Shargill, N. S., Pleta, M. and Hochstein, P. (1986) Stimulation of tyrosine-specific protein phosphorylation in the rat liver plasma membrane by oxygen radicals. *Biochem. biophys. Res. Commun.* **139:** 439–445.

Chang, P., Tamburini, J. M., Dodion, P., Riggs, C. E. and Bachur, N. R. (1983) *In vitro* metabolism of marcellomycin (M). *Proc. Am. Assoc. Cancer Res.* **24:** 258.

Chen, Z. M., Colombo, T., Conforti, L., Grazia-Donelli, M., Fierdorowicz, R. J., Marchi, S., Paolini, A., Riva, E., Zuanetti, G. and Latini, R. (1987) Effects of three new anthracyclines and doxorubicin on the rat isolated heart. *J. Pharm. Pharmac.* **39:** 947–950.

Cheng, C. C., Zbinden, G. and Zee-Cheng, R. K. Y. (1979) Comparison of antineoplastic activity of aminoethylaminoanthraquinones and anthracycline antibiotics. *J. Pharm. Sci.* **68:** 393–396.

Chesis, P. L., Levin, D. E., Smith, M. T., Ernster, L. and Ames, B. N. (1984) Mutagenicity of quinones: pathways of metabolic activation and detoxification. *Proc. natn. Acad. Sci. U.S.A.* **81:** 1696–1700.

Chevillard, S., Vielh P., Bastian, G. and Coppey, J. (1990) Adriamycin uptake and metabolism in organotypic culture of A549 human adenocarcinoma cells according to the exposure time. *J. Cancer Res. clin. Oncol.* **116:** 633–638.

Chiccarelli, F. S., Morrison, J. A. and Gautam, S. R. (1984) Biliary pharmacokinetics of ^{14}C-mitoxantrone in the rat following different intravenous doses and characteristics of drug-related material in the bile. *Fed. Proc.* **43:** 345.

Chiccarelli, F. S., Morrison, J. A., Cosulich, D. B., Perkinson, N. A., Ridge, D. N., Sum, F. W., Murdock, K. C. Woodward, D. L. and Arnold, E. T. (1986) Identification of human urinary mitoxantrone metabolites. *Cancer Res.* **46:** 4858–4861.

Chiu. Y. Y. H. and Lipscomb, W. N. (1975) Molecular and crystal structure of streptonigrin. *J. Am. Chem. Soc.* **97:** 2525–2530.

Chlebowski, R. T., Block, J. B. and Dietrich, M. (1981) Warfarin (W) and vitamin K_1 (K) enhance methotrexate (MTX) and 5-fluorouracil (FU) effects in L1210 cells. *Clin. Res.* **29:** 63A.

Chlebowski, R. T., Block, J. B., Dietrich, M. Octay, E., Barth, N., Yanagihara, R., Gota, C. and Ali, I. (1983) Inhibition of human tumor growth and DNA biosynthetic activity by vitamin K and warfarin: *in vitro* and clinical results. *Proc. Am. Assoc. Cancer Res.* **24:** 165.

Chlebowski, R. T., Dietrich, M., Akman, S. and Block, J. B. (1985) Vitamin K_3 inhibition of malignant murine cell growth and human tumor colony formation. *Cancer Treat. Rep.* **69:** 527–532.

CHOU, F., KHAN, A. H. and DRISCOLL, J. S. (1976) Potential central nervous system antitumor agents aziridinylbenzoquinones. 2. *J. Med. Chem.* **19:** 1302–1308.

COHEN, L. E., GLAUBIGER, D. L., KANN, H. E. and KOHN, K. W. (1986) Protein-associated DNA single strand breaks and cytotoxicity of dihydroxyanthracenedione (DHAD), NSC-301739 in mouse L1210 leukemia cells. *Proc. Am. Assoc. Cancer Res.* **21:** 277.

COHEN, M. M., SHAW, M. W. and CRAIG, A. P. (1963) The effects of streptonigrin on cultured human leukocytes. *Proc. natn. Acad. Sci. U.S.A.* **50:** 16–24.

COLOMBO, R. and MILZANI A. (1987) How does doxorubicin interfere with actin polymerization? *Biochim. Biophys. Acta* **968**:9–16.

COMIS, R. L., ISSELL, B. F., PITTMAN, K., GINSBERG, S. J., RUDOLPH, A., AUST, J. C., DIFINO, S. M., TINSLEY, R. W., POIESZ, B. J. and CROOKE, S. T. (1982) A Phase I and clinical pharmacology and study of intravenously administered carminomycin in cancer patients in the United States. *Cancer Res.* **42:** 2944–2948.

CONE, R., HASAN, S. K., LOWN, J. W. and MORGAN, A. R. (1976) The mechanism of the degradation of DNA by streptonigrin *Can. J. Biochem.* **54:** 219–223.

COPPINGER, G. M. and BAUER, R. H. (1963) Stability of hetero-p-benzoquinones. *J. Phys. Chem.* **67:** 2846–2848.

CORTES, E. P., LUTMAN, G., WANKA, J., PICKRON, J., WALLACE, J. and HOLLAND, J. F. (1973) Adriamycin cardiotoxicity in adults with cancer. *Clin. Res.* **21:** 412.

CORTES-FUNES, H., GOSALVEZ, M., MOYANO, A., MANAS, A. and MENDIOLA, C. (1979) Early clinical trial with quelamycin. *Cancer Treat. Rep.* **63:** 903–907.

COSBY, L. A., PARDINI, R. S., BIAGINI, R. E., LAMBERT, T. L., LIN, A. J., HUANG, Y.-M., HWANG, K. M. and SARTORELLI, A. C. (1976) Mode of action of the bioreductive alkylating agent, 2,3-bis(chloromethyl)-1,4-naphthoquinone. *Cancer Res.* **36:** 4023–4031.

CRADOCK, J. C., EGORIN, M. J. and BACHUR, N. R. (1973) Daunorubicin biliary excretion and metabolism in the rat. *Arch. Int. Pharmacodyn. Ther.* **202:** 48–61.

CRESPI, M. D., IVANIER, S. E., GENOVESE, J. and BALDI, A. (1986) Mitoxantrone affects topoisomerase activities in human breast cancer cells. *Biochem. Biophys. Res. Commun.* **136:** 521–528.

CROOKE, S. T. (1977) A review of carminomycin—a new anthracycline developed in the U.S.S.R. *J. Med.* **8:** 295–316.

CROOKE, S. T. and BRADNER, W. T. (1976) Mitomycin C: a review. *Cancer Treat. Rev.* **3:** 121–139.

CROOKE, S. T., DUVERNAY, V. H., GALVAN, L. and PRESTAYKO, A. W. (1978) Structure-activity relationships of anthracyclines relative to effects on macromolecular syntheses. *Molec. Pharmac.* **14:** 290–298.

CUMMINGS, J. (1985) Methods for the determination of 4′-deoxydoxorubicin, 4′-deoxydoxorubicin and their 7-deoxyaglycones in human serum by high-performance liquid chromatography. *J. Chromatogr.* **341:** 401–409.

CUMMINGS, J. and MCARDLE, C. S. (1986) Studies on the *in vivo* disposition of adriamycin in human tumors which exhibit different responses to the drug. *Br. J. Cancer* **53:** 835–838.

CUMMINGS, J. and MILROY, R. (1986) *In vitro* formation of a toxic aglycone metabolite of 4-demethoxydaunorubicin in conditions that parallel the stomach. *Anticancer Res.* **6:** 1177–1180.

CUMMINGS, J., MERRY, S. and WILLMOTT, N. (1986a) Disposition, kinetics of adriamycin, adriamycinol and their 7-deoxyaglycones in AKR mice bearing a subcutaneously growing Ridgway osteogenic sarcoma (ROS). *Eur. J. Cancer Clin. Oncol.* **22:** 451–460.

CUMMINGS, J., MILSTEAD, R., CUNNINGHAM, D. and KAYE, S. (1986b) Marked interpatient variation in adriamycin biotransformation to 7-deoxyaglycones: evidence from metabolites identified in serum. *Eur. J. Cancer Clin. Oncol.* **22:** 991–1002.

CURT, G. A., KELLEY, J. A., KUFTA, C. V., SMITH, B. H., KORNBLITH, P. L., YOUNG, R. C. and COLLINS, J. M. (1983) Phase II and pharmacokinetic study of aziridinylbenzoquinones [2,5-diaziridinyl-3,6-(carboethoxyamino)-1,4-benzoquinone, Diaziquone, NSC 182986] in high grade gliomas. *Cancer Res.* **43:** 6102–6105.

CUSACK, B. J., TESNOHLIDEK, D. A., LOSEKE, V. L., VESTAL, R. E., BRENNER, D. E. and OLSON, R. D. (1988) Effect of phenytoin on the pharmacokinetics of doxorubicin and doxorubicinol in the rabbit. *Cancer Chemother, Pharmac.* **22:** 294–298.

DAGHESTANI, A. N., ARLIN, Z. A., LEYLAND-JONES, B., GEE, T. S., KEMPIN, S. J., MERTELSMANN, R., BUDMAN, D., SCHULMAN, P., BARATZ, R., WILLIAMS, L., CLARKSON, B. D. and YOUNG, C. W. (1985) Phase I and II clinical and pharmacological study of 4-demethoxydaunorubicin) in adult patients with acute leukemia. *Cancer Res.* **45:** 1408–1412.

D'ALESSANDRO, N. D., DUSONCHET, L., CROSTA, L., CRESCIMANNO, M. and RAUSA, L. (1980) Does catalase play a role in adriamycin induced cardiotoxicity? *Pharmac. Res. Commun.* **12:** 441–446.

DALGLIESH, C. E. and TODD, A. R. (1949) Actinomycin. *Nature* **164:** 830.

DALTON, W. S., DURIE B. G. M., ALBERTS D. S. GERLACH, J. H. and CRESS, A. G. (1986) Characterization of a new drug-resistant human myeloma cell line that expresses P-glycoprotein. *Cancer Res.* **46:** 5125–5130.

DANESI R., DEL TACCA M., DELLA-TORRE P. and BERNARDINI C. (1986) General and cardiac toxicity of adriamycinol in rats. *Anticancer Res.* **6:** 967–972.

DANESI R., PAPARELLI A., BERNADINI N. and DEL TACCA M. (1988) Cytofluorescence localization and disposition of doxorubicin and doxorubicinol in rat cardiac tissue. *Eur. J. Cancer clin. Oncol.* **24:** 1123–1131.

DANISHEFSKY, S. J. and EGBERTSON, M. (1986) On the characterization of intermediates in the mitomycin activation cascate: A practical synthesis of an arziridinomitosene. *J. Am. Chem. Soc.* **108:** 4648–4650.

DANISHEFSKY, S. J. and GIUFOLINI, M. (1984) Leucomitomycins. *J. Am. Chem. Soc.* **106:** 6424–6425.

DAUGHERTY, J. P. and KHURANA, A. (1985) Amelioration of doxorubicin-induced skin necrosis in mice by butylated hydroxytoluene. *Cancer Chemother. Pharmac.* **14:** 243–246.

DAUGHERTY, J. P., WHEAT, M., CONLEY, S., COOLEY, E., VANZANT, C., LOGGINS, L and DURANT, J. R. (1982) Involvement of reactive oxygen species in adriamycin (ADR) cardiotoxicity. *Proc. Am. Assoc. Cancer Res.* **23:** 171.

DAVIES, K. J. A. and DOROSHOW, J. H. (Redox cycling of anthracyclines by cardiac mitochondria I. Anthracycline radical formation by NADH dehydrogenase. *J. biol. Chem.* **261:** 3060–3067.

DAVIES, K. J. A., DOROSHOW, J. H. and HOCHSTEIN, P. (1983) Mitochondrial NADH dehydrogenase-catalyzed oxygen radical production by adriamycin, and the relative inactivity of 5-iminodaunorubicin. *FEBS Lett.* **153:** 227–230.

DAVIS, H. L. and DAVIS, T. L. (1979) Daunorubicin and adriamycin in cancer treatment: analysis of their roles and limitations. *Cancer Treat. Rep.* **63:** 809–815.

DEBOER, C., DIETZ, A., LUMMUS, N. E. and SAVAGE, G. M. (1960) Porfiromycin, an antibiotic. I. Discovery and biological activities. *Antimicrobial Agents Ann.* **1960:** 17–22.

DEELEY, T. J. (1962) A clinical trial of Synkavit in the treatment of carcinoma of the bronchus. *Br. J. Cancer* **16:** 387–389.

DEESEN, P. E. and LEYLAND-JONES, B. (1984) Sensitive and specific determination of the new anthracycline analog 4′-epidoxorubicin and its metabolites by high pressure liquid chromatography. *Drug Metab. Disp.* **12:** 9–13.

DEGREGORIO, M. W., CARRERA, C. J., KLOCK, J. C. and WILBUR, J. R. (1982) Uptake and metabolism of daunorubicin by human leukemia cells. *Cancer Chemother. Pharmac.* **10:** 29–32.

DEGREGORIO, M. W., LIU, G. M., MACHER, B. A. and WILBUR, J. R. (1984) Uptake, metabolism, and cytotoxicity of doxorubicin in human Ewing's sarcoma and rhabdomyosarcoma cells. *Cancer Chemother. Pharmac.* **12:** 59–63.

DE LEONARDIS, V., NERI, B., BACALLI, S. and CINELLI, P. (1985) Reduction of cardiac toxicity of anthracyclines by L-carnitine preliminary overview of clinical data. *Int. J. clin. Pharmac. Res.* **5:** 137–142.

DE LEONARDIS, V., DE SCALZI, M., NERI, B., BARTALUCCI, S. and CINELLI, P. (1987) Echocardiographic assessment of anthracycline cardiotoxicity during different therapeutic regimens. *Int. J. clin. Pharmac. Res.* **7:** 307–311.

DEL TACCA, M., DANESI, R., DUCCI, M., BERNARDINI, C. and ROMANINI, A. (1985) Might adriamycinol contribute to adriamycin-induced cardiotoxicity? *Pharmac. Res. Commun.* **17:** 1073–1084.

DEMANT, E. J. F. (1983) NADH oxidation in submitochondrial particles protects respiratory chain activity against damage by adriamycin-Fe^{3+}. *Eur. J. Biochem.* **137:** 113–118.

DEMANT, E. J. F. (1984) Transfer of ferritin-bound iron to adriamycin. *FBS Lett.* **176:** 97–100.

DEN HARTIGH, J., MCVIE, J. G. and VAN OORT, W. J. (1982) Pharmacokinetics of mitomycin C in humans. *Cancer Res.* **43:** 5017–5021.

DESAI, M. H. and TERES, D. (1982) Prevention of doxorubicin-induced skin ulcers in the rat and pig with dimethyl sulfoxide (DMSO). *Cancer Treat. Rep.* **66:** 1371–1374.

DICKINSON, A. C., DEJORDY, J. D. and TERES, D. (1984) Absence of generation of oxygen-containing free radicals with 4′-deoxydoxorubicin iron-cardiotoxic anthracycline drug. *Proc. Am. Assoc. Cancer Res.* **25:** 296.

DICKINSON, A. C., BOUTIN, M. G., MATSUNAGA, N. and TERES, D. (1985) 4′-Deoxydoxorubicin and 4-demethoxydaunorubicin do not generate oxygen free radicals. *Proc. Am. Cancer Res.* **26:** 225.

DIFRONZO, G., GAMBETTA, R. A. and LENAZ, L. (1971) Distribution and metabolism of adriamycin in mice. Comparison with daunomycin. *Rev. Eur. Etud. Clin. Biol.* **16:** 572–576.

DIMARCO, A., GAETINI, M., DORIGOTTI, L., SOLDATTI, M. and BELLINI, O. (1963) Studi sperimentali sull'attivita' antineoplastica del neuovo antibiotico daunomicina. *Tumori* **49:** 203–217.

DIMARCO, A., BORETTI, G. and RUSCONI, A. (1967) Transformazione metabolica della daunomicina da parte di estratti di tessuti. *Farmaco [Sci.]* **22:** 535–542.

DIMONTE D., BELLOMO, G., THOR, H., NICOTERA, P. and ORRENIUS, S. (1984a) Menadione-induced cytotoxicity is associated with protein thiol oxidation and alteration in intracellular Ca^{2+} homeostasis. *Arch. Biochem. Biophys.* **235:** 343–350.

DIMONTE, D., ROSS, D., BELLOMO, G., EKLOW, L. and ORRENIUS, S. (1984b) Alterations in intracellular thiol homeostasis during the metabolism of menadione by isolated hepatocytes. *Arch. Biochem. Biophys.* **235:** 334–342.

DIONISSI, O., GALEOTTI, T., TERRANOVA, T. and AZZI, A. (1975) Superoxide radicals and hydrogen peroxide formation in mitochondria from normal and neoplastic tissues. *Biochim. biophys. Acta* **403:** 292–300.

DODION, P., BERNSTEIN, A. L., FOX, B. M., DAVIS, T. A., ENGLISCH, K. L. and BACHUR, N. R. (1984a) Enzymic catalysis of anthracyclines to non-flourescent metabolites. *Proc. Am. Assoc. Cancer Res.* **25:** 298.

DODION, P., CHANG, B. K., EGORIN, M. J., OLMAN, E. A., ENGLISCH, K. L. and BACHUR, N. R. (1984b) The disposition of the new anthracycline antibiotic, menogaril, in mice. *Drug Dispos. Metab.* **12:** 365–370.

DODION, P., DAVIS, T. A., ROZENCWEIG, M., WATTHIEU, M., CRESPEIGNE, N., BEER, M. and BACHUR, N. R. (1984c) Human pharmacokinetics of 4′-deoxydoxorubicin. *Proc. Am. Soc. Clin. Oncol.* **3:** 26.

DODION, P., EGORIN, M. J., TAMBURNI, J. M., RIGGS, C. F. and BACHUR, N. R. (1984d) The murine metabolism and disposition of marcellomycin. *Drug Metab. Disp.* **12:** 209–216.

Dodion, P., Riggs, C. E., Akmann, S. R., Tamburini, J. M., Colvin, O. M. and Bachur, N. R. (1984e) Interactions between cyclophosphamide and adriamycin metabolism in rats. *J. Pharmac. exp. Ther.* **229:** 51–57.

Dodion, P., Davis, T. A., Rozencweig, M., Crespeigne, N., Kenis, Y. and Bachur, N. R. (1985a) Human pharmacokinetics of esorubicin (4′-deoxydoxorubicin). *Invest. New Drug* **3:** 361–368.

Dodion, P., Egorin, M. J., Englisch, K. L. and Bachur, N. R. (1985b) Metabolism and disposition of menogaril (NSC 269148) in the rabbit. *Cancer Res.* **45:** 5352–5357.

Dodion, P., Egorin, M. J., Riggs, C. E., Ferraro, T. A., Tamburini, J. M. and Bachur, N. R. (1985c) Comparative murine metabolism and disposition of Class II anthracycline antibiotics. *Cancer Chemother. Pharmac.* **15:** 153–160.

Dodion, P., Rozencweig, M., Nicaise, C., Watthieu, M., Tamburini, J. M., Riggs, C. E. and Bachur, N. R. (1985d) Human pharmacokinetics of marcellomycin. *Cancer Chemother. Pharmac.* **14:** 42–48.

Dodion, P., Akmann, S. R., Tamburini, J. M., Riggs, C. E., Colvin, O. M. and Bachur, N. R. (1986a) Interactions between cyclophosphamide and doxorubicin metabolism in rats. II. Effect of cyclophosphos-phoramide on the aldoketoreductase system. *J. Pharmac. exp. Ther.* **237:** 271–274.

Dodion, P., Sessa, C., Joss, R., Crespeigne, N., Willems, Y., Kitt, M., Abrams, J., Finet, C., Brewer, J. E., Adams, W. J., Earhart, R. H., Rozencweig, M., Kenis, Y. and Cavalli, F. (1986b) Phase I study of intravenous menogaril given with an intermittent administration. *J. Clin. Oncol.* (in press).

Dodion, P., Tamburini, J. M., Fox, B. M., Riggs, C. E. and Bachur, N. R. (1986c) Comparative anthracycline metabolism in rats: loss of marcellomycin fluorescence. *Cancer Res.* **46:** 2714–2719.

Dodion, P., Bernastein, A. L., Fox, B. M. and Bachur, N. R. (1987) Loss of fluorescence by anthracycline antibiotics: effects of xanthine oxidase and identification of the nonfluorescent metabolites. *Cancer Res.* **47:** 1036–1039.

Doll, D. C., Weiss, R. B. and Issell, B. F. (1985) Mitomycin: ten years after approval for marketing. *J. Clin. Oncol.* **3:** 276–286.

Domae, N., Sawada, H., Matsuyama, E., Konishi, T. and Uchino, H. (1981) Cardiomyopathy and other chronic toxic effects induced in rabbits by doxorubicin and possible prevention of coenzyme Q10. *Cancer Treat. Rep.* **65:** 79–91.

Domagk, G., Peterson, S. and Gauss, W. (1954) Ein beitrag zur experimentellen chemotherapie der geschwülste. *Zeitschrift. Krebsforsch.* **59:** 617–622.

Doroshow, J. H. (1981) Mitomycin C enhanced superoxide and hydrogen peroxide formation in rat heart. *J. Pharmac. exp. Ther.* **218:** 206–211.

Doroshow, J. H. (1983a) Effect of anthracycline antibiotics on oxygen radical formation in rat heart. *Cancer Res.* **43:** 460–472.

Doroshow, J. H. (1983b) Anthracycline antibiotic-stimulated superoxide, hydrogen peroxide, and hydroxyl radical production by NADH dehydrogenase. *Cancer Res.* **43:** 4543–4551.

Doroshow, J. H. (1985) Oxygen radical-induced tumor cell killing by anticancer quinones: a common mechanism of cytotoxicity. *Proc. Am. Assoc. Cancer Res.* **26:** 225.

Doroshow, J. H. (1986a) Prevention of doxorubicin-induced killing of MCF-7 human breast cancer cells by oxygen radical scavengers and iron chelating agents. *Biochem. biophys. Res. Commun.* **135:** 330–335.

Doroshow, J. H. (1986b) Role of hydrogen peroxide and hydroxyl radical formation in the killing of Ehrlich tumor cells by anticancer quinones. *Proc. natn. Acad. Sci. U.S.A.* **83:** 4514–4518.

Doroshow, J. H. and Davies, K. J. A. (1983) Comparative cardiac oxygen radical metabolism by anthracycline antibiotics, mitoxantrone, bisantrene, 4′-(9-acridinylamino)-methesulfon-*m*-anisidine, and neocarzino-statin. *Biochem. Pharmac.* **32:** 2935–2939.

Doroshow, J. H. and Davies, K. J. A. (1986) Redox cycling of anthracyclines by cardiac mitochondria. II. Formation of superoxide anion, hydrogen peroxide, and hydroxyl radical. *J. biol. Chem.* **261:** 3068–3074.

Doroshow, J. H. and deVries, L. (1984) Hydroxyl radical (·OH)-induced tumor cell killing by doxorubicin (D). *Proc. Am. Assoc. Cancer Res.* **25:** 300.

Doroshow, J. H., Lockyer, G. Y. and Myers, C. E. (1980) Enzymatic defenses of the mouse heart against reactive oxygen metabolites: alterations produced by doxorubicin. *J. Clin. Invest.* **65:** 128–135.

Doroshow, J. H., Lockyer, G. Y., Ifrim, I. and Myers, C. E. (1982) Prevention of doxorubicin cardiac toxicity in the mouse by N-acetylcysteine. *J. Clin. Invest.* **68:** 1053–1064.

Doroshow, J. H., Tallent, C. and Schechter, J. E. (1985) Ultrastructural features of Adriamycin-induced skeletal and cardiac muscle toxicity. *Am. J. Path.* **118:** 288–297.

Dorr, R. T. and Alberts, D. S. (1983) Failure of DMSO and vitamin E to prevent doxorubicin skin ulceration in the mouse. *Cancer Treat. Rep.* **67:** 499–501.

Dorr, R. T., Bowden, G. T., Alberts, D. S. and Liddil, J. D. (1984) Molecular pharmacology of mitomycin C (MMC) and a polar metabolite (PM) on mammalian DNA. *Proc. Am. Assoc. Cancer Res.* **25:** 291.

Dorr, R. T., Bowden, G. T., Alberts, D. S. and Liddil, J. D. (1985) Interaction of mitomycin C with mammalian DNA detected by alkaline elution. *Cancer Res.* **45:** 3510–3516.

Dorr, R. T., Liddil, J. D., Trent, J. M. and Dalton, W. S. (1987) Mitomycin C resistant L-1210 leukemia cells: association with pleiotropic drug resistance. *Biochem. Pharmac.* **36:** 3115–3120.

Downward, J., Yarden, Y., Mayes, E., Scrace, G., Totty, N., Stockwell, P., Ullrich, A., Schlessinger, J. and Waterfield, M. D. (1984) Close similarity of epidermal growth factor receptor an v-*erb*-B oncogene protein sequences. *Nature* **307:** 521–527.

DRIEBERGEN, R. J., HOLTHUS, J. J. M., HULSHOFF, A., POSTMA-KELDER, S. J., VERBOOM, W., REINHOUDT, D. N. and LELIEVELD, P. (1986) Electrochemistry of potential bioreductive alkylating quinones: its use in the development of new aziridinylbenzoquinones. *Anticancer Res.* **6:** 605–620.

DRISCOLL, J. S., HAZARD, G. F., WOOD, H. B. and GOLDIN, A. (1974) Structure-antitumor activity relationships among quinone derivatives. *Cancer Chemother. Rep.* **4** (Part 2) 1–363.

DUBOST, M., GANTER, P., MARAL, R., NINET, L., PINNERT, S., PREU'DHOMME, J. and WERNER, G. H. (1963) Un novel antibiotique à propriètès cytostatiques: la rubidomycine. *C.R. Acad. Sci.,, Paris* **257:** 1813–1815..

DUKART, G., POSNER, L., HENRY, D. and WEISS, A. (1986) Comparative cardiotoxicity of mitoxantrone *vs* doxorubicin. *Proc. Am. Soc. Clin. Oncol.* **5:** 48.

DULHANTY, A. M., LI, M. and WHITMORE, G. F. (1989) Isolation of Chinese hamster ovary cell mutants deficient in excision repair and mitomycin C bioactivation. *Cancer Res.* **49:** 117–122.

DUSRE, L., MIMNAUGH, E. G., MYERS, C. E. and SINHA, B. K. (1989) Potentiation of doxorubicin cytotoxicity by buthionine sulfoximine in multidrug-resistant human breast tumor cells. *Cancer Res.* **49:** 511–515.

DUTHIE, S. J. and GRANT, M. H. (1989) The toxicity of menadione and mitozantrone in human liver-derived Hep G2 hepatoma cells. *Biochem. Pharmac.* **38:** 1247–1255.

DUVERNAY, V. H. and CROOKE, S. T. (1980) Effects of several anthracycline antitumor antibiotics on the transcriptional activity of isolated nucleoli. *J. Antibiot.* **33:** 1048–1053.

DUVERNAY, V. H., ESSERY, J. M., DOYLE, T. W., BRADNER, W. T. and CROOKE, S. T. (1979) The antitumor effects of anthracyclines. The importance of the carbomethoxy-group at position-10 of marcellomycin and rudolfomycin. *Molec. Pharmac.* **15:** 341–356.

EGORIN, M. J., CLAWSON, R. E., ROSS, L. A., CHOU, F. T., ANDREWS, P. A. and BACHUR, N. R. (1980) Disposition and metabolism of *N,N*-dimethyldaunorubicin and *N,N*-dimethyladriamycin in rabbits and mice. *Drug Metab. Disp.* **8:** 353–362.

EGORIN, M. J., CLAWSON, R. E., ROSS, L. A., CHOU, F. T., ANDREWS, P. A. and BACHUR, N. R. (1981) Disposition and metabolism of adriamycin octanoylhydrazone (NSC 233853) in mice and rabbits. *Drug. Metab. Disp.* **9:** 240–245.

EGORIN, M. J., VAN ECHO, D., FOX, B. M., WHITACRE, M. and BACHUR, N. R. (1982) Plasma kinetics of aclacinomycin A and its major metabolites in man. *Cancer Chemother. Pharmac.* **8:** 41–46.

EGORIN, M. J., ANDREWS, P. A., NAKAZAWA, H. and BACHUR, N. R. (1983) Purification and characterization of aclacinomycin A and its metabolites from human urine. *Drug Metab. Disp.* **11:** 167–171.

EGORIN, M. J., FOX, B. M., SPIEGEL, J. F., GUTIERREZ, P. L., FRIEDMAN, R. D. and BACHUR, N. R. (1985) Cellular pharmacology in murine and human leukemic cell lines of diaziquone (NSC 182986). *Cancer Res.* **45:** 992–999.

EGORIN, M. J., VAN ECHO, D. A., WHITACRE, M. Y., FORREST, A., SIGMAN, L. M., ENGISCH, K. L. and AISNER, J. (1986) Human pharmacokinetics, excretion, and metabolism of the anthracycline antibiotic menogaril (NSC 269148, 7-OMEN) and their correlation with clinical toxicities. *Cancer Res.* **46:** 1513–1520.

EHNINGER, G., PROKSCH, B., HARTMANN, F., GARTNER, H. V. and WILMS, K. (1984) Mitoxantrone metabolism in the isolated perfused rat liver. *Cancer Chemother. Pharmac.* **12:** 50–52.

EHNINGER, G., PROKSCH, B., HEINZEL, G., SCHILLER, E., WEIBLE, K. H. and WOODWARD, D. L. (1985a) Pharmacokinetics and metabolism of mitoxantrone in man. *Invest. New Drugs* **3:** 109–116.

EHNINGER, G., PROKSCH, B. and SCHILLER, E. (1985b) Detection and separation of mitoxantrone—plasma and urine by high-performance liquid chromatography. *J. Chromatogr.* **342:** 119–127

EKLOW, L., THOR, H. and ORRENIUS, S. (1981) Formation and efflux of glutathione disulfide studied in isolated rat hepatocytes. *FEBS Lett.* **127:** 125–128.

EKSBORG, S., EHRSSON, H. and LINDFERS, A. (1983) Liquid chromatographic determination of mitomycin C in human plasma and urine. *J. Chromatogr.* **274:** 263–270.

ELIOT, H., GIANNI, L. and MYERS, C. E. (1983) Oxidative destruction of DNA by the adriamycin-iron complex. *Biochemistry* **23:** 928–936.

ELSTNER, E., OSSWALD, W. F. and KONZE, J. R. (1980) Reactive oxygen species: electron donor-hydrogen peroxide complex instead of free OH radicals? *FEBS Lett.* **121:** 219–221.

ERNSTER, L. (1967) DT-diaphorase. *Meth. Enzymol.* **10:** 309–317.

FANTINE, E. O. and GARNIER-SUILLEROT, G. (1986) Interaction of 5-iminodaunorubicin with Fe(II) and with cardiolipin-containing vesicles. *Biochem. biophys. Acta* **856:** 130–136.

FARBER, S. (1958) Clinical and biological studies with actinomycins. In: *Ciba Foundation Symposium on Amino Acids and Peptides With Antimetabolic Activity*, pp. 138–156, WOLSTENHOLME, G. E. W. and O'CONNOR, C. M. (eds) Little, Brown and Co., Boston.

FELSTED, R., GEE, M. and BACHUR, N. R. (1974) Rat liver daunorubicin reductase. *J. biol. Chem.* **249:** 3672–3679.

FELSTED, R., RICHTER, D. R. and BACHUR, N. R. (1977) Rat liver aldehyde reductase. *Biochem. Pharmac.* **26:** 1117–1124.

FENDLER, J. H. and FENDLER, E. J. (1974) Radiation chemistry of quinones. In: *The Chemistry of Quinoid Compounds*, pp. 539–578, PATIL, S. (ed.) John Wiley, New York.

FEUN, L. G., SAVARAJ, N., LU, K., GUO, Z., RAULSTON, L. G., BENJAMIN, R. S., FIELDS, W. S. and LOO, T. L. (1983) The pharmacologic fate of 2,5-diaziridinyl-3-6-bis-(carboethoxyamine)-2,4-benzoquinone (AZQ, NSC 182986) by intracarotid or intravenous administration in beagles. *J. Neuro-Oncol.* **1:** 219–224.

FIALLO, M. M. L. and GARNIER-SUILLEROT, A. (1985) Physicochemical studies of the iron(III)-carminomycin complex and evidence of the lack of stimulated superoxide production by NADH dehydrogenase. *Biochim. biophys. Acta* **840:** 91–98.

FIALLO, M. M. L. and GARNIER-SUILLEROT, A. (1986) Metal anthracycline complexes as a new class of anthracycline derivatives. Pd(II)-adriamycin and Pd(II)-daunorubicin complexes: physicochemical characteristics and antitumor activity. *Biochemistry* **25:** 924–930.

FIESER, L. F. (1927) The alkylation of hydroxynaphthoquinone. III. A synthesis of lapachol. *J. Am. Chem. Soc.* **49:** 857–864.

FINLEY, K. T. (1974) The addition and substitution chemistry of quinones. In: *The Chemistry of Quininoid Compounds*, Part 2, pp. 877–1144, PATIL, S. (ed.) John Wiley, London.

FISHER, G. R. and GUTIERREZ P. L. (1991) The reductive metabolism of diaziquone (AZQ) in the S9 fraction of MCF-7 cells: free radical formation and NAD(P)H: quinone-acceptor oxidoreductase (DT-diaphorase) activity. *Free Rad. Biol. Med.* **10:** 359–370.

FISHER, J., RAMAKRISHNAN, K. and BECVAR, J. E. (1983) Direct enzyme catalyzed reduction of anthracyclines by reduced nicotinamide adenine dinucleotide. *Biochemistry* **22:** 1347–1355.

FISHER, J., ABDELLA, B. R. J. and MCLANE, K. E. (1985) Anthracycline antibiotic reduction by spinach ferredoxin $NADP^+$ reductase and ferredoxin. *Biochemistry*. **24:** 3562–3571.

FOLKERS, K., CHOE, J. Y. and COMBS, A. B. (1978) Rescue by coenzyme Q10 from electrocardiographic abnormalities caused by the toxicity of adriamycin in the rat. *Proc. natn. Acad. Sci. U.S.A.* **75:** 5178–5180.

FORMELLI, F., CASAZZA, A. M., DIMARCO, A., MARIANI, A. and POLLINI, C. (1979) Fluorescence assay of tissue distribution of 4-demethoxydaunorubicin and 4-demethoxydoxorubicin in mice bearing solid tumors. *Cancer Chemother. Pharmac.* **3:** 261–269.

FORMELLI, F., POLLINI, C., CASAZZA, A. M., DIMARCO, A. and MARIANI, A. (1981) Fluorescence assays and pharmacokinetic studies of 4′-deoxydoxorubicin and doxorubicin in organs of mice bearing solid tumors. *Cancer Chemother. Pharmac.* **5:** 139–144.

FORMELLI, F., CARSANA, R. and POLLINI, C. (1986a) Comparative pharmacokinetics and metabolism of doxorubicin and 4-demethoxy-4′-O-methyldoxorubicin in tumor bearing mice. *Cancer Chemother. Pharmac.* **16:** 15–21.

FORMELLI, F., CARSANA, R. and POLLINI, C. (1986b) Pharmacokinetics and metabolism of 4′-deoxy-4′-iododoxorubicin (4′-IDX) in tumor bearing mice: comparison with doxorubicin. *5th NCI/EORTC Symposium on New Drugs in Cancer Therapy*, Amsterdam, October, Abstract 915.

FORMELLI, F., CARSANA, R. and POLLINI, T. (1987) Pharmacokinetics of 4′-deoxy-4′-iodo-doxorubicin in plasma and tissues of tumor-bearing mice compared with doxorubicin. *Cancer Res.* **47:** 5401–5406.

FORNACE, A. J., LITTLE, J. B. and WEICHSELBAUM, R. R. (1979) DNA repair in a Fanconi's anemia fibroblast cell strain. *Biochim. biophys. Acta* **561:** 99–109.

FOX, T. D. (1983) Migratory DNA mitochondrial genes in the nucleus. *Nature* **301:** 371–372.

FRACASSO, P. M. and SARTORELLI, A. C. (1986) Cytotoxicity and DNA lesions produced by mitomycin C and porfiromycin in hypoxic and aerobic EMT6 and Chinese hamster ovary cells. *Cancer Res.* **46:** 3939–3944.

FRANK, W. and OSTERBERG, A. (1960) Mitomyin C (NSC 26980)—An evaluation of the Japanese reports. *Cancer Chemother. Rep.* **9:** 114–119.

FREEMAN, R. W., MACDONALD, J. S., OLSON, R. D., BOERTH, R. C., OATES, J. A. and HARBISON, R. D. (1980) Effect of sulfhydryl-containing compounds on the antitumor effects of adriamycin. *Toxicol. Appl. Pharmac.* **54:** 168–175.

FREI, B., WINTERHALTER, K. H. and RICHTER, C. (1986) Menadione-(2-methyl-1,4-naphthoquinone)-dependent enzymatic redox cycling and calcium release by mitochondria. *Biochemistry* **25:** 4438–4443.

FRIDOVICH, I. (1976) Oxygen radicals, hydrogen peroxide and oxygen toxicity. In: *Free Radicals in Biology*, p. 239, PRYOR, W. A. (ed.) Academic Press, New York.

FRY, D. W., BORITZKI, T. J., BESSERER, J. A. and JACKSON, R. C. (1985) In vitro DNA strand scission and inhibition of nucleic acid synthesis in L1210 leukemia cells by a new class of DNA complexes, the anthra[1,9-cd]pyrazol-6(2H)-ones (anthrapyrazoles). *Biochem. Pharmac.* **34:** 3499–3508.

FRYTAK, S., EAGAN, R. T., AMES, M. M., CREAGAN, E. T. and NICHOLS, W. C. (1984) Phase I study of diaziquone. *Cancer Treat. Rep.* **68:** 975–978.

FUJITA, H., OGAWA, K., TONE, H., IGUCHI, H., SHOMURA, T. and MURATA, S (1986) Pharmacokinetics of doxorubicin, (2″*R*)-4′-*O*-tetrahydropyranyl-adriamycin and aclarubicin. *Jap. J. Antibiot.* **39:** 1321–1336.

FUJITA, H. (1971) Comparative studies on the blood level, tissue distribution, excretion and inactivation of anticancer drugs. *Jpn. J. Clin. Oncol.* **12:** 151–162.

FUJITA, K., SHINPO, K., YAMADA, K., SATO, T., NIIMI, H., SHAMOTO, M., NAGATSU, T., TAKEUCHI, T. and UMEZAWA, H. (1982) Reduction of adriamycin toxicity by ascorbate in mice and guinea pigs. *Cancer Res.* **42:** 309–316.

FUJIWARA, K., SAIKUSA, H., YASUNO, M. and KITAGAWA, T. (1982) Enzyme immunoassay for quantitation of mitomycin C using β-galactosidase as a label. *Cancer Res.* **42:** 1487–1491.

FUKUYAMA, T., NAKATSUBO, F., COCUZZA, A. J. and KISHI, Y. (1977) Synthetic studies toward mitomycins. III. Total synthesis of mitomycins A and C. *Tetrahedron Lett.* 4295–4298.

FUMAGALLI, A., FACCHINETTI, T., ARRIVABENE, L., MARSIGLIO, A., GIULIANI, F. C. and CASAZZA, A. M. (1985) Distribution and pharmacokinetics of 4′-deoxydoxorubicin in mice. *Proc. Am. Assoc. Cancer Res.* **26:** 356.

GALBRAITH, W. M. and MELLETT, L. B. (1975) Disposition of [^{3}H]-actinomycin D (NSC-3053) in the rat, monkey and dog. *Cancer Chemother. Rep. Part I* **59:** 1061–1069.

GALBRAITH, W. M. and MELLETT, L. B. (1976) Disposition of [^{3}H]-actinomycin D in tumor-bearing mice. *Cancer Res.* **36:** 1242–1245.

GAMS, R. A., OSTROY, F., BENDER, J. F. and GRILLO-LOPEZ, A. J. (1985) A Phase I trial of ametantrone acetate NSC-287513. *Invest. New Drugs* **3:** 383–388.

GANT, T., D'ARCY, W., DOHERTY, M., ODOWOLE, D., SALES, K. D. and COHEN, G. M. (1986) Semiquinone anion radicals formed by reaction of quinones with glutathione and amino acids. *FEBS Lett.* **201:** 296–300.

GANZINA, F., PACCIARINI, M. A. and DIPIETRO, N. (1986) Idarubicin (4′-demethoxy-daunorubicin). A preliminary overview of preclinical and clinical studies. *Invest. New Drugs* **4:** 85–105.

GARBRECHT, M. and MÜLLERLIE U. (1986) Verapamil in the prevention of adriamycin-induced cardiomyopathy. *Klin. Wochenschr.* **64:** 132–134.

GAUSE, E. M., MONTALVO, D. A. and ROWLANDS, J. R. (1967) Electron spin resonance studies of the chloranilcysteine, dichlone-cysteine and dichlone-glutathione reactions. *Biochem. biophys. Acta* **141:** 217–219.

GAUSE, G. F. (1964) Biokhimicheskie mekhanizmy deistviga antibiotikov. *Antibiotiki.* **9:** 946–950.

GAUSE, G. F., BRAZNIKOVA, M. G. and SKORIN, V. A. (1975) A new antitumor antibiotic carminomycin (NSH 180024). *Cancer Chemother. Rep.* **58:** 255–256.

GAUSE, W. (1957) Weitere untersuchungen über äthyleniminochinone und ver wandte verbindungen. *Angew Chem.* **69:** 252–257.

GAUSE, W. (1958) The reaction of some alkoxy-*p*-benzoquinones with ethylenimide. *Chem. Ber.* **91:** 2216–2222.

GELVAN, D. and SAMUNI, A. (1988) Reappraisal of the association between adriamycin and iron. *Cancer Res.* **48:** 5645–5649.

GERHARTZ, H. (1964) Clinical results with cyclophosphamide and trisethylene iminoquinone. In: *Chemotherapy of Cancer*, pp. 62–72, PLATTNER, P. A. (ed.) Elsevier, Amsterdam.

GERONI, C., MARSIGLIO, A., FUMAGALLI, A. and GIULIANI, F. C. (1986) Intracellular metabolism of doxorubicin and daunorubicin analogs in different human tumor cell lines. *Proc. Am. Assoc. Cancer Res.* **27:** 244.

GEVAN, D., BERG, E., SALTMAN, P. and SAMUNI, A. (1990) Time-dependent modifications of ferricadriamycin. *Biochem. Pharmac.* **39:** 1289–1295.

GESSNER, T., PREISLER, H. D., AZARNIA, N., BOLANOWSKA, W., VOGLER, W. R., GRUNWALD, H., JOYCE, R. and GOLDBERG, J. (1987) Plasma levels of daunorubicin metabolites and the outcome of ANLL therapy. *Med. Oncol. Pharmacother.* **4:** 23–31.

GESSNER, T., VAUGHAN, L. A., BEEHLER, B. C., BARTELS, C. J. and BAKER, R. M. (1990) Elevated pentose cycle and glucuronyltransferase in daunorubicin-resistant P388 cells. *Cancer Res.* **50:** 3921–3927.

GEWIRTZ, D. A. and YANOVICH, S. (1986a) Metabolism of adriamycin and daunorubicin in hepatocytes from the rat and rabbit. *Proc. Am. Assoc. Cancer Res.* **27:** 241.

GEWIRTZ, D. A. and YANOVICH, S. (1986b) Metabolism of the anthracycline antibiotic daunorubicin to daunorubicinol and deoxydaunorubicinol aglycone in hepatocytes isolated from the rat and rabbit. *Biochem. Pharmac.* **35:** 4059–4064.

GEWIRTZ, D. A. and YANOVICH, S. (1987) Metabolism of adriamycin in hepatocytes isolated from the rat and the rabbit. *Biochem. Pharmac.* **36:** 1793–1798.

GIANNI, L., CORDEN , B. J. and MYERS, C. E. (1983a) The biochemical basis of anthracycline toxicity and anti-tumor activity. In: *Reviews in Biochemistry and Toxicology*, pp. 1–82, HODGSON, E., BEND, J. and PHILPOT, R. M. (eds) Elsevier/North-Holland, New York.

GIANNI, L., ZWEIR, J. L., LEVY, A. and MYERS, C. E. (1983b) Characterization of the cycle of iron-mediated electron transfer from adriamycin to molecular oxygen. *J. biol. Chem.* **260:** 6820–6826.

GILL, P., FAVRE, R., DURAND, A., ILIADIS, A., CANO, J. P. and CARCASSONNE, Y. (1983) Time dependency of adriamycin and adriamycinol kinetics. *Cancer Chemother. Pharmac.* **10:** 120–124.

GIULIANI, F. C., BORDONI, T., BARBIERI, B., GERONI, C. and BELLINI, O. (1986) Biological characterization of 4′-deoxy-4′-I-doxorubicin. *5th NCI/EORTC Symposium on New Drugs in Cancer Therapy*, Amsterdam, October, Abstract 9.06.

GLAUBIGER, D. and RAMU, A. (1982) Antitumor antibiotics. In: *Pharmacologic Principles of Cancer Treatment*, pp. 402–415, CHABNER, B. (ed.) W. B. Saunders, Philadelphia, Pennsylvania.

GOLA, A. (1979) Daunorubicin reductase activity in leukemia leukocyte homogenates. *Arch. Immunol. Ther. Exp* **27:** 815–818.

GOLD, J. (1986) Potentiation by vitamin K-3 (menadione) of antitumor effect of hydrazine sulfate in Walker 256 cardinosarcoma in rats. *Proc. Am. Assoc. Cancer Res.* **27:** 279.

GOLDENBERG, G. J., WANG, H. and BLAIR, G. W. (1986) Resistance to adriamycin: relationship of cytotoxicity to drug uptake and DNA single- and double-strand breakage in cloned cell lines of adriamycin-sensitive and -resistant P388 leukemia. *Cancer Res.* **46:** 2978–2983.

GOLDENBERG, H. (1982) Density gradient fractionation of digitonin-treated rat liver plasma membranes and subcellular localization of NADH-oxidoreductase and B-type cytochromes. *Enzyme* **27:** 227–238.

GOODMAN, J. and HOCHSTEIN, P. (1977) Generation of free radicals and lipid peroxidation by redox cycling of adriamycin and daunomycin. *Biochem. biophys. Res. Commun.* **77:** 797–803.

GOODMAN, J., BESSMAN, M. J. and BACHUR, N. R. (1974) Adriamycin and daunorubicin inhibition of mutant T4 DNA polymerase. *Proc. natn. Acad. Sci. U.S.A.* **71:** 1193–1196.

GOORMAGHTIGH, E. and RUYSSCHAERT, J. M. (1983) Evidence of a covalent linkage in the adriamycin-cardiolipid complex induced by adriamycin-mediated electron transport. *Res. Commun. Chem. Path. Pharmac.* **42:** 149–152.

GOORMAGHTIGH, E., CHATELAIN, P., CASPERS, J. and RUYSSCHAERT, J. M. (1980) Evidence of a specific complex between adriamycin and negatively-charged phospholipids. *Biochim. biophys. Acta* **597:** 1–14.

GOORMAGHTIGH, E., POLLAKIS, G. and RUYSSCHAERT, J. M. (1983) Mitochondrial membrane modifications induced by adriamycin-mediated electron transport. *Biochem. Pharmac.* **32:** 889–893.

GORDON, G. R. and KASHIWASE, D. (1981) Effects of N-substitution on the stimulation of microsomal oxygen consumption by anthracyclines. *Proc. Am. Assoc. Cancer Res.* **22:** 256.

GORMLEY, P. E., WOOD, J. H. and POPLACK, D. G. (1981) Ability of a new antitumor agent, AZQ, to penetrate into cerebrospinal fluid. *Pharmacologist* **22:** 196–198.

GOSALVEZ, M., BLANCO, M. F., HUNTER, J., MIKO, M. and CHANCE, B. (1974) Effects of anticancer agents on the respiration of isolated mitochondria and tumor cells. *Eur. J. Cancer* **10:** 567–574.

GOSALVEZ, M., BLANCO, M. F., VIVERO, C. and VALLES, F. (1978) Quelamycin, a new derivative of adriamycin with several possible therapeutic advantages. *Eur. J. Cancer* **14:** 1185–1190.

GOTTDIENER, J. S., MATHISEN, B. J., BORER, J. S., BONOW, R. D., MYERS, C. E., BARR, L. H., SCHWARTZ, P. E., BACHARACH, S. L., GREEN, M. V. and ROSENBERG, S. A. (1981) Doxorubicin cardiotoxicity: assessment of late left ventricular dysfunction by radionuclide cineangiography. *Ann. Intern. Med.* **94:** 430–435.

GREEN, M. D., SPEYER, J. L. and MUGGIA, F. M. (1984) Cardiotoxicity of anthracyclines. *Eur. J. Cancer clin. Oncol.* **20:** 293–296.

GREEN, T. R., SCHAEFER, R. E. and MAKLER, M. T. (1980) Orientation of the NADPH dependent superoxide generating oxidoreductase on the outer membrane of human PMN's. *Biochem. biophys. Res. Commun.* **94:** 262–269.

GREENE, R. F., COLLINS, J. M., JENKINS, J. F., SPEYER, J. L. and MYERS, C. E. (1983) Plasma pharmacokinetics of adriamycin and adriamycinol implications for the design of *in vitro* experiments and treatment protocols. *Cancer Res.* **43:** 3417–3421.

GREGORY, E. M. and FRIDOVICH, I. (1973) Oxygen toxicity and superoxide dismutase. *J. Bacteriol.* **114:** 1193–1197.

GRIFFIN, J. P., NEWMAN, R. A., MCCORMACK, J. J. and KRAKOFF, I. H. (1982) Clinical and clinical pharmacologic studies of aziridinylbenzoquinone. *Cancer Treat. Rep.* **66:** 1321–1325.

GRIFFIN-GREEN, E. A., ZALESKA, M. M. and ERECINSKA, M. (1988) Adriamycin-induced lipid peroxidation in mitochondria and microsomes. *Biochem. Pharmac.* **37:** 3071–3077.

GROCHOW, L. B., DONEHOWER, R. C., ETTINGER, D. S., CATES, A. E. and RICE, A. (1985) Pharmacokinetics of menogaril (MEN). *Proc. Am. Soc. Clin. Oncol.* **4:** 32.

GUPTA, R. C., GARG, A., EARLEY, K., AGARWAL, S. C., LAMBERT, B. R. and NESNOW, S. (1991) DNA adducts of the antitumor agent diaziquone. *Cancer Res.* **51:** 5198–5204.

GUPTA, V. and COSTANZI, J. J. (1987) Role of hypoxia in anticancer drug-induced cytotoxicity for Ehrlich ascites cells. *Cancer Res.* **47:** 2407–2412.

GUPTA, V. and KRISHAN, A. (1982) Effects of oxygen concentrations on the growth and drug sensitivity of human melanoma cells in soft-agar clonogenic assay. *Cancer Res.* **42:** 1005–1007.

GUTIERREZ, P. L. (1988) The influence of ascorbic acid on the free-radical metabolism of xenobiotics: the example of diaziquone. *Drug Metab. Rev.* **19:** 379–383.

GUTIERREZ, P. L. (1989) Mechanism(s) of bioreductive activation. The example of Diaziquone (AZQ). *Free Rad. Biol. Med.* **6:** 405–445.

GUTIERREZ, P. L. and BACHER, N. R. (1983) Free radicals in quinone containing antitumor agents. The nature of the diaziquone (3,6-diaziridinyl-2,5-bis-(carboethoxyamino)-1,4-benzoquinone) free radical. *Biochim. biophys. Acta* **758:** 37–41.

GUTIERREZ, P. L., FRIEDMAN, R. D. and BACHUR, N. R. (1982) Biochemical activation of AZQ [3,6-diazoiridinyl-2,5-bis(carboethoxyamino)-1,4-benzoquinone] to its free radical species. *Cancer Treat. Rep.* **66:** 339–342.

GUTIERREZ, P. L., GEE, M. V. and BACHUR, N. R. (1983) Kinetics of anthracycline antibiotic free radical formation and reductive glycosidase activity. *Arch. Biochem. Biophys.* **223:** 68–75.

GUTIERREZ, P. L., FOX, B. M., MOSSOBA, M. M. and BACHUR, N. R. (1984) Free radicals in quinone-containing antitumor agents. Electrochemical reduction of diaziquinone (2,5-diaziridinyl-3,6-bis(carboethoxyamino)-1,4-benzoquinone) and two analogues. *Molec. Pharmac.* **26:** 582–586.

GUTIERREZ, P. L., EGORIN, M. J., FOX, B. M., FRIEDMAN, R. D. and BACHUR, N. R. (1985a) Cellular activation of diaziquone [2,5-diaziridinyl-3,6-bis(carboethoxyamino)-1,4-benzoquinone] to its free radical species. *Biochem. Pharmac.* **34:** 1449–1455.

GUTIERREZ, P. L., FOX, B. M., MOSSOBA, M. M., EGORIN, M., NAKAZAWA, H. and BACHUR, N. R. (1985b) Electron spin resonance of electrochemically generated free radicals from diaziquone and its derivative. *Biophys. Chem.* **22:** 115–123.

GUTIERREZ, P. L., BISWAL, S., NARDINO, R. and BISWAL, N. (1986) Reductive activation of diaziquone and possible involvement of free radicals and the hydroquinone dianion. *Cancer Res.* **46:** 5779–5789.

GUTTERIDGE, J. M. (1983) Adriamycin-iron catalyzed phospholipid peroxidation: a reaction not involving reduced adriamycin or hydroxyl radicals. *Biochem. Pharmac.* **32:** 1949–1952.

GUTTERIDGE, J. M. (1984a) Lipid peroxidation and possible hydroxyl radical formation stimulated by the self-reduction of a doxorubicin-iron (III) complex. *Biochem. Pharmac.* **33:** 1725–1728.

GUTTERIDGE, J. M. (1984b) Streptonigrin-induced deoxyribose degradation: inhibition by superoxide dismutase, hydroxyl radical scavengers and iron chelators. *Biochem. Pharmac.* **33:** 3059–3062.

GUTTERIDGE, J. M. and QUINLAN, G. J. (1985) Free radical damage to deoxyribose by anthracycline, aureolic acid and aminoquinone antitumor antibiotics. An essential requirement for iron, semiquinones and hydrogen peroxide. *Biochem. Pharmac.* **34:** 4099–4103.

GUTTERIDGE, J. M., QUINLAN, G. J. and WILKINS, S. (1984) Mitomycin C-induced deoxyribose degradation inhibited by superoxide dismutase. A reaction involving iron, hydroxyl and semiquinone radicals. *FEBS Lett.* **167:** 37–41.

HACKMANN, C. (1952) Experimentelle untersuchungen über die wirkung von actinomycin C (HBF 386) bei bösartigen geschwülsten. *Z. Krebsforsch* **58:** 607–613.

HADLER, H. I. and MOREAU, T. L. (1969) The induction of ATP energized mitochondrial volume changes by the combination of the two antitumor agents showdomycin and lapachol. *J. Antibiot.* **22:** 513–520.

HAJDU, J. and ARMSTRONG, E. C. (1981) Interaction of metal ions with streptonigrin. I. Formation of copper (II) and zinc (II) complexes of the antitumor antibiotic. *J. Am. Chem. Soc.* **103:** 232–234.

HALLIWELL, B. and GUTTERIDGE, J. M. (1984) Oxygen toxicity, oxygen radicals, transition metals and disease. *Biochem. J.* **219:** 1–14.

HAMANA, K., KAWADA, K., SUGIOKA, K., NAKANO, M., TERO-KUBOTA, S. and IKEGAMI, Y. (1985) DNA strand scission by enzymatically reduced mitomycin C: evidence for participation of hydroxyl radical in DNA damage. *Biochem. Int.* **10:** 301–309.

HANDA, K. and SATO, S. (1975) Generation of free radicals of quinone group-containing anti-cancer chemicals in NADPH-microsome system as evidenced by initiation of sulfite oxidation. *Gann* **66:** 43–47.

HANDA, K. and SATO, S. (1976) Stimulation of microsomal NADPH oxidation by quinone group-containing anticancer chemicals. *Gann* **67:** 523–528.

HARLEY, J. B., FETTEROLF, C. J., BELLO, C. A. and FLAKS, J. G. (1982) Streptonigrin toxicity in *Escherichia coli:* oxygen dependence and the role of the intracellular oxidation-reduction state. *Can. J. Microbiol.* **28:** 545–552.

HARRIS, N. L., BRENNER, D. E., ANTHONY, L. B., COLLINS, J. C., HALTER, S. and HANDE, K. R. (1988) The influence of ranitidine on the pharmacokinetics and toxicity of doxorubicin in rabbits. *Cancer Chemother. Pharmac.* **21:** 323–328.

HARRIS, R. N. and DOROSHOW, J. H. (1985) Effect of doxorubicin-enhanced hydrogen peroxide and hydroxyl radical formation on calcium sequestration by cardiac sarcoplasmic reticulum. *Biochem. biophys. Res. Commun.* **130:** 739.

HARRIS, R. N. and SHRIEVE, D. C. (1979) Effects of adriamycin and X-rays on euoxic and hypoxic EMT-6 cells *in vitro. Int. J. Rad. Oncol. Biol. Phys.* **5:** 1245–1248.

HARRISON, R. R. (1970) Inhibition of ATP on the growth inhibitory effect of Synkavite (2-methyl-1,4-naphthoquinone bisdisodium phosphate) on mouse ascites tumor cells. *Br. J. Cancer* **24:** 807–816.

HARTLIEB, J. (1974) Untersuchungen über das wachstum von zwei tumoren des soliden Yoshida-sarkoms der ratta beim gleichentier sowie über die reakton vershieden grosser tumoren auf behandlung mit 2,3,5-trisàthylenimino-benzochinon-(1,4). *Z. Krebsforsch* **81:** 1–6.

HARTMAN, N., BASSECHES, P. J. and POWIS, G. (1982) Effect of cyclophosphamide pretreatment on the short-term disposition and biliary excretion of adriamycin and metabolites in rat. *Cancer Chemother. Pharmac.* **10:** 11–15.

HASHIMOTO, Y., SHUDO, K. and OKAMOTO, T. (1982) Alkylation of DNA with a mitomycin derivative, 7-N-(p-hydroxyphenyl)-mitomycin C. Reductive alkylation and preferential binding to adenine. *Chem. Pharmac. Bull. (Tokyo)* **30:** 2644–2646.

HASHIMOTO, Y., SHUDO, K. and OKAMOTO, T. (1983) Modification of deoxyribonucleic acid with reductivity activated mitomycin C. Structures of modified nucleotides. *Chem. Pharmac. Bull. (Tokyo)* **31:** 861–869.

HASINOFF, B. B. (1989) Self-reduction of the iron(III)-doxorubicin complex. *Free. Rad. Biol. Med.* **7:** 583–593.

HASINOFF, B. B. (1990) The iron(III) and copper(II) complexes of adriamycin promote the hydrolysis of the cardioprotective agent ICRF-187. *Agents Actions* **29:** 374–381.

HASINOFF, B. B. and DAVEY, J. P. (1988) Adriamycin and its iron(III) and copper(II) complexes. *Biochem. Pharmac.* **37:** 3663–3669.

HATA, R., SANO, Y., SUGAWARA, R., MATSUME, A., KANAMORI, K., SHIMA, T. and HOSHI, T. (1956) Mitomycin. A new antibiotic from streptomyces. I. *J. Antibiot. (Tokyo), Ser. A* **9:** 141–146.

HENDERSON, I. C., BILLINGHAM, M., ISRAEL, M., KRISHNAN, A. and FREI, E. (1978) Comparative cardiotoxicity studies with adriamycin (ADR) and AD32 in rabbits. *Proc. Am. Assoc. Cancer Res.* **19:** 158.

HENRIKSSON, R. and GRANKVIST, K. (1988) Protective effect of iron chelators on epirubicin-induced fibroblast toxicity. *Cancer Lett.* **43:** 179–183.

HENRY, D. W. (1979) Structure-activity relationships among daunorubicin and adriamycin analogs. *Cancer Treat. Rep.* **63:** 845–854.

HERMAN, E. H. and FERRANS, V. J. (1983) Influence of vitamin E and ICRF-187 on chronic doxorubicin cardiotoxicity in miniature swine. *Lab. Invest.* **49:** 69–77.

HERMAN, E. H. and FERRANS, V. J. (1986) Pretreatment with ICRF-187 provides long-lasting protection against chronic daunorubicin cardiotoxicity in rabbits. *Cancer Chemother. Pharmac.* **16:** 102–106.

HERMAN, E. J., EL-HAGE, A. N., FERRANS, V. J. and ARDALAN, B. (1985) Comparison of the severity of the chronic cardiotoxicity produced by doxorubicin in normotensive and hypertensive rats. *Toxic. Appl. Pharmac.* **78:** 202–214.

Herzog, V. and Fahimi, H. D. (1974) Microbodies (peroxisomes) containing catalase in myocardium: morphologic and biochemical evidence. *Science* **185:** 271–273.

Hickman, J., Chahwala, S. B. and Thompson, M. G. (1985) Interaction of the antibiotic adriamycin with the plasma membrane. *Adv. Enzym. Reg.* **24:** 263–274.

Himori, T., Wakui, A. and Saito, T. (1983) Clinical evaluation of anticancer alkylating agent, carboquone (NSC-134679). *Sci. Rep. Res. Inst. Tohoko Univ. C* **30:** 92–99.

Hoban, P. R., Walton, M. I., Robson, C. N., Godden, J., Stratford, I. J., Workman, P., Harris, A. L. and Hichson, I. D. (1990) Decreased NADPH—cytochrome-P-450 reductase-activity and impaired drug activation in a mammalian-cell line resistant to mitomycin C under aerobic but not hypoxic conditions. *Cancer Res.* **50:** 4692–4697.

Hochstein, P., Laszlo, J. and Miller, D. (1965) A unique dicumarol-sensitive, non-phosphorylating oxidation of DPNH and TPNH catalyzed by streptonigrin. *Biochem. biophys. Res. Commun.* **19:** 289–295.

Hodges, J. C., Remers, W. A. and Bradner, W. T. (1981) Synthesis and antineoplastic activity of mitosene analogues of the mitomycins. *J. Med. Chem.* **24:** 1184–1191.

Hodnett, E. M. and Prakash, G. (1984) *N,N'*-dihalo-1,4-benzoquinonediimines as antitumor agents. *Eur. J. Med. Chim. Ther.* **19:** 101–104.

Hodnett, E. M., Prakash, G. and Amirmoazzami, J. (1978) Nitrogen analogues of 1,4-benzoquinones. Activity against the ascitic sarcoma 180 in mice. *J. Med. Chem.* **21:** 11–16.

Hodnett, E. M., Wongweichintana, C., Dunn, W. J. and Marrs, P. (1983) Substituted 1,4-naphthoquinones vs the ascitic sarcoma 180 of mice. *J. Med. Chem.* **26:** 570–574.

Hodnick, W. F. and Sartorelli, A. C. (1991) Reductive activation of mytomycin C by NADH-cytochrome b_5 reductase. *Proc. Am. Ass. Cancer Res.* **32:** 397.

Hoey, B. M., Butler, J. and Swallow, A. J. (1988) Reductive activation of mitomycin C. *Biochemistry* **27:** 2608–2614.

Hooker, S. C. (1986) The constitution of lapachol and its derivatives. Part III. The structure of the amylene chain. *J. Chem. Soc.* **69:** 1355–1381.

Hornemann, U., Keller, P. J. and Kozlowski, J. F. (1979) Formation of 1-ethylxanthyl-2,7-diaminomitosene and 1,10-diethylxanthyl-2,7-diaminodicarbamoylmitosene in aqueous solution upon reduction-reoxidation of mitomycin C in the presence of potassium ethylxanthate. *J. Am. Chem. Soc.* **101:** 7121–7124.

Houée-Levin, C., Gardès-Albert, M. and Ferradini, C. (1984) Reduction of daunorubicin aqueous solutions by COO·-free radicals. Reactions of reduced transients with H_2O_2. *FEBS Lett.* **173:** 27–30.

Houée-Levin, C., Gardès-Albert, M., Faraggi, M. and Klapper, M. (1985) Pulse radiolysis study of daunorubicin redox cycles, reduction of eaq and COO·-free radicals. *FEBS Lett.* **179:** 46–50.

Houée-Levin, C., Gardès-Albert, M., Benzineb, K., Rouscilles, A. and Ferradini, C. (1990) One-election reduction of daunorubicin intercalated in DNA or in a protein: a α-radiolysis study. *Free Rad. Res. Commun.* **11:** 127–136.

Howland, J. L. (1963) Uncoupling and inhibition of oxidative phosphorylation by 2-hydroxy-3-alkyl-1,4-naphthoquinones. *Biochim. biophys. Acta* **77:** 659–662.

Hrushesky, W. J. M., Wood, P., Olshefski, R., Meshnick, S. and Eaton, J. W. (1985) Modifying intracellular redox balance: an approach to improving therapeutic index. *Lancet* **i:** 565–566.

Hu, E. and Howell, S. B. (1983) Pharmacokinetics of intraarterial mitomycin C in humans. *Cancer Res.* **43:** 4474–4477.

Huffman, D. H. and Bachur, N. R. (1972) Daunorubicin metabolism in acute myelocytic leukemia. *Blood* **39:** 637–643.

Huffman, D. H., Benjamin, R. S. and Bachur, N. R. (1972) Daunorubicin metabolism in acute non-lymphocytic leukemia. *Clin. Pharmac. Ther.* **13:** 895–905.

Humphrey, E. W. and Blank, N. (1961) Clinical experience with streptonigrin. *Cancer Chemother. Rep.* **12:** 99–103.

Hutchinson, F. (1957) The distance that a radical formed by ionizing radiation can diffuse in a yeast cell. *Radiation Res.* **7:** 473–483.

Iguchi, H., Tono, H., Ishikura, T., Takeuchi, T. and Umezawa, H. (1985) Pharmacokinetics and disposition of 4'-O-tetrahydropyranyladriamycin in mice by hplc analysis. *Cancer Chemother. Pharmac.* **15:** 132–140.

Ilan, Y. A., Czapski, G. and Meisel, D. (1976) The one-electron redox potentials of free radicals. 1. The oxygen superoxide system. *Biochim. biophys. Acta* **430:** 209–224.

Inouye, Y., Okada, H., Roy, S. K., Miyasaka, T., Hibino, S., Tanaka, N. and Nakamura, S. (1985) Biological properties of streptonigrin derivatives. *J. Antibiot.* **38:** 1429–1432.

Inouye, Y., Okada, H., Uno, J., Arai, T. and Nakamura, S. (1986) Effects of streptonigrin derivatives and sakyomicin A on the respiration of isolation rat liver mitochondria. *J. Antibiol.* **39:** 550–556.

Ishizu, K., Dearman, H. H., Huancy, M. T. and White, J. R. (1968) Electron paramagnetic resonance observations on biogenic semiquinone and 5-methyl phenazinium radicals. *Biochim. biophys. Acta* **165:** 283–285.

Israel, M. and Sweatman, T. W. (1983) Metabolism and elimination of N-trifluoroacetyl-adriamycin-14-*O*-hemiadipate (AD143) in the rat. *Proc. Am. Assoc. Cancer Res.* **24:** 258.

Israel, M., Pegg, W. J., Seshadri, R. and Parker, L. M. (1976) Deesterification of the side chain of

N-trifluoroacetyl-doxorubicin by serum esterases. In: *Abstracts Fifth Int. Symp. Med. Chem. Paris*, p. 63, L'Imprimerie Levert, Paris.

ISRAEL, M., WILKINSON, P. M., PEGG, W. J. and FREI, E. (1978) Hepatobiliary metabolism and excretion of adriamycin and *N*-trifluoroacetyladriamycin-14-valerate in the rat. *Cancer Res.* **38:** 365–370.

ISRAEL, M., KARKOWSKY, A. M. and KHETARPAL, V. K. (1981) Distribution of radioactivity and anthracycline-fluorescence in tissues of mice one hour after [^{14}C]-labelled AD 32 administration. *Cancer Chemother. Pharmac.* **6:** 25–30.

ISRAEL, M., SWEATMAN, T. W., SESHADRI, R. and KOSEKI, Y. (1986) Metabolic studies in rats with *N*-benzyl-adriamycin-14-valerate (AD 198), a promising new anthracycline analog. *Proc. Am. Assoc. Cancer Res.* **27:** 239.

IWAMOTO, Y., HENSEN, I. L., PORTER, T. H. and FOLKERS, K. (1974) Inhibition of coenzyme Q_{10}-enzymes, succinoxidase and NADH-oxidase, by adriamycin and other quinones having antitumor activity. *Biochem. Biophys. Res. Commun.* **58:** 633–638.

IYANAGI, T. and YAMAZAKI, I. (1969) One electron-transfer reactions in biochemical systems. III. One-electron reduction of quinones by microsomal flavin enzymes. *Biochim. biophys. Acta* **172:** 370–381.

IYANAGI, T. and YAMAZAKI, I. (1970) One-electron reductions in biochemical systems. V. Difference in the mechanism of quinone reduction by the NADH dehydrogenase and the NAD(P)H dehydrogenase (DT-diaphorase). *Biochim. biophys. Acta* **216:** 282–294.

IYENGAR, B. S. and LAL, S. K. (1982) Effect of high copper levels on actinomycin D inhibition of a rapidly proliferating cell system. *Int. J. Tissue React.* **4:** 243–245.

IYENGAR, B. S. and REMERS, W. A. (1985) A comparison of mechanisms proposed for conversion of mitomycins into mitosenes. *J. Med. Chem.* **28:** 963–967.

IYENGAR, B. S., SAMI, S. M., REMERS, W. A., BRADNER, W. T. and SCHURIG, J. E. (1983) Mitomycin C and porfiromycin analogues with substituted ethylamines at position 7. *J. Med. Chem.* **26:** 16–20.

IYENGAR, B. S., SAMI, S. M., TAKAHASHI, T., SIKORSKI, E. E., REMERS, W. A. and BRADNER, W. T. (1986) Mitomycin C analogues with increased metal complexing ability. *J. Med. Chem.* **29:** 1760–1764.

IYER, V. N. and SZYBALSKI, W. (1963) A molecular mechanism of mitomycin action: Link of complementary DNA strands. *Proc. natn. Acad. Sci. U.S.A.* **50:** 355–362.

IYER, V. N. and SZYBALSKI, W. (1964) Mitomycins and porfiromycin: chemical mechanism of activation and crosslinking of DNA. *Science* **145:** 55–58.

IZBICKI, R., AL-SARRAF, M., REED, M. L., VAUGHN, C. B. and VAITKEVICIUS, V. K. (1972) Further clinical trials with porfiromycin (NSC 56410) (Large intermittent doses). *Cancer Chemother. Rep.* **56:** 615–633.

JAENKE, R. S. (1976) Delayed and progressive mycardial lesions after adriamycin administration in the rabbit. *Cancer Res.* **36:** 2958–2966.

JAENKE, R. S., DEPREZ-DECAMPENEERE, D. and TROUET, A. (1980) Cardiotoxicity and comparative pharmacokinetics of six anthracyclines in the rabbit. *Cancer Res.* **40:** 3530–3536.

JAMIS-DOW, C. A., MYERS, C. E. and YEH, G. C. (1988) Decreased glucose-6-phosphate dehydrogenase activity associated with early stages of adriamycin resistance in human breast cancer cells. *Proc. Am. Assoc. Cancer Res.* **29:** 312.

JOHANSEN, P. B., JENSEN, S. E., RASMUSSEN, S. N. and DALMARK, M. (1984) Pharmacokinetics of doxorubicin and its metabolite doxorubicinol in rabbits with induced acid and alkaline urine. *Cancer Chemother. Pharmac.* **13:** 5–8.

JOHNSON, R. K., ZEE-CHENG, R. K. Y., LE, W. W., ACTON, E. M., HENRY, D. W. and CHENG, C. C. (1979) Experimental antitumor activity of aminoanthraquinones. *Cancer Treat. Rep.* **63:** 425–439.

JOHNSTON, J. B. and GLAZER, R. I. (1983) Cellular pharmacology of 3′-(morpholinyl) and 3′-(4-methoxy-1-p-piperidinyl) derivatives of 3′-deaminodaunorubicin in human colon carcinoma cells *in vitro*. *Cancer Res.* **43:** 1606–1610.

JOHNSTON, J. B., HABERNICHT, B., ACTON, E. M. and GLAZER, R. I. (1983) 3′-(3-Cyano-4-morpholinyl)-3′-deaminoadriamycin: a new anthracycline with potency. *Biochem. Pharmac.* **32:** 3255–3258.

JONES, D. P., THOR, H., SMITH, M. T., JEWELL, S. A. and ORRENIUS, S. (1983) Inhibition of ATP-dependent microsomal Ca^{2+} sequestration during oxidative stress and its prevention by glutathione. *J. biol. Chem.* **258:** 6390–6393.

JONES, R. (1959) Mitomycin C. A preliminary report of studies of human pharmacology and initial therapeutic trial. *Cancer Chemother. Rep.* **2:** 3–7.

JULIANE, R. L. and STAMP, D. (1978) Pharmacokinetics of liposome-encapsulated antitumor drugs. Studies with vinblastine, actinomycin D, cytosine arabinoside, and daunomycin. *Biochem. Pharmac.* **27:** 21–27.

JULICHER, R. H. M., STERRENBERG, L., BAST, A., RIKSEN, R. O. W., KOOMEN, J. M. and NOORDHOEK, J. (1986) The role of acute doxorubicin-induced cardiotoxicity studied in rat isolated heart. *J. Pharm. Pharmac.* **38:** 277–282.

KALYANARAMAN, B., PEREZ-REYES, E. and MASON, R. P. (1980) Spin-trapping and direct electron spin resonance investigations of the redox metabolism of quinone anticancer drugs. *Biochim. biophys. Acta* **630:** 119–130.

KALYANARAMAN, B., SEALY, R. C. and SINHA, B. K. (1984) An electron spin resonance study of the reduction of peroxides by anthracycline semiquinones. *Biochim. biophys. Acta* **799:** 270–275.

KANTER, P. M. and SCHWARTZ, H. S. (1979) Quantitative models for growth inhibition of human leukemia cells by antitumor anthracycline derivatives. *Cancer Res.* **39:** 3661–3672.

Kaplan, S., Sessa, C., Willems, Y., Pacciarini, M. A., Tamassia, V. and Cavalli, F. (1984) Phase I trial of 4-demethoxydaunorubicin (idarubicin) with single and doses. *Invest. New Drug* **2:** 281–286.

Karanes, C., Young, J. D., Samson, M. K., Smith, L. B., Franco, L. A. and Baker, L. H. (1983) Phase I trial of aclacinomycin A. A clinical and pharmacokinetic study. *Invest. New Drugs* **1:** 173–179.

Kennedy, K. A. and Sartorelli, A. C. (1979) Metabolic activation of mitomycin C by isolated liver nuclei and microsomes. *Fed. Proc.* **38:** 443.

Kennedy, K. A., Rockwell, S. and Sartorelli, A. C. (1980a) Preferential activation of mitomycin C to cytotoxic metabolites by hypoxic tumor cells. *Cancer Res.* **40:** 2356–2360.

Kennedy, K. A., Teicher, B. A., Rockwell, S. and Sartorelli, A. C. (1980b) The hypoxic tumor cell: a target for selective cancer chemotherapy. *Biochem. Pharmac.* **29:** 1–8.

Kennedy, K. A., Sligar, S. G., Polomski, L. and Sartorelli, A. C. (1982) Metabolic activation of mitomycin C by liver microsomes and nuclei. *Biochem. Pharmac.* **31:** 2011–2016.

Kennedy, K. A., Siegfried, J. M., Sartorelli, A. C. and Tritton, T. R. (1983) Effects of anthracyclines on oxygenated and hypoxic tumor cells. *Cancer Res.* **43:** 54–59.

Kennedy, K. A., McGurl, J. D., Leondaridis, L. and Alabaster, O. (1985a) pH Dependence of mitomycin C-induced crosslinking activity in EMT6 tumor cells. *Cancer Res.* **45:** 3541–3547.

Kennedy, K. A., Mimnaugh, E. G., Trush, M. A. and Sinha, B. K. (1985b) Effects of glutathione and ethylxanthine on mitomycin C activation by isolated rat hepatic or EMT6 mouse mammary tumor nuclei. *Cancer Res.* **45:** 4071–4076.

Kerr, D. J., Graham, J., Cummings, J., Morrison, J. G., Thompson, G. G., Brodie, M. J. and Kaye, S. B. (1986) The effect of verapamil on the pharmacokinetics of adriamycin. *Cancer Chemother. Pharmac.* **18:** 239–242.

Kessel, D. (1988) Transport of an iron: anthracycline complex by murine leukemia cells. *Cancer Lett.* **42:** 213–216.

Keyes, S. R., Fracasso, P. M., Heimbrook, D. C., Rockwell, S., Sliger, S. and Sartorelli, A. C. (1984a) Role of NADPH cytochrome c reductase and DT-diaphorase in the biotransformation of mitomycin C. *Cancer Res.* **44:** 5638–5643.

Keyes, S. R., Heimbrook, D. C., Fracasso, P. M., Rockwell, S., Sliger, S. and Sartorelli, A. C. (1984b) Chemotherapeutic attack of hypoxic tumor cells by the bioreductive alkylating agent mitomycin C. *Adv. Enz. Reg.* **23:** 291–307.

Keyes, S. R., Rockwell, S. and Sartorelli, A. C. (1985) Enhancement of mitomycin C cytotoxicity to hypoxic tumor cells by dicoumarol *in vivo* and *in vitro*. *Cancer Res.* **45:** 213–216.

Khan, A. H. and Driscoll, J. S. (1976) Potential central nervous system antitumor agents aziridinylbenzoquinones. 1. *J. Med. Chem.* **19:** 313–317.

Khan, A. H. and Ross, W. C. J. (1969) Tumor growth inhibitory nitrophenylaziridines and related compounds: structure activity relationships. *Chem. Biol. Interact.* **1:** 27–47.

Kharasch, E. D. and Novak, R. F. (1981) Anthracenedione activation of NADPH-cytochrome P-450 reductase: comparison with anthracyclines. *Biochem. Pharmac.* **30:** 2881–2884.

Kharasch, E. D. and Novak, R. F. (1982a) Inhibition of adriamycin-stimulated microsomal lipid peroxidation by mitoxantrone and ametantrone, two new anthracenedione antineoplastic agents. *Biochem. Biophys. Res. Commun.* **108:** 1346–1352.

Kharasch, E. D. and Novak, R. F. (1982b) Inhibition of microsomal oxidative drug metabolism by 1,4-bis(2-[(2-hydroxyethyl)amino]-ethylamino)-9,10-anthracenedione diacetate, a new antineoplastic agent. *Molec. Pharmac.* **22:** 471–478.

Kharasch, E. D. and Novak, R. F. (1983a) Mixtoxantrone and ametantrone: metabolic activation and effects on lipid peroxidation. *Proc. Am. Ass. Cancer Res* **24:** 257.

Kharasch, E. D. and Novak, R. F. (1983b) Structural and mechanistic differences in quinone inhibition of microsomal drug metabolism: inhibition of NADPH-cytochrome P-450 reductase activity. In: *Cytochrome P-450 Biochemistry, Biophysics and Environmental Implications*, pp. 80–97, Hietanen, J. (ed.) Elsevier/North-Holland, Amsterdam.

Kharasch, E. D. and Novak, R. F. (1983c) Bis(alkylamino)anthracenedione antineoplastic agent metabolic activation by NADPH-cytochrome P-450 reductase and NADH dehydrogenase: diminished activity relative to anthracyclines. *Arch. Biochem. Biophys.* **224:** 682–694.

Kharasch, E. D. and Novak, R. F. (1983d) Inhibitory effects of anthracenedione antineoplastic agents on hepatic and cardiac lipid peroxidation. *J. Pharmac. exp. Ther.* **226:** 500–506.

Kharasch, E. D. and Novak, R. F. (1984) Spectroscopic evidence for anthracenedione antineoplastic agent self-association and complex formation with flavin nucleotides. *Arch. Biochem. Biophys.* **234:** 497–512.

Kharasch, E. D. and Novak, R. F. (1985) Mitoxantrone and ametantrone inhibit hydroperoxide-dependent initiation and propagation reactions in fatty acid peroxidation. *J. biol. Chem.* **260:** 10645–10652.

Kikuchi, T. and Sugiura, Y. (1981) Generation of semiquinone radical from carbazilquinone by NADPH-cytochrome P-450 reductase. *Biochem. Pharmac.* **30:** 1717–1718.

Kimler, B. F. and Cheng, C. C. (1984) Modification of radiation and dihydroxyanthraquinone-induced cell lethality by cysteamine and *N*-ethylmaleimide. *Int. J. Radiat. Oncol. Biol. Phys.* **10:** 1683–1686.

Kimura, N. T., Kanematsu, T. and Baba, T. (1974) Potentiation of anticancer drug effect by cancer cell glycosis: an in vitro experiment. *Gann* **65:** 513–522.

King, C. L. and Loo, T. L. (1983) DNA damage by aziridinylbenzoquinones. *Proc. Am. Assoc. Cancer Res.* **24:** 322.

KING, C. L., HITTELMAN, W. N. and LOO, T. L. (1984a) Induction of DNA strand breaks and cross-links by 2,5-diaziridinyl-3,5-bis[carboethoxyamino]-1,4-benzoquinone in Chinese hamster ovary cells. *Cancer Res.* **44:** 5634–5637.

KING, C. L., WONG S. K. and LOO, T. L. (1984b) Alkylation of DNA by the new anticancer agent 3,6-diaziridinyl-2,5-bis(carboethoxyamino)-1,4-benzoquinone (AZQ). *Eur. J. Cancer Clin. Oncol.* **20:** 261–264.

KING, C. L., SAVARAJ, N., YEUNG, K. L. and LOO, T. L. (1984c) Mechanism of diaziquone (AZQ)-induced DNA cross-links and strand breaks. *Proc. Am. Ass. Cancer Res.* **25:** 301.

KINOSHITA, S., UZU, K., NAKANO, K., SHIMIZU, M. and TAKAHASHI, T. (1971) Mitomycin derivatives. I. Preparation of mitosene and mitosene compounds and their biological activities. *J. Med. Chem.* **14:** 103–109.

KITAMURA, I., OKI, T. and INUI, T. (1978) A sensitive analytical method for aclacinomycin A and its analogs by thin layer chromatography and fluorescence scanning. *J. Antibiot.* **31:** 919–922.

KLEYER, D. L. and KOCH, T. H. (1983) Electrophilic trapping of the tautomer of 7-deoxydaunomycin. A possible mechanism for covalent binding of daunomycin to DNA. *J. Am. Chem. Soc.* **105:** 5154–5156.

KLEYER, D. L. and KOCH, T. H. (1984) Mechanistic investigation of reduction of daunomycin and 7-deoxydaunomycinone with bi(3,5,5-trimethyl-2-oxomorpholin-3-yl). *J. Am. Chem. Soc.* **106:** 2380–2387.

KLEYER D. L., GAUDIANE, G. and KOCH, T. H. (1984) Spectroscopic and kinetic evidence for the tautomer of 7-deoxyalkavinone as an intermediate in the reductive coupling of aclacinomycin A. *J. Am. Chem. Soc.* **106:** 1105–1109.

KOBAYASHI, T., INABA, M., TSUKAGOSHI, S., SAKURAI, Y., IMAI, R. and MORIMOTO M. (1981) Comparison of the hematological toxicity and 7-*N*-(*p*-hydroxyphenyl)-mitomycin C and mitomycin C. *Gann* **72:** 950–954.

KODAMA, M., AIDA, M., NAGATA, C., OKI, T. and MATSUZAWA, Y. (1983) An electron spin resonance study on the free radicals produced from aclacinomycin A and its derivatives: analysis of hyperfine structure of the spectra by means of molecular orbital method. *Cancer Biochem. Biophys.* **6:** 243–247.

KOLODZIEJCZYK P., RESZKA K. and LOWN J. W. (1988) Enzymatic oxidative activation and transformation of the antitumor agent mitoxantrone. *Free Rad. Biol. Med.* **5:** 13–25.

KOLODZIEJCZYK P., RESZKA K. and LOWN J. W. (1989) Enzymatic oxidative acivation of 5-iminodaunorubicin—Spectrophotometric and electron paramagnetic resonance studies. *Biochem. Pharmac.* **38:** 803–809.

KOMIYAMA, T., OKI, INUI, T., TAKEUCHI, T. and UMEZAWA, H. (1978) NADH-dependent cinerulose reductase in rat liver microsomes. *Biochem. biophys. Res. Commun.* **82:** 188–195.

KOMIYAMA, T., OKI, T. and INUI, T. (1979a) A proposed reaction mechanism for the enzymatic reductive cleavage of glycosidic bond in anthracycline antibiotics. *Gann* **32:** 1219–1222.

KOMIYAMA, T., OKI, T. and INUI, T. (1979b) Activation of mitocmycin C and quinone drug metabolism by NADH-cyctochrome P-450 reductase. *J. Pharmacobio-Dynam.* **2:** 407–410.

KOMIYAMA, T., OKI, T., TAKEUCHI, T. and UMEZAWA, H. (1979c) Reduction of cinerulose in aclacinomycin-A by soluble and microsomal cinerulose reductases. *Gann* **70:** 395–401.

KOMIYAMA, T., KIKUCHI, T. and SUGIURA, Y. (1982) Generation of hydroxyl radical by anticancer quinone drugs, carbazilquinone, mitomycin C, aclacinomycin A and adriamycin, in the presence of NADPH-cytochrome P-450 reductase. *Biochem. Pharmac.* **31;** 3651–3656.

KOMIYAMA, T., SAWADA, M. T., KOBAYASHI, K. and YOSHIMOTO, A. (1985) Enhanced production of ethylene from methional by iron chelates and heme containing proteins in the system consisting of quinone compounds and NADPH-cytochrome P-450 reductase. *Biochem. Pharmac.* **34:** 977–983.

KOMIYAMA T., KIKUCHI T. and SUGIURA Y. (1986) Interactions of anticancer quinone drugs, aclacinomycin A, adriamycin, carbazilquinone, and mitomycin C, with NADPH-cytochrome P-450 reductase, xanthine oxidase and oxygen. *J. Pharmacobiodyn* **9:** 651–664.

KRAMER R. A. and ZAKHER J. (1988) Adriamycin resistance in human breast cancer cells involves both altered transport and oxygen radical detoxification mechanisms. *Proc. Am. Ass. Cancer Res.* **29,** 312.

KRAPCHO, A. P., LANDI, J. J., SHAW, K. J., PHINNEY, D. G., HACKER, M. P. and MCCORMACK, J. J. (1986) Synthesis and antitumor activities of unsymmetrically substituted 1,4-bis[(aminoalkyl)amino]anthracene-9,10-diones and related systems. *J. Med. Chem.* **29:** 1370–1373.

KREMER, W. B. and LASZLO, J. (1967) Comparison of biochemical effects of isopropylidine azastreptonigrin (NSC 62709) with streptonigrin (NSC 45383). *Cancer Chemother. Rep.* **51:** 19–24.

KREMER, W. B. and LASZLO, J. (1975) Streptonigrin. In: *Antineoplastic and Immunosuppressive Agents. Part II*, pp. 633–641, SARTORELLI, A. C. and JOHNS, D. G. (eds) Springer-Verlag, New York.

KRISHANAMURTHI, S., SHANTA, V. and SISTRI, N. (1971) Combined therapy in buccal mucosa cancers. *Radiology* **99:** 409–415.

KUANG, D. T., WHITTINGTON, R. M., SPENCER, H. H. and PANTO, M. E. (1969) Comparison of chlorambucil and streptonigrin (NSC 45383) in the treatment of malignant lymphomas. *Cancer* **23:** 1280–1283.

KUSAI, A. and UEDA, S. (1984) The stability of carboquone in aqueous solution. III. Kinetics and mechanisms of degradation of carboquone in aqueous solution. *Chem. Pharmac. Bull.* **32:** 2406–2413.

KUSAI, A., TANAKA, S. and UEDA, S. (1981) The stability of carboquone in aqueous solution. I. Kinetics and mechanisms of degradation of 2,5-diethylenimino-1,4-benzoquinone in aqueous solution. *Chem. Pharmac. Bull.* **29:** 3671–3679.

KYALWAZI, S. K. (1968) Chemotherapy of Kaposi's sarcoma: experience with trenimon. *E. Afr. Med. J.* **45:** 17–26.

LAMPIDIS T. J., GARNIER-SUILLEROT A. and TAPIERO H. (1987) Reduced toxicity of non-free radical forming adriamycin in cardiac cells. *Proc. Am. Cancer Res.* **28,** 270.

LAND, E. J., MUKHERJEE, T., SWALLOW, A. J. and BRUCE, J. M. (1983) One-electron reduction of adriamycin: properties of the semiquinone. *Arch. Biochem. Biophys.* **225:** 116–121.

LAND, E. J., MUKHERJEE, T., SWALLOW, A. J. and BRUCE, J. M. (1985) Possible intermediates in the action of adriamycin—A pulse radiolysis study. *Br. J. Cancer* **51:** 515–523.

LAU D. H. M., LEWIS A. D. and BRANIMIR I. S. (1989) Association of DNA cross-linking with potentiation of the morpholino derivative of doxorubicin by human liver microsomes. *J. natn. Cancer Inst.* **18:** 1034–1038.

LAWRENCE H. J. and GOODNIGHT S. H. (1983) Dimethylsulfoxide and extravasation of anthracycline agents. *Ann. intern. Med.* **98:** 1025–1029.

LAWRENCE H. J., WALSH D., ZAPOTOWSKI K. A., DENHAM A., GOODNIGHT S. H. and GANDRA D. R. (1989) Topical dimethylsulfoxide may prevent tissue damage from anthracycline extravasation. *Cancer Chemother. Pharmac.* **23,** 316–318.

LEA, J. S., GARNER, H. J., BUTLER J., HOEY B. M. and WARD TH (1988) The lack of correlation between toxicity and free radical formation of two diaziridinyl benzoquinones. *Biochem. Pharmac.* **37:** 2023–2025.

LE BOT, M. A., BEGUE, J. M., KERNALEGUEN, D., ROBERT, J., RATANASAVANH, D., AIRIAU, J., RICHE, C., GUILLOUZO, A. (1988) Different cytotoxicity and metabolism of doxorubicin, daunorubicin, epirubicin, esorubicin and idarubicin in cultured human and rat hepatocytes. *Biochem. Pharmac.* **37:** 3877–3887.

LEGHA, S. S., BENJAMIN, R. S., MCKAY, B., EWER, M., WALLACE, S., VALDIVIESO, M., RASMUSSEN, S. L., BLUMENSCHEIN, G. R. and FREIREICH, E. J. (1982) Reduction of doxorubicin cardiotoxicity by prolonged continuous intravenous infusion. *Ann. Intern. Med.* **96:** 133–139.

LENZHOFER, R., GANZINGER, U., RAMEIS, H. and MOSER, K. (1983) Acute cardiac toxicity in patients after doxorubicin treatment and the effect of combined tocopherol and nifedipine pretreatment. *J. Cancer Res. clin. Oncol.* **106:** 143–147.

LEVIN, M., SILBER, R., ISRAEL, M., GOLDFEDER, A., KHETARPEL, V. K. and POTMESIL, M. (1981) Protein-associated DNA breaks and DNA-protein cross-links caused by DNA nonbinding derivatives of adriamycin in L1210 cells. *Cancer Res.* **41:** 1006–1010.

LEVINE, M. and BROTHWICK, N. (1963) The action of streptonigrin on bacterial DNA metabolism and on induction of phage production in lysogenic bacteria. *Virology* **21:** 568–574.

LIN, A. J. and SARTORELLI, A. C. (1973) 2,3-Dimethyl-5,6-bis(methylene)-1,4-benzoquinone. The active intermediate of bioreductive alkylating agents. *J. Org. Chem.* **38:** 813–815.

LIN, A. J., COSBY, L. A., SHANSKY, C. W. and SARTORELLI, A. C. (1972) Potential bioreductive alkylating agents. 1. Benzoquinone derivatives. *J. Med. Chem.* **15:** 1247–1252.

LIN, A. J., PARDINI, R. S., COSBY, L. A., LILLIS, B. J., SHANSKY, C. W. and SARTORELLI, A. C. (1973) Potential bioreductive alkylating agents. 2. Antitumor effect and biochemical studies of naphthoquinone derivatives. *J. Med. Chem.* **16:** 1268–1271.

LIN, A. J., SHANSKY, C. W. and SARTORELLI, A. C. (1974) Potential bioreductive alkylating agents. 3. Synthesis and antineoplastic activity of acetoxymethyl and corresponding ethyl carbamate of benzoquinones. *J. Med. Chem.* **17:** 558–561.

LIN, A. J., TEICHER, B. A. and SARTORELLI, A. C. (1982) 2-Methylanthraquinone derivatives as potential bioreductive alkylation agents. *J. Med. Chem.* **23:** 1237–1242.

LIN, W. S. and ARMSTRONG, D. A. (1977) Glutathione mediation of papain inactivation by hydrogen peroxide and hydroxyl radicals. *Radiat. Res.* **69:** 434–441.

LIND, C., VADI, H. and ERNSTER, L. (1978) Metabolism of benzo(a)pyrene-3,6-quinone and 3-hydroxybenzo(a)pyrene in liver microsomes from 3-methylcholanthrene-treated rats. *Arch. Biochem. Biophys.* **190:** 97–108.

LIND, C., HOCHSTEIN, P. and ERNSTER, L. (1982) DT-Diaphorase as a quinone reductase: a cellular control device against semiquinone and superoxide radical formation. *Arch. Biochem. Biophys.* **216:** 178–185.

LINFORD, J. H. (1973) 2,3,5-Tris-ethyleneimino-1,4-benzoquinone (Trenimon): some chemical and biological properties. *Chem. Biol. Interact.* **6:** 149–168.

LIPSETT, M. N. and WEISSBACH, A. (1965) The site of alkylation of nucleic acids by mitomycin. *Biochemistry* **4:** 206–211.

LLESUY, S. F., MILEI, J., MOLINA, H., BOVERIS, A. and MILEI, S. (1985) Comparison of lipid peroxidation and myocardial damage induced by adriamycin and 4′-epiadriamycin in mice. *Tumori* **71:** 241–249.

LOCHER, S. E. and MEYN, R. E. (1983) Relationship between cytotoxicity and DNA damage in mammalian cells treated with anthracenedione derivatives. *Chem. Biol. Interact.* **46:** 369–379.

LONDOS-GAGLIARDI, D., BAURAIN, R., ROBERTS, J. and AUBEL-SADRON, G. (1982) Metabolism of daunorubicin in sensitive and resistant Ehrlich ascites tumor cells. Determination by high pressure liquid chromatography. *Cancer Chemother. Pharmac.* **9:** 45–48.

LONG, H. L., POWIS, G., SCHUTT, A. J., MOERTEL, C. G. and KOVACH, J. S. (1985) Menogaril by 72-hour continuous intravenous infusion: a Phase I study with pharmacokinetics. *Pro. Am. Soc. Clin. Oncol.* **4:** 28.

LOO, T. L., BENJAMIN, R. S., LU, K., BENVENUTO, J. A., HALL, S. W. and McKelvey, E. M. (1978) Metabolism and disposition of Baker's antifolate (NSC-239105), ftorafur (NSC-148958) and dichloroallyl lawsone (NSC-126771) in man. *Drug Metab. Rev.* **8:** 137–150.

LOWN, J. W. (1979) The molecular mechanism of antitumor action of the mitomycins. In: *Mitomycin C: Current Status and New Developments*, pp. 5–26, CARTER , S. K. and CROOKE, S. T. (eds) Academic Press, New York.

LOWN, J. W. (1983) The mechanism of action of quinone antibiotics. *Molec. Cell. Biochem.* **55:** 17–40.

LOWN, J. W. and CHEN, H-H. (1981) Electron paramagnetic resonance characterization and conformation of daunorubicon semiquinone intermediate implicated in anthracycline metabolism, cardiotoxicity, and anticancer action. *Can. J. Chem.* **59:** 3212–3217.

LOWN, J. W. and SIM, S. K. (1976) Studies related to antitumor antibiotics. Part VII. Synthesis of streptonigrin analogues and their single strand scission of DNA. *Can. J. Chem.* **54:** 2563–2572.

LOWN, J. W., BEGLEITER, A., JOHNSON, D. and MORGAN, R. (1976) Studies related to antitumor antibiotics V. Reaction of mitomycin C with DNA examined by ethidium fluorescence assay. *Can. J. Biochem.* **54:** 110–119.

LOWN, J. W., SIM, S.-K., MAJUMDAR, K. C. and CHANGE, R. Y. (1977) Strand scission of DNA by bound adriamycin and daunorubicin in the presence of reducing agents. *Biochem. biophys. Res. Commun.* **76:** 706–710.

LOWN, J. W., SIM, S. K. and CHEN, H. H. (1978) Hydroxyl radical production by free and DNA-bound aminoquinone antibiotics and its role in DNA degradation. Electron spin resonance detection of hydroxyl radicals by spin trapping. *Can. J. Biochem.* **56:** 1042–1047.

LOWN, J. W., CHEN, H. H., PLAMBECK, J. A. and ACTON, E. M. (1979) Diminished superoxide anion generation by reduced 5-iminodaunorubicin relative to daunorubicin and the relationship to cardiotoxicity of the anthracycline antitumor agents. *Biochem. Pharmac.* **28:** 2536–2568.

LOWN, J. W., CHEN, H. H., PLAMBECK, J. A. and ACTON, E. M. (1982) Further studies on the generation of reactive oxygen species from activated anthracyclines and the relationship to cytotoxic action and cardiotoxic effects. *Biochem. Pharmac.* **31:** 575–581.

LOWN, J. W., MORGAN, A. R., YEN, S. F., WANG, Y. H. and WILSON, W. D. (1985) Characteristics of the binding of the anticancer agents mitoxantrone and ametantrone and related structures to deoxyribonuclic acids. *Biochemistry* **24:** 4028–4035.

LU, K. and LOO, T. L. (1980) Pharmacologic disposition of 1,4-bis[2-[(2-hydroxyethyl)amino]ethylamino]-9,10-anthracenedione diacetate in the dog. *Cancer Res.* **40:** 1427–1430.

LU, K., SAVARAJ, N., YAP, B. S., BEDIKIAN, Y., FEUN, G. and LOO, T. L. (1981) Clinical pharmacology of 2,5-diaziridinyl-3,6-bis-carboethoxyamino-1,4-benzoquinone (AZQ, NSC 182986). *Proc. Am. Assoc. Cancer Res.* **22:** 180.

LU, K., SAVARJ, N., YAP, B. S., BEDIKIAN, A. Y., FEUN, L., BENJAMIN, R. S. and LOO, T. L. (1983) Clinical pharmacology of 2,5′-diaziridinyl-3,6-biscarboethoxyamino-1,4-benzoquinone (AZQ). *Eur. J. Clin. Oncol.* **19:** 603–606.

LU, K., SAVARAJ, N. and LOO, T. L. (1984) Pharmacological disposition of 1,4-dihydroxy-5-8-bis([2[(-hydroxy-ethyl)amino]ethyl]amino]-9,10-anthracenedione dihydrochloride in the dog. *Cancer Chemother. Pharmac.* **13:** 63–66.

LU, K., SAVARAJ, N., KAVANAGH, J., FEUN, L. G., BURGESS, M., BODEY, G. P. and LOO, T. L. (1986) Clinical pharmacology of 4-demethoxydaunorubicin (DMDR). *Cancer Chemother. Pharmac.* **17:** 143–145.

LUDWIG, C. U., PENG, Y. M., BEAUDRY, J. N. and SALMON, S. E. (1984) Cytotoxicity of mitomycin C on clonogenic human carcinoma cells is not enhanced by hypoxia. *Cancer Chemother. Pharmac.* **12:** 146–150.

LUDWIG, C. U., STOLL, H-R., OBRIST R., OBRECHT J-P., (1987) Prevention of cytotoxic drug induced skin ulcers with dimethylsulfoxide DMSO and α-tocopherol. *Eur. J. Cancer clin. Oncol.* **23:** 327–329.

LUSTHOF K. J., RICHTER W., DE-MOL N. J., JANSSEN L. H., VERBOOM W., REINHOUDT D. N., (1990) Reductive activation of potential antitumor bis(aziridinyl)benzoquinones by xanthine oxidase: competition between oxygen reduction and quinone reduction. *Arch. Biochem. Biophys.* **277:** 137–142.

LVSTAD, R. A., (1988) Interaction of iron-adriamycin complexes with ceruloplasmin and apotransferrin. *Int. J. Biochem.* **20:** 783–786.

LYAKHOVICH, Y., MISHIN, V. and POKROVSKY, A. (1977) A relationship between reduction of oxygen, artificial acceptors and cytochrome P-450 by NADPH-cytochrome c reductase. *Biochem. J.* **168:** 133–139.

MACPHERSON, J. S., SMYTH, J. F., CLEMENTS, J. A., RAMSAY, M. W., WARRINGTON, P. S., LEONARD, R. C. F. and WOLF, C. R. (1984) Pharmacokinetics and metabolism of mitoxantrone. *Br. J. Cancer* **50:** 252.

MAESSEN P. A., MROSS K. B., PINEDO H. M., VAN DER VIJGH W. J. (1987) Metabolism of epidoxorubicin in animals: absence of glucuronidation. *Cancer Chemother. Pharmac.* **20:** 85–87.

MAILER, K. and PETERING, D. H. (1976) Inhibition of oxidative phosphorylation in tumor cells and mitochondria by daunomycin and adriamycin. *Biochem. Pharmac.* **25:** 2085–2089.

MAJIMA, H. (1986) Clinical and pharmacologic studies of 4′-O-tetrahydropyranoyl doxorubicin (THP-ADM). *5th NCI/EORTC Symposium on New Drugs in Cancer Therapy, Amsterdam, October*, Abstract 9.50.

MALATESTA, V., PENCO, S., SACCHI, N., VALENTINI, L., VIGEVANI, A. and ARCAMONE, F. (1984) Electrochemical deglycosidation of anthracyclines: stereoelectronic requirements. *Can. J. Chem.* **62:** 2845–2850.

MALSPEIS, L., NEIDHART, J., STAUBUS, A., KEAR, T. and BOOTH, J. (1981) HPLC determination of aclacinomycin A (NSC 208734, ACM) in plasma and application to preliminary clinical pharmacokinetic studies. *Proc. Am. Assoc. Cancer Res.* **22:** 242.

MANIEZ-DEVOS, D. M., BAURAIN, R., LESNE, M. and TROUET, A. (1986a) Degradation of doxorubicin and daunorubicin in human and rabbit biological fluids. *J. Pharmaceut. Biomed. Anal.* **4:** 343–365.

MANIEZ-DEVOS, D. M., BAURAIN, R., LESNE, M and TROUET, A. (1986b) Doxorubicin and daunorubicin plasmatic, hepatic and renal disposition in the rabbit with or without enterophepatic circulation. *J. Pharmac.* **17:** 1–13.

MARAL, J., POISSON, M., PERTUISET, B. F., MASHALY, P., WEIL, M., JACQUILLAT, C. and GRILLO-LOPEZ, A. J.

(1985) Phase II evaluation of diaziquone (Cl-904, AZQ) in the treatment of human malignant glioma. *J. Neuro-Oncol.* **3:** 245–249.

MARIAM, Y. H. and GLOVER, G. P. (1986) Degradation of DNA by metalloanthracyclines: requirement for metal ions. *Biochem. biophys. Res. Commun.* **136:** 1–7.

MARINELLO, A. J., BERRIGAN, M. J., STRUCK, R. F., GUENGERICH, F. D. and GURTOO, H. L. (1981) Inhibition of NADPH-cytochrome P-450 reductase by cyclophosphamide and its metabolites. *Biochem. biophys. Res. Commun.* **99:** 399–403.

MARSHALL, R. S. and RAUTH, A. M. (1986) Modification of the cytotoxic activity of mitomycin C by oxygen and ascorbic acid in Chinese hamster ovary cells and a repair-deficient mutant. *Cancer Res.* **46:** 2709–2713.

MARSHALL, R. S., RAUTH, A. M. (1989) Deficient activation by a human cell strain leads to mitomycin resistance under aerobic but not hypoxic conditions. *Br. J. Cancer* **59:** 341–347.

MARSHALL, R. S., ERLICHMAN, C. and RAUTH, A. M. (1985) A bioassay to measure cytotoxicity of plasma from patients treated with mitomycin C. *Cancer Res.* **45:** 5939–5943.

MARTIN, B. W., IVIE, G. W. and BAILEY, E. M. (1983) The acute toxicity of 1-methylaminoanthraquinone in dogs and rabbits and its metabolism in sheep. *Arch. Environ. Contam. Toxicol.* **12:** 499–507.

MARTIN, W. M. C. and MCNALLY, N. J. (1979) The cytotoxic action of adriamycin and cyclophosphamide on tumor cells *in vitro* and *in vivo*. *Int. J. Rad. Onc. Biol. Phys.* **5:** 1309–1312.

MASON, R. P. (1979) Free radical metabolites of foreign compounds and their toxicological significance. In: *Reviews in Biochemical Toxicology*, Part 1, pp. 151–200, HODGSON, E., BEND, J. R. and PHILPOT, R. M. (eds) Elsevier, North-Holland.

MASON, R. (1982) Free radical intermediates in the metabolism of toxic chemicals. In: *Free Radicals in Biology*, Volume V, pp. 161–222, PRYOR, W. A. (ed.) Academic Press, New York.

MCGOVERN, J. P., NEIL, G. L., DENLINGER, R. H., HALL, T. L., CRAMPTON, S. L. and SWENBERG, J. A. (1979) Chronic cardiotoxicity studies in rabbits with 7-con-*O*-methylnogarol, a new anthracycline antitumor agent. *Cancer Res.* **39:** 4849–4855.

MCGOVERN, J. P., NELSON, K. G., LASSUS, M., CRADOCK, J. C., PLOWMAN, J. and CHRISTOPHER, J. P. (1984) Menogaril: a new anthracycline agent entering clinical trials. *Invest. New Drugs* **2:** 359–367.

MCKELVEY, E. M., LOMEDICO, M. LU, K., CHADWICK, M and LOO, T. L. (1979) Dichlorallyl lawsone. *Clin. Pharmac. Ther.* **25:** 586–590.

MEGURO, S., NAGATA, T., YOKOYAMA, K., CHINEN, T., YAMAZAKI, H., KOBAYASHI, T., ISOGAI, Y. and OGAWA, M. (1984) Phase I study of 7-*N*-(*p*-hydroxyphenyl)-mitomycin C. *Invest. New Drugs* **2:** 381–385.

MEIJER, C., MULDER, N. H., TIMMER-BOSSCHA, H., ZIJLSTRA, J. G. and DE VRIES, E. G. E. (1987) Role of free radicals in an adriamycin-resistant human small cell lung cancer cell line. *Cancer Res.* **47:** 4613–4617.

MEYN, R. E., JENKINS, S. F. and THOMPSON, L. H. (1982) Defective removal of DNA crosslinks in a repair deficient mutant of Chinese hamster cells. *Cancer Res.* **42:** 3106–3110.

MHATRE, R. M., HERMAN, E. H., WARAVDEKAR, V. S. and LEE, I. P. (1972) Distribution and metabolism of daunomycin, adriamycin N-acetyldaunomycin in the Syrian golden hamster. *Biochem. Med.* **6:** 445–453.

MICHAELIS, L. (1946) Review of the semiquinone problem. *Trans. Electrochem. Soc.* **71:** 17–34.

MILEI, J., VAZQUEZ, A., BOVERIS, A., LLESUY, S., MOLINA, H. A., STORINO, R. and MARANTZ, A. (1988) The role of prenylamine in the prevention of adriamycin-induced cardiotoxicity. A review of experimental and clinical findings. *J. intern. Med. Res.* **16:** 19–30.

MILLER, A. A. and SCHMIDT, C. G. (1987) Clinical pharmacology and toxicity of 4′-O-tetrahydropyranyladriamycin. *Cancer Res.* **47:** 1461–1465.

MILLER, D. S., LAZLO, J., MCCARTY, K. S., GUILD, W. R. and HOCHSTEIN, P. (1967) Mechanism of action of streptonigrin in leukemia cells. *Cancer Res.* **27:** 632–638.

MILLER, M. G., RODGERS, A. and COHEN, G. M. (1986) Mechanisms of toxicity of naphthoquinones to isolated hepatocytes. *Biochem. Pharmac.* **35:** 1177–1184.

MIMNAUGH, E. G., SIDDIK, Z. H., DREW, R., SIKIC, B. I. and GRAM, T. (1979) The effects of alpha-tocopherol on the toxicity, disposition, and metabolism of adriamycin in mice. *Toxicol. Appl. Pharmac.* **49:** 119–126.

MIMNAUGH, E. G., TRUSH, M. A. and GRAM, T. E. (1981) Stimulation of adriamycin of rat heart and liver microsomal NADPH-dependent lipid peroxidation. *Biochem. Pharmac.* **30:** 2797–2804.

MIMNAUGH, E. G., TRUSH, M. A., GINSBURG, E. and GRAM, T. E. (1982) Differential effects of anthracycline drugs on rat heart and liver microsomal reduced nicotinamide adenine dinucleotide phosphate-dependent lipid peroxidation. *Cancer Res.* **42:** 3574–3582.

MIMNAUGH, E. G., GRAM, E. G. and TRUSH, M. A. (1983) Stimulation of mouse heart and liver microsomal lipid peroxidation by anthracycline anticancer drugs: characterization and effects of reactive oxygen scavengers. *J. Pharmac. exp. Ther.* **226:** 806–816.

MIMNAUGH, E. G., KENNEDY, K. A., TRUSH, M. A. and SINHA, B. K. (1985) Adriamycin-enhanced membrane lipid peroxidation in isolated rat nuclei. *Cancer Res.* **45:** 3296–3304.

MIMNAUGH, E. G., DUSRE, L., ATWELL, J. and MYERS, C. E. (1989) Differential oxygen radical susceptibility of adriamycin-sensitive and -resistant MCF-7 human breast tumor cells. *Cancer Res.* **49:** 8–15.

MINOTTI, G., (1989) Reactions of adriamycin with microsomal iron and lipids. *Free. Rad. Res. Commun.* **7:** 143–148.

MITCHELL, J. S., BRINKLEY, D. and HAYBITTLE, J. L. (1965) Clinical trial of radiosensitizers, including Synkavit and oxygen inhaled at atmospheric pressure. *Acta Radiol. Ther. Biophys. Biol.* **3:** 329–341.

MITELMAN, F. and LEVAN, A. (1978) Clustering of aberrations to specific chromosomes in human neoplasms III. Incidence and geographic distribution of chromosome aberrations in 856 cases. *Hereditas* **89:** 207–232.

MIZUNO, N. S. (1967) Comparative effects of streptonigrin derivatives on tissue culture cells. *Biochem. Pharmac.* **16:** 933–940.

MIZUNO, N. S. and GILBOE, D. P. (1970) Binding of streptonigrin derivatives to DNA. *Biochem. biophys. Acta* **224:** 319–327.

MOORE, G. A., O'BRIEN, P. J. and ORRENIUS, S. (1986) Menadione (2-methyl-1,4-naphthoquinone)-induced Ca^{2+} release from rat liver mitochondria is caused by NAD(P)H oxidation. *Xenobiotica* **16:** 873–882.

MOORE, G. A., MCCONKEY, D. J., KASS, G. E. N., O'BRIEN, P. J. and ORRENIUS, S. (1987) 2,5-Di(*tert*-butyl)-1,4-benzohydroquinone—a novel inhibitor of liver microsomal Ca^{2+} sequestration. *FBS Lett.* **224:** 331–336.

MOORE, H. W. (1977) Bioactivation as a model for drug design bioreductive alkylation. *Science* **197:** 527–532.

MOORE, H. W. and CZERNIAK, R. (1981) Naturally occurring quinones as potenial bioreductive alkylating agents. *Med. Res. Rev.* **1:** 249–280.

MOORE, H. W., CZERNIAK, R. and HAMDAN, A. (1986) Natural quinones as quinone methide precursors—ideas in rational drug design. *Drugs Expl. Clin. Res.* **12:** 475–494.

MOORE, L., LANDON, E. J. and COONEY, D. A. (1977) Inhibition of the cardiac mitochondrial calcium pump by adriamycin *in vitro*. *Biochem. Med.* **18:** 131–138.

MORO, E., BELLOTTI, V., JANNUZZO, M. G., STEGNJAICH, S. and VLAZELLI, G. (1983) High-performance liquid chromatographic method for pharmacokinetic studies on the new anthracycline 4-demethoxydaunorubicin and its 13-dihydro derivative. *J. Chromatogr.* **274:** 281–287.

MORRISON, H., JERNSTROM, B., NORDENSKJOLD, M., THOR, H. and ORRENIUS, S. (1984) Induction of DNA damage by menadione (2-methyl-1,4-naphthoquinone) in primary cultures of rat hepatocytes. *Biochem. Pharmac.* **33:** 1763–1769.

MORRISON, H., DIMONTE, D., NORDENSKJOLD, M. and JERNSTROM, B. (1985) Induction of cell damage by menadione and benzo(a)pyrene-3,6-quinone in cultures of adult rat hepatocytes and human fibroblasts. *Toxicol. Lett.* **28:** 37-43.

MORTON, R. A. (1965) Introductory account of quinones. In: *Biochemistry of Quinones*, pp. 1–22. MORTON, R. A. (ed) Academic Press, New York.

MOSSOBA, M. M. and GUTIERREZ, P. L. (1985) Diaziquone as a potential agent for photoirradiation therapy: formation of the semiquinone and hydroxyl radicals by visible light. *Biochem. biophys. Res. Commun.* **132:** 445–452.

MOSSOBA, M. M., ALIZDEH, M. and GUTIERREZ, P. L. (1985) Mechanism for the reductive activation of diaziquinone. *J. Pharmac. Sci.* **74:** 1249–1254.

MROSS, K., MAESSEN, P., VAN DER GIJGH, W. J. F., HALL, H., BOVEN, E. and PINEDO, H. M. (1988) Pharmacokinetics and metabolism of epidoxorubicin and doxorubicin in humans. *J. clin. Oncol.* **6:** 517–526.

MUINDI, J. R., SINHA, B. K., GIANNI, L. and MYERS, C. E. (1984) Hydroxyl radical production and DNA damage induced by anthracycline-iron complexes. *FEBS Lett.* **172:** 226–230.

MUINDI, J. R. F., KATKI, A. G. and MYERS, C. E. (1985a) Role of membrane protein sulfhydryl groups in adriamycin-iron complex dependent membrane destruction. *Proc. Am. Assoc. Cancer Res.* **26:** 222.

MUINDI, J., SINHA, B., GIANNI, L. and MYERS, C. E. (1985b) Thiol-dependent DNA damage produced by anthracycline-iron complexes. The structure-activity relationships and molecular mechanisms. *Molec. Pharmac.* **27:** 356–365.

MUKHERJEE, T., LAND, E. J., SWALLOW, A. J. and BRUCE, J. M. (1989) One-electron reduction of adriamycin and daunomycin: short-term stability of the semiquinones. *Arch. Biochem. Biophys.* **272:** 450–458.

MULIAWAN, H., SCHEULEN, M. E. and KAPPUS, H. (1980) Acute adriamycin treatment of rats does not increase ethane expiration. *Res. Commun. Chem. Pathol. Pharmac.* **30:** 509–519.

MÜLLER, A., CADENAS, E., GRAF, P. and SIES, H. (1984) A novel biologically active seleno-organic compounds—1. Glutathione peroxidase-like activity *in vitro* and antioxidant capacity of PZ51 (Ebselen). *Biochem. Pharmac.* **33:** 3235–3239.

MURDOCK, K. C., CHILD, R. G., FABIO, P. F., ANGIER, R. B., WALLACE, R. E., DURR, F. E. and CITARELLA, R. V. (1979) Antitumor agents. 1. 1,4-bis[(aminoalkyl)amino]-9,10-anthraquinones. *J. Med. Chem.* **22:** 1024–1030.

MYERS, C. E. (1982) Anthracyclines. In: *Pharmacologic Principles of Cancer Treatment*, pp. 416–434, CHABNER, B. (ed.) W. B. Saunders, Philadelphia, Pennsylvania.

MYERS, C. E., MCGUIRE, W. P. and YOUNG, R. (1976) Adriamycin: amelioration of toxicity by alpha-tocopherol. *Cancer Treat. Rep.* **60:** 961–962.

MYERS, C. E., MCGUIRE, W. P., LISS, R. H., IFRIM, I., GROTZINGER, K. and YOUNG, R. C. (1977) Adriamycin: the role of lipid peroxidation in cardiac toxicity and tumor response. *Science* **197:** 165–167.

MYERS, C. E., GIANNI, L., SIMONE, C. B., KLECKER, R. and GREENE, R. (1982) Oxidative destruction of erythrocyte ghost membranes catalyzed by the doxorubicin-iron complex. *Biochemistry* **21:** 1707–1712.

MYERS, C. E., MUINDI, J. R. F., ZWEIER, J. and SINHA, B. K. (1987) 5-Iminodaunomycin—an anthracycline with unique properties. *J. biol. Chem.* **262:** 11,571–11,577.

NAFF, M. B., PLOWMAN, J. and NARYANAN, V. L. (1982) Anthracyclines in the National Cancer Institute Program. In: *Anthracycline Antiobiotics*, pp. 1–57, EL KHADEM, H. S. (ed.) Academic Press, New York.

NAGATA, C. and MATSUYAMA, A. (1970) On the mechanism of action of the carcinostatic antiobiotic mitomycin

C. Progress in Antibiotics and Anticancer Chemotherapy. *Proceedings 6th International Congress, Tokyo*, Volume II, pp. 423–427.

Nakamura, M. and Yamazaki, I. (1972) One-electron transfer reactions in biochemical systems. VI. Changes in electron transfer mechanism of lipoamide dehydrogenase by modification of sulfhydryl groups. *Biochim. biophys. Acta* **267:** 249–257.

Nakamura, M. and Yamazaki, I. (1973) One-electron transfer reactions in biochemical systems. VII. Two types of electron outlets in milk xanthine oxidase. *Biochim. biophys Acta* **327:** 247–256.

Nakamura, T., Tatsumi, K., Fukai, M., Sasada, M., Higuchi, T., Inagaki, A., Sawada, H., Shirakawa, and Wakisaka, G. (1974) Mode of action of carbazilquinone in leukemic cells. *Acta Haem. Jpn.* **37:** 1–8.

Nakane, S., Matsumoto, S., Takakura, Y., Hashida, M. and Sezaki, H. (1988) The accumulation mechanism of cationic mitomycin C-dextran conjugates in the liver: in-vivo cellular localization and in-vitro interaction with hepatocytes. *J. Pharm. Pharmac.* **40:** 1–6.

Nakao, H., Arakawa, M., Nakamura, T. and Fukushima, M. (1972) Antileukemic II. New 2,5-bis(1-aziridinyl)-*p*-benzoquinone derivatives. *Chem. Pharmac. Bull.* **20:** 1968.

Nakao, H., Arakawa, M., Shindo, H., Masuda, H. and Muramatsu, T. (1975) Carboquone, a new antitumor agent. *Ann. Sankyo Res. Lab.* **27:** 1–41.

Nakata, Y., Nakata, K. and Sakamoto, Y. (1961) On the action of mitomycin C. *Biochem. biophys. Res. Commun.* **6:** 339–343.

Nakatsubo, F., Fukuyama, T., Cocuzza, A. J. and Kishi, Y. (1977) Synthetic studies towards mitomycins 2 total synthesis of dl-porfiromycin. *J. Am. Chem. Soc.* **99:** 8115–8116.

Nakazawa, H., Chou, F. E., Gutierrez, P. and Bachur, N. R. (1980) Formation of actinomycin D (AMD) and phenoxazone free radicals. *Fed. Proc.* **39:** 310.

Nakazawa, H., Chou, F. E., Andrews, P. A. and Bachur, N. R. (1981) Chemical reduction of actinomycin D and phenoxazone analogues to free radicals. *J. Org. Chem.* **46:** 1493–1496.

Nakazawa, H., Andrews, P. A., Callery, P. S. and Bachur, N. R. (1985) Superoxide radical reactions with anthracycline antibiotics. *Biochem. Pharmac.* **34:** 481–490.

Natale, N., Brambilla, M. and Luchini, S. (1983) 4′-Epidoxorubicin and doxorubicin toxicity and pharmacokinetics in cancer patients. In: *Current Chemotherapy and Immunology*, pp. 1447–1449, The American Society for Microbiology.

Nelson, E. M., Tewey, K. M. and Liu, L. F. (1984) Mechanism of antitumor drug action: poisoning of mammalian DNA topoisomerase II on DNA by 4′-(9-acridinyl-amino)-methanesulfon-*m*-anisidide. *Proc. natn. Acad. Sci. U.S.A.* **81:** 1361–1365.

Neri, B., Cini-Neri, G. and Dalterio, M. (1984) Effect of anthracyclines and mitoxantrone on oxygen uptake and ATP intracellular concentration in rat heart slices. *Biochem. biophys. Res. Commun.* **125:** 954–960.

Netter, K. J. (1980) Inhibition of oxidative drug metabolism in microsomes. *Pharmac. Ther.* **10:** 515–535.

Nettleton, D. E., Bradner, W. T., Bush, J. A., Coon, A. B., Moseley, J. E., Myllmaki, R. W., O'Herron, F. A., Schreiber, R. H. and Vulcano, A. L. (1977) New antitumor antibiotics: musettamycin and marcellomycin from bohemic acid complex. *J. Antibiot.* **30:** 525–529.

Nguyen, B. and Gutierrez, P. P. (1990) Mechanism(s) for the metabolism of mitoxantrone: electron spin resonance and electrochemical studies. *Chem.-Biol. Interact.* **74:** 139–162.

Nguyen, B., Biswal, S. and Gutierrez, P. L. (1988) The influence of diaziquone free radicals on *the in vitro* activity of diaziquone. *Xenobiotica* **18:** 593–602.

Nickerson, W. J., Falcone, G. and Strauss, G. (1963) Studies on quinone thioethers. I. Mechanism of formation and properties of thiodone. *Biochemistry* **2:** 537–543.

Nicotera, P., Moore, M., Mirabelli, F., Bellomo, G. and Orrenius, S. (1985) Inhibition of hepatocyte plasma membrane Ca^{2+}-ATPase activity by menadione metabolism and its restoration by thiols. *FEBS Lett.* **181:** 149–153.

Nishibayashi, H., Nakai, N. and Sato, R. (1967) Specificity of naphthoquinones as cofactors for NADPH oxidation by liver microsomes. *J. Biochem. (Tokyo)* **62:** 215–222.

Nobbs, P. and Barr, R. D. (1983) Soft-tissue injury caused by antineoplastic drugs is inhibited by topical dimethyl sulphoxide and alpha-tocopherol. *Br. J. Cancer* **48:** 873–876.

Nohl, H. (1988) Identification of the site of adriamycin-activation in the heart cell. *Biochem. Pharmac.* **37:** 2633–2637.

Nohl, H. and Jordan, W. (1983) OH·-generation by adriamycin semiquinone and H_2O_2: an explanation for the cardiotoxicity of anthracycline antibiotics. *Biochem. biophys. Res. Commun.* **114:** 197–205.

Nohl, H., Jordan, W. and Youngman, R. J. (1986) Quinones in biology: Functions in electron transfer and oxygen activation. *Adv. Free Rad. Biol. Med.* **2:** 211–279.

Nooter, K., Oostrum, R. and Deurloo, J. (1987) Effects of verapamil on the pharmacokinetics of daunomycin in the rat. *Cancer Chemother. Pharmac.* **20:** 176–178.

Novak, R. F. and Kharasch, E. D. (1985) Mitoxantrone: propensity for free radical formation and lipid peroxidation—implications for cardiotoxicity. *Invest. New Drugs* **3:** 95–99.

Nudd, R. and Wilkie, D. (1983) Chemical carcinogenesis, mitochondria and glutathione. *Chem. Br.* **19:** 911–915.

Obere-Greenwood, M. A., Smith, B. H., Cooke, C., Ellis, J. R., Kornblith, P. L. and McKeever, P. E. (1983) Mitochondrial toxicity of 2,5-diaziridinyl-3,6-bis-(carboethoxyamino)-2,4-benzoquinone. *J. Natl. Cancer Inst.* **71:** 723–733.

OBERLEY, L. W. and BUETTNER, G. T. (1979) Role of superoxide dismutase in cancer: a review. *Cancer Res.* **39:** 1141–1149.

OGASAWARA, T., MASUDA, Y., GOTO, S., MORI, S. and OKI, T. (1981) High performance liquid chromatographic determination of aclacinomycin A and its related compounds. II. Reversed phase hplc determinations of aclacinomycin A and its metabolites in biological fluids using fluorescence detection. *J. Antibiot.* **34:** 52–56.

OGAWA, M., KIMURA, K., SAITO, T. and UMEZAWA, H. (1986) Phase II trial of a new anthracycline, THP-adriamycin. *5th NCI/EORTC Symposium on New Drugs in Cancer Therapy, Amsterdam, October*, Abstract 9.05.

OGAWA, Y., KONDO, T., SUGIYAMA, S., OGAWA, K., SATAKE, T. and OZAWA, T. (1987) Role of phospholipase in the genesis of doxorubicin-induced cardiomyopathy in rats. *Cancer Res.* **47:** 1239–1243.

OKI, T. (1977) New anthracycline antibiotics. *Jap. J. Antibiot.* **30**(Suppl.): S70–S84.

OKI, T., MATSUZAWA, Y., YOSHIMOTO, A., NUMATA, K., KITAMURA, I., HORI, S., TAKAMATSU, A., UMEZAWA, H., ISHIZUKA, M., NAGANAWA, H., SUDA, H., HAMADA, M. and TAKEUCHI, T. (1975) New antitumor antibiotics, aclacinomycin A and B. *J. Antibiot.* **28:** 830–834.

OKI, T., KOMIYAMA, T., TONE, H., INUI, T., TAKEUCHI, T. and UMEZAWA, H. (1977) Reductive cleavage of anthracycline glycosides by microsomal NADPH-cytochrome c reductase. *J. Antibiot. Tokyo* **30:** 613–615.

OKI, T., TAKEUCHI, T., OKA, S. and UMEZAWA, H. (1981) New anthracycline antibiotic aclacinomycin A: experimental studies and correlations with clinical trials. *Recent Res. Cancer Res.* **76:** 21–40.

OLESON, J. J., CALDERALLA, L. A., MJOS, K. J., REITH, A. R., Thie, R. S. and TOPLIN, I. (1961) The effects of streptonigrin on experimental tumors. *Antibiot. Chemother.* **11:** 158–164.

OLESON, J. J., MORRISON, R. K. and BROWN, D. E. (1967) U.S. Department of Commerce National Technical Information Service, Toxicologic and pharmacologic studies with lapachol (NSC 11905), PB-174870.

OLESON, H. M., YOUNG, D. M., PRIEUN, D. J., LEROY, A. F. and REGAN, R. L. (1974) Electrolyte and morphologic alterations of myocardium in adriamycin treated rabbits. *Am. J. Pathol.* **77:** 439.

OLSON, R. D., MCDONALD, J. S., VAN BOXTEL, C. J., BOERTH, R. C., HARBISON, R. D., SLONIM, A. E., FREEMAN, R. W. and OATES, J. A. (1980) Regulatory role of glutathione and soluble sulfhydryl groups in the toxicity of adriamycin. *J. Pharmac. exp. Ther.* **215:** 450–454.

OLSON, R. D., MUSHLIN, P. S., BRENNER, D. E., FLEISCHER, S., CUSACK, J. B., CHANG, B. K. and BOUCEK, R. J. JR (1988) Doxorubicin cardiotoxicity may be caused by its metabolite doxorubicinol. *Proc. natn. Acad. Sci. U.S.A.* **85:** 3585–3589.

OLVER, I. N., and SCHWARZ, M. A. (1983) Use of dimethylsulfoxide in limiting tissue damage caused by extravasalation of doxorubicin. *Cancer Treat. Rep.* **67:** 407–408.

OOSTERBAAN, M. J. M., DIRKS, R. J. M., VREE, T. B., VAN DER KLEIJN, E., SIMONETTI, G. S. and MCVIE, J. G. (1982) Clinical pharmacokinetics of adriamycin. *J. Drug Res.* **7:** 1372–1378.

OOSTERMAAN, M. J. M., DIRKS, R. J. M., VREE, T. B. and VAN DER KLEIJN, E. (1984) Pharmacokinetics of anthracyclines in dogs: evidence for structure-related body distribution and reduction to their hydroxy metabolites. *Pharmaceut. Res.* **1:** 33–38.

ORRENIUS, S. (1985) Biological consequences of reactive metabolite formation. 10th European Drug Metabolism Workshop (Abstract), Guildford, Surrey, England, July, 1986, p. 20.

OZOLS, R. F., CUNNION, R. E., KLECKER, R. W. JR, HAMILTON, T. C., OSTCHEGA, Y., PARRILLO, J. E. and YOUNG, R. C. (1987) Verapamil and adriamycin in the treatment of drug-resistant ovarian cancer patients. *J. clin. Oncol.* **5:** 641–647.

PAINTER, R. B. (1978) Inhibition of DNA replicon initiation by 4-nitroquinoline 1-oxide, adriamycin, and ethyleneimine. *Cancer Res.* **38:** 4445–4449.

PAN, S.-S. and BACHUR, N. R. (1980) Xanthine oxidase catalyzed reduced cleavage of anthracycline antibiotics and free radical formation. *Molec. Pharmac.* **17:** 95–99.

PAN, S.-S. and GONZALEZ, H. (1990) Mitomycin antibiotic reductive potential and related pharmacological activities. *Molec. Pharmac.* **37:** 966–970.

PAN, S.-S., GUTIERREZ, P. and BACHUR, N. R. (1980) Flavoprotein catalysis of anthracycline antibiotic reductive cleavage, free radical formation and free radical interconversions. *Fed. Proc.* **39:** 310.

PAN, S.-S., GUTIERREZ, P., NAKAZAWA, H. and BACHUR, N. R. (1981a) Formation of kinetics and interconversion of anthracycline free radicals catalyzed by flavoenzymes. *Proc. Am. Assoc. Cancer Res.* **22:** 265.

PAN, S.-S., PEDERSEN, L. and BACHUR, N. R. (1981b) Comparative flavoprotein catalysis of anthracycline antibiotic. Reductive cleavage and oxygen consumption. *Molec. Pharmac.* **19:** 184–186.

PAN, S.-S., ANDREWS, P. A., GLOVER, C. J. and BACHUR, N. R. (1984) Reductive activation of mitomycin C and mitomycin C metabolites catalyzed by NADPH-cytochrome P-450 reductase and xanthine oxidase. *J. biol. Chem.* **259:** 959–966.

PAN, S.-S., IRACKI, T. and BACHUR, N. R. (1986) DNA alkylation by enzyme-activated mitomycin C. *Molec. Pharmac.* **29:** 622–628.

PANNEERSELYAM, M., BREDEHORST, R. and VOGEL, C.-W. (1987) Cell surface cytotoxic effect immobilized doxorubicin is target cell-dependent and involves oxygen radical formation. *Proc. Am. Ass. Cancer Res.* **28:** 267.

PANNUTI, F., CAMAGGI, C. M., STROCHI, E., COMPARSI, R., ANGELELLI, B. and PACCIARINI, M. A. (1986) Low dose oral administration of 4-demethoxydaunorubicin (idarubicin) in advanced cancer patients. *Cancer Chemoher. Pharmac.* **16:** 295–299.

PATRICK, J. B., WILLIAMS, R. P., MEYER, W. E., FULMOR, W., COSULICH, D. B. BROSCHARD, R. W. and WEBB, J.

S. (1964) Aziridinomitosenes: a new class of antibiotics related to mitomycins. *J. Am. Chem. Soc.* **86:** 1889–1890.

Patterson, L. H., Gandecha, B. M. and Brown, J. R. (1983) 1,4-Bis[[2-[(2-hydroxyethyl)]aminoethylamino]-9,10-anthracenedione an anthraquinone antitumor agent with daunorubicin. *Biochem. biophys. Res. Commun.* **110:** 399–405.

Paur, E., Youngman, R. J., Lengfelder, E. and Elstner, E. F. (1984) Mechanisms of adriamycin-dependent oxygen activation catalyzed by NADPH-cytochrome c-(ferredoxin)-oxidoreductase. *Z. Naturforsch.* **39c:** 261–267.

Pedersen, J. Z., Marcocci, L., Rossi, L., Mavelli, I. and Rotilio, G. (1990) Generation of daunomycin radicals on the outer side of the erythrocyte membrane. *Biochem. biophys. Res. Commun.* **168:** 240–247.

Perlman, D., Mauger, A. B. and Weissbach, H. (1967) Microbial transformations of peptide antibiotics. I. Degradation of actinomycins by actinoplanes species. *Antimicrob. Ag. Chemother.* **16:** 581–586.

Peskin, A. V., Zbarski, I. B. and Konstantinov, A. A. (1976) Superoxide dismutase activity in neoplastic tissues. *Dokl. Akad. Nauk SSR* **229:** 751–754.

Peskin, A. V., Zharsky, I. B. and Konstantinov, A. A. (1980) A novel type of superoxide generating system in nuclear membranes from hepatoma 22a ascites cells. *FEBS Lett.* **117:** 44–48.

Peters, J. H., Gordon, G. R., Kashiwase, D., Acton, E. M. and Hunt, C. A. (1983) Metabolic disposition of *N,N*-dibenzyldaunorubicin in the rat. *Cancer Res.* **43:** 1477–1487.

Peters, J. H., Gordon, G. R., Kashiwase, D. and Acton, E. M. (1984) Metabolic disposition of 5-iminodaunorubicin in the rat. *Cancer Res.* **44:** 1453–1459.

Peters, J. H., Ross, G. G., Kashiwase, D., Lown, J. W., Yen, S. F. and Plambeck, J. A. (1986) Redox activities of antitumor anthracyclines determined by microsomal oxygen consumption and assays for superoxide anion and hydroxyl radical generation. *Biochem. Pharmac.* **35:** 1309–1323.

Peters, J. H., Streeter, D. G., Johl, J. S., Gordon, G. R. and Tracy, M. (1987) Comparative redox activities of anthracyclines by microsomes from P388 cells and rat liver. *Anticancer Res.* **7:** 1189–1192.

Peters, J. H., Gordon, G. R., Nolen, H. W. III, Tracy, M. and Thomas, D. W. (1988) Facile exchange of the cyano group a in highly potent anticancer cyanomorpholinyl anthracyclines. *Biochem. Pharmac.* **37:** 357–361.

Peterson, D. W. and Fisher, J. (1986) Autocatalytic quinone methide formation from mitomycin C. *Biochemistry* **25:** 4077–4084.

Philips, D. R. and Carlyle, G. A. (1981) The effect of physiological levels of divalent metal ions on the interaction of duanomycin with DNA. Evidence of a ternary daunomycin-Cu^{2+}-DNA complex. *Biochem. Pharmac.* **30:** 2021–2024.

Phillips, D. R., White, R. J. and Cullinane, C. (1989) DNA sequence-specific adducts of adriamycin and mitomycin C. *FEBS Lett.* **246:** 233–240.

Piccart, M., Rozencweig, M., Abele, R., Cumps, E., Dodion, P., Dupont, D., Kissner, D. and Kenis, Y. (1981) Phase I clinical trial with ametantrone (NSC 287513). *Eur. J. Cancer Clin. Oncol.* **17:** 775–779.

Pierce, R. N. and Jatlow, P. I. (1979) Measurement of adriamycin (doxorubicin) and its metabolites in human plasma using reversed-phase high-performance liquid chromatography and fluorescence detection. *J. Chromatogr.* **164:** 471–478.

Pietronigro, D. D., McGinness, J. E., Koren, M. J., Crippa, R., Seligman, M. L. and Demopoulos, H. B. (1979) Spontaneous generation of adriamycin semiquinone radicals at physiologic pH. *Physiol. Chem. Phys.* **11:** 405–413.

Pietronigro, D. D., Mignano, J. E. and Demopoulos, H. B. (1983) Direct quenching of adriamycin radicals by coenzyme Q10 and tetrazolium salts. *Biochem. Pharmac.* **32:** 1441–1444.

Pigram, W. J., Fuller, W. and Hamilton, L. D. (1972) Stereochemistry of intercalation: interaction of daunomycin with DNA. *Nature* **235:** 17–19.

Pinto, R. E. and Bartley, W. (1973) Glutathione reductase and glutathione peroxidase activities in hepatomous livers of rats treated with diethylnitrosamine. *FEBS Lett.* **32:** 307–309.

Poirier, T. I. (1986) Mitoxantrone. *Drug Intell. Clin. Pharmac.* **20:** 97–105.

Pollakis, G., Goormaghtigh, E. and Ruysschaert, J. M. (1983) Role of the quinone structure in the mitochondrial damage induced by antitumor anthracyclines. Comparison of adriamycin and 5-iminodaunorubicin. *FEBS Lett.* **155:** 267–272.

Pollakis, G., Goormaghtigh, E., Delmelle, M., Lion, Y. and Ruysschaert, J. M. (1984) Adriamycin and derivatives interaction with the mitochrondiral membrane: O_2 consumption and free radicals formation. *Res. Commun. Chem. Pathol. Pharmac.* **44:** 445–459.

Pommier, Y., Schwartz, R. E., Zwelling, L. A. and Kohn, K. W. (1985) Effects of DNA intercalating agents on topoisomerase II induced DNA strand cleavage in isolated mammalian cell nuclei. *Biochemistry* **24:** 6406–6410.

Poochikian, G. K. and Kelley, J. A. (1981) 2,5-Diaziridinyl-3,6-bis(carboethoxyamino)-1,4-benzoquinone II. Isolation and characterization of degradation products. *J. Pharmac. Sci.* **70:** 162–167.

Posner, L. E., Dukart, G., Goldbert, J., Bernstein, T. and Cartwright, K. (1985) Mitoxantrone: an overview of safety and toxicity. *Invest. New Drugs* **3:** 123–132.

Potmesil, M., Kirschenbaum, S., Israel, M., Levin, M., Khetarpal, V. K. and Silber, R. (1983) Relationship of adriamycin concentrations to the DNA lesions induced in hypoxic and euoxic L1210 cells. *Cancer Res.* **43:** 3528–3533.

POTMESIL, M., ISRAEL, M. and SILBER, R. (1984) Two mechanisms of adriamycin-DNA interaction in L1210 cells. *Biochem. Pharmac.* **33:** 3137–3140.

POTMESIL, M., ISRAEL, M., KIRSCHENBAUM, S., SWEATMAN, T. W. and SILBER, R. (1986) Kinetics of DNA protein-associated breaks induced by *N*-acyl and *N*-alkylanthracyclines as it relates to drug metabolism. *Proc. Am. Ass. Cancer Res.* **27:** 247.

POWIS, G. (1987) Anthracycline metabolism and free radical formation. In: *Metabolism and Action of Anti-Cancer Drugs*, pp. 211–260, POWIS, G. and PROUGH, R. A. (eds) Taylor and Francis, London.

POWIS, G. (1991) Toxicity of free radical forming anticancer agents in *The Toxicity of Anticancer Drugs.* pp. 106–151, POWIS, G. and HACKER, M. P. (eds) Pergamon, NY.

POWIS, G. and APPEL, P. L. (1980) Relationship of the single-electron reduction potential of quinones to their reduction by flavoproteins. *Biochem. Pharmac.* **29:** 2567–2572.

POWIS, G. and SVINGEN, B. A. (1981) Pulse radiolysis measurement of one-electron reduction potential (E^1_7) of adriamycin derivatives. *Pharmacologist* **23:** 181.

POWIS, G., SVINGEN, B. A. and APPEL, P. L. (1981) Quinone stimulated superoxide formation by subcellular fractions, isolated hepatocytes and other cells. *Molec. Pharmac.* **20:** 387–394.

POWIS, G., SVINGEN, B. A., DAHLIN, D. C. and NELSON, S. D. (1984) Enzymatic and non-enzymatic reduction of *N*-acetyl-*p*-benzoquinoneimine and some properties of *N*-acetyl-*p*-benzosemiquinoneimine radical. *Biochem. Pharmac.* **33:** 2367–2370.

POWIS, G., HODNETT, E. M., SANTONE, K.. S., LEE SEE, K. and MELDER, D. C. (1987a) The role of metabolism and redox cycling in the cytotoxicity of antitumor quinoneimines and quinonediimines. *Cancer Res.* **47:** 2363–2370.

POWIS, G., LEE SEE, K., SANTONE, K. S., MELDER, D. and HODNETT, E. M. (1987b) Quinones as substrates for quinone reductase NAD(P)H: ((quinone-acceptor)oxido-reductase) and the effect of dicumarol on their cytotoxicity. *Biochem. Pharmac.* **36:** 2473–2479.

PRAET, M., LAGHMICHE, M., POLLAKIS, G., GOORMAGHTIGH, E. and RUYSSCHAERT, J. M. (1986) *In vivo* and *in vitro* modification of the mitochondrial membrane induced by 4′-epiadriamycin. *Biochem. Pharmac.* **35:** 2923–2928.

PRAGA, C., BERETTA, G., VIGO, P. L., LENAZ, G. R., POLLINI, C., BONADONNA, G., CANETTA, R., CASTELLINI, R., VILLA, E., GALLAGHER, C. G., VON MEICHNER, H., HAYAT, M., RIBAUD, P., DE WASCH, G., MATTSON, W., HEINZ, K., WALDNER, R., KOLARIC, K., BUEHNER, R., TEN BOKKEL-HUYNINCK, W., PEREODCHIKOVA, N. I., MANZIUK, L. A., SENN, H. J. and MAYR, A. C. (1979) Adriamycin cardiotoxicity; a survey of 1273 patients. *Cancer Treat. Rep.* **63:** 827–834.

PRASAD, K. N., EDWARDS-PRASAD, J. and SAKAMOTO, A. (1981) Vitamin K_3 (menadione) inhibits the growth of mammalian tumor cells in culture. *Life Sci.* **29:** 1387–1392.

PRATT, C. B., RANSOM, J. L. and EVANS, W. E. (1978) Age-related adriamycin cardiotoxicity in children. *Cancer Treat. Rep.* **62:** 1381–1385.

PRATT, E. A. and ADAMS, W. J. (1983) Pharmacokinetics of intravenous menogaril (NSC 269148) in the beagle dog. *Proc. Am. Ass. Cancer Res.* **24:** 259.

PRATT, E. A., MCGOVERN, J. P., ADAMS, W. J. and HAMILTON, R. D. (1982) Bioavailability and pharmacokinetics of orally administered 7-con-O-methylnogarol [7-OMEN, NSC 269148] in the mouse, *Proc. Am. Ass. Cancer Res.* **23:** 171.

PREUSCH, P. C. (1986) Lapachol inhibition of DT-diaphorase (NAD(P)H:quinone dehydrogenase). *Biochem. biophys. Res. Commun.* **137:** 781–787.

PREUSCH, P. C. and SUTTIE, J. W. (1984) Lapachol inhibition of vitamin K epoxide reductase and vitamin K. *Arch. Biochem. Biophys.* **234:** 405–412.

PRITSOS, C. A. and PARDINI, R. S. (1984) A redox cycling action for 2,3-dichloro-1,4-naphthoquinone with mitochondrial membranes and the role of sulfhydryl groups. *Biochem. Pharmac.* **33:** 3771–3777.

PRITSOS, C. A. and SARTORELLI, A. C. (1986) Generation of reactive oxygen radicals through bioactivation of mitomycin antibiotics. *Cancer Res.* **46:** 3528–3532.

PRITSOS, C. A., JENSEN, D. E., PISANI, D. and PARDINI, R. S. (1982) Involvement of superoxide in the interaction of 2,3-dichloro-1,4-naphthoquinone with mitochondrial membranes, *Arch. Biochem. Biophys.* **217:** 98–109.

PRITSOS, C. A., CONSTANTINIDES, P. P., TRITTON, T. R., HEIMBROOK, D. C. and SARTORELLI, A. C. (1985) Use of high performance liquid chromatography to detect hydroxyl and superoxide radicals generated from mitomycin C. *Anal. Biochem.* **150:** 294–299.

RABKIN, S. W. and SUNGA, P. (1987) The effect of doxorubicin (adriamycin) on cytoplasmic microtubule system in cardiac cells. *J. Molec. Cell Cardiol.* **19:** 1073–1083.

RAHMAN, A., GOODMAN, A., FOO, W., HARVEY, J., SMITH, F. P. and SCHEIN, P. S. (1984) Clinical pharmacology of daunorubicin in Phase I patients with solid tumors: development of an analytical methodology for daunorubicin and its metabolites. *Semin. Oncol.* **11:** 36–44.

RALL, D. P. and ZUBROD, C. G. (1962) Mechanisms of drug absorption and excretion. Passage of drugs in and out of the central nervous system. *Ann. Rev. Pharmac.* **2:** 109–128.

RAMAKRISHNAN, K. and FISHER, J. (1983) Nucleophilic trapping of 7,11-dideoxyanthracyclinone quinone methides. *J. Am. Chem. Soc.* **105:** 7188–7192.

RAMAKRISHNAN, K and FISHER, J. (1986) 7-Deoxydaunomycinone quinone methide reactivity with thiol nucleophiles. *J. Med. Chem.* **29:** 1215–1221.

Rao, R. D. N., Takahashi, N. and Mason, R. P. (1988) Characterization of a glutathione conjugate of the 1,4-benzosemiquinone-free radical formed in rat hepatocytes. *J. biol. Chem.* **263:** 17981–17986.

Rao, G. M., Lown, J. W. and Plambeck, J. A. (1977a) Electrochemical studies of antitumor antibiotics. I. Cyclic voltammetric study of mitomycin B. *J. Electrochem. Soc.* **124:** 195–198.

Rao, G. M., Lown, J. W. and Plambeck, J. A. (1977b) Electrochemical studies of antitumor antibiotics. II. Polarographic and cyclic voltammetric studies of mitomycin C. *J. Electrochem. Soc.* **124:** 199–202.

Rao, K. V. (1974) Quinone natural products: Streptonigrin (NSC-4538J) and lapachol (NSC-11905). Structure-activity relationships. *Cancer Chemother. Rep.* **4** (Part 2, No. 4): 11–17.

Rao, K. V. and Cullen, W. P. (1960) Streptonigrin, an antitumor substance. I. Isolation and characterization. *Antibiot. Ann.* **1959–60:** 950–953.

Rao, K. V., Biemann, K and Woodward, R. B. (1963) The structure of streptonigrin. *J. Am. Chem. Soc.* **85:** 2532–2533.

Rao, R. V., McBride, T. J. and Oleson, J. J. (1968) Recognition and evaluation of lapachol as an antitumor agent. *Cancer Res.* **28:** 1952–1954.

Rauth, A. M., Mohindra, J. K. and Tannock, I. F. (1983) Activity of mitomycin C for aerobic and hypoxic cells *in vitro* and *in vivo*. *Cancer Res.* **43:** 4154–4158.

Reich, E., Shatkin, A. J. and Tatum, L. (1961) Bacteriocidal action of mitomycin C. *Biochim. biophys. Acta* **53:** 132–149.

Reich, S. D. and Gordon, S. (1977) Pharmacology of adriamycin and ferric ion-adriamycin complex. *Proc. Am. Assoc. Cancer Res.* **18:** 72.

Reich, S. D., Fandrick, S. E., Finkelstein, T. T., Schurig, J. E., Florczyk, A. P., Comis, R. L. and Crooke, S. T. (1981) Pharmacokinetics of carminomycin in dogs and humans. *Cancer Chemother. Pharmac.* **6:** 189–193.

Remers, W. A. (1979a) Actinomycins. In: *The Chemistry of Antitumor Antibiotics*, pp. 3–62. Remers, W. A. (ed.) John Wiley, New York.

Remers, W. A. (1979b) Mitomycin C and analog development. In: *Mitomycin C, Current and New Developments*, pp. 27–32, Crooke, S. K. and Crooke, S. T. (eds) Academic Press, New York.

Remers, W. A. (1979c) Mitomycins and porfiromycin. In: *The Chemistry of Antitumor Antibiotics*, pp. 221–276, Remers, W. A. (ed.) John Wiley, New York.

Remers, W. A. and Schepman, C. S. (1974) Structure–activity relationships of the mitomycins and certain synthetic analogs. *J. Med. Chem.* **17:** 729–732.

Reszka, K., Hartley, J. A., Kolodziejczyk-P. and Lown J. W. (1989) Interaction of the peroxidase-derived metabolite of mitoxantrone with nucleic acids. Evidence for covalent binding of ^{14}C-labeled drug. *Biochem. Pharmac.* **38:** 4253–4260.

Revis, N. W. and Marusic, N. (1978) Glutathione peroxidase activity and selenium concentration in the hearts of doxorubicin-treated rabbits. *J. Molec. Cell Cardiol.* **10:** 945–951.

Revis, N. W. and Marusic, N. (1979) Sequestration of $^{45}Ca^{2+}$ by mitochondria from rabbit heart, liver, and kidney after doxorubicin or digoxin/treatment. *Exp. Molec. Pathol.* **31:** 440–451.

Reynolds, D. L., Sternson, L. A. and Repta, A. J. (1981) Clinical analysis for the antineoplastic agent 1,4-dihydroxy-5,8-bis(2-[2-(2-hydroxyethyl)amino]ethyl)-amino-9,10-anthracenedione dihydrochloride (NSC 301739) in plasma. *J. Chromatogr.* **222:** 225–240.

Riggs, C. E. and Bachur, N. R. (1983) Clinical pharmacokinetics of anthracycline antibiotics. In: *Pharmacokinetics of Anticancer Agents in Humans*, pp. 229–274, Ames, M. M., Powis, G. and Kovach, J. S. (eds) Elsevier, Amsterdam.

Riggs, C. E. and Schrader, S. L. (1985) Reduction in aglycone production from the anthracycline analogs, epidabicin, esorubicin, and idarubicin, in vitro. *Proc. Amer. Cancer Res.* **26:** 219.

Rivers, S. L., Whittington, R. M. and Medrick, T. J. (1966) Treatment of malignant lymphomas with methyl ester of streptonigrin (NSC 45384). *Cancer* **19:** 1377–1385.

Robert, J., Vrignaud, P., Nguyen-Ngoc, T., Illiadis, A., Mauriac, L. and Hurteloup, P. (1985) Comparative pharmacokinetics and metabolism of doxorubicin and epirubicin in patients with metastatic breast cancer. *Cancer Treat. Rep.* **69:** 633–640.

Robert, J., Rigal-Huguet, F. and Harousseau, J. L. (1986) Pharmacokinetics of idarubicin after daily intravenous administration in leukemia patients. *5th NCI/EORTC Symposium on New Drugs in Cancer Therapy, Amsterdam, October*, Abstract 9.11.

Robert, J., David, M., Huet, S. and Chauvergne, J. (1988) Pharmacokinetics and metabolism of pirarubicin in advanced cancer patients. *Eur. J. Cancer clin. Oncol.* **24:** 1289–1294.

Robin, E. D., Murphy, B. J. and Theodore, J. (1984) Coordinate regulation of glycolysis by hypoxia in mammalia cells. *J. Cell. Physiol.* **118:** 287–290.

Roboz, J., Paciucci, P. A., Silides, D., Greaves, J. and Holland, J. F. (1984) Detection and quantification of mitoxantrone in human organs. A case report. *Cancer Chemother. Pharmac.* **13:** 67–68.

Rockwell, S., Kennedy, K. A. and Sartorelli, A. C. (1982) Mitomycin-C as a prototype bioreductive alkylating agent: in vitro studies of metabolism and cytotoxicity. *Int. J. Radiat. Oncol. Biol. Phys.* **8:** 753–755.

Rockwell, S., Keyes, S. R. and Sartorelli, A. C. (1989) Modulation of the antineoplastic efficacy of mitomycin C by dicoumarol in vivo. *Cancer Chemother. Pharmac.* **24:** 349–353.

ROSS, D., THOR, H., ORRENIUS, S. and MOLDEUS, P. (1985) Interaction of menadione (2-methyl-1,4-naphthoquinone) with glutathione. *Chem. Biol. Interact.* **55:** 177–184.

ROSS, D., THOR, H., THREADGILL, M. D., SANDY, M. A., SMITH, M. T., MOLDÉUS, P. and ORRENIUS, S. (1986) The role of oxidative processes in the cytotoxicity of substituted 1,4-naphthoquinones in isolated hepatocytes. *Arch. Biochem. Biophys.* **248:** 460–466.

ROSS, D., SIEGEL, D., GIBSON, N. W., PACHECO, D., THOMAS, D. J., REASOR, M. and WIERDA, D. (1990) Activation and deactivation of quinones catalyzed by DT-diaphorase. Evidence for bioreductive activation of diaziquone (AZQ) in human tumor cells and detoxification of benzene metabolites in bone marrow stroma. *Free Rad. Res. Commun.* **8:** 373–381.

ROSSO, R., RAVAZZONI, C., ESPOSITO, M., SALA, R. and SANTI, L. (1972) Plasma and urinary levels of adriamycin in man. *Eur. J. Cancer* **8:** 455–459.

ROUSCILLES A., HOUEE-LEVIN, D., GARDES-ALBERT, M. and FERRADINI, C. (1989) γ-Radiolysis study of the reduction by coo-free radicals of daunorubicin intercalated in DNA. *Free Rad. Biol. Med.* **6:** 37–43.

ROWLEY, D. A. and HALLIWELL, B. (1983) DNA damage by superoxide-generating systems in relation to the mechanism of action of the anti-tumor antibiotic adriamycin. *Biochim. biophys. Acta* **761:** 86–93.

RUNDGREN, M., PORUBEK, D. J., HARVISON, P. J., COTGREAVE, I. A., MOLDÉUS, P. and NELSON, S. D. (1988) Comparative cytotoxic effects of N-acetyl-p-benzoquinone imine and two dimethylated analogues. *Molec. Pharmacol.* **34:** 566–572.

SAHIN, U., HARTMANN, F., SENTER, P., POHL, C., ENGERT, A., DIEHL, V. and PFREUNDSCHUH, M. (1990) Specific activation of the prodrug mitomycin phosphate by a bispecific anti-CD30/anti-alkaline phosphatase monoclonal antibody. *Cancer Res.* **50:** 6944–6948.

SALETAN, S. (1987) Mitoxantrone an active new antitumor agent with an improved therapeutic index. *Cancer Treat. Rev.* **14,** 297–303.

SAHU, S. K., OBERLEY, L. W., STEVENS, R. H. and RILEY, E. F. (1977) Superoxide dismutase activity of Ehrlich ascites tumor cells. *J. Natl. Cancer Inst.* **58:** 1125–1128.

SAMUNI, A., CHONG, P. L. G., BARENHOLZ, Y. and THOMPSON, T. E. (1986) Physical and chemical modifications of adriamycin: iron complex by phospholipid bilayers. *Cancer Res.* **46:** 594–599.

SANTONE, K. S., OAKES, S. G., TAYLOR, S. R. and POWIS, G. (1986) Anthracycline-induced inhibition of a calcium action potential in differential neuroblastoma cells. *Cancer Res.* **46:** 2659–2664.

SARNA, G. P., CHAMPLIN, R., WELLS, J. and GALE, P. R. (1982) Phase I study of high dose mitomycin with autologous bone marrow support. *Cancer Treat. Rep.* **66:** 277–282.

SARTORELLI, A. C. (1986) The role of mitomycin antibiotics in the chemotherapy of solid tumors. *Biochem. Pharmac.* **35:** 67–69.

SATO, S., IWAIZUMI, M., HANDA, K. and TAMURA, Y. (1977) Electron spin resonance study on the mode of generation of free radicals of daunomycin, adriamycin, and carboquone in NAD(P)H-microsome system. *Gann.* **68:** 603–608.

SAVARAJ, N., LU, K., MANUEL, V. and LOO, T. L. (1982a) Pharmacology of mitoxantrone in cancer patients. *Cancer Chemother. Pharmac.* **8:** 113–117.

SAVARAJ, N., LU, K., VALDIVIESO, M., BURGESS, M., UMSAWASDI, T., BENJAMIN, R. S. and LOO, T. L. (1982b) Clinical kinetics of 1,4-dihydroxy-5,8-bis[(2-[(2-hydroxyethyl)amino]ethyl)amino]-9,10-anthracenedione. *Clin. Pharmac. Ther.* **31:** 312–316.

SAVARAJ, N., LU, K., FEUN, L. G., LEAVENS, M. E., STEWART, D., BURGESS, M. A., BENJAMIN, R. S. and LOO, T. L. (1983) Intracerebral penetration and tissue distribution of 2,5-diaziridinyl-3.6-bis(carboethoxyamino)-1,4-benzoquinone (AZQ, NSC-182986). *J. Neuro-Oncol.* **1:** 15–19.

SAWYER, D. T., ROBERTS, J. L. CALDERWOOD, T. S., TSUCHIYA, T. and STEMP, J. J. (1983) Oxygen radicals and aging. In: *Oxygen Radicals and Their Scavenger Systems*, Volume 1, pp. 8–27, COHEN, G. and GREENWALD R. A., (eds) Elsevier Science, New York.

SAZUKA, Y., YOSHIKAWA, K., TANIZAWA, H. and TAKINO Y. (1987) Effect of doxorubicin on lipid peroxide levels in tissues of mice. *Jap. J. Cancer Res.* **78:** 1281–1286.

SCHEULEN, M. E. (1985) The mechanism of antineoplastic action of the anthracyclines comparison of daunorubicin and 5-iminodaunorubicin. *J. Cancer Res. Clin. Oncol.* **109**: A45.

SCHEULEN, M. E., KAPPUS, H., NIENHAUS, A. and SCHMIDT, C. G. (1982) Covalent protein binding of reactive adriamycin metabolites in rat liver and rat heart microsomes. *J. Cancer Res. Clin. Oncol.* **103:** 39–48.

SCHEULEN, M. E., HOENSCH, H., KAPPUS, H., SEEBER S. and SCHMIDT, C. G. (1987) Positive correlation between decreased cellular uptake, NADPH-glutathione reductase activity and adriamycin resistance in Ehrlich ascites tumor lines. *Arch. Toxic.* **60:** 154-157.

SCHILCHER, R. B., YOUNG, J. D., LEICHMAN, L. P., HAAS, C. D. and BAKER, L. H. (1983) Phase I evaluation and pharmacokinetics of aziridinylbenzoquinone using a weekly intravenous schedule. *Cancer Res.* **43:** 3907–3911.

SCHILCHER, R. B., YOUNG, J. D., RATANATHARATHORN, V., KARANES, C. and BAKER, L. H. (1984) Clinical pharmacokinetics of high-dose mitomycin C. *Cancer Chemother. Pharmac.* **13:** 186–190.

SCHILSKY, R. L., KELLEY, J. A., IHDE, D. C., HOWSER, D. M., CORDES, R. S. and YOUNG, R. C. (1982) Phase I trial and pharmacokinetics of aziridinylbenzoquinones (NSC 182986) in humans. *Cancer Res.* **42:** 1582–1586.

SCHLAGER, J. J. and POWIS, G. (1988) Mitomycin C is not metabolized by, but is an inhibitor of, human kidney NAD(P)H: (quinone-acceptor) oxidoreductase. *Cancer Chemother. Pharmac.* **22:** 126–130.

Schlager, J. J. and Powis, G. (1990) Quinone cytotoxicity associated with a cell density-dependent increase in the levels of cellular quinone reductase (DT-diaphorase). *Toxicologist* **10:** 103.

Schmitt-Graff, A. and Scheulen, M. E. (1986) Prevention of adriamycin cardiotoxicity by niacin, isocitrate or N-acetyl-cysteine in mice. A morphological study. *Pathol. Res. Pract.* **181:** 168–174.

Schreiber, J., Mottley, C., Sinha, B. K., Kalyanaraman, B and Mason, R. P. (1987) One-electron reduction of daunomycin, daunomycinone, and 7-deoxydaunomycinone by the xanthine/xanthine oxidase system: detection of semiquinone free radicals by electron spin resonance. *Am. Chem. Soc.* **109:** 348–351.

Schulte, G. (1952) Erfahrungen mit neuen cytestatischen mitteln bei hämoblastosen und carcinomen und die abgrenzung ihrer wirkungen gegen röntgentherapie. *Z. Krebsforsch* **58:** 500–503.

Schwartz, E. L. and Maher, A. (1986) Molecular actions of class II anthracycline antibiotics on the human ribosomal RNA gene. *Proc. Am. Assoc. Cancer Res.* **27:** 240.

Schwartz, H. S. (1962) Pharmacology of mitomycin C: III. In vitro metabolism by rat liver. *J. Pharmac. exp. Ther.* **136:** 250–258.

Schwartz, H. S. (1975) DNA breaks in P288 tumor cells in mice after treatment with daunorubicin and adriamycin. *Res. Commun. Chem. Path. Pharmac.* **10:** 51–64.

Schwartz, H. S. (1983) Enhanced antitumor activity of adriamycin in combination with allopurinol. *Cancer Lett.* **20:** 69–74.

Schwartz, H. S. and Parker, N. B. (1981) Initial biotransformations of daunorubicin to aglycones by rat liver microsomes. *Cancer Res.* **41:** 2343–2348.

Schwartz, H. S. and Paul, B. (1984) Biotransformation of daunorubicin aglycones by rat liver microsomes. *Cancer Res.* **44:** 2480–2484.

Schwartz, H. S. and Philips, F. S. (1961) Pharmacology of mitomycin C: II. Renal excretion and metabolism by tissue homogenates. *J. Pharmac. exp. Ther.* **133:** 335–342.

Schwartz, H. S., Sodergren, J. E. and Philips, F. S. (1963) Mitomycin C: chemical and biological studies on alkylation, *Science* **142:** 1181–1183.

Schwartz, H. S., Sodergren, J. E. and Ambaye, R. Y. (1968) Actinomycin D: Drug concentrations and actions in mouse tissues and tumors. *Cancer Res.* **28:** 192–197.

Schwartz, R. G., McKenzie, W. B., Alexander, J., Sayer, P., D'Souza, A., Manatunga, A., Schwartz, P. E., Berger, H. J., Setano, J., Surkin, L., Wackers, F. J., and Zaret, B. L. (1987) Congestive heart failure and left ventricular dysfunction complicating doxorubicin therapy. *Am. J. Med.* **82:** 1110–1118.

Sciandra, J. J., Wilson, R. E. and Sutherland, R. M. (1985) Can hypoxia and/or glucose deprivation induce specific proteins which confer drug resistance. *Chemical Modifiers of Cancer Treatment.* Clearwater, Florida, *October*, Abstract 5–11.

Shaikh, I. A., Johnson, F. and Grollman, A. P. (1986) Streptonigrin. 1. Structure-activity relationships among simple bicyclic analogues. Rate dependence of DNA degradation on quinone reduction potential. *J. Med. Chem.* **29:** 1329–1340.

Schinozawa, S. and Oda, I. (1981) Determination of adriamycin (doxorubicin) and related fluorescent compounds in rat lymph and gall by high-performance liquid chromatography. *J. Chromatogr.* **212:** 323–330.

Shows, T. B. and McAlpine, P. J. (1979) The 1979 catalog of human genes and chromosome assignments. *Cytogenet. Cell Genet.* **25:** 117–127.

Shoyab, M. and Todaro, G. J. (1980) Vitamin K_3 (menadione) and related quinones, like tumor promoting phorbol esters, alter the affinity of epidermal growth factor for its membrane receptors. *J. biol. Chem.* **255:** 8735–8739.

Sieber, S. M., Mead, J. A. R and Adamson, R. H. (1976) Pharmacology of antitumor agents from higher plants. *Cancer Treat. Rep.* **60:** 1127–1139.

Siegel, D., Gibson, N. W., Preusch, P. C. and Ross, D. (1990) Metabolism of mitomycin C by DT-diaphorase: role in mitomycin C-induced DNA damage and cytotoxicity in human colon carcinoma cells. *Cancer Res.* **50:** 7485–7489.

Siegfried, J. M., Sartorelli, A. C. and Tritton, T. R. (1983) Evidence fo the lack of relationship between inhibition of nucleic acid synthesis and cytotoxicity of adriamycin. *Cancer Biochem. Biophys.* **6:** 137–142.

Silva, J. M. and O'Brien, P. J. (1989) Diaziquone-induced cytotoxicity in isolated rat hepatocytes. *Cancer Res.* **49:** 5550–5554.

Singal. P. K. and Pierce, G. N. (1986) Adriamycin stimulates low-affinity Ca^{2+} binding and lipid peroxidation but depresses myocardial function. *Am. J. Physiol.* **250:** H419–425.

Sinha, B. K. (1980) Binding specificity of chemically and enzymatically activated anthracycline anticancer agents to nucleic acids. *Chem. Biol. Interact.* **30:** 67–77.

Sinha, B. K. (1981) Irreversible binding of reductively activated streptonigrin to nucleic acids in the presence of metals. *Chem. Biol. Interact.* **36:** 179–188.

Sinha, B. K. and Chignell, C. F. (1979) Binding mode of chemically activated semiquinone free radicals from quinone anticancer agents to DNA. *Chem. Biol. Interact.* **28:** 301–308.

Sinha, B. K. and Gregory, J. L. (1981) Role of one-electron and two-electron reduction products of adriamycin and daunomycin in deoxyribonucleic acid binding. *Biochem. Pharmac.* **30:** 2626–2629.

Sinha, B. K., Motten, A. G. and Hanck, K. W. (1983) The electrochemical reduction of 1,4-bis(2-[(2-hydroxyethyl)-amino]ethylamino)-anthracenedione and daunomycin: biochemical significance in superoxide formation. *Chem. Biol. Interact.* **43:** 371–377.

SINHA, B. K., TRUSH, M. A., KENNEDY, K. A. and MIMNAUGH, E. G. (1984) Enzymatic activation and binding of adriamycin to nuclear DNA. *Cancer Res.* **44:** 2892–2896.

SINHA, B. K., MUINDI, J. R., BATIST, G. and MYERS, C. E. (1985) Hydroxyl radical formation and DNA damage by anthracycline antitumor drugs. *Proc. Am. Cancer Res.* **26:** 225.

SINHA, B. K., KATKI, A. G., BATIST, G., COWAN, K. H. and Myers, C. E. (1986) Formation of hydroxyl radicals in sensitive and resistant MCF-7 human breast tumor cells: implications for the mechanism of action. *Proc. Am. Assoc. Cancer Res.* **27:** 241.

SINHA, B. K., KATKI, A. G., BATIST, G., COWAN, K. H. and MYERS, C. E. (1987a) Adriamycin-stimulated hydroxyl radical formation in human breast tumor cells. *Biochem. Pharmac.* **36:** 793–796.

SINHA, B. K., KATKI, A. G., BATIST, G., COWAN, K. H. and MYERS, C. E. (1987b) Differential formation of hydroxyl radicals by adriamycin in sensitive and resistant MCF-7 human breast tumor cells: implications for the mechanism of actions. *Biochemistry* **26:** 3776–3781.

SINHA, B. K., DUSRE, L., COLLINS, C. and MYERS, C. E. (1989a) Resistance of paraquat and adriamycin in human breast tumor cells: role of free radical formation. *Biochim. biophys. Acta* **1010:** 304–310.

SINHA, B. K., MIMNAUGH, E. G., RAJAGOPALAN, S. and MYERS, C. E. (1989b) Adriamycin activation and oxygen free radical formation in human breast tumor cells: protective role of glutathione peroxidase in adriamycin resistance. *Cancer Res.* **49:** 3844–3848.

SKOVSGAARD, T. (1977) Transport and binding of daunorubicin, adriamycin, and rubidazone in Ehrlich ascites tumor cells. *Biochem. Pharmac.* **26:** 215–222.

SMART, R. C. and ZANNONI, V. G. (1984) DT-Diaphorase and peroxidase influence the covalent binding of the metabolites of phenol, the major metabolite of benzene. *Molec. Pharmac.* **26:** 105–111.

SMITH, D. B., MARGISON, J. M., LUCAS, S. B., WILKINSON, P. M., and HOWELL, A. (1987) Clinical pharmacology of oral and intravenous 4-demethoxydaunorubicin. *Cancer Chemother. Pharmac.* **19:** 138–142.

SMITH, E., STRATFORD, I. J. and ADAMS, G. E. (1980) Cytotoxicity of adriamycin on aerobic and hypoxic Chinese hamster V79 cells *in vitro*. *Br. J. Cancer* **42:** 568–573.

SMITH, I. E. (1983) Mitoxantrone (Novatrone): a review of experimental and early clinical studies. *Cancer Treat. Rev.* **10:** 103–115.

SMITH, P. J., MORGAN, S. A., FOX, M. E., and WATSON, J. V. (1990) Mitoxantrone-DNA binding and the induction of topoisomerase II associated DNA damage in multi-drug resistant small cell lung cancer cells. *Biochem. Pharmac.* **40:** 2069–2078.

SMITH, R. G., MILLER, A. A., BENVENUTO, J. A., VALDIVIESO, M. and LOO, T. L. (1983) Negative-ion chemical-ionization mass spectrometry of aclarubicin analogues. Characterization of two of metabolites in man. *Cancer Treat. Rep.* **67:** 351–354.

SMYTH, J. F., MACPHERSON, J. S., RAMSAY, M., WARRINGTON, P., LEONARD, R. C. F. and WOLF, C. R. (1984) Clinical pharmacology of mitoxantrone. *Proc. Am. Assoc. Cancer Res.* **25:** 162.

SMYTH, J. F., MACPHERSON, J. S. and WOLF, C. R. (1986) The clinical pharmacology of mitozantrone. *Cancer Chemother. Pharmac.* **17:** 149–152.

SOLIE, T. N. and YUNCKER, C. (1978) Adriamycin induced changes in translocation of sodium ions in transporting epithelial cells. *Life Sci.* **22:** 1907–1910.

SOMEYA, A. and TANAKA, N. (1979) DNA strand scission induced by adriamycin and aclacinomycin A. *J. Antibiot.* **32:** 839–845.

SPARANO, B. M., GORDON, G., HALL, C., IATROPOULOS, M. J. and NOBLE, J. F. (1982) Safety assessment of new anticancer compound, mitoxantrone, in beagle dogs: comparison with doxorubicin. II. Histologic and ultrastructural pathology. *Cancer Treat. Rep.* **66:** 1145–1148.

SPETH, P. A. J., LINSSEN, P. C. M., BEEX, L. V. A. M., BOEZMANN, J. B. M. and HAANEN, C. (1986A) Cellular and plasma pharmacokinetics of weekly 20-mg 4′-ep-adriamycin bolus injections in patients with advanced breast carcinoma. *Cancer Chemother. Pharmac.* **18:** 78–82.

SPETH, P. A. J., VAN DE LOO F. A. J., LINSSEN, P.C. M., WESSELS, H. M. C., and HAANEN, C., (1986B) Plasma and human leukemic cell pharmacokinetics of oral and intravenous 4-demethoxydaunomycin. *Clin. Pharmac. Ther.* **40:** 643–649.

SPEYER, J. L., GREEN, M. D., ISRAEL, M., SWEATMAN, T. W. and MUGGIA, F. (1982) The clinical pharmacology of 4′-epiadriamycin (4′EPI) administered as a 6 hour (hr) infusion. *Proc. Am. Assoc. Cancer Res.* **23:** 129.

SPEYER, J., GREEN, M., WARD, C., WERNZ, J., BLUM, R., MUGGIA, F., MEYERS, M., REY, M., SANGER, J., KRAMER, E, and EVANS, G. (1987) Rationale and preliminary results of a randomized clinical trial of ICRF 187 as a protective agent against cumulative dose-related anthracycline cardiac toxicity. *Organ-Directed Toxicities of Anticancer Drugs*, p. 13 HACKER, M. and TRITTON, T. (eds) Univ. Vermont Press, Burlington, VT.

SPEYER, J. L., GREEN, M. D., and KRAMER, E. (1988) Protective effect of ICRF-187 against doxorubicin induced cardiac toxicity in women with advanced breast cancer. *New Engl. J. Med.* **319:** 745–752.

SPEIGEL, J. F., EGORIN, M. J., COLLINS, J. M., LERNER, B. D. and BACHUR, N. R. (1982) The murine disposition and pharmacokinetics of the antineoplastic agent diaziquone (NSC 182986). *Drug Metab. Displ.* **11:** 41–46.

STANTON, G. F., RAYMOND, V., WITTES, R. E., SCHULMAN, P., BUDMAN, D., BARATZ, R., WILLIAMS, L., PETRONI, G. R., GELLER, N. L., HANCOCK, C., KREIS, W. and YOUNG, C. W. (1985) Phase I and clinical pharmacological evaluation of 4′-deoxydoxorubicin in patients with advanced cancer. *Cancer Res.* **45:** 1862–1868.

STAQUET, M. J., BYAR, D. P., GREEN, S. B. and ROSENCWEIG, M. (1983) Clinical predictivity of transplantable tumor systems in the selection of new drugs for solid tumors: rationale for a three-stage strategy. *Cancer Treat. Rep.* **67:** 753–765.

Sterrenberg, L., Julicher, R. H. M., Bast, A. and Noordhoek, J. (1984) Adriamycin stimulates NADPH-dependent lipid peroxidation in liver microsomes not ony by enhancing the production of O_2 and H_2O_2, but also by potentiating the catalytic activity of ferrous ions. *Toxicol. Lett.* **22:** 153–159.

Steven, F. S., Griffin, M. M., and Talbot, I. C. (1990) The targeting of fagmatine-liganded mitomycin C to an enzyme on the surface of tumour cells. *Anticancer Res.* **10:** 583–590.

Stevens, C. L. Taylor, K. G., Munk, M. E., Marshall, W. S., Nall, K., Shah, G. D., Shah, L. G. and Uzu, K. (1964) Chemistry and structure of mitomycin C. *J. Med. Chem.* **8:** 1–10.

Stewart, J. A., McCormack, J. J. and Krakoff, I. H. (1982) Clinical and clinical pharmacologic studies of mitoxantrone. *Cancer Treat. Rep.* **66:** 1327–1331.

Stuart, M. J., deAlarcon, P. A. and Barvinchak, M. K. (1978) Inhibition of adriamycin-induced human platelet lipid peroxidation by vitamin E. *Am. J. Hematol.* **5:** 297–303.

Sugioka, K. and Nakano, M. (1982) Mechanism of phospholipid peroxidation induced by ferric ion-ADP-adriamycin-co-ordination complex. *Biochim. biophys. Acta* **713:** 333–343.

Sugioka, K., Nakano, H., Nocuchi, T., Tsuchiya, J. and Nakano, M. (1981) Decomposition of unsaturated phospholipids by iron-ADP-adriamycin co-ordination complex. *Biochem. biophys. Res. Commun.* **100:** 1251–1258.

Sugioka, K., Nakano, H., Tsuchiya, J., Nakano, M., Sugioka, Y., Tero-Kubota, S. and Ikegami, V. (1984) Clear evidence for the participation of ·OH in gamma DNA breakage induced by the enzymatic reduction of adriamycin in the presence of iron-ADP. Importance of local ·OH concentration for DNA strand cleavage. *Biochem. Int.* **9:** 237–242.

Svingen, B. A. and Powis, G. (1981) Pulse radiolysis studies on antitumor quinones: radical lifetimes, reaction with oxygen and one-electron reduction potentials. *Arch. Biochem. Biophys.* **209:** 119–126.

Svingen, B. A., Appel, P. L. and Powis, G. (1980) Radical formation during cellular and subcellular metabolism of the chemotherapeutic agent AZQ. *Pharmacologist* **22:** 177.

Svingen, B. A., Powis, G. Appel, P. L. and Scott, M. (1981) Protection against adriamycin induced skin necrosis in the rat by dimethylsulfoxide and α-tocopherol. *Cancer Res.* **41:** 3395–3399.

Sweatman, T. W. and Israel, M. (1987) Comparative metabolism and elimination of adriamycin and 4′-epiadriamycin in the rat. *Cancer Chemother. Pharmac.* **19:** 201–206.

Sweatman, T. W., Ahmed, N. K. and Israel, M. (1986) Relative activity of daunorubicin, adriamycin and 4′-epiadriamycin with human liver reductases. *Proc. Am. Assoc. Cancer Res.* **27:** 247.

Szmigiero, L. and Kohn, K. W. (1984) Mechanisms of DNA strand breakage and interstrand crosslinking by diaziridinylbenzoquinone (Diaziquone) in isolated nuclei from human cells. *Cancer Res.* **44:** 4453–4457.

Szmigiero, L., Erickson, L. C., Ewig, R. A. and Kohn, K. W. (1984) DNA strand scission and cross-linking by diaziridinylbenzoquinone (Diaziquone) in human cells and relation to cell killing. *Cancer Res.* **44:** 4447–4452.

Szybalski, W. (1964) Structural modifications of DNA: crosslinking, circularization and single strand interruption. *Ahandl. Deut. Wiss. Berlin* **4:** 1–19.

Szybalski, W. and Iyer, V. N. (1964) Crosslinking of DNA of enzymatically or chemically activated mitomycins and profiromycins, bifunctionally "alkylating" antibiotics. *Fed. Proc.* **23:** 946–957.

Tábora, O., Lewandowski, E. and Combs, A. B. (1986) Influence of *in vitro* ubiquinone antagonists on doxorubicin toxicity *in vivo. J. Tox. Env. Hlth.* **18:** 231–240.

Takanashi, S. and Bachur, N. R. (1975) Daunorubicin metabolites in human urine. *J. Pharmac. exp. Ther.* **195:** 41–49.

Takanashi, S. and Bachur, N. R. (1976) Adriamycin metabolism in man—evidence from urinary metabolites. *Drug. Metab. Disp.* **4:** 79–87.

Talcott, R. E., Rosenblum, M. and Levin, V. A. (1983) Possible role of DT-diaphorase in the bioactivation of antitumor quinones. *Biochem. biophys. Res. Commun.* **111:** 346–351.

Tamura, Y. and Sato, S. (1977) Stimulation of a reconstituted, microsomal NADH oxidase system by carboquone, a quinoid anticancer chemical. *Gann* **68:** 353–356.

Tan, C. T. C., Hancock, C., Steinherz, P., Bacha, D. M., Steinherz, L., Luks, E., Winich, N., Meyers, P., Mondora, A., Dantis, E., Niedzwiecki, D. and Stevens, Y. W. (1987) Phase I and clinical pharmacological study of 4-demethoxydaunorubicin (idarubicin) in children with advanced cancer. *Cancer Res.* **47:** 2990–2995.

Taniguchi, S., Kimura, N. T. and Baba, T. (1981) Effects of pH on cytotoxicity of carboquone. *Jpn. J. Pharmac.* **31:** 243–247.

Tannock, I. (1982) Response of aerobic and hypoxic cells in a solid tumor to adriamycin and cyclophosphamide and interaction of the drugs with radiation. *Cancer Res.* **42:** 4291–4296.

Tannock, I. (1983) Toxicity of aziridinylbenzoquinone for aerobic and hypoxic cells of a transplanted mouse mammary tumor and interaction of the drug with radiation and adriamycin. *Cancer Res.* **43:** 2059–2062.

Tannock, I. and Guttman, P. (1981) Response of Chinese hamster ovary cells to anticancer drugs under aerobic and hypoxic conditions. *Br. J. Cancer* **43:** 245–248.

Tattersall, M. H. N., Sodergren, J. E., Senguypta, S. K., Trites, D. H., Modest, E. J. and Frei, E. (1975) Pharmacokinetics of actinomycin D in patients with malignant melanoma. *Clin. Pharmac. Ther.* **17:** 701–708.

Teicher, B. A., Lazo, J. S. and Sartorelli, A. C. (1981) Classification of antineoplastic agents by their selective toxicities toward oxygenated and hypoxic tumor cells. *Cancer Res.* **41:** 73–81.

TEWEY, K. M., ROWE, T. C., YANG, L., HALLIGAN, B. D. and LIU, L. F. (1984) Adriamycin-induced DNA damage mediated by mammalian DNA topoisomerase II. *Science* **226:** 466–468.

THAYER, W. S. (1977) Adriamycin stimulated superoxide formation in submitochondrial particles. *Chem. Biol. Int.* **19:** 265–278.

THOMAS, C. E. and AUST, S. D. (1986) Release of iron from ferritin by cardiotoxic anthracycline antibiotics. *Arch. Biochem. Biophys.* **248:** 684–689.

THOMPSON, R. H. (1971) *Naturally Occurring Quinones.* Academic Press, London.

THOR, H., SMITH, M. T., HARTZELL, P., BELLOMO, G., JEWELL, S. A. and ORRENIUS, S. (1982) The metabolism of menadione (2-methyl-l,4-naphthoquinone) by isolated hepatocytes. A study of the implication of oxidative stress cells. *J. Biol. Chem.* **257:** 12419–12425.

THORNALLEY, P. J. and DODD, N. J. F. (1985) Free radical formation from normal and adriamycin-treated rat cardiac sarcomas. *Biochem. Pharmac.* **34:** 669–674.

THORNALLEY, P. J., BANNISTER, W. H., and BANNISTER, J. V. (1986) Reduction of oxygen by NADH/NADH dehydrogenase in the presence of adriamycin. *Free Rad. Res. Common.* **2:** 163–171.

TJADEN, U. R., LANGENBERG, J. P., ENSING, K. and VAN BENNEKOM, W. P. (1982) Determination of mitomycin C in plasma, serum and urine by high-performance liquid chromatography with ultraviolet and electrochemical detection. *J. Chromatogr.* **232:** 355–367.

TOBIA, A. J., COURI, D. and SAGONE, A. (1985) The effects of the quinone type drugs on hydroxyl radical (OH·) production by rat liver microsomes. *J. Toxicol. Environ. Hlth.* **15:** 265–277.

TOMASZ, M. and LIPMAN, R. (1981) Reductive metabolism and alkylating activity of mitomycin C induced by rat liver microsomes. *Biochemistry* **20:** 5056–5061.

TOMASZ, M. and LIPMAN, R. (1979) Alkylation reactions of mitomycin C at acid pH. *J. Am. Chem. Soc.* **101:** 6063–6067.

TOMASZ, M. and LIPMAN, R. (1981) Reductive metabolism and alkylating activity of mitomycin C induced by rat liver microsomes. *Biochemistry* **20:** 5056–5061.

TOMASZ, M. MERCADO, C. M., OLSON, J. and CHATTERJIE, N. (1974) The mode of interaction of mitomycin C with deoxyribonucleic acid and other polynucleotides *in vitro*. *Biochemistry* **13:** 4878–4887.

TOMASZ, M., CHOWDARY, D., LIPMAN, R., SHIMOTAKAHARN, S., VEIRO, D., WALKER, V. and VERDINE, G. L. (1986) Reaction of DNA with chemically or enzymatically activated mitomycin C: isolation and structure of the major covalent adduct. *Proc. natn. Acad. Sci. U.S.A.* **83:** 6702–6706.

TOMASZ, M., LIPMAN, R., CHOWDARY, D., PAWLAK, J., VERDINE, G. L., and NAKANISHI, K. (1987A) Isolation and structure of a covalent cross-link adduct between mitomycin C and DNA. *Science* **235:** 1204–1208.

TOMASZ, M., LIPMAN, R., LEE, M. S., VERDINE, G. L. and NAKANISHI K. (1987b) Reaction of acid-activated mitomycin C with calf thymus DNA and model guanines: elucidation of the base-catalyzed degradation of N7-alkylguanine nucleosides. *Biochemistry* **26:** 2010-2027.

TOMASZ, M., CHAWLA, A. K. and LIPMAN, R. (1988) Mechanism of monofunctional and bifunctional alkylation of DNA by mitomycin C. *Biochemistry* **27:** 3182–3186.

TONG, G. L., HENRY, D. W. and ACTON, E. M. (1979) 5-Iminodaunorubicin reduced cardiotoxic properties in an antitumor anthracycline. *J Med. Chem.* **22:** 36–39.

TRAGANOS, F. (1983) Dihydroxyanthraquinone and related bis(substituted) aminoanthraquinones: a novel class of antitumor agents. *Phamac. Ther.* **22:** 199–214.

TRITTON, T. R., (1991) Cell surface actions of adriamycin. *Pharmac. Ther.* **49:** 293–310.

TRITTON, T. R. and HICKMAN, J. A. (1985) Cell surface membranes as chemotherapeutic target. *Cancer Treat. Rev.* **24:** 81–131.

TRITTON, T. R., MURPHREE, S. A. and SARTORELLI, A. C. (1978) Adriamycin: a proposal on the specificity of drug action. *Biochem. biophys. Res. Commun.* **84:** 802–808.

TRUMP, B. J., BEREZESKY, I. K., SATO T., LAIHO, K. U., PHELPS, P. C. and DECLARIS, N. (1984) Cell calcium, cell injury and cell death. *Env. Hlth. Perspect.* **57:** 281–287.

TRUSH, M. A., MIMNAUGH, E. G., GINSBURG, E. and GRAM, T. E. (1982) Studies on the in vitro interaction of mitomycin C, nitrofurantoin and paraquat with pulmonary microsomes. *Biochem. pharmac.* **31:** 805–814.

TULINSKY, A. (1962) The structure of mitomycin A. *J. Am. Soc.* **84:** 3188–3190.

TURNER, A. J. and HICK, P. E. (1976) Metabolism of daunorubicin by a barbiturate-sensitive aldehyde reductase from rat liver. *Biochem. J.* **159:** 819–882.

UEDA, K., MORITA, J., YAMASHITA, K. and KOMANO, T. (1980) Inactivation of bacteriophage ϕX174 by mitomycin C in the presence of sodium hydrosulfite and cupric ions. *Chem. Biol. Interact.* **29:** 145–158.

UMEZAWA, H., TAKAHASHI, Y., KINOSHITA, K., NAGANAWA, H., MASUDA, T., ISHIZUKA, M., TATSUTA, K. and TAKEUCHI, T. (1979) Tetrahydropyranyl derivatives of daunomycin and adriamycin. *J. Antibiot.* **32:** 1082–1085.

UNDERBERG, W. J. M. and LINGEMAN, H. J. (1983) Aspects of the chemical stability of mitomycin and porfiromycin in acidic solution. *J. Pharmac. Sci.* **72:** 549–553.

UNVERFERTH, D. V., LEIER, C. V., BALCERZAK, S. P. and HAMLIN, R. C. (1985) Usefulness of a free radical scavenger in preventing doxorubicin-induced heart failure in dogs. *Am. J. Cardiol.* **56:** 157–161.

UPTON, P. G., YAMAGUCHI, K. T., MYERS, S., KIDWELL, T. P. and ANDERSON, R. J. (1986) Effects of antioxidants and hyperbaric oxygen in ameliorating experimental doxorubicin skin toxicity in the rat. *Cancer Treat. Rep.* **70:** 503–507.

Uyeki, E. M., Nishio, A., Wittek, P. J. and Cheng, C. C. (1981) Antiproliferative activity of doxorubicin and aminoanthraquinone derivatives on Chinese hamster ovary cells. *J. Pharmac. Sci.* **70:** 1011–1013.

Uzuka, Y., Saito, Y., Takahashi, H. and Komatsu, M. (1982) Carboquone therapy for hematologic neoplasms. *Tohoko J. Exp. Med.* **138:** 151–160.

Van Belle, S. J. P., de Planque, M. M., Smith, I. E., van Oosterom, A. T., Schoemaker, T. J., Deneve, W. and McVie, J. G. (1986) Pharmacokinetics of mitoxantrone in humans following single-agent infusion or intra–arterial injection therapy or combined-agent infusion therapy. *Cancer Chemother. Pharmac.* **18:** 27–32.

Van Echo, D. A., Zuhowski, E., Egorin, M. J., Whitacre, M. Y., Sigman, L. M. and Forrest, A. (1986) Phase I clinical and pharmacologic study of menogaril (7-OMEN, NSC 269148) in patients (PTS) with hepatic dysfunction. *Proc. Am. Soc. Clin. Oncol.* **5:** 34.

van Hazel, G. A. and Kovach, J. S. (1982) Pharmacokinetics of mitomycin C in rabbit and human. *Cancer Chemother. Pharmac.* **8:** 182–192.

van Hazel, G. A., Scott, M., Rubin, J., Moertel, C. G., Eagan, R. T., O'Connell, M. J. and Kovach, J. S. (1983) Pharmacokinetics of mitomycin C in patients receiving the drug alone or in combination. *Cancer Treat. Rep.* **67:** 805–810.

Van Vleet, J. F., Ferrans, V. J. and Weirich, W. E. (1980) Cardiac disease induced by chronic adriamycin administration in dogs and an evaluation of vitamin E and selenium as cardioprotectants. *Am. J. Pathol.* **99:** 13–42.

Vasanthakumar, G. and Ahmed, N. K. (1985) Uptake and metabolism of daunorubicin by human myelocytic cells. *Cancer Chemother. Rep.* **15:** 35–39.

Verweij, J., den Hartigh, J., Stuurman, M., de Vries, J., and Pinedo, H. M. (1987) Relationship between clinical parameters and pharmacokinetics of mitomycin C. *J. Cancer Res. clin. Oncol.* **113,** 91–94.

Villani F., Galimberti, M., Comazzi, R., and Crippa, F. (1989) Evaluation of cardiac toxicity of idarubicin (4-demethoxydaunorubicin). *Eur. J. Cancer clin. Oncol.* **25:** 13–18.

Von Hoff, D. D., Layard, M. W. and Basa, P. (1979) Risk factors for doxorubicin-induced congestive heart failure. *Ann. Intern. Med.* **91:** 710–717.

Vrignaud, P., Eghbali, H., Hoerni, B., Iliadis, A. and Robert, J. (1985) Pharmacokinetics and metabolism of epirubicin during repetitive courses of administration in Hodgkin's patients. *Eur. J. Cancer Clin. Oncol.* **21:** 1307–1313.

Vrignaud, P., Londos-Gagliardi, D., and Robert, J. (1986) Hepatic metabolism of doxorubicin in mice and rats. *Eur. J. Drug Metab. Pharmacokinet.* **11:** 101–105.

Vromans, R. M., van de Straat, R., Groeneveld, M., and Vermeulen, N. P. (1990) One-electron reduction of mitomycin C by rat liver: role of cytochrome P-450 and NADPH-cytochrome P-450 reductase. *Xenobiotica* **20:** 967-978.

Wagner, H. U. and Gompper, R. (1974) Quinone methides. In: *The Chemistry of the Quininoid Compounds.* Volume 2, pp. 1145–1178, Patil, S. (ed.) John Wiley, New York.

Wakaki, S. (1961) Recent advance in research on antitumor mitomycins. *Cancer Chemother. Rep.* **13:** 79–86.

Wakaki, S., Marumo, H., Tomioka, K., Shimizu, G., Kato, E., Kamada, H., Kudo, S. and Fujimoto, Y. (1958) Isolation of new fractions of antitumor mitomycins. *Antibiot. Chemother.* **8:** 228–240.

Waksman, S. A. and Lechavalier, H. A. (1962) Actinomycins. In: *The Actinomycetes.* Volume III. pp. 168–178 Waksman, S. A. (ed.) Williams and Wilkins, Baltimore.

Waksman, S. A. and Woodruff, H. B. (1940) Bacteriostatic and bactericidal substances produced by a soil actinomyces. *Proc. Soc. Exp. Biol. Med.* **45:** 609–614.

Wallace, K. B. (1986a) Nonenzymatic oxygen activation and stimulation of lipid peroxidation by doxorubicin-copper. *Toxicol. Appl. Pharmac.* **86:** 69–79.

Wallace, K. B. (1986b) Aglycosylation and disposition of doxorubicin in isolated rat liver nuclei and microsomes. *Drug. Metab. Disp.* **14:** 399–304.

Wallace, K. B., and Johnson, J. A. (1987) Oxygen-dependent effect of microsomes on the binding of doxorubicin to rat hepatic nuclear DNA. *Molec. Pharmac.* **31:** 307–311.

Wallace, R. E., Murdock, K. C., Angier, R. B. and Durr, F. E. (1979) Activity of a novel anthracenedione, 1,4-dihydroxy-5,8-bis[[2-[(2-hydroxyethyl)amino]ethyl]-amino]-9,10-anthracenedione dihydrochloride, against experimental tumors in mice. *Cancer Res.* **39:** 1570–1574.

Warburg, O. (1924) Verbesserte Method zur Messung der Atmung und Glykolyse. *Biochem. Z.* **152:** 51–63.

Wardman, P. (1977) The use of nitroaromatic compounds as hypoxic cell radiosensitizers. *Curr. Topics Rad. Res. Q.* **11:** 347–398.

Webb, J. S., Cosulich, D. B., Mowat, J. H., Patrick, J. B., Broschard, R. W., Meyer, W. E., Williams, R. P., Wolfi, C. F., Fulmor, W., Pidacks, C. and Lancaster, J. E. (1962) The structure of mitomycins A, B and C and porfiromycin—Part 1. *J. Am. Chem. Soc.* **84:** 3185–3186.

Weenen. H., Lankelma, J., Penders, P. A. M., McVie, J. G., Ten Bokkel Huinink, W. A., de Planque, M. M. and Pinedo, H. M. (1983) Pharmacokinetics of 4′-epi-doxorubicin in man. *Invest. New Drugs* **1:** 59–61.

Weenen, H., Pinedo, H. M., de Planque, M. M., Ten Bokkel Huinink, W. W. T., McVie, J. G. and Lankelma, J. (1984a) Pharmacokinetics of carminomycin in man: biweekly schedule vs single dose every three weeks. *Eur. J. Cancer Clin. Oncol.* **20:** 915–918.

Weenen, H., Van Maanen, J. M. S. and de Planque, M. M. (1984b) Metabolism of 4′-modified analogs of doxorubicin. Unique glucuronidation pathway for 4′-epidoxorubicin. *Eur. J. Cancer Clin. Oncol.* **20:** 919–926.

WEFERS, H. and SIES, H. (1983) Hepatic low level chemiluminescence during redox cycling of menadione and menadione-glutathione conjugate: relation of glutathione and NADPH quinone reductase (DT-diaphorase) activity. *Arch. Biochem. Biophys.* **224:** 568–578.

WEFERS, H. and SIES, H. (1986) Generation of photoemissive species during quinone redox cycling. *Biochem. Pharmac.* **35:** 22–24.

WEISS, A. J. and MANTHEL, R. W. (1977) Experience with the use of adriamycin in combination with other anticancer agents using a weekly schedule, with particular reference to lack of cardiac toxicity. *Cancer* **40:** 2046–2052.

WEISS, R. B., SAROSY, G., CLAGETT-CARR, K., RUSSO, M., and LEYLAND-JONES, B. (1986) Anthracycline analogs: the past, present, and future. *Cancer Chemother. Pharmac.* **18,** 185–197.

WEISSBACH, A. and LISIO, A. (1965) Alkylation of nucleic acids by mitomycin C and porfirmycin. *Biochemistry* **4:** 196–200.

WEISSBACH, H., REDFIELD, B., O'CONNOR, T. and CHIRIGOS, M. A. (1966) Studies on the disposition of actinomycin D-^{3}H in virus-infected and tumor-bearing mice. *Cancer Res.* **26:** 1833–1838.

WEITZMAN, S. A., LORELL, B., CAREY, R. W., KAUFMAN, S. and STOSSEL, T. P. (1980) Prospective study of tocopherol prophylaxis for anthracycline cardiac toxicity. *Curr. Ther. Res.* **28:** 682–686.

WENDEL, A. (1981) Glutathione peroxidase. *Meth. Enzymol.* **77:** 325–333.

WESTENDORF, J., AYDIN, M., and MARQUARDT, H. (1988) Metabolism of morpholino- and cyanomorpholinoanthracyclines. *Proc. Am. Ass. Cancer Res., Exp. Ther.* **29:** 278.

WHITAKER, J. A., and AL-ISMAIL, S. A. (1984) Effect of digoxin and vitamin E in preventing cardiac damage caused by doxorubicin in actue myeloid leukemia. *Br. Med. J.* **288:** 283–284.

WHITE, H. L. and WHITE, J. R. (1966) Interaction of streptonigrin with DNA in vitro. *Biochim. biophys. Acta* **123:** 648–651.

WHITE, J. R. and DEARMAN, H. H. (1965) Generation of free radicals from phenazine methosulfate, streptonigrin and rubiflavin in bacterial suspensions. *Proc. natn. Acad. Sci. U.S.A.* **54:** 887–891.

WHITE, J. R. and WHITE, H. L. (1964) Phenethyl alcohol synergism with mitomycin C, porfiromycin and streptonigrin, *Science* **145:** 1312–1313.

WHITE, J. R., VAUGHAN, T. O. and YEH, W. S. (1971) Superoxide radical in the mechanism of action of streptonigrin. *Fed. Proc.* **30:** 1145.

WHITE, R. J. and DURR, F. E. (1985) Development of mitoxantrone. *Invest. New Drugs* **3:** 85–93.

WILSON, I., WARDMAN, P., LIN, T. S. and SARTORELLI, A. C. (1986) One-electron reduction of 2- and 6-methyl-1,4-naphthoquinone bioreductive alkylating agents. *J. Med. Chem.* **29:** 1381–1384.

WINTERBOURN, C. C. (1981) Evidence for the production of hydroxyl radicals from the adriamycin semiquinone and H_2O_2. *FEBS Lett.* **136:** 89–94.

WINTERBOURN, C. C. and SUTTON, H. C. (1984) Hydroxyl radical production from hydrogen peroxide and enzymatically generated paraquat radicals: catalytic requirements and oxygen dependence. *Arch. Biochem. Biophys.* **235:** 116–126.

WINTERBOURN, C. C., FRENCH, J. K. and CLARIDGE, R. F. C. (1978) Superoxide dismutase as an inhibitor of reactions of semiquinone radicals. *FEBS Lett.* **94:** 269–272.

WOLF, C. R., MACPHERSON, J. S. and SMYTH, J. F. (1986) Evidence for the metabolism of mitozantrone by microsomal glutathione transferases and 3-methylcholanthrene-inducible glucuronosyl transferases. *Biochem. Pharmac.* **35:** 1577–1581.

WORKMAN, P., WALTON, M. I., POWIS, G., and SCHLAGER, J. J. (1989) DT-Diaphorase: questionable role in mitomycin C resistance, but a target for novel bioreductive drugs? *Br. J. Cancer* **60:** 800–802.

WOSILAIT, W. D., and RYAN, M. P. (1987) Drug interactions affecting the elimination of doxorubicin in the rat. *Res. Commun. Chem. Path. Pharmac.* **56:** 335–348.

YAMANAKA, N., KATO, T., NISHIDA, K., FUJIKAWA, T., FUKUSHIMA, M. and OTA, K. (1979) Elevation of serum lipid peroxide level associated with doxorubicin toxicity and its amelioration by [dl]-α-tocopheryl acetate or coenzyme Q10 in mouse (doxorubicin, toxicity, lipid peroxide, tocopherol, coenzyme Q10). *Cancer Chemother. Pharmac.* **3:** 223–227.

YAMAZAKI, I. (1977) Free radicals in enzyme-substrate reactions. In: *Free Radicals in Biology*, pp. 183–215, Volume III, PRYOR, W. A. (ed.) Academic Press, New York.

YEH, G. C., OCCHIPINTI, S. J., PHANG, J. M., COWAN, K. H., CHABNER, B. A., and MYERS, C. E. (1986) Deficient glucose-6-phosphate dehydrogenase activity in adriamycin resistant tumor cells (MCF-7): a redox-dependent mechanism for adriamycin resistance. *Proc. Am. Ass. Cancer Res.* Annu. Meet. **27**:271.

YEH, G. C., OCCIPINTI, S. J., and MYERS, C. E. (1988) The regulation of glucose-6-phosphate dehydrogenase in adriamycin sensitive and resistant human breast cancer cells. *Proc. Am. Ass. Cancer Res.* **29:** 317.

YESAIR, D. W., SCHWATRZBACH, E., SHUCK, D., DENINE, E. P. and ASBELL, M. A. (1972) Comparative pharmacokinetics of daunomycin and adriamycin in several animal species. *Cancer Res.* **32:** 1177–1183.

YESAIR, D. W., THAYER, P. S., MCNITT, S. and TEAGUE, K. (1980) Comparative uptake, metabolism and retention of anthracyclines by tumors growing in vitro and in vivo. *Eur. J. Cancer* **16:** 901–907.

YODA, Y., NAKAZAWA, M., ABE, T. and KAWAKAMI, Z. (1986) Prevention of doxorubicin myocardial toxicity in mice by reduced glutathione. *Cancer Res.* **46:** 2551–2556.

YOSHIMOTO, M., MIYAZAWA, H., NAKAO, H., SHINKAI, K. and ARAKAWA, M. (1979) Quantitative structure-activity relationships in 2,5-bis(1-aziridinyl)-*p*-benzoquinone derivatives against leukemia L1210. *J. Med. Chem.* **22:** 491–496.

YOUNES, M., CORNELIUS, S. and SIEGERS, C. P. (1985) Fe^{2+}-supported in vivo lipid peroxidation induced by compounds undergoing redox cycling. *Chem. Biol. Int.* **54:** 97–103.

YOUNG, C. W. and RAYMOND, V. (1986) Clinical assessment of the structure-activity relationship of anthracyclines and related synthetic derivatives. *Cancer Treat. Rep.* **70:** 51–63.

YOUNG, R. C., OZOLS, R. F. and MYERS, C. E. (1981) Medical progress. The anthracycline antineoplastic drugs. *New Engl. J. Med.* **305:** 139–153.

YOUNGMAN, R. J. and ELSTNER, E. F. (1981) Oxygen species in paraquat toxicity: the crypto-OH radical. *FEBS Lett.* **129:** 265–268.

YOUNGMAN, R. J. and ELSTNER, E. F. (1984) On the interaction of adriamycin with DNA: investigation of spectral changes. *Arch. Biochem. Biophys.* **231:** 424–429.

YOUNGMAN, R. J., OSSWALD, W. F. and ELSTNER, E. F. (1982a) Mechanisms of oxygen activation by nitrofurantoin and relevance to its toxicity. *Biochem. Pharmac.* **31:** 3723–3729.

YOUNGMAN, R. J., OSSWALD, W. F. and ELSTNER, E. F. (1982b) Crypto-OH· radical production of nitrofurantoin. *Biochem. Pharmac.* **31:** 603–606.

ZANETTE, M. L., TIRELLI, U., ZADRO, D., SORIO, R., FIGOLI, F., SARACCHINI, S., MONFARDINI, S. and D'INCALCI, M. (1986) Pharmacokinetics of 7-con-o-methylnogarol (7-OMEN, menogaril) in cancer patients with solid tumors. *5th NCI/EORTC Symposium on New Drugs in Cancer Therapy, Amsterdam, October*, Abstract 9.28.

ZBINDEN, G., BACHMANN, E. and HOLNEGGER, C. (1978) Model systems for cardiotoxic effects of anthracyclines. *Antiot. Chemother.* **23:** 255–270.

ZEE-CHENG, R. K. Y. and CHENG, C. C. (1978) Antineoplastic agents. Structure-activity relationship; study of bis(substituted aminoalkylamino)anthraquinones. *J. Med. Chem.* **21:** 291–294.

ZEE-CHENG, R. K. Y. and CHENG, C. C. (1982) Structure-activity relationship study of anthraquinones: 1,4-dihydroxy-5,8-bis[[2-(2-hydroxyethoxy)ethyl]amino]-9,10-anthracenedione, an analog of an established antineoplastic agent. *J. Pharmaceut. Sci.* 71: 708–709.

ZEIN, N. and KOHN, H. N. (1986) Electrophilic and nucleophilic character of the carbon 10 methylene group in mitosenes revealed. *J. Am. Soc.* **108:** 296–299.

ZENEBERGH, A., BAURIN, R. and TROUET, A. (1984) Cellular pharmacology of detorubicin and doxorubicin in L1210 cells. *Eur. J. Cancer Clin. Oncol.* **20:** 115–121.

ZIMM, S., HOLCENBERG, J., BALIS, F., DOHERTY, K. and POPLACK, D. G. (1987) Intrathecal (IT) diaziquone (AZQ): a new, clinically useful agent for the treatment of meningeal neoplasia. *Proc. Am. Ass. Cancer Res.* **28:** 190.

ZINI, G., VICARIO, G. P., LAZZATI, M. and ARCAMONE, F. (1984) Radioactive species in rat urines and tissues after [^{14}C] AD 32 administration. *Cancer Chemother. Pharmac.* **12:** 154–156.

ZINI, J. L., PIERO, G., LAZZATI, M. and ARCAMONE, F. (1986) Disposition and metabolism of [14-^{14}C]-4-demethoxy daunorubicin HCl (idarubicin) and [14-^{14}C]daunorubicin HCl in the rat. *Cancer Chemother. Pharmac.* **16:** 107–115.

ZWEIER, J. L. (1983) Reduction of O_2 by iron-adriamycin, *J. biol. Chem.* **259:** 6056–6058.

ZWEIER, J. L. (1985) Iron-mediated formation of an oxidized adriamycin free radical. *Biochim. biophys. Acta* **839:** 209–213.

ZWELLING, L. A., KERRIGAN, D. and MICHAELS, S. (1982) Cytotoxicity and DNA strand breaks by 5-iminodaunorubicin in mouse leukemia L1210 cells: comparison with adriamycin and 4′-(9-acridinylamino)methanesulfon-*m*-anisidide. *Cancer Res.* **42:** 2687-2691.

Garth Powis, editor.
(1994) *Anticancer Drugs: Reactive Metabolism and Drug Interactions*,
Pergamon Press Ltd, pp. 387–396
Printed in the United Kingdom

CHAPTER 9

BLEOMYCIN HYDROLASE AND TUMOR RESISTANCE TO BLEOMYCIN

SAID M. SEBTI AND JOHN S. LAZO

Department of Pharmacology, University of Pittsburgh School of Medicine, 13th Floor, Biomedical Science Tower, Pittsburgh, PA 15261, U.S.A.

1. INTRODUCTION

Tumor resistance to antineoplastic agents remains a major obstacle to cancer treatment and the mechanism of resistance to many of these pharmacological agents is not known. Several biochemical mechanisms, such as increased DNA repair, decreased drug accumulation and increased metabolic inactivation, have been proposed to account for tumor resistance to the antitumor antibiotic bleomycin (BLM). In this article, the metabolism of BLM by a BLM-inactivating enzyme, BLM hydrolase, and its involvement in BLM resistance is reviewed.

BLM is a glycopeptide antibiotic isolated from cultures of *Streptomyces verticillus* as a copper-containing mixture of BLM analogs composed of mainly BLM A_2 and BLM B_2 (Fig. 1) (Umezawa et al., 1966; Umezawa, 1979). BLM A_2 has been chemically synthesized (Takita et al., 1982; Aoyagi et al., 1982). There are several hundred natural and synthetic BLM analogs now available; all have the fundamental glycopeptide structure of bleomycinic acid (Fig. 1). Most BLMs differ from one another at their terminal amine (R_1). For example, BLM A_2 contains a dimethylsulfonium propylamine as a terminal amine whereas BLM B_2 contains an agmatine. Peplomycin contains a phenylethyl amine and liblomycin contains a bulky lipophilic terminal amine consisting of several phenyl rings interlinked with ether bonds (Fig. 1). BLM analogs with internal modifications of the BLM molecule are also available. The talisomycins, for example, contain an additional talose sugar (R_2) whereas deglyco BLMs correspond to BLM molecules that lack the two carbohydrate groups of bleomycinic acid. Recently, we synthesized a highly fluorescent analog of talisomycin S_{10b} which may be useful for cellular drug distribution studies (Mistry et al., 1992). All BLMs contain a bithiazole moiety that confers low level intrinsic fluorescence.

The clinical mixture used in the United States and Europe to treat human malignancies comprises 55–70% BLM A_2, 25–30% BLM B_2, and small quantities of a variety of other BLMs. In the former Soviet Union and China, BLM A_5 is the predominant BLM found in the clinical mixture. Bleomycin is an essential component of regimens that are curative against germ-cell and testicular carcinomas (Einhorn and Donohue, 1977) and lymphomas (Bonadonna and Santoro, 1982; Newcomer et al., 1982). Certain types of squamous cell carcinomas also respond to a moderate degree to bleomycin containing regimens (Bennett and Reich, 1979).

One reason for the usefulness of the BLMs may relate to their ability to complement other antitumor agents. Cultured tumor cells resistant to a variety of other antineoplastic agents, such as vinblastine and doxorubicin, may be more responsive to BLM (Gupta, 1985). One of the most unusual and valuable features of the BLMs is a lack of significant bone marrow, hepatic, or renal toxicity (Bennett and Reich, 1979). Thus, overlapping toxicity between BLM and other antineoplastic drugs is uncommon. With repeated clinical doses, however, BLM does induce pulmonary fibrosis (Blum et al., 1973; Umezawa, 1979).

2. BIOCHEMISTRY OF ACTIVATION AND MECHANISM OF ACTION

Single and double strand cleavage of DNA is the mechanism by which BLM is believed to induce its toxicity. Two structural domains within the BLM molecule have been considered essential for

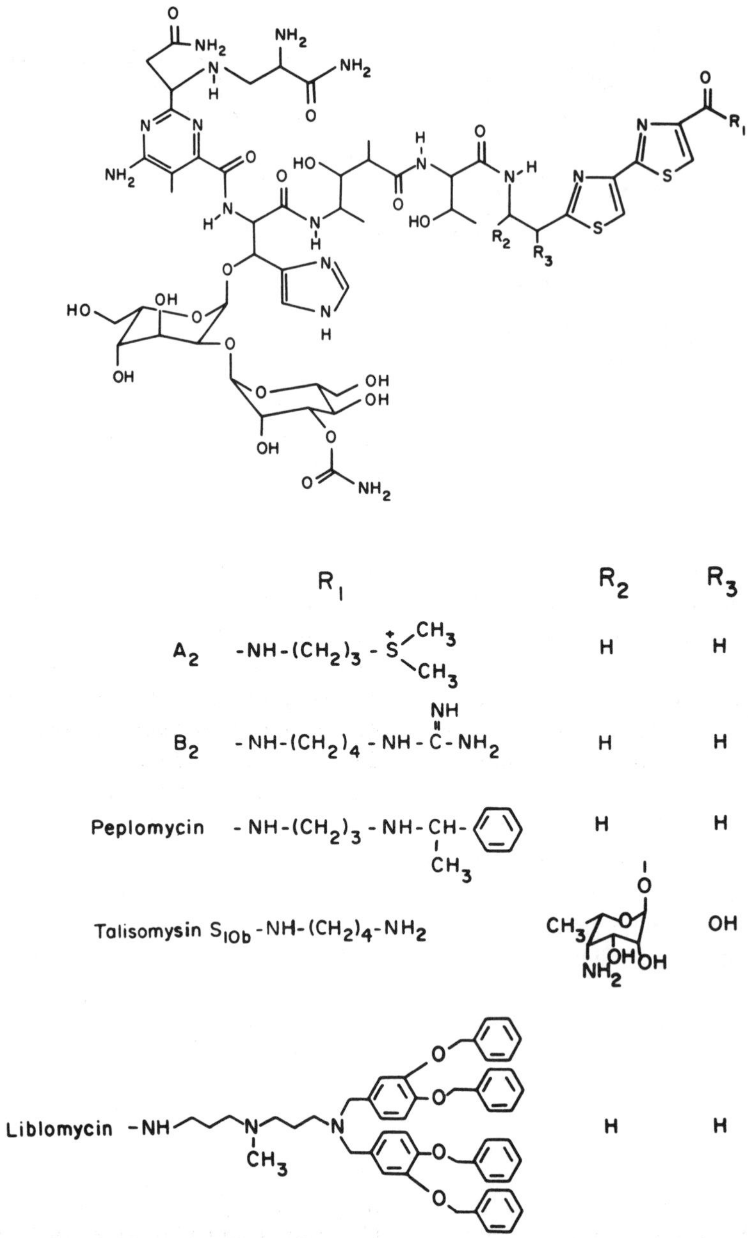

FIG. 1. Structure of bleomycin and bleomycin-like compounds.

the biological activity of these compounds. One is a DNA binding portion that consists of the terminal amine and the bithiazole moiety. The cationic character of the terminal amine and the planarity of the bithiazole are thought to dictate the affinity of bleomycin toward DNA. Recently, NMR studies with $(dC\text{-}dG)_3$ as a model showed that the bithiazole moiety of BLM partially intercalates between base pairs (Gamesik et al., 1990). The DNA binding portion of the molecule directs bleomycin to specific nucleotide sequences (e.g. 5′GC3′ and 5′GT3′). In addition to the nucleotide sequence specificity, the DNA breakage also appears to depend upon the overall DNA topology (Mirabelli et al., 1983) and possibly on the degree of DNA methylation (Hertzberg et al., 1985).

The second region contributing to the biological effect of BLM is the metal binding site between the bithiazole moiety and the beta-aminoalanine terminus. A variety of metals can bind to bleomycin, although the stability of the interaction differs in the following order: Fe(II) < Co(II) < Ni(II) < Cu(II) (Sugiura, 1980). Physicochemical studies indicate a bleomycin-

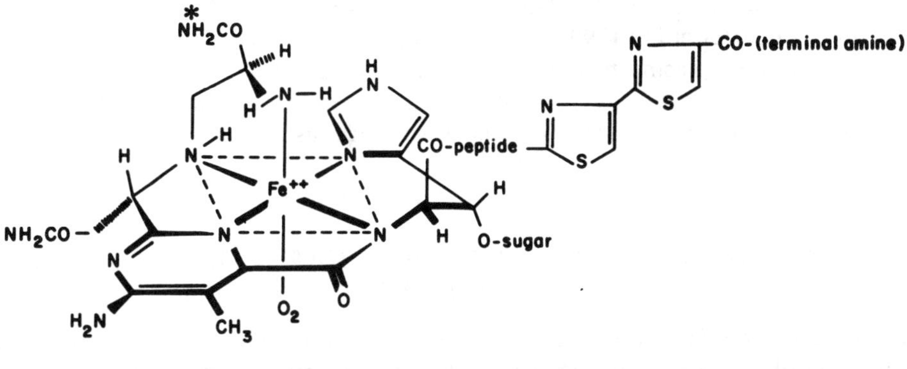

FIG. 2. The proposed metal coordination structure of bleomycin.

metal coordination construction maintaining a square-pyramidal structure with a basal plane that contains the secondary amine nitrogen, the N-4 pyrimidine ring nitrogen, the deprotonated peptide bond nitrogen of the histidine region and the histidine imidazole nitrogen (Fig. 2). The fifth axial donor has been assigned to the alpha-amino nitrogen of the beta-aminoalanine moiety of bleomycin (Sugiura, 1980). The sixth axial coordination site is thought to be occupied by exogenous oxygen. Cell-free in vitro data strongly suggest that a bleomycin–iron–oxygen complex is a biologically active species (Fig. 2). In this rigid square-pyramidal coordination environment, oxygen binding is efficient and oxygen reduction is permitted. Both hydroxyl and superoxide radicals can be formed based upon spin-trapping data (Lown and Sim, 1977), although it now seems possible that cellular injury could occur without the need for classical Fenton chemistry. DNA strand scission produced by the 'activated' iron bleomycin complex is generally thought to be responsible for cell death but it is interesting that at least three other metallobleomycins have been shown to mediate oxidative DNA strand scission in vitro (Hecht, 1986). Thus, it is possible that metal–bleomycin species other than iron–bleomycin may be important in cell damage. It is also of interest that in the absence of DNA in vitro, BLM may self-inactivate (Umezawa, 1979) pointing to the importance of rapid drug delivery to the nucleus.

The association of bleomycin with DNA allows the metal chelated portion of the molecule to perform the above mentioned radical chemistry in close proximity to DNA, which results in DNA strand scissions and base release. This is enhanced by sulphydryl compounds, ascorbate, peroxides, and phosphate-containing compounds, such as ATP (Burger et al., 1985). The chemistry of molecular oxygen bleomycin-mediated DNA strand scissions has been thoroughly studied using well defined DNA sequences and plasmid DNA (D'Andrea and Haseltine, 1978; Mirabelli et al., 1983; Hertzberg et al., 1985). Kozarich et al. (1989) showed that the rate limiting step in DNA cleavage is oxidation of deoxyribose through hydrogen abstraction at the C-4′ position by activated BLM-Fe(II)-O_2. Hydrogen abstraction is then followed by oxygen incorporation at C-4′ and formation of base propenals, which appear to have toxic properties of their own (Grollman et al., 1985).

The in vivo metal association of the clinically used bleomycin, which is metal-free upon injection, has not been well examined. Limited studies suggest that bleomycin is complexed with Cu(II) in the circulating blood (Kanao et al., 1973). The mode of bleomycin entry into cells is unknown, although a binding step has been proposed (Lymon et al., 1986). It has been hypothesized that when the Cu(II)–bleomycin complex enters cells, the cupric ion is reduced and the resulting cuprous ion is abstracted by a sulphydryl-containing macromolecule (Takahashi et al., 1977; Umezawa, 1979; Takahashi et al., 1987). Some of this metal-free drug could be inactivated and some may interact with cellular macromolecules, such as DNA. Definitive experimental data determining the biologically active form of bleomycin within cells are not available.

In addition to the DNA target, discrepancies between DNA damage and cell toxicity suggest that other sites may also be important for the antitumor properties of bleomycin (Berry et al.,

1985; Smith, 1987). BLM was shown to also bind and cleave tRNA (Magliozzo et al., 1989) and more recently mRNA (Carter et al., 1990). Bleomycin can also both bind to the plasma membrane (Fujimoto, 1974) and affect plasma membrane cellular functions (Sun and Crane, 1985), but the significance of these actions is not known. The biological targets responsible for pulmonary toxicity and the dose-limiting toxicity associated with bleomycin are also unclear.

3. IN VITRO METABOLISM OF BLM AND CHARACTERIZATION OF METABOLITES

Umezawa and coworkers (1974) identified a BLM-inactivating activity in the postmicrosomal supernatant fraction of homogenates from a variety of mouse organs. This enzyme was shown to cleave the amide bond of the beta-aminoalanine moiety of BLM resulting in a carboxylic acid. The enzyme was then termed BLM hydrolase and the metabolite deamido BLM. The chemical nature of the metabolite was deduced based upon: (a) a stoichiometric release of 1 mol of ammonia per mol of bleomycin metabolized, (b) comparison of the chemical composition of acid hydrolysis products formed with unmetabolized bleomycin and deamido bleomycin and (c) a shift in the pK of the alpha-amino group of the beta-aminoalanine moiety from 7.4 to 9.4 (Umezawa et al., 1972; Umezawa, 1979).

The conversion of the carboxyamide of the beta-aminoalamine to a carboxylic acid by the BLM-inactivating activity results in a more basic alpha-amino group on the beta-aminoalamine. Thus, at physiological pH the free carboxylic acid of the aminoalanine moiety rather than the protonated amino group occupies the fifth coordination site of the bleomycin–iron–oxygen ternary complex (Fig. 3). This leads to a marked decrease in the formation of an 'activated' bleomycin complex competent in performing radical chemistry (Huang et al., 1981; Lazo et al., 1987). The deamidated bleomycin is 1/100th as potent as the parent compound in degrading DNA (Sugiura, 1980) and at inhibiting bacterial or tumor growth (Umezawa, 1979). Lazo et al. (1987) found that BLM A_2 was 100-fold as potent as deamido bleomycin A_2 in killing murine L1210 cells in culture. Similar results have also been seen with human head and neck carcinoma A253 cells (Fig. 4). Finally, in contrast to bleomycin A_2, deamido bleomycin A_2 does not produce pulmonary fibrosis or weight loss when repeatedly administered to mice (Lazo and Humphreys, 1983). Thus, the fifth axial coordination site is essential for effective activation of BLM.

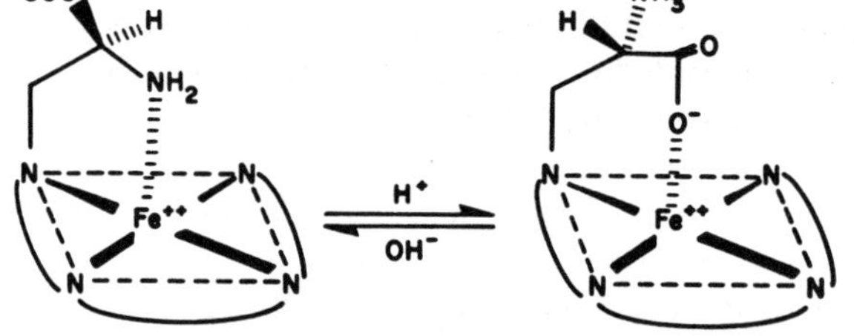

FIG. 3. A schematic proposal for the metal coordination structure of deamidobleomycin. At basic pH (left side) the primary amine of the terminal amino acid moiety of bleomycin occupies the fifth coordination site. At neutral pH (right side) the protonation of the amine moiety prevents binding and the carboxylic acid species is the preferred ligand.

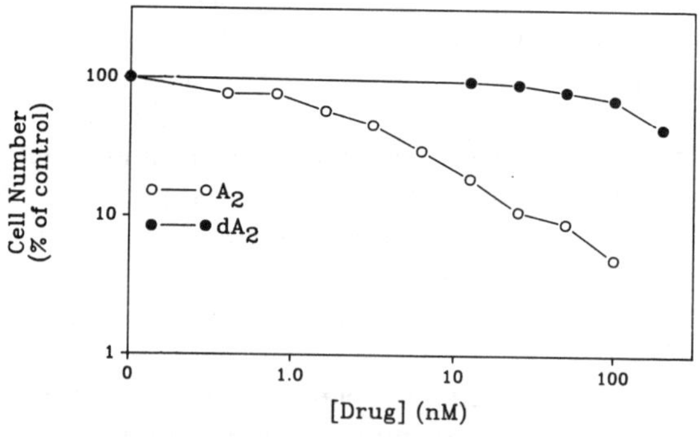

FIG. 4. Cytotoxicity of deaidobleomycin A $_2$ (dA_2, ●—●) and bleomycin A_2 (A_2, ○—○) to cultured human head and neck carcinoma A-253 cells. Cells were plated (2500 cells/well) in 96-well microtiter plates and exposed continuously to drugs. After four population doublings (96 hr) the medium and drugs were removed, the cells were stained with 0.5% methylene blue in 50% ethanol and solubolized in 1% Sarkosyl. Absorbance (600nm) was quantified using an automated plate reader.

TABLE 1. *Characteristics of Rabbit Pulmonary and Liver Bleomycin Hydrolase**

	Pulmonary	Liver
Cellular location	Cytoplasmic	Cytoplasmic
Molecular mass (native)	250 kDa	300 kDa
(denatured)	50 kDa	48 kDa
pH optimum	7.0–7.5	6.8–7.8
pI	5.3, 4.5 and 4.3	5.2
K_m (mM) (BLM B_2)	0.06	0.79
V_{max} (μmol/mg protein × hr) (BLM B_2)	1.9	38
Inhibitors	E-64	—
	Leupeptin	Leupeptin
	N-Ethylmaleimide	*N*-Ethylmaleimide
	Puromycin	TLCK
	Divalent cations	Divalent cations
Enzymatic activity	Cysteine proteinase	—

*Data for pulmonary enzyme from Sebti et al. (1987, 1989b) and for liver from Nishimura et al. (1987b).

4. CHARACTERISTICS OF BLEOMYCIN HYDROLASE

Previous attempts to characterize the biochemical properties of bleomycin hydrolase have been thwarted by the instability of the enzyme and difficulties in its purification. Umezawa et al. (1974) initially examined the enzyme in a partially purified form (27-fold) from mouse liver. They found an enzyme that had some properties similar to those of hepatic aminopeptidases. Sebti and Lazo (1987) utilized fast protein liquid chromatography to demonstrate unequivocally that bleomycin hydrolase was distinct from all detectable pulmonary aminopeptidases. In addition to charge characteristics, bleomycin hydrolase was distinguishable from aminopeptidase B based upon its enzymatic stability, molecular mass, and sensitivity to inhibitors and activators (Sebti and Lazo, 1987). Using sequential anion exchange, hydrophobic interaction, and affinity chromatography, Sebti et al. (1987) have successfully purified bleomycin hydrolase to homogeneity from rabbit lungs. The 6000-fold purified enzyme exhibited a molecular mass of 250 kDa on nondenaturing polyacrylamide gel electrophoresis and gel filtration chromatography and a single band of 50 kDa on sodium dodecylsulfate-polyacrylamide gel electrophoresis. These results suggest the enzyme normally exists in a pentameric form. Moreover, bleomycin hydrolase activity was inhibited by *N*-ethylmaleimide suggesting that it is a thiol enzyme. A summary of the relevant biochemical features of rabbit pulmonary bleomycin hydrolase are seen in Table 1.

Nishimura et al. (1987b) developed a hybridoma clone that produces an IgM monoclonal antibody to rabbit liver bleomycin hydrolase. An immunoaffinity column was prepared with this antibody and used to purify (1300-fold) rabbit liver bleomycin hydrolase. Analysis of the native form of the rabbit liver enzyme by these authors suggested that the subunits were 48 kDa and the native enzyme had a slightly larger mass (ca. 300 kDa) than that of the lung enzyme found by Sebti et al. (1987) (Table 1). It is not yet certain whether the slight differences in molecular mass between rabbit lung and liver enzyme exist or whether the assigned mass values reflect differences in preparations or analytical procedures. Nonetheless, both enzyme preparations showed similar inhibitor profiles. The use of a monoclonal antibody by Nishimura et al. (1987b) may have selected for only one of the isoforms of bleomycin hydrolase, since the liver enzyme isolated with the antibody exhibited only one pI (i.e. 5.2). The monoclonal antibody apparently recognizes only a subset of bleomycin hydrolases, since the antibody failed to immunoprecipitate bleomycin hydrolase from MH134 and Ehrlich ascites carcinoma cells. It remains possible that tumor cells may contain forms of BLM hydrolase that differ from those found in normal tissues.

The availability of purified bleomycin hydrolase has permitted our laboratories to study further the biochemical and molecular characteristics of the enzyme. Rabbit pulmonary bleomycin hydrolase was found to have a blocked amino terminus that prevented N-terminal sequence analysis. Thus, we digested bleomycin hydrolase with trypsin, isolated one major peptide by HPLC, sequenced it and found it to contain 25 amino acids. This amino acid sequence was used to construct a 36-mer oligonucleotide using the method of Lathe (1985). The 36-mer hybridizes to a single band of 2.5 kb by Northern blot analysis with rabbit liver, spleen, and lung mRNA. This

TABLE 2. K_m *and* V_{max} *of BLM Hydrolase Substrates*

	K_m (mM)	V_{max} (μmol/mg × hr)
BLM B_2	0.056	1.87
BLM A_2	0.83	4.30
Deglyco BLM A_2	0.49	16.49
Peplomycin	0.70	2.73
TLM S_{10b}	0.45	0.540
Butylamino-3-propylamino-3-propylamine BLM	2.25	8.71
Bleomycinic acid	No saturation of the enzyme was observed up to 6.5 mM	

36-mer also hybridized with a similar size mRNA species from HL-60 human promyleocytic leukemia cells and from the liver and kidneys of a variety of species. Therefore, bleomycin hydrolase appears not only to be widely distributed among cells in a given organ (Lazo et al., 1984) but also among organs of different species.

Using the 36-mer as a probe we have also isolated a partial length (832 bp) BLM hydrolase cDNA from a λgt11 rabbit liver cDNA library (Sebti et al., 1989b). Recently, we have obtained a larger (1100 bp) insert of BLM hydrolase cDNA but have been unable to isolate a full length cDNA fragment. Presently, we are cloning genomic BLM hydrolase with the hope of obtaining the entire amino acid sequence of this protein. Analysis of the predicted amino acid sequence coded by the partial length BLM hydrolase cDNA fragment revealed a 15 amino acid sequence with remarkable homology with the active site of cysteine proteinase such as cathepsin B, H and L, aleurain and papain (Sebti et al., 1989b). Biochemically, BLM hydrolase behaved as a cysteine proteinase with cathepsin H specificity and was inhibited by cysteine proteinase-specific inhibitors such as E-64 (Table 1 and Sebti et al., 1989b).

Enzyme kinetic analysis (Sebti et al., 1989a) showed that BLM hydrolase can recognize and metabolize a broad spectrum of BLM analogs. Incubation of BLM A_2, BLM B_2, talisomysin S_{10b}, peplomycin, deglycobleomycin A_2, butylamine-3-propylamino-3-propylamine bleomycin and bleomycinic acid with rabbit lung BLM hydrolase resulted in their metabolism and inactivation. Thus, BLM hydrolase can recognize and inactivate a number of structurally different BLM analogs. Kinetic studies of the above BLM analogs with rabbit lung BLM hydrolase demonstrated that the enzyme interacts with regions other than the site of metabolism of the BLM molecule. These studies indicated that the carbohydrate region dictates the rate of hydrolysis while the terminal amine region of BLM dictates the affinity of BLM analogs to BLM hydrolase. For example, removal of the carbohydrate groups from BLM A_2 resulted in deglyco BLM A_2, which had a V_{max} 4-fold higher than BLM A_2 while the K_m of both drugs were similar (Table 2). In contrast, substitution of the agmatine terminal amine in BLM B_2 by the dimethylsulfonium propylamine moiety in BLM A_2 had little effect on V_{max} but increased the K_m by 15-fold (Table 2).

5. IN VIVO METABOLIC INACTIVATION OF BLM

When Umezawa et al. (1968, 1972) injected [^{3}H]BLM subcutaneously into mice, radioactive material was found in all organs. The amount of BLM measured by radioactivity was much greater in most organ homogenates than the amount of active BLM measured by growth inhibition of *Bacillus subtillus*. In most organs a considerable fraction of the radiolabelled drug was inactive; skin and lungs were the exception where high levels of the active form of BLM were found. These data suggested the possible metabolism of BLM. Because the bioassay used by Umezawa et al. (1972) to evaluate bleomycin content could have been influenced by a variety of components in the organ homogenates (Thomas et al., 1984). Lazo and Humphreys (1983) and Lazo and Pham (1984) developed an HPLC to demonstrate unequivocally that metabolites of BLM A_2 were formed in vivo. Furthermore, they confirmed the above conclusions derived from the bioassay methods. Almost half of the radioactivity found in the kidneys, liver, and spleen of C57BL/6 mice was metabolized 1 hr after a subcutaneous drug injection. The in vivo metabolism of BLM in lung tissue was significantly less than that seen in other organs examined (Lazo and Humphreys, 1983). Significant metabolism and multiple forms of metabolites were detected (Lazo and Pham, 1984), however, when lungs were examined 12–24 hr after either an intratracheal or subcutaneous injection of [^{3}H] BLM A_2. In nonpulmonary tissues at these same times, multiple metabolites were especially obvious. Although the chemical nature of most of the peaks is unknown, the most prominent putative metabolite seen in liver and kidneys 0.5–2 hr after injection of [^{3}H] BLM A_2 comigrated on HPLC with deamido BLM A_2.

The importance of BLM hydrolase in protecting tissues against the toxic actions of BLM was first suggested by the work of Umezawa et al. (1974), Umezawa (1979), Ohnuma et al. (1974) and Yoshioka et al. (1978). Lazo and Humphreys (1983) found that lungs from a resistant species, such as the rabbit, converted a significantly greater fraction of BLM A_2 to the deamido form than did lungs from a sensitive species, mouse. Results from Schrier et al. (1983), Ekomoto et al. (1987) and Filderman and Lazo (1991) demonstrated an inbred strain variation in sensitivity to BLM-induced lung fibrosis. The level of BLM hydrolase activity in lung homogenates correlated inversely with pulmonary sensitivity to BLM (Lazo et al., 1987). Little is known, however, about the factors that control the expression or content of BLM hydrolase. Repeated BLM treatment of mice markedly decreased pulmonary BLM hydrolase levels (Filderman et al., 1988); this may render the lungs more susceptible to injury. The mechanism of this decrement in BLM hydrolase has not yet been established.

6. ROLE OF METABOLIC INACTIVATION IN TUMOR RESISTANCE TO BLM

Until recently, most studies attempting to implicate BLM metabolism to tumor resistance have been correlative and generally contradictory or inconclusive (Lazo et al., 1987; Lazo and Sebti, 1989). Some data showed a good correlation between BLM hydrolase levels in various tumor homogenates and their levels of resistance (Muller et al., 1977; Akiyama et al., 1981; Tanaka, 1984; Ueda et al., 1984), while others did not (Lazo et al., 1982; Zuckerman et al., 1986). Recently, however, more support for the involvement of BLM hydrolase in resistance was provided by Nishimura et al. (1989a) who showed that the cysteine proteinase inhibitor E-64, which inhibits BLM hydrolase activity, potentiates the cytotoxicity of peplomycin, an analog of BLM, against Chinese hamster lung cells. Furthermore, we found a human head and neck carcinoma all line (C-10E) that is highly resistant to BLM metabolized BLM A_2 to a greater extent as well as accumulated lower levels of this drug (Morris et al., 1991). Treatment of this BLM-resistant C-10E cell line with E-64 inhibited cellular BLM hydrolase and sensitized the cells to BLM (Morris et al., 1991). Using a polyclonal antibody to a specific epitope of BLM hydrolase, we have shown that the amount of BLM hydrolase in C-10E cells is higher in the corresponding parental cells (Morris et al., 1992). The lower amount of BLM hydrolase in BLM-sensitive cells as compared to BLM-resistant cells may reflect the higher instability of BLM hydrolase in the sensitive cells. In fact, Nishimura et al. (1989b) showed that BLM hydrolase in BLM-resistant Chinese hamster lung cells was degraded less rapidly than BLM hydrolase in BLM-sensitive Chinese hamster ovary cells. The 50 kDa subunit of BLM hydrolase was degraded to a 31 kDa form at a much lower rate resulting in a 3-fold higher levels of BLM hydrolase activity in the BLM-resistant cells (Nishimura et al., 1989b). The studies discussed above dealt with the involvement of BLM hydrolase in BLM resistance in vitro or in cell culture. We have recently investigated the role of BLM hydrolase in the BLM resistance of human tumors grown subcutaneously in the nude mouse xenograft model (Sebti et al., 1991). We found the BLM-resistant Daudi tumors (a human lymphoma) metabolized BLM to a much greater extent than BLM-sensitive A-253 tumors (a human head and neck squamous cell carcinoma). We have also found BLM metabolism by those two human tumors in vivo to be very complex with more than six BLM metabolites being separated by HPLC (Sebti et al., 1991). Furthermore, treatment of mice bearing Daudi xenograft with E-64, prior to BLM treatment, inhibited BLM metabolism and sensitized these tumors to BLM in vivo. Recently, we have found that solid tumors, such as human colon and lung carcinomas, that are resistant to BLM were also sensitized to BLM in vivo by E-64 (Jani et al., 1992a,b). This sensitization appears to be mediated primarily through an increase in the levels of accumulated BLM in the tumors.

Thus, studies from a number of laboratories suggest that metabolic inactivation of BLM by BLM hydrolase may be important in determining its antitumor activity. Other mechanisms, however, such as decreased BLM accumulation in some tumors may also be involved in tumor resistance to BLM.

REFERENCES

AKIYAMA, S. I., IKEZAKI, K., KURAMOCHI, H., TAKAHASHI, K. and KUWANO, M. (1981) Bleomycin-resistant cells contain increased bleomycin-hydrolase activities. *Biochem. biophys. Res. Commun.* **101:** 55–60.

AOYAGI, T., KATANO, K., SUGUNA, H., PRIMEAU, J., CHANG, L.H. and HECHT, S. M. (1982) Total synthesis of bleomycin. *J. Am. Chem. Soc.* **104:** 5537–5538.

BENNETT, J. M. and REICH, S. D. (1979) Bleomycin. *Ann. intern. Med.* **90:** 945–948.

BERRY, D. E., KILLKUSKIE, R. E. and HECHT, S. M. (1985) DNA damage induced by bleomycin in the presence of dibucaine is not predictive of cell growth inhibition. *Biochemistry* **24:** 3214–3219.

BLUM, R. H., CARTER, S. K. and AGRE, K. (1973) A clinical review of bleomycin: a new antineoplastic agent. *Cancer* **31:** 903–914.

BONADONNA, G. and SANTORO, A. (1982) ABVD chemotherapy in the treatment of Hodgkin's disease. *Cancer Treat. Rev.* **9:** 21–35.

BURGER, R. M., HORWITZ, S. B. and PEISACH, J. (1985) Stimulation of iron(II) bleomycin activity by phosphatecontaining compounds. *Biochemistry* **24:** 3623–3629.

CARTER, B. J., DE VROOM, E., LONG, E. C., VAN DER MARCEL, G. A., VAN BOOM, J. H. and HECHT, S. M. (1990) Site-specific cleavage of RNA by Fe (II) bleomycin. *Proc. natn. Acad. Sci. U.S.A.* **87:** 9373–9377.

D'ANDREA, A. D. and HASELTINE, W. A. (1978) Sequence specific cleavage of DNA by the antitumor antibiotics neocarcinostatin and bleomycin. *Proc. natn. Acad. Sci. U.S.A.* **75:** 3608–3612.

EINHORN. L. H. and DONOHUE, J. (1977) Cis-diamminedichloroplatinum, vinblastine, and bleomycin combination chemotherapy in disseminated testicular cancer. *Ann. intern. Med.* **87:** 293–298.

EKOMOTO, H., TAKADA, K., OHNUKI, T., TAKAHASHI, K., MATSUDA, A., TAKITA, T. and UMEZAWA, H. (1987) Different sensitivity to bleomycin-induced pulmonary fibrosis among various strans of mice. *J. clin. Biochem. Nutr.* **2:** 25–31.

FILDERMAN, A. E. and LAZO, J. S. (1991) Murine strain variation in bleomycin (BLM) metabolism in vitro. *Biochem. Pharmac.* **42:** 195–198.

FILDERMAN, A. E., GENOVESE, L. A. and LAZO, J. S. (1988) Alterations in pulmonary protective enzymes following systemic bleomycin treatment in mice. *Biochem. Pharmac.* **37:** 1111–1116.

FUJIMOTO, J. (1974) Radioautographic studies on the intracellular distribution of bleomycin ^{14}C in mouse tumor cells. *Cancer Res.* **34:** 2969–2974.

GAMESIK, M. P., GLICKSON, J. D. and ZON, G. (1990) NMR studies of the interaction of bleomycin with $(dC\text{-}dG)_3$. *J. Biomol. Struct. Dyn.* **7:** 1117–1133.

GROLLMAN, A. P., TAKESHITA, M., PILLAI, D. M. R. and JOHNSON, F. (1985) Origin and cytotoxic properties of base propenals derived from DNA. *Cancer Res.* **45:** 1127–1131.

GUPTA, R. S. (1985) Cross-resistance of vinblastine- and taxol-resistant mutants of Chinese hamster ovary cells to other anticancer drugs. *Cancer Treat. Rep.* **69:** 512–521.

HECHT, S. M. (1986) DNA strand scission by activated bleomycin group antibiotics. *Fed. Proc.* **45:** 2784–2791.

HERTZBERG, R. P., CARANFA, M. J. and HECHT, S. M. (1985) DNA methylation diminishes bleomycin-mediated strand scission. *Biochemistry* **24:** 5285–5289.

HUANG, C.-H., MIRABELLI, C. K., JAN, Y. and CROOKE, S. T. (1981) Single strand and double strand deoxyribonucleic acid breaks produced by several bleomycin analogs. *Biochemistry* **20:** 233–238.

JANI, J. P., MISTRY, J. S., MORRIS, G., DAVIES, P., LAZO, J. S. and SEBTI, S. M. (1992a) In vivo circumvention of human colon carcinoma resistance to bleomycin. *Cancer Res.* **52:** 2931–2937.

JANI, J. P., MISTRY, J. S., MORRIS, G., LAZO, J. S. and SEBTI, S. M. (1992b) In vivo sensitization of human lung carcinoma to bleomycin by the cysteine proteinase inhibitor E-64. *Oncol. Res.* **4**(Suppl. 2): 59–63.

KANAO, M., TOMITA, S., ISHIDA, S., MURAKAMI, A. and OKADA, H. (1973) Chelation of bleomycin with copper in vivo. *Chemotherapy (Tokyo)* **21:** 1305–1310.

KOZARICH, J. W., WORTH, L., JR, FRANK, B. L., CHRISTNER, D. F., VANDERWALL, D. E. and STUBBE, J. (1989) Sequence-specific isotope effects on the cleavage of DNA by bleomycin. *Science* **245:** 1396–1399.

LATHE, R. (1985) Synthetic oligonucleotide probes deduced from amino acid sequence data. *J. Molec. Biol.* **183:** 1–12.

LAZO, J. S. and HUMPHREYS, C. J. (1983) Lack of metabolism as the biochemical basis of bleomycin-induced pulmonary toxicity. *Proc. natn. Acad. Sci. U.S.A.* **80:** 3064–3068.

LAZO, J. S. and PHAM, E. T. (1984) Pulmonary fate of [^{3}H]bleomycin A_2 in mice. *J. Pharmac. exp. Ther.* **228:** 13–18.

LAZO, J. S. and SEBTI, S. M. (1989) Malignant cell resistance to bleomycin group antibiotics. In: *Anticancer Drug Resistance*, pp. 267–279, KESSEL, D. (ed.) CRC Press, Boca Raton, FL.

LAZO, J. S., BOLAND, C. J. and SCHWARTZ, P. E. (1982) Bleomycin hydrolase activity and cytotoxicity in human tumors. *Cancer Res.* **42:** 4026–4031.

LAZO, J. S., MERRILL, W. W., PHAM, E. T., LYNCH, T. J., MCCALLISTER, J. and INGBAR, D. H. (1984) Bleomycin hydrolase activity in pulmonary cells. *J. Pharmac. exp. Ther.* **231:** 583–588.

LAZO, J. S., SEBTI, S. M. and FILDERMAN, A. E. (1987) Metabolism of bleomycin and bleomycin-like compounds. In: *Metabolism of Anti-Cancer Drugs*, pp. 194–210, PROUGH, R. A. and POWIS, G. (eds) Taylor and Francis, Ltd., London.

LOWN, J. W. and SIM, S.K. (1977) The mechanism of the bleomycin-induced cleavage of DNA. *Biochem. biophys. Res. Commun.* **77:** 1150–1157.

LYMON, S., UJJANI, B., RENNER, K., ANTHOLINE, W., PETERING, D. H., WHETSTONE, J. W. and KNIGHT, J. M. (1986) Properties of the initial reaction of bleomycin and several of its metal complexes with Ehrlich cells. *Cancer Res.* **46:** 4472–4478.

MAGLIOZZO, R. S., PEISACH, J. and CIRIOLO, M. R. (1989) Transfer RNA is cleared by activated bleomycin. *Molec. Pharmac.* **35:** 428–432.

MIRABELLI, C. K., HUANG, C.H. and CROOKE, S. T. (1983) Role of deoxyribonucleic acid topology in altering the site/sequence specificity of cleavage of deoxyribonucleic acid by bleomycin and talisomycin. *Biochemistry* **22:** 300–306.

MISTRY, J. S., JANI, J. P., MORRIS, G., MUJUMDER, R. B., SEBTI, S. M., REYNOLDS, I. J. and LAZO, J. S. (1992) Synthesis and evaluation of a novel fluorescence-labelled derivative of talisomycin S_{10b} as a probe for identifying bleomycin-resistant cells. *Cancer Res.* **52:** 709– 718.

MORRIS, G., MISTRY, J. S., JANI, J. P., SEBTI, S. M. and LAZO, J. S. (1991) Cysteine proteinase inhibitors and bleomycin-sensitive and resistant cells. *Biochem. Pharmac.* **41:** 1559–1566.

MORRIS, G., MISTRY, J. S., JANI, J. P., MIGNANO, J. E., SEBTI, S. M. and LAZO, J. S. (1992) Neutralization of bleomycin hydrolase by an epitope-specific antibody. *Molec. Pharmac.* **42:** 57–62.

MULLER, W. E. G., SCHMIDSEDEN, R., RHODE, H. J., ZAHN, R. K. and SCHENEUMANN, H. (1977) Bleomycin sensitivity test: application for human squamous cell carcinoma. *Cancer* **40:** 2787–2791.

NEWCOMER, L. N., CADMAN, E. C., NERENBERG, M. I., CHEN, M., BERTINO, J. R., FARBER, L. R. and PROSNITZ, L. R. (1982) Randomized study comparing doxorubin, cyclophosphamide, vincristine, methotrexate with leucovorin rescue, and cytarabine (ACOMLA) with cyclophosphamide, doxorubicin, vincristine, prednisone and bleomycin (CHOP-B) in the treatment of diffuse histiocytic lymphoma. *Cancer Treat. Rep.* **66:** 1279–1284.

NISHIMURA, C., NISHIMURA, T., TANAKA, N. and SUZUKI, H. (1987a) Potentiation of the cytotoxicity of peplomycin against Ehrlich ascites carcinoma by bleomycin hydrolase inhibitors. *J. Antibiot. (Tokyo)* **40:** 1794–1795.

NISHIMURA, C., TANAKA, N., SUZUKI, H. (1987b) Purification of bleomycin hydrolase with a monoclonal antibody and its characterization. *Biochemistry* **26:** 1574–1578.

NISHIMURA, C., NISHIMURA, T., TANAKA, N., YAMAGUCHI, H. and SUZUKI, H. (1989a) Inhibition of intracellular bleomycin hydrolase activity by E-64 leads to the potentiation of the cytotoxicity of peplomycin against Chinese hamster lung cells. *Jap. J. Cancer Res.* **80:** 65– 68.

NISHIMURA, C., SUZUKI, H., TANAKA, N. and YAMAGUCHI, H. (1989) Intracellular degradation of bleomycin hydrolase in two Chinese hamster cell lines in relation to their peplomycin susceptibility. *Biochem. biophys. Acta* **1012:** 29–35.

OHNUMA, T., HOLLAND, J. F., MASUDA, H., WALIGUNDA, J. A. and GOLDBERG, G. A. (1974) Microbiological assay of bleomycin: inactivation, tissue distribution and clearance. *Cancer* **33:** 1230–1238.

SCHRIER, D. J., KUNKEL, R. G. and PHAM, S. H. (1983) The role of strain variation in murine bleomycin-induced pulmonary fibrosis. *Am. Rev. Resp. Dis.* **127:** 63–66.

SEBTI, S. M. and LAZO, J. S. (1987) Separation of pulmonary bleomycin hydrolase from pulmonary aminopeptidases. *Biochemistry* **26:** 432–437.

SEBTI, S. M., DELEON, J. C. and LAZO, J. S. (1987) Purification, characterization and amino acid composition of rabbit pulmonary bleomycin hydrolase. *Biochemistry* **26:** 4213–4219.

SEBTI, S. M., DELEON, J. C., MA, L.-T., HECHT, S. M. and LAZO, J. S. (1989a) Substrate specificity of bleomycin hydrolase. *Biochem. Pharmac.* **38:** 141–147.

SEBTI, S. M., MIGNANO, J. E., JANI, J. P., SRIMATKANDALA, S. and LAZO, J. S. (1989b) Bleomycin hydrolase: molecular cloning, sequencing and biochemical studies reveal membership in the cysteine proteinase family. *Biochemistry* **28:** 6544–6548.

SEBTI, S. M., JANI, J. P., MISTRY, J. S., GORELIK, E. and LAZO, J. S. (1991) Metabolic inactivation: a mechanism of human tumor resistance to bleomycin. *Cancer Res.* **51:** 227–232.

SMITH, P. J. (1987) Ferrous iron-mediated enhancement of DNA damage and recovery potential in bleomycin-treated human cells. *Biochem. Pharmac.* **36:** 475–480.

SUGIURA, T. (1980) Bleomycin-iron complexes. Electron spin resonance study, ligand effect, and implication for action mechanism. *J. Am. Chem. Soc.* **102:** 5208–5215.

SUN, I. L. and CRANE, F. L. (1985) Bleomycin control of transplasma membrane redox activity and proton movement in Hela cells. *Biochem. Pharmac.* **34:** 617–622.

TAKAHASHI, K., TOSKIOKA, O., MATSUDA, A. and UMEZAWA, H. (1977) Intracellular reduction of the cupric ion of bleomycin copper complex and transfer of the cuprous ion to a cellular protein. *J. Antibiot. (Tokyo) Ser. A* **30:** 861–869.

TAKAHASHI, K., TAKITA, T. and UMEZAWA, H. (1987) The nature of thiol-compounds which trap cuprous ion reductively liberated from bleomycin-Cu(II) in cells. *J. Antibiot.* **40:** 348–353.

TAKITA, T., UMEZAWA, T., SAITO, S., MORISHIMA, H., NAGANAWA, H., UMEZAWA, H., TSUCHIYA, T., MIYAKI, T., KAGEYAMA, S., UMEZAWA, S., MURAOKA, Y., SUZUKI, M., OTSUKA, M., NARITA, M., KOBAYASHI, S. and OHNO, M. (1982) Total synthesis of bleomycin A_2. *Tetrahedron Lett.* **23:** 521–524.

TANAKA, N. (1984) Studies on the mechanism of drug resistance in tumor cells and a new antitumor antibiotic. *Gan To Kagaku Ryoho* **11:** 2666–2676.

THOMAS, A. H., NEWLAND, P. and SHARMA, N. R. (1984) Chromatographic methods for the analysis of bleomycin complex. *J. Chromatog.* **291:** 219–230.

UEDA, M., NOZAWA, S., UEKI, M., SANO, T., NAGAI, S., SUGIMOTO, O. and KURIHARA, S. (1984) Peplomycin sensitivity of various types of human gynecological cultured tumor cells. *Nippon Sanka Fujinka Gakkai Zasshi* **36:** 1867–1876.

UMEZAWA, H. (1979) Advances in bleomycin studies. In: *Bleomycin: Chemical, Biochemical and Biological Aspects*, pp. 24–36, HECHT, S. M. (ed.) Springer-Verlag, New York.

UMEZAWA, H., MAEDA, K., TAKEUCHI, T. and OKAMI, T. (1966) New antibiotics, bleomycin A and B. *J. Antibiot. (Tokyo) Ser. A.* **19:** 200–209.

UMEZAWA, H., ISHIZUKA, M., HORI, S., CHIMURA, H. and TAKEUCHI, T. (1968) The distribution of [^{3}H]bleomycin in mouse tissue. *J. Antibiot. (Tokyo) Ser. A.* **21:** 638–642.

UMEZAWA, H., TAKEUCHI, T., HORI, S., SAWA, T. and ISHIZUKA, M. (1972) Studies on the mechanism of antitumor effect of bleomycin on squamous cell carcinoma. *J. Antibiot. (Tokyo) Ser. A.* **25:** 409–420.

UMEZAWA, H., HORI, S., TSUTOMU, S., TOSHIOKA, T. and TAKEUCHI, T. (1974) A bleomycin-inactivating enzyme in mouse liver. *J. Antibiot. (Tokyo) Ser. A.* **27:** 419–424.

YOSHIOKA, O., AMANO, N., TAKAHASHI, K., MATSUDA, A. and UMEZAWA, H. (1978) Intracellular fate and activity of bleomycin. In: *Bleomycin: Current Status and New Developments*, pp. 35–56, CARTER, S. K., CROOKE, S. T. and UMEZAWA, H. (eds) Academic Press, New York.

ZUCKERMAN, J. E., RAFFIN, T. A., BROWN, J. M., NEWMAN, R. A., ELIZ, B. B. and SIKIC, B. I. (1986) In vitro selection and characterization of a bleomycin-resistant sublime of B16 melanoma. *Cancer Res.* **46:** 1748–1753.

Garth Powis, editor.
(1994) *Anticancer Drugs: Reactive Metabolism and Drug Interactions*,
Pergamon Press Ltd, pp. 397–416
Printed in the United Kingdom

CHAPTER 10

METABOLIC BASIS FOR THE CHEMOSENSITIZATION OF ANTICANCER DRUG ACTION BY NITROIMIDAZOLES

FRANCIS Y. F. LEE* AND PAUL WORKMAN†

**Bristol-Myers Squibb Company, Pharmaceutical Group, Experimental Therapeutics Department, Wallingford, CT 06492, U.S.A.*

†Cancer Research Campaign, Department of Medical Oncology, CRC Beatson Laboratories, University of Glasgow, Garscube Estate, Switchback Road, Bearsden, Glasgow G61 1BD, UK

1. INTRODUCTION

In the early 1980s, an exciting new dimension was added to the area of anticancer chemotherapy research when it was demonstrated that a group of 2-nitroimidazoles, of which misonidazole (MISO) is the lead compound (see Fig. 1 for chemical structures), could enhance the antitumor action of conventional chemotherapeutic agents both in vitro (Stratford et al., 1980; Roizin-Towle and Hall, 1981) and in vivo (Rose et al., 1980; Clement et al., 1980). This phenomenon, termed chemosensitization, has been extensively studied and reported since then (see Table 1). A number of excellent reviews on various aspects of chemosensitization are available (Kennedy et al., 1980; Brown, 1982; McNally, 1982; Rauth, 1984; Siemann, 1984; Coleman et al., 1988a). In the following discussion we shall emphasize the metabolic aspects of chemosensitization in so far as they are related to the mechanisms of action of the nitroimidazole chemosensitizers.

2. THE CHEMOSENSITIZATION PHENOMENON

2.1. IN VITRO OBSERVATIONS

Chemosensitization in vitro relies on the so-called 'pre-incubation' effect (Brown, 1982). Typically this requires tumor cells to be pre-exposed to relatively high concentrations of a nitroimidazole chemosensitizer under hypoxia for a period of time, usually several hours, prior to treatment under oxic conditions with a cytotoxic agent. The resultant cell-kill due to the combination is greater than simple addition of the effects of the two agents. A large number of chemotherapeutic agents have been investigated in this manner (see Table 1), and for several of these, notably the bifunctional alkylating agents and nitrosoureas, chemosensitization has consistently been demonstrated.

2.2. IN VIVO OBSERVATIONS

Chemosensitization in vivo usually involves the treatment of tumor-bearing mice with a chemosensitizer either simultaneously with or less than 1 hr before the cytotoxic agent. The tumor response due to the combined treatment is greater than the sum of the responses of the two agents given singly. Comprehensive lists of chemotherapeutic agent–sensitizer combinations tested in this manner are shown in Tables 1–6. The greatest degree of chemosensitization in vivo has been obtained with CCNU, melphalan (MEL) and cyclophosphamide (CP), and one laboratory has also reported large chemosensitization with chlorambucil (CHL). Each of these agents will now be discussed in turn.

2.2.1. *CCNU*

The combination of MISO and CCNU is probably the most consistent of all combined regimens in producing chemosensitization in mice. Table 2 lists all available data from the literature. There

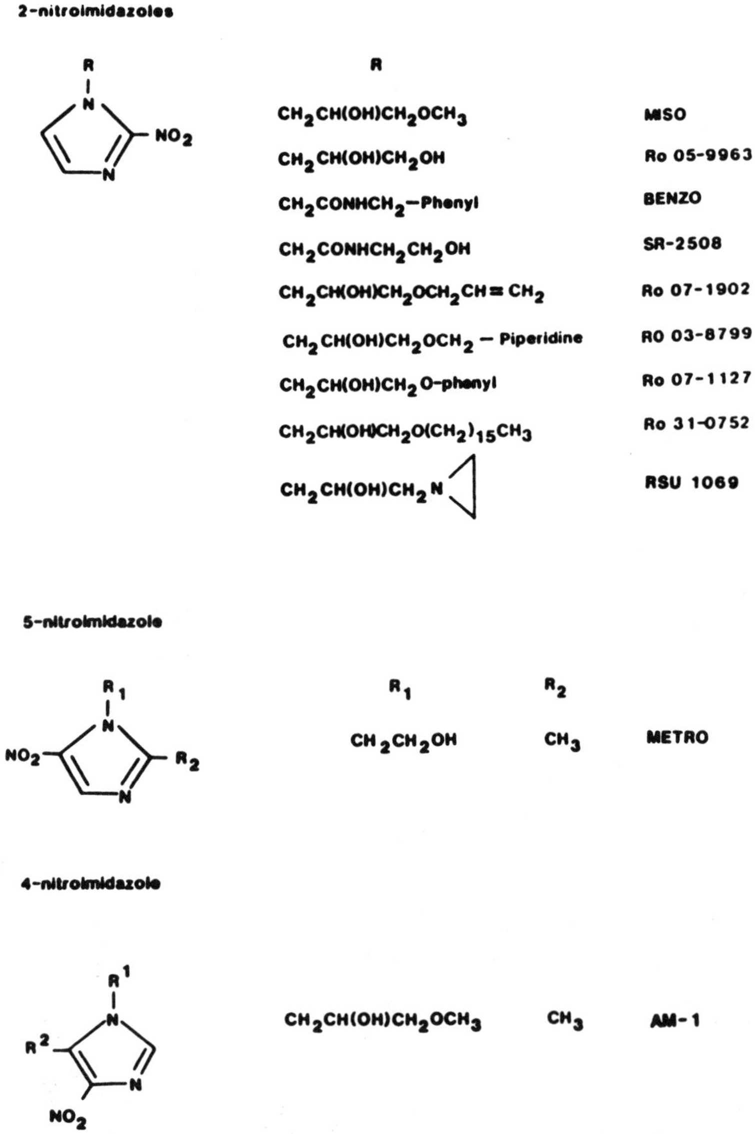

FIG. 1. Structures of the nitroimidazole chemosensitizers.

is a threshold dose of between 0.25–0.5 mg/g (1.25–2.5 mmol/kg) below which chemosensitization cannot usually be obtained. With doses between 0.5–1.0 mg/g (2.5–5.0 mmol/kg), the range of dose-modification factors (DMF) obtained for tumor response was usually >1.3 (range $= 1.0$–2.1). Normal tissue toxicity of CCNU was also enhanced but generally by a DMF of less than 1.3, thus giving therapeutic gain factors in the range 1.1–2.0 (Table 2).

Besides MISO, a range of compounds, mainly nitroimidazoles but also some others, has also been tested in combination with CCNU (Table 3). The lipophilic analog benznidazole (BENZO) had the advantage of giving a similar therapeutic gain to MISO but at lower plasma levels (Workman and Twentyman, 1982; Twentyman and Workman, 1983a). This led to a clinical trial (Roberts et al., 1984) but subsequent results were disappointing and the combination was discontinued. Of particular interest is the aziridine-substituted 2-nitroimidazole analog RSU 1069, which demonstrated superior chemosensitization activity over MISO. Most recently, newly synthesized analogs of RSU 1069 have been developed (e.g. RSU 1164 and RSU 1165) which are substantially less toxic than RSU 1069, but retain significant chemosensitizing activity. A prodrug of RSU 1069 (RB 6145) is now being developed for clinical investigation (Jenkins et al., 1990).

TABLE 1. *Potentiation of the Antitumor Activity of Various Anticancer Drugs by Misonidazole*

	Potentiated cytotoxic drugs	References	Non-potentiated cytotoxic drugs	References
In vivo	Adriamycin[1]	Tannock, 1980a	Adriamycin	Rose et al., 1980; Siemann, 1981; Randhawa et al., 1982; McNally, 1982
	BCNU	Mulcahy et al., 1981, 1982; Clutterbuck et al., 1982		
	CCNU	Stephens et al., 1981; Siemann, 1981; Hirst et al., 1982; Mulcahy et al., 1982; Siemann, 1982; Twentyman and Workman, 1982; Workman and Twentyman, 1982; Lee and Workman, 1983; Lee and Workman, 1984a; Durand and Chaplin, 1987	Bleomycin CHLZ Cis-Pt(II) MeCCNU[1] VP-16	Stephens et al., 1981 Mulcahy et al., 1982 Stephens et al., 1981 Double and Bibby, 1985 Stephens et al., 1981
	CHL	Workman and Twentyman, 1982; Lee and Workman, 1986a		
	CP	Tannock, 1980b; Twentyman 1981; Stephens et al., 1981; Law et al., 1981; Brown and Hirst, 1982; Twentyman and Workman, 1982; McNally et al., 1983; Chaplin et al., 1984; Hinchliffe and McNally, 1984; Hirst et al., 1984		
	5-Fluorouracil	Stephens et al., 1981		
	MeCCNU[1]	Stephens et al., 1981		
	MEL	Rose et al., 1980; Stephens et al., 1981; Brown and Hirst, 1982; Clutterbuck et al., 1982; Sheldon et al., 1982; McNally et al., 1983; Hinchliffe and McNally, 1984; Randhawa et al., 1985; Lee and Workman, 1986a		
	Methotrexate	Tannock, 1980a		
	Mitomycin C	Clement and Johnson, 1982		
	Nitrogen mustard	Murray and Meyn, 1984a,b		
	Vincristine	Stephens et al., 1981		
In vitro	Adriamycin[1]	Twentyman, 1982	Adriamycin[1]	West et al., 1981
	BCNU	Mulcahy, 1984	mAMSA	West et al., 1981
	Bleomycin	Roizin-Towle and Hall, 1981		
	Cis-pt(II)	Stratford et al., 1980; Roizin-Towle and Hall, 1981		
	CCNU	Twentyman, 1982; Mulcahy et al., 1984; Mulcahy 1986a,b; Durand and Chaplin, 1987		
	CHL	Twentyman, 1982		
	MEL	Stratford et al., 1980; Roizin-Towle and Hall, 1981; Smith et al., 1982; Taylor et al., 1983, 1984; Roizin-Towle, 1985		
	Monohydroxylated CCNU metabolites	Mulcahy, 1985		
	Nitrogen mustard	Twentyman, 1982; Stratford et al., 1980		

[1]Contradictory results.

TABLE 2. *Potentiation of CCNU Activity by a Single, Large Dose of Misonidazole*

Dose (mmol/kg)	Tumor	Dose-modifying factor	Therapeutic gain factor	References
1.25	KHT[1]	1.9	ND	Siemann, 1981
	KHT[2]	1.3	ND	Siemann, 1982
2.5	KHT[1]	2.1	1.7[3]	Siemann, 1981
	KHT[2]	1.5	1.4[3]	Lee and Workman, 1983
	KHT[2]	1.7	1.4[3]–1.7[4]	Siemann, 1982
	9L[1]	1.0	ND	Wheeler et al., 1984
	9L[1]	>1.0[7]	ND	Wheeler et al., 1984
	L1210[1,8]	>1.0	ND	Wheeler et al., 1984
	L1210/BCNU[1,9]	1.0	ND	Wheeler et al., 1984
	RIF-1[2]	1.3	ND	Twentyman and Workman, 1982
	MT-1[2]	1.5	1.3[3]–1.5[4]	Siemann, 1982
3.75	KHT[1]	1.7–1.8	1.1[6]–1.3[5]	Hirst et al., 1982
	SCCVII/St[1]	1.7–1.8	1.1[6]–1.3[5]	Hirst et al., 1982
	EMT6[1]	1.7–1.8	1.1[6]–1.3[5]	Hirst et al., 1982
5.0	KHT[1]	2.4	1.7[3]	Siemann, 1981
	KHT[2]	1.9	1.4[2]	Siemann et al., 1983
	KHT[2,8]	1.9	ND	Mulcahy and Siemann, 1983
	KHT/CCR[2,10]	1.9	ND	Mulcahy and Siemann, 1983
	KHT[2]	1.9	1.4[3]–1.9[4]	Siemann, 1982
	RIF-1[2]	2.0	1.4[3]–2.0[4]	Siemann, 1982

[1]Tumor response measured by clonogenic cell survival assay.
[2]Tumor response measured by regrowth delay assay.
[3]$LD_{50/7d}$ or $LD_{50/30d}$.
[4]Normal tissue toxicity assessed by peripheral white blood cell depression.
[5]Normal tissue toxicity assessed by bone marrow CFUs.
[6]Normal tissue toxicity assessed by spermatozoa counts at 29 days.
[7]Tumor made artificially hypoxic.
[8]Parent line.
[9]Cell line made resistant to BCNU.
[10]Cell line made resistant to CCNU.
ND = not determined.

In addition to CCNU, other nitrosoureas with differing lipophilicity (see Fig. 2 for chemical structures) have also been investigated (Clutterbuck et al., 1982; Mulcahy, 1982; Lee and Workman, 1984b; Wong et al., 1989, 1990). Available data show that MISO enhanced the antitumor action of lipophilic nitrosoureas (e.g. MeCCNU and BCNU) but had no effect on the hydrophilic chlorozotocin (CHLZ) (Mulcahy, 1982; Wong et al., 1990).

2.2.2. *Melphalan* (*MEL*)

Table 4 lists all the data available for large, single doses of MISO given more or less simultaneously (± 1 hr) with MEL (see Fig. 3 for chemical structure). Overall, there appears to be a threshold dose of greater than 2.5 mmol/kg for effective chemosensitization. Above the threshold dose, enhancement has been fairly consistently obtained but the magnitude of enhancement (DMF) was variable, possibly dependent on tumor type. Mainly because of the variability of the DMF for tumor response, agreement on the extent of therapeutic gain has not been universal. In several cases where DMFs were low no therapeutic gain was apparent.

Other nitroimidazole hypoxic cell radiosensitizers have also been tested (Table 5) but with only limited success. SR 2508, metronidazole (METRO) and Ro 07-9963 were generally inactive (Hinchliffe and McNally, 1984) except at very high dose (8 mmol/kg). Sheldon et al. (1982) found significant activity for relatively low doses (2.5 mmol/kg) of Ro 07-9963 and METRO in the MT tumor. BENZO and Ro 07-1902 were as effective as MISO at optimal doses (Twentyman and Workman, 1983a; Sheldon and Batten, 1982) but they also enhanced normal tissue toxicity to a similar extent (Twentyman and Workman, 1983a). The most promise was shown by RSU 1069 which was active at 10-fold lower doses than MISO (Adams et al., 1984a; Siemann et al., 1984).

TABLE 3. *Potentiation of CCNU Activity by a Single, Large Dose of Misonidazole Analogs*

Modifiers	Dose (mmol/kg)	Tumor	Dose-modifying factor	Therapeutic gain factor	References
SR 2508	2.5	KHT[2]	1.0	ND	Workman and Twentyman, 1982
	3.75	KHT[1]	1.0	ND	Hirst et al., 1983
	3.75	SCCVII/st[1]	1.0	ND	Hirst et al., 1983
	5.0	KHT[2]	1.0	ND	Siemann, 1982
	5.0	RIF-1[2]	> 1.0[7]	ND	Siemann, 1982
Ro 07-9963	2.5	KHT[2]	1.0	ND	Siemann, 1982
	5.0	KHt[2]	1.0	ND	Siemann, 1982
Metronidazole	2.5	KHT[2]	1.0	ND	Workman and Twentyman, 1982
	2.5	RIF-1[1]	1.0	ND	Twentyman and Workman, 1982
	5.0	KHT[2]	1.0	ND	Siemann, 1982
Ro 07-1902	2.5	KHT[1]	2.5	1.6[4]–1.7[3]	Twentyman and Workman, 1983a
Ro 03-8799	2.5	MT[1]	1.5	ND	Sheldon and Gibson, 1984
Benznidazole	0.3	KHT[1]	2.0	1.5[3]	Siemann et al., 1983
	0.3	KHT[2]	1.9	1.4[3]	Siemann et al., 1983
	0.3	KHT[2]	2.0	1.6[3]–1.7[4]	Twentyman and Workman, 1983a
	0.3	RIF-1[1]	1.8	1.3[3]	Siemann et al., 1983
	2.0	KHT[1]	2.7	< 0.68[5]–1.5[6]	Hirst et al., 1983
	2.0	SCC VII/st[1]	1.9	< 0.6[5]–1.1[6]	Hirst et al., 1983
RSU 1069	0.38	KHT[1]	1.9	1.6[3,4]	Siemann et al., 1985
RSU 1164	2.0	KHT[1]	1.6	1.6[5]	Siemann, 1989
RSU 1165	1.0	KHT[1]	1.5	1.5[5]	Siemann, 1989

[1]Tumor response measured by clonogenic cell survival assay.
[2]Tumor response measured by regrowth delay assay.
[3]$LD_{50/7d}$ or $LD_{50/30d}$.
[4]Normal tissue toxicity assessed by peripheral while blood cell depression.
[5]Normal tissue toxicity assessed by spermatozoa counts at 29 days.
[6]Normal tissue toxicity assessed by bone marrow CFU-S assay.
ND = not determined.

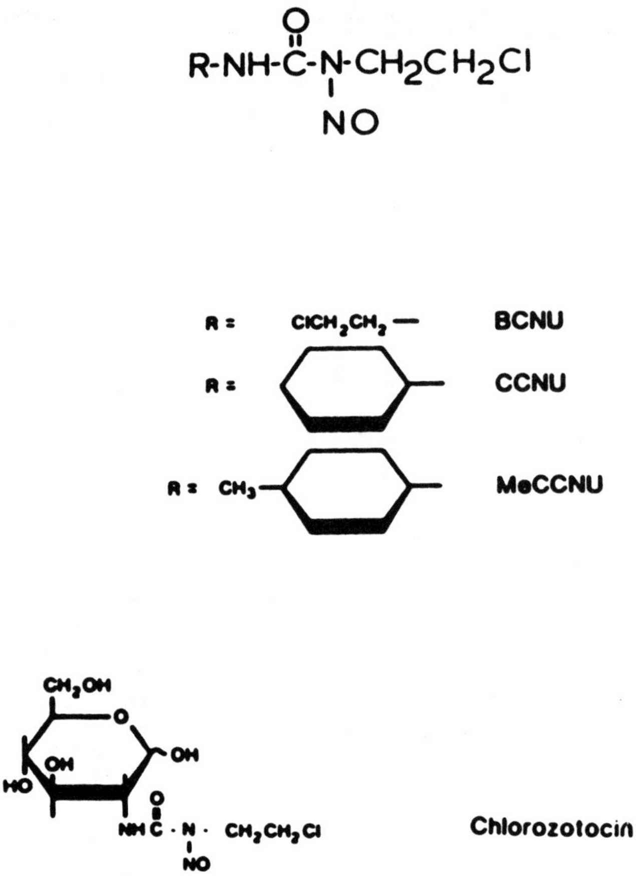

FIG. 2. Structures of the nitrosourea antitumor agents.

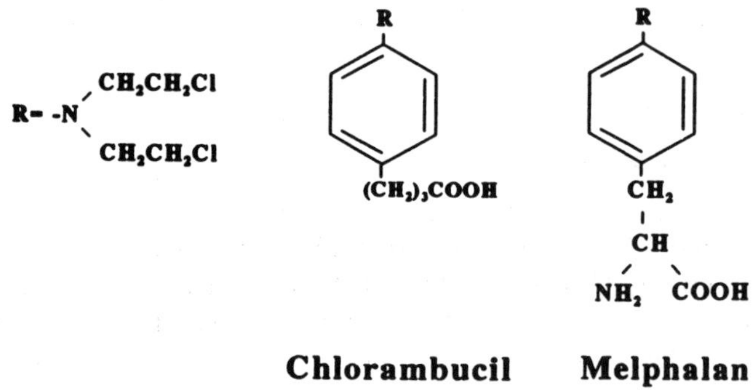

FIG. 3. Structures of the bifunctional nitrogen mustards chlorambucil and melphalan.

Evidence of enhancement of the clinical activity of melphalan by MISO was obtained in early clinical trials (Coleman et al., 1983, 1988b).

2.2.3. *Chlorambucil* (*CHL*)

Although clear enhancement of tumor response to CHL (see Fig. 3 for chemical structure) was readily achieved with 2.5 mmol/kg MISO, normal tissue toxicity was increased equally and there was no therapeutic gain (Workman and Twentyman, 1982). Since CHL and MEL are bifunctional nitrogen mustards with similar structures and mechanism of action (see Fig. 3

TABLE 4. *Potentiation of Melphalan Activity by a Single, Large Dose of Misonidazole Analogs*

Dose (mmol/kg)	Tumor	Dose-modifying factor	Therapeutic gain factor	References
1.65	Lewis lung carcinoma	>1.0	ND	Rose et al., 1980
2.5	SQ-1	1.0	ND	Fu and Phillips, 1981
	RIF-1	1.0	ND	Twentyman and Workman, 1982
	RIF-1[1]	1.0	ND	Twentyman and Workman, 1982
	KHT	1.0	ND	Twentyman and Workman, 1982
	EMT6	1.0	ND	Twentyman and Workman, 1982
	SA FA	1.4	ND	Randhawa et al., 1985
	MT[1]	1.7	ND	Sheldon et al., 1982
	KHT	1.0	1.0[2]	Lee and Workman, 1986a
3.0–5.0	M5075	1.9–2.2	1.6–1.8[4]	Clement et al., 1980
3.75	Lewis lung carcinoma	2.0	ND	Stephens et al., 1981
	RIF-1	1.4	ND	Horsman et al., 1984
4.0	CA NT	1.1–1.5	1.0[2]	Randhawa et al., 1982
	WH FIB	1.4–2.0	ND	McNally et al., 1983
	WH FIB[1]	2.7	ND	McNally et al., 1983
5.0	HX34	>1.0	ND	Clutterbuck et al., 1982
	HX47	>1.0	ND	Clutterbuck et al., 1982
	H32[1]	1.9	ND	Stephens et al., 1981
	WH FIB[1]	2.7	ND	Martin et al., 1981
	Lewis lung carcinoma[1]	2.7	1.8[3]–2.1[4]	Rose et al., 1980
	SA FA	3.1	2.1[2]	Randhawa et al., 1982
	SA FA	2.1 ± 0.2	ND	Randhawa et al., 1985
	RIF-1	1.5–2.0	1.0[2]	Twentyman and Workman, 1983a
	KHT	1.4	ND	Siemann et al., 1984
	KHT	1.35–1.55	1.0[2]	Lee and Workman, 1986a

[1]Tumor response measured by clonogenic cell survival assay.
[2]$LD_{50/7d}$ or $LD_{50/30d}$.
[3]Normal tissue toxicity assessed by bone marrow CFU-S assay.
[4]Normal tissue toxicity assessed by intestine micro-colony assay.
ND = not determined.

for chemical structures), elucidation of the reason for the differences in therapeutic gain has shed light on the mechanism of chemosensitization (Lee and Workman, 1986a).

2.2.4. *Cyclophosphamide* (*CP*)

In general, a threshold dose of 2.5 mmol/kg MISO was found to be necessary for chemosensitization (McNally, 1982). Other nitroimidazoles have also been tested including Ro 03-8799 (Sheldon and Gibson, 1984; Hinchliffe and McNally, 1984; Chaplin et al., 1984), BENZO (Twentyman and Workman, 1983a), Ro 07-9963 (McNally et al., 1983), SR 2508 (Hirst et al., 1984; Hinchliffe and McNally, 1984), Ro 07-1902 (Twentyman and Workman, 1983b; Chaplin et al., 1984) and METRO (Twentyman and Workman, 1982; Chaplin et al., 1984). In general, it has been found that none of the above was better than MISO and some were completely ineffective.

3. METABOLIC BASIS OF CHEMOSENSITIZATION

Research in the area of anticancer drug chemosensitization by nitroimidazoles and other chemical modifiers has been spurred consistently in the past by the search for the mechanism(s) of action of these agents. A variety of mechanisms of chemosensitization have been proposed (for reviews see Brown, 1982; Rauth, 1984). Compelling evidence suggests that, depending on experimental conditions, two major categories of mechanism are responsible for chemosensitization: those dependent on hypoxia and those related to pharmacokinetic modification.

TABLE 5. *Potentiation of Melphalan Activity by a Single, Large Dose of Misonidazole Analogs*

Modifiers	Dose (mmol/kg)	Tumor	Dose-modifying factor	Therapeutic gain factor	References
SR 2508	5.0	WH FIB[1]	1.0	ND	Hinchliffe and McNally, 1984
	5.0	SA F[2]	1.0	ND	Hinchliffe and McNally, 1984
Ro 07-9963	2.5	MT[1]	1.7	ND	Sheldon et al., 1982
	4.0	WH FIB[1]	1.0	ND	Hinchliffe and McNally, 1984
	8.0	WH FIB[1]	1.6	ND	Hinchliffe and McNally, 1984
Metronidazole	2.5	RIF-1[1]	1.0	N.D.	Twentyman and Workman, 1982
	2.5	RIF-1[2]	1.0	ND	Twentyman and Workman, 1982
	2.5	MT[1]	1.6	ND	Sheldon et al., 1982
Ro 07-1902	2.5	RIF-1[2]	1.5–2.0	1.0[3]	Twentyman and Workman, 1983a
Ro 03-8799	2.5	MT[1]	2.3	ND	Adams et al., 1984a
	2.5	MT[1]	2.2	ND	Sheldon et al., 1982
	2.5	MT[1]	1.5[4]	ND	Sheldon and Gibson, 1984
	2.5	MT[1]	2.0[5]	ND	Sheldon and Gibson, 1984
Benznidazole	0.3	RIF-1[2]	< 1.5	1.0[3]	Twentyman and Workman, 1983a
	0.3	KHT[1]	1.5	ND	Siemann et al., 1984
	2.5	MT[1]	2.0	ND	Sheldon et al., 1982
RSU 1069	0.38	MT[1]	3.0	ND	Adams et al., 1984a
	0.38	MT[1]	2.8	ND	Adams et al., 1984b
	0.38	KHT[1]	1.6	ND	Siemann et al., 1984

[1]Tumor response measured by clonogenic cell survival assay.
[2]Tumor response measured by regrowth delay assay.
[3]$LD_{50/7d}$ or $LD_{50/30d}$.
[4]Intramuscular tumor implant.
[5]Subcutaneous tumor implant.
ND = not determined.

3.1. Hypoxia-Dependent Mechanisms

Studies in vitro, in which cells were exposed to MISO under aerobic and anaerobic conditions for several hours before treatment with cytotoxic drugs, have demonstrated much greater sensitivity of hypoxic cells to the chemosensitizing action of MISO (Brown, 1982). Under hypoxic conditions MISO undergoes nitroreduction which generates cytotoxic metabolites such as the nitroso and hydroxylamine derivatives and other reactive intermediates (Rauth, 1984). Most investigators favor the idea that these metabolites are responsible for MISO cytotoxicity and may also be involved in chemosensitization. Evidence in support of the latter hypothesis includes, firstly, the findings of Mulcahy (1984) that the oxygen tensions required for chemosensitization by MISO were similar to those required for MISO-induced cytotoxicity. Secondly, chemosensitization in vitro by MISO required a preincubation period of several hours (Siemann, 1984) during which reductive metabolites of MISO were shown to accumulate (Taylor and Rauth, 1978; Varghese et al., 1976; Wong et al., 1978). Thirdly, it has been demonstrated that the extent of metabolic accumulation is correlated with MISO cytotoxicity (Taylor and Rauth, 1978).

Evidence for the requirement of hypoxia in vivo is more indirect. Firstly, results from studies with mouse tumors of different sizes and hypoxic fractions showed that the MISO enhancement of cytotoxic drug toxicity was lower in small tumors containing few hypoxic cells than in bigger tumors with larger hypoxic cell fractions (Martin et al., 1981; Sheldon and Batten, 1982; Spooner et al., 1982). Secondly, in the intracranially and subcutaneously implanted rat 9L tumor which lacks hypoxic cells, a large dose of MISO was shown to be ineffective in enhancing the toxicity of CCNU and BCNU (Wheeler et al., 1984). In contrast, potentiation was obtained when the tumors were made hypoxic before treatment with CCNU (Wheeler et al., 1984). Finally, cell sorting studies in the KHT mouse tumor have shown that the greatest enhancement of CCNU toxicity by MISO was found in those tumor cell subpopulations which also contained the majority of the hypoxic cells (Hill et al., 1984). This evidence does not preclude the possibility of other explanations, such as differential drug penetration in different types and sizes of tumor. In addition, whereas chemosensitization could often be demonstrated with multiple injections of nitroimidazoles to maintain low plasma levels, pharmacokinetic changes were often not seen (McNally et al., 1988; Roizin-Towle et al., 1982; Twentyman and Workman, 1983b).

3.1.1. *The Role of Reductive Bioactivation*

Many solid tumors have a poor blood supply and contain regions of extremely low oxygen tensions. Under such 'hypoxic' conditions, nitroimidazole chemosensitizers can undergo reductive bioactivation at the functional nitro group to form unstable intermediates which have been strongly implicated as the active species responsible for cytotoxicity and chemosensitization activity. These reductive reactions, which are inhibited or reversed by oxygen, are mediated by a variety of intracellular enzyme systems including the microsomal NADPH:cytochrome P450 (cytochrome c) reductase, microsomal cytochrome P450, cytosolic xanthine oxidase, aldehyde oxidase and DT-diaphorase (Josephy et al., 1981; Clarke et al., 1982; Hewick, 1982; Masana et al., 1982; McLane et al., 1983; Riley and Workman, 1992; Walton and Workman, 1987; Walton et al., 1989).

The reductive metabolism of the nitro group in nitroimidazoles to the final corresponding amine product requires the addition of up to six electrons (Wardman, 1977; Knox et al., 1983). The initial reduction pathway is assumed to involve the addition of a single electron to form the nitro radical anion (Whillans and Whitmore, 1981; Willson et al., 1974). Subsequently, several short-lived reactive intermediates, such as the hydroxylamine (Perez-Rayes et al., 1980; Sealy et al., 1978), are produced through further addition of up to five electrons to form the terminal amine derivative (McClelland et al., 1984).

Amine metabolites of nitroimidazoles have been identified in the urine of rats, dogs, monkeys and humans (Flockhart et al., 1978; Schwartz and Hofheinz, 1982). The precise molecular mechanism of nitroimidazole nitroreduction is not well documented. Using a liver microsomal enzyme system, Workman and coworkers showed that both BENZO and the dinitrophenyl azirdine CB 1954 were readily reduced to their amino derivatives (Walton and Workman, 1987; Walton et al., 1989). These nitroreduction reactions were inhibited by oxygen and required reduced cofactors (e.g.

NADPH). Further studies focused on individual enzymes using purified preparations and demonstrated a major role for cytochrome P450 reductase in the catalysis of the initial steps of BENZO reduction, while the terminal amine formation step is mediated predominantly by P450 (Walton et al., 1989).

The precise role and contribution of each reductive enzyme in the bioactivation of the nitroimidazoles in situ is still unclear, especially at the tumor cell level. Knox et al., (1988) have shown that CB 1954 is activated by DT-diaphorase purified from the drug-sensitive Walker rat tumor. Workman and colleagues further demonstrated that DT-diaphorase obtained from the human HT29 colon tumor can also catalyze the nitroreduction of CB 1954 to the highly toxic 4-hydroxylamine (Walton et al., 1992a).

3.1.2. *Depletion of Endogenous Non-Protein Thiols*

It is well established that endogenous thiols, particularly glutathione (GSH), play an important role in the cellular defence against cytotoxic insults (Arrick and Nathan, 1984). Nitroimidazoles have been shown to deplete the level of thiols in hypoxic tumor cells, an effect which has been correlated with enhanced toxicity (Roizin-Towle et al., 1982). The involvement of endogenous cellular thiols was further illustrated by the findings that exogenous thiols such as cysteamine (Roizin-Towle et al., 1982) or dithiothreitol (Smith et al., 1982) protect cells from the toxicity of MEL in vitro. In addition, agents such as diethyl maleate and buthionine sulfoximine, which deplete cellular GSH, are able to increase the chemosensitization efficacy of nitroimidazoles (Roizin-Towle, 1985; Siemann et al., 1989).

However, two major pieces of evidence suggest that depletion of thiols is not the only factor involved in chemosensitization. Firstly, for a given level of thiol depletion, enhancement of MEL toxicity was much greater following preincubation with MISO than with diethyl maleate and buthionine sulfoximine (Taylor et al., 1982, 1983; Roizin-Towle, 1985). Secondly, it was found that the effects of MISO completely disappeared when cells pretreated with MISO were allowed to recover in air for 6 hr, yet during this time only 30% of thiols were restored (Roizin-Towle et al., 1982).

3.1.3. *Enhancement of DNA Damage and Inhibition of Repair*

It has been well established that MISO preincubation can cause DNA single strand breaks in vitro (Olive and McCalla, 1977; Olive, 1980; Palcic and Skarsgard, 1978). Alkaline elution studies revealed that MISO enhanced the amount of DNA cross-linking produced by MEL in Chinese hamster ovary cells in vitro, and by nitrogen mustard (Murray and Meyn, 1984a,b) and MEL (Murray and Meyn, 1983) in a mouse tumor in vivo. Furthermore, the enhancement was greater in the tumor than in normal tissues and it was suggested that these results provided an explanation for both the enhancement of tumor response and the therapeutic gain (Murray and Meyn, 1983). However, it should be pointed out that the increase in DNA cross-linking caused by MISO can be due to either enhanced DNA damage or to decreased DNA repair, and thus it is not possible to deduce the mechanism of action of MISO by the determination of the amount of cross-linking alone (Murray and Meyn, 1983). Data from Taylor et al. (1983) suggest that inhibition of initial monoadduct repair is responsible.

Inhibition of potentially lethal damage (PLD) repair has also been implicated as a possible mechanism of chemosensitization, but mainly for the nitrosoureas. It was found for a series of nitrosoureas including CCNU, BCNU and CHLZ that the degree of chemosensitization obtained for these agents directly correlated with the extent of inhibition of PLD repair. However, similar studies carried out with CP and MEL have in the main shown no effect on PLD repair. For CP, some early results showed inhibition of PLD repair in mouse tumors by MISO (Martin et al., 1981; Law et al., 1981), but no effects on PLD repair were found subsequently by others (Siemann and Mulcahy, 1982; Spooner et al., 1982; Chaplin et al., 1984). For MEL, no effect no PLD has been found (Sheldon and Batten, 1982; Siemann and Mulcahy, 1982; Stephens et al., 1981; Horsman et al., 1984; Rose et al., 1980). Overall, it is clear that, with the possible exception of the nitrosoureas, inhibition of PLD repair probably is not responsible for chemosensitization in vivo.

TABLE 6. *The Effects of Nitroimidazole Chemosensitizers on the Pharmacokinetics of some Chemotherapeutic Agents by Nitroimidazoles*

Modified pharmacokinetics				Non-modified pharmacokinetics			
Cytotoxic agents	Sensitizers	Sensitizer dose (mmol/kg)	References	Cytotoxic agents	Sensitizers	Sensitizer dose (mmol/kg)	References
CCNU	MISO	≥ 0.3	Lee and Workman, 1983	CCNU	RSU 1069	0.24	Lee and Workman, 1984b
	Benznidazole	≥ 0.05	Lee and Workman, 1984b				
	Benznidazole	0.093	Roberts et al., 1984[1]				
	Ro 05-9963	2.5	Lee et al., 1984b				
BCNU	MISO	≥ 0.3	Lee and Workman, 1984b	CHLZ	MISO	≥ 2.5	Lee and Workman, 1984b
	MISO	2.5	Wong et al., 1989				
5-FU	MISO	2 g/m^2	McDermott et al., 1983[1]				
CHL	MISO	≤ 2.5	Lee and Workman, 1986a	CHL	Ro 05-9963	2.5	Lee and Workman, 1986a
	Benznidazole	≤ 0.3	Lee and Workman, 1986a				
	SKF 525A	0.13	Lee and Workman, 1986a				
MEL	MISO	≤ 3.0	Hinchliffe et al., 1983	MEL	SR-2508	≥ 5.0	
					MISO	≤ 0.5	Hinchliffe et al., 1983
CP	MISO	≤ 3.0	Hinchliffe et al., 1983				

[1]Human studies, otherwise data are for mice or rats.

3.2. Mechanisms Related to Modification of Cytotoxic Drug Pharmacokinetics

Nitroimidazoles contain the parent heterocycle imidazole, a functional group well known for its inhibitory effect on hepatic drug metabolizing enzymes (Testa and Jenner, 1981). Inhibition of drug metabolism by nitroimidazoles can lead to profound pharmacokinetic changes. Several groups have shown that the pharmacokinetics of anticancer drugs are altered by a single, large dose of MISO (Table 6). These alterations invariably involved the reduction of the clearance of the cytotoxic agents leading to increased drug exposure (Hinchliffe et al., 1983; Lee and Workman, 1983, 1984a; Wong et al., 1989, 1990).

3.2.1. *Nitroimidazole Structure–Activity Relationships*

A number of structure–activity relationship studies have been carried out to attempt to relate the chemical characteristics of nitroimidazoles to their chemosensitization activity (Workman and Twentyman, 1982; Hirst et al., 1984; Hinchliffe and McNally, 1984; Brown and Workman, 1980). Workman and Twentyman (1982) found that only compounds within a certain range of octanol/water partition coefficients were effective chemosensitizers. In contrast to radiosensitization, electron affinity was not an important factor. Consistent with these results was the finding that equally electron-affinic but more hydrophilic analogs such as SR 2508 and Ro 07-9963 (Table 3) were relatively ineffective chemosensitizers. Compounds more lipophilic than MISO such as BENZO and Ro 07-1902 were more potent chemosensitizers.

3.2.2. *Pharmacokinetic Basis for Selective Antitumor Activity and Therapeutic Gain*

As for chemosensitization potency, the ability of various nitroimidazole chemosensitizers to modify cytotoxic drug pharmacokinetics appeared also to be dependent on their lipophilicity. The most comprehensive studies have been with the combination of MISO and CCNU. Substantial information is also available for MEL, CHL and CP.

3.2.2.1. *CCNU.* In a series of detailed studies, Lee and Workman (1983, 1984a) reported the effects of MISO and analogs upon the pharmacokinetics of CCNU in mice. When administered alone, CCNU follows biexponential kinetics, with a rapid initial α-phase followed by a slower terminal β-phase (Fig. 4). The α and β components are normally regarded as the distribution and elimination phases, respectively. There is evidence that a considerable amount of metabolism occurs during the α-phase, and the terminal elimination may be limited by the rate of redistribution of CCNU from tissue depots back into the plasma (Lee and Workman, 1983). It has been shown unequivocally that a single dose of MISO can significantly reduce the plasma clearance of CCNU (Lee and Workman, 1983; Hill and Siemann, 1984). As shown in Fig. 4, MISO increased the half-life of the α-phase ($t_{1/2\alpha}$) from 2.3 min to 5.8 min, whereas the half-life of the β phase ($t_{\frac{1}{2}\beta}$) was not significantly changed. Peak CCNU concentration was not altered but the area under the curve ($AUC_{0-\infty}$) was increased by a factor of 1.7.

The pharmacokinetics of CCNU in two critical normal tissues, bone marrow and gut, resemble those seen in the plasma. In addition, the effects of MISO were also similar. The half-life of the α-phase was prolonged by MISO, but the terminal β-phase was not affected. Importantly, the peak concentration of CCNU was unaffected by MISO (Fig. 5). The lack of effect of MISO on peak CCNU concentration in these critical normal tissues is in marked contrast to its effect on peak tumor CCNU concentrations which were shown to be increased by MISO (Fig. 6). This difference between critical normal tissues and tumors has been proposed as a key reason for the therapeutic gain obtained with the combination of MISO and CCNU (Lee and Workman, 1984a). The differential effect of MISO is due to the fact that peak tumor concentrations lag behind the peak plasma concentrations, probably because of inadequate tumor blood supply, an effect not seen in the better perfused normal tissues. Blood flow is known to limit tissue penetration by drugs with high permeability such as CCNU (Levin et al., 1980). The reduction in the rate of CCNU clearance by MISO results in the maintenance of high plasma CCNU concentrations for a longer duration, and this in turn allows the tumor to attain a higher peak level. It is the resultant increase in tumor

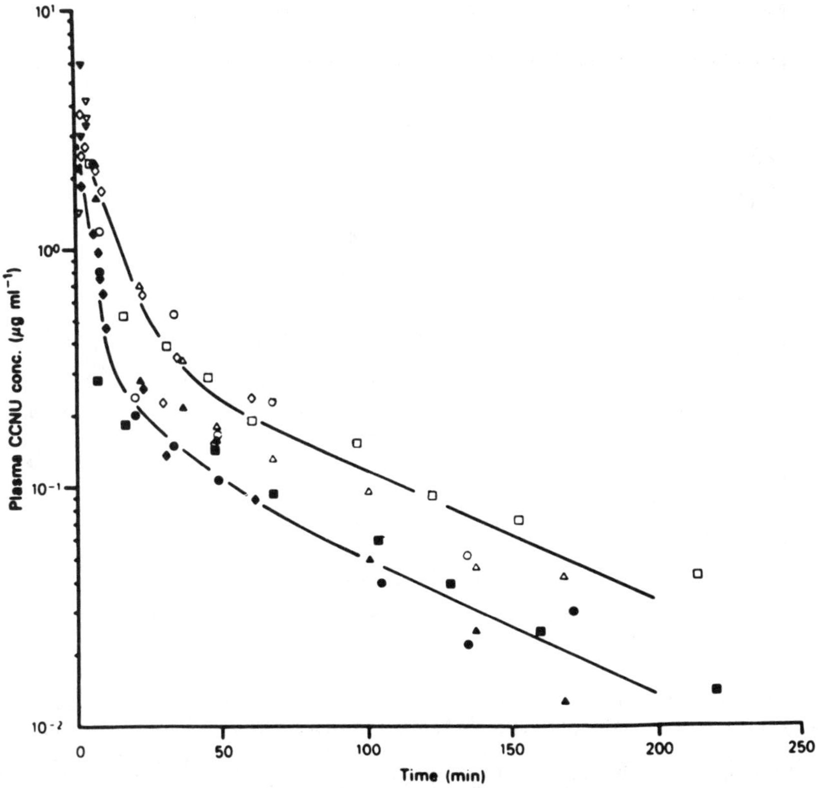

FIG. 4. The effects of 2.5 mmol/kg MISO given 30 min before on the pharmacokinetics of CCNU in mice. Solid symbols, 20 mg/kg CCNU alone; opened symbols, 20 mg/kg CCNU after MISO. Different symbols represent 5 independent experiments. Reprinted from Lee and Workman (1983), with permission of the copyright holder, Macmillan Journals Ltd., London.

CCNU concentration that is the basic cause of chemosensitization. By the same token, the lack of significant effect on CCNU concentration in critical normal tissues forms the basis for therapeutic gain.

3.2.3. *Inhibition of Hepatic P450 Monooxygenase—A Site of Sensitizer–Cytotoxic Drug Interaction*

There is considerable evidence that the nitroimidazole chemosensitizers are potent inhibitors of microsomal cytochrome P450-mediated hydroxylation of xenobiotics (Workman et al., 1983; Lee and Workman, 1986b, 1987). Inhibition can occur at concentrations of nitroimidazoles similar to those found in the plasma of mice treated with chemosensitizing doses of nitroimidazoles (Workman et al., 1986). In addition, it has been demonstrated by optical difference spectroscopy that nitroimidazoles are able to bind to cytochrome P450 (Lee and Workman, 1986b). The type II spectral change observed is indicative of the formation of nitrogenous ligands with the heme-iron of the cytochrome P450 (Jefcoate, 1978; Schenkman et al., 1981; Lee and Workman, 1986b), presumably through the free imidazole ring nitrogen.

As in the case with chemosensitization potency, the inhibitory potency of the various 2-nitroimidazoles on CCNU hydroxylation is highly dependent on lipophilicity (Fig. 7). The extremely lipophilic analogs Ro 07-1127 and benznidazole ($I_{50} \approx 0.4$ mM) were clearly the most potent inhibitors and in fact exhibited greater potency than the parent heterocycle imidazole ($I_{50} \approx 0.7$ mM). In marked contrast, the hydrophilic analog SR 2508 only showed activity at very high concentration ($I_{50} \approx 15$mM). MISO, with intermediate lipophilicity, exhibited intermediate potency ($I_{50} \approx 6$ mM).

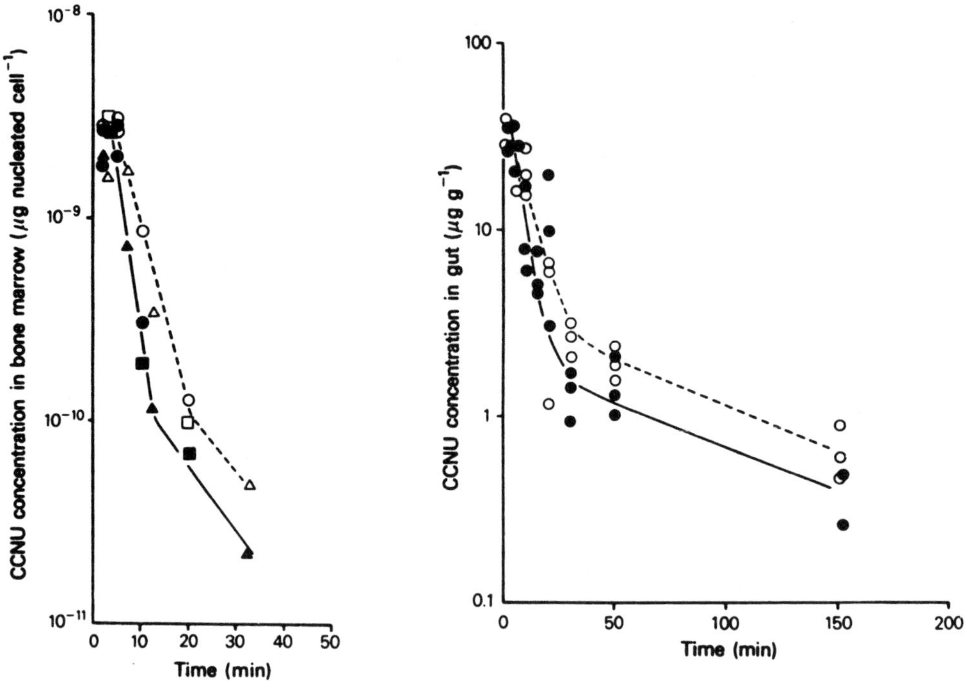

FIG. 5. Left panel. The effect of MISO (2.5 mmol/kg) on the pharmacokinetics of CCNU in the mouse bone marrow. Closed symbols, CCNU alone; opened symbols, CCNU + MISO. Right panel. The effect of MISO (2.5 mmol/kg) on the pharmacokinetics of CCNU in the mouse small intestine. Closed circles, CCNU alone; opened circles, CCNU + MISO. Reprinted from Lee and Workman (1984a), with permission of the copyright holder, Macmillan Journals Ltd., London.

4. CONCLUSIONS

Hypoxic cells in solid tumors are generally more resistant to radiotherapy and chemotherapy than their oxic counterparts. Low levels of oxygen and other nutrients encourage cells to proliferate slowly or enter a G_0-like state, thereby decreasing the response to cycle-specific drugs. Nitroimidazoles can exploit tumor hypoxia as a result of their bioreductive activation to toxic metabolites under low oxygen conditions. These metabolites can kill hypoxic tumor cells and also sensitize them to radiation and chemotherapy. This involves DNA damage, inhibition of repair and thiol depletion.

The position of chronically hypoxic cells in solid tumors, i.e. distal from the blood supply, can also lead to poor penetration of cytotoxic drugs. Hence drug levels in hypoxic tumor cells will lag behind those in the systemic circulation. By decreasing the rate of drug clearance from the blood, nitroimidazoles can allow more time for the tumor to be subjected to a higher level of drug, which in turn leads to greater killing of malignant cells.

This review has emphasized that both mechanisms can be involved in chemosensitization by nitroimidazoles, to an extent depending on the drugs concerned and the schedules of administration used. Both mechanisms could occur in humans. Hypoxia-mediated bioreductive chemosensitization is probably the preferred mechanism, since pharmacokinetic modulation introduces considerable complications. Although seen with CCNU and BENZO (Roberts et al, 1984), it is less likely with clinically-used doses of MISO and especially with the hydrophilic SR 2508.

Studies with MISO were dropped because of neurotoxicity and BENZO was also discarded after failing to show an advantage with CCNU in brain tumors. However studies with SR 2508 are continuing. In the future we are likely to see clinical trials involving combinations of cytotoxic drugs with aziridinyl nitroimidazoles such as RB 6145 and with other novel bioreductive agents such as the benzotriazine di-*N*-oxide tirapazamine (WIN 59075; SR 4233) (Zeman et al, 1986). Tirapazamine is activated by a variety of one-electron reducing enzymes under hypoxic conditions (Walton and Workman, 1990; Walton et al., 1992b) and shows promise in combination with alkylating agents and particularly cisplatin (Holden et al, 1992). Like tirapazamine, the indoloquinone EO9

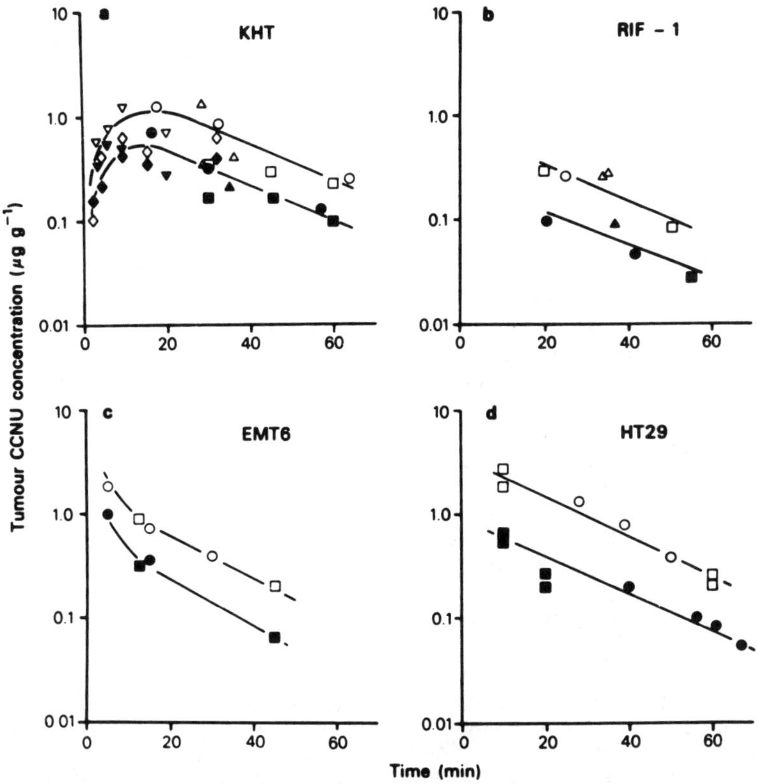

FIG. 6. The effects of 2.5 mmol/kg MISO on the concentration of CCNU in (a) KHT, (b) RIF-1, (c) EMT6 and (d) HT29 tumors. Solid symbols, 20 mg/kg CCNU alone. Opened symbols, CCNU + MISO. Each datum point is for 2 or 3 tumors. Reprinted from Lee and Workman (1983), with permission of the copyright holder, Macmillan Journals Ltd, London.

is undergoing Phase I clinical trial. This agent is activated particularly well by DT-diaphorase (Walton et al, 1991; 1992c). Since it is non-myelosuppressive (Hendriks et al, 1992), probably because of the low DT-diaphorase level in bone marrow (Lewis et al, 1993), clinical trials in combination with alkylating agents are probable. Additive killing of hypoxic and oxic populations is likely to be the major effect of such combinations but bioreductive chemosensitization is also quite feasible.

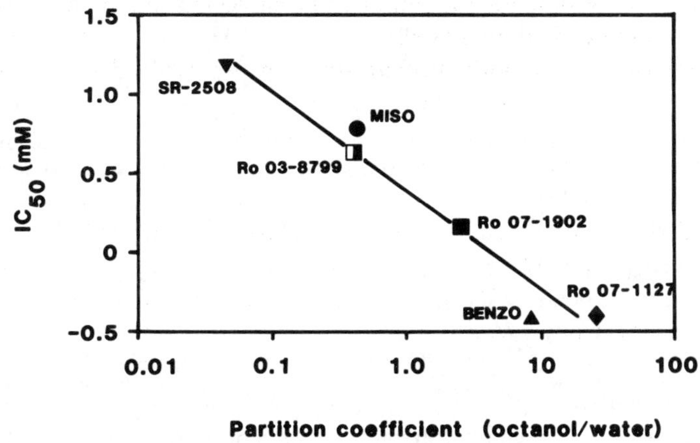

FIG. 7. The relationship between lipophilicity as measured by octanol–water (partition coefficient) and the inhibitory activity (I_{50}) of a range of 2-nitroimidazoles on CCNU metabolism.

DEDICATION

To the memory of our late friend and colleague, Dr Nic McNally.

REFERENCES

ADAMS, G. E., AHMED, I., SHELDON, P. W. and STRATFORD, I. J. (1984a) Radiation sensitization and chemopotentiation: RSU 1069, a compound more efficient than misonidazole in vivo and in vitro. *Br. J. Cancer* **49:** 571–577.

ADAMS, G. E., AHMED, I., SHELDON, P. W. and STRATFORD, I. J. (1984b) RSU 1069, a 2-nitroimidazole containing an alkylating group: high efficiency as a radio- and chemosensitizer in vivo and in vitro. *Int. J. Radiat. Oncol. biol. Phys.* **10:** 1653–1656.

ARRICK, B. A. and NATHAN, C. F. (1984) Glutathione as a determinent of therapeutic efficacy: a review. *Cancer Res.* **44:** 4224–4232.

BROWN, J. M. (1982) The mechanism of cytotoxicity and chemosensitization by misonidazole and other nitroimidazoles. *Int. J. Radiat. Oncol. biol. Phys.* **8:** 675–682.

BROWN, J. M. and HIRST, D. G. (1982) Effect of clinically relevant levels of misonidazole on the response of tumour and normal tissues in the mouse to alkylating agents. *Br. J. Cancer* **45:** 700–708.

BROWN, J. M. and WORKMAN, P. (1980) Partition coefficient as a guide to the development of radiosensitizers which are less toxic than misonidazole. *Radiat. Res.* **82:** 171–190.

CHAPLIN, D. J., SHELDON, P. W., AHMED, I. and ADAMS, G. E. (1984) Potentiation of cyclophosphamide cytotoxicity in vivo: a study with misonidazole and fifteen other 1-substituted 2-nitroimidazoles. *Int. J. Radiat. Oncol. biol. Phys.* **10:** 1647–1652.

CLARKE, E. D., GOULDING, K. H. and WARDMAN, P. (1982) Nitroimidazoles as anaerobic acceptors for xanthine oxidase. *Biochem. Pharmac.* **31:** 3237–3242.

CLEMENT, J. J. and JOHNSON, R. K. (1982) Evaluation of radiosensitizers in combination with chemotherapeutic agents in solid tumors. *Int. J. Radiat. Oncol. biol. Phys.* **8:** 631–634.

CLEMENT, J. J., GORMAN, M. S., WODINSKY, I., CUTANE, R. and JOHNSON, R. K. (1980) Enhancement of antitumor activity of alkylating agents by the radiation sensitizer misonidazole. *Cancer Res.* **40:** 4165–4172.

CLUTTERBUCK, R. D., MILLAR, J. L. and MCELWAIN, T. J. (1982) Misonidazole enhancement of the action of BCNU and melphalan against human melanoma xenografts. *Am. J. clin. Oncol.* **5:** 73–80.

COLEMAN, C. N., FRIEDMAN, M. K., JACOBS, C., HALSEY, J., IGNOFFO, R., LIEBEL, S., HIRST, V. K., GRIBBLE, M., CARTER, S. K. and PHILIPS, T. L. (1983) Phase 1 trial of intravenous L-phenylalanine mustard plus the sensitizer misonidazole. *Cancer Res.* **43:** 5022–5025.

COLEMAN, C. N., BUMP, E. A. and KRAMER, R. A. (1988a) Chemical modifiers of cancer treatment. *J. clin. Oncol.* **6:** 709–733.

COLEMAN, C. N., CARLSON, R. W., HALSEY, J., KOHLER, M., GRIBBLE, B. I. and JACOBS, C. (1988b) Enhancement of the clinical activity of melphalan by the hypoxic cell sensitizer misonidazole. *Cancer Res.* **48:** 3528–3532.

DOUBLE, J. A. and BIBBY, M. C. (1985) The effects of combinations of benznidazole and methyl CCNU on transplantable adenocarcinomas of the mouse colon. *Br. J. Cancer* **52:** 434–435.

DURAND, R. E. and CHAPLIN, D. J. (1987) Chemosensitization by misonidazole in CCNU-treated spheroids and tumours. *Br. J. Cancer* **56:** 103–109.

FLOCKHART, I. R., LARGE, P., TROUP, D., MALCOLM, S. L. and MARTEN, T. R. (1978) Pharmacokinetic and metabolic studies of the hypoxic cell radiosensitizer misonidazole. *Xenobiotica* **8:** 97–105.

FU, K. and PHILLIPS, T. L. (1981) *Proceedings of the 29th Annual Meeting of the Radiation Research Society,* p. 9091.

HENDRIKS, H. R., PIZAO, P. E., BERGER, D. P., KOOISTRA, K. L., BIBBY, M. C., BOVEN, E., DREEF-VAN DER MEULLER, H. C., HENRAR, R. E. C., FIEBIG, H. H., DOUBLE, J. A., HORNSTRA, H. W., PINEDO, H. M., WORKMAN, P. and SCHWARTSMANN, G. (1992) EO9: a novel bioreductive alkylating indoloquinone with preferential solid tumour activity and lack of bone marrow toxicity. *Eur. J. Cancer,* **29A:** 897–906.

HENWICK, D. S. (1982) Reductive metabolism of nitrogen-containing functional groups. In: *Metabolic Basis of Detoxification; Metabolism of Functional Groups,* pp. 151–170, JACOBY, W. B., BEND, J. R. and CALDWELL, J. (eds) Academic Press, New York.

HILL, S. A. and SIEMANN, D. W. (1984) Chemosensitization in vivo: no loss of sensitization with fractionation. *Br. J. Cancer* **50:** 509–517.

HILL, S. A., KENG, P. C. and SIEMANN, D. W. (1984) Survival in subpopulations of cells derived from solid KHT sarcomas by centrifugal elutriation following treatment with CCNU and MISO. *Int. J. Radiat. Oncol. biol. Phys.* **10:** 1615–1618.

HINCHLIFFE, M. and MCNALLY, N. J. (1984) A comparison of the ability of some radiosensitizers undergoing clinical trials to act as chemosensitizers. *Int. J. Radiat. Oncol. biol. Phys.* **10:** 1635–1640.

HINCHLIFFE, M., MCNALLY, N. J. and STRATFORD, M. R. L. (1983) The effect of radiosensitizers on the pharmacokinetics of melphalan and cyclophosphamide in the mouse. *Br. J. Cancer* **48:** 375–383.

HIRST, D. G., BROWN, J. M. and HAZLEHURST, J. L. (1982) Enhancement of CCNU cytotoxicity by misonidazole: possible therapeutic gain. *Br. J. Cancer* **46:** 109–116.

HIRST, D. G., BROWN, J. M. and HAZLEHURST, J. L. (1983) Effect of partition coefficient on the ability of nitroimidazoles to enhance the cytotoxicity of 1-(2-chloroethyl)-3-cyclohexyl-1-nitrosourea. *Cancer Res.* **43:** 1961–1965.

HIRST, D. G., HORSMAN, M. R., BROWN, J. M. and HAZELHURST, J. L. (1984) The effect of timing on chemosensitization by clinical levels of SR-2508. *Int. J. Radiat. Oncol. biol. Phys.* **10:** 1641–1645.

HOLDEN, S. A., TEICHER, G. A., ARA, G., HERMAN, T. S. and COLEMAN, C. N. (1992) Enhancement of alkylating agent activity by SR 4233 in the FSaIIc murine sarcoma. *J. natn. Cancer Inst.* **84:** 187–193.

HORSMAN, M. R., EVANS, J. W. and BROWN, J. M. (1984) Enhancement of melphalan-induced tumour cell killing by misonidazole: an interaction of competing mechanisms. *Br. J. Cancer* **50:** 305–316.

JEFCOATE, C. R. (1978) Measurement of substrate and inhibitor binding to microsomal cytochrome P450 by optical-difference spectroscopy. *Meth. Enzym.* **52:** 258–279.

JENKINS, T. C., NAYLOR, M. A., O'NEILL, P., THREADGILL, M. D., COLES, S., STRATFORD, I. J., ADAMS, G. E., FIELDEN, E. M. SUTO, M. J. and STIER, M. A. (1990) Synthesis and evaluation of 1-[3-(2-haloethylamino)propyl]-2-nitroimidazoles as prodrugs of RSU 1069 and its analogues, which are radiosensitizers and bioreductively activated cytotoxins. *J. med. Chem.* **33:** 2603–2610.

JOSEPHY, P. D., PALCIC, B. and SKARSGARD, L. D. (1981) Reduction of misonidazole and its derivatives by xanthine oxidase. *Biochem. Pharmac.* **30:** 849–853.

KENNEDY, K. A., TEICHER, B. A., ROCKWELL, S. and SARTORELLI, A. C. (1980) The hypoxic tumor cell: a target for selective cancer chemotherapy. *Biochem. Pharmac.* **29:** 1–8.

KNOX, R. J., KNIGHT, R. C. and EDWARDS, D. I. (1983) Studies on the action of nitroimidazole drugs: the products of nitroimidazole reduction. *Biochem. Pharmac.* **32:** 2149–2156.

KNOX, R. J., FRIEDLOS, F., JARMAN, M. and ROBERTS, J. J. (1988) A new cytotoxic, DNA interstrand crosslinking agent 5-(aziridin-1-yl)-4-hydroxylamino-2-nitrobenzamide, is formed from 5-(aziridin-1-yl)-2,4-dinitrobenzamide (CB 1954) by a nitroreductase enzyme in Walker carcinoma cells. *Biochem. Pharmac.* **37:** 4661–4669.

LAW, M. P., HIRST, D. G. and BROWN, J. M. (1981) Enhancing effect of misonidazole on the response of the RIF-1 tumour to cyclophosphamide. *Br. J. Cancer* **44:** 208–218.

LEE, F. Y. F. and WORKMAN, P. (1983) Modification of CCNU pharmacokinetics by misonidazole—A major mechanism of chemosensitization in mice. *Br. J. Cancer* **47:** 659–669.

LEE, F. Y. F. and WORKMAN, P. (1984a) Misonidazole and CCNU—further evidence for a pharmacokinetic mechanism of chemosensitization and therapeutic gain. *Br. J. Cancer* **49:** 579–585.

LEE, F. Y. F. and WORKMAN, P. (1984b) Nitroimidazoles as modifiers of nitrosourea pharmacokinetics. *Int. J. Radiat. Oncol. biol. Phys.* **10:** 1627–1630.

LEE, F. Y. F. and WORKMAN, P. (1986a) Altered pharmacokinetics in the mechanism of chemosensitization: effects of nitroimidazoles and other chemical modifiers on the pharmacokinetics, antitumour activity and acute toxicity of selected nitrogen mustards. *Cancer Chemother. Pharmac.* **17:** 30–37.

LEE, F. Y. F. and WORKMAN, P. (1986b) Interaction of nitroimidazole sensitizers with drug metabolizing enzymes—spectral and kinetic studies. *Int. J. Radiat. Oncol. biol. Phys.* **12:** 1383–1387.

LEE, F. Y. F. and WORKMAN, P. (1987) Misonidazole and benznidazole inhibition of CCNU hydroxylation by mouse liver microsome in vitro. *Biochem. Pharmac.* **36:** 1349–1355.

LEVIN, V. A., WRIGHT, D. C., LANDAHL, H. D., PATLAK, C. S. and CSEJTEY, J. (1980) In situ drug delivery. *Br. J. Cancer* **41** (Suppl. IV): 74–78.

LEWIS, A. D., HOLYOAKE, T. L., DUNLOP, D. J., PRAGNELL, J. D. and WORKMAN, P. (1993) Lack of myelosuppression with EO9 in human and mouse bone marrow: correlation with low DT-diaphorase. *Proc. Am. Ass. Cancer Res.* **34:** 345.

MARTIN, W. M. C., MCNALLY, N. J and DE RONDE, J. (1981) The enhancement of the effect of cytotoxic drugs by radiosensitizers. *Br. J. Cancer* **43:** 756–766.

MASANA, M., DE TORANZO, G. D. and CASTRI, J. A. (1982) Reductive metabolism and activation of benznidazole. *Biochem. Pharmac.* **31:** 1041–1045.

MCCLELLAND, R. A., FULLER, J. R., SEAMAN, N. E., RAUTH, A. M. and BATTATELLA, R. (1984) 2-Hydroxylaminoimidazoles—Unstable intermediates in the reduction of 2-nitroimidazoles. *Biochem. Pharmac.* **33:** 303–309.

MCDERMOTT, B. J., VAN DEN BERG, H. W., MARTIN, W. M. C. and MURPHY, R. F. (1983) Pharmacokinetic rationale for the interaction of 5-fluorouracil and misonidazole in humans. *Br. J. Cancer* **48:** 705–710.

MCLANE, K. E., FISHER, J. and RAMAKRISHNAN, K. (1983) Reductive drug metabolism. *Drug Metab. Rev.* **14:** 741–799.

MCNALLY, N. J. (1982) Enhancement of chemotherapy agents. *Int. J. Radiat. Oncol. biol. Phys.* **8:** 593–598.

MCNALLY, N. J., HINCHLIFFE, M. and DE RONDE, J. (1983) Enhancement of the action of alkylating agents by single high, or chronic low doses of misonidazole. *Br. J. Cancer* **48:** 271–278.

MULCAHY, R. T. (1982) Chemical properties of nitrosoureas: implications for interaction with misonidazole. *Int. J. Radiat. Oncol. biol. Phys.* **8:** 599–602.

MULCAHY, R. T. (1984) Effect of oxygen on misonidazole chemosensitization and cytotoxicity in vitro. *Cancer Res.* **44:** 4409–4413.

MULCAHY, R. T. (1985) Chemopotentiation of CCNU metabolites by misonidazole. *Br. J. Cancer* **51:** 733–735.

MULCAHY, R. T. (1986a) Carbamoylation, inhibition of glutathione reductase and chemopotentiation of nitrosoureas by misonidazole. *Int. J. Radiat. Oncol. biol. Phys.* **12:** 1393–1395.

MULCAHY, R. T. (1986b) Cross-link formation and chemopotentiation of EMT-6/Ro cells exposed to MISO after CCNU treatment in vitro. *Int. J. Radiat. Oncol. biol. Phys.* **12:** 1389–1392.

MULCAHY, R. T. and SIEMANN, D. W. (1983) In vivo chemosensitization by misonidazole in sensitive and resistant tumor lines. *Cancer Res.* **43:** 4709–4713.

MULCAHY, R. T., SIEMANN, D. W. and SUTHERLAND, R. M. (1981) In vivo response of KHT sarcomas to combination chemotherapy with radiosensitizers and BCNU. *Br. J. Cancer* **43:** 93–99.

MULCAHY, R. T., SIEMANN, D. W. and SUTHERLAND, R. M. (1982) Nitrosourea–misonidazole combination chemotherapy: effect on KHT sarcomas, marrow stem cells and gut. *Br. J. Cancer* **45:** 835–842.

MULCAHY, R. T., DEMBS, N. L. and UBLACKER, G. A. (1984) Enhancement of nitrosourea cytotoxicity by misonidazole in vitro: correlation with carbamoylating potential. *Br. J. Cancer* **49:** 307–313.

MURRAY, D. and MEYN, R. E. (1983) Enhancement of DNA cross-linking activity of melphalan by misonidazole in vivo. *Br. J. Cancer* **47:** 195–203.

MURRAY, D. and MEYN, R. E. (1984a) Effect of misonidazole pretreatment on nitrogen mustard-induced DNA cross-linking in mouse tissues in vivo. *Br. J. Cancer* **50:** 801–808.

MURRAY, D. and MEYN, R. E. (1984b) Enhancement of the DNA cross-linking activity of nitrogen mustard by misonidazole and diethyl maleate in a mouse fibrosarcoma tumor in vivo. *Cancer Res.* **44:** 91–96.

OLIVE, P. L. (1980) Mechanisms of the in vitro toxicity of nitroheterocycles, including Flagyl and misonidazole. In: *Radiation Sensitizers—Their Use in the Clinical Management of Cancer*, BRADY, L. W. (ed.) Masson, New York.

OLIVE, P. L. and MCCALLA, D. R. (1977) Cytotoxicity and DNA damage to mammalian cells by nitrofurans. *Chem. Biol. Interact.* **16:** 223–233.

PALCIC, B. and SKARSGARD, L. D. (1978) Cytotoxicity of misonidazole and DNA damage in hypoxic mammalian cells. *Br. J. Cancer* **37** (Suppl. III): 54–59.

PEREZ-RAYES, E., KALYANARAMAN, B. and MASON, R. P. (1980) The reductive metabolism of metronidazole and ronidazole by aerobic liver microsomes. *Molec. Pharmac.* **17:** 239–244.

RANDHAWA, V. S., STEWART, F. A. and DENEKAMP, J. (1982) Chemosensitization of mouse tumour by misonidazole. *Int. J. Radiat. Oncol. biol. Phys.* **8:** 671–674.

RANDHAWA, V. S., STEWART, F. A., DENEKAMP, J. and STRATFORD, M. R. L. (1985) Factors influencing the chemosensitization of melphalan by misonidazole. *Br. J. Cancer* **51:** 219–228.

RAUTH, A. M. (1984) Pharmacology and toxicology of sensitizers: mechanism studies. *Int. J. Radiat. Oncol. biol. Phys.* **10:** 1293–1300.

RILEY, R. J. and WORKMAN, P. (1992) DT-diaphorase and cancer chemotherapy. *Biochem. Pharmac.* **43:** 1665–1669.

ROIZIN-TOWLE, L. (1985) Selective enhancement of hypoxic cell killing by melphalan via thiol depletion: in vitro studies with hypoxic cell sensitizers and buthionine sulfoximine. *J. natn. Cancer Inst.* **74:** 151–157.

ROIZIN-TOWLE, L. and HALL, E. J. (1981) Enhanced cytotoxicity of antineoplastic agents following prolonged exposure to misonidazole. *Br. J. Cancer* **44:** 201–207.

ROIZIN-TOWLE, L., HALL, E. J., FLYNN, M., BIAGLOW, J. E. and VARNES, M. E. (1982) Enhanced cytotoxicity of melphalan by prolonged exposure to nitroimidazoles: the role of endogenous thiols. *Int. J. Radiat. Oncol. biol. Phys.* **8:** 757–760.

ROBERTS, J. T., BLEEHEN, N. M., LEE, F. Y. F., WORKMAN, P. and WALTON, M. I. (1984) A phase I study of the combination of benznidazole and CCNU in man. *Int. J. Radiat. Oncol. biol. Phys.* **10:** 1745–1748.

ROSE, C. M., MILLAR, J. L., PEACOCK, J. H. and STEPHENS, T. C. (1980) The effect of misonidazole on in vivo tumor cell kill in Lewis lung carcinoma treated with melphalan or cyclophosphamide. In: *Radiation Sensitizers—Their Use in the Clinical Management of Cancer*, BRADY, L. W. (ed.) Masson, New York.

SCHWARTZ, D. E. and HOFHEINZ, W. (1982) Metabolism of nitroimidazoles. In: *Nitroimidazoles: Chemistry, Pharmacology and Clinical Applications. Life Sci. NATO Advanced Study Institute Series, Series A*, Vol. 42, pp. 189–201, BRECCIA, A., CAVALLERI, B. and ADAMS, G. E. (eds) Plenum Press, New York.

SEALY, R. C., SWARTZ, H. M. and OLIVE, P. L. (1978) Electron spin resonance frapping. Detection of superoxide formation during aerobic microsomal reduction of nitro-compounds. *Biochem. biophys. Res. Commun.* **82:** 680–684.

SCHENKMAN, J. B., SLIGER, S. G. and CINTI, D. L. (1981) Substrate interaction with cytochrome P450. *Pharmac. Ther.* **12:** 43–71.

SHELDON, P. W. and BATTEN, E. L. (1982) Potentiation in vivo of melphalan activity by nitroimidazole compounds. *Int. J. Radiat. Oncol. biol. Phys.* **8:** 635–637.

SHELDON, P. W. and GIBSON, P. (1984) Effect of the nitromidazole Ro 03-8799 on the activity of chemotherapeutic agents against a murine tumour in vivo. *Br. J. Cancer* **49:** 291–300.

SHELDON, P. W., BATTEN, E. L. and ADAMS, G. E. (1982) Potentiation of melphalan activity against a murine tumour by nitroimidazole compounds. *Br. J. Cancer* **46:** 525–531.

SIEMANN, D. W. (1981) In vivo combination of misonidazole and the chemotherapeutic agent CCNU. *Br. J. Cancer* **43:** 367–377.

SIEMANN, D. W. (1982) Response of murine tumours to combinations of CCNU with misonidazole and other radiation sensitizers. *Br. J. Cancer* **45:** 272–281.

SIEMAN, D. W. (1984) Modification of chemotherapy by nitroimidazoles. *Int. J. Radiat. Oncol. biol. Phys.* **10:** 1585–1594.

SIEMANN, D. W. (1989) The chemosensitizing and cytotoxic effects of RSU 1164 and RSU 1165 in a murine tumor model. *Int. J. Radiat. Oncol. biol. Phys.* **16:** 1115–1118.

SIEMANN, D. W. and MULCAHY, R. T. (1982) Cell survival recovery kinetics in the KHT sarcoma following treatment with five alkylating agents and misonidazole. *Int. J. Radiat. Oncol. biol. Phys.* **8:** 619–622.

SIEMANN, D. W., MORRISSEY, S. and WOLF, K. (1983) In vivo potentiation of 1-(2-chloroethyl)-3-cyclohexyl-1-nitrosourea by the radiation sensitizer benznidazole. *Cancer Res.* **43:** 1010–1013.

SIEMANN, D. W., MADDISON, K. and WOLF, K. (1984) Potentiation of melphalan activity in the KHT sarcoma by the radiosensitizer RSU 1069. *Int. J. Radiat. Oncol. biol. Phys.* **10:** 1657–1660.

SIEMANN, D. W., ALLIET, K., MADDISON, K. and WOLF, K. (1985) Enhancement of the antitumor efficacy of Lomustine by the radiosensitizer RSU 1069. *Cancer Treat. Rep.* **69:** 1409–1414.

SIEMANN, D. W., FLAHERTY, A. A. and PENNY, D. P. (1989) Effect of thiol manipulation on chemopotentiation by nitroimidazoles. *Int. J. Radiat. Oncol. biol. Phys.* **16:** 1341–1345.

SMITH, E., STRATFORD, I. J. and ADAMS, G. E. (1982) The enhancing effect of pretreatment of cells with misonidazole in hypoxia on the subsequent response to melphalan in air. *Br. J. Cancer* **46:** 117–126.

SPOONER, D., PEACOCK, J. H. and STEPHENS, T. C. (1982) Enhancement of cytotoxic drugs by misonidazole (MISO) in Lewis lung tumours of different sizes, and in mouse bone marrow. *Int. J. Radiat. Oncol. biol. Phys.* **8:** 643–646.

STEPHENS, T. C., COURTNEY, V. D., MILLS, J., PEACOCK, J. H., ROSE, C. M. and SPOONER, D. (1981) Enhanced cell killing in Lewis lung carcinoma and a human pancreatic carcinoma xenograft by the combination of cytotoxic drugs and misonidazole. *Br. J. Cancer* **43:** 451–457.

STRATFORD, I. J., WILLIAMSON, C. and ADAMS, G. E. (1980) Combination studies with misonidazole and a cis-platinum complex: cytotoxicity and radiosensitization in vitro. *Br. J. Cancer* **41:** 517–522.

TANNOCK, I. F. (1980a) In vivo interaction of anti-cancer drugs with misonidazole or metronidazole: methotrexate, 5-fluorouracil and adriamycin. *Br. J. Cancer* **42:** 861–870.

TANNOCK, I. F. (1980b) In vivo interaction of anti-cancer drugs with misonidazole or metronidazole: cyclophosphamide and BCNU. *Br. J. Cancer* **42:** 871–880.

TAYLOR, Y. C. and RAUTH, A. M. (1978) Differences in the toxicity and metabolism of the 2-nitroimidazole misonidazole (Ro 07-0582) in HeLa and Chinese hamster ovary cells. *Cancer Res.* **38:** 2745–2752.

TAYLOR, Y. C., BUMP, E. A. and BROWN, J. M. (1982) Studies on the mechanism of chemosensitization by misonidazole in vitro. *Int. J. Radiat. Oncol. biol. Phys.* **8:** 705–708.

TAYLOR, Y. C., EVANS, J. W. and BROWN, J. M. (1983) Mechanism of sensitization of Chinese hamster ovary cells to melphalan by hypoxic treatment with misonidazole. *Cancer Res.* **43:** 3175–3181.

TAYLOR, Y. C., SAWYER, J. M., HSU, B. and BROWN, J. M. (1984) Mechanism of melphalan crosslink enhancement by misonidazole pretreatment. *Int. J. Radiat. Oncol. biol. Phys.* **10:** 1603–1608.

TESTA, B. and JENNER, P. (1981) Inhibitors of cytochrome P-450s and their mechanism of action. *Drug Metab. Rev.* **12:** 1–117.

TWENTYMAN, P. R. (1981) Modification of tumour and host response to cyclophosphamide by misonidazole and by WR 2721. *Br. J. Cancer* **43:** 745–755.

TWENTYMAN, P. R. (1982) Growth delay in small EMT6 spheroids induced by cytotoxic drugs and its modification by misonidazole pretreatment under hypoxic condition. *Br. J. Cancer* **45:** 565–570.

TWENTYMAN, P. R. and WORKMAN, P. (1982) Effect of misonidazole or metronidazole pretreatment on the response of the RIF-1 mouse sarcoma to melphalan, cyclophosphamide, chlorambucil and CCNU. *Br. J. Cancer* **45:** 447–455.

TWENTYMAN, P. R. and WORKMAN, P. (1983a) Chemosensitization by lipophilic nitroimidazoles. *Br. J. Cancer* **48:** 17–26.

TWENTYMAN, P. R. and WORKMAN, P. (1983b) An investigation of the possibility of chemosensitization by clinically achievable concentrations of misonidazole. *Br. J. Cancer* **47:** 187–194.

VARGHESE, A. J., GULYAS, S. and MOHINDRA, J. K. (1976) Hypoxia-dependent reduction of 1-(2-nitro-1-imidazolyl)-3-methoxy-2-propanol by Chinese hamster ovary cells and KHT tumour cells in vitro and in vivo. *Cancer Res.* **36:** 3761–3765.

WALTON, M. I. and WORKMAN, P. (1987) Nitroimidazole bioreductive metabolism: quantitation and characterisation of mouse tissue benzinidazole nitroreductases in vivo and in vitro. *Biochem. Pharmac.* **36:** 887–896.

WALTON, M. I. and WORKMAN, P. (1990) Enzymology of the reductive bioactivation of SR 4223: a novel benzotriazine di-*N*-oxide hypoxic cell cytotoxin. *Biochem. Pharmac.* **37:** 1735–1742.

WALTON, M. I., WOLF, C. R. and WORKMAN, P. (1989) Molecular enzymology of the reductive bioactivation of hypoxic cell cytotoxins. *Int. J. Radiat. Oncol. biol. Phys.* **16:** 983–986.

WALTON, M. I., SMITH, P. J. and WORKMAN, P. (1991) The role of NAD(P)H; quinone reductase (EC 1.6.99.2, DT-diaphorase) in the reductive bioactivation of the novel indoloquinone antitumor agent EO9. *Cancer Commun.* **3:** 199–206.

WALTON, M. I., SUGGET, N. and WORKMAN, P. (1992a) The role of human and rodent DT-diaphorase in the reductive metabolism of hypoxic cell cytotoxins. *Int. J. Radiat. Oncol. biol. Phys.* **22:** 643–648.

WALTON, M. I., WOLF, C. R. and WORKMAN, P. (1992b) The role of cytochrome P450 and cytochrome P450 reductase in the reductive bioactivation of the novel benzotiazine di-*N*-oxide 3-amino-1,2,4-benzotriazine-1,4-dioxide (SR 4233, WIN 59075) by mouse liver. *Biochem. Pharmac* **44:** 251–259.

WALTON, M. I., BIBBY, M. C., DOUBLE, J. A., PLUMB, J. A. and WORKMAN, P. (1992c) DT-diaphorase activity correlates with sensitivity to the indoloquinone EO9 in mouse and human colon carcinoma cells. *Eur. J. Cancer* **28A:** 1597–1600.

WARDMAN, P. (1977) The use of nitroaromatic compounds as hypoxic cell sensitizers. *Curr. Top. Radiat. Res. Q.* **11:** 347–398.

WEST, C., STRATFORD, I. J., BARRASS, N. and SMITH, E. (1981) A comparison of adriamycin and mAMSA in vitro: cell lethality and SCE studies. *Br. J. Cancer* **44:** 798–809.

WHEELER, K. T., WALLEN, C. A., WOLF, K. L. and SIEMANN, D. W. (1984) Hypoxic cells and in situ chemosensitization of the nitrosoureas by misonidazole. *Br. J. Cancer* **49:** 787–793.

WHILLANS, D. W. and WHITMORE, G. F. (1981) The radiation reduction of misonidazole. *Radiat. Res.* **86:** 311–324.

WILLSON, R. L., CRAMP, W. A. and INGS, R. M. J. (1974) Metronidazole ('Flagyl'): mechanisms of radiosensitization. *Int. J. Radiat. Biol.* **26:** 557–569.

WONG, K.-H., WALLEN, C. A. and WHEELER, K. T. (1989) Biodistribution of misonidazole and 1,3 bis(2-chloroethyl)-1-nitrosourea (BCNU) in rats bearing unclamped and clamped 9L subcutaneous tumors. *Int. J. Radiat. Oncol. biol. Phys.* **17:** 135–143.

WONG, K.-H., WALLEN, C. A. and WHEELER, K. T. (1990) Chemosensitization of the nitrosoureas by 2-nitroimidazoles in the subcutaneous 9L tumor model: pharmacokinetic and structure–activity considerations. *Int. J. Radiat. Oncol. biol. Phys.* **18:** 1043–1050.

WONG, T. W., WHITMORE, G. F. and GULYAS, S. (1978) Studies on the toxicity and radiosensitizing ability of misonidazole under conditions of prolonged incubation. *Radiat. Res.* **75:** 541–555.

WORKMAN, P. and TWENTYMAN, P. R. (1982) Structure–activity relationships for the enhancement by electron-affinic drugs of the antitumour effect of CCNU. *Br. J. Cancer* **46:** 249–259.

WORKMAN, P., TWENTYMAN, P. R., LEE, F. Y. F. and WALTON, M. I. (1983) Drug metabolism and chemosensitization: nitroimidazoles as inhibitors of drug metabolism. *Biochem. Pharmac.* **32:** 857–864.

WORKMAN, P., WALTON, M. I. and LEE, F. Y. F. (1986) Benznidazole: nitroreduction and inhibition of cytochrome P450 in chemosensitization of tumour response to cytotoxic drugs. *Biochem. Pharmac.* **35:** 117–119.

ZEMAN, E. M., BROWN, J. M., LEMMON, M. J., HIRST, V. K. and LEE, W. W. (1986) SR 4233: a new bioreductive agent with high selective cytotoxicity for hypoxic mammalian cells. *Int. J. Radiat. Oncol. biol. Phys.* **12:** 1239–1242.

Garth Powis, editor.
(1994) *Anticancer Drugs: Reactive Metabolism and Drug Interactions*,
Pergamon Press Ltd, pp. 417–425
Printed in the United Kingdom

CHAPTER 11

EFFECTS OF CANCER DISEASE ON THE METABOLISM OF ANTICANCER AGENTS

S. Garattini, P. Ghezzi and M. D'Incalci
Istituto di Ricerche Farmacologiche "Mario Negri", Via Eritrea, 62, 20157 Milan, Italy

1. INTRODUCTION

Anticancer agents are usually employed at the maximum tolerated doses, and their therapeutic indices are relatively low. Any variation in the metabolism (activation or inactivation) and pharmacokinetics of these compounds is particularly undesirable, because even a small decrease in drug (or active metabolite) clearance may result in intolerable side effects, and a minimal increase in their elimination rate may render treatment ineffective. In this context, knowledge of the factors most likely responsible for metabolic and kinetic variability is of great interest.

One of these factors, perhaps the most important, is the disease itself. Cancer is, in fact, a complex condition which directly or indirectly involves different organs, often significantly modifying their functions. Organs with a primary role in drug clearance, such as liver or kidney, may be the site of metastases or may be mechanically compressed by tumor masses with consequent impairment of their functions. Cancer patients may have peritoneal, pleural or pericardial effusions which can cause changes in drug distribution and elimination. The nutritional status of cancer patients, particularly the loss of adipose tissue, can also significantly alter drug distribution. In addition, qualitative and quantitative alterations of plasma protein patterns are a common feature of some neoplastic diseases and may conceivably alter the amount of drug bound to plasma proteins.

This review article summarizes some of the available experimental and clinical knowledge of the influence of these changes in host physiology on anticancer drug disposition. In addition we review some experimental evidence suggesting that factors produced by host or tumor cells may have significant effects on drug metabolism. Some of these factors have now been identified, and characterization of their properties represents a fascinating area of investigation.

2. EXPERIMENTAL STUDIES

2.1. In Vitro Metabolism

On the basis of previous evidence that some tumor extracts cause inhibition of liver catalase activity, Nakahara and Fukuoka (1949) and Kato et al. (1963) questioned whether the presence of a tumor could influence the drug metabolizing capacity of livers of tumor-bearing animals. They isolated microsomes from livers of rats with tumors and showed that these microsomal preparations, in the presence of NADPH and oxygen, oxidized strychnine, hexobarbital and meprobamate much less than did liver microsomes from normal rats. Since the animals had tumors that did not metastasize to the liver, they could exclude the presence of hepatic neoplastic deposits as causing the changes. To explain their observations they postulated that some unidentified factor(s) ('toxhormones') produced by the tumor cells had inhibitory effects on liver microsomal enzymes.

The same authors, in subsequent studies, extended their initial observations to other substrates such as hexobarbital, aminopyrine or aniline (Kato et al., 1970) and steroid hormones (progesterone, testosterone) (Kato and Takahashi, 1970). In all cases, they observed a marked reduction in the oxidative ability of liver microsomes of Walker carcinoma bearing rats compared to control rats of the same age, sex and weight, but with no tumor. They proposed as an explanation for their findings, a decrease in cytochrome P-450 content and, to a lesser extent, a lower binding capacity, of the cytochrome for the substrates. Concomitantly, this laboratory published observations concerning the reduced ability to metabolize zoxazolamine (Franchi and Rosso, 1969) and other substrates such as aniline, *p*-nitroanisole and aminopyrine (Rosso et al., 1971) by 9000 *g* preparation from livers of rats bearing different experimental tumors (Walker carcinosarcoma, Flexner-Jobling carcinoma, T-8 Guerin uterine epithelioma and sarcoma 45).

The hypothesis that some factors produced by the tumoral cells were at the basis of the depressed liver metabolism of tumor bearing rats was corroborated by some elegant experiments conducted by Boulos et al. (1972) and by Bartosek et al. (1975). When Boulos et al. (1972) used pairs of parabiotic animals (with a common circulation), one with a fibrosarcoma, hepatic drug metabolism was inhibited in the tumor-free member too. Since the fibrosarcoma used did not metastasize, the authors concluded that a circulating factor was responsible.

Bartosek et al. (1974, 1975) using the technique of isolated liver perfusion found that cyclophosphamide was metabolized less by liver from Walker carcinosarcoma-bearing rats than from normal animals. Cyclophosphamide oxidation was depressed even when livers from normal rats were perfused with blood from Walker bearing animals. These findings indicated that some circulating substance(s) was able to inhibit metabolism and was partly responsible for the reduced biotransformation of cyclophosphamide.

Other cross-experiments (normal liver perfused with blood of tumor bearing rats and vice versa) showed that blood of Walker carcinosarcoma-bearing rats inhibited the metabolism of the anticancer agent 6-mercaptopurine (Bartosek et al., 1975) and of barbiturates (Bartosek et al., 1972). Perfusion of normal liver with blood of tumor bearing rats did not influence hydrocortisone metabolism (Bartosek et al., 1973). Thus it appears that the factors produced by the tumor are not non-specific inhibitors of drug metabolism, but that their effects are specific and depend on the type of substrate involved.

Though most in vitro metabolism studies were done on rat livers, similar observations were published using liver extracts of mice (Rosso et al., 1971) or guinea pigs (Litterst et al., 1977). Of particular interest is the finding reported by Kato et al. (1982) that livers from nude mice (Balb/c-nu/nu) transplanted with human tumors contained less cytochrome P-450 and less cyclophosphamide oxidase, benzopyrene hydroxylase, aniline hydroxylase and benzphetamine *N*-demethylase activity than normal nude mice.

Another interesting question is whether neoplastic liver metabolizes drugs and, if so, how it qualitatively and quantitatively differs from normal liver. Recently, Stout and Becker (1986) investigated the activity of many enzymes that play a role in phase I or phase II metabolism of xenobiotics in spontaneous and dimethylnitrosoamine-induced mouse liver tumors. The ratios of the activity of benzopyrene monooxygenase, aminopyrene demethylase, cytochrome P-450 reductase, epoxide hydrolase and UDP glucuronosyl transferase in microsomes from spontaneous tumors relative to those from normal liver were 0.25, 0.43, 1.27, 0.90 and 0.51 respectively. Similar values were obtained with microsomes from chemically induced tumors. The ratios for activities of DT-diaphorase, glutathione reductase, glutathione S-transferase and glutathione peroxidase in cytosol from spontaneous tumors relative to cytosol from normal liver were 2.24, 2.00, 2.43 and 0.31, respectively. Similar values were obtained with cytosol from chemically induced tumors.

Powis et al. (1986) looked at the influence of infiltration of the liver by P-388 leukemic cells on mouse hepatic metabolizing activity. Six days after i.v. injection of 10^6 P-388 cells, there was no change in liver weight or in enzymatic activities, but after 8 days there was significant infiltration, with an approximately 50% increase in liver weight and decreases of approximately 60 and 20% in cytochrome P-450 and cytochrome b5 contents. Ratios for NADPH cytochrome P-450 reductase, biphenyl-2-hydroxylase and biphenyl-4-hydroxylase activities in microsomes from livers of P-388-bearing mice relative to livers of normal mice were 0.65, 0.40 and 0.68 respectively.

Studies reported by Beck et al. (1982) and by Schacter and Kurz (1982) showed that the reduced cytochrome P-450 content in liver microsomes of tumor-bearing rats is due to perturbations in heme and hemoprotein synthesis.

2.2. In Vivo Metabolism

Many studies have shown that in Walker carcinosarcoma-bearing rats the metabolism of drugs undergoing microsomal oxidation such as pentobarbital, D-amphetamine or zoxazolamine is depressed with consequent changes in their pharmacological effects (Kato et al., 1963; Rosso et al., 1968; Franchi and Rosso, 1969). The initial findings were subsequently extended to rats transplanted s.c. with other tumors such as Flexner-Jobling, T-8 Guerin, uterine epithelioma, sarcoma 45 and a rhabdomyosarcoma (Rosso et al., 1971), pituitary mammotropic tumor (Wilson, 1968) or with Yoshida AH-602 and AH-130 and Walker tumors implanted intraperitoneally (Rosso et al., 1971). In all these cases, sodium pentobarbital (25 mg/kg, i.v.) significantly prolonged sleeping time compared to control rats. The much higher drug levels in plasma and brain of the tumor bearing rats were probably one explanation of the greater pharmacological effects of pentobarbital. A substantial increase in sleeping time was also seen in male and female mice with Erlich ascites, sarcoma 180 and Yancey plasmocytoma (Beck et al., 1975). The plasma half life of unchanged pentobarbital was about four times as long in tumor-bearing mice as it was in controls. In tumor-bearing mice the sleeping time of the non-metabolizable barbiturate, barbital, was the same as in normal animals; it thus appears that the tumor affected mainly pentobarbital metabolism rather than the central nervous system substrates sensitive to barbiturates.

Relatively few published studies are available on the differences between anticancer drug pharmacokinetics in tumor-bearing and control-animals. Cyclophosphamide, a drug metabolized by hepatic cytochrome P-450, was biotransformed less in Walker carcinosarcoma bearing rats than in control as assessed by the determination of alkylating metabolites by NBP assay (Bartosek et al., 1974). Total body plasma clearance of cyclophosphamide was reduced to 53 mL/min/kg in mice that had received P-388 cells 8 days earlier, as against 97.2 mL/min/kg in controls (Powis et al., 1986).

Donelli et al. (1986) investigated the metabolism and pharmacokinetics of cyclophosphamide in two Walker sublines that differed in their cachetic properties and their drug sensitivities. Subline A, sensitive to cyclophosphamide, grew more slowly and produced metastases, whereas subline B, insensitive to cyclophosphamide, grew faster and caused anorexia, early cachexia and short survival. The plasma kinetics and distribution of cyclophosphamide appeared similar in the two sublines. Extracts of livers from Walker A-bearing animals exhibited similar abilities to biotransform cyclophosphamide. Extracts of Walker A tumor in the presence of NADPH and oxygen, however, activated the drug to species that were able to bind covalently to macromolecules.

In addition to the various aspects concerning the metabolism of anticancer agents, therefore, one must also consider the in situ metabolism in the tumor. Though negligible in comparison to the systemic metabolism, this may be important to the pharmacological effect of a drug.

Besides metabolism, drug distribution, too, may be altered in tumor-bearing animals. For example, many antitumor agents tend to distribute in metastatic deposits in large amounts, reaching concentrations much higher than in primary tumors (Donelli et al., 1984). It has also been reported that hepatic levels of BCNU, determined by differential pulse polarography, in Walker tumor-bearing rats (i.v. treated with 20 mg/kg), were significantly lower (about 10 times) than in healthy animals receiving the same i.v. dose (Bartosek et al., 1984). Other studies indicate differences in the pharmacokinetics of anticancer agents in tumor-bearing animals which apparently are not due to altered metabolism, but to different distribution as in the case of doxorubicin in rats with Brown Norway acute myeloid leukemia (Sonneveld and Van Bekkum, 1981) or in the case of cyclophosphamide in L1210 leukemia-bearing mice (Lavigne et al., 1975).

3. ENDOGENOUS MEDIATORS IN THE DEPRESSION OF CYTOCHROME P-450 IN INVASIVE DISEASES

Depression of liver cytochrome P-450 and related drug metabolizing enzymes is a frequent metabolic alteration in animal models of invasive diseases such as cancer, bacterial and viral infections and in inflammation. The metabolic derangements observed in these conditions often display similar patterns and include wasting and weight loss (Filkins, 1985; Beutler and Cerami, 1986), iron and zinc redistribution between plasma and tissue (Kampschmidt et al., 1980; Ujjani et al., 1986) and elevation of specific serum proteins such as fibrinogen (Kampschmidt et al., 1980; Poggi et al., 1977). In 1949, Nakahara and Fukuoka described a factor (termed 'toxhormone') extracted from tumors that mimicked a biochemical change typically observed in tumor-bearing animals, e.g. decrease of liver catalase. Later, 'toxhormones' from various tumors were reported to have lipolytic activity in vitro (Masuno et al., 1981), to lower plasma zinc levels by inducing liver zinc-binding to metallothionein (Ujjani et al., 1986) and to reduce plasma iron levels (Ono et al., 1960). It was also reported that cancer-associated cachexia might be mediated through humoral factors (Norton et al., 1985) and, as mentioned before, a 'toxhormone' has been implicated in the depression of liver drug metabolizing enzymes observed in tumor-bearing animals (Takahashi and Kato, 1969; Bartosek et al., 1975). To date, these putative 'toxhormones' have not been definitely characterized, possibly because of the lack of specificity and the complexity of the in vivo assay systems used. It is thus not clear whether one or more mediators are responsible for cancer-associated metabolic alterations (Fujii et al., 1964).

A clearer picture comes from the study of infectious diseases. A hormone-like substance released by macrophage stimulation with bacterial endotoxins, called 'leucocytic endogenous mediator' and later identified as the lymphocyte activating protein interleukin-1 (IL-1), has been shown to induce most of the changes (low blood iron and zinc, induction of fibrinogen and metallothionein, and fever) observed during infection, inflammation or after endotoxin injection (Dinarello, 1984). In the course of their studies on the biochemical mechanisms of cachexia in rabbits infected with *Trypanosoma brucei*, Cerami and his associates identified as endotoxin-induced, lipoprotein lipase-suppressing hormone secreted by macrophages which they termed 'cachectin' (Kawakami and Cerami, 1981). Cachectin was then sequenced and found to be identical to a macrophage tumoricidal protein known as tumor necrosis factor (Beutler et al., 1985).

The identification of two macrophage factors, IL-1 and tumor necrosis factor/cachectin (TNF/C), as mediators of most of the metabolic derangements observed in infective and inflammatory diseases goes strongly against the old idea that toxins produced by invasive agents were responsible for the metabolic changes and indicates that most of these effects are host-mediated, mainly through products of the immune system. The availability of substantial amounts of highly purified TNF/C and IL-1 produced by recombinant techniques has made it possible to study their in vivo effects on the liver. This laboratory found that administration of IL-1 or TNF/C to mice caused a depression of liver cytochrome P-450 and P-450-dependent enzymes such as ethoxycoumarin deethylase and arylhydrocarbon hydroxylase (Ghezzi et al., 1986a,b). Depression of liver drug metabolism has also been observed in mice treated with recombinant lymphotoxin, a lymphocyte-derived factor cytotoxic to tumor cells, also known as TNF-beta. Figure 1 shows the effects of various cytokines on the cytochrome P-450-dependent enzyme ethoxycoumarin deethylase.

Another endogenous mediator, interferon (IFN), which is produced by various cells in response

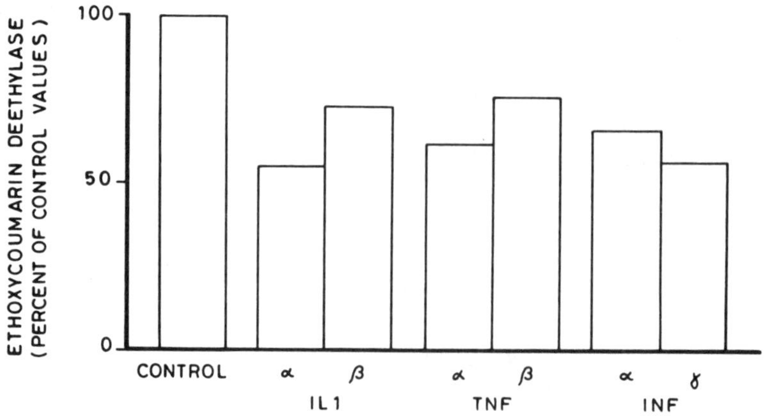

FIG. 1. Depression of liver cytochrome P-450-dependent ethoxycoumarin deethylase 24 hr after treatment with 2 μg/mouse of one of the following cytokines human IL-1 α and β, human TNF α and β (lymphotoxin), human IFN α A/D-Bgl II and murine IFN γ.

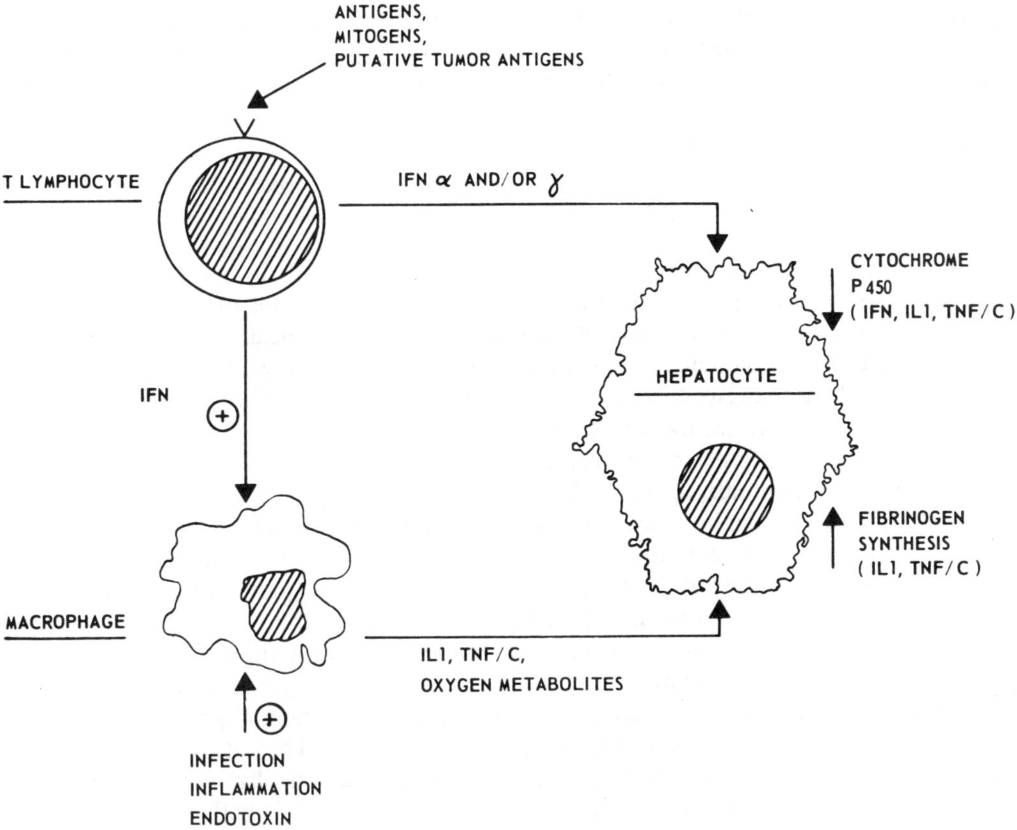

FIG. 2. Proposed scheme for the regulation of liver drug metabolism by the immune system.

to viral infections (or antigenic stimulation of T-lymphocytes in the case of IFN-gamma) was reported to depress liver drug metabolism in rats and mice (Renton and Mannering, 1976; Sonnenfeld et al., 1980; Parkinson et al., 1982; Ghezzi et al., 1985). Depression of liver drug metabolism by IFN was associated with decreased in vivo metabolism of antipyrine and increased hexobarbital sleeping time (Parkinson et al., 1982; Moore et al., 1983; Taylor et al., 1985).

IFN-mediated depression of liver cytochrome P-450 is paralleled by a pattern of biochemical changes (induction of heme oxygenase, depression of the heme-biosynthetic enzyme delta-aminolevulinate synthetase, decreased catalase, increased lipid peroxidation) almost identical to those observed in the liver of tumor-bearing animals (Mannering et al., 1980; Schacter and Kurz, 1982; Koizumi et al., 1986b; Beck et al., 1982; Boveris et al., 1985; Capel and Thornley, 1982). It is thus conceivable that impairment of liver drug metabolism in tumor-bearing animals may be mediated not only by products derived from tumors but also from the host's immune system. The proposed mechanisms of the impaired liver drug metabolism observed in invasive diseases, in terms of cellular immunology, are outlined in Fig. 2.

In this respect, the different immunogenicity of tumors may be of primary importance, since antigenic challenge is known to induce IFN-gamma, and induction of T-cell-dependent antibodies is reported to result, in some cases, in depressed cytochrome P-450 levels (Sonnenfeld et al., 1980; Koizumi et al., 1986a). Furthermore, in some acute non-lymphoblastic leukemias, malignant cells were found to secrete IL-1 (Furukawa et al., 1987); this might reasonably be expected to cause impairment of liver drug metabolism much the same way as after IL-1 administration. IL-1 production by hepatoma cells (Moore et al., 1986) and renal carcinoma (Rawlins et al., 1970) was also reported, and P-388 mouse leukemia cells which, as mentioned above, cause depression of cytochrome P-450 in vivo, are strong IL-1 producers (Mizel et al., 1978). More recently, IL-6 was found to inhibit the levels of mRNA for cytochrome P450IIC12 (Wright and Morgan, 1991). These data suggest that not only IL-I and INF but IL-6 might be implicated in the cancer-associated depression of cytochrome P-450. In fact, IL-6 bioactivity has been reported in the circulation of mice bearing a methylcholantrene-induced sarcoma (Gelin et al., 1988).

The availability of monoclonal antibodies or antagonist/inhibitors against different cytokines or their receptors will permit better characterization of the role of the immune system in cancer-associated impairment of liver functions.

4. CLINICAL STUDIES

Neoplastic disease is often associated with major functional alterations of different systems with consequent changes in drug disposition. A typical example of clinical relevance is the slowed methotrexate elimination in patients with neoplastic pleural effusions (Evans and Pratt, 1978), with consequent greater drug toxicity. Either the metastatic involvement of liver and kidney or their compression by tumor masses can affect hepatic or renal elimination of drugs in cancer patients. In addition these patients often receive prolonged nephrotoxic or hepatotoxic therapies.

Powis (1983) recently summarized the available knowledge on the clearance of anticancer agents in patients with hepatic or renal dysfunction. Much less information exists on alterations of drug metabolism and pharmacokinetics in cancer patients with apparently normal renal and hepatic function. This lack is primarily due to the fact that anticancer agents are not prescribed for conditions other than cancer so it is virtually impossible to establish control groups for adequate comparisons. However some information has been collected using antipyrine as a test drug for evaluating drug metabolism. Tschanz et al. (1977) investigated comparatively the metabolism of antipyrine in nine patients with lung cancer and in a cancer free control group of nine subjects matched for age, sex, drug intake and smoking and drinking history. The antipyrine plasma half-life was longer in the group with tumors, but the difference was not statistically significant. Elimination of the two major antipyrine metabolites 4-hydroxy antipyrine and *N*-demethylantipyrine was also similar.

Higuchi et al. (1980) found that the antipyrine half-life was significantly longer in 16 patients with pancreatic carcinoma and with disseminated gastric carcinoma than in five controls. The authors found a negative correlation between antipyrene half-life and albumin concentration, thus suggesting that nutritional status and liver function were at least partially responsible for the changes in drug metabolism.

Considering that in rodents important changes in drug metabolism become evident when tumor masses exceed approximately 10% of the body weight, it is not surprising that it is difficult to detect changes in drug metabolism in cancer patients unless very advanced cases are analyzed. In fact, even though we have no really reliable methods to quantitate tumor masses precisely in patients, it is reasonable to assume that only in rare circumstances does tumor burden ever achieve 10% of the body weight. One could perform pharmacokinetic studies stratifying patients affected by the same tumor according to their clinical stage and residual tumor after surgery and evaluate whether there is any correlation between tumor burden and metabolism of anticancer agents. This would perhaps be feasible, but would require a very large case-list, particularly considering the generally large intersubject variability of drug kinetics in cancer patients.

A further complication arises from the fact that the determination of drugs in plasma can give misleading data in relation to the concentrations achieved in the tumor, where the drugs exert their antitumor effects. An example of how unpredictable the tumor concentrations are in cancer patients is given in Fig. 3. Doxorubicin plasma concentrations were similar in both patients whereas doxorubicin concentrations achieved in the breast tumor itself were much higher in case No. 1 than in case No. 2 at 24 and 48 hr after drug injection.

The reasons for these differences in distribution were not elucidated but data obtained in rodent tumors indicate that doxorubicin reaches much higher concentrations in better-vascularized tumors (Donelli et al., 1984). Another reason for the differences in anticancer drug pharmacokinetics in cancer patients may be the abnormal number of circulating blood cells. For example, the low hematocrit often seen in cancer patients may significantly affect the plasma concentrations of drugs which tend to concentrate differently in different cellular blood elements and in plasma. Piazza et al. (1981) investigated this aspect for doxorubicin and found significantly higher concentrations in

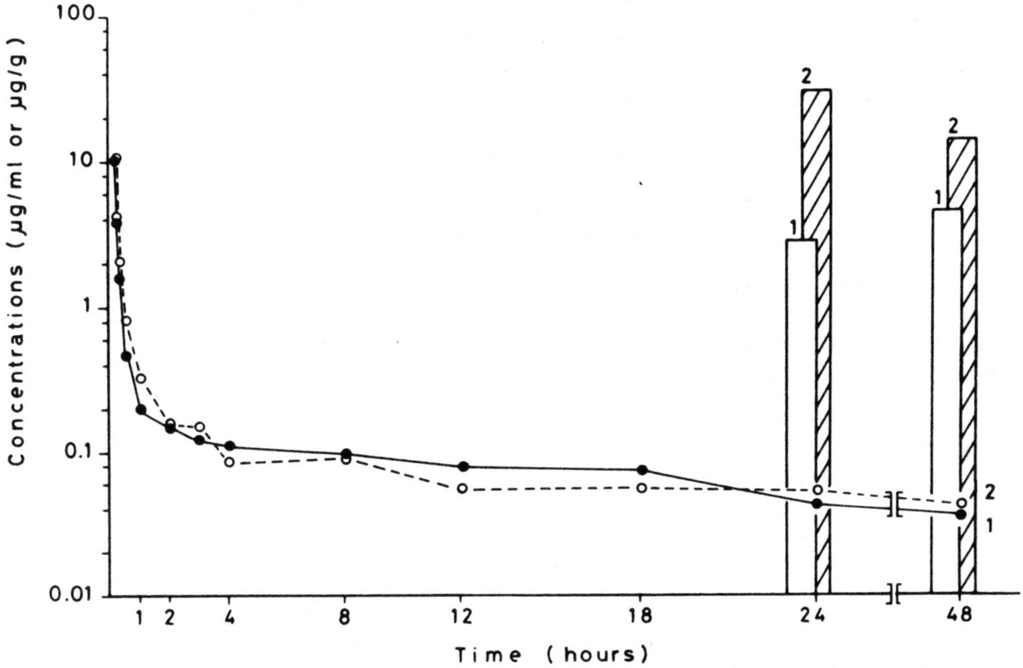

FIG. 3. Plasma and tumor doxorubicin (Dx) concentrations in two breast cancer patients. Dx was given i.v. at a dose of 75 mg/m^2. Plasma levels were essentially the same but tumor drug concentrations were markedly different. For details of the analytical methods used for the determination of Dx in plasma and tumor see Broggini et al. (1984).

plasma of anemic patients, with possible consequences on the rate of drug distribution in these cases.

Acknowledgement—The generous contribution of the Italian Association for Cancer Research, Milan, Italy, is gratefully acknowledged.

REFERENCES

BARTOSEK, I., GUAITANI, A. and DONELLI, M. G. (1972) Prolonged metabolism of pentobarbital in isolated perfused liver of tumor bearing rats. *Biochem, Pharmac.* **21:** 2359–2362.

BARTOSEK, I., MARC, V., GUAITANI, A. and GARATTINI, S. (1973) Accelerated catabolism of hydrocortisone in isolated perfused liver of tumor-bearing rats. *Biochem. Pharmac.* **22:** 2429–2431.

BARTOSEK, I., DONELLI, M. G. and GUAITANI, A. (1974) Modification of drug metabolism induced in the host by the presence of a tumor. In: *Recent Results in Cancer Research*, pp. 95–100, MATHÉ, G. and OLDHAM, R. K. (eds) Springer, Berlin.

BARTOSEK, I., DONELLI, M. G., GUAITANI, A., COLOMBO, T., RUSSO, R. and GARATTINI, S. (1975) Differences of cyclophosphamide and 6-mercaptopurine metabolic rates in perfused liver of normal and tumour-bearing animals. *Biochem. Pharmac.* **24:** 289–291.

BARTOSEK, I., RUSSO, R. G. and CATTANEO, M. T. (1984) Pharmacokinetics of nitrosoureas: Levels of 1,3-bis(2-chloroethyl)-1-nitrosourea (BCNU) in organs of normal and Walker 256/B carcinoma bearing rats after i.v. bolus. *Tumori* **70:** 491–498.

BECK, W. T., MANDEL, H. G. and FABRO, S. (1975) Physiological disposition of pentobarbital in tumour-bearing mice. *Cancer Res.* **35:** 1333–1340.

BECK, W. T., DEDMON, M. L. and OULLETTE, M. A. (1982) Biochemical basis for impaired drug metabolism in tumor-bearing rats. Evidence for altered regulation of hepatic microsomal hemeprotein synthesis. *Biochem. Pharmac.* **31:** 1535–1543.

BEUTLER, B. and CERAMI, A. (1986) Cachectin and tumour necrosis factor as two sides of the same biological coin. *Nature* **320:** 584–588.

BEUTLER, B., GREENWALD, D., HULMES, J. D., CHANG, M., PAN, Y.-C. E., MATHISON, J., ULEVITCH, R. and CERAMI, A. (1985) Identity of tumour necrosis factor and the macrophage-secreted factor cachectin. *Nature* **316:** 552–554.

BOULOS, B. M., MACDOUGALL, M., SHOEMAN, D. W. and AZARNOFF, D. L. (1972) Evidence that inhibition of hepatic drug oxidation by tumors is mediated by a circulating humor. *Proc. Soc. exp. Biol. Med.* **139:** 1353–1355.

BOVERIS, A., LLESUY, S. F. and FRAGA, C. G. (1985) Increased liver chemiluminescence in tumor-bearing mice. *J. Free Radicals Biol. Med.* **1:** 131–138.

BROGGINI, M., ITALIA, C., COLOMBO, T., MARMONTI, L. and DONELLI, M. G. (1984) Activity and distribution of i.v. and oral 4-demethoxydaunorubicin in murine experimental tumors. *Cancer Treat. Rep.* **68:** 739–747.

CAPEL, I. D. and THORNLEY, A. C. (1982) Superoxide dismutase activity, caeruloplasmin activity and lipoperoxide levels in tumour and host tissues of mice bearing the Lewis lung carcinoma. *Eur. J. Cancer clin. Oncol.* **18:** 507–513.

DINARELLO, C. A. (1984) Interleukin-1. *Rev. Infect. Dis.* **6:** 51–95.

DONELLI, M. G., D'INCALCI, M. and GARATTINI, S. (1984) Pharmacokinetic studies of anticancer drugs in tumor-bearing animals. *Cancer Treat. Rep.* **68:** 381–400.

DONELLI, M. G., GUAITANI, A., TORTI, L., DAMIA, G., CORTI, F., BIANCHI, M., TORTORETO, M., PANTAROTTO, C. and BARTOSEK, I. (1986) Different sensitivity of two Walker 256 carcinoma lines to cyclophosphamide: Correlation with drug distribution, biotransformation and macromolecule binding. *Oncology* **43:** 257–263.

EVANS, W. E. and PRATT, C. B. (1978) Effect of pleural effusion on high-dose methotrexate kinetics. *Clin. Pharmac. Ther.* **23:** 68–72.

FILKINS, J. P. (1985) Monokines and the metabolic pathophysiology of septic shock. *Fed. Proc.* **44:** 300–304.

FRANCHI, G. and ROSSO, R. (1969) Metabolic fate of zoxazolamine in tumor bearing rats. *Biochem. Pharmac.* **18:** 236–238.

FUJII, S., YUASA, A., KAWACHI, T., OKAMURA, Y., WAKASUGI, H. and YAMAMURA, Y. (1964) Purification of toxohormone by carboxymethyl-cellulose column chromatography. *Gann* **55:** 67–71.

FURUKAWA, Y., OHTA, M., MIURA, Y. and SAITO, M. (1987) Interleukin-1 producing ability of leukaemia cells and its relationship to morphological diagnosis. *Br. J. Haemat.* **65:** 11–15.

GELIN, J., MOLDAWER, L. L., LONNROTH, C., DEMAN, P., SVANBORG-EDEN, C., LOWRY, S. F. and LUNDHOLM, K. G. (1988) Appearance of hybridoma growth factor/interleukin-6 in the serum of mice bearing a methylcholanthrene-induced sarcoma. *Biochem. biophys. Res. Commun.* **157:** 575–579.

GHEZZI, P., BIANCHI, M., GIANERA, L., LANDOLFO, S. and SALMONA, M. (1985) Role of reactive oxygen intermediates in the interferon-mediated depression of hepatic drug metabolism and protective effect of *N*-acetylcysteine in mice. *Cancer Res.* **45:** 3444–3447.

GHEZZI, P., SACCARDO, B. and BIANCHI, M. (1986a) Recombinant tumor necrosis factor depresses cytochrome P450-dependent microsomal drug metabolism in mice. *Biochem. biophys. Res. Commun.* **136:** 316–321.

GHEZZI, P., SACCARDO, B., VILLA, P., ROSSI, V., BIANCHI, M. and DINARELLO, C. A. (1986b) Role of interleukin-1 in the depression of liver drug metabolism by endotoxin. *Infections Immun.* **54:** 837–840.

HIGUCHI, T., NAKAMURA, T. and UCHINO, H. (1980) Antipyrine metabolism in cancer patients. *Cancer* **45:** 541–544.

KAMPSCHMIDT, R. F., PULLIAM, L. A. and UPCHURCH, H. F. (1980) The activity of partially purified leukocytic endogenous mediator in endotoxin-resistant C3H/HeJ mice. *J. Lab. clin. Med.* **95:** 616–623.

KATO, R. and TAKAHASHI, A. (1970) Decreased hydroxylation of steroid hormones by liver microsomes from rats bearing Walker carcinosarcoma 256. *Cancer Res.* **30:** 2346–2352.

KATO, R., FRONTINO, G. and VASSANELLI, P. (1963) Decreased activities of liver microsomal drug-metabolizing enzymes in the rats bearing Walker carcinosarcoma. *Experientia* **19:** 31–32.

KATO, R., TAKANAKA, A. and TAKAHASHI, A. (1970) Decrease in the substrate interaction with cytochrome P-450 in drug hydroxylation by liver microsomes from rats bearing Walker 256 carcinosarcoma. *Gann* **61:** 359–365.

KATO, R., YAMAZOE, Y., MITA, S., KAMATAKI, T., KUBOTA, T., HANATANI, Y. and MAHEJIMA, K. (1982) Decrease in the activity of hepatic microsomal drug-metabolizing enzymes in tumor-bearing nude mice. *Gann* **73:** 907–911.

KAWAKAMI, M. and CERAMI, A. (1981) Studies of endotoxin-induced decrease in lipoprotein lipase activity. *J. exp. Med.* **154:** 631–639.

KOIZUMI, A., HASEGAWA, L., THOMAS, I. K. and IAMAMURA, T. (1986a) Effect of induction of T-cell-dependent antibody with sheep red blood cells on P-450-dependent and -independent xenobiotic metabolizing enzymes. *Biochem. Pharmac.* **35:** 2743–2748.

KOIZUMI A., WALFORD, R. L. and IMAMURA, T. (1986b) Treatment with poly i.c. enhances lipid peroxidation and the activity of xanthine oxidase, and decreases hepatic P-450 content and activities in mice and rats. *Biochem. biophys. Res. Commun.* **134:** 632–637.

LAVIGNE, J.-G., BARRY, A., D'AUTEUIL, C. and DELAGE, J. M. (1975) Increase in the gastrointestinal absorption and in tissue storage of cyclophosphamide in L-1210 leukaemic mice at an advanced stage of the disease. *Br. J. Cancer* **32:** 720–729.

LITTERST, C. L., MIMNAUGH, E. G. and GRAM, T. E. (1977) Effect of strain differences and tumor presence on microsomal drug metabolism in the guinea pig. *J. natn. Cancer Inst.* **59:** 1737–1739.

MANNERING, G. J., RENTON, K. W., EL AZHARY, R. and DELORIA, L. B. (1980) Effects of interferon-inducing agents on hepatic cytochrome P-450 drug metabolizing systems. *Ann. N.Y. Acad. Sci.* **350:** 314–331.

MASUNO, H., YAMASAKI, N. and OKUDA, H. (1981) Purification and characterization of a lipolytic factor (toxohormone-L) from cell-free fluid of ascites sarcoma 180. *Cancer Res.* **41:** 284–288.

MIZEL, S. B., ROSENSTREICH, D. L. and OPPENHEIM, J. J. (1978) Phorbol myristic acetate stimulates LAF production by the macrophage cell line P388D. *Cell. Immun.* **40:** 230–235.
MOORE, J. A., MARAFINO, B. J., JR and STEBBING, N. (1983) Influence of various purified interferons on effects of drugs in mice. *Res. Commun. Chem. Path. Pharmac.* **39:** 113–125.
MOORE, W. M., WESTER, W. N. and SPILBURG, C. A. (1986) Production of interleukin 1 by SK hepatoma tumor cells. *Biochemistry* **25:** 7696–7701.
NAKAHARA, W. and FUKUOKA, F. (1949) Toxohormone: A characteristic toxic substance produced by cancer tissue. *Gann* **40:** 45–69.
NORTON, J. A., MOLEY, J. F., GREEN, M. V., CARSON, R. E. and MORRISON, S. D. (1985) Parabiotic transfer of cancer anorexia/cachexia in male rats. *Cancer Res.* **45:** 5547–5552.
ONO, T., OHASHI, M. and YAGO, N. (1960) The effect of toxohormone on iron metabolism. *Gann* **51:** 213–221.
PARKINSON, A., LASKER, J., KRAMER, M. J., HUANG, M. T., THOMAS, P. E., RYAN, D. E., REIK, L. M., NORMAN, R. L., LEVIN, W. and CONNEY, A. H. (1982) Effects of three recombinant human leukocyte interferons on drug metabolism in mice. *Drug Metab. Dis.* **10:** 579–585.
PIAZZA, E., BROGGINI, M., TRABATTONI, A., NATALE, N., LIBRETTI, A. and DONELLI, M. G. (1981) Adriamycin distribution in plasma and blood cells of cancer patients with altered hematocrit. *Eur. J. Cancer clin. Oncol.* **17:** 1089–1096.
POGGI, A., POLENTARUTTI, N., DONATI, M. B., DEGAETANO, G. and GARATTINI, S. (1977) Blood coagulation changes in mice bearing Lewis lung carcinoma, a metastasizing tumor. *Cancer Res.* **37:** 272–277.
POWIS, G. (1983) Effects of disease states on pharmacokinetics of anticancer drugs. In: *Pharmacokinetics of Anticancer Agents in Humans*, pp. 363–397, AMES, M. M., POWIS, G. and KOVACH, J. S. (eds) Elsevier, Amsterdam.
POWIS, G., HARRIS, R. N., BASSECHES, P. J. and SANTONE, K. S. (1986) Effects of advanced leukemia on hepatic drug-metabolizing activity in the mouse. *Cancer Chemother, Pharmac.* **16:** 43–49.
RAWLINS, M. D., LUFF, R. H. and CRANSTON, W. I. (1970) Pyrexia in renal carcinoma. *Lancet* **1:** 1371–1373.
RENTON, K. W. and MANNERING, G. J. (1976) Depression of hepatic cytochrome P-450-dependent monooxygenase systems with administered interferon inducing agents. *Biochem. biophys. Res. Commun.* **73:** 343–348.
ROSSO, R., DOLFINI, E. and DONELLI, M. G. (1968) Prolonged effect of pentobarbital in tumor bearing rats. *Eur. J. Cancer* **4:** 133–135.
ROSSO, R., DONELLI, M. G., FRANCHI, G. and GARATTINI, S. (1971) Impairment of drug metabolism in tumor-bearing animals. *Eur. J. Cancer* **7:** 565–577.
SCHACTER, B. A. and KURZ, P. (1982) Alterations in hepatic and splenic microsomal electron transport system components, drug metabolism, heme oxygenase activity, and cytochrome P-450 turnover in Murphy–Sturm lymphosarcoma-bearing rats. *Cancer Res.* **42:** 3557–3564.
SONNENFELD, G., HARNED, C. L., THANIYAVARN, S., HUFF, T., MANDEL, A. D. and NERLAND, D. E. (1980) Type II interferon induction and passive transfer depress the murine cytochrome P-450 drug metabolism system. *Antimicrob. Agents Chemother.* **17:** 969–972.
SONNEVELD, P. and VAN BEKKUM, D. W. (1981) Different distribution of adriamycin in normal and leukaemic rats. *Br. J. Cancer* **43:** 464–470.
STOUT, D. L. and BECKER, F. F. (1986) Xenobiotic metabolizing enzymes in genetically and chemically initiated mouse liver tumors. *Cancer Res.* **46:** 2693–2696.
TAKAHASHI, A. and KATO, R. (1969) Effect of toxohormone in microsomal cytochromes and hydroxylating systems of rat liver. *J. Biochem. Tokyo* **65:** 325–327.
TAYLOR, G., MARAFINO, B. J., JR, MOORE, J. A., GURLEY, V. and BLASCHKE, T. F. (1985) Interferon reduces hepatic drug metabolism in vivo in mice. *Drug Metab. Dis.* **13:** 459–463.
TSCHANZ, C., HIGNITE, C. E., HUFFMAN, D. H. and AZARNOFF, D. L. (1977) Metabolic disposition of antipyrine in patients with lung cancer. *Cancer Res.* **37:** 3881–3886.
UJJANI, B., KRAKOWER, G., BACHOWSKI, G., KREZOSKI, S., SHAW, C. F., III and PETERING, D. H. (1986) Host zinc metabolism and the Ehrlich ascites tumour. Zinc redistribution during tumour-related stress. *Biochem. J.* **233:** 99–105.
WILSON, J. T. (1968) An investigation of the decrease in the metabolism of hexobarbital, aminopyrine and *p*-nitrobenzoic acid by liver from rats bearing a pituitary mammotropic tumor. *J. Pharmac. exp. Ther.* **160:** 179–188.
WRIGHT, K. and MORGAN, E. T. (1991) Regulation of cytochrome P450IIC12 expression by interleukin-1alpha, interleukin-6, and dexamethasone. *Molec. Pharmac.* **39:** 468–474.

Garth Powis, editor.
(1994) *Anticancer Drugs: Reactive Metabolism and Drug Interactions*,
Pergamon Press Ltd, pp. 427–438
Printed in the United Kingdom

CHAPTER 12

EFFECTS OF ANTICANCER DRUGS ON DRUG METABOLISM

JARLE AARBAKKE* AND LARS SLØRDAL†*
**Department of Pharmacology, Institute of Medical Biology, University of Tromsø, N-9001 Tromsø, Norway*
†Clinical Pharmacology Laboratory, The Norwegian Radium Hospital, N-0310 Oslo 3, Norway

1. INTRODUCTION

Drug interactions are pharmacological responses due to two or more drugs acting simultaneously. Such interactions are classified as pharmacodynamic or pharmacokinetic. Pharmacokinetic interactions may take place at the level of drug absorption, distribution, excretion and metabolism. Drug metabolism changes the physicochemical properties of a drug and may increase or decrease its biological activity. The metabolism of one compound can be inhibited or induced by other drugs. This review is confined to interactions effected by anticancer drugs at the level of drug metabolism.

The concept of combining anticancer drugs, administered concomitantly or sequentially, has proven its usefulness in the treatment of neoplastic diseases for decades. The combinations employed are, for the most part, chosen empirically, with a potential for changes in pharmacological response due to metabolic interactions. In addition, cytotoxic combinations often cause severe toxicity which, together with the underlying malignant disease, requires therapy with drugs such as antiemetics, antibiotics, analgesics and psychotropic agents, thus increasing the probability for interactions to occur.

Rational predictions of interindividual variations, genetic polymorphism and drug–drug interactions should be facilitated by identification of the cytochrome P450 enzymes that are metabolizing anticancer drugs. Only recently has the identity of anticancer drug-metabolizing enzymes been addressed. Relling et al. (1989) investigated the effect of a number of extensively metabolized anticancer agents on two well-defined cytochrome P450 polymorphisms of oxidative metabolism; mephenytoin and debrisoquine hydroxylation. The chemotherapeutic compounds studied were cyclophosphamide, teniposide, vinblastine, etoposide, flavone acetic acid and ifosphamide. Clinically relevant concentrations of teniposide and high levels of flavone acetic acid demonstrated a potential for interactions at the (S)-mephenytoin 4-hydroxylation site, whereas vinblastine interacted with debrisoquine hydroxylation (Relling et al., 1989).

It is not surprising that reports of unexpected effects of drug combinations with anticancer compounds frequently appear. The paucity of data finally available for this review is explained by the principles applied for the selection of information:

(1) Traditional anticancer drugs, radiosensitizers and some hormones are included as effectors, while effects of noncytostatic drugs on the metabolism of anticancer drugs are beyond the scope of this review.

(2) Interactions with a likely pharmacokinetic mechanism are included and interactions taking place at effector sites, i.e. pharmacodynamic interactions, are excluded.

(3) Pharmacokinetic interactions with a likely effect on drug biotransformation are included, whereas effects on drug absorption, distribution and excretion are not dealt with.

Some important or illustrative interactions that are not within this scope will, however, be dealt with briefly. For example, phenobarbital, probably the best characterized inducer of hepatic mixed function oxidase activity and with no reported anticancer effect, may serve as a model compound for studies of interactions with drug metabolism. Such studies may also serve as sources for estimating the magnitude of changes to be expected. Data collected from phenobarbital studies further demonstrate the complexity of the issue. Phenobarbital pretreatment may shorten the half life of an anticancer drug that has to be metabolically activated and increase the formation of active metabolites. Yet, the cytotoxic effect may be unaffected due to a concomitant increase in the clearance of active metabolites.

2. INTERACTIONS BY ANTICANCER DRUGS

2.1. CYCLOPHOSPHAMIDE

Cyclophosphamide is in itself inactive. The drug is hydroxylated by the hepatic mixed function oxidase system, resulting in the primary metabolites, 4-hydroxy-cyclophosphamide and aldo-phosphamide, which are cytotoxic in vivo and possibly represent transport forms of the active alkylating moiety, phosphoramide mustard (Colvin et al., 1976). At least 50% of an administered dose of cyclophosphamide is eliminated by metabolism in man, yielding multiple metabolites of varying cytotoxic activity (Grochow and Colvin, 1979).

Cyclophosphamide is used as the racemic mixture. Animal studies have given evidence of a highly stereoselective first pass microsomal metabolism of cyclophosphamide and investigations in man are in progress (Holm et al., 1990).

The effect of continued cyclophosphamide administration on its own metabolism has been investigated in a number of studies in man, using various doses and treatment periods. A report on three patients treated each morning for five days with cyclophosphamide as a single drug showed that the mean half life on day five was reduced from 6.1 to 4.3 hr, while the peak plasma levels of metabolites were increased by 73% on the third day of therapy (Bagley et al., 1973). In six patients treated for myeloma with a regimen of cyclophosphamide, prednisolone and melfalan, significant increases in cyclophosphamide clearance from 61 $\pm$ 25 to 97 $\pm$ 36 mL/min (mean $\pm$ SD) were demonstrated after three months (Edwards et al., 1980). When cyclophosphamide (50 mg/kg/day) was given as intravenous doses for four successive days in five patients, the half life of the drug was found to decrease from a mean of 5.1 hr at day 1 to 2.6 hr at day 4, whereas the volume of distribution was not altered significantly (Graham et al., 1983). A decrease in cyclophosphamide half life of approximately 50% in most patients has also been demonstrated in children administered comparable daily cyclophosphamide doses (Sladek et al., 1980). In a study of 16 patients given 100 mg/day of cyclophosphamide for over one year, re-examination of pharmacokinetic variables after more than six months demonstrated a significant reduction in mean cyclophosphamide half life from 7.3 to 4.9 hr, indicating increased metabolism (D'Incalci et al., 1979). The volume of distribution, however, was also decreased. Using their data for estimations of clearance values, a reduction of the mean clearance of 25% in the 16 patients is suggested.

High-dose cyclophosphamide rapidly enhanced its own clearance in 9 patients from a mean of 93 $\pm$ 27 mL/min on the first day to 178 $\pm$ 83 mL/min (mean $\pm$ SD) on the second day, accompanied by an increase in the formation of the pharmacologically active metabolite phosphoramide mustard (Moore et al., 1988).

The clearance of dexamethazone was increased from 369 to 526 mL/min (mean) after high-dose cyclophosphamide in 9 patients, probably due to a rapid enzyme induction (Moore et al., 1988).

Two reports (Jao et al., 1972; Mouridsen et al., 1976) have shown that cyclophosphamide disposition did not change during therapy. However, it nevertheless seems established that cyclophosphamide changes its own metabolism after repeated administration in humans.

Animal data are partly contrasting to the observations in man. Cyclophosphamide administered as a single dose to rats caused a dose-dependent decrease in hepatic NADPH cytochrome P450 reductase activity of 48% and a reduction of microsomal mixed function oxidase activity of 67%, measured four days after the injection (Marinello et al., 1981). The data suggest that cyclophosphamide may affect its own metabolism as well as the metabolism of other drugs.

Adriamycin is metabolized to the active alcohol, adriamycinol, by cytoplasmic aldoketoreductase and, further, to an inactive aglycone by NADPH cytochrome P450 reductase (Evans et al., 1983). Microsomes from rats pre-treated four days before sacrifice with cyclophosphamide (180 mg/kg i.p. as a single dose) showed a significant reduction of NADPH cytochrome P450 reductase activity from 3.4 ± 1.6 to 2.6 ± 1.4 U/mg protein (mean ± SD), accompanied by a mean decrease of 62% in formation of the inactive 7-deoxyadriamycinol aglycone (Dodion et al., 1984). In vitro studies suggest that cyclophosphamide has no effect on a cytosolic carbonyl reduction system for anthracycline antibiotics but inhibits a microsomal anthracycline carbonyl reductase (Dodion et al., 1986). Cyclophosphamide significantly decreased adriamycin clearance in rats from 125 ± 12 to 48 ± 17 mL/min/kg (mean ± SEM) (Hartman et al., 1982). Consistent with the latter result, concomitantly administered cyclophosphamide delayed adriamycin and adriamycinol clearance in children (Evans et al., 1980).

Cyclophosphamide, in combination with methotrexate, increased the elimination half life of 5-fluorouracil in rats (de Bruijn et al., 1987).

Studies with antipyrine, which is eliminated by oxidative metabolism in the rat (Aarbakke, 1978), showed that cyclophosphamide treatment for five days in rats neither changed antipyrine clearance in vivo (Høyem-Johansen et al., 1980) nor antipyrine oxidation in rat liver microsomes in vitro (Slørdal et al., 1983).

Experimental studies in animals show convincingly that the metabolism of cyclophosphamide can be altered by the use of inducers such as phenobarbital and inhibitors such as SKF 525A and cimetidine. Phenobarbital pretreatment accelerated the rate of cyclophosphamide metabolism and the rate of elimination of active metabolites in mice, causing a 30% reduction of the area under curve (AUC) of the plasma alkylating metabolites (Alberts and van Daalen Wetters, 1976). In mice, Bus et al. (1973) reported a decrease in half life of cyclophosphamide and metabolites, measured as total radioactivity, from 8.8 to 8.2 hr, which is in agreement with the results of Field et al. (1972). Similar effects have been demonstrated in both mice and rats by Sladek (1972).

However, the effects of changes of cyclophosphamide metabolism on tumor cell kill, animal survival and therapeutic index are less clear. A correlation between enhanced metabolism, resulting in a decrease in total circulating active metabolites and a decrease in cyclophosphamide antitumor activity following phenobarbital pretreatment, has been demonstrated in leukemia-bearing mice (Field et al., 1972; Alberts and van Daalen Wetters, 1976). In newborn mice without tumors, the increase in cyclophosphamide metabolism induced by phenobarbital pretreatment was accompanied by a near 4-fold increase in mortality during the first 10 days of treatment, while SKF 525A decreased cyclophosphamide half life from 8.8 to 11.5 hr and mortality to almost control values (Bus et al., 1973). Although increased metabolism of cyclophosphamide was observed in rats pretreated with phenobarbital, no effect on the ED_{50} of cyclophosphamide effect on growth of Walker 256 carcinosarcoma cells was seen (Sladek, 1972). When phenobarbital was given to four patients as a daily oral dose of 180 mg for 10 consecutive days and cyclophosphamide kinetics were studied one day prior to and one day after treatment, the elimination rate constant increased 2- to 3-fold after treatment and there was no change in the volume of distribution of cyclophosphamide (Jao et al., 1972). Since comprehensive studies in animals have failed to demonstrate unequivocal effects of phenobarbital pretreatment on the cyclophosphamide chemotherapeutic index and there are indications that plasma alkylating metabolites declined more rapidly in patients who were administered metabolic inducers such as phenobarbital (Bagley et al., 1973), it seems reasonable to predict that the therapeutic outcome of cyclophosphamide treatment should not be significantly altered by phenobarbital administration. It should also be borne in mind that proper interpretation of longitudinal interaction studies, such as those cited above, is dependent on detailed information on baseline cyclophosphamide kinetics.

Cyclophosphamide i.v., in a dose of 200 mg daily for 15 days, caused a mean fall of pseudocholinesterase levels of 50% (Mone and Mathie, 1967) and an inhibition of human plasma cholinesterase in vitro with an IC_{50} of 4×10^{-4} M. A reduction in enzyme levels of this magnitude is not usually associated with very prolonged apnea (Foldes et al., 1963; Harris, 1964) and the clinical significance of this interaction is not established.

2.2. Thiotepa

In vitro, thiotepa inhibited human plasma pseudocholinesterase with an IC_{50} value of 7.9×10^{-3} M, demonstrating a lower potency than that of cyclophosphamide (Zsigmond and Robins, 1972). It is unknown whether this depression is sufficient to prolong the effect of succinylcholine in humans. No decrease in plasma pseudocholinesterase level was seen in one patient who received 225 mg thiotepa intravesically (Mone and Mathie, 1967).

2.3. PROCARBAZINE

Procarbazine undergoes hepatic conversion to alkylating intermediates, involving enzymes subjected to induction (Weinkam and Shiba, 1982). The antitumor activity and the rate of microsomal metabolism of procarbazine were increased by pretreatment of L-1210 leukemia-bearing mice with phenobarbital, as well as by treatment with procarbazine itself, thus supporting the concept of autoinductive properties of this drug (Shiba et al., 1979). Procarbazine by itself also inhibited microsomal metabolism of pentobarbital and aminopyrine, indicating that it may have important interactions with cytotoxic drugs that undergo microsomal metabolism in man, such as dacarbazine (DTIC) and cyclophosphamide (Chabner and Myers, 1989).

Originally synthesized as a potential monoamine oxidase inhibitor, procarbazine has been reported to augment the effects of central nervous system depressants (Oliverio, 1982) and centrally acting depressants should therefore be administered with care in patients receiving this drug. Furthermore, a disulfiram-like reaction may occur following ethanol ingestion in patients receiving procarbazine (Oliverio, 1982).

2.4. METHOTREXATE

In humans, methotrexate administered i.v. together with an i.v. dose of cyclophosphamide inhibited the elimination of cyclophosphamide, whereas oral treatment with methotrexate for nine days had inconsistent effects on cyclophosphamide metabolism (Mouridsen et al., 1976). In rats, methotrexate treatment for five days significantly decreased antipyrine clearance from 12.9 ± 1.8 to 4.2 ± 2.7 mL/min/kg (mean $\pm$ SD) (Høyem-Johansen et al., 1980).

High-dose methotrexate (2 g/m^2) administered in combination with prednisone (40 mg/m^2/day), vincristine (1.5 mg/m^2/week), asparaginase (10,000–15,000 U/m^2/dose), teniposide (150–200 mg/m^2/dose), ara-C (300 mg/m^2/dose) and, in some patients, daunorubicin (25 mg/m^2/week), as induction therapy for acute lymphocytic leukemia in 14 children, significantly increased antipyrine clearance from 0.65 to 0.95 mL/min/kg and lorazepam clearance from 0.93 to 1.20 mL/min/kg within approximately 6 weeks, while indocyanine green clearance was unaffected (Relling et al., 198). In this study, antipyrine, lorazepam and indocyanine green were used as model compounds for detection of alterations in hepatic oxidation, glucuronidation and hepatic blood flow, respectively. The observed increases in hepatic clearance of antipyrine and lorazepam were not a consequence of altered protein binding of these drugs. It is suggested that oxidative and conjugative pathways were enhanced after therapy, while liver blood flow was unchanged (Relling et al., 1987). Whether these changes are related to eradication of hepatic leukemic infiltrations or other mechanisms remains to be determined.

2.5. AMSACRINE

Following intravenous administration, methotrexate is in part metabolized to 7-hydroxy-methotrexate in man (Breithaupt and Kuenzlen, 1982; Wang and Fujimoto, 1984; Slørdal et al., 1986). This metabolite may contribute to the renal (Jacobs et al., 1977) and hepatic (Bremnes et al., 1991a) toxicity of high-dose methotrexate regimens. In the rabbit, the aldehyde oxidase inhibitor amsacrine has been demonstrated to decrease the fractional rate conversion from methotrexate from 0.6% to 0.4%, the AUC for 7-hydroxy-methotrexate from 9215 to 6765 $\mu M \times$ min and cumulative urinary excretion of 7-hydroxy-methotrexate from 52–35 mg, without affecting pharmacokinetic variables of the parent compound (Lee and Chan, 1986).

The rat appears, however, to be a more appropiate choice than the rabbit as a model animal for methotrexate hydroxylation studies in humans. The rat liver aldehyde oxidase closely resembles the human enzymes with respect to stability and specific activity (Stanulovic and Chaykin, 1971). In the presence of amsacrine, there was a substantial reduction in 7-hydroxy-methotrexate formation in intact rats, rat-derived liver cells and liver homogenates (Bremnes et al., 1991c).

Until the identity of the enzyme(s) responsible for methotrexate metabolism is firmly established

(Newton and Blakley, 1984), the clinical implications of this inhibition of methotrexate hydroxylation are unclear.

2.6. 5-Fluorouracil

5-Fluorouracil undergoes intracellular conversion to active metabolites and the liver is the primary site of fluorouracil catabolism (Chabner et al., 1977). 5-Fluorouracil demonstrates dose-dependent kinetics with apparent saturation of enzymes at higher doses (Collins et al., 1980). 5-Fluorouracil did not change antipyrine metabolism in vivo or in vitro in the rat (Høyem-Johansen et al., 1980; Slørdal et al., 1983).

2.7. Thymidine

Thymidine has been used either alone in high doses (Chiuten et al., 1980) or as an enhancer of 5-fluorouracil antitumor efficacy (Ohnuma et al., 1980; Au et al., 1982). Rat hepatocytes exposed to 5-fluorouracil and thymine, to which thymidine is rapidly metabolized in vivo, produced a novel metabolite, identified as a 5-fluorouracil glucuronide conjugate (Sommadossi et al., 1985). Thymine decreased 5-fluorouracil clearance in dogs to approximately 50% of control values at a steady state level of 20 μM thymine and to 20% at 100 μM thymine (Covey and Straw, 1983). In 7 patients, thymidine increased elimination half lives of 5-fluorouracil 260–525 mg/m^2/day in the postdistributional phase (Kirkwood et al., 1980). Without thymidine, the half life was 37 ± 15 min at day 1 and with thymidine it was 77 ± 25 min, whereas the corresponding values after 5 days of treatment were 43 ± 13 min and 59 ± 10 min (mean $\pm$ SEM) (Kirkwood et al., 1980). Consistent with these results, Au et al. (1982) showed a 7-fold reduction in 5-fluorouracil clearance in patients when thymidine was administered concomitantly.

2.8. Mercaptopurine

Mercaptopurine therapy repeatedly led to increased warfarin requirements in anticoagulation therapy in one patient during two treatment periods separated by 16 months (Spiers and Mibashan, 1974). No extensive measures were taken to elucidate the possible mechanism of action, but enzyme induction cannot be ruled out, despite the fact that the rise in warfarin requirement was seen very shortly after the onset of mercaptopurine treatment.

The pharmacokinetics of mercaptopurine and its active intra-cellular metabolite 6-thioguanine mononucleotide display great interindividual variation (Lennard and Lilleyman, 1989). The activity of the RBC thiopurine methyltransferase, an alternative catabolic route regulating the cytotoxic effect of 6-mercaptopurine (Lennard et al., 1990), is subject to genetic polymorphism (Weinshilboum and Sladek, 1980) and interethnic variation (Klemetsdal et al., 1992). The decrease in thiopurine methyltransferase activity after withdrawal of chemotherapy suggests that the enzyme may be prone to induction, although the chemotherapy component(s) responsible presently remain(s) unknown (Lennard et al., 1990).

2.9. Azathioprine

Azathioprine, an imidazole precursor of 6-mercaptopurine, reversed neuromuscular blockade by D-tubocurarine and potentiated the succinylcholine blockade in the in vivo cat soleus muscle preparation (Dretchen et al., 1976). In vitro, azathioprine inhibited phosphodiesterase with an IC_{50} of 2×10^{-5} M, being 5 times more potent than theophylline in the same preparation. Neither compound inhibited cholinesterase activity in vitro (Dretchen et al., 1976). Accumulation of cyclic AMP, resulting in enhanced influx of calcium ions and release of transmitter, could be a possible explanation for the reversal of neuromuscular blockade of D-tubocurarine by azathioprine.

The activity of thiopurine methyltransferase also regulates the pharmacokinetics of azathioprine, the metabolism of which may also be changed by ongoing chemotherapy.

2.10. VINDESINE

Concomitant vindesine may reduce steady-state methotrexate levels during 24 hr methotrexate infusions (Lena et al., 1984). In 10 patients with head and neck cancer given high-dose methotrexate alone or high-dose methotrexate and vindesine simultaneously, vindesine significantly decreased the mean AUC for 7-hydroxy-methotrexate from 10.7 to 7.6 μM hr (Bore et al., 1986).

The effect of vindesine on 7-OH-methotrexate serum levels was reproduced in rats in vivo, but was shown by studies in isolated rat hepatocytes and liver cell homogenates to be due to interference with hepatocellular transport of methotrexate (Bremnes et al., 1991b). This finding in non-transformed cells, and the synergistic action of vindesine and methotrexate cytotoxicity in malignant cell lines (Chello and Sirotnak, 1981; Sirotnak et al., 1983), makes vindesine an interesting agent for inclusion in combination chemotherapy regimens with methotrexate.

2.11. ETOPOSIDE

In a study of five patients receiving combination chemotherapy for lymphoma or small cell lung cancer, Cummings et al. (1986) found that etoposide increased the volume of distribution of the central compartment for adriamycin up to 3-fold, decreased the AUC for adriamycin up to 2-fold and increased its clearance by the same magnitude. Also, etoposide increased renal excretion of adriamycin. Notably, these effects could be ascribed to the action of the non-ionic surfactant polysorbate 80 (Tween 80), which, due to the relative aquenous insolubility of etoposide, is an additive to its intravenous preparation. In vitro, however, etoposid inhibited (S)-mephenytoin hydroxylation by 25% at 200 μM in human liver microsomes from kidney transplant donors (Relling et al., 1989).

2.12. TENIPOSIDE

Teniposide competitively inhibited the 4-hydroxylation of (S)-mephenytoin, with a K_i of 12 μM for a reaction with a K_m of 65 μM (Relling et al., 1989).

2.13. STREPTOZOTOCIN

Streptozotocin, a nitrosourea gluco-derivative, was administered to 10 patients at doses of 500 $mg/m^2/24$ hr i.v. on days 1–5 every three weeks, in combination with 60 mg/m^2 adriamycin i.v. on day 1 every three weeks (Chang et al., 1976). Streptozotocin altered adriamycin pharmacokinetics with the AUC increasing by 100–210% with drug concentrations determined by fluorescence and radioimmunoassay, respectively, and caused a significant increase in clinical and biochemical evidence of adriamycin-related toxicity (Chang et al., 1976).

2.14. STEROIDS

Glucocorticoids may affect the mixed function oxidase system in a complex manner. Using a photometric assay which measured alkylating capacity, Hayakawa et al. (1969) demonstrated that addition of prednisolone inhibited cyclophosphamide activation in vivo in rats and in rat liver slices. Faber et al. (1974) studied cyclophosphamide metabolism in six patients one day prior to and 12–15 days after 50 mg orally-administered prednisone daily. A statistically significant reduction of the mean half life from 443 min before to 360 min after treatment was observed with no concomitant change in the volume of distribution. The area under the serum metabolite curve was increased by 24%. In this study, an immediate prolongation of the cyclophosphamide half life was observed in both prednisone pretreated and untreated patients when, 2 hr after the i.v. cyclophosphamide injection, 60 mg prednisone succinate was injected. Hanasono and Fisher (1972) found no effect on cyclophosphamide activation after 10 days pretreatment with prednisolone in rats and Bagley et al. (1973) observed no effect on cyclophosphamide kinetics from simultaneous prednisolone administration in man. Therefore, the hypothesis that concomitant corticosteroid administration acutely inhibits cyclophosphamide metabolism and chronically causes enzyme induction needs further examination. Since no clinical variables have been measured, the question as to clinical significance remains unanswered.

2.15. Antiestrogens

Tamoxifen is a potent inhibitor of some mixed function oxidases in vitro (Meltzer et al., 1984). Life-threatening interactions between tamoxifen and warfarin have been reported (Lodwick et al., 1987; Ritchie and Grant, 1989; Tenni et al., 1989). Tamoxifen further influences digitoxin pharmacokinetics, resulting in elevated digitoxin plasma levels (Middeke et al., 1986).

2.16. Aromatase Inhibitors

Aminogluthetimide is a well known inducer of mixed function oxidases. Aminogluthetimide increased the formation rate of metabolites of dexamethazone (Santen et al., 1974), antipyrine, theophylline, digitoxin (Lønning et al., 1984) and warfarin (Lønning et al., 1986) in man. Administration of aminogluthetimide reduces plasma levels of progestins (van Deijk et al., 1985; Lundgren et al., 1990) and tamoxifen (Lien et al., 1990). Progestins and tamoxifen should be administrated in increased doses if they are used together with aminogluthetimide in clinical settings.

2.17. High-dose Progestins

Some studies suggest that progestins may increase plasma levels of warfarin (Lundgren et al., 1986). Medroxyprogesterone acetate therapy reduced tamoxifen demethylation in patients on combined tamoxifen treatment (Cammagi et al., 1985, Reid et al., 1992).

2.18. Radiosensitizers

High doses (800 mg/kg) of the radiosensitizer, misonidazole, enhanced the retention of active metabolites of cyclophosphamide when the two drugs were administered simultaneously to mice (Hinchliffe et al., 1983). Twentyman and Workman (1982) found only marginal response with lower doses of the sensitizers misonidazole and metronidazole on cyclophosphamide effects in RIF-1 mouse sarcoma. Addition of misonidazole has been shown to alter lomustine pharmacokinetics by decreasing clearance of the drug in mice by almost 50% (Lee and Workman, 1983) and high doses of concomitantly administered misonidazole caused an increase in the mean half life of melphalan from 21 to 50 min in the mouse (Hinchliffe et al., 1983).

Administered with 1000 mg/m^2 5-fluorouracil in five patients, 1750–2000 mg/m^2 misonidazole significantly reduced 5-fluorouracil clearance and increased the elimination half life from 2.8 ± 0.4 to 3.3 ± 0.4 hr of the drug (mean $\pm$ SEM) (McDermott et al., 1983). In contrast to cyclophosphamide and several other alkylating agents, which undergo microsomal metabolism, 5-fluorouracil is catabolized at mitochondrial and cytosolic sites and these data suggest that chemosensitizers can affect several metabolic pathways (McDermott et al., 1983).

Although it has been proposed that the in vivo interaction between misonidazole and cytotoxic drugs is unlikely to be the result of pharmacokinetic effects of misonidazole (McNally, 1982), Siemann (1982) concluded that altered pharmacokinetics appear to be involved in chemopotentiation by hypoxic cell radiation sensitizers. The observations that misonidazole and related compounds prolonged pentobarbital sleeping time and zoxazolamine paralysis time in mice and reduced the clearance of pentobarbital, aminopyrine and chlorambucil without any effect on renal function and protein binding, strongly support the theory that inhibition of metabolism of anticancer agents is a significant mechanism for chemosensitization (Workman et al., 1983).

Several clinical studies have shown that the combination of misonidazole and 5-fluorouracil results in a reduction of the therapeutic index of 5-fluoruracil with increased toxicity and no increase in therapeutic effect (Bardkji et al., 1986; Spooner et al., 1981).

3. INTERACTIONS CAUSED BY CONCOMITANT TREATMENT AND CONCOMITANT DISEASE

Drugs used in the treatment of symptoms and accompanying disease in cancer patients may affect the metabolism of anticancer agents. Allopurinol has been demonstrated to alter 6-mercaptopurine metabolism in man (Zimm et al., 1983, 1985). Although similar interactions have not been reported in humans, cimetidine, but not ranitidine, enhanced bioactivation of cyclophosphamide in mice (Dorr and Alberts, 1982; Dorr et al., 1986). In a study of 15 patients with carcinoma, pretreatment with cimetidine (1000 mg daily for 4 weeks) increased peak concentrations and AUC for 5-fluorouracil with no alterations in half life, probably due to a combination of inhibition of drug metabolism and reduced liver blood flow (Harvey et al., 1984).

Hyperthermia, as part of cancer treatment, may influence anticancer drug metabolism in man. This is suggested by studies in rats, where hyperthermia reduced the activation of cyclophosphamide (Clawson et al., 1981) and affected the disposition of adriamycin in perfused liver, possibly through a decrease in bile flow (Riggs et al., 1982; Skibba et al., 1982).

In dogs, whole body hyperthermia markedly increased adriamycin clearance and apparent volume of distribution (Wilke et al., 1991).

The risk of adverse drug reactions, presumably including those orginating from metabolic interactions, has been shown to increase with the number of drugs administered (May et al., 1977). Although, to our knowledge, such studies have not been undertaken with cytostatic drugs, it seems reasonable to assume that this principle might be applicable to anticancer agents as well.

The liver is the main site of metabolism for most drugs, including anticancer agents. Since hepatotoxicity is a feature of many antineoplastic compounds (for review see Menard et al., 1980), cancer treatment regimens frequently include one or more potentially hepatotoxic drugs. Any liver impairment, such as in patients with solid tumors or advanced leukemia (Powis et al., 1986), may in principle affect the fate of drugs and drug combinations usually metabolized by the liver, thus modulating pharmacological effects.

The effect of hepatic resection, not infrequently carried out in concert with anticancer therapy for hepatocellular carcinoma, has received little attention with regard to its impact on drug metabolism. Hall and coworkers (1990) have reported that partially hepatectomized rats showed a 2-fold increase in 4-epidoxorubicin AUC, without a change in terminal half life, as compared with sham-operated controls.

The present review shows that only limited information is available as to effects of anticancer drugs on drug metabolism. Where data are scarce or lacking, some general principles may be of help. Penicillins, cephalosporins and aminoglycoside antibiotics are not metabolized to a significant degree. Metoclopramide, salicylates, acetaminophen and opioids are conjugated in the liver (Bateman et al., 1980; Gilman et al., 1990) and, thus, seem less prone to metabolic induction or inhibition by anticancer drugs. Minor tranquilizers, neuroleptics, tricyclic antidepressants and barbiturates are to a large extent metabolized by mixed function oxidases (Gilman et al., 1990). The anticancer agents cyclophosphamide, melphalan, lomustine (CCNU), carmustine (BCNU), procarbazine and dacarbazine are also biotransformed by mixed function oxidases (Chabner and Myers, 1989; Menard et al., 1980; Balis et al., 1983), whereas this metabolic pathway is of no or minor significance for the clearance of methotrexate, cytarabine (Ara-C), 5-fluorouracil, thiopurines, vinca-alkaloids and epipodophyllotoxins (Chabner and Myers, 1989; Menard et al., 1980; Balis et al., 1983; Philips and Lauper, 1983; Sinkule, 1984). Interactions, where the pharmacokinetics of either drug in principle might be affected, should be expected when anticancer drugs metabolized by mixed function oxidases are employed in combination with drugs eliminated by this pathway.

4. CONCLUSION

Anticancer drugs affect drug metabolism in vitro and in vivo in several species, including humans. Limited data are available from systematic studies designed to obtain information on the pharmacokinetic and therapeutic consequences of interactions caused by cytostatics. Until more information is presented from well-planned studies in man, the clinician should, at least in principle, be prepared for potential interactions with almost any combination of anticancer drugs. Pending further studies, investigations of compounds metabolized by mixed function oxidases have shown these drugs to be likely candidates for interactions at the level of drug metabolism.

Acknowledgements—The expert secretarial help of Jorunn Karlstad is gratefully acknowledged. The authors further acknowledge the support from the Norwegian Cancer Society.

REFERENCES

AARBAKKE, J. (1978) Disposition and oxidative metabolism of antipyrine in the rat. *Acta Pharmac. Toxic.* **43:** 64–68.

ALBERTS, D. S. and VAN DAALEN WETTERS, T. (1976) The effect of phenobarbital on cyclophosphamide antitumor activity. *Cancer Res.* **36:** 2785–2789.

AU, J. L.-S., RUSTUM, Y. M., LEDESMA, E. J., MITTELMAN, A. and CREAVEN, P. J. (1982) Clinical pharmacological studies of concurrent infusion of 5-fluorouracil and thymidine in treatment of colorectal carcinomas. *Cancer Res.* **42:** 2930–2937.

BAGLEY, C. M., JR, BOSTICK, F. W. and DEVITA, V. T., JR (1973) Clinical pharmacology of cyclophosphamide. *Cancer Res.* **33:** 226–233.

BALIS, F. M., HOLCENBERG, J. S. and BLEYER, W. A. (1983) Clinical pharmacokinetics of commonly used anticancer drugs. *Clin. Pharmacokin.* **8:** 202–232.

BARDKJI, Z., JOLIVET, J., LONGELIER, Y., BRESNER, J. G. and AYOB, J. (1986) 5-fluorouracil metronidazole combination therapy in metastatic colorectal cancer. *Cancer Chemother. Pharmac.* **18:** 140–144.

BATEMAN, D. N., KAHN, C. and DAVIES, D. S. (1980) The pharmacokinetics of metoclopramide in man with observations in the dog. *Br. J. clin. Pharmac.* **9:** 371–377.

BORE, P., LENA, N., IMBERT, A. M., FAVRE, R., CANO, J. P., MEYER, G. and CARCASSONNE, Y. (1986) Methotrexate–vindesine association in head and neck cancer: modification of methotrexate's hydroxylation in presence of vindesine. *Cancer Chemother. Pharmac.* **17:** 171–176.

BREITHAUPT, H. and KUENZLEN, E. (1982) Pharmacokinetics of high-dose methotrexate treatment in children. *Eur. J. clin. Pharmac.* **14:** 143–147.

BREMNES, R. M., SMELAND, E., HUSEBY, N.-E., EIDE, T. J. and AARBAKKE, J. (1991a) Acute hepatotoxicity after high-dose methotrexate administration to rats. *Pharmac. Toxic.* **69:** 132–139.

BREMNES, R. M., SMELAND, E., SLØRDAL, L., WIST, E. and AARBAKKE, J. (1991b) The effect of vindesine on methotrexate hydroxylation in the rat. *Biochem. Pharmac.* **42:** 1561–1568.

BREMNES, R. M., SMELAND, E., WILLASSEN, N.-P., WIST, E. and AARBAKKE, J. (1991c) Inhibition of 7-hydroxy-methotrexate formation by amsacrine. *Cancer Chemother. Pharmac.* **28:** 377–383.

BUS, J. S., SHORT, R. D. and GIBSON, J. E. (1973) Effect of phenobarbital and SKF 525A on the toxicity, elimination and metabolism of cyclophosphamide in newborn mice. *J. Pharmac. Exp. Ther.* **184:** 749–756.

CAMAGGI, C. M., STROCCHI, E., COSTANTI, B., BEGHELLI, P., FERRARI, P. and PANNUTI, F. (1985) Medroxy-progesterone acetate bioavailability after high-dose intraperitoneal administration in advanced cancer. *Cancer Chemother. Pharmac.* **14:** 232–234.

CHABNER, B. A. and MYERS, C. E. (1989) Clinical pharmacology of cancer chemotherapy. In: *Cancer. Principles and Practice of Oncology*, pp. 301–347, DEVITA, V. T., HELLMAN, S. and ROSENBERG, S. A. (eds) J. B. Lippincott Co., Philadelphia.

CHABNER, B. A., MYERS, C. E. and OLIVERIO, V. T. (1977) Clinical pharmacology of anticancer drugs. *Semin. Oncol.* **4:** 165–191.

CHANG, P., RIGGS, C. E., JR, SCHEERER, M. T., WIERNIK, P. H. and BACHUR, N. R. (1976) Combination chemotherapy with adriamycin and streptozotocin. II. Clinicopharmacologic correlation of augmented adriamycin toxicity caused by streptozotocin. *Clin. Pharmac. Ther.* **20:** 611–616.

CHELLO, P. L. and SIROTNAK, F. M. (1981) Increased schedule-dependent synergism of vindesine versus vincristine in combination with methotrexate against L1210 leukemia. *Cancer Treat. Rep.* **65:** 1049–1053.

CHIUTEN, D. F., WIERNIK, P. H., ZAHARKO, D. S. and EDWARDS, L. (1980) Clinical phase I–II and pharmaco-kinetic study of high-dose thymidine given by continuous intravenous infusion. *Cancer Res.* **40:** 818–822.

CLAWSON, R. E., EGORIN, M. J., FOX, B. M., ROSS, L. A. and BACHUR, N. R. (1981) Hyperthermic modification of cyclophosphamide metabolism in rat hepatic microsomes and liver slices. *Life Sci.* **28:** 1133–1137.

COLLINS, J. M., DEDRICK, R. L., KING, F. G., SPEYER, J. L. and MYERS, C. E. (1980) Nonlinear pharmacokinetic models for 5-fluorouracil in man: intravenous and intraperitoneal routes. *Clin. Pharmac. Ther.* **28:** 235–246.

COLVIN, M., BRUNDRETT, R. B., KAN, M. N. N., JARDINE, I. and FENSELAU, C. (1976) Alkylating properties of phosphoramide mustard. *Cancer Res.* **36:** 1121–1126.

COVEY, J. M. and STRAW, J. A. (1983) Nonlinear pharmacokinetics of thymidine, thymine and fluorouracil and their kinetic interactions in normal dogs. *Cancer Res.* **43:** 4587–4595.

CUMMINGS, J., FORREST, G. J., CUNNINGHAM, D., GILCHRIST, N. L. and SOUKOP, M. (1986) Influence of polysorbate 80 (Tween 80) and etoposide (VP-16-213) on the pharmacokinetics and urinary excretion of adriamycin and its metabolites in cancer patients. *Cancer Chemother. Pharmac.* **17:** 80–84.

DE BRUIJN, E. A., DRIESSEN, O., LEEFLANG, P., VAN STRIJEN, E., VAN DEN BOSCH, N. and HERMANS, J. (1987)

Interactions of methotrexate and cyclophosphamide with the pharmacokinetics of 5-fluorouracil in an animal model. *Cancer Treat. Rep.* **71:** 1267–1269.

D'INCALCI, M., BOLIS, G., FACCHINETTI, T., MANGIONI, C., MORASCA, L., MORAZZONI, P. and SALMONA, M. (1979) Decreased half life of cyclophosphamide in patients under continual treatment. *Eur. J. Cancer* **15:** 7–10.

DODION, P., RIGGS, C. E., AKMAN, S. R., TAMBURINI, J. M., COLVIN, O. M. and BACHUR, N. R. (1984) Interactions between cyclophosphamide and adriamycin metabolism in rats. *J. Pharmac. exp. Ther.* **229:** 51–57.

DODION, P., AKMAN, S. R., TAMBURINI, J. M., RIGGS, C. E., COLVIN, O. M. and BACHUR, N. R. (1986) Interaction between cyclophosphamide and doxorubicin. Metabolism in rat, effect of cyclophosphamide aldoketoreductase system. *J. Pharmac. exp. Ther.* **237:** 271–274.

DORR, R. T. and ALBERTS, D. S. (1982) Cimetidine enhancement of cyclophosphamide antitumor activity. *Br. J. Cancer* **45:** 35–43.

DORR, R. T., SOBLE, M. J. and ALBERTS, D. S. (1986) Interaction of cimetidine but not ranitidine with cyclophosphamide in mice. *Cancer Res.* **46:** 1795–1799.

DRETCHEN, K. L., MORGENROTH, V. H., III, STANDAERT, F. G. and WALTS, L. F. (1976) Azathioprine: effects on neuromuscular transmission. *Anesthesiology* **45:** 604–609.

EDWARDS, G., CALVERT, R. T., CROWTHER, D., BRAMWELL, V. and SCARFFE, H. (1980) Repeated investigations of cyclophosphamide disposition in myeloma patients receiving intermittent chemotherapy. *Br. J. clin. Pharmac.* **10:** 281–285.

EVANS, W. E., CROM, W. R., YEE, G. C., GREEN, A. A., HAYES, F. A., PRATT, C. B. and AVERY, T. L. (1980) Adriamycin pharmacokinetics in children. *Proc. Am. Ass. Cancer Res.* **21:** 176.

EVANS, W. E., CROM, W. R., SINKULE, J. A., YEE, G. C., STEWART, C. F. and HUTSON, P. R. (1983) Pharmacokinetics of anticancer drugs in children. *Drug Metab. Rev.* **14:** 847–886.

FABER, O. K., MOURIDSEN, H. T. and SKOVSTED, R. (1974) The biotransformation of cyclophosphamide in man: influence of prednisone. *Acta Pharmac. Toxic.* **35:** 195–200.

FIELD, R. B., GANG, M., KLINE, I., VENDITTI, J. M. and WARAVDEKAR, V. S. (1972) The effect of phenobarbital or 2-diethylaminoethyl-2,2-diphenylvalerate on the activation of cyclophosphamide in vivo. *J. Pharmac. exp. Ther.* **180:** 475–483.

FOLDES, F. F., FOLDES, V. M., SMITH, J. C. and ZSIGMOND, E. K. (1963) The relation between plasma cholinesterase and prolonged apnea caused by succinylcholine. *Anesthesiology* **24:** 208–216.

GILMAN, A. G., RALL, T. W., NIES, A. S. and TAYLOR, P. (EDS) (1990) *The Pharmacological Basis of Therapeutics.* Macmillan Publishing Co., New York.

GRAHAM, M. I., SHAW, I. C., SOUHAMI, R. L., SIDAU, B., HARPER, P. G. and MCLEAN, A. E. M. (1983) Decreased plasma halflife of cyclophosphamide during repeated high-dose administration. *Cancer Chemother. Pharmac.* **10:** 192–193.

GROCHOW, L. B. and COLVIN, M. (1979) Clinical pharmacokinetics of cyclophosphamide. *Clin. Pharmacokin.* **4:** 380–394.

HALL, K. S., ENDRESEN, L., SCHJERVEN, L. and RUGSTAD, H. E. (1990) The influence of partial hepatectomy on the pharmacokinetics of preoperatively injected 4′epidoxorubicin in rats. *Cancer Chemother. Pharmac.* **26:** 444–448.

HANASONO, G. K. and FISCHER, L. J. (1972) Plasma levels and urinary excretion of [^{14}C]cyclophosphamide and its radioactive metabolites in rats pretreated with prednisolone. *Biochem. Pharmac.* **21:** 272–276.

HARRIS, H. (1964) Enzymes and drug sensitivity. The genetics of serum cholinesterase 'deficiency' in relation to suxamethonium apnoea. *Proc. R. Soc. Med.* **57:** 503–506.

HARTMAN, N., BASSECHES, P. J. and POWIS, G. (1982) Effect of cyclophosphamide pretreatment on the short-term disposition and biliary excretion of adriamycin metabolites in rat. *Cancer Chemother. Pharmac.* **10:** 11–15.

HARVEY, V. J., SLEVIN, M. L., DILLOWAY, M. R., CLARK, P. I., JOHNSTON, A. and LANT, A. F. (1984) The influence of cimetidine on the pharmacokinetics of 5-fluorouracil. *Br. J. Clin. Pharmac.* **18:** 421–430.

HAYAKAWA, T., KANAI, N., YAMADA, R., KURODA, R., HIGASHI, H., MOGAMI, H. and JINNAI, D (1969) Effect of steroid hormone on activation of endoxan (cyclophosphamide). *Biochem. Pharmac.* **18:** 129–135.

HINCHLIFFE, M., MCNALLY, N. J. and STRATFORD, M. R. L. (1983) The effect of radiosensitizers on the pharmacokinetics of melphalan and cyclophosphamide in the mouse. *Br. J. Cancer* **48:** 375–383.

HOLM, K. A., KINDBERG, C. G., STOBAUGH, J. F., SLAVIK, M. and RILEY, C. R. (1990) Stereoselective pharmacokinetics and metabolism of the enantiomers of cyclophosphamide. Preliminary results in humans and rabbits. *Biochem. Pharmac.* **39:** 1375–1384.

HØYEM-JOHANSEN, T., SLØRDAL, L., HØYLANDSKJBR, A. and AARBAKKE, J. (1980) The effect of antineoplastic drugs on the pharmacokinetics of antipyrine in the rat. *Acta Pharmac. Toxic.* **47:** 279–284.

JACOBS, S. A., STOLLER, R. G., CHABNER, B. A. and JOHNS, D. G. (1977) Dose dependent metabolism of methotrexate in man and rhesus monkeys. *Cancer Treat. Rep.* **61:** 651–656.

JAO, J. Y., JUSKO, W. J. and COHEN, J. L. (1972) Phenobarbital effect on cyclophosphamide pharmacokinetics in man. *Cancer Res.* **32:** 2761–2764.

KIRKWOOD, J. M., ENSMINGER, W., ROSOWSKY, A., PAPATHANASOPOULOS, N. and FREI, E., III (1980) Comparison of pharmacokinetics of 5-fluorouracil and 5-fluorouracil with concurrent thymidine infusions in a phase I trial. *Cancer Res.* **40:** 107–113.

KLEMETSDAL, B., TOLLEFSEN, E., LOENNECHEN, T., JOHNSEN, K., UTSI, E., GISHOLT, K., WIST, E. and AARBAKKE, J. (1992) Interethnic difference in thiopurine methyltransferase activity. *Clin. Pharmac. Ther.* **51:** 24–31.

LEE, F. Y. F. and WORKMAN, P. (1983) Modification of CCNU pharmacokinetics by misonidazole—a major mechanism of chemosensitization in mice. *Br. J. Cancer* **47:** 659–669.

LEE, Y. J. and CHAN, K. K. (1986) Metabolic interaction between methotrexate (MTX) and MAMSA in the rabbit. *Proc. Am. Ass. Cancer Res.* **27:** 258.

LENA, N., IMBERT, A. M., PIGNON, T., FAVRE, R., MEYER, G., CANO, J. P. and CARCASSONNE, Y. (1984) Methotrexate–vindesine association in the treatment of head and neck cancer: influence of vindesine on methotrexate's pharmacokinetic behaviour. *Cancer Chemother. Pharmac.* **12:** 120–124.

LENNARD, L. and LILLEYMAN, J. S. (1989) Variable mercaptopurine metabolism and treatment outcome in childhood lymphoblastic leukemia. *J. clin. Oncol.* **7:** 1816–1823.

LENNARD, L., LILLEYMAN, J. S., VAN LOON, J. and WEINSHILBOUM, R. M. (1990) Genetic variation in response to 6-mercaptopurine for childhood acute lymphoblastic leukaemia. *Lancet* **336:** 225–229.

LIEN, E. A., ANKER, G., LØNNING, P. E., SOLHEIM, E. and UELAND, P. M. (1990) Decreased serum concentrations of tamoxifen and its metabolites induced by aminoglutethimide. *Cancer Res.* **50:** 5851–5857.

LODWICK, R., MCCONKEY, B., BROWN, A. M. and BEELEY, L. (1987) Life threatening interactions between tamoxifen and warfarin. *Br. Med. J.* **295:** 1141.

LØNNING, P. E., KVINNSLAND, S. and BAKKE, O. M. (1984) Effect of aminoglutethimide on antipyrine, theophylline and digitoxin disposition in breast cancer. *Clin. Pharmac. Ther.* **36:** 796–802.

LØNNING, P. E., UELAND, P. M. and KVINNSLAND, S. (1986) The influence of a graded dose schedule of aminoglutethimide on the disposition of the optical enantiomers of warfarin in patients with breast cancer. *Cancer Chemother. Pharmac.* **17:** 177–181.

LUNDGREN, S., KVINNSLAND, S., UTAAKER, E., BAKKE, O. M. and UELAND, P. M. (1986) Effect of oral high dose progestins on the disposition of antipyrine, digitoxin and warfarin in patients with advanced breast cancer. *Cancer Chemother. Pharmac.* **18:** 270–275.

LUNDGREN, S., LØNNING, P. E., AAKVAAG, A. and KVINNSLAND, S. (1990) Influence of aminoglutethimide on the metabolism of medroxy-progesterone acetate and megestrol acetate in postmenopausal patients with advanced breast cancer. *Cancer Chemother. Pharmac.* **27:** 101–105.

MARINELLO, A. J., BERRIGAN, M. J., STRUCK, R. F., GUENGERICH, F. P. and GURTOO, H. L. (1981) Inhibition of NADPH–cytochrome P450 reductase by cyclophosphamide and its metabolites. *Biochem. biophys. Res. Commun.* **99:** 399–406.

MAY, F. E., STEWART, R. B. and CLUFF, L. E. (1977) Drug interactions and multiple drug administration. *Clin. Pharmac. Ther.* **22:** 322–328.

MCDERMOTT, B. J., VAN DEN BERG, H. W., MARTIN, W. M. C. and MURPHY, R. F. (1983) Pharmacokinetic rationale for the interaction of 5-fluorouracil and misonidazole in humans. *Br. J. Cancer* **48:** 705–710.

MCNALLY, N. J. (1982) Enhancement of chemotherapy agents. *Int. J. Radiat. Oncol. Biol. Phys.* **8:** 593–598.

MELTZER, N. M., STANG, P. and STERNSON, L. A. (1984) Influence of tamoxifen and its *N*-desmethyl and 4-hydroxy metabolites on rat liver microsomal enzymes. *Biochem. Pharmac.* **33:** 115–123.

MENARD, D. B., GISSELBRECHT, C., MARTY, M., REYES, F. and DHUMEAUX, D. (1980) Antineoplastic agents and the liver. *Gastroenterology* **78:** 142–164.

MIDDEKE, M., REMIEN, C., LOHMØLLER, G., HOLZGREVE, H. and ZØLLNER, N. (1986) Interaction between tamoxifen and digitoxin? *Klinische Wochenschrift* **64:** 1211.

MONE, J. G. and MATHIE, W. E. (1967) Qualitative and quantitative defects of pseudocholinesterase activity. *Anaesthesia* **22:** 55–68.

MOORE, M. J., HARDY, R. W., THIESSEN, J. J., SOLDIN, S. J. and ERLICHMAN, C. (1988) Rapid development of enhanced clearance after high-dose cyclophosphamide. *Clin. Pharmac. Ther.* **44:** 622–628.

MOURIDSEN, H. T., FABER, O. and SKOVSTED, L. (1976) The metabolism of cyclophosphamide. Dose dependency and the effect of long-term treatment with cyclophosphamide. *Cancer* **37:** 665–670.

NEWTON, P. A. and BLAKLEY, R. L. (1984) 7-Hydromethotrexate formation in a human lymphoblastic cell line. *Biochem. biophys. Res. Commun.* **122:** 1212–1217.

OHNUMA, T., ROBOZ, J., WAXMAN, S., MANDEL, E., MARTIN, D. S. and HOLLAND, J. F. (1980) Clinical pharmacological effects of thymidine plus 5-FU. *Cancer Treat. Rep.* **64:** 1169–1177.

OLIVERIO, V. T. (1982) Derivatives of triazenes and hydrazines. In: *Cancer Medicine*, pp. 850–860, HOLLAND, J. F. and FREI, E., III (eds) Lea and Febiger, Philadelphia.

PHILLIPS, N. C. and LAUPER, R. D. (1983) Review of etoposide. *Clin. Pharm.* **2:** 112–119.

POWIS, G., HARRIS, R. N., BASSECHES, P. J. and SANTONE, K. S. (1986) Effects of advanced leukemia on hepatic drug-metabolizing activity in the mouse. *Cancer Chemother. Pharmac.* **16:** 43–49.

REID, A. D., HOROBIN, J. M., NEWMAN, E. L. and PREECE, P. E. (1992) Tamoxifen metabolism is altered by simultaneous administration of medroxyprogesterone acetate in breast cancer patients. *Breast Cancer Res. Treat.* **22:** 153–156.

RELLING, M. V., CROM, W. R., PIEPER, J. A., CUPIT, G. C., RIVERA, G. K. and EVANS, W. E. (1987) Hepatic drug clearance in children with leukemia: changes in clearance of model substrates during remission therapy. *Clin. Pharmac. Ther.* **41:** 651–660.

RELLING, M. V., EVANS, W. E., FONNE-PFISTER, R. and MEYER, U. A. (1989) Anticancer drugs as inhibitors of two polymorphic cytochrome P450 enzymes, debrisoquin and mephenytoin hydroxylase, in human liver microsomes. *Cancer Res.* **49:** 68–71.

RIGGS, C. E., JR, EGORIN, M. J., AKMAN, S. R., ANGELOU, J. E., VAN ECHO, D. A., WHITACRE, M. and BACHUR, N. R. (1982) Doxorubicin metabolism is altered by combination therapy with cyclophosphamide and whole body hyperthermia. *Proc. Am. Soc. clin. Oncol.* **22:** 26.

RITCHIE, L. D. and GRANT, S. M. T. (1989) Tamoxifen–warfarin interaction: the Aberdeen hospitals drug file. *Br. Med. J.* **298:** 1253.

SANTEN, R. J., LIPTON, A. and KENDALL, J. (1974) Successful medical adrenalectomy with aminoglutethimide. *J. Am. Med. Ass.* **230:** 1661–1665.

SHIBA, D. A., WEINKAM, R. J. and LEVIN, V. A. (1979) Metabolic activation of procarbazine: activity of the intermediates and the effects of pretreatment. *Proc. Am. Ass. Cancer Res.* **20:** 139.

SIEMANN, D. W. (1982) Potentiation of chemotherapy by hypoxic cell radiation sensitizers—a review. *Int. J. Radiat. Oncol. Biol. Phys.* **8:** 1029–1034.

SINKULE, J. A. (1984) Etoposide: a semisynthetic epipodophyllotoxin. Chemistry, pharmacology, pharmacokinetics, adverse effects and use as an antineoplastic agent. *Pharmacotherapy* **4:** 61–73.

SIROTNAK, F. M., SCHMID, F. A., TEMPLE, C. and MONTGOMERY, J. A. (1983) Optimum scheduling during combination chemotherapy of murine leukemia. Additional examples of schedule-dependent synergism between S-phase-specific antimetabolites and agents inducing mitotic or pre-mitotic (G_2) arrest. *Cancer Chemother. Pharmac.* **11:** 205–207.

SKIBBA, J. L., JONES, F. E. and CONDON, R. E. (1982) Altered hepatic disposition of doxorubicin in the perfused rat liver at hyperthermic temperatures. *Cancer Treat. Rep.* **66:** 1357–1363.

SLADEK, N. E. (1972) Therapeutic efficacy of cyclophosphamide as a function of its metabolism. *Cancer Res.* **32:** 535–542.

SLADEK, N. E., PRIEST, J., DOEDEN, D., MIROCHA, C. J., PATHRE, S. and KRIVIT, W. (1980) Plasma half life and urinary excretion of cyclophosphamide in children. *Cancer Treat. Rep.* **64:** 1061–1066.

SLØRDAL, L., HØYEM-JOHANSEN, T. and AARBAKKE, J. (1983) Microsomal metabolism of antipyrine in rats treated with antineoplastic drugs. *Pharmacology* **26:** 95–99.

SLØRDAL, L., KOLMANNSKOG, S., PRYTZ, P. S., MOE, P. J. and AARBAKKE, J. (1986) Pharmacokinetics of methotrexate and 7-hydroxy-methotrexate after high-dose (33.6 g/m^2) methotrexate therapy. *Pediat. Hematol. Oncol.* **3:** 127–134.

SOMMADOSSI, J.-P., GEWIRTZ, D. A., CROSS, D. S., GOLDMAN, I. D., CANO, J.-P. and DIASIO, R. B. (1985) Modulation of 5-fluorouracil catabolism in isolated rat hepatocytes with enhancement of 5-fluorouracil glucuronide formation. *Cancer Res.* **45:** 116–121.

SPIERS, A. S. D. and MIBASHAN, R. S. (1974) Increased warfarin requirement during mercaptopurine therapy: a new drug interaction. *Lancet* **ii:** 221–222.

SPOONER, D., BERGDEN, R. D., PECKHAM, M. J. and WIST, E. A. (1981) The combination of 5-fluorouracil with misonidazole in patients with advanced colorectal cancer. *Int. J. Rad. Oncol. Biol. Physics* **8:** 387–389.

STANULOVIC, M. and CHAYKIN, S. (1971) Metabolic origins of the pyridones of N^1-methylnicotinamide in man and rat. *Arch. Biochem. Biophys.* **145:** 35–42.

TENNI, P., LALICH, D. L. and BYRNE, M. J. (1989) Life threatening interaction between tamoxifen and warfarin. *Br. J. Med.* **298:** 93.

TWENTYMAN, P. R. and WORKMAN, P. (1982) The effect of radiosensitizer pretreatment on the response of the RIF-1 mouse sarcoma to cytotoxic drugs. *J. Radiat. Oncol. Biol. Phys.* **8:** 611–613.

VAN DEIJK, W. A., BLIJHAM, G. H., MELLINK, W. A. M. and MEULENBERG, P. M. M. (1985) Influence of aminoglutethimide on plasma levels of medroxyprogesterone acetate: its correlation with serum cortisol. *Cancer Treat. Rep.* **69:** 85–90.

WANG, Y.-M. and FUJIMOTO, T. (1984) Clinical pharmacokinetics of methotrexate in children. *Clin. Pharmacokin.* **9:** 335–348.

WEINKAM, R. J. and SHIBA, D. A. (1982) Procarbazine. In: *Pharmacologic Principles of Cancer Treatment*, pp. 340–362, CHABNER, B. A. (ed) W. B. Saunders and Co., Philadelphia.

WEINSHILBOUM, R. M. and SLADFK, S. L. (1980) Mercaptopurine pharmacogenetics; monogenic inheritence of erythrocyte thiopurine methyltransferase activity. *Am. J. Hum. Genet.* **32:** 651–662.

WILKE, A. V., JENKINS, C., MILLIGAN, A. J., LEGENDRE, A. and FRAZIER, D. L. (1991) Effect of hyperthermia on normal tissue toxicity and on adriamycin pharmacokinetics in dogs. *Cancer Res.* **51:** 1680–1683.

WORKMAN, P., TWENTYMAN, P. R., LEE, F. Y. F. and WALTON, M. I. (1983) Drug metabolism and chemosensitization. Nitroimidazoles as inhibitors of drug metabolism. *Biochem. Pharmac.* **32:** 857–864.

ZIMM, S., COLLINS, J. M., O'NEILL, D., CHABNER, B. A. and POPLACK, D. G. (1983) Inhibition of first-pass metabolism in cancer chemotherapy: interaction of 6-mercaptopurine and allopurinol. *Clin. Pharmac. Ther.* **34:** 810–817.

ZIMM, S., ETTINGER, L. J., HOLCENBERG, J. S., KAMEN, B. A., VIETTI, T. J., BELASCO, J., COGLIANO-SHUTTA, N., BALIS, F., LAVI, L. E., COLLINS, J. M. and POPLACK, D. G. (1985) Phase I and clinical pharmacological study of mercaptopurine administered as a prolonged intravenous infusion. *Cancer Res.* **45:** 1869–1873.

ZSIGMOND, E. K. and ROBINS, G. (1972) The effect of a series of anti-cancer drugs on plasma cholinesterase activity. *Can. Anaesth. Soc. J.* **19:** 75–82.

INDEX